Pediatric
and
Adolescent
Gynecology

Pediatric
and
Adolescent
Gynecology

Second Edition

JOSEPH S. SANFILIPPO, M.D.
Professor of Obstetrics, Gynecology, and Reproductive Sciences
Vice Chairman, Reproductive Sciences
University of Pittsburgh School of Medicine
Magee Women's Hospital
Pittsburgh, Pennsylvania

DAVID MURAM, M.D.
Professor of Obstetrics and Gynecology
State University of New York–Downstate
Brooklyn, New York
Senior Clinical Research Physician
Eli Lilly and Company
Indianapolis, Indiana

JOHN DEWHURST, F.R.C.O.G., F.R.C.S.
Emeritus Professor
University of London
Queen Charlotte's and Chelsea Hospital
London, United Kingdom

PETER A. LEE, M.D., Ph.D.
Pennsylvania State University College of Medicine
Chief, Division of Pediatric Endocrinology/Diabetes
Penn State College of Medicine
The Milton S. Hershey Medical Center
Hershey, Pennsylvania

W.B. SAUNDERS COMPANY
A Harcourt Health Sciences Company
Philadelphia London New York St. Louis Sydney Toronto

W.B. SAUNDERS COMPANY
A Harcourt Health Sciences Company

The Curtis Center
Independence Square West
Philadelphia, Pennsylvania 19106

Library of Congress Cataloging-in-Publication Data

Pediatric and adolescent gynecology / Joseph S. Sanfilippo . . . [et al.].—2nd ed.

p.   ; cm.

Includes bibliographical references and index.

ISBN 0–7216–8346–0

1. Pediatric gynecology.   2. Adolescent gynecology.   I. Sanfilippo, J. S.
  (Joseph S.)   [DNLM: 1. Genital Diseases, Female—Adolescence.
  2. Genital Diseases, Female—Child.   3. Adolescent Medicine.
  4. Pediatrics.   WS 360 P3707 2001]

RJ478 .P43 2001   618.92′098—dc21   00–058859

Acquisitions Editor: Judith Fletcher
Developmental Editor: Heather Krehling
Project Manager: Tina Rebane
Production Manager: Norman Stellander
Illustration Specialist: Lisa Lambert
Book Designer: Steven Stave
Indexer: Angela Holt

PEDIATRIC AND ADOLESCENT GYNECOLOGY   ISBN 0–7216–8346–0

Printed in the United States of America.

Last digit is the print number: 9   8   7   6   5   4   3   2   1

Contributors

PAUL F. AUSTIN, M.D.
Assistant Professor, Department of Surgery
(Urology), Washington University School of
Medicine; Physician, St. Louis Children's
Hospital, St. Louis, Missouri
Urologic Problems

KUNWAR P. BHATNAGAR, M.SC., PH.D.
Professor, Anatomical Sciences and
Neurobiology, School of Medicine, University of
Louisville, Louisville, Kentucky; Research
Associate, Carnegie Museum of Natural History,
Pittsburgh, Pennsylvania
Embryology and Normal Anatomy

ROBERT T. BROWN, M.D.
Professor, Clinical Pediatrics and Clinical
Obstetrics/Gynecology, The Ohio State
University Colleges of Medicine and Public
Health; Chief, Adolescent Health, Children's
Hospital, Columbus, Ohio
Adolescent Sexuality

JOSÉ F. CARA, M.D.
Section Head, Henry Ford Hospital, Detroit,
Michigan
Androgens and the Adolescent Girl

ANTHONY J. CASALE, M.D.
Associate Professor, Department of Urology,
Indiana University School of Medicine,
Indianapolis, Indiana
Urologic Problems

JOHN DEWHURST, F.R.C.O.G., F.R.C.S.
Emeritus Professor, University of London,
Queen Charlotte's and Chelsea Hospital,
London, United Kingdom
Rectovaginal Fistulas and Associated Anomalies

MILENA DORTA, M.D.
Assistant Professor, Department of Obstetrics
and Gynecology, University of Verona, Verona,
Italy
Diagnostic Imaging

**D. KEITH EDMONDS, F.R.C.O.G.,
F.R.A.N.Z.C.O.G.**
Consultant Obstetrician and Gynaecologist,
Queen Charlotte's and Chelsea Hospital,
London, United Kingdom
*Sexual Developmental Anomalies and Their
Reconstruction: Upper and Lower Tracts*

S. BETH EDWARDS, PHARM.D. CANDIDATE
University of Kentucky, Lexington, Kentucky
*Appendices: Commonly Used Medications;
Commonly Used Oral Contraceptives*

THOMAS E. ELKINS, M.D. (DECEASED)
Department of Obstetrics and Gynecology,
Johns Hopkins University School of Medicine,
Baltimore, Maryland
*Reproductive Health Care Needs of the
Developmentally Disabled*

LUIGI FEDELE, M.D.
Chairman, Department of Obstetrics and
Gynecology, University of Verona, Verona, Italy
Diagnostic Imaging

THOMAS P. FOLEY, JR., M.D.
Professor of Pediatrics, School of Medicine, and
Professor of Epidemiology, Graduate School of
Public Health, University of Pittsburgh;
Professor of Pediatrics, Division of
Endocrinology, Metabolism, and Diabetes
Mellitus, Department of Pediatrics, Children's
Hospital of Pittsburgh, Pittsburgh, Pennsylvania
*Effects of the Thyroid on Gonadal and
Reproductive Function During Childhood and
Adolescence*

GILBERT B. FORBES, M.D.
Professor of Pediatrics, Emeritus, and
Biophysics, University of Rochester School of
Medicine and Dentistry; Pediatrician, Emeritus,
Strong Memorial Hospital, Rochester, New York
Nutrition, Growth, and Development

GITA P. GIDWANI, M.D.
Consultant Staff Physician, Departments of
Gynecology/Obstetrics and Pediatrics, Cleveland
Clinic, Cleveland, Ohio
Dysmenorrhea and Pelvic Pain

ANGELA M. HAGY, M.S.P.H.
Program Manager, University of Alabama at
Birmingham, Birmingham, Alabama
Human Immunodeficiency Virus in Adolescents

KEITH HANSEN, M.D.
Professor, Department of Obstetrics and
Gynecology, Section of Reproductive
Endocrinology, University of South Dakota
School of Medicine, Sioux Falls, South Dakota
Future Perspectives

S. PAIGE HERTWECK
Assistant Professor, Department of Obstetrics and Gynecology, Division of Pediatric and Adolescent Gynecology, University of Louisville School of Medicine; Chief of Gynecology, Kosair Children's Hospital, Louisville, Kentucky
Vaginal Bleeding in Childhood and Menstrual Disorders in Adolescence

MICHAEL L. HICKS, M.D.
Assistant Professor of Reproductive Biology, Case Western Reserve University, Cleveland, Ohio; Staff Gynecologic Oncologist, Henry Ford Hospital, Detroit, and The Michigan Cancer Institute, Pontiac, Michigan
Oncologic Problems

RAYMOND L. HINTZ, M.D.
Professor of Pediatrics, Stanford University School of Medicine and Medical Center, Stanford, California
Abnormalities of Growth

CYNTHIA HOLLAND, M.D., M.P.H.
Assistant Professor of Clinical Pediatrics, Ohio State University College of Medicine and Public Health, Section of Adolescent Medicine, Children's Hospital, Columbus, Ohio
Depression, Suicide, and Drug Abuse

BARBARA R. HOSTETLER, M.D.
Instructor, Department of Obstetrics and Gynecology, University of Tennessee–Memphis, Memphis, Tennessee
Appendices: Growth Charts; Tanner Staging; Normal Laboratory Values; Temperature Conversion; Commonly Used Medications

NATALIE PIERRE JOSEPH, M.D., M.P.H.
Assistant Professor of Pediatrics/Adolescent Medicine and Co-Director, Teen-Tot Clinic, Boston University School of Medicine and Medical Center; Instructor in Pediatrics/ Adolescent Medicine, Children's Hospital, Boston, Massachusetts
Pregnancy in Adolescence

MARSHA KAY, M.D.
Staff Physician, Department of Pediatric Gastroenterology and Nutrition, The Cleveland Clinic Foundation, Cleveland, Ohio
Dysmenorrhea and Pelvic Pain

PETER A. LEE, M.D., PH.D.
Pennsylvania State University College of Medicine; Chief, Division of Pediatric Endocrinology/Diabetes, Penn State College of Medicine, The Milton S. Hershey Medical Center, Hershey, Pennsylvania
Neuroendocrinology of Puberty; Precocious Puberty; Delayed Puberty; Abnormal Sexual Differentiation and Hypogonadism: Management and Therapy

DIANE F. MERRITT, M.D.
Professor of Obstetrics and Gynecology, Washington University School of Medicine; Director of Pediatric and Adolescent Gynecology, St. Louis Children's Hospital, Barnes Jewish Hospital, and Missouri Baptist Medical Center, St. Louis, Missouri
Genital Injuries in Pediatric and Adolescent Girls

KRISTI MORGAN MULCHAHEY, M.D.
Private practice, Atlanta, Georgia
Sexually Transmissible Diseases in Childhood

DAVID MURAM, M.D.
Professor of Obstetrics and Gynecology, State University of New York–Downstate, Brooklyn, New York; Senior Clinical Research Physician, Eli Lilly and Company, Indianapolis, Indiana
Vulvovaginitis in Children and Adolescents; Vaginal Bleeding in Childhood and Menstrual Disorders in Adolescence; Sexually Transmitted Diseases in Adolescents; Child Sexual Abuse; Delayed Consequences of Childhood Malignancies; Reproductive Health Care Needs of the Developmentally Disabled; Genital Injuries in Pediatric and Adolescent Girls; Sexual Developmental Anomalies and Their Reconstruction: Upper and Lower Tracts; Commonly Used Oral Contraceptives

PAMELA J. MURRAY, M.D., M.H.P.
Associate Professor of Pediatrics and Obstetrics, Gynecology and Reproductive Health Sciences, University of Pittsburgh School of Medicine; Division Chief, Adolescent Medicine, Children's Hospital of Pittsburgh, Pittsburgh, Pennsylvania
Depression, Suicide, and Drug Abuse

LOUIS S. O'DEA, M.D., B.CH., B.A.O., F.R.C.P.
Executive Medical Director, Reproduction and Growth Division, Serono Labs, Inc., Norwell, Massachusetts
Delayed Puberty

PAOLA A. PALMA SISTO, M.D.
Assistant Professor of Pediatrics, Medical College of Wisconsin, Milwaukee, Wisconsin
Neuroendocrinology of Puberty

GEETA N. PANDYA, M.B.B.S., D.(OBST.)R.C.O.G., F.R.C.O.G., F.I.C.S.
Gynecologic Endocrinologist, Jaslok Hospital and Research Centre, Breach Candy Hospital and Research Centre, Mumbai (Bombay), India
Pubertal Aberrancy in the Third World

M. STEVEN PIVER, M.D.
Professor of Gynecology, State University of
New York at Buffalo, and Senior Gynecologic
Oncologist, Sisters of Charity Hospital, Buffalo,
New York
Oncologic Problems

LEO PLOUFFE, JR., M.D.
Medical Director, US Women's Health and
Reproductive Medicine, Eli Lilly and Company,
Indianapolis, Indiana
Future Perspectives

SUSAN F. POKORNY, M.D.
Formerly Assistant Professor of Obstetrics and
Gynecology and Pediatrics, Baylor College of
Medicine; Chief of Gynecology, Texas
Children's Hospital, and Director of Obstetrics
and Gynecology, Outpatient Clinics, Ben Taub
General Hospital, Houston, Texas
*Genital Examination of Prepubertal and
Peripubertal Females*

ANTONELLA PORTUESE, M.D.
Assistant Professor, Department of Obstetrics
and Gynecology, University of Verona, Verona,
Italy
Diagnostic Imaging

PAULINE S. POWERS, M.D.
Professor of Psychiatry and Behavioral
Medicine, College of Medicine, Health Sciences
Center, University of South Florida, Tampa;
Medical Director, Eating Disorder Program,
Fairwinds Residential Treatment Center,
Clearwater, Florida
Eating Disorders

FREDERICK J. RAU, M.D.
Assistant Clinical Professor, Obstetrics and
Gynecology and Pediatrics, University of
Connecticut School of Medicine, Farmington;
Director, Division of Gynecology, Connecticut
Children's Medical Center, Hartford,
Connecticut
Vulvovaginitis in Children and Adolescents

ROBERT W. REBAR, M.D.
Associate Executive Director, American Society
for Reproductive Medicine, Birmingham,
Alabama
Sports-Related Problems in Reproductive Function

EDWARD O. REITER, M.D.
Professor of Pediatrics, Tufts University School
of Medicine, Boston; Chairman, Department of
Pediatrics, Baystate Medical Center Children's
Hospital, Springfield, Massachusetts
Neuroendocrinology of Puberty

C. MARJORIE RIDLEY, M.A., F.R.C.P.
Honorary Consultant and Senior Lecturer in
Dermatology, St. John's Institute of
Dermatology, St. Thomas' Hospital, London,
England, United Kingdom
Dermatologic Conditions of the Vulva

MARY E. RIMSZA, M.D.
Professor of Pediatrics, University of Arizona
Health Science Center, Tucson, Arizona
Genital Injuries in Pediatric and Adolescent Girls

ROBERT L. ROSENFIELD, M.D.
Professor of Pediatrics and Medicine, University
of Chicago Pritzker School of Medicine;
Pediatric Endocrinologist, University of Chicago
Children's Hospital, Chicago, Illinois
Androgens and the Adolescent Girl

JOSEPH S. SANFILIPPO, M.D.
Professor of Obstetrics, Gynecology, and
Reproductive Sciences, and Vice Chairman,
Reproductive Sciences, University of Pittsburgh
School of Medicine, Magee Women's Hospital,
Pittsburgh, Pennsylvania
*Vaginal Bleeding in Childhood and Menstrual
Disorders in Adolescence; Chronic Pelvic
Pain—Medical and Surgical Approaches*

BETSY SCHROEDER, M.D.
Instructor, Department of Obstetrics/
Gynecology, MCP/Hahnemann School of
Medicine; Director, Pediatric and Adolescent
Gynecology, Allegheny General Hospital,
Pittsburgh, Pennsylvania
*Chronic Pelvic Pain—Medical and Surgical
Approaches*

LEE P. SHULMAN, M.D.
Professor, Obstetrics and Gynecology; Director,
Division of Reproductive Genetics; Deputy
Head, Department of Obstetrics and
Gynecology, University of Illinois, Chicago,
Chicago, Illinois
Molecular Biology and Genetics Aspects

PATRICIA S. SIMMONS, M.D.
Associate Professor of Pediatrics,
Mayo Medical School and Mayo Clinic,
Rochester, Minnesota
Breast Disorders

JOE LEIGH SIMPSON, M.D.
Professor and Chairman, Department of
Obstetrics and Gynecology, Baylor College of
Medicine, Houston, Texas
Disorders of Sexual Differentiation

RAMONA I. SLUPIK, M.D.
Assistant Professor, Department of Gynecology
and Obstetrics, Northwestern University
Medical School; Head of Pediatric and
Adolescent Gynecology, Children's Memorial
Hospital, Chicago, Illinois
Adolescent Contraception

STEVEN R. SMITH, M.S., J.D.
Dean and Professor, California Western School
of Law, San Diego, California
Legal Issues in Treating Minors

DENNIS M. STYNE, M.D., PH.D.
Professor and Chief, Pediatrics Endocrinology,
University of California, Davis, Medical Center,
Sacramento, California
Normal Growth and Pubertal Development

CLAIRE TEMPLEMAN, M.D.
Clinical Associate, Reproductive Specialty
Centre, Milwaukee, Wisconsin
*Vaginal Bleeding in Childhood and Menstrual
Disorders in Adolescence*

MARLAH TOMBOC, M.D.
Fellow, Pediatric Endocrinology, Children's
Hospital of Pittsburgh, University of Pittsburgh
School of Medicine, Pittsburgh, Pennsylvania
Precocious Puberty

STEN H. VERMUND, M.D., PH.D.
Professor and Division Director, Geographic
Medicine; Professor, Epidemiology and
International Health, University of Alabama at
Birmingham, Birmingham, Alabama
Human Immunodeficiency Virus in Adolescents

STEPHEN S. WACHTEL, PH.D.
Professor, Obstetrics and Gynecology, and Chief
of Research for Reproductive Genetics,
University of Tennessee, Memphis, Tennessee
Molecular Biology and Genetics Aspects

SELMA FELDMAN WITCHEL, M.D.
Associate Professor of Pediatrics, University of
Pittsburgh School of Medicine; Physician,
Children's Hospital of Pittsburgh, Pittsburgh,
Pennsylvania
*Precocious Puberty; Abnormal Sexual
Differentiation and Hypogonadism: Management
and Therapy*

Foreword

The new edition of *Pediatric and Adolescent Gynecology* is here, and one can comfortably say that the previous edition of this textbook was just a taster for this new edition. This is the defining text in this important area of clinical medicine. For readers who enjoy the convenience of a single clinical discipline neatly bound in a single volume, this textbook, stitched together seamlessly by the editor Joe Sanfilippo, is without peer. The organization of the text reflects the long-time experience of the editor in the area of pediatric and adolescent gynecology. The composition of the book illustrates how important it is to cross disciplines and reach out to enlist contributors who have unusual expertise and experience. The clinical specialty of pediatric and adolescent gynecology is laid bare by a series of exceptionally qualified experts.

The book starts with the embryology and anatomy of the neonatal female genital tract by Kunwar Bhatnagar and finishes with a look into the future by Leo Plouffe. It is important to note that an array of standard growth charts and reference ranges for a large number of analytes are part of the appendices (A to D). This information and the standard drug dosing regimens for pediatric and adolescent patients, presented in Appendices E and F, make the text a virtual "point of care" commodity. Between the Preface by Doctor Sanfilippo and the appendices by Barbara Hostetler and others are a series of 39 different stations that address the most common gynecologic problems that one might encounter in a female child or adolescent. The chapters are succinct and guaranteed not to intensify the information glut faced by today's clinicians. However, each chapter contributes the necessary solid background information on the topic coupled with clinical problem solving.

Every topic and category seems to be covered in the text, and the effects are cumulative. There are no loose ends. The area of neuroendocrinology is nicely updated by three very expert authors. The three authors together (Peter Lee, Edward Reiter, and Paola A. Palma Sisto) represent years of experience probing the neuroendocrine system. The fact that they were able to reach a consensus is remarkable and worth reading, if for no other reason than to know what constitutes a consensus on this dynamic topic. Doctor Simpson's chapter on abnormal sexual development is as close to the "Bible" as one will ever come in a textbook of clinical medicine. He

writes just as well as before he was Joe Leigh Simpson. The chapter by Lee Shulman and Stephen Wachtel gently and painlessly brings the hesitant reader into the modern area of molecular biology. Gilbert Forbes has written a chapter on nutrition, growth, and development that should be required in every textbook of pediatric and adolescent gynecology. The clinical problems related to examination, vulvovaginitis, vaginal bleeding, dysmenorrhea, and pelvic pain are well written and illustrated. In the chapter on vulvar disorders by C. Marjorie Ridley, even the "old hands" in the discipline will see photos and descriptions of disorders that are infrequently seen or have been infrequently recognized. The chapter on "Androgens and the Adolescent Girl" by Bob Rosenfield and José Cara is a classic that deserves rereading. Bob Brown's chapter on adolescent sexuality and Ramona Slupik's chapter on adolescent contraception provide a stunning breadth of new perspectives on both of these important subjects. David Muram's chapters on child sexual abuse and sexually transmitted diseases are written in his imitable style and worth reading on several different occasions. It is invaluable to have a chapter on eating disorders in a text book of this type. Pauline Powers is a psychiatrist, who seems to have a grasp of the wide variety of clinical phenotypes resulting from eating aberrations and their sometimes subtle clinical manifestations.

More and more clinicians are dealing with technologies that have been developed outside of their discipline or outside of medicine altogether. It is critical that they understand the scope and limitations of this technology and be in a position to make their own assessment of the results. The chapter on diagnostic imaging by Drs. Luigi Fedele, Milena Dorta, and Antonella Portuese from Verona is just what the "clinician reader" needs in this day and age of ever-increasing technology. The chapter on puberty aberrancy in the third world by Geeta N. Pandya is fascinating and reawakens our memories of pelvic tuberculosis from many years back. The chapters by Susan Pokorny, Mary Rimsza, and others on examination of the prepubertal child and sexual trauma help to clear much of the "fog" in this area of clinical and forensic medicine.

Many of the chapters in this book will be part of mainstream discussions in pediatric and adolescent gynecology for many years to come. I started out scanning the text to write this foreword and ended up reading the entire book. The most compelling aspects of this text-reference book are the comprehensiveness of the material, the quality of the presentations, and the diverse backgrounds of the contributors. It makes one want to meet each of them personally and have the benefit of a private quiz session. Reading this textbook can make one think that one has found the "black book" on pediatric and adolescent gynecology, or, if not the "black book," at least one that has a more holistic view of this challenging area of medicine where anatomy, develop-mental biology, genetics, endocrinology, and clinical medicine intersect. By providing a listing of the links to searchable archives and other resources in the area of pediatric and adolescent gynecology, the textbook retains the essential character and scope of pediatric and adolescent gynecology, while adapting to the electronic exigencies of modern scholarly discourse. This is a textbook that not only leads the way, but is the way for those who have a continuing interest in the gynecologic problems of children. It deserves to be in our office right next to the computer.

Paul G. McDonough
Professor, Obstetrics and Gynecology,
Medical College of Georgia

Preface

Pediatric and adolescent gynecology has reached a new plateau since the publication of our previous edition in 1994. From a global perspective, new societies focusing on the pediatric adolescent gynecologic patient have emerged. These include the British Society for Pediatric and Adolescent Gynecology (BRITSPAG) and the continued expansion of the relatively new society, the South American Society for Pediatric and Adolescent Gynecology (ALOGIA), both of which complement the well-established societies of the North American Society for Pediatric and Adolescent Gynecology and the International Society for Pediatric and Adolescent Gynecology (FIGIJ).

The American College of Obstetricians and Gynecologists and the American Academy of Pediatrics, as well as the American Academy of Family Practice, continue to affirm the importance of our specialized area of medicine with new initiatives designed to facilitate access to the health care system. Methods of making an office "adolescent friendly" have led to more and more clinicians seeking opportunities to reach out to this age group. A key objective of the current edition of this textbook is to provide clinicians all over the world access to updated, leading-edge information in a readily accessible manner. Each subsection editor has called on experts with extensive clinical acumen to provide for the reader information readily applicable to the clinical setting. Complementing the textbook chapters is an expanded appendix that allows readers information at their fingertips, including an armamentarium of medications with dosages that can facilitate addressing the immediate problem at hand.

I am indebted to each and every author for their extensive literature review, communication skills, and sharing of their clinical experience. This has created the environment for a comprehensive textbook addressing virtually all challenging situations that a clinician is likely to encounter.

Joseph S. Sanfilippo, M.D.

Contents

Section III
SURGICAL PROBLEMS
JOSEPH S. SANFILIPPO

Appendices

Color
Figures

Color Figures 15–1 to 15–7 are courtesy of the North American Society for Pediatric Adolescent Gynecology.

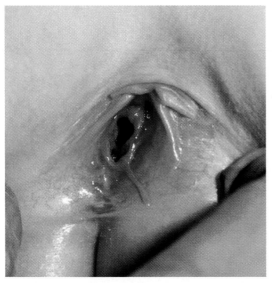

Color Figure 14–1. Hymenal polyp noted on gynecologic examination of a newborn.

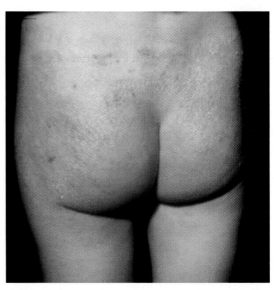

Color Figure 14–2. Diaper dermatitis. Note the clear demarcation of the diaper area with the irritation.

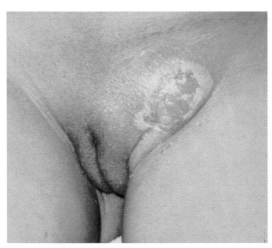

Color Figure 14–5. Infantile gluteal granuloma located in the left inguinal area.

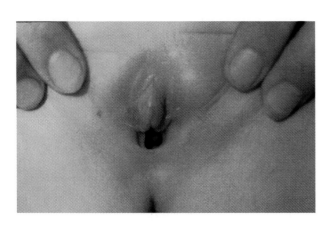

Color Figure 14–8. *D*, An intact hymen and introitus with lateral displacement of the adherent area.

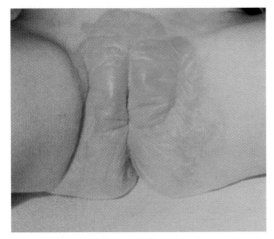

Color Figure 14-11. Epidermolysis bullosa involving the vulvar area.

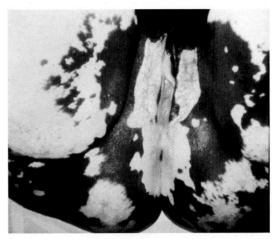

Color Figure 14-13. Vitiligo. Note the depigmented areas of the vulva.

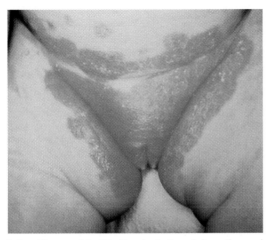

Color Figure 14-15. Psoriasis involving the vulvovaginal area.

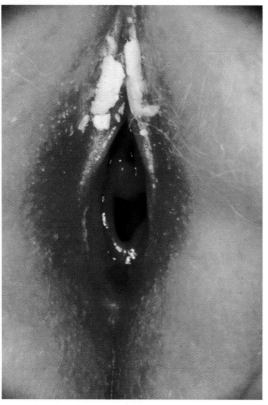

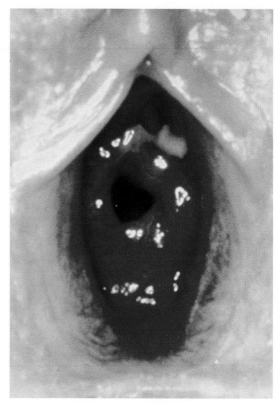

Color Figure 15–1. Vulvitis in a prepubertal girl. Vulvar erythema present.

Color Figure 15–2. Streptococcal vaginitis in a prepubertal girl. Note the purulent material near the urethra. Gross erythema of the hymen obscures the normal vascular pattern.

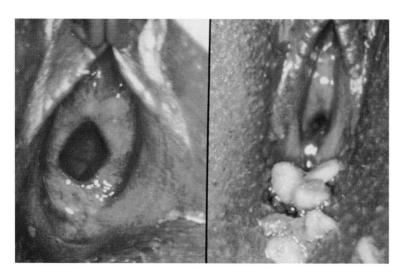

Color Figure 15–3. The cause of vaginal discharge and bleeding was initially puzzling. After vaginal irrigation, it was revealed to be small pieces of toilet paper.

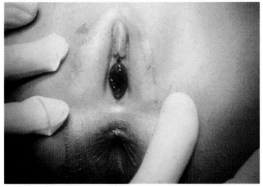

Color Figure 15–4. Urethral prolapse in a pre-pubertal girl.

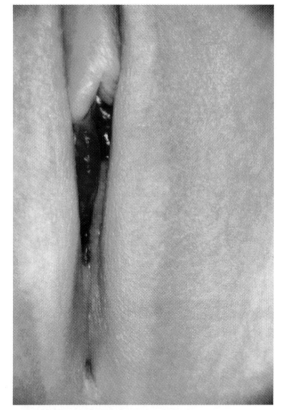

Color Figure 15–5. Lichen sclerosus in a young girl. Note the pale labia majora and ecchymosis of the labia minora.

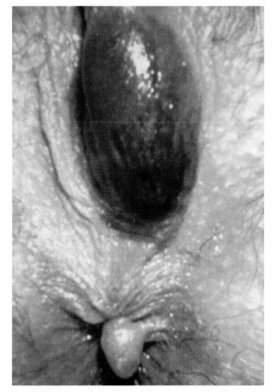

Color Figure 15–6. Straddle injury to the vulva resulted when a girl fell on the middle bar of a boys' bicycle. The hymen was spared in this case.

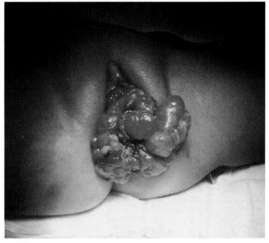

Color Figure 15–7. Lesions of sarcoma botryoides (vulvovaginal rhabdomyosarcoma) protrude from the vagina of a 3-year-old girl.

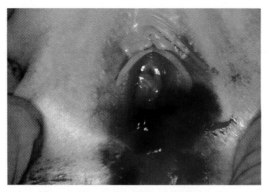

Color Figure 33–1. Straddle injury. Ecchymoses and abrasions were sustained in a fall onto a bicycle crossbar.

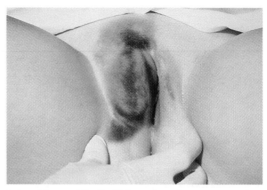

Color Figure 33–3. This vulvar hematoma does not distort the perineal anatomy. If the patient can void spontaneously, she can be managed conservatively with ice packs and bed rest.

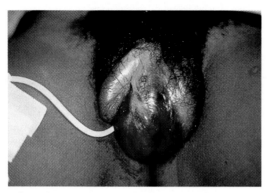

Color Figure 33–4. A large expanding vulvar hematoma distorts the anatomy and should be drained.

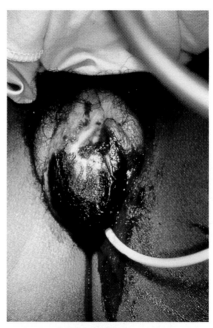

Color Figure 33–5. Failure to decompress the expanding hematoma can lead to tissue necrosis and eschar formation. This can be avoided by surgical drainage.

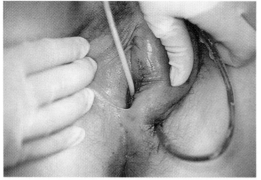

Color Figure 33–6. Vulvar hematoma that has been incised and drained. Note incision on medial aspect of left labium, which has been closed with absorbable sutures. A urethral catheter is in place for bladder decompression and closed suction drain exits the most dependent aspect of vulva.

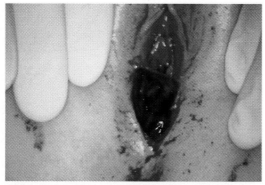

Color Figure 33–9. Impalement injury. This young girl leapt into a swimming pool and impaled herself on a broom handle. The entry wound is seen here, just beneath the introitus; the exit wound was in the rectum.

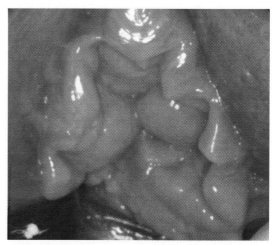

Color Figure 33–10. Vaginal-hymenal tear secondary to sexual abuse. Note the disruption of the hymen at the lower margin of the photograph.

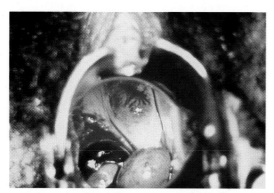

Color Figure 33–11. Evisceration injury. Lacerations of the posterior fornix may extend into the peritoneal cavity. In this young patient, loops of small bowel are seen in the vagina.

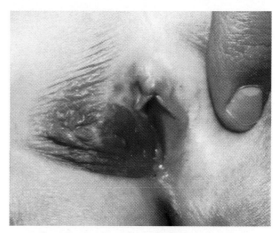

Color Figure 33–13. Vulvar hemangioma.

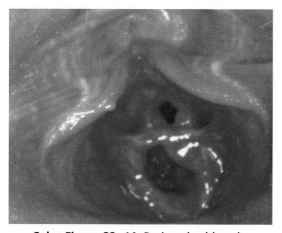

Color Figure 33–14. Periurethral bands.

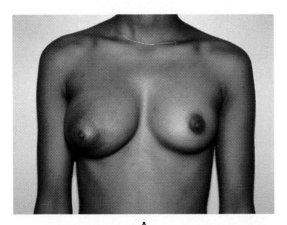

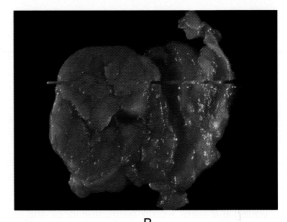

A

B

Color Figure 36–3. *A,* Unilateral fibroadenoma. *B,* Surgical specimen of a fibroadenoma.

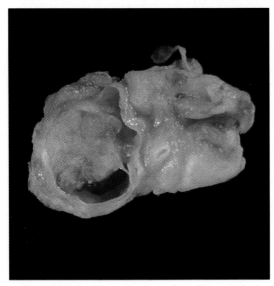

Color Figure 36–7. Biopsy of a fibrocystic lesion.

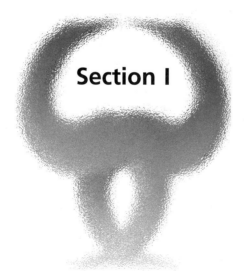

Section I

Growth and Development

ASSOCIATE EDITOR: PETER A. LEE

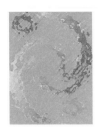

Chapter 1

Embryology and Normal Anatomy

Kunwar P. Bhatnagar

Ovaries apparently are not necessary for primary female sexual development. In embryos with no gonads or ovaries, most of the internal and external genitalia develop like those in females. Conversely, testes are essential for male sexual development. In the early embryo (week 4), three sets of renal excretory organs develop: the pronephroi, the mesonephroi, and the metanephroi. In the male, the mesonephros and its duct, the mesonephric (wolffian) duct, develop into the ductal structures of the internal male reproductive tract, whereas in the female only nonfunctional remnants develop from the regressing mesonephric duct (Table 1–1). In the female, the paramesonephric (müllerian) duct, another paired structure, develops lateral to the mesonephric duct and forms the major internal female reproductive organs, whereas in the male the paramesonephric duct regresses, leaving a few nonfunctional remnants (see Table 1–1). Thus, although the gonads differentiate into the ovaries in the female, the uterine tubes, the uterus, and the upper portion of the vagina develop independently of ovarian influence. In the constitutive development of the external genitalia in the female, the undifferentiated fetal external genitalia become the vulva. The developmental history of the female genital system is systematically presented in this chapter followed by applied embryology.

PRIMORDIAL GERM CELLS

The primordial germ cells are relatively large cells, 12 to 20 μm in diameter, with vesicular, centrally located nuclei and distinct nuclear membranes.[1] Yolk granules persist in these cells much longer than in the somatic cells and become a diagnostic feature. The cytoplasm is rich in glycogen. Spindle-shaped germ cells are seen in the interstitial tissue, whereas the germ cells resting beneath or between the coelomic epithelial germ cells are round or oval. These (mesothelial) cells are first recognized in the 13-somite, 4-week human embryo, when as many as 30 of them are seen in the endoderm and the splanchnic mesoderm near the base of the allantois and the adjacent yolk sac. These primordial germ cells are believed to be derived from the endoderm. Migrating through the dorsal mesentery, they reach the medial mesonephric ridges, the sites for gonadal development. These sex cells become incorporated into the primary sex cords during the sixth week. Some of them may not reach the sex cords, and such ectopically oriented primordial germ cells may be the source for extragonadal teratomas and seminoma-like tumors.[2]

The ultrastructural characteristics of germ cells are unique.[1] A few pseudopodia extend from the cell surface. The round nucleus contains one or two nucleoli, finely dispersed chromatin, and numerous nuclear pores. In the cytoplasm are seen juxtanuclear Golgi complexes, centrioles, ribosomes, round mitochondria with vesicular cristae, some elements of rough endoplasmic reticulum, lysosome-like granules, lipid droplets, and pinocytotic vesicles (Fig. 1–1). Glycogen particles aggregate and monofilament bundles are conspicuous. Microtubules and chromatoid bodies are not observed. Occasional desmosomes are noted between germ cells and the surrounding coelomic epithelial or interstitial cells.

ULTRASTRUCTURE OF THE MATURE HUMAN OOCYTE

The normal mature human oocyte (Fig. 1–2) is large and is enveloped by follicular cells. The nucleus is large, spherical, and eccentric in location with a large nucleolus. Chromatin is mostly dispersed, and nuclear pores are numerous. A cluster of fine filaments is attached to the nuclear

Table 1–1. Homologies of the Female and the Male Genital Systems*[6, 8, 10, 11]

Female	Undifferentiated	Male
Oocytes	*Primordial germ cells*	Spermatozoa
Ovary	*Gonad*	Testis
Proper ovarian ligament and round ligament of the uterus	*Gubernacular cord*	Gubernaculum testis
Epoöphorantic (Gartner's) duct	*Mesonephric (wolffian) duct*	Duct of epididymis and ductus deferens (distal)
No homologue		Ductus deferens (proximal); ejaculatory duct and seminal vesicle
Appendices vesiculosae (?)	*Mesonephric tubules*	Appendix of epididymis (?)
Epoöphoron		Efferent ductules
		Lobules of epididymis
Paroöphoron		Paradidymis (tubuli)
		Paradidymis
		Aberrant ductules
Ostium abdominale of uterine tube	*Paramesonephric (müllerian) duct*	Appendix of testis
Uterus		No homologue
Vagina (? lower portion)		No homologue
Vagina (upper portion)		Prostatic utricle
Urethra	*Urogenital sinus*	No homologue
Greater vestibular glands		Urethra (except navicular fossa)
Urethral and paraurethral glands		Bulbourethral glands
		Prostate gland
		Remaining urethra and glands
Vestibule	—	Rest of urethra to glans
Labia minora	*Genital folds*	Penis, urethral surface
Labia majora	*Labioscrotal swellings*	Scrotum
Hymen	*Sinus tubercle*	Seminal colliculus
Urachus (median umbilical ligament)	*Allantois*	Urachus (median umbilical ligament)
Rectum and upper anal canal	*Dorsal cloaca*	Rectum and upper anal canal
Most of the bladder and the urethra	*Ventral cloaca*	Most of the bladder; part of prostatic urethra
Ureter, pelvis, calyces, and collecting tubules	*Metanephric diverticulum (ureteric bud)*	Ureter, pelvis, calyces, and collecting tubules
Broad ligament	*Peritoneal fold*	No homologue

Generalized mesoderm (Phallus)

Mesovarium	Mesorchium
Clitoris	Penis
Glans clitoridis	Glans penis
Corpora cavernosa clitoridis	Corpora cavernosa penis
Bulbs of the vestibule	Corpus spongiosum penis
Mons pubis	No named homologue; this region is similar to the mons pubis of the female†

*Corresponding male structures are given for comparison.

†In the *Nomina Anatomica*,[11] the term *mons pubis* has been listed both as a general surface feature and under the female external genitalia. No such listing occurs with the scrotum. On the basis of surface anatomy, the mons pubis (the rounded fleshy prominence over the symphysis pubis) should be a valid landmark in both sexes. The question remains whether males have either a mons pubis or at least its homologue. *Mons veneris* is the name of the prominence in the female. I suggest *mons martialis* as the term for this yet to be specified region in the human male.

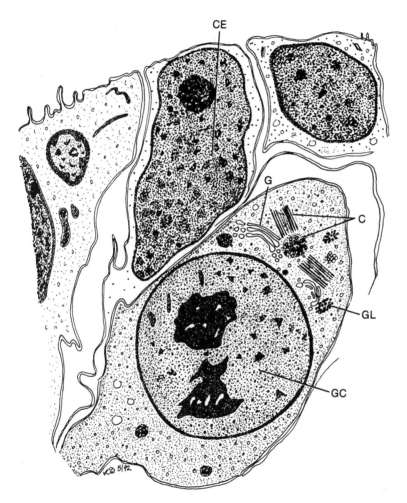

Figure 1–1. A diagrammatic illustration of the ultrastructure of a human primordial germ cell (GC) located beneath the coelomic epithelium (CE). The nucleus is round and contains two irregular and prominent nucleoli. The juxtanuclear cytoplasm shows the Golgi complex (G), centrioles (C), and glycogen particles (GL). (Modified from Fukuda T: Ultrastructure of primordial germ cells in human embryo. Virchows Arch [Cell Pathol] 1976; 20:85–89.)

Figure 1–2. A diagrammatic illustration of the ultrastructure of a normal human oocyte in contact with the first polar body. Notice the cluster of cell organelles in the paranuclear complex of Balbiani's body (vitelline body). AL, annulate lamellae; CA, compound aggregates; CG, cortical granules; FI, filaments; G, Golgi complexes; MV, microvilli; NL, nucleolus; PB1, first polar body; V, vesicles. (Modified from Lentz TL: Cell Fine Structure. An Atlas of Drawings of Whole-Cell Structure. Philadelphia: WB Saunders, 1971, and VanBlerkom J: Occurrence and developmental consequences of aberrant cellular organization in meiotically mature human oocytes after exogenous ovarian hyperstimulation. J Electron Microsc Technol 1990; 16:324–346.)

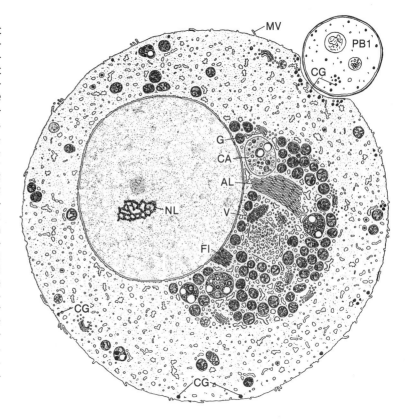

envelope. Attached to the nucleus is an aggregate of cytoplasmic organelles that corresponds to Balbiani's vitelline body[3, 4]; this consists of multiple Golgi complexes; a single stack of annulate lamellae; randomly distributed mitochondria; lipid droplets; dilated, smooth-surfaced endoplasmic reticulum; a centrosome; fine filaments; small aggregates of dense amorphous material; dispersed or aggregated vesicles; short and irregular tubules; multivesicular bodies; and a few membrane-attached and free ribosomes (see Fig. 1–2). The rest of the cytoplasm has a uniform texture with fewer of the organelles. The entire circumference of the subplasmalemmal cytoplasm of the oocyte and the cytocortical region of the first polar body show a heavy population of cortical granules.[5] Microvilli cover the entire oocyte surface, with the exception of the region in contact with the first polar body. The metaphase II spindle is characteristically organized.[5]

DEVELOPMENT OF THE FEMALE INTERNAL ORGANS

Female sexual development does not depend on the presence of ovaries. The gonad, in an undifferentiated stage, begins to develop in the fifth week as a region of multilayered coelomic epithelium (mesothelium), on the entire medial aspect of the gonadal (mesonephric) ridge. The coelomic epithelium is only one to two cells thick elsewhere on the mesonephric ridge. Primary sex cords, consisting of fingerlike extensions of the epithelial cords, grow into the mesenchyme. An outer cortex and an inner medulla result. In embryos with 46,XX chromosomes, the cortex develops into the ovary, and the medulla regresses. In male embryos, this is reversed, with the medulla differentiating into the testis and the cortex regressing. A tunica albuginea develops in both sexes, but in the female it develops at a later stage and is a much thinner layer than in males.

The developing ovary differentiates slowly. Very few primary sex cords invade the medulla, and nearly all of them remain in the cortex. After the regression of the medulla, the primary sex cord clusters surround the primordial ova, which at this time are differentiated as primary oocytes that are in the prophase of the first meiotic division. The follicular cells proliferate from the coelomic epithelium. A full complement of primary oocytes—estimated to be 2 million—are present in the ovaries of a newborn. Regression occurs during childhood, and by puberty some 40,000 primary oocytes are said to remain.[6] Of these, only approximately 400 will develop into secondary oocytes by completing the first meiotic division, one by one, shortly before ovulation each month. Virtually always, only one follicle matures and ruptures at midcycle each month. This continues until about 51.4 years of age, which is the average age when menopause occurs.[5]

During the early fetal period, the ovaries are juxtarenal. They gradually descend into the lesser pelvis. Rarely, when the gubernaculum fails to unite with the uterine fundus, the ovarian and round ligaments become continuous, fail to lengthen, and as a result pull the ovary into the labia majora. In the newborn the ovaries are triangular in a cross section made centrally through the longest plane and are rounded at the ends.[7–9] Surface furrows disappear within months after birth.[9]

MESONEPHRIC (WOLFFIAN) DUCTS AND FORMATION OF NONFUNCTIONAL REMNANTS

The urogenital organs develop from the intermediate mesoderm (Fig. 1–3). They are closely associated with each other during early development. The fetal renal excretory system consists of three organs that develop chronologically into the pronephros, the mesonephros, and the metanephros.[6] Only the mesonephros and its duct participate in the formation of the female genital ducts (see Table 1–1). Excluding the most cranial one or two tubules and the associated mesonephric, or wolffian duct, some five or six cranial mesonephric tubules form the epoöphoron, a vestigial structure associated with the ovary. The

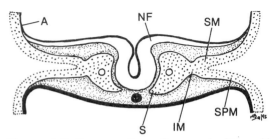

Figure 1–3. Cross section of an early (3-week) embryo showing the three divisions of the mesoderm. A, amnion; IM, intermediate mesoderm; NF, neural fold; S, somite (paraxial mesoderm); SM, somatic mesoderm; SPM, splanchnic mesoderm. (Redrawn from Moore KL, Persaud TVN: The Developing Human. Clinically Oriented Embryology, 6th ed. Philadelphia: WB Saunders, 1998.)

more caudal mesonephric tubules give rise to the paroöphoron, an inconsistent group of coiled tubules seen between the layers of the mesosalpinx. The paroöphoron usually disappears before adulthood. Additionally, one or more stalked, oval, pea-sized cysts known as the *appendices vesiculosae epoöphorontis* (hydatids of Morgagni) are found near the epoöphoron and close to the ostium of the uterine tube. The vestigial remains of the lower portion of the mesonephric (wolffian) duct may be identified laterally on the upper half of the vagina as a minute tube or fibrous cord, the epoöphorantic duct (duct of Gartner). Occasionally, this duct forms into a cyst (Figs. 1–4, 1–5).

PARAMESONEPHRIC (MÜLLERIAN) DUCTS AND FORMATION OF THE UTERINE TUBES AND UTERUS

The paired paramesonephric ducts develop as an invagination of the coelomic epithelium on the lateral aspect of the cranial end of the mesonephric ridge. The caudal end of this ridge grows blindly, subsequently acquires a lumen as it lengthens, and remains lateral to the mesonephric duct (see Figs. 1–4, 1–5). At the caudal end of the mesonephros, the paramesonephric duct turns medially and, crossing ventrally to the mesonephric duct, enters the genital cord, where it bends caudally, juxtaposed with its companion on the opposite side by the third month of gestation. The blind ends of the two ducts produce an elevation on the dorsal wall of the urogenital sinus, the sinus (müllerian) tubercle. Each duct consists of vertical cranial and caudal segments with an intermediate horizontal section (Fig. 1–6). The cranial segment forms the uterine tube, with its coelomic invagination forming the ostium of the tube; the caudal vertical segments fuse to form the uterovaginal primordium, which develops into the lower uterine segment and, while enlarging, incorporates the horizontal aspects to give rise to the fundus and the body of the uterus. The endometrial stroma and myometrium develop from the surrounding mesenchyme.

ADNEXA

The ovary traverses a short distance while descending to occupy its place in the ovarian fossa. It does not enter the inguinal canal. Through the mesovarium the ovary is attached to the medial aspect of the mesonephric fold.

The inguinal fold attaches it to the ventral abdominal wall. A gubernaculum develops in the inguinal fold and later attaches to the uterus laterally near the entrance of the uterine tube. The lower part of the gubernaculum becomes the round ligament of the uterus, whereas the upper part becomes the ovarian ligament. The processus vaginalis peritonei (saccus vaginalis) also develops as a temporary peritoneal evagination. Usually its prolongation into the inguinal canal is completely obliterated. When patent (known as the *canal of Nuck*), it may form the sac of a potential inguinal hernia. The urethral and paraurethral glands remain rudimentary. The greater vestibular glands develop from the urogenital sinus.

ACCESSORY STRUCTURES AND CONGENITAL MALFORMATIONS

Supernumerary ovaries have been reported to occur in the mesovarium, in the broad ligament, and, very rarely, in association with a third uterine tube. Bilateral absence of ovaries is rare. Unilateral absence has been associated with the absence of the corresponding uterine tube. Divided ovaries are common. Ectopically, an ovary can be drawn through the inguinal canal into the labia majora.

The uterus, fallopian tubes, and vagina are often absent in those with severe congenital malformations such as in sympodia or sirenomelia. Unilateral absence of the paramesonephric duct, resulting in severe anomalies, has been reported. The anomalies of the female genital system result from faulty union or lack of the two paramesonephric (müllerian) ducts. This may result in either incomplete or complete duplication of the uterus combined with duplication of the vagina. Many variations between the two extremes are seen. The bicornuate uterus is a common condition in which a single vagina and cervix occur with duplication of the body of the uterus.

Hypospadias in the female, in which the urethra opens in the vagina, is quite different from that in the male. Epispadias in females is very rare and is similar to that in males. Usually there is an associated bifid clitoris and prepuce. A deep groove separates the two halves, and the urethral orifice may be in the clitoris or ventral to it.

Errors in sexual development result in ambiguous genitalia. These may be the result of defective genetic direction, steroidogenesis, abnormal hormonal influences, or dyssynchrony during organogenesis. These disorders are discussed in Chapters 7 and 8.

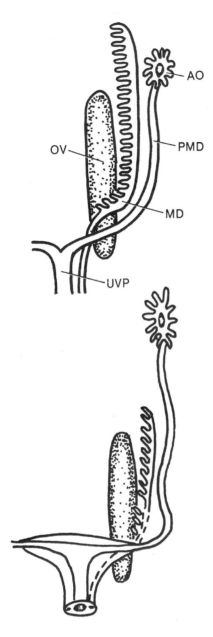

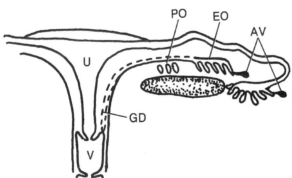

Figure 1–4. Transformation of the mesonephric (wolffian) and paramesonephric (müllerian) ducts into definitive structures. AO, abdominal ostium; AV, appendices vesiculosae (hydatids of Morgagni); EO, epoöphoron; GD, Gartner's duct; MD, mesonephric (wolffian) duct; OV, ovary; PMD, paramesonephric (müllerian) duct; PO, paroöphoron; U, uterus; UVP, uterovaginal primordium; V, vagina. (Modified from Anson BJ [ed]: Morris' Human Anatomy. A Complete Systematic Treatise, 12th ed. New York: McGraw-Hill, 1966. Modified with permission of McGraw-Hill, Inc.)

Figure 1–5. Persisting remnants of the mesonephric (wolffian) duct at puberty drawn in relation to the uterine tubes, uterus, and vagina. AV, appendices vesiculosae; CMD, cranial mesonephric duct remnants; CTM, cranial mesonephric tubules; EO, epoöphoron (cranial mesonephric tubule remnants); GDC, Gartner's duct cysts (caudal mesonephric duct remnants); PO, paroöphoron (caudal mesonephric tubule remnants). (Modified from Anson BJ [ed]: Morris' Human Anatomy. A Complete Systematic Treatise, 12th ed. New York: McGraw-Hill, 1966. Modified with permission of McGraw-Hill, Inc.)

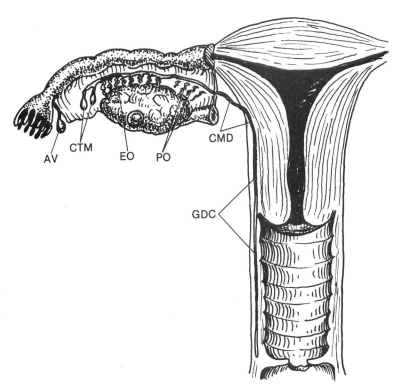

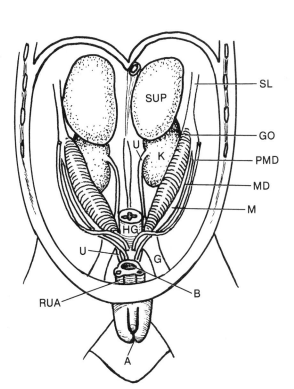

Figure 1–6. Dissection of a 26-mm human embryo at the end of the embryonic period (about 56 days) showing the developing mesonephric and paramesonephric ducts. A, anus; B, bladder; G, gubernaculum in inguinal fold; GO, gonad; HG, hindgut; K, kidney; M, mesonephros; MD, mesonephric duct; PMD, paramesonephric duct; RUA, right umbilical artery; SL, atrophying suspensory ligament; SUP, suprarenal gland; U, ureter. (Redrawn from Hamilton WJ, Boyd JD, Mossman HW: Human Embryology, 4th ed. Baltimore: Williams & Wilkins, 1972.)

DEVELOPMENT OF THE FEMALE EXTERNAL GENITALIA

The mons pubis, the rounded fleshy prominence over the symphysis pubis, is formed from subcutaneous adipose tissue. It remains devoid of hair until puberty, when it becomes covered by coarse hair limited above by a horizontal boundary.

The external genitalia initially develop in an undifferentiated state, and it is not possible to identify the sex externally before 12 weeks of gestation (Fig. 1–7, Table 1–2). At the end of the embryonic period (about 8 weeks), the genital tubercle appears as a surface elevation at the cranial end of the cloacal membrane and lengthens into the phallus (Figs. 1–8, 1–9). Within it, the urethral plate grows toward the tip. The lower end of the plate abuts the ectoderm-lined primary urethral groove, which concomitantly develops along the caudal surface of the phallus. The margins of the groove are the genital folds that surround the urogenital membrane and proximally terminate near the ventral end of the anus. The urogenital membrane ruptures at about 6 weeks, providing a common perineal space (the future vestibule) for the urinary and genital openings at the base of the phallus, bounded by the genital folds, which develop into labia minora. Two genital (labioscrotal) swellings form laterally and become the labia majora. The vestibule develops from the remains of the uro-

genital sinus. The urethral meatus, vaginal opening, the ducts of the greater and lesser vestibular glands, and the bulbs of the vestibule are found in the floor of the vestibule (Fig. 1–10).

The phallus, which in the early stages is longer in the female than in the male, forms the clitoris. The prepuce develops first as a ridge proximal to the glans and extending forward. Over the dorsum and the sides of the glans clitoridis, the shallow preputial sac is formed, but the ventral side remains free. Only in this manner does preputial development differ from the male homologue. The homologies of the external (and internal) genital organs are shown in Table 1–1.[8, 10, 11]

DEVELOPMENT OF THE VAGINA AND HYMEN

In the tenth week of gestation an epithelial proliferation from the dorsal lining of the urogenital sinus begins in the region of the sinus tubercle. The hymen develops later at this site of proliferation. It is not known whether the proliferating epithelium is derived from the sinus tubercle or from the mesonephric duct. The proliferating epithelium extends cranially and forms a solid, flattened plate inside the tubular uterovaginal primordium. The fibromuscular vagina develops from this solid plate by recanalization in a caudocranial direction. The caudal end of the paramesonephric duct recedes until its junc-

Table 1–2. Chronology of the Appearance of the Components of the Genital System

Fertilization Age	Crown-Rump Length (mm)	Developmental Event
Days		
Zero time	—	Chromosomal sex established
24–25	2.5–4.5 (13–20 somites)	Primordial germ cells; genital tubercle develops at the cranial end of the cloacal membrane
33–36	7.0–9.0	Undifferentiated gonad
41–43	11.0–14.0	Primordial germ cells incorporated in the primary sex cords; paramesonephric (müllerian) duct; nipples; urorectal septum fuses with the cloacal membrane; urogenital membrane ruptures (15-mm embryo)
56	27.0–31.0	Anal membrane ruptures; despite the fetus's human appearance, the external genitalia are still ambiguous
Weeks		
10	61	Ovary and vagina differentiate
12	87	External genitalia distinguished
16	140	Primordial follicles
18	160	Clitoris relatively large
Perinatal period	—	Hymen may rupture
Newborn	—	2 million primary oocytes in the ovaries
Childhood, puberty	—	Regression of primary oocytes; some 40,000 remain at puberty
Reproductive period (15–50 yr)	—	Only about 400 become secondary oocytes and are expelled, one at a time, at ovulation
After menopause	—	Internal reproductive organs gradually regress

Data from Moore KL, Persaud TVN: The Developing Human. Clinically Oriented Embryology, 6th ed. Philadelphia: WB Saunders, 1998.

Figure 1–7. A series of diagrams illustrating the developing female external genitalia. *A, B,* The undifferentiated stages, 4 to 8 weeks. *C–E,* At 9, 11, and 12 weeks, respectively. A, anus; AM, anal membrane; CM, cloacal membrane; DGC, developing glans clitoridis; FLSS, fused labioscrotal swellings; GC, glans clitoridis; GT, genital tubercle; HY, hymen; LMA, labia majora; LMI, labia minora; LSS, labioscrotal swelling; MP, mons pubis; PLC, posterior labial commissure; UF, urogenital fold; UG, urethral groove; UM, urogenital membrane; UO, urethral orifice; VV, vestibule of vagina. (Redrawn from Moore KL, Persaud TVN: The Developing Human. Clinically Oriented Embryology, 6th ed. Philadelphia: WB Saunders, 1998.)

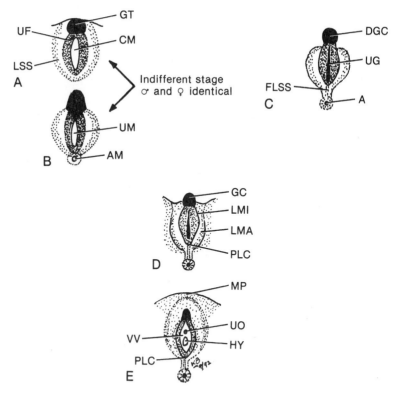

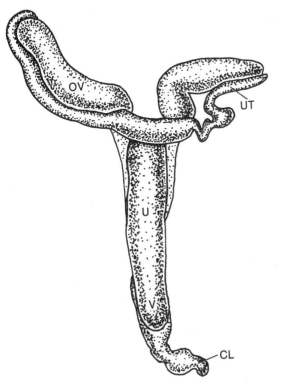

Figure 1–8. The female internal genitalia at 13 weeks (crown-rump length, 101 mm). CL, clitoris; OV, ovary; U, uterus; UT, uterine tube; V, vagina. (Redrawn from England MA: Color Atlas of Life Before Birth. Normal Fetal Development. London: Mosby–Year Book Europe Ltd., 1983.)

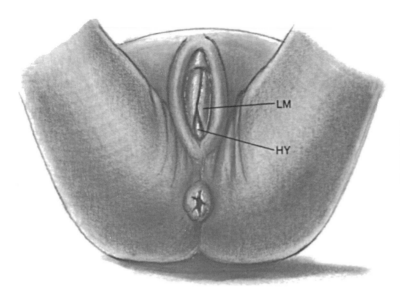

Figure 1–9. The perineum of a female fetus in the third trimester (crown-rump length, 254 mm). HY, pouting hymen; LM, labia minora.

tion with the sinus epithelium reaches the cervical canal. Vaginal fornices develop from the upper end of the vaginal plate, growing around the cervix. At the lower end, the plate around the hymenal orifice forms the hymen by trapping a thin layer of mesoderm. The walls of the vagina are seen through the hymenal orifice; the rugae in the lower part of the anterior wall of the vagina immediately beneath the urethra are more prominent in young females and in virgins.

The hymen is lined on its superior (vaginal) surface by the vaginal epithelium and by the sinus epithelium on its inferior (vestibular) surface. In later development the inferior hymenal surface and most of the vestibule are lined by an epithelium similar to that of the vagina. The urogenital sinus shortens to form the vaginal vestibule, which opens on the surface between the genital folds. The vaginal epithelium hypertro-

phies greatly in the fetus under the influence of maternal hormones but remains unproliferated after birth and through childhood.

The hymen, a fold of vascularized mucous membrane, lies within the vaginal orifice and separates the vagina from the vestibule. It shows great variations in thickness and in the size and shape of the hymenal opening. The more commonly observed hymenal variations are described and illustrated in Table 1–3.

GENITAL SYSTEM OF THE FEMALE NEWBORN AND THE CHILD

The average weight of a full-term newborn infant is about 3300 gm (7 lb), and the average crown-to-heel length is about 50 cm (20 in). In

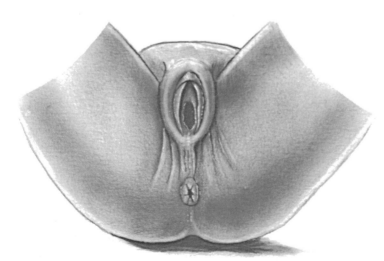

Figure 1–10. The perineum of a newborn female.

Table 1–3. Commonly Observed Hymenal Types*

Hymen	Hymenal Opening(s)	Illustrations†
i. Annular; circular; lunar	Circular or moon-shaped	GC, UM, LM, HY
ii. Bifenestratus; biforis	Two side-by-side openings with an intervening septum between them	
iii. Crescentic	Half moon–shaped	
iv. Cribriform; fenestrated	Many small openings	
v. Denticular; fringed	Serrate-edged (as in a parous condition)	
vi. Falciform	Sickle-shaped	
vii. Imperforate	None; vaginal orifice completely closed	
viii. Infundibuliform	Centrally open with sloping sides	
ix. Septate	Opening divided by a narrow septum	
x. Subseptate	Opening partially blocked by a septum growing out of one edge but not reaching the other	

*After coitus the remnants of the torn hymen are known as hymenal caruncles.

†All illustrations (i–x) depict the hymenal condition in a 3-year-old child. The labia minora (LM) are pulled widely apart; the hymenal openings (HY) are diagrammatically exaggerated. GC, glans clitoridis; UM, urinary meatus.

Data partly from Anson BJ (ed). Morris' Human Anatomy. A Complete Systematic Treatise, 12th ed. New York: McGraw-Hill, 1966, p 1523.

general, the newborn female is slightly smaller and weighs less than the newborn male.[9] Water constitutes 80% of the total body weight, as compared with 60% at puberty. The newborn has 45% of water as extracellular fluid and 35% as intracellular fluid (as compared with 17% and 43%, respectively, at puberty). The development of the various components of the female genital system is described in Table 1–2.

In the newborn, the relatively large labia majora are bound inferiorly by a posterior labial commissure. Superiorly, they merge into the mons pubis (see footnote in Table 1–1). The labia minora are relatively larger at birth. The clitoris is also relatively larger and more prominent in the newborn than in the adult. The hymen in late fetal life and at birth consists of a membranous fold, which may protrude between the labia minora (see Fig. 1–9). The vaginal orifice has a circumference of about 5 cm and can permit speculum examination of the vagina. During early childhood the orifice is more deeply positioned. The rugae of the anterior vaginal wall are prominent and are seen through the vaginal orifice (Fig. 1–11; see Table 1–3). The vaginal wall is thin until puberty and has a much redder appearance than in the adult. At puberty, Döderlein's bacillus (*Lactobacillus acidophilus*), a large gram-positive microorganism, appears in the vagina and breaks down glycogen in desquamated cells to form lactic acid. This protective phenomenon changes the pH of vaginal secretions from alkaline to acidic, thus reducing the incidence of vaginitis. Mucous glands are absent in the vagina; cervical gland mucus keeps the vagina moist. Pubic hair appears at puberty; the labia minora remain devoid of hair.

The vaginal vestibule is the cleft between the labia minora into which open the urethra, the vagina, and many lesser vestibular glands. The greater vestibular glands open by a duct in the groove between the hymen and the labium minus on either side at the posterior or inferior aspect of the vaginal orifice (Fig. 1–12). Between the vaginal orifice and the frenulum of the labia minora is a shallow vestibular fossa. The hymen surrounds the vaginal orifice, which appears as an opening into it. The hymen shows great variation (see Table 1–3). The bulbs of the vestibule, the homologue of the corpus spongiosum penis, are paired erectile bodies on both sides of the vaginal orifice and are united in front of it by a commissura bulborum or pars intermedia. Poste-

riorly they are in contact with the greater vestibular glands, and their anterior ends are joined to one another by a commissure and to the glans clitoridis by two bands of erectile tissue.

The form, size, position, and histologic appearance of the internal genital organs vary greatly between birth and the attainment of puberty (Table 1–4).[9] Before birth, the uterus projects above the lesser pelvis, and the cervix is much larger than the fundus. The uterus is piriform at puberty and weighs 14 to 17 gm. Usually the fundus is below the superior pelvic aperture, but its position depends on the contents of the bladder and the rectum. The organ is somewhat enlarged during menstruation because of increased vascularity. The ovaries are very large in the fetus, extending nearly the entire length of the uterine tubes (see Fig. 1–8).[7] After birth, subsequent development reduces their overall dimension, and they reach the adult size at puberty, gradually regressing after menopause.

APPLIED EMBRYOLOGY

IN VITRO TECHNIQUES TO AID FERTILIZATION

In recent years several new methods are being successfully applied to ensure fertilization and implantation, thus bridging the gap between ste-

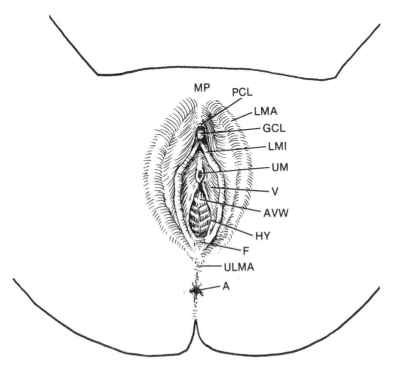

Figure 1–11. Illustration of the perineum of a 10-year-old female with labia separated. A, anus; AVW, anterior vaginal wall; F, fourchette; GCL, glans clitoridis; HY, hymen; LMA, labia majora; LMI, labia minora; MP, mons pubis; PCL, prepuce of the clitoris; ULMA, union of labia majora, posterior commissure; UM, urethral meatus; V, vestibule. (Redrawn from Snell RS: Atlas of Clinical Anatomy. Boston: Little, Brown, 1978.)

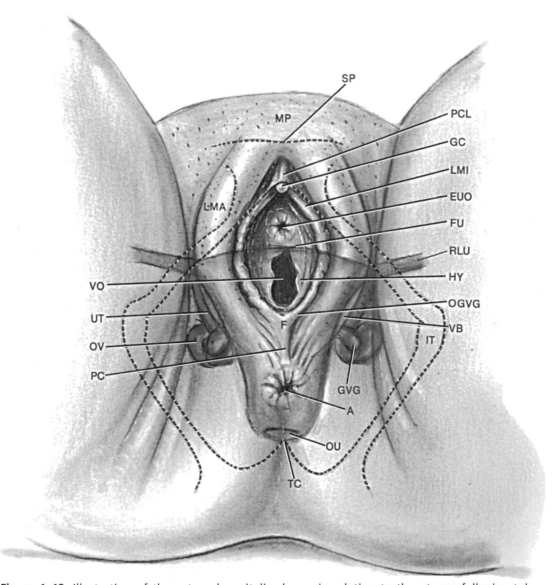

Figure 1–12. Illustration of the external genitalia shown in relation to the uterus, fallopian tubes, and ovaries, and the bony pelvis in a 10-year-old female. These internal structures are shown superimposed from an examining physician's view. A, anus; EUO, external urethral opening; F, fourchette; FU, fundus uteri; GC, glans clitoridis; GVG, greater vestibular gland; HY, hymen; IT, ischial tuberosity; LMA, labia majora; LMI, labia minora; MP, mons pubis; OGVG, opening of the greater vestibular gland; OU, ostium uteri; OV, ovary; PC, posterior commissure; PCL, prepuce of the clitoris; RLU, round ligament of the uterus; SP, pubic symphysis; TC, tip of coccyx; UT, fallopian (uterine) tube; VB, vestibular bulb; VO, vaginal orifice. (Modified from Anson BJ [ed]: Morris' Human Anatomy. A Complete Systematic Treatise, 12th ed. New York: McGraw-Hill, 1966. Modified with permission of McGraw-Hill, Inc.)

Table 1–4. Data on the Female Reproductive Organs[8, 9]

	Ovaries	Uterine (Fallopian) Tubes	Uterus	Vagina†
Combined weight				
In the newborn	0.3 gm	—	3–4 gm	—
First 6 weeks postnatally	0.6 gm	—	—	—
Increase between birth and adulthood	5.0 gm°	—	— 14–17 gm (adult weight)	—
Size				
At birth	13 mm long, 6 mm wide, 4 mm thick[8]	3.0 cm long, 5.0 mm wide	2.5–5.0 cm long, 2.0 cm wide, 1.3 cm thick	2.5–3.5 cm long, 1.5 cm wide; only potential cavity
In the adult	2.5–3.5 cm long, 2.0 cm wide, 1.0 cm thick	10 cm long, 0.1–3.0 mm wide	7.5 cm long, 5 cm wide, 2.5 cm thick, weighs 30–40 gm (1 kg at term)[8]	Anterior wall, 7.5 cm long; posterior wall, 9.0 cm long; circumference, about 4–5 cm†
Long axis				
At birth	Vertical	—	—	—
During descent after birth	Horizontal	—	—	—
In ovarian fossa	Vertical	—	—	—
Epithelium				
Fetal	—	—	—	Greatly hypertrophic
During childhood	—	—	—	Remains inactive, growing slowly

°The ovaries weigh 11.3 gm at maturity, a 32- to 37-fold increase from the birth weight.[10]
†The stated circumference of the orifice is about 5 cm.[9]

rility and fertility. Some of these new procedures are the following:

1. Intracytoplasmic Sperm Injection: A single sperm is injected into the cytoplasm of a mature oocyte in cases where in vitro fertilization has failed or where too few sperm are available.

2. In Vitro Fertilization (IVF) and Embryo Transfer (ET): Transfer of the cleaving stages into the uterus after the IVF procedure (zygote intrafallopian transfer, ZIFT) has been successfully employed for women sterile because of tubal occlusion. The first such IVF baby, Louise Brown, was born in England.[12] For details of these procedures see Edwards and Brody.[13]

3. Assisted In Vivo Fertilization: Superovulated oocytes are retrieved and laparoscopically placed with the sperm into the uterine tubes for the gamete intrafallopian transfer (GIFT) procedure.

4. Cryopreservation of Early Embryonic Stages: Blastocysts and cleaving stages of about eight cells can be preserved by freezing in glycerol for long periods and transferred to the uterus after thawing.

5. Partial Zona Drilling (PZD): A tiny hole is drilled through the zona pellucida for unobstructed passage of the sperm into the oocyte cytoplasm.

6. Surrogacy: A woman who underwent hysterectomy still produces viable oocytes. In such cases IVF procedures are applied, and early-stage embryos or cleaving fertilized oocytes are transferred to the uterus of a surrogate mother for further development.

CHORIONIC VILLUS SAMPLING

Chorionic villus biopsy specimens are obtained via one of several approaches (abdominal, transcervical). These are of great value for detecting chromosomal evaluations, X-linked disorders, and inborn errors of metabolism. This procedure can be performed around the seventh week after fertilization.

MOLECULAR BIOLOGY AS APPLIED TO HUMAN DEVELOPMENT

Molecular biological approaches such as recombinant DNA technology, transgenic animals, and chimeric models are important tools that examine specific gene expressions, their regulation of morphogenesis, and how various cells form specific embryonic parts. Homeobox-containing *(HOX)* genes are reported to control pattern formation during embryonic development.

REFERENCES

1. Fukuda T: Ultrastructure of primordial germ cells in human embryo. Virchows Arch [Cell Pathol] 1976; 20:85–89.
2. Turner JH, Bloodworth JMB Jr: The testis. In: Bloodworth JMB Jr (ed): Endocrine Pathology. Baltimore: Williams & Wilkins, 1968, pp 430–477.
3. Hertig AT: The primary human oocyte: Some observations on the fine structure of Balbiani's vitelline body and the origin of the annulate lamellae. Am J Anat 1968; 122:107–138.
4. Lentz TL: Cell Fine Structure. An Atlas of Drawings of Whole-Cell Structure. Philadelphia: WB Saunders, 1971, p 269.
5. VanBlerkom J: Occurrence and developmental consequences of aberrant cellular organization in meiotically mature human oocytes after exogenous ovarian hyperstimulation. J Electron Microsc Technol 1990; 16:324–346.
6. Moore KL, Persaud TVN: The Developing Human. Clinically Oriented Embryology, 6th ed. Philadelphia: WB Saunders, 1998.
7. England MA: Color Atlas of Life Before Birth. Normal Fetal Development. Chicago: Year Book Medical, 1983.
8. Williams PL, Bannister LH, Barry MM, Collins P, Dyson M, Dussek JE, Ferguson MWJ: Gray's Anatomy, 38th ed. Edinburgh: Churchill Livingstone, 1995.
9. Crelin ES: Functional Anatomy of the Newborn. New Haven, CT: Yale University Press, 1973.
10. Anson BJ (ed): Morris' Human Anatomy. A Complete Systematic Treatise, 12th ed. New York: McGraw Hill, 1966.
11. International Anatomical Nomenclature Committee: Nomina Anatomica, 6th ed. Baltimore: Williams & Wilkins, 1989.
12. Steptoe PC, Edwards RG: Birth after the reimplantation of a human embryo. Lancet 1978; 2:366.
13. Edwards RG, Brody SA: Principles and Practice of Assisted Human Early Embryonic Reproduction. Philadelphia: WB Saunders, 1995.

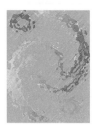

Chapter 2

Normal Growth and Pubertal Development

Dennis M. Styne

Growth in stature comprises distinct phases, each of which is controlled by a different mix of endocrine factors. Growth can be suppressed by a multitude of disorders, but it can be augmented by rather few conditions. Sexual precocity figures prominently in the diagnoses to be entertained in such a situation. The normal physiology of growth and pubertal development is the focus of this chapter.

GROWTH

THE MEASUREMENT OF GROWTH

Measurement of stature is the most cost-effective procedure available in the pediatric office and is exceptionally important. Failing to measure a child limits the assessment of the health of the patient. A growth deficiency can be missed for several visits, and the diagnosis of a systemic disorder that may cause such a growth failure as its first outward manifestation may be delayed. Mismeasurements are responsible for numerous incorrect referrals for short stature. Alternating measurements with and without shoes on or allowing the child to slouch causes many such errors (of omission or commission).

It is difficult to obtain an accurate measurement of an infant's length; measuring an infant always requires the assistance of two adults. The child must be laid on a flat surface fitted with a device that has another flat surface horizontal to the plane of the top of the child's head and yet another parallel to the first, in the plane of the child's feet. The two planes should be at a 90-degree angle to a ruler which forms the back of the device and on which the child's height is read. A device such as an "Infantometer" is used for this technique. Common errors occur with the most often used method for infant measurements when a single observer makes a mark on the paper covering the soft examining table at

the foot of the child and another mark at the head. Unfortunately, the distance between the mark at the head and the mark at the feet will vary owing to the flexibility of the paper, and the movement of a conscious child restrained by only one person will make such measurements meaningless. Again, it takes two adults to measure one infant using correct technique.

The measurement of a patient older than 2 years is taken with the child standing. The change from lying to standing measurements is responsible for a large number of inappropriate referrals owing to the 1- to 2-cm decrease in height that occurs when switching from lying to standing. The position used for measuring should be indicated on the chart next to the numerical value for children between 2 and 4 years to avoid this mistake. The child must be measured with shoes off; if the child is measured in shoes one time and without them another time, the technique is guaranteed to cause 2- to 4-cm discrepancies in height measurements every year.

The device used to measure standing height must be a variation of a stadiometer (Fig. 2–1). The child must stand with the back to a wall or another hard surface with the back straight, and heels and back pressed to the surface. The head is level in the Frankfort plane (i.e., a line connecting the outer canthus of the eye with the external auditory meatus intersects the long axis of the trunk at a 90-degree angle). The bare feet must be on a horizontal plane made of a hard surface, which is considered to be the lower border of the measurement; the top or upper border of the distance of height must be delineated by a firm plate precisely horizontal to the plane of the feet, and the measurement must be read from a stationary ruler placed at right angles to the planes at the feet and head. A Harpenden stadiometer (available from Seritex Inc., 450 Barell Ave., Carlsbad, NM 88220) is the most accurate of such devices, but a simpler apparatus that meets the criteria will give accurate meas-

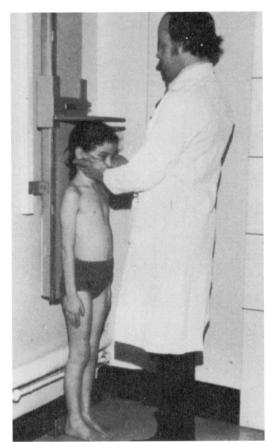

Figure 2–1. Measuring stature using a Harpenden stadiometer. The head is held with the external auricular meatus and outer canthus of the eye in a Frankfort plane (horizontal). Upward pressure is applied to the mastoid processes in order to encourage the child to stand up straight and thus eliminate changes in posture and bearing. The counter to the right of the moving platform is read when the child has taken a deep breath and exhaled. This equipment can be obtained from Jeritax Inc., Carlstadt, NJ. (From Hindmarsh PC, Brook CGD: Normal growth and its endocrine control. *In* Brook CGD [ed]: Clinical Paediatric Endocrinology. 2nd ed. Oxford: Blackwell Scientific Publications, 1989, p 59.)

urements. Unfortunately, the useless device attached to a common office scale is found in many offices. The plate at the top of the pole cannot be guaranteed to be horizontal to the floor and usually can angle up and down, thus introducing errors in the measurement. Without the means to straighten the back against a straight surface, the child may slouch and confound the measurement. This flexible measuring arm attached to the common office scale must not be used to measure children.

All measurements should be taken in metric units. The tendency to round off numbers becomes troublesome when an inch is the unit of measure; an inaccuracy of an inch or a half-inch due to rounding off is a more serious error than a mistake of 1 or 0.5 cm: a half-inch (1.25-cm) rounding error over a 6-month period, when annualized to 2.5 cm, means the difference between 4-cm growth per year, which is abnormal, and 6.5-cm/year, which is normal in middle childhood. Careful measurement by either method described earlier should allow three measurements made at the same office visit to differ by no more than 0.2 to 0.3 cm (Fig. 2–2).

After the measurement is obtained, it must be displayed graphically on a growth chart (see Fig. 2–2). Physicians evaluating growth in the United States use charts derived from a National Center for Health Statistics (NCHS) survey of children's heights (see www.cdc.gov/hchs/about/major/nhanes/growthcharts/charts.htm).[1] Other available charts are based on theoretical constructs which explain different aspects of growth. For example, Tanner has constructed growth curves utilizing longitudinal data derived from the NCHS and calculated data from theoretical growth curves thereafter.[2] The age of the child must be accurately plotted; it is useless to plot a child of 10 years and 4 months as a 10-year-old. The exact numeric measurement should be recorded on the patient's medical chart, but an abnormality of stature or growth is more obvious to an observer on a chart than as a number on a table. A decrease in growth rate in which the child "falls away from the curve" becomes obvious much more quickly on the graphic display. Growth rate velocity charts that demonstrate growth in centimeters per 6 months or per year make variations in growth rate extremely obvious earlier than it is apparent on the more common stature growth chart (Fig. 2–3).[3]

Growth charts are available for a few diseases and more are being developed. For example, charts are available to assess the progress of a child with Turner syndrome,[4] achondroplasia, and Down syndrome. It is important, therefore, to realize that children with one of these syndromes can have another complicating, possibly treatable, condition that can further impair their growth. A patient with Down syndrome may have hypothyroidism, which will make the child extremely short for a patient with Down syndrome.

A convenient method of comparing the height of a child to those of the biologic parent is provided by the use of target heights. In the United States the mid-parental height, the average height of the parents ([mother's height + father's height]/2), is plotted on the growth chart

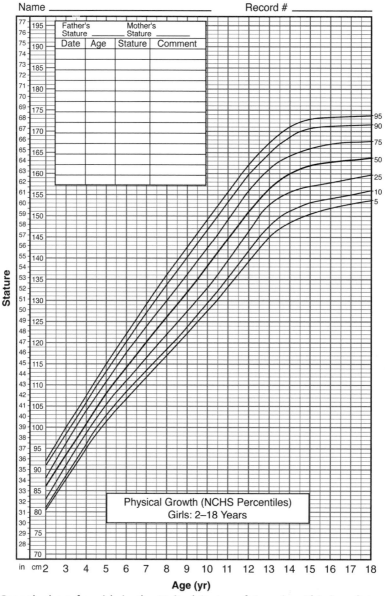

Figure 2–2. *A,* Growth chart for girls in the United States of America. This is a distance chart which displays height at a given chronological age. The fact that the lower limit of the curve is set at the 5th percentile is arbitrary and does not mean per se that a child below the 5th percentile requires medical evaluation; children with true growth disorders usually have stature well below the 5th percentile. (Data from 1976 study of the National Center for Health Statistics, Hyattsville, MD; and Hamill PVV, et al: Physical growth: National Center for Health Statistics percentiles. Am J Clin Nutr 1979; 32:607. Reproduced from Styne DM: Growth. *In* Greenspan FP [ed]: Basic and Clinical Endocrinology, 3rd ed. Los Altos, CA: Lange, 1991. Redrawn by Appleton & Lange and reprinted with permission of Ross Laboratories, Columbus, OH 43216 and Appleton & Lange, San Mateo, CA. 1991, Ross Laboratories.)

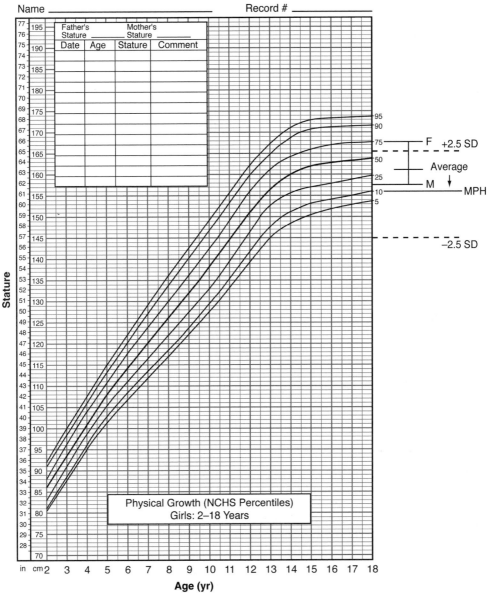

Figure 2–2 *Continued. B*, Parent-specific adjustment of the growth curve is noted for a girl of 10 years of age with a height of 125 cm (the circled point) which puts her below the 5th percentile for the U.S. population. Her mother is plotted at M with a height of 62 inches (adults usually bring in their historical heights in inches). Her father's height is 66 inches at F. Both parents are at about the 10th percentile for their sex. The average of the parents' heights is 64 inches. After subtracting 2.5 inches from this average, the adjusted mid-parental height is 61.5 inches, at the 10th percentile on a U.S. girl's chart at 18 years of age (noted as MPH). If we were to extrapolate these boundaries back to 10 years, following the standard growth curve we would find that her height is well within the normal range for this family, and if we were to consider the adjusted mid-parental height as the 50th percentile for this family, we would see that she is actually at about the 25th percentile for this family. The bounds of ±2.5 SD from mean is approximately 4 inches above and 4 inches below the adjusted mid-parental height. Thus, the target height for the girl and the boundaries of 2.5 SD is about 61.5 inches for the mean, 57.5 inches for the lower boundary and 65.5 inches for the upper boundary (boundaries noted by dashed lines). We would expect a healthy girl of this height in this family to reach a height between these boundaries.

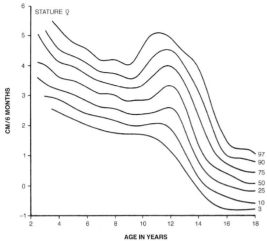

Figure 2–3. Growth velocity chart for girls in the United States. This chart demonstrates the amount of growth achieved over a 6-month period. Note the pubertal growth spurt. Growth velocity decreases before stature decreases in disorders of growth and is a more sensitive indication of a problem. This chart has a lower limit of the 3rd percentile compared to the 5th percentile limit in Figure 2–2. (Roche AF, Himes JH: Incremental growth charts. Am J Clin Nutr 1980; 33:2041. © American Society for Clinical Nutrition.)

at 18 years, after it is adjusted for gender. Thus, 2.5 inches is *subtracted from* the mid-parental height before plotting on a daughter's chart but is *added to* the mid-parental height to plot it on a son's chart. The resulting corrected mid-parental height represents the 50th percentile for this family. The 5th percentile for this family is represented by drawing a line at 2 SD below this mean (subtract 4 inches from the mid-parental height in the United States) and the 95th percentile by drawing another line at 2 SD above this mean (add 4 inches from the mid-parental height in the United States). Extrapolating these lines back to the height of the child along the standard growth curve will determine whether the height of the child is appropriate for the genetic characteristics of this family. If the parents grew up in poverty or in a war zone or if they suffered from chronic disease or malnutrition, their heights might be spuriously decreased.

It is possible to revise the percentile height of a child based on the parents' heights. Roche developed tables to determine whether an American child's height should be revised upward or downward owing to the influence of the biologic parents' heights.[5] Thus, a child with a height at the 5th percentile on the U.S. growth chart who

has short parents might have an adjusted height raised to, for example, the 20th percentile, eliminating worry about abnormal growth, whereas another child of the same age and same height with tall parents might have height adjusted down significantly, so that concern about stature is increased.

The upper to lower segment ratio (U/L) is useful in determining causes of growth deviations. *U/L* is defined as the length from the top of the pubic ramus to the top of the head divided by the distance from the top of the pubic ramus to the floor. Owing to the elongation of the extremities during puberty, U/L changes markedly during the prepubertal and early pubertal periods. The gain in length of the legs is similar to that in growth of the upper torso due to the growth of the spine, although the legs grow longer before the trunk does. Thus there is an increase in sitting height during puberty. The mean U/L of children at birth is 1.7, of a 1-year-old is 1.4, and that of white adults is 0.92 ± 0.4 (SD) and that of African American adults is 0.85. There is no difference in U/L between the sexes.[6] "Eunuchoid proportions" are identified in hypogonadal patients, whose delayed epiphyseal fusion leads to lengthened extremities, and a decreased U/L, and an increased arm span relative to height.

Fetal Growth[7]

The growth of a fetus to parturition is a remarkable event: a human fetus begins as a single fertilized cell that differentiates into more than 200 cell types. The length of the human conceptus increases 5000-fold, the surface area by 61 × 10[6],[8] the weight by 6 × 10[12].[9] The growth of the fetus is promoted by the availability of adequate oxygen and nutrition in concert with the effects of growth factors, all operating according to a basic plan dictated by the genes (which is especially important early in gestation) and influenced by the maternal environment, which is most important late in gestation.

Peak growth velocity in the fetus approaches 12 cm/month (approximately 12 times peak velocity (Fig. 2–4) during the pubertal growth spurt) at 4 to 6 months of gestation, only to decrease toward term owing to limitations of space within the uterus.[10] The brief increase in growth in the months after parturition is probably due to catch-up growth after release from uterine constraints. Weight increases later than growth in the fetus—after 30 weeks of gestation—as most adipose tissue is added during

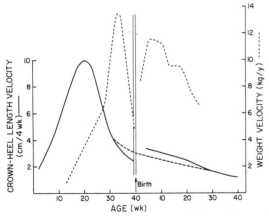

Figure 2–4. Fetal and neonatal length and weight velocity curves. The solid line indicates growth velocity (in cm/4 weeks) and shows the remarkable peak at midgestation. The heavy dashed line shows what growth velocity would have been if uterine restraint were eliminated, thereby allowing increased growth in utero toward term and less catch-up growth after release from the uterine environment in the neonatal period. Weight velocity is indicated by the dotted line. (Redrawn by Underwood and Van Wyk in Foster and Wilson [eds]: Williams Textbook of Endocrinology, Philadelphia: WB Saunders, 1985, from data in Tanner JM: Fetus into Man. Cambridge: Harvard University Press, 1978.)

the third trimester. Fetal size is more closely related to maternal influences than to paternal ones (e.g., the birth size of singletons is proportional to maternal size rather than paternal size). Multiple births reduce the space available in the uterus and multiple-birth newborns are smaller for gestational age than age-matched singletons.

Genetic influences affect birth weight. Many syndromes associated with disorders of chromosome number (e.g., trisomies) or structure (e.g., abnormalities of the X chromosome) lead to poor fetal growth and low birth weight. There is a difference in the range of birth weights between ethnic groups demonstrating genetic influence.[11]

The placenta is an endocrine organ that influences all aspects of fetal growth. It also ensures the supply of adequate nutrition and oxygen for the fetus and regulates hormones and growth factors that affect growth.[12] Embryonic growth is controlled in the individual organs by nutrient supply and locally active growth factors during the first trimester of pregnancy. Thereafter, fetal growth depends essentially upon maternalplacental cooperation in delivering nutrients to the fetus.[13]

Placental weight is usually directly related to birth weight. Infections or vascular abnormalities affecting placental circulation and nutrient delivery impair fetal growth: the size of the placenta decreases with fetal weight.[14] The surface area for exchange between the maternal and fetal circulation is important in normal pregnancies as it is reduced with preeclampsia, when birth weight is reduced.[15] Severe diabetes mellitus, cigarette smoking, and abuse of certain drugs decrease placental blood flow and retard fetal growth. Uterine circulation will be impaired by placental infarction, infection or the development of fistulas, hemangiomas, among other conditions. Infections such as toxoplasmosis, rubella, cytomegalovirus, herpes, and syphilis are well-documented causes of decreased fetal growth and birth weight.

The classic definition of intrauterine growth retardation or intrauterine growth restriction (IUGR) is a birth weight below the 10th percentile (or 2500 gm for a term baby in the United States). This definition has been criticized as being too inclusive, *too small for gestational age* is the suggested designation for those whose weight is below the 10th percentile and *IUGR* is reserved for those lower than the 3rd percentile.[16] IUGR is classified as *symmetric* when the head and the body are small and as *asymmetric* when the head is relatively spared. The latter group show catch-up growth more frequently than the former, but some 10% to 30% of IUGR infants remain short as children and adults, in contrast to infants appropriate for gestational age, who generally have catch-up growth in the first 2 years.[17] Several investigators suggest that symmetric IUGR is simply more severe than asymmetric IUGR. There is evidence from several studies that growth hormone treatment of IUGR infants increases their growth rate.[18–20] IUGR is a very costly condition, in emotional, social, and financial terms, because the consequences persist long after birth.

Growth in Infancy

During the first year of life, a normal child doubles birth weight and increases length 50% over the measurements at birth. Thus, an infant grows faster than at any other time after delivery. Male infants have advanced bone development and grow faster than girls for the first 3 to 6 months of life, a period contemporaneous with the episodic increases in testosterone secretion characteristic of infant boys.

Although most healthy babies tend to cluster in their birth weights about the population mean, during the 2 years after birth infants will find the growth channel they are to occupy until puberty.[21, 22] Those destined genetically to achieve taller stature but of below average birth weight (perhaps because of a smaller mother) will increase their growth velocity until a stature above average is reached. Conversely, those of above average birth length but with a genetic endowment to achieve a shorter than average stature will have a slower than average growth rate during this period. Those children who will ultimately have constitutional delay in growth decrease their position on the growth curves. This is the period that Smith called "the era of changing growth rate."[21] It must be emphasized that these gentle changes in percentiles of stature are quite different than the more dramatic changes characteristic of pathologic conditions.

Growth in Childhood

Karlberg divides growth into distinct phases—infant, childhood, and pubertal (ICP) growth—and relates them to the endocrine milieu by the ICP growth curves (Fig. 2–5).[23] The infancy period is considered to be a manifestation of the continuation of the decreasing growth rate seen in the fetus after mid-gestation. Thus, the growth rate is very fast during the first 12 to 18 months, but shows a consistent downward trend until the infancy influence on total growth disappears between age 18 and 48 months. The infancy period is considered to be relatively growth hormone–independent. The childhood component becomes prominent at about 3 to 4 years of age and is related to the importance of growth hormone–responsive growth. There is an overlap of these two phases of growth hormone–independent and growth hormone–dependent growth. Thus, at 6 to 12 months of age, many children demonstrate an increase in growth rate (the infancy-childhood growth spurt), which is growth hormone–dependent and does not occur in growth hormone–deficient patients. After the infancy period ends, the growth rate is relatively stable, with a slow deceleration of linear growth and weight gain during childhood until the onset of puberty and the influence of sex steroids increase. A mid-childhood growth spurt has been described at about 7 years of age in 60% of children which causes an upward inflection of the stable growth rate of childhood.

Adolescent Growth Spurt

During the pubertal period, growth in stature is greater than in any postnatal period after in-

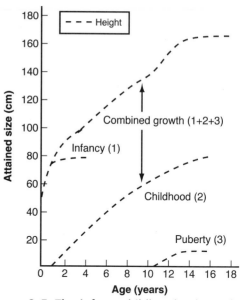

Figure 2–5. The infancy-childhood-puberty (ICP) model for girls for attained height, sitting height, and leg length. Three phases of growth combine into the cumulative curve depicted. Initially, there is the remarkable growth velocity in infancy which tapers off by 18 months. There is relatively stable growth during childhood, but the growth spurt of puberty adds to this baseline, leading to an upward trend until epiphyseal fusion finally stops all growth. The combined chart is the equivalent of the 50th percentile line on Figure 2–2. The mean functions are plotted for each component as well as for the mean combined growth. The average age at peak velocity was used to time the function for the mean puberty component. (From Karlberg J, Fryer JG, Engstrom I, Karlberg P: Analysis of linear growth using a mathematical model. II. From 3 to 21 years of age. Acta Paediatr Scand (Suppl) 1987; 337:13.)

fancy. The striking pubertal growth spurt was divided into three stages by Tanner: age at takeoff, which is the time of minimal growth velocity in peripuberty; peak height velocity (PHV), which is the time of most rapid growth; and the stage of decreased velocity and cessation of growth at epiphyseal fusion.[24] Because boys reach PHV approximately 2 years later than girls, they are taller at take-off than girls; PHV occurs during stage 5 of puberty in more than 95% of boys. On the average, males grow 28 cm and females 25 cm between take-off and cessation of growth. Thus, the mean height difference (13 cm) between adult men and women results from two factors: the fact that boys are taller than girls at age of take-off and the greater male height gain during the spurt.[25]

The pubertal growth spurt is an early pubertal event for girls. In fact, it is the first manifestation of puberty in most, although breast development is more obvious.[26] PHV occurs in 50% of girls during breast stage 3, although about a quarter experience it in stage 2 and a quarter in stage 4. There is limited growth potential in a postmenarcheal girl, because girls reach PHV before menarche and growth rate decelerates thereafter.

The pubertal growth spurt causes impressive increases in height but also signals the beginning of the end of the growing period, as marked by epiphyseal fusion, cessation of growth, and the attainment of final adult height. Several methods are available to predict final height during childhood and adolescence. The Bailey Pinneau charts in the Greulich and Pyle atlas utilize height and bone age to predict final height in children with a bone age over 6 years.[27] The Roche-Wainer-Thissen method utilizes recumbent length, bone age, mid-parental height, and weight to predict final height in children over 2 years of age.[28] Last, the HAPO method is based upon the ICP growth charts.[23] When children deviate from the normal growth pattern due to disease or constitutional delay, the predictive values of these methods decrease.

ENDOCRINE CONTROL OF GROWTH

A combination of endocrine and paracrine factors mediate growth with a differing mix in the prenatal period than the postnatal phase and further changes in the mix during various phases of postnatal growth.

Growth Hormone

Growth hormone (GH) is a 191–amino acid protein that increases linear growth via the stimulation of insulin-like growth factor 1 (IGF-1). GH is released from the pituitary gland due to stimulation by hypothalamic GH–releasing hormone (GhRH) and inhibited by hypothalamic somatostatin or GH release–inhibiting factor (SRIF or SS). During most of a 24-hour period, GH concentrations are low, but several peaks occur, most notably during sleep. Thus, random sampling of GH concentrations for diagnosis is useless. Stimulatory tests to diagnose GH deficiency utilize such secretagogues as alpha-adrenergic agents, beta-adrenergic blocking agents, insulin, or GRF (see Chapter 3).

Serum GH concentrations rise during pubertal development, owing in large part to increased secretion of gonadal sex steroids, but secretion of GH decreases after the end of pubertal development.[29] During puberty in adolescents of normal height, there is an inverse relationship between weight and GH levels. Thus, obese persons secrete less GH than the normal population without being GH-deficient, an important issue in diagnosis.[30]

The aromatization of testosterone to estradiol is the major stimulus to GH secretion in puberty.[31, 32] The administration of exogenous estrogen increases the peak GH after insulin-induced hypoglycemia, exercise, and arginine.[33] A class of 6– and 7–amino acid peptides (growth hormone–releasing peptides or GhRPs) stimulate GH release independently in a manner additive to GhRH, and these molecules are being developed for clinical use in diagnosis and therapy.[34]

Growth hormone–binding protein (GhBP) has the same amino acid sequence as the extracellular component of the GH receptor and is directly related to the amount of cellular GH receptors. In normal children, GhBP is inversely related to 24-hour GH secretion.[35] In subjects who lack growth receptors, such as "Laron dwarfs," the GhBP is decreased or undetectable.

Growth Factors

Growth factors are small peptides (smaller than 30 kd) that are produced in many cells and organs and affect numerous aspects of cellular growth and development. These peptides are hydrophilic and lipid-insoluble and interact with membrane-bound receptors on target cells. The occupied receptors have a classic structure: (1) an extracellular domain which attaches to the stimulating growth factor, (2) a seven-transmembrane domain, and (3) an intracellular domain, which causes the final cellular effects of the growth factor. These receptors characteristically evoke autophosphorylation of tyrosine kinase activity in the intracellular domain to initiate a response.[36] Activated second messenger systems then lead to the characteristic growth factor activity involving amino acid transport, glucose uptake, RNA and protein synthesis followed by DNA synthesis, and cell replication in most cells. In spite of the general designation *growth factors*, some of these molecules inhibit growth and development.

Different growth factors affect different portions of the cell cycle. Competence factors such as fibroblast growth factor (FGF) and platelet-derived growth factor (PDGF) cause the cell to move out of the quiescent GO phase into the v or midpoint of the G1 phase, during which the cell prepares for DNA synthesis.[37] Progression of the cell farther into the second half of the G1 phase and into the DNA synthesis phase, or S phase, requires progression factors such as epidermal growth factor (EGF) or IGF-1. The development of an organ ultimately requires a balance of all of these effects as well as the action of inhibitory factors. In some cell systems, a given growth factor may have both competence and progression effects; the same growth factor may serve several roles, depending on its concentration and interactions with other growth factors.

Insulin-like Growth Factor

IGF-1 (previously called *somatomedin*) is the growth factor most closely associated with linear growth. The IGFs are single-chain polypeptides with three intrachain disulfide bonds and have 40% homology with insulin.[38, 39] There is 60% homology in the amino acid sequences between human IGF-1 and IGF-2. IGF-1 synthesis is directly regulated after birth by the effects of GH, nutrition, sex steroids, and thyroid hormone, among other agents. IGF-1 exerts effects on postnatal linear growth by stimulation of chondrogenesis (somatogenic action), by stimulation of protein synthesis (anabolic action) and inhibition of protein degradation (anticatabolic function). In addition, IGF-1 regulates protein turnover and insulin sensitivity. IGF-1 is the universal progression factor in the cell cycle necessary for the cell to enter the S phase of DNA synthesis, but IGF-1 can also promote cell differentiation.[40] Most tissues express IGF-1, which leads to the concept that this molecule exerts autocrine (exerting effects on the cell of origin) and paracrine (exerting effects on neighboring cells) effects rather than acting solely by endocrine mechanisms (i.e., effects induced after being released into the circulation at a distance from the cell of origin).

IGFs exert their effects through four different cell membrane receptors that have functions (noted earlier) for growth factors: The type 1 receptor (1) and the insulin receptors (2) are structurally homologous, as each has two alpha and two beta subunits. Type 2 receptor (3) is structurally identical to the mannose 2 phosphate receptor. Last, hybrid receptors (4) are heterodimers consisting of parts of the insulin and IGF-1 receptors.[41] Types 1, 2, and 4 serve as receptors utilized by IGF-1, and type 2 receptors are occu-

pied by IGF-2. The beta subunits of the type 1 IGF receptor, the insulin receptor, and the hybrid receptors have tyrosine kinase activity and the ability to autophosphorylate, two properties shared with other receptors for factors important in growth. A soluble form of the type 2 IGF/mannose-6-phosphate receptor is derived from the type 2 receptor and may serve as a circulating binding protein for IGF-2. Concentrations of this circulating protein in amniotic fluid decrease with advancing gestation, and values in serum decrease progressively from highest levels in preterm cord blood to lower values in term cord blood to postnatal months, with the lowest values of all found in the adult.[42]

IGFs circulate in association with IGF-binding proteins (IGFBPs), six of which have so far been described (with more presumably to be found). Very little IGF is in the free state, although it is the free IGF that appears to exert metabolic effects.[43] The binding proteins are produced in various tissues and found in different locations, some in the circulation, others attached to tissues, and some in both forms. IGFBP-1 is identical to placental protein 12, a product of the decidua; in amniotic fluid concentrations of this protein are higher earlier in gestation than later. In the postnatal subject, IGFBP-1 is inversely related to insulin secretion and negatively related to GH secretion and is inhibitory to the growth and metabolic effects of IGF-1, especially inhibiting the tendency of IGF-1 to cause hypoglycemia. IGFBP-3 is regulated positively by GH secretion and nutritional status. IGFBP-3 combines with a 53-d acid-labile subunit (ALS) and IGF-1 to create a 150-kd ternary compound which contains most of the circulating IGF and which probably serves as a readily available reservoir for IGF-1. Specific IGFBP proteases attack the binding proteins themselves, thus leading to another layer of control over IGF action.

Insulin-like Growth Factors in Normal and Abnormal Fetal Growth

IGFs have several roles in normal fetal growth.[44-55] IGF-1 has the ability to regulate partitioning of nutrients between the placenta and fetus, leading to anabolism in the fetus and reduction in placental uptake of nutrients preferentially shunting them to the fetus.[45] IGF stimulates the growth of human fetal fibroblasts, myoblasts, chondrocytes, osteoblasts, hepatocytes, glia cells, adrenal cells, and IGFs also effect the differentiation of fetal cells, including muscle, cartilage, and growth retardation, especially those associated with specific evidence of reduced uteroplacental blood flow. Thus, levels of IGFBP-1 appear to be a sensitive indicator of fetal nutrition and of the short- or long-term response to reduced fetal nutrition.

Serum IGF-2 concentrations are higher in human fetuses than in adults, although adult values remain higher than those of any other protein hormone. In postnatal life, IGF-2 is less dependent on GH, insulin, and nutritional factors, and it is less active in regulating growth and anabolism than is IGF-1.

Endocrine Control of Postnatal Growth and the Pubertal Growth Spurt

The pubertal growth spurt is controlled by multiple factors, and recent information points out surprising insight into the relative importance of some of these factors. The pubertal growth spurt is created by the concerted action of sex steroids, thyroid hormone, and GH. Patients who lack some or all of these hormones do not have a pubertal growth spurt.

IGF-1 concentrations are low at birth but increase through the later stages of childhood. IGF-1 rises during puberty to values higher than those of prepubertal or adult subjects, remains elevated past the time of peak height velocity, and then falls to normal adult levels.[56-60] The increase in estradiol during the progression of puberty correlates with the rise in IGF-1. Sex steroids directly increase IGF-1 production within the growing cartilage of the long bones, but sex steroids alone are not a direct cause of the increase in serum IGF-1. Increased sex steroid secretion with subsequent aromatization of androgens to estrogen plays a major role in augmenting release of GH, thereby increasing IGF-1 generation. GH secretion approximately doubles during puberty, a phenomenon reflected by increased GH pulse amplitude, but not frequency. Children with true precocious puberty have plasma IGF-1 values and GH secretion characteristic of children in the same stage of normal puberty, rather than values of children of the patient's chronologic age.[59, 61] After several months of therapy with a superactive LRF agonist, IGF-1 values in patients with precocious puberty decrease along with the secretion of GH. Alternatively, patients with constitutional delay in puberty have concentrations of IGF-1 characteristic of their bone age rather than their chronologic age. The pattern of the growth hormone–

dependent IGFBP-3 in pubertal development is similar to that of serum IGF-1.[62]

There is no pubertal growth spurt in children who have severe primary or secondary hypogonadism. In the face of deficient adrenal androgen secretion, children with chronic adrenal insufficiency usually have a normal growth spurt, indicating the minimal role of adrenal androgens in stimulating normal pubertal growth. Hypopituitary patients with GH and gonadotropin deficiencies do not have an adolescent growth spurt when only one replacement hormone is given, as both GH and sex steroids (stimulated by gonadotropins) are necessary. Phenotypic females with 46XY genotypes who have the complete form of familial androgen insensitivity (testicular feminization) despite virtually complete insensitivity to androgens (but not to estrogen) have a pubertal growth spurt. This observation demonstrates a role for estrogen in the adolescent growth spurt in girls.[63]

The role of estrogen in the maturation of skeletal development has only recently become clear through the study of two types of patients. A single male patient 28 years of age was found still to be growing in stature and to have a 15-year-old bone age (not yet fused) with a normal male phenotype. He had an estrogen receptor defect, and the failure of estrogen effects explained the failure of his epiphyses to fuse and the continued lengthening of his long bones.[64] Several families recently reported with aromatase deficiency could not convert androgens to estrogens. While the males had a normal male phenotype, females had ambiguous genitalia and reproductive difficulties. None had fused epiphyses, and all were of tall stature and continued to grow into young adulthood.[65, 66] These patients demonstrate the important effect that estrogen has in skeletal development and highlight the effects of unopposed androgen in stimulating prolonged growth in stature.

BONE AGE

Skeletal development is a better indicator of physiologic maturity than chronologic age. For example, bone age is closely associated with menarche and is better correlated with the onset of secondary sexual development in delayed puberty than is chronologic age. Bone age is determined by comparing radiographs of the hand, the knee, or the elbow with standards of maturation in a normal population as presented in photographic atlases such as the Greulich and Pyle atlas, the one used most frequently in the United

States.[27] Ossification centers appear early in life then mold to fit with surrounding bones, until, finally, the epiphyses or growth plates fuse with their shafts. The delay or advancement in bone age is expressed in standard deviations from the mean reading for chronologic age. A bone age more than 2 SD in either direction from the mean for chronologic age is a significant deviation. Bone age, height, and chronologic age are used to predict final adult height from the Bayley-Pinneau tables in the Greulich and Pyle atlas,[27] the Roche Whitehouse Tanner (RWT),[28] or HAPO technique.[23] Because osseous maturation is more advanced in females than in males of the same chronologic age, separate standards are used for boys and girls. For example, the bone ages of 11 years in girls and 13 years in boys (i.e., of early puberty in each sex) represent equivalent stages of bone maturation. While bone age determinations can *help* to identify various conditions, they do not, by themselves, establish a diagnosis.

SKELETAL DENSITY

Bone mineral density increases throughout childhood, but the major increases occur during the first 3 years of life and the critical growth phase of puberty and "plateau" at or after the end of puberty.[67–71] A peak of bone mineral density is reached at 17.5 years for boys and 15.8 years for girls, after the peak height increase of puberty, a factor that may result in a period of increased fragility and susceptibility to trauma.[72, 73] Weight is a principal determinant of bone density in postpubertal females.[74] While bone density accrual is related to calcium intake,[75, 76] the calcium intake of girls during puberty is estimated to be well below recommended levels, and even those recommended levels may be too low for optimal mineralization.[77, 78] African-American children retain more calcium than Caucasians, and their bones are thicker.[79] The difference in vertebral bone density appears to develop by late puberty, as in prepuberty there is no difference between the groups.[80] Exogenous calcium administration may increase bone accretion and may safely be accomplished by increasing consumption of dairy products,[81–83] though the effect of increased ingestion of calcium may last only as long as the calcium is actually administered.[84]

Deficiencies of pubertal development impair bone accretion in both sexes, mainly as a consequence of estrogen deficiency due to either decreased secretion or peripheral aromatization of androgens, for example, loss of bone density occurs in girls with anorexia nervosa, hypothalamic amenorrhea, or ovarian failure.[85, 86] Children with precocious puberty have increased bone density but successful treatment with GnRH agonist decreases bone density again.[87, 88] Testosterone administration to normal prepubertal boys increases calcium retention and bone growth, an effect mediated mainly by peripheral aromatization to estradiol, including in skeletal tissue.[89]

A correlation between the bone density of children and parents with osteoporosis suggests the importance of the pubertal period of bone accretion. Indeed, there is a relationship of bone density between generations if the effects of age and puberty are eliminated.[90, 91]

BODY COMPOSITION

Changes in body composition occur during puberty and are a reflection of much of the dichotomy in physique between men and women. By the end of puberty, men have 1.5 times the lean body mass and almost 1.5 times the skeletal mass of women, whereas women have twice as much body fat as men.

Abdominal fat accumulates in girls with progression through pubertal development and leads to the differences in the generalized distribution of fat in males (central fat, or apple-shaped, *android*) and females (lower body fat predominance or pear-shaped, *gynecoid*).[92, 93] Hips enlarge with pubertal development in girls, but, as there is no change in waist circumference, the waist-hip ratio drops. Different ethnic groups exhibit different patterns of the waist-hip ratio.[94]

The accumulation of fat mass in childhood has recently taken on increased importance. There is an epidemic of childhood and adolescent overweight and obesity in the United States. Obesity is partially due to genetic factors (said to be between 40% and 60%), but the recent increase in obesity in the population is clearly due to a combination of changes in eating behavior and lifestyle. Treatment too frequently is unsuccessful; prevention is the key to the problem.

By age 9 to 10 years, African-American females tend to have a higher calorie intake because they consume more fat and are less physically active than Caucasian girls. By age 9 to 10 years, the prevalence of obesity is already higher in African-American girls.[95] At 10 years of age, there is a demonstrable difference in girls' concerns about eating and weight gain as compared with boys'.[96] African-American and Caucasian girls are equally likely to diet, but African-American girls more frequently attempt to *gain* weight; this has been attributed to parental influence,[97] possibly related to the average 20-pound greater weight of the African-American girls' mothers in the study.[98] It is now clear that being overweight in childhood correlates with adult mortality.[99]

Leptin is a peptide hormone produced in adipose tissue that has many metabolic effects, the most prominent being its ability to feedback and decrease excessive eating behavior in leptin deficient animals and humans.[100] Leptin-deficient mice do not secrete gonadotropin and have hypogonadal hypogonadism, a condition that is reversed with the administration of leptin. This pattern was documented in one 9-year-old child with leptin deficiency who was extremely obese but did not exhibit advanced bone age or pubertal gonadotropin secretion, as would be expected in such an obese child.[101] With leptin treatment, gonadotropin secretion rose and eating behavior and weight gain abated.[102] Some studies suggest an active role for leptin in inducing the onset of puberty, but others believe it to be more a reflection of the pubertal process in human beings. At present, it appears that leptin is necessary but not sufficient for the onset of puberty.

EVALUATION OF GROWTH

The evaluation of a patient with a growth abnormality must start with a comprehensive history. Prenatal history, including the health of the mother and her exposure to toxins or drugs, can explain some cases of growth deficiency. Birth history—difficulties of delivery, evidence of anoxia, and the infant's length and weight at birth—can point to acquired hormonal deficiencies or "small for gestational age" syndromes. The height of all family members, age at onset of puberty and growth spurt will point to genetic tendencies toward short stature or constitutional delay of puberty.

Review of systems is essential to search for a disease that affects growth: headaches or vision problems can suggest a central nervous system problem; nocturia or enuresis may suggest diabetes insipidus; gastrointestinal symptoms may point to celiac disease, which can suppress a child's growth rate and delay puberty; pulmonary, renal, or cardiac symptoms that might be associated with disease in any of those systems. All such information will suggest an avenue of investigation for diagnosis of the cause of short stature.

A detailed and complete physical examination is necessary for the evaluation of every patient

with a growth disorder. A search for midline defects of the skull, face, optic nerves, or palate, which can be related to hypothalamic deficiencies, is essential. Evidence of hypothyroidism, Cushing disease, Prader-Willi syndrome, or pseudohypoparathyroidism should be noted. Any girl of short stature must be assumed to have Turner syndrome until this diagnosis is eliminated. The signs can be subtle. Signs of chronic disease that can interfere with good nutrition and energy balance, among other manifestations, may direct the examiner toward a diagnosis that is not likely related to the endocrine system.

PUBERTAL DEVELOPMENT

TIMING OF PUBERTY

The statistics on age of onset of puberty were first developed in Europe and were extrapolated to the United States. In fact, no large-scale, systematic survey of the ages of puberty in the United States was published until 1997. A large cross-sectional study sponsored by the American Academy of Pediatrics of 17,070 girls visiting the office of a pediatrician across the United States and evaluated by trained observers started with girls aged 3 years. Because it followed them only to age 12, it excluded normal children who entered puberty at a later age, but it *is* useful for puberty of females at the youngest ages.[103] In this study, 3.0% of Caucasian girls had stage 2 breast development by 6 years and 5.0% by 7 years, whereas 6.4% of African-Americans had stage 2 breast development by 6 years and 15.4% by 7 years. The mean age of breast development for Caucasian girls was 10.6 years (2.5 SD or 6.7 to 14.5 years), and 8.9 years was the mean age for African-American girls (2.5 SD or 6 to 13 years). These findings confirm what some clinicians surmised: a substantial number of normal girls undergo pubertal development earlier than the (generally stated) 2.5 SD years below the mean of 8 years. The decision to embark on an evaluation of precocious puberty must be based on the presence of signs of disease in the central nervous system or elsewhere or on the rapidity of development, but such an evaluation is not categorically indicated for every child who exhibits pubertal development before 8 years of age (Fig. 2–6).

The average age of menarche in industrialized European countries has decreased between 2 to 3 months per decade over the past 150 years,[104, 105] but this trend has ceased in "developed countries" such as the United States. Although me-

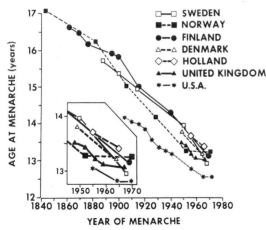

Figure 2–6. Changes in age at menarche between 1840 and 1978. (From Tanner JM, Eveleth PB: Onset of puberty. *In* Berenberg SR [ed]: Puberty: Biologic and Social Components. Leiden, The Netherlands: HE Stenfert Kroese Publishers, 1975, p 256. Reprinted by permission of Kluwer Academic Press.)

narche is a middle-puberty event, it is used as an indicator, since approximately 1940, of the general trend in pubertal development. According to a survey by the U.S. National Center for Health Statistics from the 1970s,[1] the age of menarche in the United States is 12.8 years. This was confirmed in the recent study of pubertal development in the 17,070 girls cited earlier.[103] Age of onset of pubertal development is earlier for African-American girls than for Caucasian girls by about 1 year, even though in the cross-sectional study the difference in average age of menarche was only 8.5 months (12.2 years for African-Americans and 12.9 for Caucasians).

Socioeconomic conditions, nutrition, and general health and well-being affect the age of onset of pubertal development and its progression. In countries where standards of living have not improved over the last century, the age of onset of puberty may not have changed.[106]

Other influences also affect the age of puberty. Delayed puberty is a feature of chronic disease and of malnutrition. Strenuous physical activity in girls can delay or arrest puberty, especially when associated with a thin habitus.[107] Moderate obesity (up to 30% above normal weight for age) is associated with earlier menarche, although delayed menarche is common with severe obesity.

When socioeconomic and environmental factors lead to good nutrition and good general health, the age of onset of puberty is determined largely by genetic factors. This is demonstrated by similar ages of menarche in members of an ethnic population and in mother-daughter pairs.[108]

PHYSICAL AND HORMONAL CHANGES IN PUBERTY

Secondary Sexual Characteristics

An objective method of the maturation of secondary sexual characteristics allows the observer to describe whether puberty begins at a normal age and progresses at a normal rate. The standards Tanner proposed are accepted as universal (Fig. 2–7).[26]

Breast development is mainly under control of estrogens secreted by the ovaries, whereas growth of pubic and axillary hair is under the influence of androgens secreted by both the ovaries and the adrenal glands. The classification of the stages of breast development depends on specific characteristics common to all females but does not include size or inherent shape of the breasts, features determined by genetic and nutritional factors. It is important to realize that initial breast development may be unilateral for several months and this may cause undue concern for girls or parents. Girls have been referred for breast biopsy because this fact was overlooked. Changes in areola papilla diameter are also used as an indication of pubertal development (Table 2–1, Fig. 2–8).[109]

In normal girls, the stage of breast develop-

Table 2–1. Cross-Sectional and Longitudinal Papillary Diameter at Each Stage of Pubertal Development

Stage	Nipple Size (mm)[*]	
	Cross-Sectional	*Longitudinal*
BI	2.89 (0.81)	3.00 (0.77)
BII	3.28 (0.89)	3.37 (0.96)
BIII	4.07 (1.32)	4.72 (1.40)[†]
BIV	7.74 (1.64)[†]	7.25 (1.46)[†]
BV	9.94 (1.38)[†]	9.41 (1.45)[†]
PH1	2.95 (1.02)	3.14 (1.31)
PH2	3.32 (0.91)	3.69 (1.34)
PH3	4.11 (1.54)	4.44 (1.17)[†]
PH4	7.15 (1.81)[†]	6.54 (1.47)[†]
PH5	9.66 (1.59)[†]	8.98 (1.56)[†]

[*]Results are means ± SD (in parentheses).
[†]Significantly different from previous state, $P < .05$.
From Rhone RD. Papilla (nipple) development during female puberty. J Adolesc Health Care 1982; 2:217.

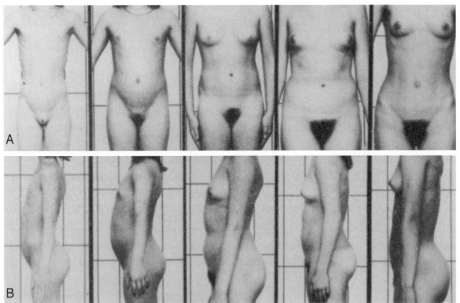

Figure 2–7. *A,* Pubertal development of female pubic hair. Stage 1: There is no pubic hair. Stage 2: There is sparse growth of long, slightly pigmented, downy hair, straight or only slightly curled, primarily along the labia. Stage 3: The hair is considerably darker, coarser, and more curled and spreads sparsely over the junction of the pubes. Stage 4: The hair, now adult in type, covers a smaller area than in the adult and does not extend onto the thighs. Stage 5: The hair is adult in quantity and type, with extension onto the thighs. *B,* Pubertal development of female breasts. Stage 1: The breasts are preadolescent. There is elevation on the papilla only. Stage 2: Breast bud stage. A small mound is formed by the elevation of the breast and papilla, and the areolar diameter enlarges. Stage 3: There is further enlargement of breasts and areola with no separation of their contours. Stage 4: There is a projection of the areola and papilla to form a secondary mound above the level of the breast. Stage 5: The breasts resemble those of a mature female as the areola has recessed to the general contour of the breast. (From Brook CGD, Stanhope R: Normal puberty: Physical characteristics and endocrinology. *In* Brook CGD [ed]: Clinical Paediatric Endocrinology, 2nd ed. Oxford: Blackwell Scientific Publications, 1989, p 172.)

ment is *usually* consonant with the stage of pubic hair development. Nevertheless, since two different endocrine organs cause these two different physical manifestations, the two stages should be classified individually, to increase accuracy of assessment. Dulling of the surface of the vaginal mucosa from the reddish prepubertal appearance is the result of cornification due to estrogen stimulation, and secretion of clear or whitish discharge increases in the months just before menarche. The vaginal pH drops as menarche approaches. Thickening, protrusion, and rugation of the labia majora and minora are features of puberty. The pubertal thickening of the hymen has been reported to antedate other physical changes of puberty.

Standards have been published for the shape and volume of the uterus and the ovaries by age.[110–112] By ultrasonography, the uterus is largest in the neonatal period and at puberty.[112] Ultrasonographic studies show that the corpus of the uterus grows during pubertal progression

from a tubular shape to a bulbous structure; that the length of the uterus increases from 2 to 3 cm to 5 to 8 cm,[113] and the volume from 0.4 to 1.6 ml to 3 to 15 ml.[114] The upper limit of uterine length in the prepubertal state is 3.5 cm.[110] Further, a uterine volume of greater than 1.8 ml is quite specific for the onset of puberty while increased ovarian volume is less specific for the onset of puberty.[114] Enlargement of the uterus on ultrasonography (volume >1.8 ml, length >36 mm) is rare in association with premature thelarche; patients with premature thelarche were indistinguishable from controls. Measurement of the ellipsoid volume of the uterus (V = longitudinal diameter × anteroposterior diameter × transverse diameter 0.523) is said to be the most sensitive and specific discriminator between premature thelarche and early true precocious puberty.[114, 115]

During prepuberty, on ultrasound scans, ovarian volume is 0.2 to 1.6 ml, and, after the onset of puberty, it increases to 2.8 to 15 ml.[114, 116] The

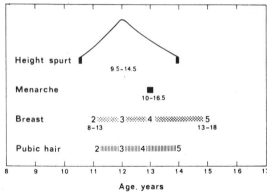

Figure 2–8. A graphic depiction of the ages at which girls reach the stage of normal pubertal development. The data is from Britain, and the ages are older than those of girls in the United States, especially with the latest information about the age of onset of breast development in the United States, but the general pattern of development is constant between the countries. (From Marshall WA, Tanner JM. Variation in the pattern of pubertal changes in girls. Arch Dis Child 1969; 44:291–303.)

multicystic ultrasound appearance of the ovaries that progresses throughout puberty should not be considered a sign of disease.[115, 117] Cysts may be found in the ovaries in true precocious puberty or GnRH independent isosexual precocity, but usually the cysts are smaller than 9 mm in the former and greater than 9 mm in the latter.[118]

Hormonal Changes in Puberty

GONADOTROPINS

During the first 1 to 2 years of life, plasma levels of LH and FSH intermittently rise to adult values. Subsequently, the plasma concentrations remain low until the onset of puberty. New ultrasensitive LH and FSH assays allow accurate determination of basal levels of serum LH and FSH, and the results are lower than previous assays allowed. The basal values of serum LH and FSH, measured by immunochemiluminometric assay are reported to predict the onset of pubertal development as well as the GnRH testing that was necessary in the past. Laboratories' standards vary, but a serum LH value greater than the lower limit of standard for stage 2 of puberty *in that laboratory* is consistent with the onset of puberty.[119, 120] When ultrasensitive assays are used to determine concentration of LH and FSH in urine during puberty, a pattern of a five-

fold rise in urinary FSH in boys and girls, a 50-fold rise in urinary LH in boys, and a 100-fold rise in urinary LH in girls is noted.[121, 122]

TESTOSTERONE

In females, the peripheral conversion of ovarian and adrenal androstenedione accounts for most of the circulating testosterone. Prepubertal boys and girls have plasma testosterone concentrations of less than 10 ng/dl. While there is a greater rise in testosterone in boys during puberty, there is a smaller but definite increase in its concentrations in girls between pubertal stages 1 and 4. Measurement of free testosterone is a useful method for detecting abnormal androgen production in girls.

ESTROGENS

In the fetus and at term, estrogen values are extremely high (approximately 5000 pg/ml at term) because of the conversion by the placenta of fetal and maternal C19 steroid precursors to estrogen. In term male and female infants, breast budding is the physical manifestation of these high concentrations of circulating estrogen, but breast budding soon ceases in all but some of those girls, ones who may be destined to experience premature thelarche. Plasma levels of placenta-derived estrogen drop precipitously in the first few days after delivery. There are episodic peaks of LH and FSH in the months after birth. Plasma estrogens rise owing to these gonadotropin peaks but gradually fall during the first year and remain low until puberty; estradiol falls to less than 7 pg/ml; and estrone to less than 20 pg/ml. These estrogen levels are so low in prepuberty that detection has been difficult with standard techniques, but a highly sensitive bioassay demonstrated measurable serum concentrations of estradiol in both boys and girls before puberty (higher in girls).[123] The higher estrogen levels in girls may be an important factor in their more advanced levels of skeletal maturation and the earlier onset of sexual maturation. Plasma estradiol levels rise through the stages of puberty until maturity; estrone levels rise early and reach a plateau by mid-puberty.[124, 125] In early pubertal girls, the daily peak of estradiol occurs about 6 to 9 hours after the nightly peaks of serum LH, probably a reflection of the time necessary for ovarian synthesis of estradiol.[126]

ADRENAL ANDROGENS

Both boys and girls demonstrate a progressive increase in the plasma delta-5 steroids dehydro-epiandrosterone (DHEA) and dehydroepiandrosterone sulfate (DHEAS) that starts by age 8 years (skeletal age 6 to 8 years) and continues through ages 13 to 15 years. This increase in the secretion of adrenal androgen is known as *adrenarche*. Although the cause of adrenarche is not known, it is clear that adrenocorticotropin (ACTH) is necessary to the process. This increase in the secretion of adrenal androgens precedes the increased secretion of gonadal sex steroids (gonadarche) and the increased pulsatile secretion of gonadotropins by approximately 2 years. Plasma DHEAS shows less variation than DHEA and is a useful biochemical marker of adrenarche. Those children who have early increases in DHEA secretion soon follow with the appearance of pubic hair, axillary hair or mild acne characteristic of premature adrenarche.[127]

INHIBIN, ACTIVIN, FOLLISTATIN

Inhibin and follistatin inhibit, and activin stimulates, FSH-β subunit expression and, therefore, FSH biosynthesis and secretion. It is now recognized that both are synthesized in a variety of tissues, aside from the gonads, and have various activities apart from those that affect the reproductive apparatus.

Inhibin, a heterodimeric glycoprotein product of the Sertoli cells of the testes and of the ovarian granulosa cells (as well as the placenta and other tissues), exerts a negative feedback action on the secretion of FSH from the pituitary. Inhibin is composed of an α subunit and one of two β subunits, βA or βB, which form inhibin A or inhibin B, respectively, dimers with apparently identical function. Inhibin is a member of the transforming growth factor β superfamily that includes antimüllerian hormone (AMH, also called *müllerian factor*) and the dimers of two inhibin subunits, activin A and activin B, which stimulate release of FSH from pituitary cells. Synthesis and secretion of gonadal inhibin are induced by FSH.[128] Inhibin plays a role in the feedback regulation of FSH secretion during puberty, in males and females.[129] Thus, while LH remains predominantly under the control of GnRH, FSH depends less on GnRH.[130] Serum inhibin A and B increase early in puberty in girls; inhibin B is predominant in the follicular phase and inhibin A during the luteal phase.

SEX HORMONE–BINDING GLOBULIN

Some 97% to 99% of circulating testosterone and estradiol is reversibly bound to sex hormone–binding globulin (SHBG); the free steroid is the only physiologically active moiety.[131] SHBG is a glycoprotein hormone of 90 to 100 kd and consists of heterogeneous monomers and one steroid-binding site per dimeric molecule.[132] Levels of SHBG in boys and girls are approximately equal before puberty. SHBG decreases with advancing prepubertal age, which effect leads to an increase in the free sex steroids. At puberty, there is a small decrease of SHBG in girls but a greater decrease in boys, so that adult males have half the SHBG concentration of adult females. While the plasma concentration of testosterone is 20 times greater in men than in women, the concentration of free testosterone is 40 times greater because of these differences.[131, 133–135]

PROLACTIN

Prepubertal boys have mean plasma prolactin concentrations similar to those of girls.[136] Because of elevations of estradiol concentration, late pubertal girls and adult women have higher concentrations of prolactin, whereas the mean concentrations in adult men are similar to those of prepubertal children.

INSULIN

Serum fasting insulin concentrations increase two- to threefold at peak height velocity, and, after a glucose load, insulin secretion increases over prepubertal levels, demonstrating a degree of insulin resistance during puberty.[137–140] Insulin sensitivity is related to pubertal stage and body mass index (BMI). In a longitudinal study, insulin sensitivity inversely correlated with BMI, decreased progressively from pubertal stage 2 to stage 3, and was lower in girls than in boys at stage 2 and stage 3.[141] This impairment of insulin-stimulated glucose metabolism, which can be demonstrated by the euglycemic insulin clamp technique,[139] is more striking in adolescents with diabetes mellitus. Hyperglycemic clamp studies indicate that puberty compensates for this deficit by increasing insulin secretion and suggest that the physiologic phenomena of insulin resistance does not involve the effect of insulin on amino acid metabolism.[142, 143] Insulin resistance has been attributed, at least in part, to increased fat oxidation at puberty which correlates with rising serum IGF-1 and which may be linked to increased GH secretion.[144] Adolescents with insulin-dependent diabetes mellitus (IDDM) have lower serum concentrations of IGF-1 than controls.[145] The elevated GH levels are associated with low serum concentrations of IGF-1 and GHBP, and the usual reciprocal relationship between serum GH and GHBP no longer holds.[145–147] At puberty, patients with type I (insulin-dependent) diabetes mellitus usually require larger doses of insulin for glycemic control.[137, 148]

Insulin resistance is present early in Turner syndrome.[149] For children whose insulin-dependent diabetes mellitus is well-controlled, the growth rate may slow slightly and transiently in the 10 years after diagnosis; bone maturation likewise slows during this period, leading to a transient slowing of development. The effect of diabetes on growth is, however, smaller than the genetic influence of parental height. Whereas growth rate accelerates again (mainly during puberty), weight gain increases even more during puberty in affected children, the result being a higher incidence of obesity in children with IDDM than what would be expected from family patterns.[150] Unfortunately, some adolescents with IDDM (predominantly girls) reduce their insulin doses to lose weight—with dire consequences. A retrospective study found a decrease in final height when the diagnosis of IDDM was made before age 5 years, but not when it was made later. The pubertal growth rate was reduced in all patients, but girls were more affected than boys.[151]

While type 2 or non–insulin-dependent diabetes mellitus (NIDDM) has long been recognized in children and adolescents, the incidence is increasing, probably owing to the increase in obesity in these age groups. Classic NIDDM of early onset with impaired insulin secretion is prevalent among the Native American and Mexican-American populations but the rate is rising also among African-Americans. NIDDM should be considered in subjects manifesting acanthosis nigricans as a marker for insulin resistance. In young persons, NIDDM is a heterogeneous disorder, and obesity, while common, is a variable feature.[152–154] Several variations of maturity-onset diabetes of the young (MODY) have been described. All are characterized by slowly progressive loss of pancreatic beta cell function and are inherited as an autosomal-dominant trait in individuals that need not be obese. Type 2 MODY appears linked to a mitochondrial defect in glucokinase.

In several syndromes of insulin resistance hyperglycemia and virilization always occur together.[155] The Kahn type A syndrome features include a lean, muscular adolescent female phenotype with acanthosis nigricans, hirsutism, oligomenorrhea or amenorrhea, and ovarian hyperthecosis with stromal hyperplasia, all associated with abnormalities of the insulin receptor gene. The syndrome of hyperandrogenism, insulin resistance, and acanthosis nigricans and polycystic ovary syndrome are less severe than Kahn type A and usually are manifested in adolescent females. Robson-Mendenhall is a syndrome of severe insulin resistance (possibly leading to diabetic ketoacidosis), dysmorphic facies, acanthosis, nigricans, thickened nails, hirsutism, dental dysplasia, abdominal distention, and phallic or clitoral enlargement. The Robson-Mendenhall syndrome, like the Donahue leprechaunism syndrome, which shares some features, is attributed to homozygous or compound heterozygous defects in the insulin receptor gene. Kahn type B syndrome is due to inhibitory or stimulatory antibodies to the insulin receptor, sometimes with acanthosis nigricans and ovarian hyperandrogenism. This syndrome can be associated with ataxia-telangiectasia syndrome in otherwise normal adolescents. Seip-Berardinelli syndrome combines lipodystrophy, severe insulin resistance, and complete or partial absence of subcutaneous fat with increased growth and skeletal maturation, muscle hypertrophy, acanthosis nigricans, hypertrichosis, organomegaly, and mild hypertrophy of the external genitalia. Most of these NIDDM syndromes can be treated initially with oral hypoglycemic agents; as the disorder progresses, patients may require exogenous insulin.

Obese teenage girls with predominantly abdominal adiposity have insulin resistance, and, since, for them, puberty and menarche are often early, their exposure to an endocrine profile that predisposes to breast cancer is relatively prolonged.[156, 157] Plasma insulin values for obese adolescents have certain correlates: for boys, fasting plasma glucose, plasma triglycerides, uric acid, and systolic blood pressure are directly related; whereas, for girls, the direct correlates are plasma triglycerides and systolic and diastolic blood pressure. Plasma insulin correlated negatively with high-density lipoprotein cholesterol in both boys and girls.[158]

MENARCHE

With respect to the menstrual cycle, it is appropriate to point out the high incidence of anovulatory cycles in the first years after menarche. Even 5 years later, one in five girls may be anovulatory.[159] While the majority of pubertal subjects are infertile, in terms of pregnancy risk, a substantial number *are* fertile. It is possible to become pregnant well before the end of puberty, and, in fact, a woman can become pregnant even before her first menstrual period.

CONSTITUTIONAL DELAY IN PUBERTY

In the United States, delayed puberty is usually of more concern to boys and their parents than to girls and their parents. Nevertheless, a girl older than 13 years with no evidence of pubertal development requires consideration of potential diagnoses. In the absence of signs or symptoms of central nervous system disease, or chronic conditions, or interference with nutrition *and* if the child seems quite healthy in general, constitutional delay in puberty should be considered. Affected children are usually short and have been shorter than average throughout childhood, although their growth rate remains normal for bone age. There is a family history of pubertal delay in a parent or sibling in about 50% of such cases. Skeletal development is delayed two or more standard deviations and is a *sine qua non* of the diagnosis. Biochemical tests including sex steroid and gonadotropin values are prepubertal as are serum chemistries and IGF-1 concentrations. In fact, this variation of normal tempo of development cannot reliably be diagnosed by any given test but, rather, is confirmed after normal pubertal development occurs at an advanced age. While, generally, constitutional delay in puberty is considered not a true disease, but, rather, a variation of normal, new information indicates that families with hypogonadotropic hypogonadism and anosmia (Kallmann syndrome) may have members whose constitutional delay in growth by all methods of evaluation suggests that, at least in some cases, constitutional delay in puberty is, truly, a form of gonadotropin deficiency.[160] If the patient's psychological or educational situation is affected, and if constitutional delay seems a serious consideration, low-dose estrogen may be offered for a 3-month period to advance physical development cosmetically and to improve self-esteem.

REFERENCES

1. Hamil P: Physical growth: National Center for Health Statistics percentiles. Am J Clin Nutr 1979; 32:607.
2. Tanner JM, Davies PSW: Clinical longitudinal standards for height and height velocity for North American children. J Pediatr 1985; 107:317–329.
3. Roche AF, Himes JH: Incremental growth charts. Am J Clin Nutr 1980; 333:2041.
4. Brook CGD, Murset G, Zachmann M: Growth in children with 45,XO Turner's syndrome. Arch Dis Child 1974; 73:789–795.
5. Himes JH, Roche AF, Thissen D: Parent Specific Adjustments for Assessment of Recumbent Length and Stature. Basel: Karger, 1981.
6. McKusick VA: Heritable Disorders of Connective Tissue. St. Louis: CV Mosby, 1972, p 73.
7. Styne DM: Fetal growth. Perinatol Clin North Am 1998; 25(4):917–938.
8. Corliss LE: Patten's Human Embryology: Elements of Clinical Development. New York: McGraw-Hill, 1976.
9. Hod M, Langer O: Fuel metabolism in deviant fetal growth in offspring of diabetic women. Obstet Gynecol Clin North Am 1996; 23:259–277.
10. Underwood LE, Van Wyk J: Normal and abnormal growth. In Wilson JE, Foster DW (eds): Williams Textbook of Endocrinology. Philadelphia: WB Saunders, 1994, pp 1079–1138.
11. Morton NE: The inheritance of human birth weight. Ann Hum Genet 1955; 20:125–134.
12. Garnica AD, Chan WY: The role of the placenta in fetal nutrition and growth (see Comments). J Am Coll Nutr 1996; 15:206–222.
13. Evain-Brion D: Hormonal regulation of fetal growth. Horm Res 1994; 42:207–214.
14. Bassett JM: Current perspectives on placental development and its integration with fetal growth. Proc Nutr Soc 1991; 50:311–319.
15. Aherne W: Morphometry. In The Placenta and Its Maternal Supply Line. Gruenwald P (ed): London: Medical and Technical Publishers, 1975, pp 80–97.
16. Warshaw J: Intrauterine Growth Retardation. In Lifshitz F (ed): Pediatric Endocrinology. New York: Marcel Dekker, 1996, pp 95–102.
17. Albertsson-Wikland K, Karlberg J: Postnatal growth of children born small for gestational age. Acta Paediatr Suppl 1997; 436:193–195.
18. de Zegher FK, Albertsson-Wikland P, Wilton P, et al: Growth hormone treatment of short children born small for gestational age: Metanalysis of four independent, randomized, controlled, multicentre studies. Acta Paediatr Suppl 27–31.
19. de Zegher F, Francois I, van Helvoirt M, Van den Berghe G: Clinical review 89: Small as fetus and short as child: From endogenous to exogenous growth hormone. J Clin Endocrinol 1997; 82(7)2021–2026.
20. Azcona C, Albanese A, Bareille P, Stanhope R: Growth hormone treatment in growth hormone–sufficient and –insufficient children with intrauterine growth retardation/Russell-Silver syndrome. Horm Res 1998; 50:22–27.
21. Smith DW: Growth and Its Disorders: Basics and Standards. Philadelphia: WB Saunders, 1977.
22. Tanner JM, Whitehouse RH, Takaishi M: Standards from birth to maturity for height, weight, height velocity, and weight velocity, British children. Arch Dis Child 1966; 44:454–471.
23. Karlberg J, Fryer JG, Engstrom I, Karlberg P: Analysis of linear growth using a mathematical model. II. From 3 to 21 years of age. Acta Paediatr Scand Suppl 1987; 337:12–29.
24. Tanner JM, Whitehouse RH, Marubini E, Resele LF: The adolescent growth spurt of boys and girls of the Harpenden growth study. Ann Hum Biol 1976; 3:109–126.

25. Largo RH, Gasser TH, Prader A: Analysis of the adolescent growth spurt using smoothing spline functions. Ann Hum Biol 1978; 5:421–434.

26. Marshall WA, Tanner JM: Variations in pattern of pubertal changes in girls. Arch Dis Child 1969; 44:291–303.

27. Greulich WS, Pyle SI: Radiographic Atlas of Skeletal Development of the Hand and Wrist. Stanford: Stanford University Press, 1959.

28. Roche AF, Wainer H, Thissen D: The RWT method for the prediction of adult stature. Pediatrics 1975; 56:1026–1033.

29. Martha PMJ, Rogol AD, Veldhuis JD, et al: Alterations in the pulsatile properties of circulating growth hormone concentrations during puberty in boys. J Clin Endocrinol Metab 1989; 69:563–570.

30. Albertsson-Wikland K, Rosberg S, Karlberg J, Groth T: Analysis of 24-hour growth hormone profiles in healthy boys and girls of normal stature: Relation to puberty. J Clin Endocrinol Metab 1994; 78:1195–1201.

31. Eakman GD, Dallas JS, Ponder SW, Keenan BS: The effects of testosterone and dihydrotestosterone on hypothalamic regulation of growth hormone secretion. J Clin Endocrinol Metab 1996; 81:1217–1223.

32. Metzger DL, Kerrigan JR: Estrogen receptor blockade with tamoxifen diminishes growth hormone secretion in boys: Evidence for a stimulatory role of endogenous estrogens during male adolescence. J Clin Endocrinol Metab 1994; 79:513–518.

33. Marin G, Domene HM, Barnes KM, et al: The effects of estrogen priming and puberty on the growth hormone response to standardized treadmill exercise and arginine-insulin in normal girls and boys. J Clin Endocrinol Metab 1994; 79:537–541.

34. Mericq V, Cassorla F, Garcia H, et al: Growth hormone (GH) responses to GH-releasing peptide and to GH-releasing hormone in GH-deficient children. J Clin Endocrinol Metab 1995; 80:1681–1684.

35. Martha PMJ, Rogol AD, Blizzard RM, et al: Growth hormone–binding protein activity is inversely related to 24-hour growth hormone release in normal boys. J Clin Endocrinol Metab 1991; 73:175–181.

36. Dohlman HG, Caron MG, Lefkowitz RJ: A family of receptors coupled to guanine nucleotide regulatory proteins. Biochemistry 1987; 26:2657–2664.

37. Leof EB, Van Wyk J, O'Efe EJ: Epidermal growth factor (EGF) is required only during the traverse of early G1 in PDGF stimulated density arrested BALB/c 3T3 cells. 1983; 107–115.

38. Rinderknecht E, Humbel RE: The amino acid sequence of human insulin like growth factor 1 and its structural homology with proinsulin. J Biol Chem 1978; 253:2769–2776.

39. Rinderknecht E, Humbel RE: Primary structure of insulin like growth factor II. FEBS Lett 1978; 89:283–286.

40. Leof EB, Wharton W, Van Wyk J: Epidermal growth factor and somatomedin-C regulate G1 progression in competent BALB/c 3T3 cells. Exp Cell Res 1982; 141:107–115.

41. Gluckman PD: Insulin-like growth factors and their binding proteins. *In* Hanson MA, Spencer JAD, Rodeck CH (eds): Growth. Cambridge: Cambridge University Press, 1995, pp 97–115.

42. Xu Y, Papageorgiou A, Polychronakos C: Developmental regulation of the soluble form of insulin-like growth factor-II/mannose 6-phosphate receptor in human serum and amniotic fluid. J Clin Endocrinol Metab 1998; 83:437–442.

43. Ranke MB, Elminger M: Functional role of insulin-like growth factor binding proteins. Horm Res 1997; 48:9–15.

44. Gluckman PD, Gunn AJ, Wray A: Congenital growth hormone deficiency associated with prenatal and early postnatal growth failure. International Board of the Kabi Pharmacia International Growth Study. Pediatrics 1992; 121:920–923.

45. Gluckman PD, Harding JE: Fetal growth retardation: Underlying endocrine mechanisms and postnatal consequences. Acta Paediatr Suppl 1997; 422:69–72.

46. Holmes R, Montemagno R, Jones J, et al: Fetal and maternal plasma insulin-like growth factors and binding proteins in pregnancies with appropriate or retarded fetal growth. Early Hum Dev 1997; 49:7–17.

47. Pirazzoli P, Cacciari E, De Iasio R, et al: Developmental pattern of fetal growth hormone, insulin-like growth factor I, growth hormone binding protein and insulin-like growth factor binding protein-3. Arch Dis Child Fetal Neonatal Ed 1997; 77:F100–F104.

48. Hills FA, English J, Chard T: Circulating levels of IGF-I and IGF-binding protein-1 throughout pregnancy: Relation to birthweight and maternal weight. J Endocrinol 1996; 148:303–309.

49. Giudice LC, de Zegher F, Gargosky SE, et al: Insulin-like growth factors and their binding proteins in the term and preterm human fetus and neonate with normal and extremes of intrauterine growth. J Clin Endocrinol Metab 1995; 80:1548–1555.

50. Klauwer D, Blum WF, Hanitsch S, et al: IGF-I, IGF-II, free IGF-I and IGFBP-1, -2 and -3 levels in venous cord blood: Relationship to birthweight, length and gestational age in healthy newborns. Acta Paediatr 1997; 86:826–833.

51. Baker J, Liu JP, Robertson EJ, Efstratiadis A: Role of insulin-like growth factors in embryonic and postnatal growth. Cell 1993; 75:73–82.

52. De Chiara TM, Efstratiadis A, Robertson EJ: A growth deficiency phenotype in heterozygous mice carrying an insulin-like growth factor-II gene disrupted by targeting. Nature 1990; 78–80.

53. Liu JP, Baker J, Perkins AS: Mice carrying null mutations of the genes encoding insulin-like growth factor I (IGF-I) and type I IGF receptor (IGFIr). Cell 1993; 75:59–72.

54. Murphy LJ, Rajkumar K, Molnar P: Phenotypic manifestations of insulin-like growth factor–binding protein-1 IGFBP-1 and IGFBP-3 overexpression in transgenic mice. Progr Growth Factor Res 1995; 6:425–432.

55. Gay E, Seurin D, Babajko S, et al: Liver-specific expression of human insulin-like growth factor binding protein-1 in transgenic mice: Repercussions on reproduction, ante- and perinatal mortality and postnatal growth. Endocrinology 1997; 138:2937–2947.

56. Juul A, Bang P, Hertel NT, et al: Serum insulin-like growth factor-I in 1030 healthy children, adolescents, and adults: Relation to age, sex, stage of puberty, testicular size, and body mass index. J Clin Endocrinol Metab 1994; 78:744–752.

57. Luna AM, Wilson DM, Wibbelsman CJ, et al: Somatomedins in adolescence: A cross-sectional study of the effect of puberty on plasma insulin-like growth factor I and II levels. J Clin Endocrinol Metab 1983; 57:268–271.

58. Bala RM, Lopatka J, Leung A: Serum immunoreactive somatomedin levels in normal adults, pregnant women at term, children at various ages, and children with constitutionally delayed growth. J Clin Endocrinol Metab 1981; 52:508–512.

59. Harris DA, Van Vliet G, Egli CA, et al: Somatomedin-C in normal puberty and in true precocious puberty before and after treatment with a potent luteinizing hormone–releasing hormone agonist. J Clin Endocrinol Metab 1985; 61:152–159.

60. Argente J, Barrios V, Pozo J, et al: Normative data for insulin-like growth factors (IGFs), IGF-binding proteins, and growth hormone–binding protein in a healthy Spanish pediatric population: Age- and sex-related changes. J Clin Endocrinol Metab 1993; 77:1522–1528.

61. Attie KM, Ramirez NR, Conte FA, et al: The pubertal growth spurt in eight patients with true precocious puberty and growth hormone deficiency: Evidence for a direct role of sex steroids. J Clin Endocrinol Metab 1990; 71:975–983.

62. Juul A, Dalgaard P, Blum WF, et al: Serum levels of insulin-like growth factor (IGF)-binding protein-3 (IGFBP-3) in healthy infants, children, and adolescents: The relation to IGF-I, IGF-II, IGFBP-1, IGFBP-2, age, sex, body mass index, and pubertal maturation. J Clin Endocrinol Metab 1995; 80:2534–2542.

63. Zachman M, Prader A, Sobel E, et al: Pubertal growth in patients with androgen insensitivity: Indirect evidence for the importance of estrogens in pubertal growth of girls. J Pediatr 1997; 108:694–697.

64. Smith EP, Boyd J, Frank GR, et al: Estrogen resistance caused by a mutation by the estrogen receptor in a man. N Engl J Med 1994; 331:1056–1061.

65. Morishima A, Grumbach MM, Simpson ER, et al: Aromatase deficiency in male and female siblings caused by a novel mutation and the physiological role of estrogens. J Clin Endocrinol Metab 1995; 80:3689–3698.

66. Conte FA, Grumbach MM, Ito Y, et al: A syndrome of female pseudohermaphroditism, hypergonadotropic hypogonadism and multicystic ovaries associated with missense mutations in the gene encoding aromatase (P450 atom). J Clin Endocrinol Metab 1994; 78:1287–1292.

67. Weaver CM, Peacock M, Martin BR, et al: Calcium retention estimated from indicators of skeletal status in adolescent girls and young women. Am J Clin Nutr 1996; 64:67–70.

68. Carrie Fassler AL, Bonjour JP: Osteoporosis as a pediatric problem. Pediatr Clin North Am 1995; 42:811–824.

69. Matkovic V, Jelic T, Wardlaw GM, et al: Timing of peak bone mass in Caucasian females and its implication for the prevention of osteoporosis. Inference from a cross-sectional model. J Clin Invest 1994; 93:799–808.

70. Bachrach LK: Bone mineralization in childhood and adolescence. Curr Opin Pediatr 1993; 5:467–473.

71. Theintz G, Buchs B, Rizzoli R, et al: Longitudinal monitoring of bone mass accumulation in healthy adolescents: Evidence for a marked reduction after 16 years of age at the levels of lumbar spine and femoral neck in female subjects. J Clin Endocrinol Metab 1992; 75:1060–1065.

72. Lu PW, Briody JN, Ogle GD, et al: Bone mineral density of total body, spine, and femoral neck in children and young adults: A cross-sectional and longitudinal study. J Bone Miner Res 1994; 9:1451–1458.

73. Bonjour JP, Theintz G, Law F, et al: Peak bone mass. Osteoporos Int 1994; 4 Suppl 1:7–13.

74. Rico H, Revilla M, Villa LF, et al: Determinants of total-body and regional bone mineral content and density in postpubertal normal women. Metabolism 1994; 43:263–266.

75. Rubin K, Schirduan V, Gendreau P, et al: Predictors of axial and peripheral bone mineral density in healthy children and adolescents, with special attention to the role of puberty. J Pediatr 1993; 123:863–870.

76. Sentipal JM, Wardlaw GM, Mahan J, Matkovic V: Influence of calcium intake and growth indexes on vertebral bone mineral density in young females. Am J Clin Nutr 1991; 54:425–428.

77. Abrams SA, Stuff JE: Calcium metabolism in girls: Current dietary intakes lead to low rates of calcium absorption and retention during puberty. Am J Clin Nutr 1994; 60:739–743.

78. Matkovic V: Calcium metabolism and calcium requirements during skeletal modeling and consolidation of bone mass. Am J Clin Nutr 1991; 54:245S–260S.

79. Anderson JJ, Pollitzer WS: Ethnic and genetic differences in susceptibility to osteoporotic fractures. Adv Nutr Res 1994; 9:129–149.

80. Gilsanz V, Roe TF, Mora S, et al: Changes in vertebral bone density in black girls and white girls during childhood and puberty. Am J Med Genet 1991; 41:313–318.

81. Chan GM, Hoffman K, McMurry M: Effects of dairy products on bone and body composition in pubertal girls. J Pediatr 1995; 126:551–556.

82. Johnston CCJ, Miller Z, Slemenda CW, et al: Calcium supplementation and increases in bone mineral density in children. N Engl J Med 1992; 327:82–87.

83. Matkovic V: Calcium and peak bone mass. J Intern Med 1992; 231:151–160.

84. Lee WT, Leung SS, Leung DM, Cheng JC: A follow-up study on the effects of calcium-supplement withdrawal and puberty on bone acquisition of children. Am J Clin Nutr 1996; 64:71–77.

85. Hergenroeder AC: Bone mineralization, hypothalamic amenorrhea, and sex steroid therapy in female adolescents and young adults. J Pediatr 1995; 126:683–689.

86. Fabbri G, Petraglia F, Segre A, et al: Reduced spinal bone density in young women with amenorrhoea. Eur J Obstet Gynecol Reprod Biol 1991; 41:117–122.

87. Saggese G, Bertelloni S, Baroncelli GI, et al: Reduction of bone density: An effect of gonadotropin releasing hormone analogue treatment in central precocious puberty. Eur J Pediatr 1993; 152:717–720.

88. Neely EK, Bachrach LK, Hintz RL, et al: Bone mineral density during treatment of central precocious puberty. J Pediatr 1995; 127:819–822.

89. Mauras N, Haymond MW, Darmaun D, et al: Calcium and protein kinetics in prepubertal boys. Positive effects of testosterone. J Clin Invest 1994; 93:1014–1019.

90. Lonzer MD, Imrie R, Rogers D, et al: Effects of heredity, age, weight, puberty, activity, and calcium intake on bone mineral density in children. Clin Pediatr (Phila) 1996; 35:185–189.

91. McKay HA, Bailey DA, Wilkinson AA, Houston CS: Familial comparison of bone mineral density at the proximal femur and lumbar spine. Bone Miner 1994; 24:95–107.

92. Garn SM: Fat weight and fat placement in the female. Science 1957; 125:1091–1092.

93. Kissebah AH, Krakower GR: Regional adiposity and morbidity. Physiol Rev 1994; 74:761–811.

94. Hammer LD, Wilson DM, Litt IF, et al: Impact of pubertal development on body fat distribution among white, Hispanic, and Asian female adolescents. J Pediatr 1991; 118:975–980.

95. Obesity and cardiovascular disease risk factors in black and white girls: The NHLBI Growth and Health Study. Am J Public Health 1992; 82:1613–1620.

96. Ohzeki T, Otahara H, Hanaki K, et al: Eating attitudes test in boys and girls aged 6–18 years: Decrease in concerns with eating in boys and the increase in girls with their ages. Psychopathology 1993; 26:117–121.

97. Schreiber GB, Robins M, Striegel-Moore R, et al: Weight modification efforts reported by black and white preadolescent girls: National Heart, Lung, and Blood Institute Growth and Health Study. Pediatrics 1996; 98:63–70.

98. Falkner F: Obesity and cardiovascular disease risk factors in prepubescent and pubescent black and white females. Crit Rev Food Sci Nutr 1997; 33:397–402.

99. Javier Nieto F, Szklo M, Comstock GW: Childhood weight and growth rate as predictors of adult mortality. Am J Epidemiol 1992; 136:201–213.

100. Caro JF, Sinha MK, Kolaczynski JW, et al: Leptin: The tale of an obesity gene. Diabetes 1996; 45:1455–1462.

101. Montague CT, Farooqi IS, Whitehead JP, et al: Congenital leptin deficiency is associated with severe early-onset obesity in humans. Nature 1997; 387:903–908.

102. Montague CT, Farooqi IS, Whitehead JP, et al: Program of the International Congress of Obesity (Abstract).

103. Herman-Giddens ME, Slora EJ, Wasserman RC, et al: Secondary sexual characteristics and menses in young girls seen in office practice: A study from the Pediatric Research in Office Settings network. Pediatrics 1997; 99:505–512.

104. Tanner JM, Eveleth PB: Onset of puberty. In Bierich JR (ed): Puberty: Biologic and Social Components. Leiden: HE Stenfert Kroese, 1975, p 256.

105. Tanner JM: The trend toward earlier menarche in London, Oslo, Copenhagen, the Netherlands and Hungary. Nature 1973; 243:95.

106. Kill V: Stature and growth of Norwegian men during past 200 years. Skr Nor Vidensk Akad 1939; 2(6):1–175.

107. Constantini NW, Warren MP: Special problems of the female athlete. Baillieres Clin Rheumatol 1994; 8:199–219.

108. Zacharias L, Wurtman RJ: Age at menarche. N Engl J Med 1969; 280:868–875.

109. Rhone RD: Papilla (nipple) development during female puberty. J Adolesc Health Care 1982; 2:217.

110. Ivarsson SA, Nilsson KO, Persson PH: Ultrasonography of the pelvic organs in prepubertal and postpubertal girls. Arch Dis Child 1983; 58:352–354.

111. Griffin IJ, Cole TJ, Duncan KA: Pelvic ultrasound measurements in normal girls. Acta Paediatr 1995; 84:536–543.

112. Haber HP, Mayer EI: Ultrasound evaluation of uterine and ovarian size from birth to puberty. Pediatr Radiol 1994; 24:11–13.

113. Fleischer AC, Shawker TH: The role of sonography in pediatric gynecology. Clin Obstet Gynecol 1987; 30:735–746.

114. Haber HP, Wollmann HA, Ranke MB: Pelvic ultrasonography: Early differentiation between isolated premature thelarche and central precocious puberty. Eur J Pediatr 1995; 154:182–186.

115. Salardi S, Orsini LF, Cacciari E, et al: Pelvic ultrasonography in girls with precocious puberty, congenital adrenal hyperplasia, obesity, or hirsutism. J Pediatr 1988; 112:880–887.

116. Salardi S, Orsini LF, Cacciari E, et al: Pelvic ultrasonography in premenarcheal girls: Relation to puberty and sex hormone concentrations. Arch Dis Child 1985; 60:120–125.

117. Bridges NA, Cooke A, Healy MJ, et al: Standards for ovarian volume in childhood and puberty. Fertil Steril 1993; 60:456–460.

118. King LR, Siegel MJ, Solomon AL: Usefulness of ovarian volume and cysts in female isosexual precocious puberty. J Ultrasound Med 1993; 12:577–581.

119. Neely EK, Hintz RL, Wilson DM, et al: Normal ranges for immunochemiluminometric gonadotropin assays. J Pediatr 1997; 127:40–46.

120. Garibaldi LR, Picco P, Magier S, et al: Serum luteinizing hormone concentrations, as measured by a sensitive immunoradiometric assay, in children with normal, precocious or delayed pubertal development. J Clin Endocrinol Metab 1991; 72:888–898.

121. Demir A, Dunkel L, Stenman UH, Voutilainen R: Age-related course of urinary gonadotropins in children. J Clin Endocrinol Metab 1995; 80:1457–1460.

122. Demir A, Voutilainen R, Juul A, et al: Increase in first morning voided urinary luteinizing hormone levels precedes the physical onset of puberty. J Clin Endocrinol Metab 1996; 81:2963–2967.

123. Klein KO, Baron J, Colli MJ, et al: Estrogen levels in childhood determined by an ultrasensitive recombinant cell bioassay. J Clin Invest 1994; 94:2475–2480.

124. Grumbach MM: Onset of puberty. In Berenberg SR (ed): Puberty, Biologic and Social Components. Leiden: H. E. Stenfert Kroese, 1975, pp 1–21.

125. Jenner MR, Kelch RP, Kaplan SL, Grumbach MM: Hormonal changes in puberty. IV. Plasma estradiol, LH, and FSH in prepubertal children, pubertal females, and in precocious puberty, premature thelarche, hypogonadism, and in a child with a feminizing ovarian tumor. J Clin Endocrinol Metab 1972; 34:521–530.

126. Goji K: Twenty-four-hour concentration profiles of gonadotropin and estradiol (E2) in prepubertal and early pubertal girls: The diurnal rise of E2 is opposite the nocturnal rise of gonadotropin. J Clin Endocrinol Metab 1993; 77:1629–1635.

127. Sklar CA, Kaplan SL, Grumbach MM: Evidence for dissociation between adrenarche and gonadarche: Studies in patients with idiopathic precocious puberty, gonadal dysgenesis, isolated gonadotropin deficiency, and constitutionally delayed growth and adolescence. J Clin Endocrinol Metab 1980; 51:548–556.

128. Vale W, Bilezikjian LM, Rivier C: Reproductive and other roles of inhibins and activins. In Knobil E, Neil JD (eds): Physiology of Reproduction. New York: Raven, 1994, pp 1861–1878.

129. De Jong FH: Inhibin. Physiol Rev 1988; 68:555–607.

130. Yen SS, Apter D, Butzow T, Laughlin GA: Gonadotrophin releasing hormone pulse generator activity before and during sexual maturation in girls: New insights. Hum Reprod 1993; 8 (Suppl 2):66–71.

131. Anderson DC: Sex hormone–binding globulin. Clin Endocrinol 1974; 3:69–95.

132. Lindstedt G, Lundberg P, Hammond GL: Sex hormone binding globulin—still many questions. Scand J Clin Lab Invest 1985; 45:1–6.

133. Horst HJ, Bartsch W, Dirksen-Thiedens I: Plasma testosterone, sex hormone binding globulin binding capacity and per cent binding of testosterone and 5 alpha-dihydrotestosterone in prepubertal, pubertal and adult males. J Clin Endocrinol Metab 1977; 45:522–527.

134. Bartsch W, Horst HJ, Derwahl DM: Interrelationships between sex hormone-binding globulin and 17 beta-estradiol, testosterone, 5 alpha-dihydrotestosterone, thyroxine, and triiodothyronine in prepubertal and pubertal girls. J Clin Endocrinol Metab 1980; 50:1053–1056.

135. August GP, Tkachuk M, Grumbach MM: Plasma testosterone-binding affinity and testosterone in umbilical cord plasma, late pregnancy, prepubertal children and adults. J Clin Endocrinol Metab 1969; 29:891–899.

136. Aubert ML, Sizonenko PC, Kaplan SL, et al: The ontogenesis of human prolactin from fetal life to puberty. In Crosignani PG, Robyn C (eds): Prolactin and Human Reproduction. New York: Academic Press, 1977, pp 9–20.

137. Amiel SA, Caprio S, Sherwin RS, et al: Insulin resistance of puberty: A defect restricted to peripheral glucose metabolism. J Clin Endocrinol Metab 1991; 72:277–282.
138. Bloch CA, Clemons P, Sperling MA: Puberty decreases insulin sensitivity. J Pediatr 1987; 110:481–487.
139. Amiel SA, Sherwin RS, Simonson DC, et al. Impaired insulin action in puberty. A contributing factor to poor glycemic control in adolescents with diabetes. N Engl J Med 1986; 315:215–219.
140. Hindmarsh P, Di Silvio L, Pringle PJ, et al: Changes in serum insulin concentration during puberty and their relationship to growth hormone. Clin Endocrinol (Oxf) 1988; 28:381–388.
141. Travers SH, Jeffers BW, Bloch CA, et al: Gender and Tanner stage differences in body composition and insulin sensitivity in early pubertal children. J Clin Endocrinol Metab 1995; 80:172–178.
142. Caprio S, Clin G, Boulware S, et al: Effects of puberty and diabetes on metabolism of insulin-sensitive fuels. Am J Physiol 1994; 266:E885–E891.
143. Amiel SA, Caprio S, Sherwin RS, et al: Insulin resistance of puberty: A defect restricted to peripheral glucose metabolism. J Clin Endocrinol Metab 1991; 72:277–282.
144. Arslanian SA, Kalhan SC: Correlations between fatty acid and glucose metabolism. Potential explanation of insulin resistance of puberty. Diabetes 1994; 43:908–914.
145. Normann EK, Evald U, Dahl-Jorgensen K, et al: Decreased serum insulin-like growth factor I during puberty in children with insulin dependent diabetes mellitus (IDDM). Uppsala J Med Sci 1994; 99:147–154.
146. Pal BR, Matthews DR, Edge JA, et al: The frequency and amplitude of growth hormone secretory episodes as determined by deconvolution analysis are increased in adolescents with insulin dependent diabetes mellitus and are unaffected by short-term euglycaemia. Clin Endocrinol (Oxf) 1993; 38:93–100.
147. Menon RK, Arslanian S, May B, et al: Diminished growth hormone–binding protein in children with insulin-dependent diabetes mellitus. J Clin Endocrinol Metab 1992; 74:934–938.
148. Rosenbloom AL, Wheeler L, Bianchi R, et al: Age-adjusted analysis of insulin responses during normal and abnormal glucose tolerance tests in children and adolescents. Diabetes 1975; 4:820–828.
149. Caprio S, Amiel SA, Merkel P, Tamborlane WV: Insulin-resistance syndromes in children. Horm Res 1993; 39(Suppl 3):112–114.
150. Holl RW, Heinze E, Seifert M, et al: Longitudinal analysis of somatic development in paediatric patients with IDDM: Genetic influences on height and weight. Diabetologia 1994; 37:925–929.
151. Brown M, Ahmed ML, Clayton KL, Dunger DB: Growth during childhood and final height in type 1 diabetes. Diabet Med 1994; 11:182–187.
152. Glaser NS: Non–insulin-dependent diabetes mellitus in childhood and adolescence. Pediatr Clin North Am 1997; 44:307–337.
153. Glaser N, Jones KL: Non–insulin-dependent diabetes mellitus in children and adolescents. Adv Pediatr 1996; 43:359–396.
154. Todd JA: Transcribing diabetes. Nature 1996; 384:407–408.
155. Glaser NS: Non–insulin-dependent diabetes mellitus in childhood and adolescence. Pediatr Clin North Am 1997; 44:307–337.
156. Stoll BA: Obesity and breast cancer. Int J Obes Rel Metab Disord 1996; 20:389–392.
157. Stoll BA, Vatten LJ, Kvinnsland S: Does early physical maturity influence breast cancer risk? Acta Oncol 1994; 33:171–176.
158. Islam AH, Yamashita S, Kotani K, et al: Fasting plasma insulin level is an important risk factor for the development of complications in Japanese obese children—results from a cross-sectional and a longitudinal study. Metabolism 1995; 44:478–485.
159. Apter D, Vihko R: Serum pregnenolone, progesterone, 17-hydroxyprogesterone, testosterone and 5 alpha-dihydrotestosterone during female puberty. J Clin Endocrinol Metab 1977; 45:1039–1048.
160. Seminara SB, Hayes FJ, Crowley WFJ: Gonadotropin-releasing hormone deficiency in the human (idiopathic hypogonadotropic hypogonadism and Kallmann's syndrome): Pathophysiological and genetic considerations (Abstract). Endocr Rev 1999;19:521–539.

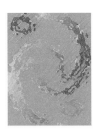

Chapter 3
Abnormalities of Growth

R. L. HINTZ

CONTROL OF GROWTH

OVERVIEW

The control of growth is a complex process involving many hormonal and nonhormonal components (Fig. 3–1). Many of the hormonal components of growth are controlled via the hypothalamic-pituitary axis.[1] Thus, the secretion of growth hormone (GH), which leads to the secretion of insulin-like growth factors (IGF), is under the control of hypothalamic neuropeptide hormones known as *growth hormone–releasing factor* (GHRF) and *somatostatin*, or *somatotropin release–inhibiting factor* (SRIF). Similarly, the secretion of thyroid-simulating hormone (TSH or thyrotropin), follicle-stimulating hormone (FSH), luteinizing hormone (LH), and adrenocorticotrophic hormone (ACTH), all of which play major roles in the control of growth, are themselves under the control of hypothalamic neurohormones. In addition, the secretion of insulin, which is not directly under pituitary control, also plays an important role in the control of cell growth.[2] Of course, many nonhormonal factors play major roles in the control of growth. Foremost among these is nutrition, since without substrate no cell could grow or divide. There are also underlying genetic factors that determine the potential for growth, not only for the whole organism but for each organ and tissue. In addition, there are a host of tissue growth factors, such as epidermal growth factor (EGF) and nerve growth factor (NGF), whose roles in the overall control of growth are only beginning to be understood.[3] The interaction of these hormonal and nonhormonal factors leads to the normal growth and development of children, and it is abnormalities of these mechanisms that lead to disorders in growth that cause children to be

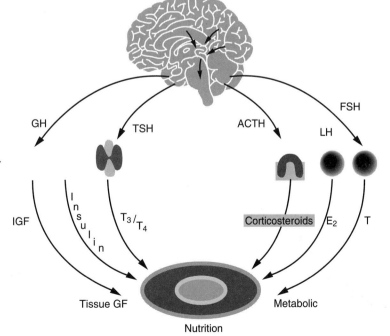

Figure 3–1. Control of cellular growth.

brought to a physician. In this chapter, we review our current understanding of the physiology of growth and the application of that understanding to the clinical problems of short stature and tall stature in children and adolescents.

THE GROWTH HORMONE–INSULIN-LIKE GROWTH FACTOR AXIS

Growth Hormone

GH is a 191–amino acid polypeptide secreted by special cells in the anterior pituitary gland called *somatotropes*. Neurohormones control these cells through the hypophyseal portal system, and are both a positive effector and an inhibitor of GH secretion exist.[4] Present data indicate that GHRF is responsible for the rapid pulses of GH secretion seen mainly during the nighttime hours and in response to meals and exercise, whereas the inhibitor of GH secretion, SRIF, appears to be responsible for the underlying tone of GH secretion. There are two major forms of GH synthesized, stored, and secreted by the somatotropes.[5] The most abundant form (approximately 90%) is the 22-kd molecular weight form. In addition, alternative splicing of the GH mRNA leads to a minor, 20-kd form of GH whose physiological role is not known.

It has been known for some time that GH secretion, like that of many other polypeptide hormones, is pulsatile.[6] In addition, GH has a striking predilection for secretion in association with sleep. A large number of brain centers and neurotransmitters have been implicated in the control of GH. In addition, there is evidence that one of the GH-stimulated peptides, IGF-I, plays a feedback role in the secretion of GH at the levels of both the hypothalamus and the somatotropes.[7]

The secretion of GH leads to a complex chain of events illustrated in Figure 3–2, which ultimately leads to the stimulation of growth at the endocrine level. After GH is released into the bloodstream, a large proportion of it binds to a specific GH-binding protein.[8] Recent advances have led to better understanding of the molecular character of this GH protein. It is now clear that it represents the extracellular portion of the GH receptor site. Like many receptors for polypeptide hormones, the receptor site for GH consists of three polypeptide domains: an extracellular domain that contains all of the three-dimensional structure necessary for the recognition of the hormone; a transmembrane domain that is highly hydrophobic; and, finally, an intra-

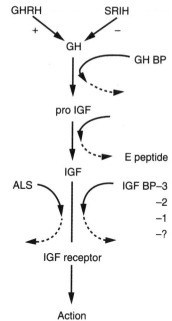

Figure 3–2. The chain of growth hormone action.

cellular domain that contains the three-dimensional structure necessary to lead to the biological action in the cell. In humans, it appears that there is proteolytic cleavage of the extracellular domain of the GH receptor that leads to a soluble, circulating polypeptide that plays a major role in protein binding of GH in the serum. The exact biological role of this binding protein is unclear; however, it does seem that it will serve as a useful index to the level of GH receptors in the body. GH receptors are widely distributed throughout tissues in the body, and it is the binding of the GH ligand to these receptors that leads to the biological events within the cells themselves. Of the many direct biological events ascribed to GH activity, clearly, one of the most important is the control of the production of yet another polypeptide hormone, IGF-I.

Insulin-like Growth Factors

IGF messenger RNA is widely distributed throughout the body and is under GH control, not only in the liver, as would have been predicted by the original somatomedin hypothesis (the original description called *somatomedin*) but in other tissues as well.[9] There are two distinctly different types of IGF, IGF-I and IGF-II. The two bear strong homology—to each other and to insulin. Of the two polypeptides, IGF-I is more closely related to GH secretion and action. Two forms of IGF-I prohormone are predicted, and thus far only one is predicted for IGF-II. All of these prohormone forms contain long carboxyl terminal extensions beyond the known structure of the active hormone, which are known as *E regions*. It appears that, in normal circumstances, these E regions are cleaved off very efficiently before IGF is secreted; however, in certain circumstances such as renal failure and tumor-associated hypoglycemia, both circulating prohormone forms and E peptide segments have been demonstrated.[10]

IGFs circulate tightly bound to proteins known as IGF-binding proteins (IGFBPs).[11] In most normal circumstances, little or no free IGF-I or IGF-II polypeptide circulates. Six distinct but homologous IGFBPs are now known (Table 3–1). By far the most abundant form of IGFBP in normal serum is IGFBP-3, a glycosylated protein of approximately 40 kd molecular weight. The combined IGF-peptide–IGFBP-3 complex binds to yet another protein known as *acid-labile subunit* (ALS) to form a 150-kd, three-subunit protein complex, which is the major circulating form of the IGFs. In most circumstances, this 150-kd complex contains well over 90% of the total IGF in the serum. A smaller proportion of the IGF in serum circulates bound to the other forms of IGFBP—IGFBP-1, -2, -4, -5, and -6). In addition, these other IGFBPs are major components of certain body fluids, such as IGFBP-1 in amniotic fluid, IGFBP-2 in joint fluid, and IGFBP-5 in cerebrospinal fluid. The exact biological purpose of this complex system for controlling the amount and distribution of IGF in the serum and extracellular fluid spaces is not known for certain; however, it does prolong the circulating time of IGFs in plasma and may participate in modulating the delivery of the IGF peptides to the receptor sites on cells.

Biological Activity

Just as there is more than one form of IGF, there is more than one form of IGF receptor on the surface of cells.[12] The type 1 IGF receptor has the strongest affinity for IGF-I and weaker affinity for IGF-II and insulin. The type 1 receptor resembles the insulin receptor itself in its subunit construction and amino acid sequence and appears to have been derived from the insulin receptor during evolution. The type 2 IGF receptor has greatest affinity for IGF-II and somewhat less for IGF-I. Unlike the situation with the type 1 receptor or with the insulin receptor, the type 2 IGF receptor has no affinity for insulin itself. The molecular corollary of this observation has been that there is no structural relationship between the type 2 receptor and either the type 1 receptor or the insulin receptor. Rather, the type 2 receptor appears to be a bifunctional receptor with ligand specificity for both IGF peptides and for mannose-6 phosphate. The role of the type 2 receptor in the control of growth is unclear and still controversial. Most of the observed biological actions of GH on the control of growth appear to be subserved by the chain of actions initiated by GH. This leads to the production of IGF-I and its delivery to the IGF type 1 receptor sites in the tissues (see Fig. 3–2). It is this chain of action that has been most clearly linked to the anabolic and growth-promoting events we associate with GH in the entire organism.

THYROID HORMONE

Thyroid hormone also plays an extremely important role in the control of growth. As in the GH-IGF axis, there is a hypothalamic control

Table 3–1. Insulin-like Growth Factor–Binding Proteins

Designation	Characteristics	Source	Amino-Terminal Amino Acid* (Human)
IGFBP-1	Growth hormone (GH) independent; insulin dependent; high in utero	Amniotic fluid Hep G-2 media	APWQ<u>C</u>APCSAEKLAL
IGFBP-2	GH independent; insulin dependent; high in utero	Joint fluid MDBK media BRL 3A media	EVLFR<u>CPPC</u>TPERLA
IGFBP-3	GH dependent; insulin independent; major IGFBP in serum postnatally	Serum (150-kd complex)	GASSGGLGPVVR<u>CEP</u>
IGFBP-4	"Inhibitory" IGFBP	Serum, osteosarcoma	DEAIH<u>CPPC</u>SEEKLA
IGFBP-5	High in joint fluid	Serum, cerebrospinal fluid, human bone extract	LGSFVH<u>CEPC</u>DEKAL
IGFBP-6	Cerebrospinal fluid–binding protein	Serum, cerebrospinal fluid, transformed and fetal fibroblasts	ALAR<u>CPGC</u>GQVQAGC

*The new terminology, characteristics, and the amino-terminal amino acid sequences of the insulin-like growth factor–binding proteins are summarized here. The homologous C**C regions of the amino-terminal amino acid sequences are underlined.

mechanism: neurohormone thyrotropin-releasing hormone (TRH) being secreted by specialized neurons into the hypophyseal portal system and leading to the release of a pituitary hormone TSH.[13] TSH then leads to the production and release of the final hormones in the chain, thyroid hormones thyroxine (T_4) and triiodothyronine (T_3). Like the IGFs, the thyroid hormones are almost totally bound to plasma proteins, which control their half-lives and delivery to tissue. Thyroid hormone action is subserved by the thyroid hormone receptor sites, which are widely distributed throughout cells in the body. These receptor sites are located within the cells, like those of steroid hormones, and the ligand-T_3 complex binds to chromatin and DNA to initiate mRNA synthesis. Without thyroid hormone action through its receptor sites, GH and IGFs are unable to stimulate anabolic and growth responses. Furthermore, there is a close relationship between thyroid hormone and GH secretion.[14] In persons with hypothyroidism, GH secretion from the pituitary gland is decreased in response to both pharmacologic and physiologic stimulation.

SEX HORMONE

The sex hormones estrogen and androgen play extremely important roles in the control of growth during puberty. Secretion of these hormones is relatively low after the perinatal period until an increase in the gonadotropins (LH and FSH) occurs, before the clinical onset of puberty.[15] It is the secretion of estrogens and androgens under the control of the pituitary gonadotropins that leads to the development of the secondary sex characteristics that are so closely associated with the events of puberty. Estrogens and androgens have been associated with growth stimulation, both directly and indirectly. Both androgens and estrogens have been shown to affect the secretion of GH at puberty.[16] This increase in GH secretion at puberty is thought to play a major part in the pubertal growth spurt. Direct end-organ effects of both androgens and estrogens have also been demonstrated in a variety of experimental systems. In addition to their direct and indirect roles in the stimulation of growth, androgens and estrogens also play major roles in the maturation of bones and the ultimate disappearance of the epiphyseal plates.[17] It is this event that results in the cessation of growth in stature at the end of puberty. Like the thyroid hormones, the sex hormones appear to act by diffusing into the cell and binding to the specific

receptor sites of the steroid-TSH category. The binding of androgens and estrogens to their respective receptor sites initiates changes in the three-dimensional structure which allows the interaction of these activated receptors with chromatin and the chromosomal DNA, which in turn leads to the production of specific mRNA and secretion of specific proteins that produce the biologic action observed.[18]

ADRENAL HORMONES

In addition to the other hormonal factors, clearly, adrenal hormones also play a role in the control of growth. Adrenal androgens appear to have an important adjunctive role in the events of puberty and act in concert with androgens from the testes and ovaries to stimulate growth by both direct and indirect means and the maturation of the bones.[19] In addition, the adrenal glucocorticoids appear to have bimodal action in the control of growth. Experimental evidence suggests that a minimal level of glucocorticoids is necessary for cells to function, grow, and divide. On the other hand, many observations have shown that an excess of glucocorticoids renders cells unresponsive to the other hormonal growth-stimulating agents reviewed earlier.[20]

OTHER FACTORS

In addition to the hormones that control growth, there are many extremely important nonhumoral factors. It is intuitively obvious that, without adequate nutrients, and therefore without adequate substrate for cells, no effective growth can occur. This is seen most clearly in the clinical disorders of kwashiorkor and marasmus,[21] but is also manifested in many more subtle clinical disorders of nutrition. Genetics also plays an extremely important role in determining growth potential. The potential limits of growth for three related primates, the gorilla, the human, and the chimpanzee, are genetically determined. On a more subtle level, it is clear that the differences in stature among humans depend to a large extent on individual genetic constitution. So far, our best, but relatively crude, way of determining these underlying genetic factors is to look at the heights of the parents and other family.[22] Tissue growth factors, such as EGF, clearly play a critical, though largely unknown, role in the control of growth (Table 3–2).[3] Further work will be necessary to relate these individual growth factors to clinical growth disorders. Finally, the role

Table 3–2. Families of Tissue Growth Factors

Insulin related
    Insulin-like growth factor-I (IGF-I)
    Insulin-like growth factor-II (IGF-II)
    Nerve growth factor (NGF)
Epidermal growth factor related
    Epidermal growth factor (EGF)
    Transforming growth factor-alpha (TGF-alpha)
Transforming growth factor-beta related
    Transforming growth factor-beta (TGF-β)
    Müllerian-inhibiting factor (MIF)
    Inhibin
    Activin
Platelet-derived growth factor
Fibroblast growth factor cytokines
    Erythropoietin
    Granulocyte/monocyte colony–stimulating
      factor (GM-CSF)
    Granulocyte-CSF (G-CSF)
    Monocyte-CSF (M-CSF)
    Multi-CSF
Interleukins
    Interleukin 1 through 9
    Tumor necrosis factor (TNF)
Interferons

of systemic disease in the growth of children and adolescents cannot be overstated. Even in the presence of normal hormonal, nutritional, and genetic factors, underlying systemic disease such as inflammatory bowel disease can interfere with growth potential.[23] Short or tall stature in an affected patient is an important clue to the underlying condition of the patient.

SHORT STATURE

As might be expected from the multiplicity of control mechanisms for growth, there are many causes of short stature (Table 3–3).

NONPATHOLOGIC SHORT STATURE

Clinically significant short stature is defined as height below the third percentile for age as compared with accepted standards. Using this definition, it is clear that the vast majority of children with short stature do not have underlying hormonal or genetic disease. Such children are frequently described as having *normal variant short stature* (NVSS). Many come from "short families" and might be said to exhibit *familial short stature*. Others are from average-height families and have retarded bone maturation and so could be classified as having constitutional delay. The reality in clinical practice, however, is that many children have a combination

of these features, and subcategorization of NVSS is not often very helpful. Hidden within this large number of basically normal children are some who may have clinically important disorders. As a group, children with NVSS secrete smaller average amounts of GH and have lower mean levels of circulating IGF-I than age-matched controls. This observation has led to the suggestion that some of these children have subtle abnormalities of GH secretion or action and might benefit from treatment with GH.[24] In addition to NVSS, nutritional disorders (including maternal malnutrition and anorexia and bulimia) can certainly cause children to be short for their age.

GROWTH HORMONE–RELATED SHORT STATURE

Clinical abnormalities of GH secretion or action are clearly associated with short stature. The most apparent of these is GH deficiency, which is either a disorder of the hypothalamic control of GH or inability of the pituitary gland to secrete GH.[25] The consequences of classic GH deficiency are reflected not only in low levels of circulating GH as assessed by both physiologic and pharmacologic stimulation, but also in extremely low levels of IGF-I and, consequently, a decrease in the growth rate. These children almost invariably respond to GH treatment with a marked increase in growth rate.[26] An interesting though rare disorder of the chain of GH action is

Table 3–3. Causes of Short Stature

Normal variant short stature (NVSS)
    Constitutional delay
    Familial
    Nutritional
Growth hormone (GH)-related causes
    GH deficiency
    GH resistance syndrome (Laron syndrome)
Hypothyroidism
Sex hormone–related causes
    Delayed puberty
    Hypogonadotropic hypogonadism (Kallmann syndrome)
Glucocorticoid excess
    Cushing syndrome
    Exogenous administration
Genetic causes
    Chromosomal
      Turner syndrome (XO and variants)
      Down syndrome (21 trisomy)
    Syndromes
      Pseudohypoparathyroidism
      Prader-Willi syndrome
      Lawrence-Moon-Biedl syndrome
      Skeletal dysplasias
      Miscellaneous (e.g., Russell-Silver, Seckel)

Laron syndrome (also known as *GH insensitivity syndrome*). This disorder, originally described in Ashkenazi Jews, is now known to be ethnically and geographically more widely distributed.[27] Laron syndrome is a group of genetic disorders of the GH receptor that render it incapable of binding GH. This results in an increase in circulating GH levels (secondary to failure of IGF feedback), a decrease in the level of circulating GH-binding protein derived from the GH receptor, markedly decreased levels of IGF-I, and extremely slow growth rates. Early results suggest that children with Laron syndrome will respond to treatment with synthetic IGF-I with accelerated growth (thus validating the somatomedin hypothesis).[28] It is possible that more subtle abnormalities of the GH-binding protein or GH receptor are underlying causes in some of the undiagnosed cases of poor growth.[29]

THYROID HORMONE–RELATED SHORT STATURE

Because of the important role of thyroid hormone in both the secretion and endocrine actions of GH, it is clear that hypothyroidism of any degree would reduce the growth rate and eventually result in short stature.[30] Figure 3–3 demonstrates the remarkable decrease in growth rate seen with severe hypothyroidism and the rapid increase in growth after thyroid therapy is instituted. Some patients with severe hypothyroidism actually present with a peculiar form of precocious puberty known as *overlap syndrome*, in which there is a premature activation of the FSH receptor, apparently associated with the high levels of TSH secretion.[31] On the other hand, the treatment of hypothyroidism can lead to rapid onset of true puberty which leads to an accelerated advance in bone age and may limit the final height achieved despite thyroid therapy.

SEX HORMONE–RELATED SHORT STATURE

Short stature relative to that expected for age can also result from undersecretion of sex hormone. This is most common in boys who have delayed puberty, but some girls also have a significant delay. Treatment with short courses of androgen has been used in boys with long delayed puberty.[32] Many times, the delay is physiologic; however, it can also be associated with hypogonadotropic hypogonadism, in both boys and girls. Affected children may present in the

ACQUIRED HYPOTHYROIDISM

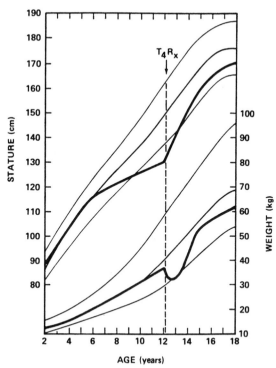

Figure 3–3. Growth in hypothyroidism before and after treatment.

early pubertal stage with short stature, which is due to the lack of sex hormone secretion and failure of the pubertal growth spurt, even though their final adult height may not be "short." A relatively common form of hypogonadotropic hypogonadism in both boys and girls is Kallmann syndrome, in which the hypogonadotropic hypogonadism is associated with anosmia.[33] These patients can be treated with androgens or estrogens, as appropriate.

ADRENAL HORMONE–RELATED SHORT STATURE

Short stature can also be associated with hypersecretion of glucocorticoids caused by an increase in ACTH secretion (Cushing disease)[34] or by a functioning adrenal tumor. These patients need to be treated by controlling their excessive glucocorticoid secretion. Of course, the most common cause of glucocorticoid excess leading to growth failure is the treatment of steroid-responsive diseases with pharmacologic doses of glucocorticoids. For these patients the obvious treatment of reducing the dose or stopping the therapy may, in practice, be very difficult to accomplish because of exacerbation of the underlying disease.

SHORT STATURE OF GENETIC CAUSES

In girls, by far the most common genetic disorder that leads to short stature is Turner syndrome.[35] The mechanism by which Turner syndrome leads to short stature is not yet clear, but it does not appear to be directly related to GH. These girls have relatively slow growth during childhood, which leads to a progressive decrease in their average height relative to those of normal girls of the same age (Fig. 3–4). In addition, they fail to enter puberty because of the ovarian failure associated with Turner syndrome and thus achieve very short adult stature (average height approximately 4 ft 7 in [140 cm]). GH treatment has had some success in increasing growth rates and final height in girls with Turner syndrome.[36] Although the vast majority of these children have delayed puberty, a significant percentage secrete enough estrogen from their ovaries to develop

secondary sex characteristics and even to menstruate. Thus, it cannot be too strongly recommended that any physician who treats a girl who is pathologically short and has no established diagnosis should always order a chromosomal evaluation, regardless of the presence or absence of secondary sex characteristics.

Other genetic causes of severe short stature include Down syndrome, pseudohypoparathyroidism, Lawrence-Moon-Biedl syndrome, Weaver syndrome, and Prader-Willi syndrome.

TALL STATURE

Just like short stature, tall stature has many causes (Table 3–4).

TALL STATURE OF NONPATHOLOGIC BENIGN CAUSES

Most children with clinically significant tall stature (above the 97th percentile of height for age) do not have a defined disease, and most are

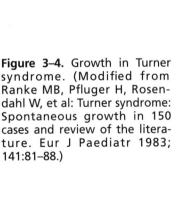

Figure 3–4. Growth in Turner syndrome. (Modified from Ranke MB, Pfluger H, Rosendahl W, et al: Turner syndrome: Spontaneous growth in 150 cases and review of the literature. Eur J Paediatr 1983; 141:81–88.)

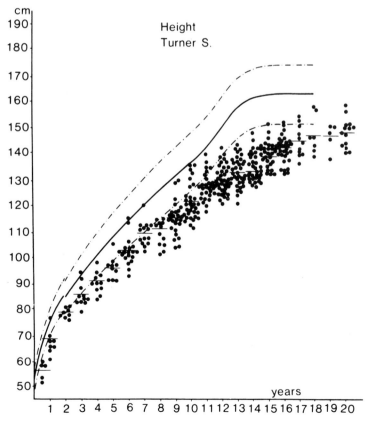

Table 3–4. Causes of Tall Stature

Normal variant tall stature
  Genetic/familial
  Obesity
Pituitary gigantism
Hyperthyroidism
Sex hormone–related causes
  Precocious puberty
  Hypogonadotropic hypogonadism
  Primary hypogonadism
Adrenal hormone–related causes
  Precocious adrenarche
  Adrenogenital syndrome
  Adrenal tumors
Genetic causes
  Disorder of sex chromosomes
    Klinefelter syndrome (XXY)
    Extra Y (e.g., XYY, XYYY)
  Genetic syndromes
    Marfan syndrome
    Homocystinuria
    Cerebral gigantism (Sotos syndrome)
    Weaver syndrome

from tall families or tall genetic groups. Studies of these children have, however, suggested that, as a group, they may have higher rates of GH secretion and higher levels of IGF-I.[37] These findings suggest that at least one of the underlying reasons for "normal variant" tall stature is a genetically determined increase in GH secretion or activity. Another common cause of relatively tall stature is overnutrition leading to exogenous obesity. Studies of obesity in childhood have demonstrated that almost all of the patients are above the 50th percentile of height for age, regardless of their genetic background, and a large proportion of them are above the 97th percentile. Owing to ill-defined neuroendocrine mechanisms, these obese children have relatively low secretion of GH, as determined by both physiologic and pharmacologic stimulation.[38]

TALL STATURE OF GROWTH HORMONE–RELATED CAUSES

There are well-documented instances of pituitary tumors with excess GH secretion leading to tall stature, including the famous Alton giant,[39] but as a cause of tall stature such tumors are exceedingly rare in most endocrinologists' experience. It is important to exclude this possibility in rapidly growing children, and a serum level of IGF-I is probably an adequate screen for excessive pituitary secretion of GH.

TALL STATURE OF THYROID–RELATED CAUSES

In addition to growth hormone-related causes, hyperthyroidism has been associated with tall stature in childhood.[40] These patients may grow rapidly under the influence of high levels of thyroid hormone, but they also mature their epiphyseal centers faster so that they finish their growth prematurely.

TALL STATURE OF SEX HORMONE–RELATED CAUSES

Precocious puberty is well-known to be associated with relatively tall stature for age[41] and is the best clinical illustration of the role of sex hormone secretion in growth. The disorder of precocious puberty is covered in more detail in Chapter 5. Somewhat paradoxically, delayed puberty due to hypogonadotropic hypogonadism or Kallmann syndrome can also be associated with tall stature. The explanation is that, although these children grow relatively slowly during the time that other children their age are having their pubertal growth spurt, they continue to grow long after the majority of children are through puberty, and they can eventually attain tall stature. In fact, even children with "physiologic" delayed puberty can end up tall for age, as illustrated by the growth data on the eighteenth-century German poet Schiller.[42]

ADRENAL HORMONE–RELATED TALL STATURE

Adrenal causes of tall stature in childhood are also common. Children with precocious adrenarche, in which increased secretion of adrenal androgens early in childhood is associated with the other events of puberty, can grow fast and develop clinically significant tall stature. Children with adrenogenital syndrome can also present with tall stature plus signs of adrenal stimulation and early development of secondary sex characteristics.[43] Of course, this syndrome of early development and relatively tall stature for age can also be seen with functioning adrenal tumors leading to androgen secretion. Patients with tall stature secondary to hypersecretion of androgens exhibit early epiphyseal fusion and have short or low-normal adult height.

TALL STATURE OF GENETIC CAUSES

The genetic influence on tall stature of benign causes, including familial and the racial group–related causes, have already been discussed. In addition, Klinefelter syndrome (XXY karyotype) patients and genetic males with extra Y chromosomes (e.g., XYY, XYYY) can attain tall stature.[44] Marfan syndrome, homocystinuria, and cerebral gigantism (Sotos syndrome) are also relatively common genetic syndromes that are associated with tall stature.

SUMMARY AND CONCLUSIONS

Physicians who treat children and adolescents should always be alert for abnormalities in growth as an important clue to the patient's underlying health. Advances in understanding the control of growth have led to better diagnosis and therapy of growth disorders. Many growth disorders are associated with disorders of pubertal development and therefore may present to clinicians who deal with pediatric and adolescent gynecologic problems.

REFERENCES

1. Lechan RM: Neuroendocrinology of pituitary hormone regulation. Endocrinol Metab Clin North Am 1987; 16:475–501.
2. Van Assche FA, Holemans K, Aerts L: Fetal growth and consequences for later life. J Perinat Med 1998; 26:337–346.
3. Hintz RL: Growth factors. Curr Opin Pediatrics 1990; 2:786–793.
4. Reichlin S: Neuroendocrinology. In Wilson JD, Foster DW (eds): Williams Textbook of Endocrinology, 9th ed. Philadelphia: WB Saunders, 1998, pp 165–248.
5. Baumann G: Growth hormone heterogeneity: Genes, isohormones, variants, and binding proteins. Endocrine Rev 1991; 12:424–449.
6. Muller EE, Locatelli V, Cocchi D: Neuroendocrine control of growth hormone secretion. Physiol Rev 1999; 79:511–607.
7. Chapman IM, Hartman ML, Pezzoli SS, et al: Effect of aging on the sensitivity of growth hormone secretion to insulin-like growth factor-I negative feedback. J Clin Endocrinol Metab 1997; 82:2996–3004.
8. Spencer SA, Leung DW, Godowski PJ, et al: Growth hormone receptor and binding protein. Recent Prog Horm Res 1990; 46:165–181.
9. Hintz RL: The somatomedin hypothesis of growth hormone action. In Kostyo J, Goodman HM (eds): Handbook of Physiology. Section 7: The Endocrine System. Volume V: Hormonal Control of Growth. New York: Oxford University Press, 1999, pp 481–500.
10. Powell DR, Lee PDK, Chang D, et al: Antiserum developed for the E peptide region of human IGF-IA prohormone recognizes a 13–19 kilodalton serum protein. J Clin Endocrinol 1987; 65:868–875.
11. Hintz RL: The role of growth hormone and insulin-like growth factor–binding proteins. Hormone Res 1990; 33:105–110.
12. Rechler MM, Nissley SP: Insulin-like growth factor (IGF)/somatomedin receptor subtypes: structure, function, and relationships to insulin receptors and IGF carrier proteins. Horm Res 1986; 24:152–159.
13. Morley JE: Neuroendocrine control of thyrotropin secretion. Endocr Rev 1981; 2:396–436.
14. Giustina A, Wehrenberg WB: Influence of thyroid hormones on the regulation of growth hormone secretion. Eur J Endocrinol 1995; 133:646–653.
15. August GP, Grumbach MM, Kaplan SL: Hormonal changes in puberty III. Correlation of plasma testosterone, LH, FSH, testicular size and bone age with male pubertal development. J Clin Endocrinol Metab 1972; 34:319–326.
16. Rose SB, Municchi G, Barnes KM, et al: Spontaneous growth hormone secretion increases during puberty in normal girls and boys. J Clin Endocrinol Metab 1991; 73:428–435.
17. Greulich WW, Pyle SI: Radiographic Atlas of Skeletal Development of the Hand and Wrist, 2nd ed. Stanford: Stanford University Press, 1959.
18. O'Malley BW, Tsai SY, Bagchi M, et al: Molecular mechanisms of action of a steroid hormone receptor. Rec Prog Hormone Res 1991; 47:1–24.
19. Tanner JM: Growth and endocrinology of the adolescent. In Gardner L (ed): Endocrine and Genetic Disease of Childhood, 2nd ed. Philadelphia: WB Saunders, 1975, pp 14–64.
20. Robyn JA, Koch CA, Montalto J, et al: Cushing's syndrome in childhood and adolescence. J Paediatr Child Health 1997; 33:522–527.
21. Hintz RL, Suskind R, Amatayakul K, et al: Somatomedin and growth hormone in children with protein-calorie malnutrition. J Pediatr 1978; 92:153–156.
22. Tanner JM, Goldstein H, Whitehouse RH: Standards for children's height at ages 2–9 years allowing for height of parents. Arch Dis Child 1970; 45:755–762.
23. Savage MO, Beattie RM, Camacho-Hubner C, et al: Growth in Crohn's disease. Acta Paediatr Suppl 1999; 88:89–92.
24. Hintz RL, Attie KM, Baptista J, Roche A: Effect of growth hormone treatment on adult height of children with idiopathic short stature. Genentech Collaborative Group. N Engl J Med 1999; 340:502–507.
25. Hintz RL: Growth hormone deficiency. In Kelnar CJH, Savage MO, Stirling HF, Saenger P (eds): Growth Disorders: Pathophysiology and Treatment. London: Chapman & Hall Medical, 1998.
26. Kaplan SL, Underwood LE, August GP, et al: Clinical studies with recombinant DNA–derived methionyl-hGH in GH deficient children. Lancet 1986; 1:697–700.
27. Fielder PJ, Guevara-Aguirre J, Rosenbloom AL, et al: Expression of serum insulin-like growth factors, IGF binding proteins, and the growth hormone–binding protein in heterozygote relatives of Ecuadorian GH-receptor deficiency patients. J Clin Endocrinol Metab 1992; 74:743–750.
28. Backeljauw PF, Underwood LE: Prolonged treatment with recombinant insulin-like growth factor-I in children with growth hormone insensitivity syndrome—a clinical research center study. GHIS Collaborative Group. J Clin Endocrinol Metab 1996; 81:3312–3317.
29. Goddard AD, Dowd P, Chernausek S, et al: Partial growth-hormone insensitivity: The role of growth-hor-

mone receptor mutations in idiopathic short stature. J Pediatrics 1997; 131:S51–S55.

30. Rivkees SA, Bode HH, Crawford JD: Long-term growth in juvenile acquired hypothyroidism: The failure to achieve normal stature. N Engl J Med 1988; 318:599–602.

31. Anasti JN, Flack MR, Froehlich J, et al: A potential novel mechanism for precocious puberty in juvenile hypothyroidism. J Clin Endocrinol Metab 1995; 80:276.

32. Wilson DM, Kei J, Hintz RL, Rosenfeld RG: Effects of testosterone enanthate treatment for pubertal delay. Am J Dis Child 1988; 142:96–99.

33. Seminara SB, Hayes FJ, Crowley WF Jr: Gonadotropin-releasing hormone deficiency in the human (idiopathic hypogonadotropic hypogonadism and Kallmann's syndrome): pathophysiological and genetic considerations. Endocrinol Rev 1998; 19:521–539.

34. McArthur RG, Cloutier MD, Hayles AB, Sprague RE: Cushing's disease in children. Findings in 13 cases. Mayo Clin Proc 1972; 47:318–326.

35. Ranke MB, Pfluger H, Rosendahl W, et al: Turner syndrome: Spontaneous growth in 150 cases and review of the literature. Eur J Paediatr 1983; 141:81–88.

36. Hintz RL, Attie KM, Compton PG, Rosenfeld RG: Multifactorial studies of GH treatment of Turner syndrome: The Genentech National Cooperative Growth Study. In Albertsson-Wikland K, Lippe B (eds): Turner Syndrome

in a Life-Span Perspective. Amsterdam: Elsevier, 1995, pp 167–173.

37. Albertsson-Wikland K, Rosberg S: Analysis of 24-hour growth hormone profiles in childhood: Relation to growth. J Clin Endocrinol Metab 1988; 67:493–500.

38. Veldhuis JD, Iranmanexh A, Ho KK, et al: Dual defects in pulsatile growth hormone secretion and clearance subserve the hyposomatotropism of obesity in man. J Clin Endocrinol Metab 1991; 72:51–59.

39. Behrens LH, Barr DP: Hyperpituitarism beginning in infancy. The Alton giant. Endocrinology 1932; 16:120–128.

40. Sotos JF, Romsche CM: Gigantism and acromegaly. In Gardner L (ed): Endocrine and Genetic Disease of Childhood, 2nd ed. Philadelphia: WB Saunders, 1975, p 158.

41. Neely EK, Hintz RL, Parker B, et al: Two year results of treatment with depot leuprolide acetate therapy for central precocious puberty. J Pediatr 1992; 121:634–640.

42. Tanner JM: A History of the Study of Human Growth. Cambridge: Cambridge University Press, 1981, pp 106–112.

43. New MI, Newfield RS: Congenital adrenal hyperplasia. Curr Ther Endocrinol Metab 1997; 6:179–187.

44. Robinson A, Lubs HA, Bergsma D: Summary of clinical findings: Profiles of children with 47,XXY, 47,XYY, and 47,XXX karyotypes. Birth Defects 1982; 18:1–5.

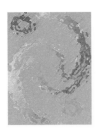

Chapter 4

Neuroendocrinology of Puberty

PAOLA A. PALMA SISTO, EDWARD O. REITER,
AND PETER A. LEE

Puberty is the transitional stage of development during which an individual matures from childhood to sexual and reproductive maturity. This period is characterized by the maturation of the hypothalamus, pituitary gland, and gonads (primary sexual characteristics) and by the development and maturation of sexual hair, breasts, and genitalia (secondary sexual characteristics), accompanied by a dramatic growth spurt. Profound psychological changes take place that lead to mental and emotional maturity.

These changes result from the direct and indirect effects of the sex steroids, principally estradiol in females and testosterone in males. These steroids, secreted mostly by the gonads, are initially stimulated by the pituitary gonadotropins, luteinizing hormone (LH) and follicle-stimulating hormone (FSH). Both LH and FSH are necessary for the increased activity of the ovary, including steroidogenesis and follicular maturation leading to ovulation. Among males, LH is the gonadotropin primarily responsible for testicular steroidogenesis, whereas LH and FSH plus testosterone stimulate spermatogenesis. Inhibin B, produced by the seminiferous tubule unit, is indicative upon FSH release of sperm production and feedback. Pituitary gonadotropin secretion, in turn, is regulated by the hypothalamic neuropeptide, gonadotropin-releasing hormone (GnRH). Each member of this intricately organized hypothalamic-pituitary-gonadal system exerts effects on the other, culminating in fine tuning of the reproductive system.

NEUROENDOCRINE SYSTEM

The basic components of the neuroendocrine system involved in reproduction include these[1-3]:

1. Suprahypothalamic sites, higher cortical centers, and the limbic system, which influence production and release of GnRH by neurons within the hypothalamus.

2. The arcuate nucleus of the medial basal hypothalamus, which controls GnRH release, which occurs in intermittent bursts from the median eminence into the hypothalamic-hypophyseal portal circulation (considered one area of the GnRH "pulse generator").[4]

3. The LH- and FSH-secreting cells (gonadotropes) located in the pituitary, which respond to regular episodic GnRH stimulation in a similar pulsatile release of LH and FSH into the petrosal sinus.

The end result of the neuroendocrine component is upregulation and activation by gonadotropins of specific target receptors within the gonad, stimulating synthesis and secretion of gonadal steroids and peptides, and maturation of germinal tissue.

REGULATION OF GnRH

The GnRH neuronal system is a unique member of the neuroendocrine system. Neurons destined to secrete GnRH originate in the olfactory placode and, during early fetal development, migrate through the forebrain to occupy positions scattered throughout the hypothalamus.[5-9] Axons project from these neurons to the primary capillary plexus of the pituitary portal system in the median eminence (Table 4–1).[5]

Since the identification and cloning of the GnRH gene,[10] its role in reproduction and in the disease processes affecting reproduction has been studied extensively. The study of a naturally occurring murine model led researchers to find a deletion in the GnRH gene, which was identified as the cause of idiopathic hypogonadotropic hypogonadism (IHH) in hypogonadal mice.[11, 12]

51

Table 4–1. Genes Involved in Reproduction and Their Mutation

Gene	Chromosome Location	Mutations	Phenotype
GnRH	8p11	None	? IHH
KAL	Xp22.3	Inactivating	IHH and anosmia
DAX-1	Xp21	Inactivating	AHC and IHH
GnRH receptor	4q21.2	Inactivating	IHH
α-Subunit	6q	None	? IHH and hypothyroidism
LH-β	19q13.3	Inactivating	Isolated LH deficiency
hCG-β	19q13.3	None	?
FSH-β	11p13	Inactivating	Isolated FSH deficiency
LH/hCG receptor	2p21	Activating	Familial precocious puberty; no effect on females
		Inactivating	Undermasculinization of genetic males; secondary amenorrhea in females
FSH receptor	2p21	Inactivating	Premature ovarian failure in females; oligospermia in males
		Activating	? Increased sperm

GnRH = gonadotropin-releasing hormone; KAL = Kallmann syndrome; DAX-1 = *Dosage-sensitive sex reversal, Adrenal hypoplasia congenita, critical region of X chromosome, gene 1*; LH = luteinizing hormone; FSH = follicle-stimulating hormone; hCG = human chorionic gonadotropin; AHC = adrenal hypoplasia congenita; IHH = idiopathic hypogonadotropic hypogonadism.

In contrast, no evidence for a GnRH gene mutation was found among patients with IHH.[13–16]

However, when the genotypes of patients who had an X-linked recessive disorder of hypogonadotropic hypogonadism with anosmia (*Kallmann syndrome*) were studied, a subset of them were found to have a defect in a gene, now called the KAL gene, located in the pseudoautosomal region of the short arm of the X chromosome.[17, 18] The protein derived from this gene is found to have neural cell adhesion molecule properties and is likely involved in directing the migration of the GnRH neurons from the olfactory placode to their normal position in the hypothalamus.[17, 18]

Regulators of GnRH production and secretion from transcription of the gene to release of the mature peptide are partially understood. Modulators have included catecholamines, norepinephrine, dopamine, opiates, and both stimulatory factors (such as glutamate) and inhibitory factors (such as gamma aminobutyric acid [GABA]).[19–22] The role of neuropeptide Y (NPY),[23–25] and its possible link to leptin,[26–28] a protein derived from adipocytes and involved in controlling food intake at a central level, has reactivated the issue of the role of body size and composition in relation to pubertal onset. NPY is synthesized in the arcuate nucleus of the hypothalamus and appears to be involved in the control of metabolic functions such as food intake and temperature regulation.[29] NPY gene expression has been shown to decrease with the pubertal increase in GnRH production and release. These phenomena may be involved in the timing of puberty, in terms of attainment of adequate fat mass.[26] Leptin and NPY are also being evaluated to help to explain the delays in sexual development secondary to underweight such as that associated with intensive athletic training or eating disorders (such as anorexia nervosa[26]) and in the syndrome of constitutional delay of growth maturation.[30]

GONADOTROPINS

The gonadotropes are located in the anterior pituitary gland. Originating from the ectodermal evagination from the oropharynx, called *Rathke's pouch*, the anterior pituitary gland has its population of gonadotropes (which comprise approximately 10% to 15% of its cells) scattered throughout the anterior lobe.[19] A complex cascade of homeobox genes, phylogenetically related to *Drosophila* segmentation genes, encoding multiple nuclear transcription factors, direct its temporal and anatomic development.

The gonadotropins contain a common alpha subunit encoded by a single gene and a specific beta subunit.[31] FSH-β and LH-β are products of single genes located on chromosomes 11 and 19, respectively.[32–34] A gene knockout mouse containing a mutation in the alpha-subunit gene exhibits severe growth deficiency and infertility as a result of deficiencies of gonadotropin and TSH (which also shares the same alpha subunit).[35] No human alpha-subunit mutations have been described to date.

Only one true mutation of the LH-β gene has been described. The patient was a 17-year-old male with delayed puberty and small, bilateral, undescended testes.[36] A woman found to have an FSH-β gene mutation had delayed puberty and an undetectable level of FSH.[37] She ovulated and conceived after having received exogenous FSH. As predicted, follicle development, estradiol production, and oocyte maturation were impaired.

Disorders involving gonadotropin receptor defects have been well characterized, especially *familial male precocious puberty*, previously known as *testotoxicosis*.[38] Affected boys typically present in early childhood with signs of complete precocious puberty, adult levels of testosterone, and prepubertal levels of gonadotropins secondary to constitutive activation of the LH receptor.[38, 39] This mutation is silent in females, as both gonadotropins are needed for ovarian steroidogenesis.

To help shed light on the fundamental role FSH may play in ovarian development, investigators in Finland studied women with primary amenorrhea who were subsequently diagnosed with hypergonadotropic ovarian dysgenesis.[40] These patients frequently had hypoplastic or streak ovaries but normal karyotypes. In several of these patients, a mutation was found in the FSH-receptor gene in the extracellular ligand-binding domain. This evidence suggests that FSH may play a crucial role in the development of normal ovaries.

Studies aimed at understanding gonadotropin regulation have involved the GnRH receptor and its expression on the gonadotropes,[40, 41] in addition to more recent discoveries of other regulators, such as *DAX-1*.[42] DAX-1 is a transcription factor associated with X-linked congenital adrenal hypoplasia and is important in maintaining appropriate synthesis and secretion of both GnRH at the hypothalamic level and of the gonadotropins at the pituitary level.[42–45]

THE OVARY AS A NEUROENDOCRINE ORGAN

Many ovarian factors are involved in the control of follicular development, acting as hormones involved in modulating gonadotropin release or as paracrine or autocrine factors that affect the ovarian response to gonadotropins.[46, 47] Inhibins provide a model for this. The inhibins are glycoproteins composed of alpha and beta subunits joined by disulfide bonds and are present in two forms, inhibin A and inhibin B. Ovarian inhibin (also found in many other organs) is produced primarily by the granulosa and luteal cells. Its target organ is the pituitary gland. It inhibits the synthesis and release of FSH by gonadotropes in vitro.[46, 47] Inhibin also decreases gonadotropic sensitivity to GnRH activity (likely at the GnRH receptor level), thus modulating GnRH's effect on gonadotropin secretion.[48] LH, FSH, and other paracrine factors modulate inhibin in the ovary. Ovarian secretion of inhibin, and its effect on FSH release, seems to be an important mechanism by which the follicle may control its own development.

THE NEUROPHYSIOLOGY OF PUBERTY

What basic mechanism (gonadostat) "turns on" the process of puberty is largely unknown. It is known that the GnRH pulse generator, the complex interplay of synchronously secreting GnRH neurons, is actively driving the fetal pituitary by mid-gestation.[19] GnRH pulse generator activity is robustly expressed during the initial months after birth, as evidenced by the elevated and equally pulsatile LH and FSH values. By the end of the first year of life, the GnRH pulse generator is turned down, as the child enters a period of physiologic hypogonadotropism, until puberty begins with the resurgence of the pulse generator (Fig. 4–1).[49, 50]

It is well-known that the gonadal steroids exert negative feedback on GnRH and gonadotropin secretion. While this system appears to be extra sensitive in prepubertal children, the main level of constraint is central in origin.[19] Suppression of gonadotropins during mid-childhood, in the face of the absence of gonadal steroids among functionally agonadal girls (such as those with Turner syndrome),[51] provide strong evidence for this concept. The central control of gonadotropin suppression is further supported by studies of the effects of GnRH on the pituitary axis in the prepubertal stage. GnRH stimulation testing with a single bolus of GnRH results in a characteristic prepubertal, pubertal (including central precocious puberty), or hypogonadotropic response (Fig. 4–2). Administration of exogenous pulses of GnRH, however, results in pubertal LH and FSH responses in prepubertal subjects.[52, 53] Studies demonstrating release of GnRH and gonadotropins in response to excitatory amino acids, namely *N*-methyl-D-aspartate (a known stimulator of GnRH, LH, and FSH secretion) in prepubertal subjects confirm the capability of prepubertal subjects to secrete adult levels of those hormones when so stimulated.[54]

Patterns of gonadotropin secretion in children during mid-childhood are characterized by nocturnal low-amplitude, low-frequency, pulsatile

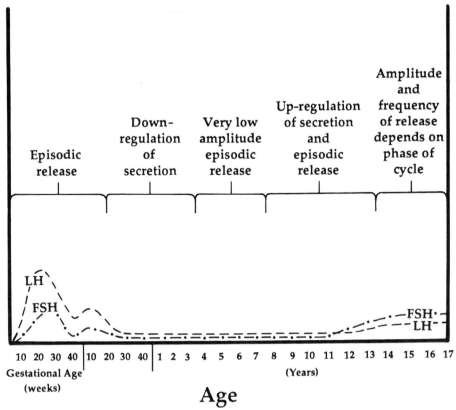

Figure 4–1. Profile of relative mean levels of circulating luteinizing hormone (LH) and follicle-stimulating hormone (FSH) during fetal life, infancy, childhood, and puberty. Episodic release, first apparent before birth, persists into early infancy, becomes less frequent during childhood, and then resurges to stimulate puberty.

gonadotropin secretion, girls having much higher FSH concentrations than boys.[55] These gonadotropin pulses have been demonstrated to be GnRH dependent.[55]

An increase in gonadotropin concentration anticipates the onset of puberty. Prepubertal girls who develop thelarche (breast budding) within 6 months were found to have higher gonadotropin concentrations, during both sleep and waking periods, as compared with girls who took longer to exhibit the first physical signs of puberty.[55] The onset of puberty is marked by a dramatic increase in amplitude of gonadotropin pulses that is most prominent during sleep (Fig. 4–3). The accentuation of sleep-enhanced gonadotropin secretion, particularly increased amplitude of pulsatile LH release, is characteristic of puberty.[19, 55]

As puberty progresses, one sees the emergence of regular daytime LH pulses, as nocturnal accentuation of the pulses becomes less prominent. This finding is closely associated with increases in serum estradiol, androstenedione, and testosterone concentrations.[55] These increasing

steroid concentrations in turn induce the appearance of secondary sexual characteristics and synergize the GH/IGF system in producing the adolescent growth spurt. The regulation of the rate of pubertal progress, the so-called tempo, remains unknown.

There are distinct disparities between the patterns of LH and FSH secretion in different age groups. The most striking difference is in the prepubertal group, where the FSH level is 10- to 20-fold higher than that of LH.[55] This disparity diminishes by postmenarche. A possible explanation for this disparity between age groups may involve the gonadal feedback effect.[56] FSH secretion seems to be more GnRH dependent before ovarian activation than afterward, when estradiol and inhibin may exert their modulatory effects on FSH. Overall, there is an approximately 70-fold increase in gonadotropin production between prepuberty and full maturity.

There are important sex differences in pubertal gonadotropin secretion; ratios of LH and FSH responses to GnRH stimulation at the onset of

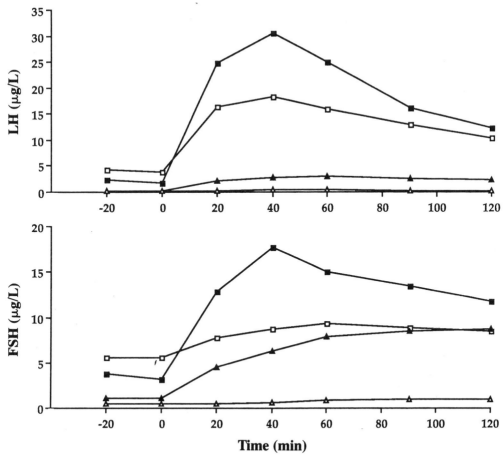

Figure 4–2. Gonadotropin-releasing hormone (GnRH) stimulation testing showing the release of luteinizing hormone (LH) and follicle-stimulating hormone (FSH) after 100 μg of GnRH at time 0. Responses are depicted for a 6-year-old girl with central sexual precocity (■), a 14-year-old girl with normal pubertal development (□), a 5-year-old prepubertal girl (△), and a 16-year-old girl (▲) with hypothalamic-pituitary destruction secondary to a craniopharyngioma, after treatment.

puberty are different in males and in females. Also, ratios of bioactive and immunoactive go-nadotropins change with puberty and may also differ by gender.[57] In females, LH pulses occur every 60 to 90 minutes in the follicular and early luteal phases of the menstrual cycle. During the late luteal phases, the frequency of LH pulses drops to every 3 to 4 hours.[57]

This adult pattern of gonadotropin secretion, as determined by GnRH secretion, is seen in children with true or central precocious puberty. If this intermittent pattern of GnRH secretion is replaced by a consistent high level of GnRH at the pituitary level, gonadotropin synthesis and secretion are downregulated and a hypogonado-tropic or prepubertal state is restored.[58–61]

The mature reproductive cycle in human fe-males is marked by a midcycle gonadotropin surge exerted by increasing levels of gonadal ste-roids, or *positive feedback*.[19] The midcycle LH and FSH surges are the result of positive feed-back induced by estradiol, in adequate concen-tration for a certain interval (usually more than 36 hours), at the end of the follicular phase of the menstrual cycle. This does not occur before midpuberty, because the negative feedback sys-tem is very sensitive. The hormonal milieu also requires FSH priming of the ovarian follicle to sustain adequate estradiol secretion, and GnRH priming of the pituitary sufficient to allow storage of pools of releasable gonadotropins adequate to produce a surge.[1, 19]

Although the cyclic nature of gonadotropins and estrogen-induced positive feedback has been demonstrated by midpuberty, the positive feed-back loop does not appear to be completely ma-ture at this stage.[62] The ovary is not responsive enough or is insufficiently primed to secrete

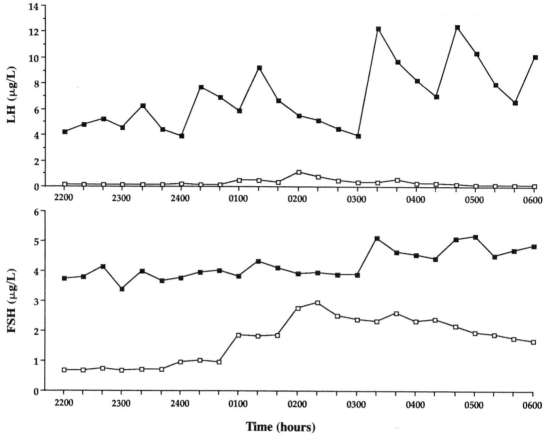

Figure 4–3. Serum luteinizing hormone (LH) and follicle-stimulating hormone (FSH) levels measured by fluoroimmunoassay of samples obtained at 20-minute intervals between 10:00 PM and 6:00 AM from a 7-year-old prepubertal female (□) and a 13-year-old pubertal, premenarcheal female (■). Note the episodic release, particularly of LH in the pubertal girl.

enough estradiol long enough to induce an LH surge, even though the pituitary contains sufficient stores of readily releasable gonadotropin. This likely explains why, during the first few years after menarche, the majority of cycles are anovulatory.[63, 64]

Many of the components of neuroendocrine regulation have been described, but most of the pieces of the puzzle are still missing. A greater understanding of the anatomic and molecular associations involved in this system will progress in the understanding of both the physiologic changes associated with puberty and the disorders surrounding the (early or late) attainment of pubertal changes.

REFERENCES

1. Reiter EO, Grumbach MM: Neuroendocrine control mechanisms and the onset of puberty. Annu Rev Physiol 1982; 44:595.

2. Lee PA: Pubertal neuroendocrine maturation. Early differentiation and stages of development. Adolesc Pediatr Gynecol 1988; 1:3.
3. Lee PA: Neuroendocrinology of puberty. Semin Reprod Endocrinol 1988; 1:3.
4. Knobil E: The GnRH pulse generator. Am J Obstet Gynecol 1990; 153:1721.
5. Silverman A-J, Jhamandas J, Renaud LP: Localization of luteinizing hormone–releasing hormone (LHRH) neurons that project to the median eminence. J Neurosci 1987; 7:2312.
6. Jennes L: Prenatal development of the gonadotropin-releasing hormone–containing systems in rat brain. Brain Res 1989; 482:97.
7. Schwanzel-Fukuda M, Pfaff DW: Origin of luteinizing hormone–releasing hormone neurons. Nature 1989; 338:161.
8. Wray S, Grant P, Garner H: Evidence that cells expressing luteinizing hormone–releasing hormone mRNA in the mouse are derived from progenitor cells in the olfactory placode. Proc Nat Acad Sci USA 1989; 86:8132.
9. Ronnekliev OK, Resko JA: Ontogeny of gonadotropin-releasing hormone–containing neurons in early fetal development of the rhesus macacques. Endocrinology 1990; 126:498.
10. Adelman JP, Mason AJ, Hatflick JS, et al: Isolation of the

gene and hypothalamic cDNA for the common precursor of gonadotropin-releasing hormone and prolactin release–inhibiting factor. Proc Natl Acad Sci USA 1986; 83:179.

11. Krieger DT, Perlow MJ, Gibson MJ, et al: Brain grafts reverse hypogonadism of gonadotropin-releasing hormone deficiency. Nature 1982; 298:468.

12. Mason AJ, Hayflick JS, Zoeller T, et al: A deletion truncating the gonadotropin-releasing hormone gene is responsible for hypogonadism in the hpg mouse. Science 1986; 234:1366.

13. Weiss J, Crowley WF Jr, Jameson JL: Normal structure of the gonadotropin-releasing hormone (GnRH) gene in patients with GnRH deficiency and idiopathic hypogonadotropic hypogonadism. J Clin Endocrinol Metab 1989; 69:299.

14. Layman LC, Wilson JT, Huey LO, et al: Gonadotropin-releasing hormone, follicle-stimulating hormone beta, and luteinizing hormone–beta gene structure in idiopathic hypogonadotropic hypogonadism. Fertil Steril 1992; 57:42.

15. Nakayama Y, Wondisford FE, Lash RW, et al: Analysis of gonadotropin-releasing hormone gene structure in families with familial central precocious puberty and idiopathic hypogonadotropic hypogonadism. J Clin Endocrinol Metab 1990; 70:1233.

16. Weiss J, Adams E, Whitcomb RW, et al: Normal sequence of the gonadotropin-releasing hormone gene in patients with idiopathic hypogonadotropic hypogonadism. Biol Reprod 1991; 45:74.

17. Franco B, Guioli S, Pragiola A, et al: A gene deleted in Kallmann's syndrome shares homology with neural cell adhesion and axonal path-finding molecules. Nature 1991; 353:529.

18. Legouis R, Hardelin J, Levilliers J, et al: The candidate gene for the X-linked Kallmann syndrome encodes a protein related to adhesion molecules. Cell 1991; 67:423.

19. Grumbach MM, Styne DM: Puberty. Ontogeny, neuroendocrinology, physiology and disorders. *In* Wilson JD, Foster DW (eds): William's Textbook of Endocrinology, 9th ed. Philadelphia: WB Saunders, 1997.

20. Plant TM: Puberty in primates. *In* Knobil E, Neill J (eds): The Physiology of Reproduction, vol. 2, 2nd ed. New York: Raven Press, 1994, p 443.

21. Ramirez VD, Feder HH, Sawyer CH: The role of brain catecholamines in the regulation of LH secretion: A critical inquiry. *In* Martini L, Ganaong WF (eds): Frontiers in Neuroendocrinology, vol. 8. New York: Raven Press, 1984, p 27.

22. Ojeda SR, Ma YJ: Epidermal growth factor tyrosine kinase receptors and the neuroendocrine control of puberty. Molec Cell Endocrinol 1998; 140(1–2):101.

23. Aubert ML, Pierroz DD, Gruaz NM, et al: Metabolic control of sexual function and growth: Role of neuropeptide Y and leptin. Molec Cell Endocrinol 1998; 140:107.

24. Gruaz NM, Pierroz DD, Rohner-Jeanrenaud F, et al: Evidence that neuropeptide Y could represent a neuroendocrine inhibitor of sexual maturation in unfavorable metabolic conditions in the rat. Endocrinology 1993; 133:1891.

25. Rohner-Jeanrenaud F, Cusin I, Sainsbury A, et al: The loop system between neuropeptide Y and leptin in normal and obese rodents. Horm Metab Res 1996; 28:642.

26. Ahima RS, Prabakaran D, Mantzoros C, et al: Role of leptin in the neuroendocrine response to fasting. Nature 1996; 382:250.

27. Chehab F, Lim M, Lu R: Correction of the sterility defect in homozygous obese female mice by treatment with the human recombinant leptin. Nat Genet 1996; 12:318.

28. Zhang Y, Proenca R, Maffei M, et al: Positional cloning of the mouse obese gene and its human homologue. Nature 1994; 372:425.

29. Pierroz DD, Catzeflis C, Aebi AC, et al: Chronic administration of neuropeptide Y into the lateral ventricle inhibits both the pituitary-testicular axis and growth hormone and insulin-like growth factor-I secretion in intact adult male rats. Endocrinology 1996; 137:3.

30. Cunningham MJ, Clifton DK, Steiner RA: Leptin's actions on the reproductive axis: Perspectives and mechanisms. Biol Reprod 1999; 60:216.

31. Layman LC: The genetics of gonadotropin genes and the GnRH/GAP gene. Semin Reprod Endocrinol 1991; 9:22.

32. Jameson JL, Lindell CM: Isolation and characterization of the human chorionic gonadotropin β-subunit (CGβ) gene cluster:regulation of a transcriptionally active CGβ gene by cyclic AMP. Molec Cell Biol 1988; 8:5100.

33. Talmadge K, Vamvakopoulos NC, Fiddes JC: Evolution of the genes for the β subunits of human chorionic gonadotropin and luteinizing hormone. Nature 1984; 307:37.

34. Policastro P, Ovitt CE, Hoshina M, et al: The β-subunit of human chorionic gonadotropin is encoded by multiple genes. J Biol Chem 1983; 258:11492.

35. Kendall SK, Samuelson LC, Saunders TL, et al: Targeted disruption of the pituitary glycoprotein hormone alpha-subunit produces hypogonadal and hypothyroid mice. Genes Dev 1995; 9:2007.

36. Weiss J, Axelrod L, Whitcomb RW, et al: Hypogonadism caused by a single amino acid substitution in the β subunit of luteinizing hormone. N Engl J Med 1992; 326:179.

37. Matthews CH, Borgato S, Beck-Peccoz P, et al: Primary amenorrhea and infertility due to a mutation in the β-subunit of follicle-stimulating hormone. Nat Genet 1993; 5:83.

38. Rosenthal SM, Grumbach MM, Kaplan SL: Gonadotropin independent familial sexual precocity with premature Leydig and germinal cell maturation (familial testotoxicosis): Effects of a potent luteinizing hormone releasing hormone agonist and medroxyprogesterone acetate therapy in four cases. J Clin Endocrinol Metab 1983; 57:571.

39. DiMeglio LA, Pescovitz OH: Disorders of puberty: Inactivating and activating molecular mutations. J Pediatr 1997; 131:S8.

40. Aittomaki K, Lucena JLD, Pakarinen P, et al: Mutation in the follicle-stimulating hormone receptor gene causes hereditary hypergonadotropic hypogonadism. Cell 1995; 82:959.

41. Layman LC, Cohen DP, Jin M, et al: Mutations in the gonadotropin-releasing hormone gene cause hypogonadotropic hypogonadism. Nat Genet 1998; 18:14.

42. Zanaria E, Muscatelli F, Bardoni B, et al: An unusual member of the nuclear hormone receptor superfamily responsible for X-linked adrenal hypoplasia congenita. Nature 1994; 372:635.

43. Muscatelli F, Strom TM, Walker AP, et al: Mutations in the DAX-1 gene give rise to both X-linked adrenal hypoplasia congenita and hypogonadotropic hypogonadism. Nature 1994; 372:672.

44. Habiby RL, Boepple P, Nachtigall L, et al: Adrenal hypoplasia congenita with hypogonadotropic hypogonadism: Evidence that DAX-1 mutations lead to combined hypothalamic and pituitary defects in gonadotropin production. J Clin Invest 1996; 98:1055.

45. Guo W, Mason JS, Stone CG, et al: Diagnosis of X-linked adrenal hypoplasia congenita by mutation analysis of the DAX1 gene. JAMA 1995; 274:324.

46. Genazzani AR, Petraglia F, Gamba O, et al: Neuroendo-

crinology of the menstrual cycle. Ann NY Acad Sci 1997; 816:143.

47. Ying HY: Inhibins, activins, and follistatins: Gonadal proteins modulating the secretion of follicle-stimulating hormone. Endocrinol Rev 1988; 9:267.

48. Culler MD, Negro-Vilar A: Endogenous inhibin suppresses only basal follicle-stimulating hormone secretion but suppresses all parameters of pulsatile luteinizing hormone secretion in diestrous female rat. Endocrinology 1989; 124:2944.

49. Wu FCW, Butler GE, Kelnar CJH, et al: Patterns of pulsatile luteinizing hormone secretion before and during the onset of puberty in boys: A study using an immunoradiometric assay. J Clin Endocrinol Metab 1990; 70:629.

50. Drop SLS, de Muinck Keizer-Scharama SMPF: Pubertal development and gonadal function. Curr Opinion Pediatr 1991; 3:701.

51. Winter JSD, Faiman C: Serum gonadotropin levels in agonadal children and adults. J Clin Endocrinol Metab 1972; 35:561.

52. Wildt L, Marshall GR, Knobil E: Experimental induction of puberty in the female rhesus monkey. Science 1980; 207:1373.

53. Stanhope R, Brook CGD, Adams PPJ, Jacobs HS: Induction of puberty by pulsatile gonadotropin releasing hormone. Lancet 1987; 2:552.

54. Medhamurthy R, Dichek HL, Plant TM, et al: Stimulation of gonadotropin secretion in prepubertal monkeys after hypothalamic excitation with aspartate and glutamate. J Clin Endocrinol Metab 1990; 71:1390.

55. Apter D, Butzow TL, Laughlin GA, et al: GnRH pulse generator activity during pubertal transition in girls: Pulsatile and diurnal patterns of circulating gonadotropins. J Clin Endocrinol Metab 1993; 76:940.

56. Yen SSC: The human menstrual cycle: Neuroendocrine regulation. *In* Yen SSC, Jaffe RB (eds): Reproductive Endocrinology, 3rd ed. Philadelphia: WB Saunders, 1991; p 273.

57. Filicori M, Butler JP, Crowley WF Jr: Neuroendocrine regulation of the corpus luteum in the human. J Clin Invest 1984; 74:1638.

58. Oerter KE, Uriarte MM, Rose SR, et al: Gonadotropin secretory dynamics during puberty in normal girls and boys. J Clin Endocrinol Metab 1990; 70:1082.

59. Kaplan SL, Grumbach MM: Pathophysiology and treatment of sexual precocity. J Clin Endocrinol Metab 1990; 71:785.

60. Rosenfield RL: Puberty and its disorders in girls. Endocrinol Metab Clin North Am 1991; 20:15.

61. Wheeler MD, Styne DM: The treatment of precocious puberty. Endocrinol Metab Clin North Am 1991; 20:183.

62. Reiter EO, Kulin HE, Hamwood SM: The absence of positive feedback between estrogen and luteinizing hormone in sexually immature girls. Pediatr Res 1974; 8:740.

63. Apter D, Vihko R: Serum pregnenolone, progesterone, 17-hydroxyprogesterone, testosterone and 5-dihydrotestosterone during female puberty. J Clin Endocrinol Metab 1977; 45:1039.

64. Winter JSD, Faiman C: Pituitary-gonadal relations in female children and adolescents. Pediatr Res 1973; 7:948.

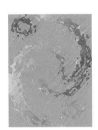

Chapter 5

Precocious Puberty

MARLAH TOMBOC, SELMA FELDMAN WITCHEL, AND PETER A. LEE

Normal puberty is initiated by the reemergence of the episodic gonadotropin-releasing hormone (GnRH) stimulation from the hypothalamus, resulting in an increase in the frequency and magnitude of the episodic release of pituitary gonadotropins, especially luteinizing hormone (LH). This leads to increased stimulation of the gonads, subsequently causing pubertal development and spermatogenesis or follicular maturation. Multiple other factors, which are not fully understood, are involved in pubertal maturation.

The statistical norms for the age of onset of puberty and for the rate of progression through its stages differ among countries and even among ethnic groups and social classes within a population. It is difficult to ascertain the early age limit for the onset of puberty among females and males because complete current data are lacking. Generally, puberty begins between the ages of 8 and 13 years in girls and 9 and 14 years in boys. However, it is apparent that some girls have early breast changes before the traditional early cut-off of 8 years.[1, 2] Fifteen percent of black girls and 5% of white girls were reported to have Tanner stage 2 or greater breast development at 7 years of age, without associated early menarche.[2] Abnormalities in the process of sexual maturation may be classified as (1) premature or precocious, (2) late or delayed, or (3) dyssynchronous (e.g., when physical changes are not followed by the onset of menses after an appropriate interval). In this chapter we focus on both boys and girls, to allow for appropriate comparisons.

Since precocious puberty, by definition, is based on early onset of puberty, the lack of complete data concerning the early age limit for the normal onset of puberty makes its diagnosis difficult. While the diagnosis of precocious puberty can be based on the traditional ages of 8 years for girls and 9 to 9.5 years for boys, the extent of diagnostic assessment and any consideration of therapy should be tempered by the results of screening tests and progression of pubertal changes. In girls, usually the first sign is breast development, followed by growth acceleration. Menarche before age 10 years is also considered precocious. In boys, testicular enlargement or pubic hair development before age 9 years is precocious. Precocious puberty can be classified as (1) central precocious puberty (CPP), also known as gonadotropin-dependent or true precocious puberty; (2) peripheral precocious puberty (PPP), also called gonadotropin-independent precocious puberty (GIP); or (3) incomplete precocious puberty (IPP) or isolated partial early development (e.g., premature thelarche and premature pubarche). Borderline early onset of puberty may fall into the category that has been referred to as *nonprogressive precocious puberty* or *slowly progressive precocious puberty*[3] and may simply be a normal variant. Isosexual development is appropriate, respectively, for girls or boys.

CENTRAL PRECOCIOUS PUBERTY

CPP is physiologically normal pubertal development that is chronologically early and results from hypothalamic GnRH-stimulated episodic gonadotropin secretion. There is often no demonstrable underlying pathology, particularly among females (thus, it is idiopathic). It may also be associated with a central nervous system (CNS) lesion such as congenital defect, tumor, trauma, or inflammation. The causes of CPP are listed in Table 5–1.

As in normal puberty, the first changes among girls are usually breast development and increased growth rate, followed by other pubertal events, including menarche. In boys, the first change is testicular enlargement, followed by penile growth and the appearance of pubic hair. Accelerated growth and advanced skeletal maturation are observed. A pubertal gonadotropin response (LH-predominant) to exogenous GnRH stimulation occurs inappropriately early.

Table 5–1. Causes of Precocious Puberty

I. Central GnRH-dependent precocious puberty
  A. Idiopathic
  B. Central nervous system dysfunction
    1. Congenital defects
      a. Septooptic dysplasia
    2. Destruction from tumors
      a. Craniopharyngiomas
      b. Dysgerminomas
      c. Ependymomas
      d. Ganglioneuromas
      e. Optic gliomas
    3. Destruction from other space-occupying lesions
      a. Arachnoid cysts
      b. Suprasellar cysts
    4. Excessive exposure to sex steroids
      a. Congenital adrenal hyperplasia
      b. McCune-Albright syndrome
    5. Excessive pressure
      a. Hydrocephalus
    6. Infection/inflammation
      a. Brain abscess
      b. Encephalitis
      c. Granulomas
      d. Meningitis
    7. Injury
      a. Head trauma
      b. Irradiation
    8. Redundant GnRH-secreting tissues
      a. Hypothalamic hamartomas
    9. Syndromes/phakomatoses
      a. Neurofibromatosis
      b. Prader-Willi syndrome
      c. Tuberous sclerosis
II. Peripheral (GnRH-independent) precocious puberty
  A. Exogenous sex steroids/gonadotropins
  B. Chronic primary hypothyroidism
  C. Ovarian tumors
    1. Granulosa cell
    2. Granulosa-theca cell
	3. Mixed germ cell
	    4. Cystadenoma
	    5. Gonadoblastoma
	    6. Lipoid
	  D. Ovarian cysts
	  E. McCune-Albright syndrome
	  F. Feminizing adrenal tumors
	  G. Familial male-limited gonadotropin-independent
	     precocious puberty
	III. Incomplete precocious puberty
	  A. Premature breast development
	    1. Premature thelarche
	    2. Initial presentation: precocious puberty
	    3. Nonprogressive precocious puberty
	    4. Exogenous sex steroids
	  B. Premature pubarche
	    1. Premature adrenarche
	    2. Congenital adrenal hyperplasia
	    3. Adrenal tumors
	    4. Ovarian tumors
	      a. Arrhenoblastoma
	      b. Lipoid tumors
	  C. Isolated vaginal bleeding
	    1. Exogenous sex steroids
	    2. Foreign body
	    3. Hemorrhagic cystitis
	    4. Hypothyroidism
	    5. McCune-Albright syndrome
	    6. Ovarian cyst
	    7. Sexual abuse/child abuse
	    8. Trauma
	    9. Tumor
	      a. Rhabdomyosarcoma
	      b. Clear cell
	      c. Endodermal carcinoma
	      d. Mesonephric carcinoma
	   10. Urethral prolapse
	   11. Vulvovaginitis

CAUSES OF CENTRAL PRECOCIOUS PUBERTY

CPP is more common in girls than in boys. Among females, most cases are idiopathic and attributed to premature enhancement of the hypothalamic GnRH pulsatile release. Males are more likely to have an underlying CNS abnormality. Hypothalamic hamartoma is a congenital malformation consisting of a heterotropic mass of nerve tissue that contains GnRH neurosecretory neurons attached to the tuber cinereum or the floor of the third ventricle. Neither the size nor the shape of such tumors changes significantly over time. It is the most common type of CNS tumor that causes precocious puberty.[4] With improved imaging techniques, more cases of precocious puberty are being attributed to hypothalamic hamartomas. Such tumors can be classified

as *parahypothalamic* (i.e., being attached only to the floor of the third ventricle or suspended from the floor by a peduncle) or "intrahypothalamic," (i.e., enveloped by the hypothalamus and distorting the third ventricle). The parahypothalamic type is generally associated with precocious puberty, but not with seizures or developmental delay, whereas the intrahypothalamic type is generally associated with seizures.[5] Rapidly progressive CPP in a child younger than 2 years suggests this cause. Removal of pedunculated hamartomas that secrete GnRH can be expected to result in regression of the precocious pubertal development[6, 7]; however, the majority of hamartomas are not pedunculated and pose a much greater surgical risk without the prospect of complete cure and regression. Recent data showed that GnRH therapy provides satisfactory and safe treatment for most children with CPP due to hypothalamic hamartomas.[8, 9] Thus, medical treatment may be appropriate management even for pedunculated forms.

Other tumors associated with precocious puberty include optic gliomas, which may occur in association with neurofibromatosis.[10] CNS radiation therapy for treatment of intracranial tumors or prophylaxis against malignancies is associated with CPP. Affected children may have concomitant growth hormone deficiency, which can be masked by the accelerated growth characteristic of CPP.[11] Previous head trauma, CNS infections, and arachnoid cysts have also been identified with CPP. Although septo-optic dysplasia is more often associated with hypopituitarism, it can also occur with sexual precocity.[12] Children with neurodevelopmental disabilities are also at increased risk for central precocious puberty.[13] Finally, CPP secondary to prolonged excessive sex steroid exposure (indicated by extremely advanced bone age) may be a consequence of congenital adrenal hyperplasia (CAH) or adrenal or ovarian tumors.

PERIPHERAL PRECOCIOUS PUBERTY

GIP is pubertal development resulting from stimulation with a hormone other than hypothalamic GnRH. Causes include inappropriate sex steroid hormone secretion and exposure to exogenous steroids (see Table 5–1). Circulating LH and follicle-stimulating hormone (FSH) concentrations are low or at prepubertal levels owing to suppression of pituitary gonadotropins by the autonomous or exogenous steroids. This form may present with some or all of the physical changes of CPP. Breast development or vaginal bleeding suggests increased estrogen stimulation, whereas pubic hair, acne, genital enlargement, and adult-type body odor suggest increased androgenic hormone effect.

CAUSES OF GnRH–INDEPENDENT PRECOCIOUS PUBERTY

Categories of GIP or PPP include pubertal development resulting from any abnormal secretion of gonadotropin (tumors in boys that secrete LH or human chorionic gonadotropin [hCG]) or sex steroid (congenital adrenal hyperplasia, adrenal or gonadal tumors). Mutations that affect gonadal hormone production (e.g., LH-activating receptor mutation in males, activating mutations of the alpha subunit of G protein in the McCune-Albright syndrome) can also cause GIP.

It has been thought that, in the absence of FSH, hCG does not produce precocious puberty in girls, and this has been cited as an explanation for the rarity of precocious puberty in girls with hCG-secreting brain tumors. (An hCG-secreting suprasellar immature teratoma has been described in a girl who presented with precocious puberty.[14]) Resolution of breast budding was observed with normalization of serum hCG after chemotherapy. It has also been reported that hCG has weak FSH-like activity. Thus, some speculate that a very high level of serum hCG can produce precocious puberty in girls.

Ovarian tumors are uncommon and rarely present with sexual precocity. Some 70% of children with granulosa cell and theca cell tumors present with precocious puberty.[15] Mixed germ cell–sex cord tumors may present with isosexual precocity and are usually benign, but malignant transformation has been described.[16] Presenting features may consist of rapid progression of breast development, vaginal bleeding, or abdominal pain. On physical examination, a palpable abdominal mass and dulling of the vaginal mucosa may be detected. Estradiol levels are often excessively elevated while gonadotropin levels are undetectable. Imaging studies such as ultrasonography, computed tomography (CT), and magnetic resonance imaging (MRI) are helpful in confirming the diagnosis of an ovarian lesion. The treatment of choice is surgical resection. Regression of secondary sexual characteristics often follows removal of the tumor.

Other rare ovarian tumors, such as cystadenomas, gonadoblastomas, and lipoid tumors of the ovary, may produce estrogen, androgen, or both. Children with Peutz-Jeghers syndrome (PJS) have a particular predisposition to ovarian lipid-rich Sertoli cell tumor, which has been associated with isosexual precocious puberty.[17] The PJS gene on chromosome 19p13.3, which encodes the serine/threonine kinase LKB1, was recently cloned. It has been proposed that the loss of the kinase activity of LKB1 is probably responsible for the development of PJS phenotypes.[18] Twelve novel LKB1/STK11 mutations were recently reported among PJS families.[19] Other functioning ovarian tumors include epitheliomas and dysgerminomas. Functional ovarian cysts may occur in prepubertal girls.[20] Such cysts can secrete estrogen and may cause premature breast development. When the cysts rupture or resolve, the estrogen withdrawal may produce vaginal bleeding. Sexual maturation is not progressive and can be expected to wane. Small cysts are not uncommon in prepubertal ovaries; usually one or two are present in each ovary, ranging in size from 5 to 7 mm.[21] When an isolated functioning ovarian cyst is identified by ultrasonography, no therapy is indicated unless rupture is considered likely. Surgical intervention should be avoided if at all possible. Clinical observation and repeat sonography in 2 to 3 months will likely verify regression.

The McCune-Albright syndrome is characterized by patchy cutaneous hyperpigmentation (*café au lait* spots), polyostotic fibrous dysplasia, and several endocrine disorders (including toxic multinodular goiter, pituitary gigantism, amenorrhea-galactorrhea, Cushing syndrome, and precocious puberty). Premature sexual development can occur at any time from a few months after birth to late childhood. It is gonadotropin independent and cannot be arrested by treatment with GnRH analogue. The defect underlying this syndrome was identified to be mutations (Arg201His or Arg201Cys) within exon 8 of the Gs-alpha gene. These mutations result in constitutive activation of the encoded Gs-alpha protein. Given that the action of gonadotropins is mediated by Gs alpha, the precocious puberty of McCune-Albright syndrome is due to constitutive activation of gonadotropin signaling.[22–25] Menses, fertility, and adult stature may be normal.

Male-limited, gonadotropin-limited precocious puberty (MGIP), also called *familial male precocious puberty* or *testotoxicosis*, is an autosomal-dominant disorder that is due to autonomous testicular testosterone secretion sustained by constitutive activation of the LH receptor. Patients are heterozygous for an activating missense mutation of the LH receptor gene. Seven different mutations of the LH receptor gene were recently detected.[26] Boys with MGIP present with enlarged penis and testes, pubic hair, rapid growth, advanced bone age, acne, increased muscle mass, voice deepening, and spontaneous erections. Testicular volume is increased to a size that is less than expected for the degree of sexual development. Current therapies are based on diminishing androgen production or inhibiting its peripheral effects. It was shown that cyproterone acetate, which inhibits androgens at the receptor level, does not enhance final height. Ketoconazole seems to reduce testosterone secretion, but its effect on final height cannot yet be determined.[27] Other treatment options include medroxyprogesterone acetate, spironolactone, and the aromatase inhibitor testolactone. Addition of testolactone to spironolactone has been noted to control precocity, but not to improve predicted adult height.

Exogenous medications such as oral contraceptives, topical estrogens, or postmenopausal estrogen agents or the overuse of vaginal estrogen creams in prepubertal girls induce early pubertal development.

PPP associated with hypothyroidism may manifest itself as breast development (with or without galactorrhea) and vaginal bleeding. It has been proposed that the high levels of thyrotropin (TSH) in patients with juvenile hypothyroidism can act through the FSH receptor (FSH-R) to cause the associated gonadal stimulation.[28] Unlike some forms of precocious puberty, findings are reversible by treatment with thyroid hormone.

INCOMPLETE PRECOCITY

Incomplete early puberty consists of partial sexual development, including isolated development of the breasts (premature thelarche) and pubic hair (premature pubarche), and isolated vaginal bleeding (premature menarche). It is characterized by partial—often transient and minimal—pubertal development in the absence of other stigmata of puberty. Slow progression, no change, or waning (as in premature thelarche during infancy) of the physical findings may be observed.

PREMATURE THELARCHE

Premature thelarche refers to premature onset of breast enlargement in the absence of other signs of sexual maturation. The unilateral or bilateral breast development is nonprogressive and is not associated with areolar development. Most frequently, premature thelarche occurs before age 2 years, a period of relative but decreasing activity of the hypothalamic-pituitary-ovarian (HPO) axis. By history, breast tissue may be persistent from early infancy or even birth. Other constitutional changes of puberty, such as sexual hair, acne, and accelerated growth are absent. Skeletal maturation is not advanced for the girl's chronologic age.

Estradiol levels can be significantly higher than those of normal prepubertal girls.[29] Although the vaginal mucosa is usually pink and shiny, showing little estrogen effect, some evidence of estrogen stimulation may be found on vaginal smear. LH levels are prepubertal, whereas immunoactive and bioactive FSH levels may be normal or elevated for age. The prepubertal response to GnRH testing should distinguish this entity from CPP. Ultrasonography shows a prepubertal uterus and ovaries. However, differentiation may sometimes be difficult, and some girls appear to have a slowly progressive or attenuated form of CPP, which suggests partial activation or incomplete suppression of the HPO axis. Typically, such patients are referred between 12 and 24 months of age.

Longitudinal follow-up should distinguish premature thelarche from CPP and regression of the breast tissue is usually observed over 2 to 4 years.[30] Consequently, no therapy is indicated. Subsequently, normal puberty occurs at an appropriate age, and adult height and development of reproductive capacity are normal.[31] A rare patient slowly progresses toward precocious puberty, but final adult stature is not compromised.[32]

PREMATURE PUBARCHE

Commonly, *premature pubarche* is defined as the appearance of pubic hair before age 8 years in girls and 9 years in boys (although, in black girls, pubarche may occur several months earlier and, usually, just before or synchronous with thelarche). This phenomenon is attributed to early maturation of the normal pubertal adrenal androgen secretory mechanism (adrenarche). With adrenarche comes increased production and secretion of the adrenal androgens dehydroepiandrosterone (DHEA), dehydroepiandrosterone sulfate (DHEAS), and androstenedione (AND).[33] DHEA and AND are relatively weak androgens but can peripherally be converted to testosterone. Although pubarche may be the first manifestation of adrenarche to be noted, other signs (adult-type body odor, axillary hair, acne, oily hair and skin) sometimes antedate pubarche. Thus, premature pubarche is evidence of premature adrenarche in the absence of activation of the HPO axis. Breast development is absent, although slightly accelerated growth velocity, tall stature, and advanced skeletal maturation may be present. Gonadotropin responses to GnRH are prepubertal. Whereas some individuals show elevated basal adrenal hormone levels, responses to adrenocorticotropin (ACTH)-stimulation tests rule out inherited defects of steroidogenesis (i.e., virilizing CAH). Over time, growth of pubic hair can be minimal to moderate. Subsequently, puberty occurs normally and at an appropriate age, and adult height is not compromised. Premature adrenarche is a diagnosis of exclusion, and disorders that induce sexual precocity and excessive androgen production (e.g., the virilizing CAH and androgen-secreting tumors) should be eliminated from the differential diagnosis. An ACTH-stimulation test may be necessary to rule out CAH.

Some girls who present with typical premature pubarche secondary to premature adrenarche develop clinical features and hormonal evidence of excessive ovarian androgen synthesis in adolescence.[14] One retrospective study showed progression from premature pubarche to polycystic ovary syndrome (PCOS) in approximately half of the subjects.[34] Premature pubarche is associated with hyperinsulinemia and increased serum triglycerides, very low-density lipoprotein cholesterol, and low-density–high-density lipoprotein ratios, as compared with pubertal control subjects. Such findings demonstrate that the cluster of highly metabolic abnormalities typical of syndrome X are present in childhood.[35–38] It has also been suggested that girls with premature pubarche are at increased risk for anovulation from late adolescence onward.[39]

Hyperandrogenism and insulin resistance are characteristic features of PCOS (also known as *functional ovarian hyperandrogenism* and *chronic anovulatory hyperandrogenism*).[40] Familial clustering of PCOS supports a role for genetic factors in the pathogenesis of this common disorder.[41, 42] Evidence to date suggests that heterozygosity for 21-hydroxylase may be one genetic factor associated with premature adrenarche and functional adolescent hyperandrogenism[43–46]; but it cannot be the sole genetic factor that favors the development of PCOS, because the majority of obligate heterozygotic carriers of 21-hydroxylase mutations show minimal signs of hyperandrogenism, if any.[47] Presumably, an admixture of genetic and environmental factors influences outcome and risk for progression from premature pubarche to persistent hyperandrogenism. Some girls who initially present with CPP show an exaggerated adrenal response to ACTH stimulation and, in late adolescence, develop persistent hyperandrogenism.[48]

The virilizing forms of CAH include decreased activity of the enzymes 21-hydroxylase, 11 beta-hydroxylase, and 3 beta-hydroxysteroid dehydrogenase. In these autosomal-recessive disorders, increased ACTH secretion to maintain adequate cortisol production results in overproduction of adrenal androgens. These disorders range in severity from the classical forms that present in the first few years of life to late-onset or nonclassical forms, which become evident during adolescence or young adulthood. At the molecular level, the causes of these disorders have been well-characterized.[49–53] Because random steroid hormone concentrations may be normal,

ACTH-stimulation tests may be necessary to detect mild forms of CAH.

To perform an ACTH-stimulation test, a pharmacologic dose (0.25 mg) of synthetic ACTH (cosyntropin) is administered after a basal blood sample has been obtained. Another sample is collected some 30 to 60 minutes after cosyntropin is administered. Basal levels, incremental elevations (the difference between the stimulated and basal levels), and hormone ratios provide important information. Levels or responses slightly above the normal range do not, in themselves, constitute evidence of mild virilizing adrenal hyperplasia. This diagnosis should be reserved for patients who exhibit clear evidence of hyperandrogenism. In addition, therapy for these disorders should generally be restricted to patients with excessive androgenization or frank virilization, with significantly advanced skeletal maturation, or with androgen levels greater than the upper limit for normal adult females. Elevated plasma levels of 17-hydroxyprogesterone, AND, and DHEA are characteristic of 21-hydroxylase deficiency. Approximately 50% of obligate heterozygotes demonstrate increased incremental 17-hydroxyprogesterone elevations after ACTH stimulation. For most 17-hydroxyprogesterone assays, stimulated values less than 500 ng/dl are normal; 500 to 1200 ng/dl may indicate heterozygosity for CYP21 mutation; and values greater than 1200 ng/dl are diagnostic for late-onset CAH.[54]

Glucocorticoid therapy should not be initiated unless the manifestations are severe enough to justify its possible consequences (i.e., adrenal suppression, the need for supplemental therapy during times of stress, required monitoring of adequacy of therapy, and the risk of excessive glucocorticoid effects). It is important to note that CPP can occur secondary to late diagnosis or inadequate treatment of CAH and that some patients with true precocious puberty may be heterozygous for CYP21 mutation.[55] Whether heterozygosity of CYP21 is related to the premature activation of the hypothalamic-pituitary-gonadal axis remains to be determined.

STEROID-PRODUCING TUMORS

In contrast to the mild adrenal hyperplasias, adrenocortical and androgen-secreting ovarian tumors produce noticeable and progressive evidence of androgen excess (virilization in girls and pseudoprecocious puberty in boys). Such androgenic tumors are rare, but they tend to occur more often in girls than in boys. DHEAS, DHEA, and testosterone levels are usually elevated. Although serum cortisol levels and urinary cortisol excretion may be elevated, the typical features—glucocorticoid excess, short stature, growth deceleration, and delayed skeletal maturation—are sometimes masked by hyperandrogenism.[56]

Adrenal tumors generally function autonomously and usually are not suppressed after dexamethasone administration. Useful imaging techniques are sonography, CT, and MRI.[57] Clinical features, imaging studies, and even histologic findings may not distinguish adenoma from carcinoma, because pleomorphism and capsular invasion have been noted in tumors whose clinical behavior was benign.[58] It was recently proposed that tumor size is important in assessing malignant potential. Tumors measuring 5 cm in diameter are usually benign, whereas those larger than 10 cm are very often associated with malignancy.[59] Pulmonary metastases may already exist at the time of presentation and should be sought in malignant tumors. Surgical resection of the adrenal tumor is the treatment of choice for both benign and malignant disease and requires perioperative and postoperative glucocorticoid replacement. In patients with multiple metastases, treatment with adrenolytic agents o,p'-dihydroxynaphthyl disulfide (o,p'-DDD) or mitotane may be beneficial in suppressing hormone secretion and ameliorating symptoms of the tumor.[57] Survival may be prolonged by therapy, and initiation of therapy in the immediate postoperative period is suggested. Nonetheless, the prognosis remains poor. Other agents reported variably to be helpful in the management of this disease are spironolactone, ketoconazole, and RU-486. Feminizing adrenal tumors are rare causes of GIP.[60] Adrenal sex steroid–secreting tumors can also secrete glucocorticoids and androgens, so such patients often present with virilization or evidence of Cushing syndrome. The development of breasts can be explained by the elevated level of estradiol. LH-secreting adrenal tumor has also been reported as a cause of precocious puberty.[61]

Virilizing ovarian tumors, arrhenoblastomas, and lipoid cell tumors may present in preadolescence. A palpable mass may or may not be present. Both testosterone and AND levels may be elevated, but DHEA and DHEAS are not. Serum gonadotropin concentrations are at prepubertal levels. Increased urinary 17-ketosteroid values do not eliminate an ovarian source. Frequently, androgen-secreting tumors of the ovary are small and difficult to visualize by ultrasound, CT, or MRI.

Testosterone concentrations greater than 200 ng/dl suggest that the patient should be carefully examined for an ovarian tumor.

PREMATURE MENARCHE

Premature menarche (vaginal bleeding) may occur normally in the immediate postnatal period, as a result of estrogen withdrawal. In the absence of other signs of puberty in prepubertal girls, vaginal bleeding is otherwise uncommon. Nonendocrine causes, such as vulvovaginitis, trauma, a foreign body, or child abuse, may be associated with a bloody, foul vaginal discharge and must be excluded from the differential diagnosis, as must bleeding from the urinary tract. Genital tumors such as rhabdomyosarcoma, endodermal carcinoma, and clear cell adenocarcinoma are sometimes manifested as isolated vaginal bleeding.[62]

Spontaneous regression of an ovarian cyst may induce isolated vaginal bleeding. Hypothyroidism can also cause vaginal bleeding without other evidence of pubertal development. In hypothyroid patients, skeletal maturation is generally delayed. The McCune-Albright syndrome, a condition characterized by the development and regression of estrogen-producing ovarian cysts, can be associated with isolated vaginal bleeding. Typically, although ovarian cysts may be visualized, uterine size is prepubertal. Gonadotropin levels are prepubertal, whereas estradiol levels vary. Generally, skeletal maturation is not advanced. Often, by the time ultrasonography is performed, the cyst can no longer be visualized.

The goal of evaluating patients with isolated vaginal bleeding is to rule out serious causes of bleeding. To do so requires a detailed physical examination, including (unless the cause is apparent) a pelvic examination, which may require anesthesia. Culture material should be obtained to seek sexually transmitted diseases. Pelvic ultrasonography, bone-age radiography, and determination of gonadotropin and estradiol levels may be indicated to differentiate CPP from PPP. There do not appear to be long-term consequences of premature menarche for subsequent puberty and fertility.[63]

EVALUATION OF THE PATIENT WITH SEXUAL PRECOCITY

For a girl who presents with signs of precocity, the age of onset and the duration and progression of signs and symptoms constitute valuable historical information. Breast development is at least Tanner stage 2, the areolae having a broadened, darkened, "stimulated" appearance. Genital changes may include fullness of the labia and pink dulling of the vaginal mucosa, reflections of estrogen-induced thickening of the vaginal mucosa. Increased vaginal leukorrhea may be found. Dark, coarse pubic hair—true sexual hair as opposed to the fine hair of childhood—may be present. Additional androgen-dependent findings include acne and adult-type body odor. In girls, enhancement of general growth is coincident with onset of estrogen-stimulated changes, and accelerated growth velocity, tall stature for age, and advanced skeletal maturation may be found.

The differentiation of CPP from PPP necessitates demonstration of pubertal gonadotropin secretion. The diagnostic evaluation required to document early pubertal development and to differentiate central from peripheral causes is outlined in Table 5–2. Findings in the patient's history consistent with central cause include previous CNS trauma or infection, symptoms of associated neurologic or neuroendocrine dysfunction, or a family history of early puberty. It should also be determined whether exposure to exogenous sex steroids in cosmetics, food, or medications may have occurred.

Physical findings suggestive of synchronous normal puberty are consistent with central precocity but do not rule out a peripheral cause. Particular attention should be paid to the neurologic examination and to any signs of neuroendocrine or endocrine dysfunction. Evidence of hypothyroidism, hyperadrenalism, or significant virilization implies a peripheral cause. Useful laboratory studies include determinations of serum LH, FSH, estradiol, DHEA, or DHEAS, TSH, thyroxine (T_4), and hCG levels. Levels of LH and FSH may be measured by a variety of tests, including radioimmunoassay (RIA), newer, more sensitive immunoradiometric assay (IRMA), and immunochemiluminometric and immunofluorimetric (ICMA, IFMA) assays. Before values can be interpreted, it is necessary to know the levels and responses typical in prepubertal and pubertal subjects for any particular assay. DHEA or DHEAS levels may indicate adrenarche, and, when markedly elevated, suggest an adrenal origin of PPP. Abnormal results on thyroid function tests and elevated hCG levels suggest one of the rare forms of nonpituitary gonadotropin-stimulated early puberty associated with chronic primary hypothyroidism and gonadotropin-secreting tumors.

Basal levels of LH and FSH, GnRH-stimulated gonadotropin responses, or periodic sam-

Table 5–2. Physical Findings and Laboratory Results in Precocious Puberty

History and Physical Findings	Central Precocious Puberty	Peripheral Precocious Puberty	Premature Thelarche	Premature Adrenarche
Breast Tanner stage	≥ 2	≥ 2	≥ 2	1
Pubic hair stage	≥ 1	≥ 1	≥ 1	≥ 2
Stature for age	Tall	Tall	Normal or slightly elevated	Normal or slightly elevated
Growth rate	Accelerated	Accelerated	Normal or slightly elevated	Normal or slightly elevated
Adult-type body odor	Present	Generally absent	Absent	Sometimes present
Laboratory Studies				
LH and FSH	Pubertal >1	Prepubertal <1	Prepubertal <1	Prepubertal <1
LH-FSH ratio	Pubertal	Prepubertal	Prepubertal	Prepubertal
Estradiol	Prepubertal	Prepubertal	Prepubertal	Pubertal
DHEAS	Pubertal	Prepubertal or suppressed	Prepubertal	Prepubertal
GnRH stimulation	Advanced	Advanced	Normal or slightly elevated	Normal or slightly increased
Skeletal age	Pubertal ovaries	Prepubertal, adrenal tumor or ovarian tumor	May be used to assess for ovarian cysts	Not indicated
Pelvic ultrasound	Helpful			
MRI of CNS		Not indicated	Not indicated	Not indicated

LH, luteinizing hormone; FSH, follicle-stimulating hormone; DHEAS, dehydroepiandrosterone sulfate; GnRH, gonadotropin-releasing hormone; MRI, magnetic resonance imaging; CNS, central nervous system.

pling of LH and FSH can be used to assess for pubertal gonadotropin secretion. Random LH and FSH values may provide sufficient information about gonadotropin status to preclude GnRH-stimulation testing. Low LH level (an LH-FSH ratio of less than 1), is suggestive of prepubertal gonadotropin secretion. Conversely, an LH-FSH ratio greater than 1 is indicative of pubertal gonadotropin response. Therefore, if the patients have LH levels above the prepubertal range and the LH-FSH ratio suggest pubertal status, the diagnosis of CPP can be made without GnRH testing.

The definitive diagnostic test for CPP is GnRH stimulation of gonadotropin release. GnRH-stimulation testing may involve collecting only a single sample 20 to 40 minutes after giving 100 μg of GnRH intravenously. Prepubertal status is suggested when the FSH level is greater than the LH level and the LH rise is minimal (approximately less than 7 μ/l for third-generation assays and less than 10 IU/ml for traditional assays). Pubertal responses are characterized by an LH peak above the upper limit of the prepubertal range and an LH level greater than the FSH level. Periodic sampling is expensive and

generally is not necessary to determine pubertal gonadotropin secretion. Accurate interpretation of the GnRH-stimulation test results requires the establishment of the normal ranges for the populations being studied and for the particular assay method.

All patients should undergo a baseline skeletal-age radiograph, which reflects the degree of excessive hormone stimulation. Bone-age radiography helps to estimate additional growth potential and to gauge pubertal progression. The most common method of determining bone age is comparison with standards in the Greulich and Pyle's *Atlas of Skeletal Maturation*. CT or MRI of the hypothalamic-pituitary region should be considered in all cases of suspected central precocity, to exclude a structural abnormality, especially when neurologic symptoms antedate pubertal development, but also in suspected PPP of uncertain origin. Abdominopelvic ultrasonography may be performed to document ovarian, uterine, and adrenal size and symmetry. In CPP, the ovaries may be significantly enlarged.[64] Small ovarian cysts may be present, although this finding is not abnormal for prepubertal and premenarchal girls.[65] The uterus is enlarged for age but appropriate for pubertal stage. A vaginal smear is a quick and simple bioassay of the current level of estrogen stimulation, particularly when the estradiol level is prepubertal. Estrogen exposure of the prepubertal vaginal mucosa increases the number of cornified cells with small pyknotic nuclei. The results are expressed as a percentage of basal cells (deeply staining round or oval basal cells), intermediate cells (transitional cells), and superficial cells (flattened, poorly stained squamous cells). The greater the percentage of superficial cells, the greater is the estrogen effect.

TREATMENT OF CENTRAL PRECOCIOUS PUBERTY

Indications for treatment of CPP include extreme tall stature during childhood or projected severely foreshortened adult height. Avoidance or amelioration of the psychosocial consequences of increased size, advanced pubertal development, or unrealistic adult expectations are also important considerations. Each indication should be carefully considered. A child, who in comparison with age peers exhibits early puberty, accelerated growth, and advanced skeletal age is a candidate for therapy. Usually, a child with pubertal changes of early onset, but without indications that puberty is advancing in an early (and untimely) fashion, should be followed rather than treated. Unsustained or slowly progressive puberty in young girls does not warrant therapy with GnRH agonists.[66]

The treatment of choice for CPP is a GnRH analogue (GnRHa). Such analogues are modifications of the native hormone, usually at position six and at the carboxyl-terminal end, that have greater resistance to degradation and increased affinity for the pituitary GnRH receptor. Competitive inhibition by the GnRH agonist induces down-regulation of receptor function and of gonadotropin secretion, resulting in temporary, reversible inhibition of the HPO axis as reflected by minimal or no response to GnRH stimulation and regression of the manifestations of puberty.[67]

Management of CPP by GnRHa decreases gonadotropins and sex steroids to prepubertal or hypogonadal levels, which effects are followed by stabilization or regression of secondary sexual characteristics.[68, 69] The goal of GnRH therapy in North America and Europe is *complete suppression* of gonadotropin secretion, as demonstrated by the absence of significant gonadotropin response to GnRH stimulation during analogue therapy. (This is intended to prevent intervals of gonadotropin release that would stimulate puber-

tal progression.) Even "complete" suppression of gonadotropin may not lower the estradiol level to the prepubertal range.[70] Periodic assessment is indicated to determine continued suppression on GnRHa therapy. The definitive test is GnRH-stimulation testing with lack of LH and FSH response. Prepubertal level of estradiol in females and testosterone in males is indicative of suppression. Although pretreatment urinary excretion may be consistent with elevated gonadotropin secretion secondary to CPP, single urine samples may lack the sensitivity and specificity to assess the adequacy of HPG axis suppression and, thus, the appropriateness of GnRHa dosage.[71]

The adult height of patients given GnRH therapy is taller than that of untreated patients[72–75] and exceeds pretreatment stature projection.[76–79] Changes in height prediction during therapy are directly related to skeletal age at onset of therapy; however, reports to date find adult heights to be less than either target height and predicted height at the end of therapy.[75, 80] Recent study also showed that the prognosis for stature, with respect to target height, is generally most favorable for patients who, at the end of treatment, are tallest and have the lowest bone age–chronologic age ratio.[75] The robust resurgence of puberty secondary to the potent secretion of sex steroids leads to "catch-down" growth and rapid—and disproportional—skeletal advancement. A subset of patients with the slowly progressive variant of CPP do not require treatment, because they generally have good statural outcome.[66]

Treatment is continued until the progress of puberty is age-appropriate and consistent with emotional maturity, current height, and height potential. As far as the optimal timing for discontinuation of treatment is concerned, the best statural outcome can be achieved by patients who stop treatment at a bone age of 12 to 12½ years. If therapy is discontinued too early for pubertal levels of sex steroids to affect skeletal development, height potential will be lost. Such premature discontinuation of therapy is detrimental and is not recommended if the therapeutic goal is to maximize adult stature. Final height may also be compromised, however, if treatment is discontinued too late—after bone age of 13 years.[80] One study showed that the addition of growth hormone to GnRH in children with severe impairment in predicted adult height results in significant improvement in adult height.[81]

Resumption of puberty occurs after discontinuation of GnRHa therapy and proceeds at a pace similar to normal.[82] Pubertal LH and FSH responses to GnRH stimulation resume within 3 to 6 months in the majority of patients.[83] Recent data showed that, 1 year after therapy is withdrawn, peak LH and FSH levels are within the ranges for normal pubertal stage 4 or 5 girls.[84] It is not clear whether this is a consequence of prolonged suppression of the pituitary gonadotropes or represents the natural history of early maturation of the hypothalamic-pituitary-gonadal unit. After treatment, mean ovarian volume in girls with CPP tends to increase progressively and, after 4 to 5 years, to be significantly greater than that of normal girls. Ovulatory menstrual cycles sometimes develop within a matter of months after discontinuation of GnRHa treatment; for other girls, they may not occur until as long as 5 years later. Females who experienced menarche before therapy usually resume menses within 12 to 18 months. Several females who were treated with GnRHa for CPP have become pregnant and have borne normal infants.[84] Bone mineral density is increased for age among patients with precocious puberty, since pubertal hormones are important to the accrual of bone mass. Reports on the effects of GnRH therapy on bone mineral density differ. Using different methods, various investigators have observed either a decrease or no change during treatment.[85, 86] A recent study that used dual-energy absorptiometry determined that children have normal bone mineral density for *chronologic* age but below-average density for *skeletal* age after 2 years of treatment with GnRHa.[87] It is presumed that accretion will resume and peak at the appropriate age after therapy. For girls with precocious puberty, calcium supplementation may reverse or prevent the reduction in bone mineral density during GnRH therapy.[88]

Children who develop sexual precocity secondary to a CNS lesion or its treatment, particularly those who receive CNS radiotherapy for cancer, should be assessed and followed for growth hormone deficiency. The diagnosis may not be readily apparent, because the accelerated growth associated with precocity sometimes masks clinical evidence of such a deficiency. Growth rate and levels of insulin-like growth factor are greater in growth hormone–deficient patients with sexual precocity than in those with isolated growth hormone deficiency.[89] With initiation of GnRHa therapy, growth rates drop precipitously. Treatment with *both* growth hormone and GnRHa is indicated for these patients.

The principal known side effects of long-acting GnRH are (1) a local injection reaction and (2) the development of sterile abscesses. These reactions appear to be responses to the inert polymer that is used as a vehicle.[90] Prolonged vaginal bleeding, sometimes massive and recurrent, has also been reported; however, most episodes resolve spontaneously and need no further treatment.[91]

If GnRHa cannot be used to treat CPP, medroxyprogesterone may be used. This treatment may suppress progression of puberty and menses. Importantly, however, no effect on growth velocity, skeletal maturation, or adult height has been conclusively demonstrated.[92] Medroxyprogesterone is particularly useful in girls with complete precocity that is a complication of a neurologic disorder associated with profound mental retardation and whose menstrual hygiene is a management problem for caretakers.

Because precocious pseudopuberty is gonadotropin independent, GnRH analogues are not effective treatment. The appropriate therapy depends on the underlying disorder. Occasionally, GnRH analogues are useful as adjunctive therapy when the underlying disorder has also caused premature maturation of the hypothalamic-pituitary-gonadal axis.

PSYCHOSOCIAL CONSEQUENCES OF PRECOCITY

Children with precocious puberty are often noticeably taller and more developed at the time of diagnosis and may, therefore, appear older than their peers. Parents, teachers, and others in authority may respond negatively to this age-appearance disparity and unwittingly increase the risk of adjustment reactions. Excessive growth and early pubertal changes may result in the child's perceiving herself or himself as different, although this does not appear to produce long-term psychological abnormalities and most girls with CPP do well psychologically. No documentation that CPP is accompanied by significant psychosocial problems has been published. Concern is frequently expressed about the early initiation into heterosexual activity of such girls, but little evidence exists to support this concern. One study reported few effects of hormone administration on sexual behaviors and responses in hypogonadal adolescents, a finding that suggests that pubertal hormone levels alone would not be expected to bring about adolescent sexual activity.[93] Appropriate sex education is recommended—with particular emphasis on avoiding being victimized by sexual abusers—as advanced sexual maturity, combined with childlike responses to expressions of caring, often place these children at greater risk for sexual abuse.

REFERENCES

1. Elders MJ, Scott CR, Frindik JP, et al: Clinical workup for precocious puberty. Lancet 1997; 350:457.
2. Herman-Giddens ME, Slora EJ, Wasserman RC, et al: Secondary sexual characteristics in young girls seen in office practice: A study from the pediatric research in office settings network. Pediatrics 1997; 99:505.
3. Fontoura M, Brauner R, Prevot C, et al: Precocious puberty in girls: Early diagnosis of a slowly progressing variant. Arch Dis Child 1989; 64:1170.
4. Ghai K, Rosenfield RL: Disorders of pubertal development: Too early, too much, or too little. Adolesc Med 1994; 5:19.
5. Arita K, Ikawa F, Kurisu K, et al: The relationship between magnetic resonance imaging findings and clinical manifestations of hypothalamic hamartoma. J Neurosurg 1999; 91:212.
6. Price RA, Lee PA, Albright AL, et al: Treatment of sexual precocity by removal of a luteinizing hormone–releasing hormone-secreting hamartoma. JAMA 1984; 251:2247.
7. Starceski PJ, Lee PA, Albright AL, et al: Hypothalamic hamartomas and sexual precocity. Am J Dis Child 1990; 144:225.
8. Stewart L, Steinbok P, Daaboul J: Role of surgical resection in the treatment of hypothalamic hamartomas causing precocious puberty. J Neurosurg 1998; 88:340.
9. de Brito VN, Latronico AC, Arnhold IJP, et al: Treatment of gonadotropin-dependent precocious puberty due to hypothalamic hamartoma with gonadotropin-releasing hormone agonist depot. Arch Dis Child 1999; 80:231.
10. Carmi D, Shohat M, Metzker A, et al: Growth, puberty, and endocrine functions in patients with sporadic or familial neurofibromatosis type 1: A longitudinal study. Pediatrics 1999; 103:1257.
11. Rappaport R, Brauner R: Growth and endocrine disorders secondary to cranial irradiation. Pediatr Res 1989; 25:561.
12. Hanna CE, Mandel SH, LaFranchi SH: Puberty in the syndrome of septo-optic dysplasia. Am J Dis Child 1989; 143:186.
13. Siddiqi SU, Van Dyke DC, Donohoue P, et al: Premature sexual development in individuals with neurodevelopmental disabilities. Develop Med Child Neurol 1999; 41:392.
14. Kitanaka C, Matsutani M, Sora S, et al: Precocious puberty in a girl with an hCG-secreting suprasellar immature teratoma. Case report. J Neurosurg 1994; 81:601.
15. Cronje HS, Niemand I, Bam RH, et al: Granulosa and theca cell tumors in children: A report of 17 cases and literature review. Obstet Gynecol Survey 1998; 53:240.
16. Lacson AG, Gillis DA, Shawwa A: Malignant mixed germ cell–sex cord–stromal tumors of the ovary associated with isosexual precocious puberty. Cancer 1988; 61:2122.
17. Zung A, Shoham Z, Open M, et al: Sertoli cell tumor causing precocious puberty in a girl with Peutz-Jeghers syndrome. Gynecol Oncol 1998; 70:421.
18. Mehenni H, Gehrig C, Nezu J, et al: Loss of LKB1 kinase activity in Peutz-Jeghers syndrome, and evidence for allelic and locus heterogeneity. Am J Hum Genet 1998; 63:1641.
19. Westerman AM, Entius MM, Boor PP, et al: Novel mutations in the LKB1/STK11 gene in Dutch Peutz-Jeghers families. Hum Mutat 1999; 13:476.
20. Eberly SM: Pediatric adolescent gynecologic imaging: Precocious puberty and hormone-producing neoplasms. Adolesc Med 1994; 5:111.
21. Cohen HL, Eisenberg P, Mandel F, et al: Ovarian cysts are common in premenarchal girls: A sonographic study of 101 children 2–12 years old. AJR 1992; 159:89.
22. Adashi EY, Hennebold JD: Single-gene mutations resulting in reproductive dysfunction in women. N Engl J Med 1999; 340:709.
23. Weinstein LS, Shenker A, Gejman PV, et al: Activating mutations of the stimulatory G protein in the McCune-Albright syndrome. N Engl J Med 1991; 325:1688.
24. Levine MA: The McCune-Albright syndrome. N Engl J Med 1991; 325:1738.
25. Olsen BR: A rare disorder, yes; an unimportant one, never. J Clin Invest 1998; 101:1545.
26. Kremer H, Martens JW, van Reen M, et al: A limited repertoire of mutations of the luteinizing hormone (LH) receptor gene in familial and sporadic patients with male LH-independent precocious puberty. J Clin Endocrinol Metab 1999; 84:1136.
27. Bertelloni S, Baroncelli GI, Lala R, et al: Long-term outcome of male-limited gonadotropin-independent precocious puberty. Horm Res 1997; 48:235.
28. Anasti JN, Flack MR, Froehlick J, et al: A potential novel mechanism for precocious puberty in juvenile hypothyroidism. J Clin Endocrinol Metab 1995; 80:276.
29. Klein KO, Mericq V, Brown-Dawson JM, et al: Estrogen levels in girls with premature thelarche compared with normal prepubertal girls as determined by an ultrasensitive recombinant cell bioassay. J Pediatr 1999; 134:190.
30. Mills JL: Premature thelarche—natural history and etiologic investigation. Am J Dis Child 1981; 135:743.
31. Van Winter JT, Noller KL, Zimmerman D, et al: Natural history of premature thelarche in Olmstead County, Minnesota, 1940–1984. J Pediatr 1990; 116:278.
32. Salardi S, Cacciari E, Mainetti B, et al: Outcome of premature thelarche: Relation to puberty and final height. Arch Dis Child 1998; 79:173.
33. Korth-Schutz S, Levine LS, New MI: Serum androgens in normal prepubertal and pubertal children and in children with precocious adrenarche. J Clin Endocrinol Metab 1976; 42:117.
34. Ibañez L, Potau N, Virdis R, et al: Postpubertal outcome in girls diagnosed of premature pubarche during childhood: Increased frequency of functional ovarian hyperandrogenism. J Clin Endocrinol Metab 1993; 76:1599.
35. Ibañez L, Potau N, Chacon P, et al: Hyperinsulinaemia, dyslipaemia, and cardiovascular risk in girls with a history of premature pubarche. Diabetologia 1998; 41:1057.
36. Ibañez L, Potau N, Zampolli M, et al: Hyperinsulinemia in postpubertal girls with a history of premature pubarche and functional ovarian hyperandrogenism. J Clin Endocrinol Metab 1996; 81:1237.
37. Ibañez L, Potau N, Zampolli M, et al: Hyperinsulinemia and decreased insulin-like growth factor–binding protein-1 are common features in prepubertal and pubertal girls with a history of premature pubarche. J Clin Endocrinol Metab 1997; 82:2283.
38. Apter D, Bützow T, Laughlin GA, Yen SSC: Metabolic features of polycystic ovary syndrome are found in adolescent girls with hyperandrogenism. J Clin Endocrinol Metab 1995; 80:2966.
39. Ibañez L, de Zegher F, Potau N: Anovulation after precocious pubarche: Early markers and time course in adolescence. J Clin Endocrinol Metab 1999; 84:2691.
40. Dunaif A: Insulin resistance and the polycystic ovary syndrome: Mechanism and implications for pathogenesis. Endocrinol Rev 1997; 18:774.

41. Legro RS, Driscoll D, Strauss JF, et al: Evidence for a genetic basis for hyperandrogenemia in the polycystic ovary syndrome. Proc Natl Acad Sci 1998; 95:14956.

42. Urbanek M, Legro RS, Driscoll DA, et al: Thirty-seven candidate genes for polycystic ovary syndrome: Strongest evidence for linkage is with follistatin. Proc Natl Acad Sci 1999; 96:8573.

43. Witchel SF, Lee PA, Suda-Hartman M, Hoffman EP: Hyperandrogenism and manifesting heterozygotes for 21-hydroxylase deficiency. Biochem Molec Med 1997; 62:151.

44. Blanché H, Vexiau P, Clauin S, et al: Exhaustive screening of the 21-hydroxylase gene in a population of hyperandrogenic women. Hum Genet 1997; 101:56.

45. Ostlere LS, Rumsby G, Holownia P, et al: Carrier status for steroid 21-hydroxylase deficiency is only one factor in the variable phenotype of acne. Clin Endocrinol 1998; 48:209.

46. Dacou-Voutetakis C, Dracopoulou M: High incidence of molecular defects of the CYP21 gene in patients with premature adrenarche. J Clin Endocrinol Metab 1999; 84:1570.

47. Knochenhauer ES, Cordet-Rudelli C, Cunningham RD, et al: Carriers of 21-hydroxylase deficiency are not at increased risk for hyperandrogenism. J Clin Endocrinol Metab 1997; 82:479.

48. Lazar L, Kauli R, Bruchis C, et al: Early polycystic ovary–like syndrome in girls with central precocious puberty and exaggerated adrenal response. Eur J Endocrinol 1995; 133:403.

49. Wedell A: Molecular genetics of congenital adrenal hyperplasia (21-hydroxylase deficiency): Implications for diagnosis, prognosis, and treatment. Acta Paediatr 1998; 87:159.

50. Speiser PW, White PC: Congenital adrenal hyperplasia due to steroid 21-hydroxylase deficiency. Clin Endocrinol 1998; 49:411.

51. Hughes IA: Congenital adrenal hyperplasia—a continuum of disorders. Lancet 1998; 352:752.

52. Geley S, Kapelari K, Johrer K, et al: CYP11B1 mutations causing congenital adrenal hyperplasia due to 11-beta hydroxylase deficiency. J Clin Endocrinol Metab 1996; 81:2896.

53. Simard J, Rhéaume E, Sanchez R: Molecular basis of congenital adrenal hyperplasia due to 3β-hydroxysteroid dehydrogenase deficiency. Molec Endocrinol 1993; 7:716.

54. Moran C, Knochenhauer ES, Azziz R: Non-classic adrenal hyperplasia in hyperandrogenism: A reappraisal. J Endocrinol Invest 1998; 21:707.

55. Cisternino M, Dondi E, Martinetti M, et al: Exaggerated 17-hydroxyprogesterone response to short-term adrenal stimulation and evidence for CYP21B gene point mutations in true precocious puberty. Clin Endocrinol 1998; 48:555.

56. Lee PDK, Winter RJ, Green OC: Virilizing adrenocortical tumors in childhood: Eight cases and a review of the literature. Pediatrics 1985; 76:437.

57. Daneman A: Adrenal neoplasms in children. Semin Roentgenol 1988; 23:205.

58. Mayer SK, Oligny LL, Deal C, et al: Childhood adrenocortical tumors: Case series and reevaluation of prognosis—a 24-year experience. J Pediatr Surg 1997; 32:911.

59. Wolthers OD, Cameron FJ, Scheimberg I, et al: Androgen secreting adrenocortical tumours. Arch Dis Child 1999; 80:46.

60. Comite F, Schiebinger RJ, Alberton BD, et al: Isosexual precocious pseudopuberty secondary to a feminizing adrenal tumor. J Clin Endocrinol Metab 1984; 58:435.

61. Romer TE, Sachnowska K, Savage MO, et al: Luteinizing hormone–secreting adrenal tumor as a cause of precocious puberty. Clin Endocrinol 1998; 48:367.

62. Cowan BD, Morrison JC: Management of abnormal genital bleeding in girls and women. N Engl J Med 1991; 324:1710.

63. Muram D: Premature menarche: A follow-up study. Arch Dis Child 1983; 58:142.

64. Jensen A-MB, Brocks V, Holm KK, et al: Central precocious puberty in girls: Internal genitalia before, during, and after treatment with long-acting gonadotropin–releasing hormone analogues. J Pediatr 1998; 132:105.

65. Buzi F, Pilotta A, Dordoni D, et al: Pelvic ultrasonography in normal girls and in girls with pubertal precocity. Acta Paediatr 1998; 87:1138.

66. Palmert MR, Malin HV, Boepple PA: Unsustained or slowly progressive puberty in young girls: Initial presentation and long-term follow-up of 20 untreated patients. J Clin Endocrinol Metab 1999; 84:415.

67. Conn PM, Crowley WF Jr: Gonadotropin-releasing hormone and its analogues. N Engl J Med 1991; 324:93.

68. Lee PA, Page JG: The Leuprolide Study Group: Effects of leuprolide in the treatment of central precocious puberty. J Pediatr 1989; 114:321.

69. Tanaka T, Hibi I, Kato K, et al: A dose finding study of a super long–acting luteinizing hormone–releasing hormone analog (leuprolide acetate depot, TAP-144-SR) in the treatment of central precocious puberty. Endocrinol Jpn 1991; 38:369.

70. Klein KO, Baron J, Barnes KM, et al: Use of an ultrasensitive recombinant cell bioassay to determine estrogen levels in girls with precocious puberty treated with a luteinizing hormone–releasing hormone agonist. J Clin Endocrinol Metab 1998; 83:2387.

71. Witchel SF, Baens-Bailon RG, Lee PA: Treatment of central precocious puberty: Comparison of urinary gonadotropin excretion and gonadotropin-releasing hormone (GnRH) stimulation tests in monitoring GnRH analog therapy. J Clin Endocrinol Metab 1996; 81:1353.

72. Kauli R, Galatzer A, Kornreich L: Final height of girls with central precocious puberty: Untreated versus treated with cyproterone acetate or GnRH analogue. Horm Res 1997; 47:54.

73. Paul D, Conte FA, Grumbach MM, et al: Long term effect of gonadotropin-releasing hormone agonist therapy on final and near-final height in 26 children with true precocious puberty treated at a median age of less than 5 years. J Clin Endocrinol Metab 1995; 80:546.

74. Galluzi F, Salti R, Bindi G, et al: Adult height comparison between boys and girls with precocious puberty after long-term gonadotropin-releasing hormone analogue therapy. Acta Paediatr 1998; 87:521.

75. Arrigo T, Cisternino M, Galluzzi F, et al: Analysis of the factors affecting auxological response to GnRH agonist treatment and final height outcome in girls with idiopathic central precocious puberty. Eur J Endocrinol 1999; 141:140.

76. Brauner R, Adan L, Malandry F, et al: Adult height in girls with idiopathic true precocious puberty. J Clin Endocrinol Metab 1994; 79:415.

77. Cacciari E, Cassio A, Balsamo A, et al: Long-term follow-up and final height in girls with central precocious puberty treated with luteinizing hormone–releasing hormone analogue nasal spray. Arch Pediatr Adolesc Med 1994; 148:1194.

78. Kletter G, Kelch RP: Effects of gonadotropin-releasing hormone analog therapy on adult stature in precocious puberty. J Clin Endocrinol Metab 1994; 79:331.

79. Oostdijk W, Rikken B, Schreuder S, et al: Final height

in central precocious puberty after long-term treatment with slow-release GnRH agonist. Arch Dis Child 1996; 75:292.

80. Bertelloni S, Baroncelli GI, Sorrentino MC, et al: Effect of central precocious puberty and gonadotropin-releasing hormone analogue treatment on peak bone mass and final height in females. Eur J Pediatr 1998; 157:363.

81. Pasquino AM, Pucarelli I, Segni M, et al: Adult height in girls with central precocious puberty treated with gonadotropin-releasing hormone analogues and growth hormone. J Clin Endocrinol Metab 1999; 84:449.

82. Manasco P, Pescovitz OH, Feuillan PP, et al: Resumption of puberty after long term luteinizing hormone–releasing hormone agonist treatment of central precocious puberty. J Clin Endocrinol Metab 1988; 67:368.

83. Jay N, Mansfield MJ, Blizzard RM, et al: Ovulation and menstrual function of adolescent girls with central precocious puberty after therapy with gonadotropin-releasing hormone agonists. J Clin Endocrinol Metab 1992; 75:890.

84. Feuillan PP, Jones JV, Barnes K, et al: Reproductive axis after discontinuation of gonadotropin-releasing hormone analog treatment of girls with precocious puberty: Long term follow-up comparing girls with hypothalamic hamartoma to those with idiopathic precocious puberty. J Clin Endocrinol Metab 1999; 84:44.

85. Saggese G, Bertelloni S, Baroncelli GI, et al: Reduction of bone density: An effect of gonadotropin releasing hormone analogue treatment in central precocious puberty. Eur J Pediatr 1993; 152:717.

86. Antoniazzi F, Bertoldo F, Zamboni G, et al: Bone mineral metabolism in girls with precocious puberty during gonadotropin-releasing hormone agonist testing. Eur J Endocrinol 1995; 133:412.

87. Boot A, de Muinck Keizer-Schrama SMPF, Pols HAP, et al: Bone mineral density and body composition before and during treatment with gonadotropin-releasing hormone agonist in children with central precocious puberty. J Clin Endocrinol Metab 1998; 83:370.

88. Antoniazzi F, Bertoldo F, Lauriola S, et al: Prevention of bone mineralization by calcium supplementation in precocious puberty during gonadotropin-releasing hormone agonist treatment. J Clin Endocrinol Metab 1999; 84:1992.

89. Cara JF: Growth hormone deficiency impedes the rise in plasma insulin-like growth factor I levels associated with precocious puberty. J Pediatr 1989; 115:64.

90. Manasco P, Neely EK: Local reactions to depot leuprolide therapy for central precocious puberty. J Pediatr 1993; 123:334.

91. Yeshaya A, Kauschansky A, Orvieto R, et al: Prolonged vaginal bleeding during central precocious puberty therapy with a long-acting gonadotropin-releasing hormone agonist. Acta Obstet Gynecol Scand 1998; 77:327.

92. Lee PA: Medroxyprogesterone therapy for sexual precocity in girls. Am J Dis Child 1981; 135:443.

93. Finkelstein JW, Susman EJ, Chinchilli VM, et al: Effects of estrogen or testosterone on self-reported sexual responses and behaviors in hypogonadal adolescents. J Clin Endocrinol Metab 1998; 83:2281.

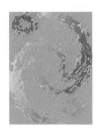

Chapter 6
Delayed Puberty

Louis S. O'Dea and Peter A. Lee

Delayed puberty is defined as the failure to exhibit the physical signs of puberty within the expected time period for puberty in the normal human population. Either absence of evidence of the onset of puberty or failure of normal progression through puberty constitutes pubertal delay. For boys, absence of testicular enlargement by 14 years of age is considered delayed development. For girls, delayed puberty means the absence of thelarche by age 13 and of menarche by age 16. Using a 99% confidence interval (SD 2.57), 0.62% of normal males and females in the general population will be, by inference, delayed in their development. Boys, however, present more frequently than girls for assessment of pubertal delay. Delayed linear growth and absence of physical maturity are the common presentations in boys and are often recognized in relation to performance in physical sports and to the accelerating development of their peers. Girls most frequently present with questions related to sexual development and, specifically, delayed menarche.

Pubertal delay often reflects a lag in the timing of normal pubertal development, owing to delayed reactivation of the hypothalamic-pituitary-gonadal axis. Conversely, pubertal delay may be a sign of a more significant underlying abnormality including failure of hypothalamic activation, failure of pituitary transmission of the hypothalamic signal, or inability of the gonad to respond appropriately to the pituitary message; all of these may present as delayed pubertal development.

CATEGORIES

The three broad diagnostic categories of pubertal delay are (1) hypergonadotropic hypogonadism or delayed puberty due to an unresponsive gonad, (2) hypogonadotropic hypogonadism or delayed puberty due to failure of hypothalamic or pituitary function, and (3) physiologic or constitutional delay of development due to late activation of the hypothalamic-pituitary-gonadal axis, frequently a diagnosis of exclusion (Table 6–1). In addition, serious systemic illness, malnutrition, and untreated endocrine diseases may also reversibly delay or alter the course of puberty. This discussion pertains to patients who are otherwise disease-free or whose illness is adequately treated.

HYPERGONADOTROPIC HYPOGONADISM

Hypergonadotropism occurs with primary gonadal failure. The most common cause of primary amenorrhea associated with primary gonadal failure is Turner syndrome. The classic findings of Turner syndrome (Fig. 6–1) are short stature and primary hypogonadism associated with a 45,X karyotype, although clinical features and karyotype vary. Mosaic karyotypes and structural abnormalities of the X chromosome occur. Sensitive molecular techniques have revealed that some girls with Turner syndrome carry Y chromosome material.[1]

Turner Syndrome

Turner syndrome may manifest at birth with low birth weight and lymphedema, in childhood with short stature, or in adolescence with short stature and delayed puberty or primary amenorrhea. The lymphedema may be asymmetric or limited to only a portion of the body. Additional clinical features include low posterior hairline, webbed neck, cubitus valgus, short fourth metacarpals, high-arched palate, congenital heart disease, multiple nevi, and renal abnormalities. The frequency of autoimmune disorders is increased in girls with Turner syndrome. During infancy and after age 7 to 8 years, gonadotropin levels, especially follicle-stimulating hormone (FSH), are elevated.[2] Turner syndrome and its variants are discussed in greater detail in Chapter 8.

Table 6–1. Origins of Delayed Puberty

I. Delayed puberty: No signs of pubertal development
  A. Hypergonadotropic hypogonadism
    1. Autoimmune oophoritis
    2. Galactosemia
    3. Gonadal agenesis (XX or XY)
    4. Gonadal dysgenesis, mixed
    5. "Resistant ovaries" syndrome
    6. Secondary to destruction of ovaries
      a. Chemotherapy
      b. Infection
      c. Irradiation
      d. Surgery
      e. Bilateral torsion
      f. Trauma
      g. Sickle cell disease
    7. Errors in steroidogenesis
      a. Mutations in CYP17
      b. Mutations in StAR
  B. Hypogonadotropism
    1. Permanent hypothalamic-pituitary defects
      a. Autoimmune disease
      b. Craniopharyngioma
      c. Granulomatous disease
      d. Hypothalamic tumors
      e. Idiopathic hypopituitarism
      f. Female Kallmann syndrome
      g. Pituitary tumor
      h. Septooptic dysplasia
      i. Syndromes
        i. Laurence-Moon-Biedl
        ii. Prader-Willi
      j. Secondary to:
        i. Irradiation
        ii. Surgery

    2. Immature or reversible hypogonadotropism
      a. Anorexia nervosa
      b. Chronic illness
        i. Inflammatory bowel disease
        ii. Sickle cell disease
        iii. Cystic fibrosis
        iv. Rheumatoid arthritis
      c. Constitutional delay of puberty
      d. Endocrinopathies
        i. Cushing's syndrome
        ii. Diabetes mellitus
        iii. Growth hormone deficiency
        iv. Hyperprolactinemia
        v. Hypothyroidism
II. Breast development with primary amenorrhea
  A. Hypergonadotropic
    1. Androgen insensitivity syndrome
  B. Normal or low gonadotropins
    1. Anatomic
      a. Imperforate hymen
      b. Mayer-Rokitansky-Kuster-Hauser syndrome
    2. Pituitary
      a. Hyperprolactinemia
      b. Hypothyroidism
      c. Cushing's disease
III. Delayed puberty with virilization
  A. Deficiency of 5α-reductase
  B. Congenital adrenal hyperplasia
  C. Virilizing tumors
  D. Mixed gonadal dysgenesis
  E. 17βHSD3

Mixed Gonadal Dysgenesis

Humans with mixed gonadal dysgenesis may have somatic features typical of Turner syndrome, especially short stature. The most common karyotype is 45,X/46,XY. The external and internal genitalia reflect the extent of testosterone exposure in utero and, thus, may be female, ambiguous, or male. The gonads may vary from symmetric streak ovaries or dysgenetic testes to asymmetric gonads with a streak ovary on one side and a dysgenetic testis on the opposite side. Often, the external genital development appears asymmetric. The presence of the Y chromosome increases the chance of gonadal tumors, especially gonadoblastoma. Virilization may occur at puberty, and, for these reasons, such gonads should be removed before puberty. Estrogen replacement is required to induce puberty. Spontaneous breast development suggests an estrogen-secreting gonadoblastoma. When the physical finding of ambiguous genitalia leads to the diagnosis of mixed gonadal dysgenesis, the decision on gender assignment, or sex of rearing, should be carefully and thoroughly discussed with the parents and should rest on, among other considerations, the potential for the external genitalia to fulfill a male or female sexual role later in life.

46,XX Gonadal Dysgenesis

Normal or tall stature and hypergonadotropic hypogonadism are observed in pure gonadal dysgenesis. Characteristics associated with 46,XX gonadal dysgenesis include delayed puberty, bilateral streak gonads, and normal female internal genitalia. A report of 46,XX and 46,XY sisters with gonadal agenesis provides evidence for involvement of an autosomal locus in gonadal differentiation.[3] Perrault syndrome is XX gonadal dysgenesis and sensorineural deafness.[4]

46,XY Gonadal Dysgenesis

Delayed puberty is a typical presentation for 46,XY complete gonadal dysgenesis. Ambiguous internal and external genitalia or some pubertal changes may be noted in incomplete or partial

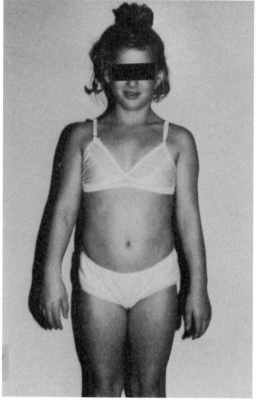

Figure 6–1. A 9-year-old girl with short stature and a karyotype of 45,X (Turner syndrome with minimal stigmata). Elevated gonadotropin levels indicated ovarian failure. This patient was treated with growth hormone to stimulate linear growth before institution of sex steroid replacement therapy.

forms of 46,XY gonadal dysgenesis. Mutations in the *SRY* gene have been identified in some patients with gonadal dysgenesis.[5, 6] Familial gonadal dysgenesis has been described in which the phenotype and sex of rearing differed between family members despite a common mutation in the *SRY* gene in all affected family members.[7] The *SRY* gene appears to be normal in the majority of subjects with 46,XY gonadal dysgenesis, however. Another genetic cause of 46,XY sex reversal is duplication of portions of the short arm of the X chromosome that include the gene *DAX1*.[8] Gonadectomy is generally recommended because dysgenetic gonads show an increased risk to develop dysgerminoma or gonadoblastoma.

Gonadal Damage

Prepubertal or pubertal gonadal injury may result in hypergonadotropic hypogonadism, al-

though the ovary is less vulnerable than the testis to most toxins, the seminiferous tubules being more susceptible than Leydig cells. Chemotherapy for cancer or immune-mediated disorders can damage the gonads; nitrogen mustard compounds are particularly toxic in this regard. The degree of injury is greater when chemotherapy occurs during, rather than before, puberty.[9] Pelvic irradiation may also affect reproductive function, yet many girls treated for acute lymphocytic leukemia appear to retain ovarian function.[10]

Autoimmune and Other Gonadal Failure

Autoimmune oophoritis can occur in type I autoimmune polyglandular syndrome, which is characterized by hypoparathyroidism, Addison disease, vitiligo, hypothyroidism, and pernicious anemia. Galactosemia is associated with ovarian failure.[11] *Resistant ovary syndrome* (gonadotropin-resistant ovary) is the term applied to the state of anovulation in the presence of elevated gonadotropin levels and numerous primordial follicles identified on ovarian biopsy that fail to respond appropriately to endogenous or exogenous gonadotropins. The mechanism of this disorder is unclear but may involve deficient gonadotropin receptor function. The syndrome remains controversial, however. In many cases, it progresses to true premature ovarian failure. Thus, for some patients the resistance may simply reflect a stage along the path to ovarian failure.

Described Genetic Mutations

Hypergonadotropic hypogonadism may also be associated with recently described mutations of the luteinizing hormone (LH) receptor. In XX females, the presentation has been primary amenorrhea in a girl with normal female genitalia and secondary sexual characteristics.[12] Endocrine assessment reveals elevated serum LH and low estradiol levels. XY males with LH receptor mutations have presented with male pseudohermaphroditism, a condition characterized by female external genitalia, absence of müllerian structures, and failure of breast development. Biopsy on the inguinal gonads of such males has revealed absence of Leydig cells but evidence of Sertoli cells, spermatogonia, and primary spermatocytes.[12] Such patients have demonstrated a limited response to exogenous human chorionic gonadotropin (hCG).[13] Earlier descriptions of male pseudohermaphroditism (Leydig cell hypoplasia) with amenorrhea, inguinal testes, and elevated LH levels may reflect the same disorder.[14] That mutations in the LH receptor gene were not detected in several patients with a similar phenotype suggests that other genes may be involved in Leydig cell differentiation.[15]

Mutations in the follicle-stimulating hormone (FSH)–receptor gene have been identified in women with primary amenorrhea. Additional phenotypic features include normal breast development and elevated FSH. Histologic examination of ovary specimens shows numerous small follicles up to the antral stage but disruption of later stages.[16, 17]

HYPOGONADOTROPIC HYPOGONADISM

Isolated Gonadotropin Deficiency

Isolated gonadotropin deficiency (IGD), or idiopathic hypogonadotropic hypogonadism (IHH), is the most common form of hypogonadotropic hypogonadism. It is estimated to occur in only 1 in 50,000 women, a rate that is one fifth that for males.[18] Although autosomal-recessive, autosomal-dominant, and X-linked modes of inheritance have been described, most cases appear to be sporadic.[19, 20] A single case report of direct father-son inheritance after treatment of the father suggests alternative mechanisms in addition to the X-linked hypothesis.[21] Mother-daughter transmission has not been reported.

Normal gonadotropin-releasing hormone (GnRH) gene structure was reported in men with IHH by Weiss and coworkers.[22] Deletion involving the Kallmann syndrome interval gene 1 (KALIG-1), in the region of Xp22.3 has been reported in men with an X-linked familial form of Kallmann syndrome. In addition to anosmia and hypogonadism, affected persons may have other clinical features, such as neurologic deficits, mental retardation, unilateral kidney agenesis, or cryptorchidism.[23, 24] The structure of this gene suggests that it is a neural cell–adhesion molecule gene.[25, 26] Thus, it has been suggested that its deletion accounts for the association of failed axonal migration and anosmia with Kallmann syndrome. High-resolution magnetic resonance imaging (MRI) has demonstrated hypoplasia of the olfactory bulbs in affected persons.[27] Another report of 21 cases of sporadic nonfamilial IHH that showed evidence of KALIG-1 deletion in only one subject suggests genetic heterogeneity.[28] Recent genetic investigations have focused on mutations of the GnRH receptor gene, which, if they contribute to the disease, should result in failure of response to exogenous GnRH.[29] However, while rarely detected in affected families, and more rarely in isolated affected patients, its overall contribution to the incidence of IHH remains, as yet, unknown. In summary, therefore, IHH is most commonly sporadic. The familial forms appear to result from mutation at one of several different loci, rather than being a single-gene disorder. One other recognized locus is the DAX1 gene mapped to the short arm of the X chromosome. Mutations in DAX1 are associated with congenital adrenal hypoplasia and hypogonadotropic hypogonadism.[30] The variability of the associated disorders points, again, to a more complex genetic cause.

Not all patients with hypogonadotropic hypogonadism have Kallmann syndrome. Low-frequency and low-amplitude pulses are found in many persons with IHH who do not have Kallmann syndrome and in those with constitutional delayed puberty (discussed later).[31] Indeed, in males whose IHH is associated with initiated but arrested puberty, clear nocturnal enhancement of LH pulsatility is apparent.[32] Thus, Kallmann syndrome is a more profound form of IHH, usually associated with flat pulse studies and failure to respond to GnRH stimulation testing (Fig. 6–2). Therefore, unless there is strong evidence that Kallmann syndrome is present, pulse studies have limited usefulness in the differentiation or prognostication of pubertal delay, in terms of IHH.

Mutations of the FSH-beta gene have also been associated with the presentation of primary amenorrhea in otherwise normal XX females. Deletion of two nucleotides in exon 3 caused a frame shift in the codon reading and resulted in a truncated FSH-beta. Endocrine findings, which have included elevated serum LH levels and low or undetectable immuno and bio FSH levels,[33] confirm the structural abnormality of the FSH molecule. Consistent with the nature of the abnormality, and in contrast to receptor defects, such patients exhibit a normal response to exogenous FSH.

Multiple Hormone Deficiencies: Congenital and Acquired

Hypogonadotropic hypogonadism may also occur in association with other anterior pituitary hormone deficiencies. These congenital or acquired disorders may predominantly affect the

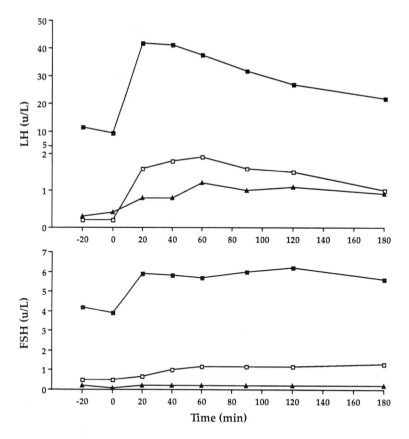

Figure 6–2. Gonadotropin responses to GnRH stimulation testing in patients suspected to have hypogonadotropism. ■, A normal pubertal response in a 13-year-old female patient with growth hormone deficiency secondary to an eosinophilic granuloma who subsequently had normal spontaneous pubertal development. □, Lack of response in a 15-year-old female without pubertal development who had a brother with Kallmann syndrome; this patient had the same diagnosis. ▲, Lack of response in a 14-year-old female with a history of a craniopharyngioma and panhypopituitarism. Height at various ages for these patients is plotted in Figure 6–3.

hypothalamus, the pituitary, or both. Congenital hypopituitarism may be associated with structural abnormalities such as midline facial defects, septo-optic dysplasia, or ectopic location of the posterior pituitary at the base of the hypothalamus.[34] Most commonly, GH deficiency is the associated endocrine defect. Structural abnormalities of the hypothalamus may include craniopharyngiomas, hamartomas, gliomas, and hypothalamic cysts. Histiocytosis X, sarcoidosis, and radiation therapy are causes of acquired hypopituitarism. Granulomatous infiltrates may interfere with GnRH, LH, and FSH release. The coexistence of more than one tropic hormone deficiency (except in idiopathic hypopituitarism diagnosed in early childhood) strongly suggests an anatomic lesion. Diabetes insipidus or hyperprolactinemia in association with pubertal delay is particularly suggestive of a central lesion.

Gonadotropin Insufficiency of Other Causes

Prolactinomas may present with either delayed puberty or arrested pubertal development and with primary or secondary amenorrhea.[35, 36]

Galactorrhea is not a constant finding. Gonadotropin levels are usually low. Clinically, some patients resemble those with anorexia nervosa because of poor appetite, weight loss, and delayed pubertal progression. Although most prolactinomas are responsive to bromocriptine therapy, transsphenoidal surgery or pituitary irradiation is occasionally necessary.[37, 38]

Hemochromatosis leading to pituitary infiltration, whether idiopathic or secondary (e.g., to sickle cell disease or thalassemia), may also result in gonadotropin deficiency because of the preferential affinity of iron for the gonadotropin-producing cells. Affected girls may have delayed puberty.[39] In persons with an idiopathic or familial form of the disease, reversal of the pituitary gonadotropin deficiency and recovery of reproductive function may follow aggressive phlebotomy and chelation therapy.[40] The pituitary gonadotropin deficiency may occur in a similar fashion in Wilson disease.

Anorexia nervosa is often associated with delayed puberty, slowing of normal pubertal progression, and primary or secondary amenorrhea. Osteopenia is often a serious and persistent complication of anorexia nervosa that appears to be associated with a major effect on osteoblast function.[41] Delayed puberty may also be observed in athletes and in patients with chronic illnesses.[42] Failure to supply the requisite increased calorie intake for normal accelerated pubertal growth frequently contributes to physiologic delay.[43] Frequently, in participants in certain sports (e.g., ballet, gymnastics, track), pubertal delay is a consequence of hypothalamic hypofunction resulting from strenuous exercise, stress-related or intentional calorie restriction, or even an eating disorder. The chronic illnesses frequently associated with delayed puberty (i.e., inflammatory bowel disease, cystic fibrosis, chronic renal disease, and poorly controlled diabetes mellitus) are characterized by undernutrition. Serum gonadotropin levels are low, reflecting the absence or altered frequency of the normal GnRH pulsatile pattern.[44]

It is not clear whether these heterogeneous causes of functional hypogonadotropic hypogonadism share a common pathophysiologic mechanism. Altered neuroendocrine dynamics are described in functional hypothalamic amenorrhea.[45] Hypercortisolism and blunted cortisol responses to corticotropin-releasing hormone (CRH) detected in women with hypothalamic amenorrhea suggest involvement of the hypothalamic-pituitary-adrenal axis.[46] Pubertal hormone secretion and menstrual periods usually ensue after correction of the energy imbalance and weight gain.[46] Conversely, progressive exercise and calorie output have been shown to predictably and progressively attenuate HPO function.[47]

Hypothyroidism retards growth and skeletal maturation. In addition to growth failure, cold intolerance, constipation, and dry skin are suggestive of hypothyroidism. On physical examination, mild obesity for height, goiter, sluggishness, delayed reflexes, and cool, dry skin may be noted. Hypothyroidism delays maturation and thus, when present during childhood, may interfere in the pubertal process. Onset during or after pubertal development is associated with menstrual disorders, primary or secondary amenorrhea, and menometrorrhagia. Hypothyroidism during childhood may result in a final height deficit.[48]

Among children or adolescents, glucocorticoid excess, either endogenous or exogenous, is associated with growth failure, pubertal delay, amenorrhea, and low gonadotropin levels. The most common cause of Cushing syndrome in the pediatric and adolescent population is exogenous steroid therapy for a chronic illness. Cushing syndrome may manifest with moon face, obesity, myopathy, striae, ecchymoses, hypertension, and hypercortisolemia in association with growth failure and pubertal delay. Typical laboratory findings of Cushing disease include loss of diurnal variation, elevated urinary free cortisol excretion, inadequate cortisol suppression following dexamethasone, and inappropriately elevated simultaneous adrenocorticotropin (ACTH) and cortisol concentrations.[49]

Syndromes Associated with Gonadotropin Deficiency

Several syndromes are characterized by hypogonadotropic hypogonadism. The Laurence-Moon-Biedl syndrome involves retinitis pigmentosa, polydactyly, obesity, mental retardation, and hypogonadism. Typical signs of the Bardet-Biedl subgroup of this syndrome are retinal dystrophy, dystrophic extremities (polydactyly, syndactyly, brachydactyly), obesity, and retinal disease. At least five distinct gene loci have been identified for this autosomal-recessive disorder.[50] Hypogonadism is more common in males, although it can occur in females. Hirsutism and elevated LH levels appear to be more common in girls.[51]

Typical features of Prader-Willi syndrome include short stature, hypotonia, hyperphagia, and obesity. By history, affected infants are typically poor feeders in the neonatal period because of the hypotonia. Hypogonadotropic hypogonadism may occur. A microdeletion at 15q 11-q13 or maternal disomy of chromosome 15 has been identified in many patients.[52, 53] Other unusual syndromes such as Alstrom, Rud, and Bloom syndromes may also be associated with pubertal delay. Frohlich syndrome is simply the association of obesity and hypothalamic hypogonadism, not a separate entity in this spectrum of disorders.

CONSTITUTIONAL DELAY OF GROWTH AND DEVELOPMENT

Constitutional delay of puberty, although a common cause for lack of timely pubertal development among boys, is rare among girls. Thus, this diagnosis should not be assigned until other causes of pubertal delay have been sought. The onset of puberty correlates better with skeletal maturity than with chronologic age; however, there may be underlying pathologic causes of pubertal delay. With constitutional delay of puberty, bone age is delayed but progresses, and puberty begins at the appropriate skeletal age. When there is underlying disease, skeletal age may not advance. Children with constitutional delay are otherwise healthy but typically of short stature. Their growth rate during childhood is normal to slow normal, with more pronounced deceleration than usual just before the onset of puberty. Other family members, such as the same-sex parent, may have had similarly delayed pubertal development.

Constitutional delay is a diagnosis of exclusion. Commonly, there is already some physical evidence of the onset of puberty at presentation. To confirm the diagnosis, a short period of follow-up may be all that is required. Therapy may be indicated when a diagnosis of constitutional delay is strongly suspected but unconfirmed, especially when the delay is marked or psychosocial stress is intense. Therapy may be begun with low-dose estrogen, with cyclical progestin added after 6 to 12 months, depending on the progress of physical development or when breakthrough bleeding occurs. For a person with a tentative diagnosis of constitutional delay therapy is usually reassessed after 4 to 6 months by interrupting treatment to determine whether pubertal hormonal activity has commenced.

DELAYED PUBERTY OF OTHER CAUSES

Defects of Steroidogenesis

Decreased activity of steroidogenic enzymes can delay puberty. Deficiency of 17α-hydroxylase/17,20-lyase (cytochrome P450c17) affects both the adrenal glands and the gonads. Affected persons are unable to synthesize sex steroid hormones, whether androgens or estrogens.[54] At birth, affected 46,XX infants appear to be normal girls, and they present during adolescence with delayed puberty. Impaired testosterone biosynthesis leads to undervirilization of affected 46,XY fetuses. With *complete* loss of function mutations, affected 46,XY infants are generally assigned female sex of rearing and present in adolescence with delayed puberty. As testicular secretion of müllerian inhibitory hormone (MIH) is unaffected, müllerian ducts regress in affected 46,XY children. Affected 46,XY children with *partial* loss of function mutations may present in infancy with ambiguous genitalia. Both 46,XX and 46,XY affected individuals show hypergonadotropic hypogonadism. Hypertension may occur.

This disorder is due to mutations in the 17α-hydroxylase/17,20-lyase gene *(CYP17)*. This single gene codes for the enzyme that catalyzes both activities.[55] The majority of affected persons show both impaired 17α-hydroxylase and 17,20-

lyase activity. Two unrelated persons have been described who have lost approximately 95% of 17,20-lyase activity while retaining approximately 65% of 17α-hydroxylase activity.[56] Laboratory findings include elevated gonadotropins, 11-deoxycorticosterone, and corticosterone concentrations with low androgen, estrogen, and cortisol concentrations. Glucocorticoid and sex steroid replacement therapies are typically required. Inheritance is autosomal-recessive.

Another cause of sexual ambiguity and delayed puberty is 17β-hydroxysteroid dehydrogenase deficiency, a defect of testosterone biosynthesis. Impaired conversion of androstenedione to testosterone results in undervirilization of 46,XY fetuses. At birth, the external genitalia are female or ambiguous, and testes are usually palpable in the inguinal canal. The presence of (MIH) leads to regression of the müllerian structures, so, often, there is only a blind vaginal pouch. At puberty, affected individuals exhibit virilization and/or primary amenorrhea. Laboratory studies show low testosterone and variable estradiol concentrations. Gonadotropin levels are generally, but not always, elevated. Basal androstenedione concentrations are typically 10 times normal. An elevated androstenedione-testosterone ratio is found following hCG administration.

Virilization and nearly normal testosterone concentrations at puberty are characteristic of this rare autosomal-recessive disorder. Mutations in the 17β-hydroxysteroid dehydrogenase type 3 *(17βHSD3)* gene have been identified in affected individuals.[57–59] Measurable testosterone presumably results from the conversion of androstenedione to testosterone catalyzed by one of the unaffected 17β-hydroxysteroid dehydrogenase isozymes. Sisters of affected persons who are either homozygous or compound heterozygous for the same mutations as their affected 46,XY siblings show no clinical abnormalities.[60]

Some 46,XY affected individuals initially raised as girls elect to change to male gender identity when virilization occurs at puberty, whereas others continue in a female gender identity.[57, 61] The high frequency of gender role reversal necessitates comprehensive explanation and evaluation, including psychological assessment prior to gonadectomy.[61]

Sharing some clinical features with 17β-hydroxysteroid dehydrogenase deficiency is the syndrome of 5α-reductase deficiency. This enzyme catalyzes the conversion of testosterone to dihydrotestosterone. Defective enzyme activity in utero results in poor virilization of the genital tubercle and limited development of the penile urethra and fusion of the labioscrotal folds, a form of pseudohermaphroditism also described as *pseudovaginal perineoscrotal hypospadias*. The presence of a normal testis secreting MIH in utero induces regression of müllerian structures. At puberty, further virilization of the external genitalia occurs as a result of increased testosterone secretion, and phallic growth is sufficient so that some persons adopt a male sexual role. Peripheral effects of testosterone on muscle mass and linear growth are also seen in these patients at puberty. Severe hypospadias may not be an absolute barrier to fertility but frequently the vasa deferentia may be incomplete and result in azoospermia. Normal to high serum testosterone levels are the rule, with low dihydrotestosterone and mildly elevated or normal gonadotropin levels, whereas decreased conversion of testosterone to dihydrotestosterone occurs in cultured skin fibroblasts. Inheritance is autosomal-recessive, and the disorder is more common in certain ethnic groups.[62] Several mutations in the 5α-reductase (*SRD5A2*) gene have been described.[63] The normal activity of the type 1 isozyme (*SRD5A1*) likely contributes to the pubertal virilization. As for those with 17β-hydroxysteroid dehydrogenase type 3 deficiency, comprehensive evaluation, including psychological assessment, may be valuable for clinical management.

Defects of Androgen Activity

Complete androgen insensitivity occurs as the result of an androgen receptor defect and is characterized by a female phenotype with primary amenorrhea, a short vagina, absent uterus, and absent sexual hair in the presence of an XY karyotype. Less commonly, an incomplete defect or partial androgen insensitivity may occur with some degree of androgenization and virilization of the external genitalia. The functional testes, often detected as labial masses or associated with inguinal hernias, produce MIH, which induces müllerian regression in utero. Wolffian duct development is not stabilized because of androgen insensitivity. In adolescence, serum gonadotropin and testosterone levels are usually elevated. Increased conversion of testosterone to estrogens contributes to feminization at puberty with spontaneous breast development. Some patients present for evaluation of primary amenorrhea. There is an increased incidence of gonadal tumors in persons with androgen insensitivity, and therefore gonadectomy is recommended, usually by the end of the second decade of life after pubertal development has occurred spontaneously. Partial forms of androgen receptor insensitivity

syndromes may manifest, not only at birth, with varying degrees of sexual ambiguity, but also at puberty, with some degree of virilization. Infertility and gynecomastia in adult men are clinical features of partial androgen insensitivity. Affected individuals raised as females require estrogen replacement therapy to promote breast development. Those with partial androgen insensitivity who are raised as males may benefit from exogenous testosterone.

Androgen insensitivity is due to mutations in the androgen receptor (*AR*) gene,[64] which is located at Xq11-12 and contains 8 exons. Exon 1 codes for the amino-terminal transactivation domain. Exons 2 and 3 code for the DNA-binding domain. Exons 4 through 8 code for the ligand-binding domains. Genital skin fibroblast-binding studies are normal for mutations in exons 1 through 3 and abnormal for mutations in exons 4 through 8. More than 200 different mutations have been described.[65]

DELAYED MENARCHE

Menarche may be delayed in the presence of normal secondary sexual development and may be related to anatomic obstruction of the outflow tract or to abnormalities of ovarian or adrenal steroidogenesis, commonly characterized by hyperandrogenism.

Anatomic Causes

Anatomic causes of primary amenorrhea should be excluded in girls who have full secondary sexual characteristics. Menarche occurs at a mean age of 12½ years and usually at a time when breast and pubic hair development have reached Tanner stage IV. Failure of menarche at a bone age of 13 or with Tanner IV pubertal development should prompt a search for an anatomic cause of the delayed menarche.

Mayer-Rokitansky-Kuster-Hauser syndrome is vaginal agenesis with or without uterine agenesis. It occurs in 1 in every 4000 to 10,000 female births. Remnants of müllerian structures may be palpable on rectoabdominal examination as a midline band of tissue. Magnetic resonance imaging and ultrasonography are useful.[66] Cyclic abdominal pain may occur in those patients who have a partial endometrial cavity.[67] Severe unrecognized mittelschmerz sometimes is manifested as a possible "acute abdomen." Renal abnormalities, especially ectopic kidneys or unilateral renal agenesis, occur in approximately one third of such patients. Skeletal anomalies, especially spinal malformations, are also common and are often discovered serendipitously on radiologic studies. Vaginal development adequate for sexual function is occasionally present, but, commonly, a vaginal dilator, with or without vaginoplasty, is necessary to achieve full sexual capability.[68] The patient's motivation is critical to the success of therapy.

An imperforate hymen is an easily detected and correctable cause of primary amenorrhea in pubertal females with normal secondary sexual characteristics. Endocrine testing shows a normal female ovulatory profile, and ultrasound studies demonstrate normal müllerian structures.

Functional Causes

Primary or secondary amenorrhea may be associated with hyperandrogenism, particularly with the more severe forms. Acne, hirsutism, and clitoromegaly are clinical manifestations of androgen excess. Increased androgen production may occur primarily, through the adrenal gland or the ovary, or secondarily, through peripheral conversion of weakly androgenic precursors. Biochemical confirmation of hyperandrogenism should be obtained before an extensive diagnostic evaluation is undertaken.

HYPERANDROGENISM

Hyperandrogenism of Ovarian Origin

Polycystic ovarian syndrome (PCOS) is a heterogeneous disorder characterized by oligomenorrhea, chronic anovulation, hirsutism, and hyperandrogenism. It has been estimated that 8% of reproductive-aged women suffer from PCOS.[69] The spectrum of severity ranges from milder forms to the classic syndrome described by Stein and Leventhal. Owing to tremendous phenotypic heterogeneity, only some symptoms may be manifested in any individual. PCOS may manifest as primary or secondary amenorrhea and is a common cause of menstrual disturbance in adolescents.[70] Notably, the presence of polycystic ovaries is not required for diagnosis. Hyperinsulinemia and/or insulin resistance are typically present. Consensus diagnostic criteria are hirsutism, ovulatory dysfunction, hyperandrogenism, and exclusion of other disorders such as congenital adrenal hyperplasia, Cushing's syndrome, and hyperprolactinemia.[71] Premature pubarche appears to be an early manifestation of PCOS, especially in obese girls.[72] Investigation of affected adolescent girls has demonstrated hyperandrogenism, hyperinsulinemia or insulin resistance, increased LH-FSH ratio, and decreased sex hormone–binding globulin.[73, 74] Among girls previously evaluated for premature pubarche who develop PCOS, anovulation appears to develop several years after menarche rather than during the early pubertal years.[75]

Affected women are at increased risk to develop impaired glucose tolerance and diabetes mellitus.[76] Several studies suggest increased risk for coronary artery disease and endometrial cancer.[77] An increased frequency of type 2 diabetes mellitus and evidence of impaired glucose tolerance has also been noted in first-degree relatives of girls with premature pubarche.[78]

Familial clustering of cases has led to investigation of the genetic factors associated with PCOS. The extensive phenotypic heterogeneity of PCOS even within a single family has complicated identification of "PCOS" genes. Biochemical phenotyping based on serum testosterone and DHEAS concentrations has demonstrated that first-degree relatives of women with PCOS show a greater risk for hyperandrogenemia than do controls.[79] Candidate gene studies have focused on genes involved in steroidogenesis, insulin action, and obesity.[80] For one candidate gene, *CYP21*, the observed frequency of heterozygosity for mutations in the 21-hydroxylase gene is greater than expected in some populations[81]; however, the frequency of PCOS is not increased among female obligate heterozygote carriers.[82] Thus, additional factors must influence the development of hyperandrogenism in the subset of manifesting heterozygotic carriers of 21-hydroxylase mutations. Available evidence is consistent with the hypothesis that hyperinsulinism, insulin resistance, and obesity magnify a genetic tendency toward hyperandrogenism, leading to excessive ovarian and/or adrenal androgen secretion. This excessive ovarian and/or adrenal androgen secretion influences gonadotropin secretion such that vicious circles of increased LH secretion, decreased FSH secretion, increased androgen secretion, and chronic anovulation ensue. PCOS appears to be a complex trait influenced by multiple genetic and environmental factors.

Laboratory findings typically show elevated basal androstenedione and/or testosterone concentrations. LH is often elevated relative to FSH. Testing with ACTH, GnRH analogue, or human chorionic gonadotropin may be necessary to distinguish chronic anovulatory syndromes from mild congenital adrenal hyperplasia, particularly where DHEAS and basal 17-hydroxyprogesterone levels are slightly elevated.[83] One caveat is that basal and stimulated steroid hormone responses do not clearly distinguish between ovarian and adrenal hyperandrogenism.[84]

Low-dose combination oral contraceptives offer a number of therapeutic advantages in PCOS, in addition to contraception: regulation of menstrual function, suppression of the ovarian androgen production, increased sex hormone–binding globulin production with reduction of free androgen levels, and often improvement of the other manifestations of hyperandrogenism, such as acne and hirsutism. Use of the least androgenic progestin is desirable. Spironolactone can be used to decrease the effects of circulating androgens. Improved insulin sensitivity through weight loss or the use of insulin-sensitizing drugs is also associated with clinical improvement. Although metformin therapy has been beneficial for some women with PCOS,[85] its role as a standard treatment remains to be determined.[86]

Hyperandrogenism of Adrenal Origin

Mild congenital adrenal hyperplasias may manifest in the peripubertal period with premature adrenarche, hirsutism, or oligomenorrhea or amenorrhea. The virilizing congenital adrenal hyperplasias include 21-hydroxylase deficiency ($P450_{C21}$), 11β-hydroxylase deficiency ($P450_{C11}$), and 3β-hydroxysteroid dehydrogenase deficiency. Approximately 90% of cases are due to 21-hydroxylase deficiency, which is caused by loss of function mutations in the 21-hydroxylase (*CYP21*) gene. The most common type of 21-hydroxylase deficiency is the nonclassical (NC-CAH) or late-onset form.[87, 88] Measurement of basal and ACTH-stimulated adrenal 17-hydroxyprogesterone concentrations may be needed to confirm the diagnosis. Correlation of biochemical responses with molecular genotype analysis has shown that most individuals with NC-CAH show an ACTH-stimulated 17-hydroxyprogesterone concentration greater than 1200 ng/dl.

Both 11β-hydroxylase and 3β-hydroxysteroid dehydrogenase deficiency are rare causes of virilizing congenital adrenal hyperplasia. Indeed, nonclassical congenital adrenal hyperplasia due to either 11β-hydroxylase or 3β-hydroxysteroid dehydrogenase deficiency is extremely rare.

Deficiency of 11β-hydroxylase is due to mutations in the 11β-hydroxylase (*CYP11B1*) gene.[89, 90] Hypertension is often detected.[91] Laboratory findings include elevated 11-deoxycortisol concentrations and suppressed peripheral renin activity. The 3β-hydroxysteroid dehydrogenase deficiency is secondary to mutations in the type 2 3β-hydroxysteroid dehydrogenase (*3βHSD2*) gene.[92] The majority of the mutations reported to date are associated with classical forms of 3β-hydroxysteroid dehydrogenase deficiency.[93]

Treatment of the virilizing congenital adrenal hyperplasias involves glucocorticoid therapy to suppress the excessive adrenal androgen secretion. The goal of therapy is to prevent features of androgen excess while maintaining normal linear growth and bone maturation. With appropriate suppressive therapy, regular menses generally occur, although some affected women's androgen concentrations are not adequately suppressed without concomitant ovarian suppression. All patients receiving glucocorticoid suppression should be instructed how to increase their glucocorticoid treatment for acute physiologic stress and should have ready access to injectable hydrocortisone for emergencies.

EVALUATION OF THE PATIENT WITH DELAYED PUBERTY

The sequence for evaluation is determined by the patient's history and physical examination (Table 6–2). Thorough questioning about past medical illnesses is important to assess for chronic conditions. A history of central nervous system, ocular, olfactory, pelvic, gonadal, and genital abnormalities should be obtained. Age of onset of pubertal development in both parents and siblings should be elicited. Linear growth for age should be carefully plotted (Fig. 6–3).

Height, weight, and the extent of any evidence of pubertal development should be noted. Physical findings consistent with estrogen and androgen effects should be noted. Longitudinal growth data may be very helpful in the evaluation of pubertal delay. For example, a short girl with delayed puberty requires a determination of karyotype to exclude Turner syndrome in addition to an evaluation for endocrine disorders (e.g., growth hormone deficiency, thyroid hormone deficiency, or hypercortisolism). The presence of breast development and primary amenorrhea suggests testicular feminization as well as Mayer-Rokitansky-Kuster-Hauser syndrome. In contrast, primary amenorrhea and hirsutism are more suggestive of hyperandrogenism.

Useful laboratory studies include determinations of LH, FSH, prolactin, DHEAS, and estradiol levels. Hypothyroidism should be excluded

Table 6–2. Findings in Delayed Puberty

Diagnosis	Breast	Sexual Hair	Stature	BA	LH	FSH	Estrogens	Androgens	Pelvic
Hypergonadotropic									
Turner syndrome	A	±	↓↓	↓	↑↑	↑↑	↓	N or ↓	Streak
Mixed gonadal dysgenesis	A	±	N or ↓	N or ↓	↑	↑	↓	N, ↓, or ↑	Streak
Pure gonadal dysgenesis	A	±	↑	N or ↓	↑	↑	↓	N, ↓, or ↑	Streak
Primary ovarian failure	A	±	N	N or ↓	↑	↑	↓	N or ↓	Variable
Hypogonadotropic									
Constitutional delay	A	A	N or ↓	↓	↓	↓	↓	↓	Normal
Female Kallmann syndrome	A	A	N or ↑	↓	↓	↓	↓	↓	Normal
Miscellaneous									
Chronic disease	±	±	N or ↓	N or ↓	↓	↓	↓	↓	Normal
Anorexia nervosa	±	±	N	N or ↓	↓	↓	↓	↓	Normal
Hypothyroidism	±	±	N or ↓	↓	↓	↓	↓	N	Normal
Cushing syndrome	±	± or ↑	N or ↓	↓	↓	↓	↓	N or ↑	Normal
Virilizing errors in steroidogenesis	±	↑	N or ↓	↑	↓	↓	↓	↑	N/cyst
Androgen insensitivity	P	↓	N or ↑	N	↑	↑	↑	↑	No uterus
Mayer-Rokitansky-Kuster-Hauser syndrome	P	P	N	N	N	N	N	N	Abnormal

±, Absent or present; ↓, decreased; ↑, increased; A, absent; cyst, polycystic ovaries; N, normal; P, present; streak, streak gonad.

with measurements of thyroxine and thyrotropin levels. Bone age radiographs can be used to document degree of delay, monitor subsequent development, and provide an estimate of adult height. Elevated gonadotropin levels confirm a diagnosis of gonadal failure unless puberty is so long delayed that the bone age is less than 10 to 11 years. A progesterone withdrawal test may be helpful in girls with primary amenorrhea to assess estrogenization of the uterus and patency of the uterovaginal outflow tract. After ensuring that the patient is not pregnant, oral progesterone (10 mg daily) can be administered for 10 days. Withdrawal bleeding generally occurs within 72 hours of completing the progesterone treatment.

Differentiating constitutional delay from hypogonadotropic hypogonadism is often difficult unless coincident disorders make hypothalamic-pituitary dysfunction probable. Low gonadotropin levels are present in both constitutional delay and permanent hypogonadotropic hypogonadism. Serum levels of adrenal androgens such as DHEAS indicate evidence of adrenarche and usually correlate with pubertal development. Therefore, prepubertal androgen levels are the usual finding in constitutional delay, whereas pubertal androgen levels in the absence of evidence of puberty may be more consistent with hypogonadotropic hypogonadism.

Responses to GnRH stimulation in both constitutional delay and hypogonadotropic hypogonadism are similar and have no prognostic value in cases of constitutional delay. Responses to GnRH may be useful in differentiating gonadotropin sufficiency from gonadotropin insufficiency in patients with other known pituitary disease or evidence of Kallmann syndrome (see Fig. 6–2). No single blood test, imaging technique, or stimulation study fully distinguishes between these two entities. The variability of gonadotropin pulse patterns in individuals with pubertal delay and those with hypogonadotropic hypogonadism limits the utility of these studies. Even the apparent lack of pubertal sleep-enhanced gonadotropin secretion and poor synchronization of LH and FSH pulses in hypogonadotropic hypogonadal persons may fail to differentiate the two conditions.[31] Longitudinal observation remains the best means to distinguish between these diagnoses.

TREATMENT OF DELAYED PUBERTY

For induction of the secondary sexual changes of puberty in girls, estrogen replacement therapy may be given as ethinyl estradiol (5 to 10 mg daily), conjugated equine estrogens (0.3 mg daily), or transdermal 17β-estradiol (Estraderm, 0.025 mg). Because of first-pass hepatic effects, oral agents are associated with greater levels of sex hormone and other carrier proteins and renin substrate. High-density lipoprotein cholesterol levels are also greater. Transdermal systems pro-

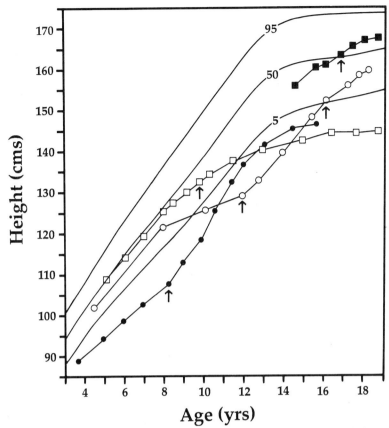

Figure 6–3. Height according to age for four females who presented with delayed puberty. □, A patient with panhypopituitarism and severe mental deficit secondary to the presence and treatment of an astrocytoma. Diagnosis was made and the tumor treated at the point designated by the arrow. Because of mental deficit, the parents elected not to treat with growth hormone or pubertal hormones. Note the extreme short stature. ○, A girl with growth hormone and gonadotropin deficiency secondary to a craniopharyngioma in whom growth hormone therapy was begun at age 12 *(arrow)* and sex steroid therapy at age 16 *(arrow)*. Note acceptable adult height. ●, A patient with growth hormone deficiency in whom growth hormone therapy was begun at age 8 years and who subsequently had spontaneous pubertal development. ■, A patient with Kallmann syndrome first treated with sex steroids at age 17 years. Note normal stature for age.

vide the added advantage of measurable blood levels of estradiol and have been successfully utilized in hypogonadal girls.[94, 95] After 12 to 18 months of unopposed estrogen therapy or after vaginal bleeding occurs, a progestin should be added; for long-term replacement programs, the estrogen may be increased. Oral progestin, usually medroxyprogesterone acetate (Provera, 5 or 10 mg daily), can be added to the estrogen regimen in a sequential fashion. Oral contraceptive therapy is an additional option for long-term replacement, particularly in sexually active patients, recognizing that this approach to estrogen replacement therapy is less physiologic. Replacement treatment is also indicated to reduce the risk of osteoporosis.[96]

Height for age and growth potential, as projected by height, chronologic age, and skeletal age, should be major considerations in the timing and intensity of sex steroid therapy, particularly when treatment with other growth-promoting hormones is indicated (see Fig. 6–3). Untimely treatment or large doses may disproportionately accelerate skeletal maturation and further shorten adult height.

Although this text focuses primarily on girls, similar considerations apply to boys. Intramuscular testosterone enanthate or testosterone cypionate can be used to induce pubertal development. The initial dose is 50 to 100 mg administered monthly. When constitutional delay cannot be clearly differentiated from hypogonadotropic hypogonadism, a course of hormone replacement therapy to induce secondary sexual characteristics, followed by a period of observation off therapy, may be beneficial for psychosocial reasons.

PSYCHOSOCIAL ASPECTS OF DELAYED PUBERTY

Significant delay in pubertal development may be associated with poor self-esteem and reduced academic performance and socialization with peers. Parents' and teachers' attitudes are partly determined by the physical maturity of the adolescent and, therefore, the difficulties of adolescence may be compounded, particularly when short stature is associated, and lead to prolonged dependency on parents.[97]

REFERENCES

1. Kocova M, Siegel SF, Wenger SL, et al: Detection of Y chromosome sequences in Turner's syndrome by Southern blot analysis of amplified DNA. Lancet 1993; 342:140.
2. Conte FA, Grumbach MM, Kaplan SL: A diphasic pattern of gonadotropin secretion in patients with the syndrome of gonadal dysgenesis. J Clin Endocrinol Metab 1975; 40:670.
3. Mendonca BB, Barbosa AS, Arnhold IJP, et al: Gonadal agenesis in XX and XY sisters: Evidence for the involvement of an autosomal gene. Am J Med Genet 1994; 52:39.
4. Bosze P, Skripeczky K, Gaal M, et al: Perrault's syndrome in two sisters. Am J Med Genet 1983; 16:237.
5. Jager RJ, Anvret M, Hall K, Scherer G: A human XY female with a frame shift mutation in the candidate testis-determining gene SRY. Nature 1990; 348:452.
6. Veitia R, Ion A, Barbaux S, et al: Mutations and sequence variants in the testis-determining region of the Y chromosome in individuals with a 46,XY female phenotype. Hum Genet 1997; 99:648.
7. Vilain E, McElreavey K, Jaubert F, et al: Familial case with sequence variant in the testis-determining region associated with two sex phenotypes. Am J Hum Genet 1992; 50:1008.
8. Bardoni B, Zanaria E, Guioli S, et al: A dosage sensitive locus at chromosome Xp21 is involved in male to female sex reversal. Nat Genet 1994; 7:497.
9. Rivkees SA, Crawford JD: The relationship of gonadal activity and chemotherapy-induced gonadal damage. JAMA 1988; 259:2123.
10. Poplack DG: Acute lymphoblastic leukemia. In Pizzo PA, Poplack DG (eds): Principles and Practice of Pediatric Oncology. Philadelphia: JB Lippincott, 1989, p. 323.
11. Gibson JB: Gonadal function in galactosemics and in galactose-intoxicated animals. Eur J Pediatr 1995; 154:S14.
12. Stavrou SS, Zhu YS, Cai LQ, et al: A novel mutation of the human luteinizing hormone receptor in 46XY and 46XX sisters. J Clin Endocrinol Metab 1998; 83:2091.
13. Latronico AC, Chai Y, Arnhold IJ, et al: A homozygous microdeletion in helix 7 of the luteinizing hormone receptor associated with familial testicular and ovarian re-

14. el-Awady MK, Temtamy SA, Salam MA, Gad YZ: Familial Leydig cell hypoplasia as a cause of male pseudohermaphroditism. Hum Hered 1987; 37:36.
15. Zenteno JC, Canto P, Kofman-Alfaro S, Mendez JP: Evidence for genetic heterogeneity in male pseudohermaphroditism due to Leydig cell hypoplasia. J Clin Endocrinol Metab 1999; 84:3803.
16. Beau I, Touraine P, Meduri G, et al: A novel phenotype related to partial loss of function mutations of the follicle stimulating hormone receptor. J Clin Invest 1998; 102:1352.
17. Touraine P, Beau I, Gougeon A, et al: New natural inactivating mutations of the follicle-stimulating hormone receptor: Correlations between receptor function and phenotype. Molec Endocrinol 1999; 13:1844.
18. Jones JR, Kemmann E: Olfacto-genital dysplasia in the female. Obstet Gynecol Ann 1976; 5:443.
19. Waldstreicher J, Seminara SB, Jameson JL, et al: The genetic and clinical heterogeneity of gonadotropin-releasing hormone deficiency in the human. J Clin Endocrinol Metab 1996; 81:4388.
20. White BJ, Rogol AD, Brown KS: The syndrome of anosmia with hypogonadotropic hypogonadism: A genetic study of 18 new families and a review. Am J Med Genet 1983; 15:417.
21. Merriam GR, Beitins IZ, Bode HH: Father-to-son transmission of hypogonadism with anosmia. Am J Dis Child 1977; 131:1216.
22. Weiss J, Crowley WF Jr, Jameson JL: Normal structure of the gonadotropin-releasing hormone (GnRH) gene in patients with GnRH deficiency and idiopathic hypogonadotropic hypogonadism. J Clin Endocrinol Metab 1989; 69:299.
23. Bick D, Franco B, Sherins RJ, et al: Brief report: Intragenic deletion of the Kalig-1 gene in Kallmann's syndrome. N Engl J Med 1992; 326:1752.
24. Hardelin J-P, Levilliers J, Young J, et al: Xp22.3 deletions in isolated familial Kallmann's syndrome. J Clin Endocrinol Metab 1993; 76:827.
25. Franco B, Guioli A, Pragliola A, et al: A gene deleted in Kallmann's syndrome shares homology with neural cell adhesion and axonal path-finding molecules. Nature 1991; 353:529.
26. Legouis R, Hardelin J-P, Levilliers J, et al: The candidate gene for the X-linked Kallmann syndrome encodes a protein related to adhesion molecules. Cell 1991; 67:423.
27. Bimbacher R, Wandl-Vergesslich K, Frisch H: Diagnosis of X-recessive Kallmann syndrome in early infancy. Eur J Pediatr 1994; 153:245.
28. Georgopoulos NA, Pralong FP, Seidman CE, et al: Genetic heterogeneity evidenced by low incidence of Kal-I gene mutations in sporadic cases of gonadotropin-releasing hormone deficiency. J Clin Endocrinol Metab 1997; 82:213.
29. de Roux N, Young J, Brailly-Tabard S, et al: The same molecular defects of the gonadotropin-releasing hormone receptor determine a variable degree of hypogonadism in affected kindred. J Clin Endocrinol Metab 1999; 84:567.
30. Habiby RL, Boepple P, Nachtigall L, et al: Adrenal hypoplasia congenita with hypogonadotropic hypogonadism. Evidence that DAX-1 mutations lead to combined hypothalamic and pituitary defects in gonadotropin production. J Clin Invest 1996; 98:1055.
31. Wu FCW, Butler GE, Kelnar CJH, et al: Patterns of pulsatile luteinizing hormone and follicle-stimulating hormone secretion in prepubertal (midchildhood) boys

and girls and patients with idiopathic hypogonadotropic hypogonadism (Kallman's syndrome): A study using an ultrasensitive time-resolved immunofluorometric assay. J Clin Endocrinol Metab 1991; 72:1229.

32. Spratt DI, Carr DB, Merriam GR, et al: The spectrum of abnormal patterns of gonadotropin-releasing hormone secretion in men with idiopathic hypogonadotropic hypogonadism: Clinical and laboratory correlations. J Clin Endocrinol Metab 1987; 64:283.

33. Matthews CH, Borgato S, Beck-Peccoz P, et al: Primary amenorrhoea and infertility due to a mutation in the β-subunit of follicle-stimulating hormone. Nat Genet 1993; 5:83.

34. Root AW: Magnetic resonance imaging in hypopituitarism. J Clin Endocrinol Metab 1991; 72:10.

35. Sadeghi-Nejad A, Wolfsdorf JI, Biller BJ, et al: Hyperprolactinemia causing primary amenorrhea. J Pediatr 1981; 99:802.

36. Huseman CA, Kelch RP, Hopwood NJ, Zipf WB: Sexual precocity in association with septo-optic dysplasia and hypothalamic hypopituitarism. J Pediatrics 1978; 92:748.

37. Cheyne KL, Lightner ES, Comerci GD: Bromocriptine-unresponsive prolactin macroadenoma in a prepubertal female. J Adolesc Health Care 1988; 9:331.

38. Howlett TA, Wass JAH, Grossman A, et al: Prolactinomas presenting as primary amenorrhea and delayed or arrested puberty: Response to medical therapy. Clin Endocrinol 1989; 30:131.

39. De Sanctis V, Vullo C, Katz M, et al: Gonadal function in patients with thalassaemia major. J Clin Pathol 1988; 41:133.

40. Kelly TM, Edwards CO, Meikle AW, Kushner JP: Hypogonadism in hemochromatosis: Reversal with iron depletion. Ann Intern Med 1984; 101:629.

41. Soyka LA, Grinspoon S, Levitsky LL, et al: The effects of anorexia nervosa on bone metabolism in female adolescents. J Clin Endocrinol Metab 1999; 84:4489.

42. Mansfield MJ, Emans SJ: Anorexia nervosa, athletics, and amenorrhea. Pediatr Clin North Am 1989; 36:533.

43. Pugliese MT, Lifshitz F, Grad G, et al: Fear of obesity. A cause of short stature and delayed puberty. N Engl J Med 1983; 309:513.

44. Veldhuis JD, Evans WS, Demers LM, et al: Altered neuroendocrine regulation of gonadotropin secretion in women distance runners. J Clin Endocrinol Metab 1985; 61:557.

45. Berga SL, Mortola JF, Girton L, et al: Neuroendocrine aberrations in women with functional hypothalamic amenorrhea. J Clin Endocrinol Metab 1989; 68:301.

46. Biller BMK, Federoff HJ, Koenig JI, Klibanski A: Abnormal cortisol secretion and responses to corticotropin-releasing hormone in women with hypothalamic amenorrhea. J Clin Endocrinol Metab 1990; 70:311.

47. Bullen BA, Skrinar GS, Beitins IZ, et al: Induction of menstrual disorders by strenuous exercise in untrained women. N Engl J Med 1985; 312:1349.

48. Pantsiotou S, Stanhope R, Uruena M, et al: Growth prognosis and growth after menarche in primary hypothyroidism. Arch Dis Child 1991; 66:838.

49. Ross RJ, Trainer PJ: Endocrine investigation: Cushing's syndrome. Clin Endocrinol 1998; 49:153.

50. Young T-L, Woods MO, Parfrey PS, et al: A founder effect in the Newfoundland population reduces the Bardet-Diedl syndrome (BBS1) interval to 1 cM. Am J Hum Genet 1999; 65:1680.

51. Green JS, Parfrey PS, Harnett JD, et al: The cardinal manifestations of Bardet-Biedl syndrome, a form of Laurence-Moon-Biedl syndrome. N Engl J Med 1989; 321:1002.

52. Couper R: Prader-Willi syndrome. J Paediatrics Child Health 1999; 35:331.

53. Jones KL: Prader-Willi syndrome. *In* Smith's Recognizable Patterns of Human Malformation, 4th ed. Philadelphia: WB Saunders, 1988, p 170.

54. Winter JSD, Couch RM, Muller J, et al: Combined 17-hydroxylase and 17,20-desmolase deficiencies: Evidence for synthesis of a defective cytochrome P450$_{c17}$. J Clin Endocrinol Metab 1989; 68:309.

55. Yanase T, Simpson ER, Waterman MR: 17α-hydroxylase/17,20 lyase deficiency: From clinical investigation to molecular definition. Endocrinol Rev 1991; 12:91.

56. Geller DH, Auchus RJ, Mendonca BB, Miller WL: The genetic and functional basis of isolated 17,20-lyase activity. Nat Genet 1997; 17:201.

57. Geissler WM, Davis DL, Wu L, et al: Male pseudohermaphroditism caused by mutations of testicular 17β-hydroxysteroid dehydrogenase 3. Nat Genet 1994; 7:34.

58. Andersson S, Geissler WM, Wu L, et al: Molecular genetics and pathophysiology of 17β-hydroxysteroid dehydrogenase 3 deficiency. J Clin Endocrinol Metab 1996; 81:130.

59. Boehmer ALM, Brinkmann AO, Sandkuijl LA, et al: 17β-Hydroxysteroid dehydrogenase-3 deficiency: Diagnosis, phenotypic variability, population genetics, and worldwide distribution of ancient and de novo mutations. J Clin Endocrinol Metab 1999; 84:4713.

60. Mendonca BB, Arnhold IJP, Bloise W, et al: 17β-hydroxysteroid dehydrogenase 3 deficiency in women. J Clin Endocrinol Metab 1999; 84:802.

61. Wilson JD: The role of androgens in male gender role behavior. Endocrin Rev 1999; 20:726.

62. Imperato-McGinley J, Guerrero L, Gautier T, Peterson RE: Steroid 5α-reductase deficiency in man: An inherited form of male pseudohermaphroditism. Science 1974; 186:1213.

63. Thigpen AE, Davis DL, Milatovich A, et al: Molecular genetics of steroid 5α-reductase 2 deficiency. J Clin Invest 1992; 90:799.

64. Quigley CA, DeBellis A, Marschke KB, et al: Androgen receptor defects: Historical, clinical, and molecular perspectives. Endocrinol Rev 1995; 16:271.

65. Gottlieb B, Lehvaslaiho H, Beitel LK, et al: The androgen receptor gene mutations database. Nucleic Acids Res 1998; 26:234.

66. Hugosson C, Jorulf H, Bakri Y: MRI in distal vaginal atresia. Pediatr Radiol 1991; 21:281.

67. Griffin JE, Edwards C, Madden JD, et al: Congenital absence of the vagina—the Mayer-Rokitansky-Kuster-Hauser syndrome. Ann Intern Med 1976; 85:224.

68. Ellis CEG, Dewhurst J: A simplified approach to management of congenital absence of the vagina and uterus. Pediatr Adolesc Gynecol 1984; 2:25.

69. Knochenhauer ES, Key TJ, Kashar-Miller M, et al: Prevalence of the polycystic ovary syndrome in unselected Black and White women of the Southeastern United States: A prospective study. J Clin Endocrinol Metab 1998; 83:3678.

70. Van Hooff MHA, Voorhorst FJ, Kaptein MBH, et al: Endocrine features of polycystic ovary syndrome in a random population sample of 14–16 year old adolescents. Hum Reprod 1999; 14:2223.

71. Dunaif A, Givens JR, Haseltine FP, et al: Polycystic Ovary Syndrome: Current Issues in Endocrinology and Metabolism. Boston: Blackwell Scientific, 1992.

72. Ibanez L, Potau N, Virdis R, et al: Postpubertal outcome in girls diagnosed of premature pubarche during childhood: Increased frequency of functional ovarian hyperandrogenism. J Clin Endocrinol Metabol 1993; 76:1599.

73. Ibanez L, Potau N, Zampolli M, et al: Hyperinsulinemia and decreased insulin-like growth factor—binding protein-1 are common features in prepubertal and pubertal girls with a history of premature pubarche. J Clin Endocrinol Metabol 1997; 82:2283.

74. Apter D, Butzow T, Laughlin GA, Yen SS: Accelerated 24-hour luteinizing hormone pulsatile activity in adolescent girls with ovarian hyperandrogenism: relevance to the developmental phase of polycystic ovarian syndrome. J Clin Endocrinol Metab 1994; 79:119.

75. Ibanez L, de Zegher F, Potau N: Anovulation after precocious pubarche: Early markers and time course in adolescence. J Clin Endocrinol Metab 1999; 84:2691.

76. Legro RS, Kunselman AR, Dodson WC, Dunaif A: Prevalence and predictors of risk for type 2 diabetes mellitus and impaired glucose tolerance in polycystic ovary syndrome: A prospective, controlled study in 254 affected women. J Clin Endocrinol Metab 1999; 84:165.

77. Solomon CG: The epidemiology of polycystic ovary syndrome: prevalence and associated disease risk. Endocrinol Metab Clin North Am 1999; 28:247.

78. Ibanez L, Castell C, Tresserra R, Potau N: Increased prevalence of type 2 diabetes mellitus and impaired glucose tolerance in first-degree relatives of girls with a history of precocious puberty. Clin Endocrinol 1999; 51:395.

79. Legro RS, Driscoll D, Strauss JF III, et al: Evidence for a genetic basis for hyperandrogenemia in the polycystic ovary syndrome. Proc Natl Acad Sci 1998; 98:14956.

80. Urbanek M, Legro RS, Driscoll DA, et al: Thirty-seven candidate genes for polycystic ovary syndrome: Strongest evidence for linkage is with follistatin. Proc Natl Acad Sci 1999; 96:8573.

81. Witchel SF, Lee PA, Suda-Hartman M, Hoffman EP: Hyperandrogenism and manifesting heterozygotes for 21-hydroxylase deficiency. Biochem Molec Med 1997; 62:151.

82. Knochenhauer ES, Cortet-Rudelli C, Cunnigham RD, et al: Carriers of 21-hydroxylase deficiency are not at increased risk for hyperandrogenism. J Clin Endocrinol Metab 1997; 82:479.

83. Witchel SF, Lee PA: Human chorionic gonadotropin stimulation to assess for ovarian hyperandrogenism. J Pediatr Adolesc Gynecol 1998; 11:73.

84. Escobar-Morreale HF, San Millan JL, Smith RR, et al: The presence of the 21-hydroxylase deficiency carrier status in hirsute women: Phenotype-genotype correlations. Fertil Steril 199; 72:629.

85. Nestler JE, Jakubowicz DJ, Evans WS, Pasquali R: Effects of metformin on spontaneous and clomiphene-induced ovulation in the polycystic ovary syndrome. N Engl J Med 1998; 338:1876.

86. Ehrmann DA, Cavaghan MK, Imperial J, et al: Effects of metformin on insulin secretion, insulin action, and ovarian steroidogenesis in women with polycystic ovary syndrome. J Clin Endocrinol Metab 1997; 82:524.

87. Pang S, Wallace MA, Holman L, et al: Worldwide experience in newborn screening for classical congenital adrenal hyperplasia due to 21-hydroxylase deficiency. Pediatrics 1988; 81:866.

88. Miller WL, Morel Y: Molecular genetics of 21-hydroxylase deficiency. Annu Rev Genet 1989; 23:371.

89. Curnow KM, Slutsker L, Vitek J, et al: Mutations in the CYP11B1 gene causing congenital adrenal hyperplasia and hypertension cluster in exons 6, 7, and 8. Proc Natl Acad Sci 1993; 90:4552.

90. Merke DP, Tajima T, Chhabra A, et al: Novel CYP11B1 mutations in congenital adrenal hyperplasia due to steroid 11β-hydroxylase deficiency. J Clin Endocrinol Metab 1999; 83:270.

91. Zachmann P, Tassinari D, Prader A: Clinical and biochemical variability of congenital adrenal hyperplasia due to 11α-hydroxylase deficiency. A study of 25 cases. J Clin Endocrinol Metab 1983; 56:222.

92. Rhéaume E, Simard J, Morel Y, et al: Congenital adrenal hyperplasia due to point mutations in the type II 3β-hydroxysteroid dehydrogenase gene. Nat Genet 1992; 1:239.

93. Moisan AM, Ricketts ML, Tardy V, et al: New insight into the molecular basis of 3β-hydroxysteroid dehydrogenase deficiency: Identification of eight mutations in the HSD3B2 gene in eleven patients from seven new families and comparison of the functional properties of twenty-five mutant enzymes. J Clin Endocrinol Metab 1999; 84:4410.

94. Chetkowski RJ, Meldrum DR, Steingold KA, et al: Biologic effects of transdermal estradiol. N Engl J Med 1986; 314:1615.

95. Illig R, DeCampo C, Lang-Muritano MR, et al: A physiological mode of puberty induction in hypogonadal girls by low dose transdermal 17β-oestradiol. Eur J Pediatr 1990; 150:86.

96. Emans SJ, Grace E, Hoffer FA, et al: Estrogen deficiency in adolescents and young adults: Impact on bone mineral content and effects of estrogen replacement therapy. Obstet Gynecol 1990; 76:585.

97. Mazur T, Clopper RR: Pubertal disorders—psychology and clinical management. Endocrinol Metab Clin North Am 1991; 20:211.

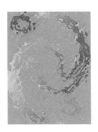

Chapter 7
Disorders of Sexual Differentiation

Joe Leigh Simpson

EMBRYOLOGY OF THE REPRODUCTIVE SYSTEM

Primordial germ cells originate in the endoderm of the yolk sac and migrate to the genital ridge to form the indifferent gonad. Initially, 46,XY and 46,XX gonads are indistinguishable. Indifferent gonads develop into testes when the embryo, or more specifically the gonadal stroma, is 46,XY. This process begins about 43 days after conception. Testes become morphologically identifiable 7 to 8 weeks after conception (9 to 10 gestational or menstrual weeks).

TESTICULAR DIFFERENTIATION

Sertoli cells are the first cells to become recognizable in testicular differentiation, organizing the surrounding cells into tubules. Both Leydig cells[1] and Sertoli cells[2] function in dissociation from testicular morphogenesis, consistent with their directing gonadal development rather than the converse. These two cell types secrete different hormones that, in aggregate, direct subsequent male differentiation (Fig. 7–1).

Fetal Leydig cells produce an androgen, testosterone, that stabilizes wolffian ducts and permits differentiation of the vasa deferentia, epididymides, and seminal vesicles. After conversion by 5α-reductase to dihydrotestosterone (DHT), external genitalia are virilized. These actions can be mimicked by administering testosterone to female or castrated male embryos (as demonstrated clinically in teratogenic forms of female pseudohermaphroditism). Fetal Sertoli cells produce anti-Müllerian hormone (AMH, or Müllerian inhibitory substance [MIS]), a glycoprotein that diffuses locally to produce regression of müllerian derivatives (uterus and fallopian tubes). This hormone also has functions related to gonadal development. When AMH is overexpressed in XX transgenic mice, oocytes fail to persist, tubulelike structures develop in gonads, and müllerian differentiation is abnormal.[3] AMH also exerts an inhibitory effect on oocyte meiosis and plays a role in the descent of the testes.[4] AMH is detectable in the serum of males throughout life but is not measurable in females until the second decade of life; thus, the presence of AMH can be a sensitive marker for the presence of testicular tissue in patients with male pseudohermaphroditism or true hermaphroditism.[5]

OVARIAN DIFFERENTIATION

In the absence of a Y chromosome, the indifferent gonad develops into an ovary. Transformation into fetal ovaries begins at 50 to 55 days of embryonic development. Germ cells are initially present in 45,X embryos[6] but atresia is more rapid than in normal 45,XX embryos.

DUCTAL AND GENITAL DIFFERENTIATION

Independent of gonadal differentiation is the development of ductal and external genitalia. In the absence of testosterone and AMH, external genitalia develop in female fashion. Müllerian ducts form the uterus and fallopian tubes; wolffian ducts regress. Such changes occur in normal XX embryos and in XY animals that were castrated as embryos before testicular differentiation.

GENETIC CONTROL OF SEX DIFFERENTIATION

Both sex chromosomes (X and Y) and autosomes contain loci that must remain intact for normal sexual development to occur. The chro-

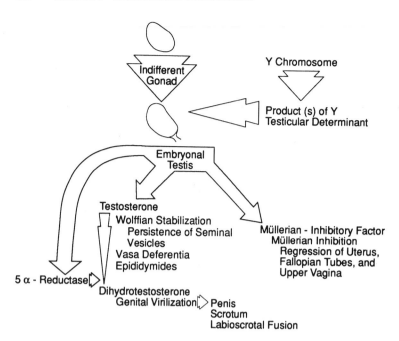

Figure 7–1. Schematic diagram illustrating embryonic differentiation in the normal male. (From Simpson JL: Genetics of sexual differentiation. *In* Rock JA, Carpenter SE [eds]: Pediatric and Adolescent Gynecology. New York: Raven Press, 1992.)

mosomal location of these loci is important for clinical management, because autosomal factors that influence sexual development would be predicted to be perturbed by autosomal rearrangements.

GENETICS OF TESTICULAR DEVELOPMENT

Y Chromosome

That 46,X,i(Yq) individuals were female in appearance was the first indication that the major testicular determinants (testis-determining factor or TDF) were localized to the Y short arm (Yp). Since those observations were first made, 30 years ago, various genes have been proposed as the TDF. First, the region was localized to the distal Y short arm just below the pseudoautosomal boundary. In the 1980s, first H-Y antigen (HYA) and later ZFY were considered strong candidates. Since the early 1990s, the consensus

has been that the gene SRY (sex-determining region Y) is the testicular determinant.[7, 8]

Identification of SRY came as result of mapping in 46,XX males and sporadic 46,XY phenotypic females (gonadal dysgenesis). The cause of most (80%) 46,XX males involves interchange of not just the usual pseudoautosomal regions of Xp and Yp, but also the contiguous proximal nonpseudoautosomal region. In XX males, SRY was present in the smallest translocated region compatible with male differentiation. That SRY, and not ZFY, was pivotal was shown by the fact that some 46,XX males show SRY but not ZFY. Moreover, 10% to 15% of persons with sporadic XY gonadal dysgenesis (phenotypic females) show point mutations within SRY.[9]

The SRY gene is composed of two open reading frames consisting of 99 and 273 amino acids (Fig. 7–2), respectively. Judging from females with XY gonadal dysgenesis who have mutations involving SRY,[9–12] the key sequence involves a high-mobility group box that shares characteristics with other DNA-binding sequences. When XY gonadal dysgenesis is associated with a point

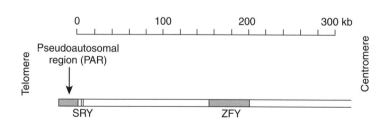

Figure 7–2. Schematic diagram illustrating the SRY gene.

mutation or deletion in SRY, the mutant sequence has always been located in the high-mobility group box. SRY is also expressed before testicular differentiation is manifested.[7] Transgenic XX mice with SRY, predictably, show testicular differentiation.[13]

X Chromosome

In addition to genes on the Y chromosome, various clinical disorders indicate that testicular differentiation also requires loci on X. The importance of genes on the X chromosome was first evidenced by an X-linked recessive form of XY gonadal dysgenesis.[14, 15] Xp also contains a region that, when duplicated, suppresses testicular development despite the presence of SRY. First recognized by Bernstein and coworkers,[16] this phenomenon has since been observed in more than a dozen other cases.[17–20] The duplicated gene responsible for this phenomenon[21] has been called *dose-sensitive sex reversal* (DSS). The sex reversal (male to female despite an intact Y) appears to be the result of Xp duplication, not disruption, given molecular analysis showing breakpoints encompassing the entire region believed to include the gene. The locus is near that for adrenal hypoplasia (AHC), but the exact relationship to DSS remains obscure.

Autosomes

Autosomal loci are pivotal for testicular differentiation. Several autosomal regions have generated special interest—9p, 10q, 11p, 17q. The gene responsible for camptomelic dysplasia and XY gonadal dysgenesis (sex reversal), localized to 17q24.3→q25.1, has been studied especially extensively.[22] Pathogenesis involves SOX9, like SRY a DNA protein with an HMG box;[23] however, analysis of SOX9 in camptomelic dysplasia has not always shown correlations with sex reversal,[24] suggesting genetic heterogeneity.

The Wilms tumor–suppressor gene (WT-1), located on 11p, is associated with gonadal and genital abnormalities (male pseudohermaphroditism);[25, 26] however, WT-1 is apparently rarely (if ever) deleted in XY gonadal dysgenesis.[27] Deletions of 10q have also been associated with XY gonadal dysgenesis.[28]

The autosomal region that is most pivotal could be 9p.[29, 30] Perhaps 70% of 46,XY persons with del(9p) show sex reversal,[31] and increasing numbers of XY gonadal dysgenesis cases are associated with del(9p).[30, 32, 33] Vegetti and coworkers[30]

found that five of nine XY gonadal dysgenesis cases showed 9p deletions.

Other syndromes deleteriously affecting testicular differentiation are heritable in autosomal fashion but have not been localized to a specific chromosomal region. These include agonadia,[34] rudimentary testes syndrome,[35] and the syndrome of germ cell hypoplasia in both males (germinal cell aplasia) and females (streak gonads).[36–40] Another line of evidence that autosomal regions control male differentiation is the existence of XX true hermaphrodites, who almost always lack SRY.

GENETICS OF OVARIAN DEVELOPMENT

In the absence of a Y chromosome, the indifferent gonad develops into an ovary. Germ cells exist in 45,X human fetuses[6] and 39,X mice;[41] thus, presumably the pathogenesis of germ cell failure involves increased germ cell attrition, not failure of formation. If two intact X chromosomes are not present, 45,X ovarian follicles usually degenerate by birth. The second X chromosome is therefore responsible for ovarian *maintenance*, as opposed to ovarian *differentiation*.

Ovarian maintenance can be deduced (phenotype-karyotype correlations) to exist on both Xp and Xq.[42–48] Each arm probably has several distinct regions of differential importance for ovarian development, a topic that will be discussed at length later. In addition to regions on the X chromosome, autosomal loci are essential for normal ovarian development. It has been accepted for more than 30 years that an autosomal-recessive gene causes gonadal dysgenesis in XX individuals,[14, 49] and, more recently, other related yet genetically distinct entities have been recognized.[48]

MONOSOMY X (TURNER SYNDROME)

The complement most frequently associated with ovarian dysgenesis is 45,X. The proportion of 45,X individuals in a given sample depends on the method of ascertainment. Fewer 45,X individuals are detected if primary amenorrhea is used as the presenting complaint than if short stature or other somatic anomalies are used. Primary amenorrhea is more likely to be the presenting complaint in 45,X women identified by gynecologists, whereas short stature is more likely in children identified by pediatricians.

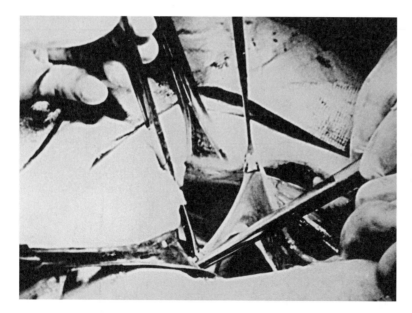

Figure 7–3. A streak gonad. (From Simpson JL: Disorders of Sexual Differentiation: Etiology and Clinical Delineation. New York: Academic Press, 1976.)

Overall, about 50% of all patients with gonadal dysgenesis have a 45,X complement; 25% have sex chromosome mosaicism with a structural abnormality (e.g., 45,X/46,XX). Far fewer have a structurally abnormal X or Y chromosome.[50, 51]

In 80% of cases, the paternally derived X is not present.[52] With one possible exception to be noted, the phenotype does not differ between 45,X^m and 45,X^P cases (X^m,X, maternal origin; X^P,X, paternal origin). In structurally abnormal X chromosomes, it is also the paternal X that is lost.[53, 54] This suggests that X^m and X^P chromosomes are lost randomly.[55] Assuming that 45,Y is lethal, the theoretical percentage of 45,X^m cases would be 67%, not much different from the 80% actually observed.

GONADS

In most 45,X adults with gonadal dysgenesis, the normal gonad is replaced by a white fibrous streak, 2 to 3 cm long and about 0.5 cm wide, located in the position ordinarily occupied by the ovary (Fig. 7–3). Histologically, a streak gonad is characterized by interlacing waves of dense fibrous stroma that are indistinguishable from normal ovarian stroma (Fig. 7–4). That germ cells are usually completely absent in adults but present in 45,X embryos has inspired the conclusion that the pathogenesis of germ cell failure is increased atresia, not failure of germ cell formation. Ovarian rete tubules, which probably originate from either mesonephric tubules or medullary sex cords, are present in the medial portion of most streak gonads. Hilar cells are usually detected in streak gonads of patients past the age of expected puberty.

That 45,X humans have streak gonads is not so obvious as one might expect. Relatively normal ovarian development occurs in many other monosomy X mammals (e.g., mice). The likely explanation is that in humans not all loci on the normal heterochromatic (inactive) X are inacti-

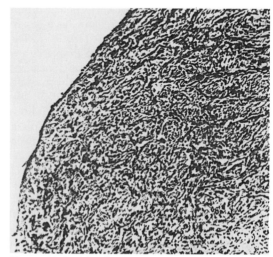

Figure 7–4. Histologic appearance of a streak gonad demonstrating absence of oocytes. (From Simpson JL: Disorders of Sexual Differentiation: Etiology and Clinical Delineation. New York: Academic Press, 1976.)

vated. In addition, X inactivation never exists in oocytes: X reactivation of germ cells antedates entry in meiotic oogenesis.[56] X inactivation could also occur only after some crucial point in differentiation, beyond which only a single euchromatic (active) X is necessary for continued oogenesis.

SECONDARY SEXUAL DEVELOPMENT

Although streak gonads are usually present in 45,X humans, about 3% of affected adults menstruate spontaneously and 5% show breast development (Table 7–1). Occasionally, the interval between menstrual periods appears normal in 45,X patients, and fertile patients have been reported. Although an occult 46,XX cell line should always be suspected in menstruating 45,X patients, it is plausible that a few 45,X individuals could be fertile, inasmuch as germ cells are present in 45,X embryos.

The rare offspring of 45,X women are probably not at greatly increased risk for chromosomal abnormalities,[57, 58] although, theoretically, they should be. Some authors disagree with this statement,[59] and some studies utilizing X-specific FISH probes to score large numbers of interphase nuclei suggests that low-grade 45,X/46, XX mosaicism may be more common in women who experience repeated abortions.[60] Nevertheless, menstruation and fertility are so rare that 45,X patients should be counseled to anticipate primary amenorrhea and sterility. Once hormone therapy is instituted in such women, uterine size becomes normal. This permits 45,X women to carry pregnancies in their own uterus after receipt of donor embryos or donor oocytes fertilized in vitro with the husband's sperm.

SOMATIC ANOMALIES

Genotypic 45,X individuals not only are short (less than 4 ft 10 in) but also often exhibit many Turner stigmata (Table 7–2). No single Turner stigma is pathognomonic, although, in aggregate, a characteristic spectrum exists that is more likely to occur in those with a 45,X complement than in persons with most other sex chromosome abnormalities. Assessment of renal, vertebral, cardiac, and auditory function is obligatory.

The molecular basis for short stature and Turner stigmata is indeterminate, although the distal X short arm has long been known to be

Table 7–1. Somatic Features Associated with 45,X Chromosome Complement

Growth
  Decreased birth weight
  Decreased adult height (141–146 cm)
Intellectual function
  Verbal IQ> performance IQ
  Cognitive deficits (space-form blindness)
Craniofacial
  Premature fusion of sphenooccipital and other sutures, producing brachycephaly
  Abnormal pinnae
  Retruded mandible
  Epicanthal folds (25%)
  High-arched palate (36%)
  Abnormal dentition
  Visual anomalies, usually strabismus (22%)
  Auditory deficits, sensorineural or secondary to middle ear infections
Neck
  Pterygium colli (46%)
  Short, broad neck (74%)
  Low nuchal hair (71%)
Chest
  Rectangular contour (shield chest) (53%)
  Apparent widely spaced nipples
  Tapered lateral ends of clavicles
Cardiovascular
  Coarctation of aorta or ventricular septal defect (10%–16%)
Renal (38%)
  Horseshoe kidneys
  Unilateral renal aplasia
  Duplication of ureters
Gastrointestinal
  Telangiectasias
Skin and lymphatics
  Pigmented nevi (63%)
  Lymphedema (38%) due to hypoplasia of superficial vessels
Nails
  Hypoplasia and malformation (66%)
Skeletal
  Cubitus valgus (54%)
  Radial tilt of trochlear surface of humerus
  Clinodactyly V
  Short metacarpals, usually IV (48%)
  Decreased carpal arch (mean angle 117 degrees)
  Deformities of medial tibial condyle
Dermatoglyphics
  Increased total digital ridge count
  Increased distance between palmar triradii a and b
  Distal axial triradius in position t'

Modified from Simpson JL: Gonadal dysgenesis and abnormalities of the human sex chromosomes: Current status of the phenotypic-karyotypic correlations. Birth Defects 1975; 11(4):23.

integral to normal somatic development. Fisher and associates[61] suggested that absence of a specific DNA sequence may cause Turner stigmata. DNA sequence RPS4Y is present on the Y short arm, and homologous sequence RPS4X on the X. These sequences differ at only 19 of 263

Table 7–2. Ovarian Failure (Percentage) in X-Deletions*

	Complete (Primary Amenorrhea or Streak Gonads)	Partial (Secondary Amenorrhea or Abnormal Menses)	None (Presumed normal)
Monosomy X (45,X)	88%	12%	0
Short-arm deficiency			
del (X)(p11)	50	45	5
del (X)(p21-22.2)	13	25	62
del (X)(p22.3)	0	0	100
i(Xq)	91	9	0
idic(Xq)	80	20	0
Long-arm deficiency			
del(X)(q13-21)	69	31	0
del(X))q22-25)	31	56	13
del(X)(q26-28)	8	67	25
idic(Xp)	73	27	0

*Ovarian function as tabulated on basis of cases reviewed in 1995 by Ogata and Matsuo.[55] Ogata and Matsuo provided data in first two columns, the assumption being that remainder of cases have normal ovarian function, e.g., 5% in del(X)(p11). Publications surveyed overlap in large part those used for analysis of Simpson.

amino acid residues. RPS4X is not inactivated; thus, monosomy X individuals are deficient at this locus. Fisher's group[61] believe the number of ribosomes per cell is reduced when an RPS4X sequence is lacking, as it is in monosomy X.

GROWTH

Persons with a 45,X genotype have low birth weight.[62] Total body length at birth is less than normal, but often is close to the 50th percentile. Height gain before puberty generally lies in the 10th to 15th percentile,[63] however, and the mean height of 45,X adults (16 years and older) is between 141 and 146 cm.[50, 64]

Various treatments for short stature in 45,X patients have been proposed: growth hormone, anabolic steroids, and low-dose estrogen. Growth hormone abnormalities have long been posited; however, their existence is a matter of debate, and they may simply be secondary to gonadal inactivity.[65] Nevertheless, each of the treatment regimens listed above shows some benefit, at least in the first few years of therapy. Effect on ultimate height is still not clear, but the consensus is that final height is increased by 6 to 8 cm[66] with growth hormone therapy. Pediatric endocrinologists favor recombinant DNA–derived human growth hormone. Blunting of the effect of growth hormone treatment may be unavoidable, however, because epiphyses of patients with a 45,X complement are structurally abnormal. Not only are long bones abnormal but so are the teeth[67] and skull.[68] Thus, those with a 45,X karyotype could be said to have a skeletal dysplasia.

INTELLIGENCE

Most 45,X patients have normal intelligence, but any given one has a slightly higher chance than a 46,XX person of being retarded.[50] Performance IQ is lower than verbal IQ, the latter being similar to those of 46,XX matched controls, and 45,X individuals may also have a cognitive defect that is characterized by poor spatial-processing skills ("space-form blindness"). When psychosocial deficits are associated, they primarily involve immaturity and social relationships.[69, 70]

X CHROMOSOMAL MOSAICISM: 45,X/46,XX AND 45,X/47,XXX

The most common form of mosaicism associated with gonadal dysgenesis is 45,X/46,XX. A 45,X/46,XX complement, predictably, is associated with fewer anomalies than is 45,X. Simpson[50] determined that 12% of one series of 45,X/46,XX individuals menstruated, as compared with only 3% of 45,X subjects. Some 18% of 45,X/46,XX individuals exhibit breast development, as compared with 5% for the 45,X genotype. Mean adult height is greater with a 45,X/46,XX complement than with 45,X; more mosaic (25%) than nonmosaic (5%) patients reach adult heights greater than 152 cm.[50] Somatic anomalies are less likely with 45,X/46,XX than with 45,X.

Although 45,X/47,XXX occurs less often, it is phenotypically similar to 45,X/46,XX. Individuals with 45,X/46,XY may also have bilateral streak gonads, but, more often, they have a unilateral streak gonad and a contralateral dysgenetic testis (mixed gonadal dysgenesis).

X SHORT ARM DELETIONS

DELETION OF 46,X,DEL(Xp) OR 45,X/46,X, DEL(Xp)

Deletions of the short arm of the X chromosome produce a variety of phenotypes, depending on the amount of Xp that persists. The most common breakpoint for terminal deletions is Xp11 (Fig. 7–5). In 46,X,del(X)(p11) only proximal Xp remains; the del(Xp) chromosome thus appears acrocentric or telocentric. Chromosomes whose breakpoint is elsewhere have been reported: Xp21, 22.1, 22.3. Although, today, poly-

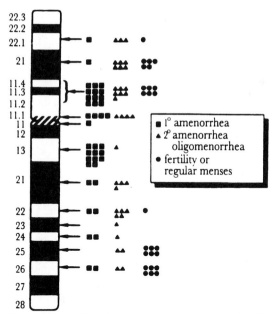

Figure 7–6. Ovarian function associated with simple deletions of the X chromosome. All cases are characterized by banding studies and reasonable exclusion of mosaicism. (From Simpson JL: Genetic programming in ovarian development and oogenesis. *In* Lobo RA, et al [eds]: Menopause. New York: Academic Press, 2000.)

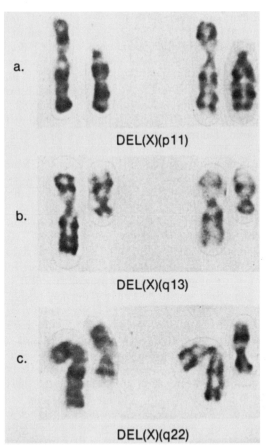

DEL(X)(p11)

DEL(X)(q13)

DEL(X)(q22)

Figure 7–5. A normal X chromosome and deletions of the X chromosome derived from three different persons. (From Simpson JL, LeBeau MN: Gonadal and statural determinants on the X chromosome and their relationship to *in vitro* studies showing prolonged cell cycles in 45,X; 46,X,del(X)(p11); 46,X,del(X)(q13); and 46,X,del(X)q(22) fibroblasts. Am J Obstet Gynecol 1981; 141:930.)

morphic DNA markers allow precise determination of breakpoints in terminal deletions, relatively few cases have been subjected to refined molecular analysis.

Approximately half the reported 46,X, del(Xp)(p11) individuals show primary amenorrhea and gonadal dysgenesis. Others menstruate—and usually show breast development. In one early tabulation by this author, 12 of 27 reported del(X)(p11.2→11.4) subjects menstruated spontaneously, but their menstruation was rarely normal.[71] More recent compilation have not materially altered these conclusions.[45, 48, 72] Ogata and Matsuo[55] estimate that 50% of del(X)p11 persons have primary amenorrhea and 45% secondary amenorrhea. Ovarian function is thus observed more often in those who have a del(Xp11) chromosome than in 45,X individuals. Women with more distal deletions—del(X)(p21.1 to p22.1.22)—menstruate more often, but, still, many are infertile or even have secondary amenorrhea (Fig. 7–6). Thus, Xp [X(pter→ p21)] retains a role in ovarian development.[45, 48, 72] The distal region of importance must involve Xp21,22.1 or 22.2, because del(X)(p22.3) is not associated with primary amenorrhea.

Most women with deletions of Xp are short in stature. Thus, Xp must bear stature determinant(s) (i.e., regions with genes). Given that del(Xp) women may menstruate but still be short, regions on Xp that are responsible for ovarian and statural determinants must, respectively, be separate.[45, 48, 72–74] Clinically, it is important to realize that del(Xp) women may be short even when they manifest normal ovarian function.

ISOCHROMOSOMES FOR Xq

Almost always, 46,X,i(Xq) individuals have streak gonads and primary amenorrhea. Occasionally, they menstruate, but recent surveys continue to agree with findings published by this author[50] more than 25 years ago that menstruation is rare.[55] The nearly complete lack of gonadal development in 46,X,i(Xq) contrasts to that in 46,X, del(X)(p11) individuals, about half of whom menstruate or develop breasts. Phenotypic differences could be explained if gonadal determinants were present at several different locations on Xp and if one locus were deficient in i(Xq) but were retained in del(X)(p11). Alternatively, 46,XX cells may be associated with del(Xp) more often than we generally appreciate. Nevertheless, duplication of Xq—that is, i(Xq)—fails to compensate for deficiency of Xp. One explanation is that gonadal determinants on Xq and Xp have different functions. Another is that *all* loci on i(Xq) chromosomes are completely inactivated, even those not inactivated when present on an intact X. It seems unlikely that duplication of Xq per se produces abnormalities, given that, usually, 47,XXX women are clinically "normal."

Almost all reported 46,X,i(Xq) patients are short (i.e., mean height usually less than that of 45,X subjects). The mean height of nonmosaic 46,X,i(Xq) patients is 136 cm,[50] and many somatic features of the Turner stigmata are observed.[50] Somatic anomalies occur as frequently in 46,X,i(Xq) as in 45,X, and, in general, the spectra of anomalies associated with the two complements are similar.

X LONG-ARM DELETIONS

46,X,DEL(Xq) AND 45,X/ 46,X,DEL(Xq) DELETIONS

Deletions of the X long arm are well-known[43, 45, 48, 72] and, like del(Xp), they vary in composition. If the breakpoint that leads to a terminal deletion originates at band Xq13, the derivative chromo-

some resembles No. 17 or No. 18; a breakpoint at band Xq21 produces a chromosome resembling No. 16 (see Fig. 7–5).

Almost all deletions originating at Xq13 are associated with primary amenorrhea, absence of breast development, and complete ovarian failure.[72] Xq13 thus seems to be an important region for ovarian maintenance. Key loci could lie in proximal Xq21, but not more distal given that del(X)(q21) to (q24) individuals menstruate far more often (see Fig. 7–6). Menstruating del(X)(q21) women may have retained a region that contained an ovarian maintenance gene, whereas del(X)(q13 or 21) women with primary amenorrhea may have lost such a locus.[72]

Molecular attempts at mapping the region of Xq that is most integral to ovarian development were recently reported. Sala and colleagues[75] studied seven subjects with X/autosome translocations involving Xq21–22, five of whom had primary amenorrhea. In all seven cases, a 15-mb region of Xq encompassed breakpoints. Breakpoints in four X-autosome translocations studied by Philippe and coworkers[76] were also localized to the same region. The YAC contig encompassing these breakpoints spanned most of the Xq21 region and extended between DXS233 and DXS1171.[77] That breakpoints associated with ovarian failure spanned this entire large Xq21 region makes it unlikely that a single gene causes ovarian failure, unless, in these balanced X/autosome translocations, ovarian failure is the result, not of disruption of a gene per se, but rather of generalized cytologic perturbation.

With more distal Xq deletions, the more common phenotype is not primary amenorrhea but premature ovarian failure.[45, 48, 78, 79] Whereas distal Xq seems less important than proximal Xq for ovarian maintenance, the former must still have regions that are important for ovarian maintenance.

Not infrequently, distal Xq deletions are familial. Some familial Xq deletions are a derivative of Xq autosome translocations, but familial terminal or interstitial deletions are also possible.[47] Familial Xp terminal or interstitial deletions have been characterized by breakpoints ranging between Xq25 and Xq28. Breakpoints near or in Xq27 seem most common. Some families have been identified for reasons other than premature ovarian failure; a case reported by our group was noticed after amniotic fluid analysis in a fetus.[80] This finding suggests that more families would be detected were prometaphase analysis or polymorphic molecular studies more routinely performed in premature ovarian failure (POF).

Distal Xq deletions seem to have a less severe

effect on stature than do proximal deletions. Somatic anomalies of the Turner stigmata are uncommon—and perhaps no more common than in the general population.

Currently, the only genuine candidate gene for a role in ovarian maintenance is the human homologue of the *Drosophila melanogaster* gene *diaphanous* (dia). This gene causes sterility in male and female *Drosophila* flies.[81] Sequence comparisons between *dia* and the relevant human expressed sequence tag (EST) DRE25 show significant homology. DRE25 maps to human Xq22,[81] a region key to ovarian maintenance. *Drosophila dia* is a member of a family of proteins that help to establish cell polarity, govern cytokinesis, and reorganize the actin cytoskeleton. In a study of familial POF, an Xq21/autosome translocation (alluded to earlier)[82] was found to be associated with disruption of DRE25.[83] Perturbation involving the last intron produced a human DIA characterized by truncated transcripts; these transcripts were unstable and could not be translated.

AUTOSOMAL GENES CAUSING OVARIAN FAILURE

XX GONADAL DYSGENESIS

Gonadal dysgenesis histologically similar to that in persons with an abnormal sex chromosome complement may be present in 46,XX individuals, as I first observed more than 25 years ago.[14] Mosaicism has been reasonably excluded in affected individuals, although mosaicism restricted to the embryo can never be excluded. The general term *XX gonadal dysgenesis* can be applied to those persons.

Many different forms of 46,XX gonadal dysgenesis exist, but the prototypical form of XX gonadal dysgenesis *not* associated with somatic anomalies is clearly an autosomal-recessive inherited condition. Affected persons are of normal stature (mean height 165 cm),[84] and Turner stigmata are usually absent. Frequent reports of consanguinity have long made it clear that autosomal-recessive genes are responsible. More recent segregation analysis by the author and colleagues revealed the segregation ratio to be 0.16 for female sibs.[85] Thus, two thirds of gonadal dysgenesis cases in 46,XX individuals are genetic. The third of cases that are not genetic (but are phenocopies) could be attributable to infection, infarction, or infiltrative or autoimmune phenomena.

Of considerable clinical interest is the variability of expression. In some families, one sibling has streak gonads whereas another affected individual has primary amenorrhea and extreme ovarian hypoplasia (presence of a few oocytes).[14, 49, 86–88] If the mutant gene responsible for XX gonadal dysgenesis is capable of variable expression, some sporadic cases of POF may also be attributable to it.

The mechanism underlying failure of germ cell persistence in most forms of XX gonadal dysgenesis is not known, but several hypotheses seem reasonable. One is perturbation of meiosis. In plants and lower mammals, meiosis is known to be under genetic control. Surely, this is true in humans, too. Thus it might be reasonable to predict mutations that would be manifested as ovarian failure and infertility in otherwise normal women. Other possibilities include interference with germ cell migration, abnormal connective tissue milieu, and gonadotropin receptor perturbation (see below).

The murine gene *germ cell deficiency* (gcd)[89] is an especially attractive model. This autosomal-recessive murine gene reduces production of germ cells in both ovaries and testes. Its human homologue could be responsible for some cases of XX gonadal dysgenesis. Even more plausibly, *gcd* could be responsible for the syndrome of germ cell deficiency, which affects both sexes.

PERRAULT SYNDROME (XX GONADAL DYSGENESIS WITH NEUROSENSORY DEAFNESS)

A distinct variant of XX gonadal dysgenesis associated with neurosensory deafness is called *Perrault syndrome*. Like XX gonadal dysgenesis without deafness, Perrault syndrome is an autosomal recessive condition.[85, 90–93]

XX GONADAL DYSGENESIS DUE TO FOLLICLE-STIMULATING HORMONE RECEPTOR MUTATION

In Finland, Aittomaki and colleagues,[49, 88] searched hospitals and cytogenetic laboratories and were able to identify 75 patients (countrywide) who had XX gonadal dysgenesis (defined as 46,XX women with primary or secondary amenorrhea and serum follicle-stimulating hormone (FSH) $\geq$ 40 mIU/ml). These 75 included 57 sporadic cases and 18 women (from seven families) who had affected relatives. Most women lived in north-central Finland, a sparsely populated part of the country. The overall frequency of the disorder in Finland was 1 per 8300 liveborn females, a relatively high incidence that was attributed to a founder effect. A segregation ratio of 0.23 for female sibs was consistent with autosomal-recessive inheritance, as was the consanguinity rate of 12%.

Next, sib pair analysis using polymorphic DNA markers localized the gene to chromosome 2p, a region that had been known to contain genes for both the FSH receptor (FSHR) and the luteinizing hormone (LH) receptor (LHR). One specific mutation—C566T, or alanine to valine—in exon 7 was observed in six families.[88, 94]

That C566T was not found in all Finnish XX gonadal dysgenesis cases indicates genetic heterogeneity. C566T-negative Finnish patients might have the same disorder discussed earlier—XX gonadal dysgenesis with no somatic anomalies. Consistent with this idea is the finding that the C566T mutation is rarely detected in samples of women with 46,XX ovarian failure who reside outside Finland. Layman and associates[95] found no mutations in the FSHR gene in 35 46,XX women who had hypergonadotropic hypogonadism. Of the 35, 15 had primary amenorrhea and 20 had secondary amenorrhea. Liu and colleagues[96] found no sequence abnormalities in one multigeneration POF family, four of whom had sporadic POF and two, hypergonadotropic hypogonadism.

Aittomaki and coworkers[94] later contrasted the phenotype of C566T XX gonadal dysgenesis with that of non-C566T XX gonadal dysgenesis. Subjects with the former phenotype were more likely to exhibit ovarian follicles on ultrasonography. Thus, C566T XX gonadal dysgenesis shows *some* features expected of gonadotropin resistance (Savage syndrome); however, the FSH level is clearly elevated and the phenotype is, in general, far more reminiscent of prototypical XX gonadal dysgenesis and bilateral streak gonads.

INACTIVATING LUTEINIZING HORMONE RECEPTOR MUTATIONS

Another trophic hormone receptor gene whose mutation causes gonadal dysgenesis in 46,XX genotypes is the LHR gene. Most LHR mutations have been associated with the 46,XY genotype, but 46,XX cases have been identified in sibships when an affected 46,XY male had Leydig cell hypoplasia.[97] Latronico and associates[98] reported primary amenorrhea in a 22-year-old woman. In that family, three males and one

female had a homozygous nonsense (stop) mutation at codon 554 (C554X). The resulting stop codon produced a truncated protein that had five, rather than seven, transmembrane domains. The affected woman had breast development but only a single episode of menstrual bleeding at age 20 years; the LH value was 37 mIU/ml, FSH 9 mIU/ml. The mutation reduced signal transduction activity of the LHR gene. In another 46,XX case, reported by Toledo and associates,[99] secondary amenorrhea occurred; LH and FSH were 10 and 9 mIU/ml, respectively. The mutations resulted in alanine, rather than proline, at amino acid position 593.

Activating LHR mutations seem to have little effect in females, but males experience precocious puberty.[97]

XX GONADAL DYSGENESIS AND MULTIPLE MALFORMATION SYNDROMES

Mutant genes that act on multiple organ systems are said to be *pleiotropic*. The pleiotropic gene that causes XX gonadal dysgenesis and neurosensory deafness *(Perrault syndrome)* earlier received comment. Other pleiotropic syndromes include XX gonadal dysgenesis and cerebellar ataxia;[100] XX gonadal dysgenesis, microcephaly, and arachnodactyly;[101] XX gonadal dysgenesis and epibulbar dermoid;[102] and XX gonadal dysgenesis, short stature, and metabolic acidosis.[103] Presumably, these four disorders are distinctive and autosomal-recessive, judging from multiple affected sibs.

One autosomal-dominant syndrome, blepharophimosis-ptosis, long has been recognized as being associated with ovarian failure.[104, 105] From the study of several large kindreds, sib-pair analysis using polymorphic DNA variants[106] localized the blepharophimosis-ptosis gene to 3q21–24. This region contains no obvious candidate genes. Surprisingly, Fraser and coworkers[107] reported that in one blepharophimosis-ptosis case ovaries were unresponsive to gonadotropins.

In each of the multiple malformation syndromes associated with ovarian failure, underlying biologic questions must be posed. Does the seemingly pleiotropic gene cause both the somatic anomalies and the ovarian failure? Do the somatic and nonsomatic phenotypes involve only closely linked genes (i.e., contiguous gene syndrome)? Could unrecognized parental chromosomal rearrangements be involved? Do any of these genes play pivotal roles in normal ovarian differentiation and maintenance, or is the perturbation of ovarian development merely secondary, perhaps to a generalized disturbance of connective tissue?

GALACTOSEMIA

In galactosemia, enzyme deficiencies prevent synthesis of glucose from galactose. Several enzymes and their mutant alleles, usually *autosomal*-recessive ones, may be responsible. Of special interest is the form of galactosemia caused by deficiency of galactose 1-phosphate uridyl transferase (GALT), controlled by a gene on 9p. In addition to renal, hepatic, and ocular damage, ovarian failure may be associated. Initially, Kaufman and coworkers[108] reported 12 of 18 galactosemic women had premature POF. Waggoner and associates[109] later reported that 8 of 47 (17%) females with galactosemia had ovarian failure. The pathogenesis presumably involves galactose toxicity after birth, given that maternal enzymes should be protective in utero. Consistent with this idea is the finding that a neonate with galactosemia showed normal ovarian histology.[110]

Given the clinical severity of galactosemia and the necessity for childhood dietary treatment, it seems highly unlikely that undiagnosed galactosemia would prove to be the cause of ovarian failure in women who present solely with primary amenorrhea or POF. Of greater general interest, therefore, was the report in 1989 by Cramer and coworkers[111] that GALT heterozygotes were at increased risk for POF,[112] although, later, the same authors failed to observe GALT abnormalities in another sample of women with early menopause.[111, 112] Kaufman and colleagues[113] likewise failed to confirm. Moreover, not all homozygotes for human galactosemia are abnormal, nor are all transgeneic mice whose GALT is inactivated.[114] In summary, homozygous (but probably not heterozygous) GALT deficiency is associated with ovarian failure.

OTHER CAUSES OF 46,XX OVARIAN FAILURE

Other disorders exist, and a more complete discussion of this topic is provided elsewhere. Specifically discussed elsewhere in this chapter are several disorders that must be included in the differential diagnosis of 46,XX individuals with gonadal failure: 17α-hydroxylase deficiency, aromatase defects, and agonadia.

GERM CELL FAILURE IN BOTH SEXES

In several sibships, both males and females have shown germinal cell failure. Affected females show streak gonads, whereas males show germ cell aplasia (Sertoli cell only syndrome or del Castillo phenotype; see later). In two of these families, parents were consanguineous, and neither exhibited any somatic anomalies.[37, 38] In three other families, characteristic patterns of somatic anomalies were observed, suggesting distinctive entities. Hamet and associates[36] reported germ cell failure, hypertension, and deafness; Al-Awadi and colleagues[39] reported germ cell failure and alopecia; Mikati's group[40] reported germ cell failure, microcephaly, short stature, and minor anomalies.

These families demonstrate that a single autosomal gene can deleteriously affect germ cell development in both sexes. Presumably the gene(s) acts either at a site common to early germ cell development or through a mechanism that produces meiotic perturbation. Elucidating such genes could have profound implications for understanding normal developmental processes.

XY GONADAL DYSGENESIS

Gonadal dysgenesis may occur in persons with an apparently normal male (46,XY) chromosomal complement. Loss of testicular tissue before 7 to 8 weeks of embryonic life would be expected to produce such a female phenotype, as Jost[115] showed in rabbits. In at least some cases, the gonads of these persons appeared to have been ovaries during embryonic development.[116]

Individuals with XY gonadal dysgenesis show female external genitalia, a uterus, and fallopian tubes, but at puberty they fail to develop secondary sexual characteristics. Height is normal and somatic anomalies are usually absent, although there is a relationship between XY gonadal dysgenesis and renal failure.[117–119]

Approximately 20% to 30% of XY gonadal dysgenesis patients develop dysgerminoma or gonadoblastoma.[120] Often, the neoplasm arises in the first or second decade of life. Because of the relatively high probability of neoplastic transformation, gonads should be extirpated from persons with XY gonadal dysgenesis. Uterus and fallopian tubes should *not* be removed, however, because pregnancy through donor oocytes or donor embryos might still be possible. Usually, laparoscopic removal of gonads or even a gona-doblastoma is possible.[121, 122]

The XY gonadal dysgenesis phenotype may result from a mutation within the SRY HMG box;[11, 12] however, only 10% to 15% of sporadic cases show perturbations of SRY.[9] One form of XY gonadal dysgenesis segregates in the fashion expected of an X-linked recessive condition.[14, 84, 117, 123–125] That the responsible X-linked gene is related to the postulated DSS gene on Xp21 is a consideration; however, only 1 of 27 "46,XY sex-reversal females" studied by Bardoni and associates[21] showed submicroscopic duplication of the region (Xp21.2→22.1) containing DSS.

Genetic heterogeneity is illustrated by the existence of at least four syndromes: (1) XY gonadal dysgenesis and camptomelic dysgenesis;[126, 127] (2) XY gonadal dysgenesis and ectodermal anomalies;[128] (3) genitopalatocardiac (Gardner-Silengo-Wachtel) syndrome;[129] and (4) spastic paraplegia, optic atrophy, and microcephaly but normal intelligence.[130]

FEMALE PSEUDOHERMAPHRODITISM

Female pseudohermaphrodites have a 46,XX genotype but fail to develop the external genitalia expected of normal females because of excess androgens in utero. The most common cause is congenital adrenal hyperplasia resulting from deficiencies of the various enzymes required for steroid biosynthesis (Fig. 7–7): 21-hydroxylase, 11β-hydroxylase, and 3β-ol-dehydrogenase. The common pathogenesis involves decreased production of adrenal cortisol, which regulates secretion of adrenocorticotropic hormone (ACTH) through negative feedback inhibition. If cortisol production is decreased, ACTH secretion is not inhibited. Elevation of ACTH leads to increased quantities of steroid precursors, from which androgens are synthesized.

Syndromes of adrenal hyperplasia must be excluded quickly when assessing an individual with genital ambiguity, because cortisol and corticosterone deficiencies result in sodium wasting that can be life-threatening. Even if cortisol administration is begun immediately after birth, patients with adrenal hyperplasia usually grow only to a height between the third and 15th percentile.[131] If cortisol is not administered, affected persons initially experience increased growth during early childhood; however, premature epiphyseal closure limits overall growth.

DEFICIENCY OF 21-HYDROXYLASE

Clinical

Deficiency of 21-hydroxylase is the most common cause of genital ambiguity among 46,XX individuals. If 21-hydroxylase is deficient, this cytochrome P450 enzyme fails to convert 17α-hydroxyprogesterone (17α-OHP) to 11-deoxycortisol (see Fig. 7–7). Serum cortisol and deoxycortisol are decreased; 17α-OHP, androstenedione,

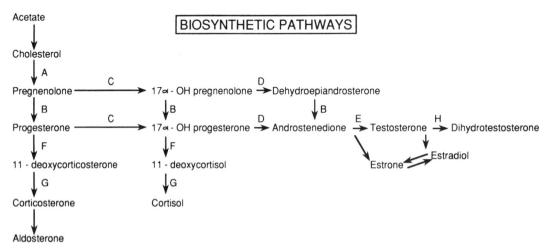

Figure 7–7. Important adrenal and gonadal biosynthetic pathways. Letters designate enzymes required for the appropriate conversions. *A*, 20α-hydroxylase and 20,22-desmolase; *B*, 3β-ol-dehydrogenase; *C*, 17α-hydroxylase; *D*, 17,20-desmolase; *E*, 17-ketosteroid reductase; *F*, 21-hydroxylase; *G*, 11β-hydroxylase. (From Simpson JL: Disorders of Sexual Differentiation: Etiology and Clinical Delineation. New York: Academic Press, 1976.)

estrone, and testosterone are increased. Increased 17α-OHP in either serum (affected neonate) or amniotic fluid (affected fetus) provides the basis for diagnosis.

Females deficient for 21- or 11β-hydroxylase show clitoral hypertrophy, labioscrotal fusion, and displacement of the urethral orifice to a site more nearly that expected in a male. The extent of virilization may vary among individuals who have the same enzyme deficiency. Wolffian derivatives (vasa deferentia, seminal vesicles, epididymides) are absent, probably because fetal adrenal function begins too late in embryogenesis to stabilize the wolffian ducts. Müllerian derivatives develop normally, as would be expected in the absence of AMH (MIS). Ovaries likewise develop normally. Scrotal and areolar hyperpigmentation may occur, presumably as a result of proopiomelanocortin (POMC), the parent hormone of both melanocyte-stimulating hormone (MSH) and ACTH occurs. In fact, hyperpigmentation suggests 21- or 11β-hydroxylase deficiency in males whose genitalia are normal at birth. If not detected before birth, these enzyme deficiencies may go unrecognized until age 2 years or later. At that time, genital enlargement, pubic hair, and prematurely tall stature are usually noted.

Sodium wasting may or may not occur in 21-hydroxylase deficiency. In the form of 21-hydroxylase deficiency that is not associated with sodium wasting (non–sodium-wasting 21-hydroxylase deficiency), it is assumed that increased ACTH secretion results in levels of aldosterone and cortisol sufficient to prevent sodium wasting. Mineralocorticoid and sodium chloride must be administered to correct hyperkalemia and restore fluid-electrolyte balance. If it is not treated, hyponatremia, hyperkalemia, dehydration, and death may occur. Cortisol administration must be continued into adulthood, although, after infancy, requirements (per unit of weight) may diminish. Long-term replacement with sodium-retaining hormone (e.g., fluorinated hydrocortisone) may also be necessary.

Molecular

Located in mitochondria, 21-hydroxylase is a cytochrome P450 enzyme. Its gene (CYP21) is coded on chromosome 6p21, closely linked to human leukocyte antigen (HLA). This linkage facilitates heterozygote identification and antenatal diagnosis. The CYP21 gene is unusual in that it is arranged in tandem with the gene for the C4 component of complement. In addition, this entire arrangement is repeated. The actual sequence is C4A-CYP21P-C4B-CYP21, oriented with the sense strand reading left to right. It is presumed that this CYP21/C4 tandem configuration arose by gene duplication through recombination. The configuration is the same in mice, great apes, and cattle, but not in all mammals. Although both complement genes (C4A and C4B) are active, only a single CYP21 gene is active. The other is a pseudogene (CYP21P), an 8bp deletion in exon 3 having produced an altered reading frame and, thus, a truncated nonfunctional protein. The CYP21 and CYP21P genes are each about 5 kb long.

As a result of the CYP21/C4 tandem arrangement, there is a predisposition to unequal crossover owing to chromosomal misalignment. This may lead to unusual molecular perturbations, specifically one chromosome having a duplication and its homologue being deleted. A related phenomenon is gene conversion, in which nonreciprocal recombination results in CYP21 being "converted" to a CYP21P. Regardless, deletions (25%) and gene conversion (15%) are less unusual explanations for 21-hydroxylase deficiency than single-point mutations.

The relative frequency of various CYP mutations varies among ethnic groups and by phenotypes associated with 21-hydroxylase deficiency. Simple virilizing 21-hydroxylase deficiency is associated with a nucleotide substitution, whereas the salt-wasting form is more likely to be associated with deletions, frame shifts, and nonsense mutations, although the phenotype cannot always be predicted from the molecular mutation.

DEFICIENCY OF 11β-HYDROXYLASE

Much less common than 21-hydroxylase deficiency, 11β-hydroxylase deficiency is also an autosomal-recessive condition. It is characterized by decreased conversion of 11-desoxycortisol to cortisol and 11-deoxycorticosterone to corticosterone. Therefore, the principal metabolite of 11-deoxycortisol, tetrahydrocortisol, is more plentiful. Because deoxycortisol and deoxycorticosterone are potent sodium-retaining hormones, increased levels may lead to hypervolemia and, thus, to hypertension. Infants with 11β-hydroxylase deficiency manifest not only the genital virilization characteristic of 21-hydroxylase deficiency but also hypertension.

There are two 11β-hydroxylase genes that code for the mitochondrial cytochrome P450 enzymes CYP11B1 and CYP11B2. The latter is expressed only in zona glomerulosa and is important for aldosterone synthesis. CYP11B1 is abnormal in female pseudohermaphrodites. The gene is located on 8q22, and the most common perturbations are point mutations.[132–134]

DEFICIENCY OF 3β-HYDROXYSTEROID-DEHYDROGENASE (3β-HSD)

In 3β-ol-dehydrogenase (see Fig. 7–7) deficiency, the principal androgen synthesized is dehydroepiandrosterone (DHEA). This relatively weak androgen cannot be converted to either androstenedione or testosterone. Females with 3β-ol-dehydrogenase deficiency are thus less virilized than females with 21- or 11β-hydroxylase deficiencies. DHEA is such a weak androgen that males with 3β-ol-dehydrogenase deficiency fail to masculinize completely (male pseudohermaphroditism). Thus, 3β-ol-dehydrogenase deficiency is the only form of adrenal hyperplasia that produces genital ambiguity in both males and females. In embryonic testes, 3β-ol-dehydrogenase activity reaches its maximum earlier in embryogenesis (third month) than the adrenals and ovaries (fourth month). Otherwise, one might expect the external genitalia to be identical in affected males and affected females.

Complete deficiency of 3β-ol-dehydrogenase results in severe sodium wasting secondary to deficiency of sodium-retaining hormones. Sodium wasting is often so pronounced that affected infants die precipitantly; however, less severe deficiencies are compatible with long-term survival. The condition is autosomal recessive. It is best diagnosed on the basis of serum steroids measured before and after ACTH stimulation.[135] The gene is located on chromosome 1, and, unlike CYP21 and CYP11B, it is not mitochondrial but microsomal; that is, 3β-ol-dehydrogenase is not a cytochrome P_{450} enzyme. There are two 3BH-SHD genes (I and II), both located on chromosome 1 (p11–13) and both consisting of four exons. Type II is expressed in gonads and adrenals. Point mutations are the most common molecular perturbations in 3β-ol-dehydrogenase deficiency.[136–139]

17α-HYDROXYLASE/17,20-lyase (CYP17) DEFICIENCY

Deficiency of the cytochrome P450 enzyme 17α-hydroxylase/17,20-lyase results in failure of pregnenolone to be converted to 17α-hydroxypregnenolone. If the enzyme defect were complete, cortisol, androstenedione, testosterone, and estrogens could not be synthesized; however, 11-deoxycorticosterone and corticosterone could. As ACTH secretion compensatorily increases, 11-deoxycorticosterone and corticosterone increase. The result is hypernatremia, hypokalemia, and hypervolemia. Clinically, hypertension is evident. Aldosterone levels are decreased, presumably because hypervolemia suppresses the renin-angiotensin system.

Females with 17α-hydroxylase/17,20-lyase deficiency have normal external genitalia, but at puberty they fail to undergo normal secondary sexual development (primary amenorrhea). Thus, these cases are encountered in differential diagnosis of XX gonadal dysgenesis. Hypertension is a major diagnostic clue. Oocytes appear incapable of reaching a diameter greater than 2.5 mm.[140] Oocytes are capable of responding to exogenous gonadotropins.[141] Affected males usually have ambiguous genitalia (male pseudohermaphroditism).

Deficiency of 17α-hydroxylase/17,20-lyase is autosomal recessive. The gene (CYP17) is localized to 10q 24–25. A single gene is responsible for the action of 17α-hydroxylase and 17,20-desmolase/lyase activity. Most individuals with 17α-hydroxylase mutations are male pseudohermaphrodites; thus, more detailed discussion of molecular changes in the CYP17α gene is deferred until later discussion of male pseudohermaphroditism.

TERATOGENIC FORMS

Administration of testosterone and other androgens to pregnant women may masculinize female fetuses, producing phallic enlargement, labioscrotal fusion, displacement of the urogenital sinus invagination, and wolffian duct development. These forms of female pseudohermaphroditism are now rare, but important because these causes are preventable.

To interfere with genital differentiation, a teratogen must also exert its action during organogenesis. Before that time, no organ-specific structure can be affected. In humans, the genital tubercle first becomes evident at about 5 weeks of embryogenesis (7 weeks' gestation). If an androgenic teratogen is administered before 12 weeks of gestation, labioscrotal fusion may occur. After 12 weeks, an androgenic teratogen may cause clitoral enlargement, but not labioscrotal fusion. Excessive androgen production predictably does not affect Müllerian differentiation or ovarian differentiation.

Androgen-induced female pseudohermaphroditism was more common decades ago, when women were more frequently treated during pregnancy with high doses of synthetic progestins. Virilized female offspring often resulted.[142, 143] Administration of progestins during pregnancy, especially in high doses, is now rarely indicated;[144] thus, the problem arises only rarely.

Testosterone, ethinyl testosterone, norethindrone acetate, norethindrone, and danocrine are potent teratogens that are sometimes administered to women of childbearing age. If doses are administered therapeutically to women pregnant with female embryos, female pseudohermaphroditism may result.[51, 142] Norethynodrel, medroxyprogesterone, and 17α-hydroxyprogesterone caproate have rarely been implicated. Large doses are required to produce virilization. A single oral contraceptive pill taken daily should specifically not produce teratogenic female pseudohermaphroditism.

Fetal masculinization has been reported in pregnancies associated with Sertoli cell tumors (arrhenoblastoma), Leydig cell tumors, luteomas of pregnancy, and certain adenocarcinomas that metastasize to the ovary (e.g., Krukenberg tumor). Frequently cited in texts as a cause for masculinizing female fetuses, androgen-secreting tumors in pregnant women are actually an extraordinarily rare cause of female pseudohermaphroditism. Moreover, patients with preexisting androgen-secreting tumors rarely become pregnant. In 1973, Verhoeven and associates[145] collected only 45 reports of virilizing tumors associated with pregnancy. Among the offspring were 18 females whose external genitalia were described; nine had clitoral or labial hypertrophy, but only one had labioscrotal fusion.

Marked clitoral enlargement of unexplained origin sometimes results from hemangiomas, neurofibromas, or tumors. In other cases, enlargement seems to be idiopathic and may reflect end-organ hyperresponsiveness.

OTHER FORMS OF FEMALE PSEUDOHERMAPHRODITISM

Two siblings had clitoral hypertrophy, a single perineal orifice leading anteriorly to a urethra and posteriorly to a vagina, and numerous skeletal anomalies (hypoplasia of the mandible and maxilla, brachycephaly, narrow vertebral bodies, relatively long, slender bones, dislocation of fusion of the radial heads leading to abnormal-looking elbows, coxa valga, and phalangeal fusion of several toes).[146, 147] Müllerian derivatives and ovaries were normal. Both siblings developed breasts and pubic hair but failed to menstruate. Their parents were consanguineous; thus, autosomal-recessive inheritance seems probable.

Female pseudohermaphroditism of unknown origin can also be associated with one or more of the following anomalies: absence or duplication of the uterus; renal absence, duplication, or hydronephrosis; and imperforate anus.[148] Short stature, mental retardation, deafness, ear and nose malformation, and a blind colon are less often associated; the ovaries are usually normal.

Genital abnormalities may also result from maldevelopment of the genital tubercle, cloacal membrane, urogenital membrane, or the entire hind end of the embryo (i.e., caudal regression syndrome). With some of these malformations the external genitalia may be so abnormal that the sex of rearing is in doubt. These rare disorders, discussed elsewhere in detail,[51] include exstrophy of the bladder, exstrophy of the cloaca, and sirenomelia.

MALE PSEUDOHERMAPHRODITISM

Male pseudohermaphrodites are individuals with a Y chromosome whose external genitalia fail to fully develop as expected for normal males. Some authors apply the term only to those whose external genitalia are sufficiently ambiguous to confuse the sex of rearing; however, applying the term more liberally seems more useful clinically. Cytogenetic forms of male pseudohermaphroditism (45,X/46,XY and variants) will also be discussed in this section, to contrast their phenotype with genetic forms of male pseudohermaphroditism.

TERATOGENIC FORMS

Several agents would be expected to produce incompletely developed male external genitalia when given in sufficiently high doses in the first trimester to a woman pregnant with a male fetus. These drugs include cyproterone acetate, whose mode of action involves blocking androgen receptor, and finasteride, whose mode of action involves inhibition of 5α-reductase. Later in this section the consequence of agents with these actions will become clear. Both agents are approved in the United States for treatment of hirsutism.

Controversy exists concerning whether administration of progestins or progesterones to women having male fetuses can produce hypospadias. In my opinion, the weight of evidence indicates that these agents do not produce this defect.[149]

CYTOGENETIC FORMS

Persons with a 45,X/46,XY genotype have both a 45,X cell line and at least one cell line containing a Y chromosome. Based on cohort studies of 45,X/46,XY cases detected without bias in utero (prenatal genetic diagnosis), well over 90% of cases are normal males.[150] Cases identified postnatally differ, manifesting a variety of phenotypes: almost normal males with cryptorchidism or penile hypospadias, genital ambiguity, or females indistinguishable from those with 45,X Turner syndrome.[51, 151, 152] Different phenotypes presumably reflect different tissue distributions of the various cell lines. Not infrequently, a Y chromosome is structurally abnormal. Since many structurally abnormal chromosomes (e.g., dicentric) are unstable, it is likely that the 45,X line arises secondarily after loss of the structurally abnormal Y.

45,X/46,XY with Female External Genitalia

The 45,X/46,XY genotype may be associated with Turner stigmata and affected persons may be clinically indistinguishable from 45,X individuals. Such individuals usually are normal in stature and show no somatic anomalies. As with other types of gonadal dysgenesis, the external genitalia, vagina, and Müllerian derivatives remain unstimulated at puberty because of the absence of sex steroids. Breasts fail to develop, and pubic and axillary hair is sparse. If breast development occurs in a 45,X/46,XY individual, an estrogen-secreting tumor like gonadoblastoma or dysgerminoma should be suspected.[153] Virilization has also been claimed to result from gonadotropin stimulation of dysgenetic gonads.[154]

Although streak gonads of 45,X/46,XY individuals are usually histologically indistinguishable from streak gonads of 45,X individuals, gonadoblastomas or dysgerminomas develop in about 15% to 20% of 45,X/46,XY individuals.[120] Neoplasia may develop in the first or second decade of life. Despite the possibility that a region (locus) on Yq may protect against neoplasia,[155] gonadal extirpation is recommended for all 45,X/46,XY persons who have female external genitalia. The uterus should be retained because pregnancy

may be achieved through donor oocytes or donor embryos. Gonadectomy can usually be accomplished by laparoscopy.[122] It is preferable to remove only gonads, but technically it may be necessary to remove the adnexa as well. Only rarely should laparotomy prove necessary.

45,X/46,XY with Ambiguous External Genitalia

The term *asymmetric* (or *mixed*) *gonadal dysgenesis* is applied to individuals with one streak gonad and one dysgenetic testis. These individuals typically have ambiguous external genitalia and a 45,X/46,XY complement, and, usually, a uterus. Occasionally, only 45,X or only 46,XY cells are demonstrable. Many investigators believe that the phenotype is invariably associated with 45,X/46,XY mosaicism. "Nonmosaic" cases most likely reflect merely the inability to sample enough tissues.

Usually, 45,X/46,XY individuals with ambiguous external genitalia have Müllerian derivatives (e.g., a uterus). A uterus is a very important diagnostic sign, because that organ is absent in almost all the genetic (mendelian) forms of male pseudohermaphroditism discussed elsewhere in this section. If an individual has ambiguous external genitalia, bilateral testes, and a uterus, it is reasonable to infer 45,X/46,XY mosaicism, regardless of whether both lines can be demonstrated cytogenetically. Occasionally the uterus is rudimentary or a fallopian tube fails to develop ipsilateral to a testis.

45,X/46,XY with Nearly Normal Male External Genitalia

Mosaicism of 45,X/46,XY may be detected in persons with nearly normal male external genitalia. In fact, this phenotype has the highest incidence, based on follow-up of most fetuses of 45,X/46,XY genotype identified at amniocentesis; most (90%) have a normal male phenotype.[156] That 45,X/46,XY neonates far more often show genital ambiguity reflects ascertainment bias.

It seems that 45,X/46,XY individuals who have almost normal male external genitalia do not develop neoplasia as often as 45,X/46,XY individuals with female or frankly ambiguous genitalia do.[120] Gonadal extirpation may not be necessary if male sex of rearing is chosen, provided the gonads can be assessed periodically within the scrotum by ultrasound or palpation.[120]

DEFICIENCIES IN TESTOSTERONE BIOSYNTHESIS

Male pseudohermaphroditism may result from deficiencies of 17α-hydroxylase, 3β-ol-dehydrogenase, 17-ketosteroid reductase, and 17,20-desmolase, as well as the enzymes required to convert cholesterol to pregnenolone (congenital adrenal lipoid hyperplasia; see Fig. 7–7). Deficiencies of 21- or 11β-hydroxylase, the most common causes of female pseudohermaphroditism, do not cause male pseudohermaphroditism; instead, males (46,XY) show precocious masculinization (see earlier).

Defects of adrenal biosynthesis should be suspected when levels of testosterone or its metabolites are decreased. Diagnosis of the various conditions to be discussed later is not difficult in older children, but detection may be difficult during infancy because neonatal testosterone levels are naturally low. The postnatal rise of testosterone between 6 and 12 weeks of age may be helpful, however. Provocative tests (e.g., human chorionic gonadotropin [hCG] stimulation) may facilitate diagnosis.

Congenital Adrenal Lipoid Hyperplasia

Male pseudohermaphrodites with congenital adrenal lipoid hyperplasia show ambiguous or gynecoid external genitalia and severe sodium wasting. Adrenals are characterized by foamy-looking cells filled with cholesterol.[157, 158] Accumulation of cholesterol has long indicated that cholesterol cannot be converted to pregnenolone (see Fig. 7–7). Inheritance has been presumed to be autosomal-recessive, on the basis of increased parental consanguinity.

The cytochrome P450 enzyme responsible for converting cholesterol to pregnenolone is called P450scc (side chain cleavage); the gene is CYP11A. P450scc converts cholesterol to pregnenolone via 20α-hydroxylase, 22α-hydroxylase, and 20,22-desmolase. A large gene located on chromosome 15, CYP11A is 20 kb long with nine exons.

Surprisingly, perturbations of CYP11A have never been demonstrated in association with congenital adrenal lipoid hyperplasia.[159] Rather, the disorder results from perturbation steroidogenic acute regulatory protein (StAR). The StAR protein delivers precursors for cholesterol side chain cleavage, and, predictably, its perturbation has profound effects on processes that require steroids. The StAR gene is located on chromosome 8 (p11.2). It consists of seven exons and is 8 kb long. Mutations in StAR have been reported in congenital lipoid hyperplasia.[160] This mutation results in the production of a nonfunctional protein. The usual molecular defects are point mutations producing stop condons or exon-intron splicing errors that yield large deletions or truncated gene products. In either case the protein is nonfunctional.

3β-Hydroxysteroid Dehydrogenase (3β-HSD)(3β-ol-Dehydrogenase) Deficiency

Already mentioned in the section on female pseudohermaphroditism, this enzyme deficiency is inherited in autosomal-recessive fashion. Synthesis of both androgens and estrogens is decreased (see Fig. 7–7).[161] The major androgen produced is DHEA, which is a weaker androgen than testosterone and, thus, not capable of adequately virilizing a male fetus. The diagnosis is usually established on the basis of serum DHEA levels before and after ACTH stimulation. In addition to genital abnormalities, 3β-ol-dehydrogenase deficiency is associated with severe sodium wasting, as a result of reductions in both aldosterone and cortisol.

Incompletely developed external genitalia of males with 3β-HSD deficiency are clinically similar to the external genitalia of most other male pseudohermaphrodites: small phallus, urethral opening proximal on the penis, and incomplete labioscrotal fusion. Testes and wolffian ducts differentiate normally.

Unlike 21- or 11β-hydroxylase, 3β-HSD is a microsomal enzyme. The relevant gene is located on 1p 13.1, and is the type II enzyme. Type I is expressed in placenta, skin, and breasts; type II in adrenal cortex and gonads. Male pseudohermaphroditism resulting from type II 3β-HSD mutations usually are point mutations.[138]

17α-Hydroxylase and 17,20-Desmolase (Lyase) Deficiency

The enzyme 17α-hydroxylase/17,20-lyase is cytochrome P450 gene (CYP17), located on 10q24–25. The gene product has both 17α-hydroxylase and 17,20 desmolase (lyase) activity. Males deficient in 17α-hydroxylase/17,20 desmolase (lyase) usually have ambiguous external genitalia. Severely affected males may even have gynecoid external genitalia.[162] Both males and females are affected, inheritance being autosomal-recessive.

When it became evident that a single enzyme serves both 17α-hydroxylase and 17,20-desmolase functions, considerable genetic and nosologic confusion was generated.[163] That a single gene and enzyme are responsible for both these functions was a surprise, because some studies had suggested two genetically distinct conditions involving two separate genes. Recent reports of mutations that affect only the 17,20-lyase function may compound the confusion.[164, 165] On the other hand, this phenomenon might help explain the family described by Zachmann's group.[166] Two maternal cousins had genital ambiguity, bilateral testes, and no Müllerian derivatives; a maternal "aunt" was said to have abnormal external genitalia and bilateral testes. The deficient enzyme in this family was thought to be 17,20-desmolase (lyase), on the basis of both cousins' showing low plasma testosterone and DHEA levels despite normal urinary excretion of pregnanediol, pregnanetriol, and 17-hydroxycorticoids. In testicular tissue, testosterone could be synthesized from androstenedione or DHEA; this finding ruled out 17-ketosteroid reductase deficiency (see later) but suggested isolated 17,20-desmolase deficiency.

The single P450c17 enzyme is coded by a gene (CYP17) on chromosome 10q24–25. Consisting of eight exons, CYP17 is structurally reminiscent of its CYP21 cousin 21-hydroxylase; however, no pseudogene coexists. Point mutations are the typical molecular perturbation. Deletions and gene conversions are uncommon.[167–169]

Deficiency of 17β-Hydroxysteroid Dehydrogenase (17-Ketosteroid Reductase)

Inability to convert androstenedione to testosterone is the result of deficiency of this microsomal enzyme (see Fig. 7–7).[170] Plasma testosterone is usually decreased; androstenedione and DHEA are increased. Affected males have ambiguous external genitalia, bilateral testes, and no Müllerian derivatives. Breast development may or may not be present, apparently depending on the estrogen-testosterone ratio.[171] Pubertal virilization is greater than with many other enzyme deficiencies, and sometimes gynecomastia is not even evident.[172] In one report, the sex of rearing of an affected person was changed from female to male after puberty.[171]

The 17-β-hydroxysteroid dehydrogenase gene (17HSD-3) is located on chromosome 9 and consists of 11 exons. This gene is microsomal, like 3β-HSD, reflecting its principal action involving gonads. Molecular perturbations typically involve single amino acid substitutions,[173, 174] but disruption of the splice junction involving intron 3 is not uncommon. Exon or intron 3 is most often involved, but mutations may also occur in exons 2, 8, 9, 10, 11, and 12. Missense mutations may result in negligible levels of testosterone secondary to complete impairment of the enzyme.

COMPLETE ANDROGEN INSENSITIVITY (COMPLETE TESTICULAR FEMINIZATION)

Persons with complete androgen insensitivity (CAI) have a 46,XY genotype and bilateral testes, female external genitalia, a blind vagina, and no Müllerian derivatives (Fig. 7–8). These findings are entirely predictable, given that the underlying mechanism is the inability to respond to testosterone. AMH is synthesized as in normal testes. The body responds normally to AMH, for which reason, and predictably, no uterus is present. Because the testes synthesize estrogen,

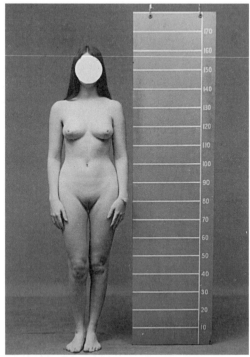

Figure 7–8. Photograph of patient with complete testicular feminization. (From Simpson JL: Disorders of Sexual Differentiation: Etiology and Clinical Delineation. New York: Academic Press, 1976. Courtesy of Dr. Charles Hammond.)

affected persons develop breasts and exhibit pubertal feminization.

Despite pubertal feminization, some individuals with androgen insensitivity show clitoral enlargement and labioscrotal fusion. The term *incomplete* (or *partial*) *androgen insensitivity* (PAI) or *incomplete testicular feminization* is applied to their condition. At the most benign end of the spectrum are only males who have gynecomastia and oligospermia or azoospermia. Complete, incomplete (partial), and mild androgen insensitivity are all inherited in X-linked recessive fashion, and, in fact, all result from mutations of the androgen receptor gene on the X long arm (Xq11).

As adults, persons with CAI may be quite attractive and show excellent breast development. Despite the traditional textbook description, most are actually similar in appearance to unaffected women in the general population. Breasts contain normal ductal and glandular tissue, but areolae are often pale and underdeveloped. Pubic hair and axillary hair are usually sparse (only vellus hair present), but scalp hair is normal. The vagina is blind, and sometimes shorter than usual. Occasionally, it is only 1 to 2 cm long or is merely a dimple. Surgery to create a neovagina or use of dilators may be necessary, but vaginal length is usually adequate without intervention. Neither a uterus nor fallopian tubes are ordinarily present, but there may be fibromuscular remnants, rudimentary fallopian tubes, or, rarely, even a uterus.[175]

Testes are usually normal in size. They may be located in the abdomen, inguinal canal, labia, or anywhere along the path of embryonic testicular descent. When located in the inguinal canal, the testes may produce inguinal hernias. Half of all individuals with testicular feminization have inguinal hernias. It is therefore worthwhile to determine the cytogenetic status of prepubertal girls with inguinal hernias, although most are 46,XX. Height is slightly greater than that of normal women, but is unremarkable as compared with 46,XY males.

The frequency of gonadal neoplasia is increased, but not so much as was once assumed.[176] The actual risk is probably no greater than 5%.[120, 143] The risk of malignancy is low before 25 to 30 years of age. Benign tubular adenomas (Pick adenomas) are common in postpubertal patients, probably as a result of increased LH secretion. Orchiectomy is eventually necessary, but it is acceptable to leave the testes in situ until spontaneous pubertal feminization is completed. However, if herniorrhaphy proves necessary before puberty, most surgeons perform orchiectomy at the same time. There may also be some psychological benefit to prepubertal orchiectomy.

The androgen receptor gene, localized to Xq11-Xq12, consists of eight exons. Exons 2 and 3 are the DNA-binding domains, whereas exons 4 through 8 are androgen-binding domains (Fig. 7–9).[177] Many different mutations have been reported,[178] but no single perturbation has proved paramount. Deletions and insertions are rare,[179] and point mutations in general far more common. These include deletion of three nucleotides with preservation of an open reading frame, single-nucleotide changes resulting in substitution of an unscheduled amino acid, or changes generating a stop codon, which would result in premature message termination and production of a nonfunctional protein. Mutations are found throughout the gene, but particularly in exons 4 through 8 (the androgen-binding domain). In

Exons, Binding Domains of the hAR

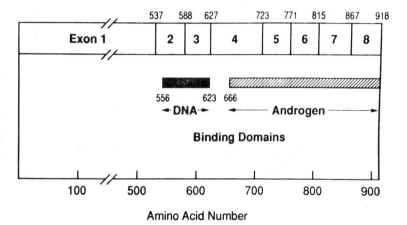

Figure 7–9. Schematic diagram showing androgen-binding gene. Exons 2 through 4 relate to DNA binding, whereas exons 5 through 7 confer androgen binding. Sites of some reported mutations are noted. (Adapted from a diagram of Dr. Leonard Pinsky's, Montreal, Quebec.)

exons 5 to 8 the preponderance of mutations are missense. Mutations in exon 1 usually cause complete androgen insensitivity, and mutations in exons 2 and 3 (the DNA-binding domain) produce either CAI or PAI. In general and predictably, large deletions and mutations resulting in premature termination (stop codon) produce no functional receptor and cause CAI.[180] Point mutations resulting from single-nucleotide substitutions have a similar phenotype but may also be compatible with production of some androgen receptor. The receptor may nevertheless be unstable or display poor binding.[180]

INCOMPLETE OR PARTIAL ANDROGEN INSENSITIVITY (INCOMPLETE TESTICULAR FEMINIZATION AND REIFENSTEIN SYNDROME)

At puberty, certain 46,XY individuals develop breasts, whereas their external genitalia are characterized by phallic enlargement and partial labioscrotal fusion (Fig. 7–10). These persons have incomplete or partial androgen insensitivity (PAI; incomplete testicular feminization). PAI and CAI share many features: bilateral testes with Leydig cell hyperplasia, no müllerian derivatives, pubertal breast development, failure of pubertal virilization, normal (male) plasma testosterone, and androgen unresponsiveness.[181] Cellular pathogenesis involves decreased numbers or qualitative defects of androgen receptors.[182–184]

Incomplete androgen insensitivity must be excluded before a male sex of rearing can be assigned. Demonstration of response by androgen receptors or of a clinical response to exogenous androgen rules out the condition; demonstration of a specific molecular defect in the androgen receptor gene would be useful only if the mutation in an index case were already available or the phenotype of that specific nucleotide change were known.

As in CAI, molecular analysis reveals mutations. Molecular analysis has revealed many different mutations in the DNA and androgen-binding domains. Aside from the generalizations cited earlier, correlation between phenotype and the involved exon or sequence is poor.

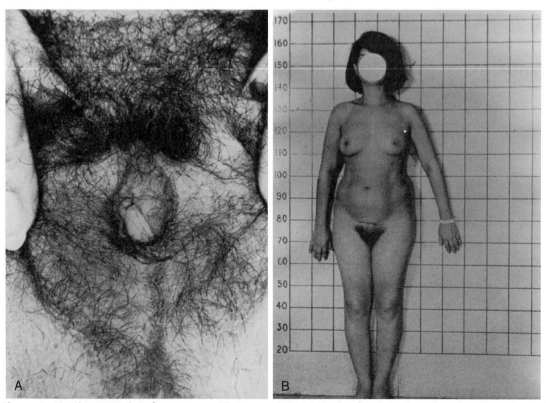

Figure 7–10. Photographs of a person with incomplete testicular feminization. Despite the enlarged phallus and labioscrotal fusion, *A*, breasts developed at puberty, *B*. (From Park IJ, Jones HW: Familial male hermaphroditism with ambiguous external genitalia. Am J Obstet Gynecol 1970; 108:1197.)

5α-REDUCTASE DEFICIENCY (PSEUDOVAGINAL PERINEOSCROTAL HYPOSPADIAS)

For decades it has been recognized that some genetic males who show ambiguous external genitalia at birth undergo virilization at puberty as normal males do—phallic enlargement, increased facial hair, muscle hypertrophy, and voice deepening, but no breast development. Their external genitalia consist of a phallus that resembles a clitoris more than a penis, a perineal urethral orifice, and, usually, a separate, blind perineal orifice that resembles a vagina (pseudovagina; Fig. 7–11).

Initially called *pseudovaginal perineoscrotal hypospadias* (PPSH), this trait was shown in 1971 to be inherited in autosomal-recessive fashion.[185, 186] This disorder later proved to result from deficiency of 5α-reductase,[187–189] an enzyme that converts testosterone to dihydrotestosterone (DHT). That intracellular 5α-reductase deficiency results in the PPSH phenotype is consistent with virilization of the external genitalia during embryogenesis requiring dihydrotestosterone; wolffian differentiation requires only testosterone. Pubertal virilization can also be accomplished by testosterone alone. Females (46,XX) deficient in 5α-reductase show normal ovarian function.[190]

Diagnosis is most easily made on the basis of an elevated testosterone-DHT ratio after administration of hCG or testosterone propionate.[191] The ratio of the respective urinary metabolites of testosterone and DHT (i.e., etiocholanolone and androsterone) is also elevated. In infants, baseline levels of testosterone and DHT are so low that distinguishing normal from affected individuals may be difficult. An elevated urinary tetrahydrocortisol–5α-tetrahydrocortisol ratio is also diagnostic.[192]

A caveat: 5α-reductase activity is higher in some tissues than in others. Thus, it is preferable to assay cells derived from genital tissue (e.g., foreskin). Considerable variability in 5α-reductase activity is observed among control genital tissue samples, however, with near overlap between controls and individuals recognized on other grounds to be deficient in 5α-reductase. Presence of 5α-reductase in cultural genital fibroblasts thus excludes 5α-reductase deficiency, whereas absence of 5α-reductase makes the diagnosis less conclusive. Diagnosis may be especially vexing in infants because baseline levels of T and DHT are so low and distinguishing normal from affected individuals may be difficult.

Two 5α-reductase (SRD5) genes exist. The type I gene is located on chromosome 5 (SRD5A1), type II (SRD5A2) on chromosome 2p23. Only type II is expressed in gonads; thus, of the two isoforms type II is deficient in male pseudohermaphroditism. Consisting of five exons,[193] the SRD5A2 gene has been shown to have undergone deletions far less[194] often than point mutations.[195] Different ethnic groups show different mutations (founder effect) scattered among the five exons. The molecular basis can be exploited for prenatal diagnosis and genetic counseling in kindreds, but usually only after one affected case has been detected.

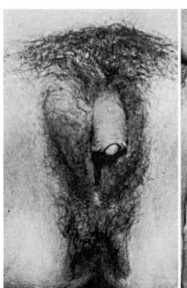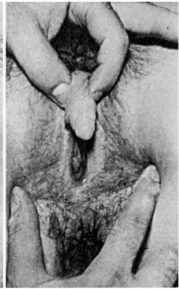

Figure 7–11. Photographs of the external genitalia of a person with pseudovaginal perineoscrotal hypospadias. At puberty, phallic enlargement occurred and breast development did not. Some with this phenotype have 5α-reductase deficiency. (From Opitz JM, Simpson JL, Sarto GE, et al: Pseudovaginal perineoscrotal hypospadias. Clin Genet 1972; 3:1.)

AROMATASE MUTATIONS (CYP19 DEFICIENCY)

Conversion of androgens (Δ4-androstenedione) to estrogens (estrone) requires cytochrome P450 aromatase, an enzyme that is the gene product of a single 40-kb gene located on chromosome 15q21.1.[196] The gene consists of 10 exons. Although Ito and associates[197] reported a mutation in this cyp19 (P450 arom) gene in an 18-year-old, 46,XX woman with primary amenorrhea and cystic ovaries, deficiency of the aromatase enzyme is more often associated with genital ambiguity.

Shozu and colleagues[198] detected *placental* aromatase deficiency manifested as maternal virilization during the third trimester. The 46,XX infant had ambiguous genitalia (female pseudohermaphroditism). Adrenal enzyme defects were not evident. The molecular basis of the mutation was an 87-bp insert in exon 6 of the aromatase gene, altering the splice junction site to produce a novel protein with 29 additional amino acids. Aromatase mutation in 46,XX female infants has been associated with genital ambiguity[197] or clitorimegaly.[199] In the latter cases, clitoral enlargement occurred at puberty, but breast development did not. Multiple ovarian follicular cysts were evident. FSH was elevated, estrone and estradiol low. Estrogen and progesterone therapy produced a growth spurt, decreased FSH, decreased androstenedione and testosterone, breast development, menarche, and fewer follicular cysts. Molecular studies demonstrated compound heterozygosity for CYP19 point mutations.

ESTROGEN RECEPTOR DEFECTS

The estrogen receptor gene consists of eight exons and is coded on chromosome 6q24→27. Like the much better-studied androgen receptor gene, the gene contains a DNA-binding region (exons 2 and 3) and an estrogen-binding domain (exons 4 through 8).

An estrogen receptor mutation described by Lubahn and coworkers[200] was found in a 28-year-old man who showed normal male sexual development. Incomplete epiphyseal closure led to tall stature. Serum gonadotropin and estrogen levels were elevated, and neither decreased after exogenous estrogen administration. The molecular basis proved to be a homozygous transition in exon 2 that resulted in a premature stop codon.[201]

AGONADIA (TESTICULAR REGRESSION SYNDROME)

In agonadia, gonads are absent, external genitalia are normal, and all but rudimentary Müllerian or wolffian derivatives are absent. External genitalia usually consist of a phallus about the size of a clitoris, underdeveloped labia majora, and nearly complete labioscrotal fusion. A persistent urogenital sinus is often present. By definition, gonads are undetectable. Ordinarily, neither normal Müllerian derivatives nor normal wolffian derivatives are present; however, rudimentary structures may be present along the lateral pelvic wall. Somatic anomalies (craniofacial or vertebral anomalies or mental retardation) sometimes co-exist.[202]

The pathogenesis of agonadia must take into account not only the absence of gonads but also abnormal external genitalia and absence of internal ducts. Two explanations seem plausible:

1. Fetal testes functioned long enough during development to inhibit müllerian development but not long enough to allow complete normal male sexual differentiation. Believing this explanation to be valid, some prefer the appellation *testicular regression syndrome.*
2. Alternatively, gonadal, ductal, and genital systems all could have developed abnormally as a result of defective primordium, defective connective tissue, or a teratogen. Coexistence of somatic anomalies is most consistent with this second hypothesis.

Several sibships of affected males have been reported,[34] suggesting autosomal-recessive inheritance. The presence of SRY indicates that pathogenesis does not involve gross perturbation of that gene.[9, 203, 204] Kwok and coworkers[203] found no mutations in the sequence 2kb 5' to the SRY-coding region.

LEYDIG CELL HYPOPLASIA

With complete absence of Leydig cells,[205, 206] 46,XY persons have female external genitalia, no uterus, and bilateral testes lacking Leydig cells. Epididymides and vasa deferentia are present, and serum LH is elevated. Affected siblings have been reported[207, 208] and parental consanguinity observed.[204] Thus, autosomal-recessive inheritance has long been accepted.

More recently, a molecular basis was elucidated, a mutation in the LHR gene located on chromosome 2 near the FSHR gene. Kremer and colleagues[209] reported two siblings (of consanguineous parents) who were homozygous for a missense mutation (Ala[(593)]→Pro). In another case, Salameh's group[210] detected a deletion in exon 11. Leydig cells presumably fail to develop because LH cannot exert its effect during embryogenesis. This is reminiscent of ovarian failure due to FSHR mutation (see earlier).

Activating mutations cause precocious puberty in males. In females, LHR-activating mutations do not result in any clinical abnormality.

TRUE HERMAPHRODITISM

True hermaphrodites have both ovarian and testicular tissue. They may have a discrete ovary and a discrete testis, but more often they have one or more ovotestes. Most true hermaphrodites (60%) have a 46,XX chromosome complement; however, a majority have 46,XX/46,XY, 46,XY, 46,XX/47,XXY, or another one.[211] Phenotype may reflect karyotype,[211, 212] but it is preferable here only to generalize about the phenotype of all true hermaphrodites.

CLINICAL

If no medical intervention were to occur (today, obviously, a rarity in most venues), two thirds of true hermaphrodites would be raised as males.[51] By contrast, external genitalia are usually ambiguous or predominantly female. Breast development usually occurs at puberty, even in those with predominantly male external genitalia.

Gonadal tissue may be located in the ovarian, inguinal, or labioscrotal region. A testis or an ovotestis is more likely to be present on the right than on the left side. Spermatozoa are rarely present;[213] however, apparently normal oocytes often are, even in ovotestes (Fig. 7–12). A few 46,XX true hermaphrodites have become pregnant,[214, 215] usually, though not always, after removal of testicular tissue.

The greater the proportion of testicular tissue in an ovotestis, the greater is the likelihood of gonadal descent. In 80% of ovotestes, testicular and ovarian components are juxtaposed end to end.[216] An ovotestis may thus be detectable by inspection or palpation because testicular tissue is softer and darker than ovarian tissue. Accurate identification by ultrasound or magnetic resonance is necessary if the inappropriate portion of the ovotestis is to be extirpated. Both gonadal neoplasia and breast carcinoma have been reported.[153, 211] The former probably reflects the risks associated with intra-abdominal testicular tissue.

A uterus is usually present although sometimes bicornuate or unicornuate. Absence of a uterine horn usually indicates an ipsilateral testis or ovotestis. The fimbriated end of the fallopian tube may be occluded ipsilateral to an ovotestis, and squamous metaplasia of the endocervix may occur.[216] Menstruation is not uncommon and may be manifested as cyclic hematuria.[217]

Presence of a uterus is diagnostically useful in true hermaphroditism and particularly invaluable in the rare 46,XY cases. Among those with ambiguous genitalia who have a Y chromosome,

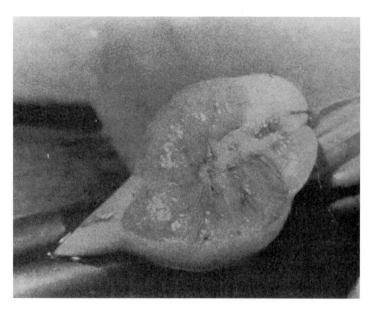

Figure 7–12. A bisected ovotestis from a patient of Van Niekerk's. The patient had a 46,XX complement. The ratio of ovarian to testicular tissue is about 1:4; ovarian tissue is present in the upper right. The testicular portion appeared yellowish brown, whereas the ovarian portion was white, although, in this photograph, the color difference cannot be appreciated. The ovarian portion was firmer than was the testicular portion. In 80% of ovotestes, just as in this patient, ovarian and testicular tissues are arranged end to end. (From Van Niekerk WA: True Hermaphroditism. New York: Harper & Row, 1974.)

only 46,XY hermaphrodites and 45,X/46,XY mosaics have a uterus.

Diagnosis is usually made only after excluding male and female pseudohermaphroditism. If a female sex of rearing is chosen, extensive surgery may or may not be necessary. If a male sex of rearing is chosen, genital reconstruction and selective gonadal extirpation are invariably indicated.

46,XX/46,XY AND 46,XY FORMS

True hermaphroditism is heterogeneous in origin. Usually, 46,XX/46,XY true hermaphroditism is caused by chimerism, the presence in a single individual of two or more cell lines, each derived from a different zygote. Some 46,XY cases are unrecognized chimeras.[211] Chimerism is not the likely explanation for 46,XX true hermaphrodites, however. Explanations for the presence of testes in individuals who ostensibly lack a Y have focused on (1) translocation of SRY from the paternal Y to the paternal X during meiosis, (2) translocation of SRY from the paternal Y to a paternal autosome, (3) undetected mosaicism or chimerism, and (4) autosomal sex reversal genes.

46,XX FORM

The 46,XX true hermaphrodites fail to show SRY on DNA sequences from their fathers' Y chromosomes.[218] This contrasts with 46,XX males, 80% of whom show SRY. Detection of the SRY sequence in one 46,XX true hermaphrodite and a 46,XX male sibling did give a strong clue that Y/X translocation can be involved,[12] but, overall, mendelian factors seem more likely explanations for the reported sibships with XX true hermaphroditism.[211] Occurrence of 46,XX males and 46,XX true hermaphrodites in the same kindred has also been reported. The 46,XX males in these kindreds usually have ambiguous genitalia, unlike typical 46,XX males.

REFERENCES

1. Patsavoudi E, Magre S, Castinior M, et al: Dissociation between testicular morphogenesis and functional differentiation of Leydig cells. J Endocrinol 1985; 28:235.
2. Magre S, Jost A: Dissociation between testicular morphogenesis and endocrine cytodifferentiation of Sertoli cells. Proc Natl Acad Sci USA 1984; 81:783.
3. Behringer RR, Cate RL, Froelick GJ, et al: Abnormal sexual development in transgenetic mice chronically expressing Müllerian inhibiting substance. Nature 1990; 345:16.
4. Lee MM, Donahoe PK: Müllerian inhibiting substance: A gonadal hormone with multiple functions. Endocrinol Rev 1993; 14:152.
5. Gustafson ML, Lee MM, Asmundson L, et al: Müllerian inhibiting substance in the diagnosis and management of intersex and gonadal abnormalities. J Pediatr Surg 1993; 28:439.
6. Jirasek J: Principles of reproductive embryology. In Simpson JL (ed): Disorders of Sexual Differentiation. San Diego: Academic Press, 1976, p 51.
7. Gubbay J, Collignon J, Koopman P, et al: A gene mapping to the sex-determining region of the mouse Y chromosome is a member of a novel family of embryonically expressed genes. Nature 1991; 346:245.
8. Sinclair AH, Berta PH, Palmer MS, et al: A gene from the human sex-determining region encodes a protein with homology to a conserved DNA-binding motif. Nature 1990; 346:240.
9. Pivnick EK, Wachtel S, Woods D, et al: Mutations in the conserved domain of SRY are uncommon in XY gonadal dysgenesis. Hum Genet 1992; 90:308.
10. Berta P, Hawkins JR, Sinclair AH, et al: Genetic evidence equating SRY and the testis-determining factor. Nature 1990; 348:448.
11. Hawkins JR, Taylor A, Berta P, et al: Mutational analysis of SRY: Nonsense and missense mutations in XY sex reversal. Hum Genet 1992; 88:471.
12. Jager RJ, Anvret M, Hall K, et al: A human XY female with a frame shift mutation in the candidate testis-determining gene SRY. Nature 1990; 348:452.
13. Koopman P, Gubbay J, Vivian N, et al: Male development of chromosomally female mice transgenic for Sry. Nature 1991; 351:117.
14. Simpson JL, Christakos AC, Horwith M, et al: Gonadal dysgenesis associated with apparently chromosomal complements. Birth Defects 1971; 7(6):215.
15. German J, Simpson JL, Chaganti RSK, et al: Genetically determined sex-reversal in 46,XY humans. Science 1978; 205:53.
16. Bernstein R, Jenkins T, Dawson T, et al: Female phenotype and multiple abnormalities in siblings with a Y-chromosome and partial X-chromosomal duplication: H-Y antigen and Xg blood group findings. J Med Genet 1980; 17:291.
17. Ogata T, Hawkins JR, Taylor A, et al: Sex reversal in a child with a 46,X,Yp + karyotype: Support for the existence of a gene, located in distal Xp, involved in testis formation. J Med Genet 1992; 29:226.
18. Ogata T, Tomita K, Hida A, et al: Chromosomal localization of a Y specific growth gene(s). J Med Genet 1995; 32:572.
19. Arn P, Chen H, Tuck-Muller CM, et al: SRVX, a sex reversing locus in Xp21.2→p22.11. Hum Genet 1994; 4:389.
20. Rao PN, Klinepeter K, Stewart W, et al: Molecular cytogenetic analysis of a duplication Xp in a male: Further delineation of a possible sex influence region on the X chromosome. Hum Genet 1994; 94:149.
21. Bardoni B, Xanaria E, Guioli S, et al: A dose sensitive locus at chromosome Xp21 is involved in male to female sex reversal. Nat Genet 1994; 7:497.
22. Tommerup N, Schempp W, Meinecke P, et al: Assignment of an autosomal sex reversal locus (SRA1) and campomelic dysplasia (CMPD1) to 17q24.3-q25.1. Nat Genet 1993; 4:170.
23. Foster JW, Dominguez-Steglich MA, Guioli S, et al: Campomelic dysplasia and autosomal sex reversal caused by mutations in an SRY-related gene. Nature 1994; 372:525.

24. Meyer J, Sudbeck P, Held M, et al: Mutational analysis of the SOX9 gene in campomelic dysplasia and autosomal sex reversal: Lack of genotype/phenotype correlations. Hum Mol Genet 1997; 6(1):91.

25. Pelletier J, Bruening W, Li FP, et al: WT1 mutations contribute to abnormal genital system development and hereditary Wilms' tumour. Nature 1991; 353:431.

26. Pelletier J, Bruening W, Kashtan CE, et al: Germline mutations in the Wilms' tumor suppressor gene are associated with abnormal urogenital development in Danys-Drash syndrome. Cell 1991; 67:437.

27. Nordenskjold Á, Fricke G, Anvret M: Absence of mutations in the WT1 gene in patients with XY gonadal dysgenesis. Hum Genet 1995; 96:102.

28. Wilkie AOM, Campbell FM, Daubeney P, et al: Complete and partial XY sex reversal associates with terminal deletion of 10q: Report of cases and literature review. Am J Med Genet 1993; 46:597.

29. Bennett CP, Docherty Z, Robb SA, et al: Deletion 9p and sex reversal. J Med Genet 1993; 30:518.

30. Vegetti W, Grazia Tibiletti M, Testa G, et al: Inheritance in idiopathic premature ovarian failure: Analysis of 71 cases. Hum Reprod 1998; 13:1796.

31. Schinzel A: Phocomelia and additional anomalies in two sisters. Hum Genet 1990; 84:539.

32. Ferguson-Smith MA, Sanoudou D, Lee C: Microdeletion of DMT1 at 9p24.3 is the commonest cause of 46,XY females. Am J Hum Genet 1998; 63:A162.

33. McDonald MT, Flejter W, Sheldon S, et al: XY sex reversal and gonadal dysgenesis due to 9p24 monosomy. Am J Med Genet 1997; 73:321.

34. de Grouchy J, Gompel A, Salmon-Bernard Y: Embryonic testicular regression syndrome and severe mental retardation in sibs. Ann Genet 1985; 28:154.

35. Najjar SS, Takla RJ, Nassar VH: The syndrome of rudimentary testes: Occurrence in five siblings. J Pediatr 1974; 84:119.

36. Hamet P, Kuchel O, Nowacynski JM, et al: Hypertension with adrenal, genital, renal defects, and deafness. A new familial syndrome. Arch Intern Med 1973; 131:563.

37. Smith A, Fraser IS, Noel M: Three siblings with premature gonadal failure. Fertil Steril 1979; 32:528.

38. Granat M, Amar A, Mor-Yosef S, et al: Familial gonadal germinative failure: Endocrine and human leukocyte antigen studies. Fertil Steril 1983; 40:215.

39. Al-Awadi SA, Farag TI, Geebie AS, et al: Primary hypergonadism and partial alopecia in three sibs with Müllerian hypoplasia in the affected females. Am J Med Genet 1985; 22:619.

40. Mikati MA, Samir SN, Sahil IF: Microcephaly, hypergonadotropic hypogonadism, short stature and minor anomalies. A new syndrome. Am J Med Genet 1985; 22:599.

41. Burgoyne PS, Baker TG: Perinatal oocyte loss in XO mice and its implication for the etiology of gonadal dysgenesis in XO women. J Reprod Fertil 1987; 75:633.

42. Simpson JL: Phenotypic-karyotypic correlations of gonadal determinants: Current status and relationship to molecular studies. *In* Sperling K, Vogel F (eds): Proceedings of the 7th International Congress, Human Genetics, Berlin, 1986. Heidelberg: Springer-Verlag, 1987, p 224.

43. Simpson JL: Genetic control of sexual development. *In* Ratnam SS, Teoh ED (eds): Advances in Fertility and Sterility: Releasing Hormones and Genetics and Immunology in Human Reproduction, vol 3. Proceedings of the 12th World Congress on Fertility and Sterility, Singapore, 1986. Lancaster, UK: Parthenon Press, 1987, p 165.

44. Simpson JL: Genetic control of sex determination. *In* Iizuka R, Seem K, Ohno T (eds): Human Reproduction—Current Status, Future Prospects. Proceedings of the 6th World Congress on Human Reproduction, Tokyo, 1987. Amsterdam: Elsevier Scientific, 1988, p 19.

45. Simpson JL: Genetics of female infertility. *In* Filicori M, Flamigni C (eds): Proceedings of the Conference, Treatment of Infertility: The New Frontiers. Boca Raton, Florida, Communications Media for Education, Inc., 1998, p 37.

46. Zinn AR, Tonk VS, Chen Z, et al: Evidence for a Turner syndrome locus or loci Xp11.2-p22.1. Am J Hum Genet 1998; 63:1757.

47. Tharapel AT, Anderson KP, Simpson JJ, et al: Deletion (X)(q26.1→q28) in a proband and her mother: Molecular characterization and phenotypic-karyotypic deduction. Am J Hum Genet 1993; 52:463.

48. Simpson JL: Genetics of oocyte depletion. *In* Lobo RA (ed): Perimenopause. Serono Symposia USA Norwell, Massachusetts. New York: Springer, 1998, p 36.

49. Aittomaki K: The genetics of XX gonadal dysgenesis. Am J Hum Genet 1994; 54:844.

50. Simpson JL: Gonadal dysgenesis and abnormalities of the human sex chromosomes: Current status of the phenotypic-karyotypic correlations. Birth Defects 1975; 11(4):23.

51. Simpson JL: Disorders of sexual differentiation: Etiology and clinical delineation. New York: Academic Press, 1976, p 259.

52. Loughlin SAR, Redha A, McIver J, et al: Analysis of the origin of Turner's syndrome using polymorphic DNA probes. J Med Genet 1991; 28:156.

53. James RS, Dalton P, Gustashaw K, et al: Molecular characterization of isochromosomes of Xq. Ann Hum Genet 1997; 61:485.

54. James RS, Coppin B, Dalton P, et al: A study of females with deletions of the short arm of the X chromosome. Hum Genet 1988; 102:507.

55. Ogata T, Matsuo N: Turner syndrome and female sex chromosome aberrations: Deduction of the principal factors involved in the development of clinical features. Hum Genet 1995; 95:607.

56. Migeon BR, Jelalian K: Evidence for two active X chromosomes in germ cells of female before meiotic entry. Nature 1977; 269:242.

57. Simpson JL: Pregnancies in women with chromosomal abnormalities. *In* Schulman JD, Simpson JL (eds): Genetic Disease in Pregnancy. New York: Academic Press, 1981.

58. Dewhurst J: Fertility in 47,XXX and 45,X patients. J Med Genet 1978; 15:132.

59. Singh DN, Hara S, Foster HW, et al: Reproductive performance in women with sex chromosome mosaicism. Obstet Gynecol 1980; 55:608.

60. Ishikawa M, Hidaka E, Wakui K, et al: Habitual abortion and low frequent X chromosome monosomy mosaicism: Detection by interphase FISH analyses of buccal mucosa cells and lymphocytes. 48th Annual Meeting, American Society of Human Genetics. Am J Hum Genet 1998; 63:A108.

61. Fisher EM, Beer-Romero P, Brown LG, et al: Homologous ribosomal protein genes on the human X and Y chromosomes: Escape from X inactivation and possible implications for Turner syndrome. Cell 1990; 63:1205.

62. Chen YC, Woolley PV Jr: Genetic studies on hypospadias in males. J Med Genet 1971; 8:153.

63. Brook CGD, Wagner H, Zachman M, et al: Familial occurrence of persistent Müllerian structures in otherwise normal males. BMJ 1973; 1:771.

64. Ranke MB, Pfluger H, Rosendahl W, et al: Turner's syndrome spontaneous growth in 150 cases and review of the literature. Eur J Pediatr 1983; 181:141.

65. Ranke MB, Blum WF, Hang F, et al: Growth hormone, somatomedin levels and growth regulation in Turner's syndrome. Acta Endocrinol (Copenh) 1987; 116:305.

66. Rosenfeld RG, Grumbach MM: Turner Syndrome. New York: Marcel Dekker, 1990.

67. Filippson R, Lindsten J, Almqvist S: Time of eruption of the permanent teeth, cephalometric and tooth measurement and sulphation factor activities in 45 patients with Turner's syndrome with different types of X chromosome aberrations. Acta Endocrinol (Copenh) 1965; 48:91.

68. Lindsten J, Fraccaro M: Turner's syndrome. *In* Rashad MN, Morton WRN (eds): Genital Anomalies. Springfield, Ill: Charles C Thomas, 1969, p 396.

69. McCauley E, Sybert VP, Ehrhardt A: Psychological adjustments of adult women with Turner syndrome. Clin Genet 1986; 29:284.

70. McCauley E, Kay T, Ito I, et al: The Turner syndrome: Cognitive defects, affective discrimination and behavior problems. Child Dev 1987; 58:464.

71. Simpson JL: Genetic control of sexual development. *In* Teoh ES, Ratnam SS, Goh VHH (eds): Fertility and Sterility Series. Lancaster, UK: Parthenon Press, 1987, p 165.

72. Simpson JL: Ovarian maintenance determinants on the X chromosome and on autosomes. *In* Coutifaris C, Mastroianni L (eds): New Horizons in Reproductive Medicine—Proceedings of the IXth World Congress on Human Reproduction. Philadelphia: 1996; 1997, p 439.

73. Fraccaro M, Maraschio P, Pasquali F, et al: Women heterozygous for deficiency of the (Xpter→ X21) region of the X chromosome are fertile. Hum Genet 1977; 39:283.

74. Simpson JL, LeBeau MM: Gonadal and statural determinants on the X chromosome and their relationship to *in vitro* studies showing prolonged cell cycles in 45,X; 46,X,del(X)(p11); 46,X,del(X)(q13); and 46,X,del(X)q(22) fibroblasts. Am J Obstet Gynecol 1981; 141:930.

75. Sala C, Arrigo G, Torri G, et al: Eleven X chromosome breakpoints associated with premature ovarian failure (POF) map to a 15-Mb YAC contig spanning Xq21. Genomics 1997; 40:123.

76. Philippe C, Arnould C, Sloan F, et al: A high-resolution interval map of the q21 region of the human X chromosome. Genomics 1995; 27:539.

77. Willard HF, Cremers FP, Mandel JL, et al: Report of the Fifth International Workshop on Human X Chromosome Mapping. Cytogenet Cell Genet 1994; 67:295.

78. Krauss CM, Turkray RN, Atkins L, et al: Familial premature ovarian failure due to interstitial deletion of the long arm of the X chromosome. N Engl J Med 1987; 317:125.

79. Fitch N, de Saint VJ, Richer CL, et al: Premature menopause due to small deletion in long arm of the X chromosome: A report of three cases and a review. Am J Obstet Gynecol 1982; 142:968.

80. Jones MH, Furlong RA, Burkin H, et al: The *Drosophila* developmental gene fat facets has a human homologue in Xp11.4 which escapes X-inactivation and has related sequences on Yp11.2. Hum Mol Genet 1996; 5:1695.

81. Castrillon DH, Wasserman SA: *Diaphanous* is required for cytokinesis in *Drosophila* and shares domains of similarity with the products of the limb deformity gene. Development 1994; 120:3367.

82. Philippe C, Cremers FPM, Chery M, et al: Physical mapping of DNA markers in the q13-q22 region of the human X chromosome. Genomics 1993; 17:147.

83. Bione S, Sala C, Manzini C, et al: A human homologue of the *Drosophila melanogaster* diaphanous gene is disrupted in a patient with premature ovarian failure: Evidence for conserved function in oogenesis and implications for human sterility. Am J Hum Genet 1998; 62:533.

84. Simpson JL: Gonadal dysgenesis and sex chromosome abnormalities. Phenotypic/karyotypic correlations. *In* Vallet HL, Perter IH (eds): Genetic Mechanisms of Sexual Development. New York: Academic Press, 1979, p 365.

85. Meyers CM, Boughman JA, Rivas M, et al: Gonadal dysgenesis in 46,XX individuals: Frequency of the autosomal recessive form. Am J Med Genet 1996; 63:518.

86. Boczkowski K: Pure gonadal dysgenesis and ovarian dysplasia in sisters. Am J Obstet Gynecol 1970; 106:626.

87. Portuondo JA, Neyro JL, Benito JA, et al: Familial 46,XX gonadal dysgenesis. Int J Fertil 1987; 32:56.

88. Aittomaki K, Dieguez Luccena JL, Pakarinen P, et al: Mutation in the follicle-stimulating hormone receptor gene causes hereditary hypergonadotropic ovarian failure. Cell 1995; 82:959.

89. Pellas TC, Ramachandran B, Duncan M, et al: Germ-cell deficient (gcd), an insertional mutation manifested as infertility in transgenic mice. Proc Natl Acad Sci USA 1991; 88:8787.

90. Christakos AC, Simpson JL, Younger JB, et al: Gonadal dysgenesis as an autosomal recessive condition. Am J Obstet Gynecol 1969; 104:1027.

91. Pallister PD, Opitz JM: The Perrault syndrome: autosomal recessive ovarian dysgenesis with facultative, non–sex-limited sensorineural deafness. Am J Med Genet 1979; 22:629.

92. McCarthy DJ, Opitz JM: Perrault syndrome in sisters. Am J Med Genet 1985; 22:629.

93. Nishi Y, Hamamoto K, Kajiyama M, et al: The Perrault syndrome: Clinical report and review. Am J Med Genet 1988; 31:623.

94. Aittomaki K, Herva R, Stenman UH, et al: Clinical features of primary ovarian failure caused by a point mutation in the follicle-stimulating hormone receptor gene. J Clin Endocrinol Metab 1996; 81:3722.

95. Layman LC, Amede S, Cohen DP, et al: The Finnish follicle-stimulating hormone receptor gene mutation is rare in North American women with 46,XX ovarian failure. Fertil Steril 1998; 69:300.

96. Liu JY, Gromoll J, Cedars MI, et al: Identification of allelic variants in the follicle-stimulating hormone receptor genes of females with or without hypergonadotropic amenorrhea. Fertil Steril 1998; 70:326.

97. Sultan LH, Lumbroso S: LH receptor defects. *In* Kempers RD, Cohen J, Haney AF, Younger JB (eds): Fertility and Reproductive Medicine—Proceedings of the XVIth World Congress on Fertility and Sterility. Amsterdam: Elsevier Science, 1998, p 769.

98. Latronico AC, Anasti J, Arnhold IJ, et al: Brief report: Testicular and ovarian resistance to luteinizing hormone caused by inactivating mutations of the luteinizing hormone–receptor gene. N Engl J Med 1996; 334:507.

99. Toledo SP, Brunner HG, Kraaij R, et al: An inactivating mutation of the luteinizing hormone receptor causes amenorrhea in a 46,XX female. J Clin Endocrinol Metab 1996; 81:3850.

100. Skre H, Bassoe HH, Berg K, et al: Cerebellar ataxia and hypergonadotropic hypogonadism in two kindreds. Chance concurrence, pleiotropism or linkage? Clin Genet 1976; 9:234.

101. Maximilian C, Ionescu B, Bucur A: Deux soeurs avec dysgenesie gonadique majeure, hypotrophie staturale, microcephalie, arachnodactylie et caryotype 46,XX. J Genet Hum 1970; 10:26.

102. Quayle SA, Copeland KC: 46,XX gonadal dysgenesis with epibulbar dermoid. Am J Med Genet 1991; 40:75.

103. Pober BR, Zemel S, Hisama F: 46,XX gonadal dysgenesis, short stature and recurrent metabolic acidosis in two sisters. 48th Annual Meeting, The American Society of Human Genetics. Am J Hum Genet 1998; 63:652, A117.

104. Zlotogora J, Sagi M, Cohen T: The blepharophimosis-ptosis, and epicanthus inversus syndrome: Delineation of two types. Am J Hum Genet 1983; 33:1020.

105. Panidis D, Rousso D, Vavilis D, et al: Familial blepharophimosis with ovarian failure. Hum Reprod 1994; 9:2034.

106. Harrar HS, Jeffrey S, Patton MA: Linkage analysis in blepharophimosis-ptosis syndrome confirms localization to 3q21–24. J Med Genet 1995; 32:774.

107. Fraser IS, Shearman RP, Smith A, et al: An association among blepharophimosis, resistant ovary syndrome, and true premature menopause. Fertil Steril 1988; 50:747.

108. Kaufman FR, Kogut MD, Donnell GN, et al: Hypergonadotropic hypogonadism in female patients with galactosemia. N Engl J Med 1981; 304:994.

109. Waggoner DD, Buist NR, Donnell GN: Long-term prognosis in galactosaemia: Results of a survey of 350 cases. J Inherit Metab Dis 1990; 13:802.

110. Levy HL, Driscoll SG, Porensky RS, et al: Ovarian failure in galactosemia. N Engl J Med 1984; 310:50.

111. Cramer DW, Xu H, Harlow BL: Family history as a predictor of early menopause. Fertil Steril 1995; 64:740.

112. Cramer DW, Harlow BL, Barbieri RL, et al: Galactose-1-phosphate uridyl transferase activity associated with age at menopause and reproductive history. Fertil Steril 1989; 51:609.

113. Kaufman FR, Devgan S, Donnell GN: Results of a survey of carrier women for the galactosemia gene. Fertil Steril 1993; 60:727.

114. Leslie ND, Yager K, Bai S: A mouse model for transferase deficiency galactosemia. Am J Hum Genet 1995; 57:191, A38.

115. Jost A: Problems of fetal endocrinology. The gonadal and hypophyseal hormones. Recent Prog Horm Res 1953; 8:379.

116. Cussen LK, McMahon R: Germ cells and ova in dysgenetic gonads of a 46,XY female dizygote twin. Arch Dis Child 1979; 133:373.

117. Simpson JL, Blagowidow N, Martin OA: XY gonadal dysgenesis: Genetic heterogeneity based upon clinical observations. H-Y antigen status and segregation analysis. Hum Genet 1981; 58:91.

118. Simpson JL, Chaganti RSK, Mouradian J, et al: Chronic renal disease, myotonic dystrophy, and gonadoblastoma in an individual with XY gonadal dysgenesis. J Med Genet 1982; 19:73.

119. Haning RV Jr, Chesney RW, Moorthy AV, et al: A syndrome of chronic renal failure and XY gonadal dysgenesis in young phenotypic females without genital ambiguity. Am J Kidney Dis 1985; 6:40.

120. Simpson JL, Photopulos G: The relationship of neoplasia to disorders of abnormal sexual differentiation. Birth Defects 1976; 12(1):15.

121. Wilson EE, Vuitch F, Carr BR: Laparoscopic removal of dysgenetic gonads containing a gonadoblastoma in a patient with Swyer syndrome. Obstet Gynecol 1992; 79:842.

122. Pisarska MD, Simpson JL, Zepeda DE, et al: Laparo-

scopic removal of streak gonads in 46,XY or 45,X/46,XY gonadal dysgenesis. J Gynecol Tech 1998; 4:95.

123. Sternberg WH, Barclay DL, Kloepfer HW: Familial XY gonadal dysgenesis. N Engl J Med 1968; 278:695.

124. Espiner EA, Veale AMO, Sands VE, et al: Familial syndrome of streak gonads and normal male karyotype in five phenotypic females. N Engl J Med 1970; 238:6.

125. Mann JR, Corkery JJ, Fisher HJW, et al: The X-linked recessive form of XY gonadal dysgenesis with high incidence of gonadal cell tumours: Clinical and genetic studies. J Med Genet 1983; 20:264.

126. Bricarelli FD, Fraccaro M, Lindsten J, et al: Sex-reversed XY females with campomelic dysplasia are H-Y negative. Hum Genet 1981; 57:15.

127. Puck SM, Haseltine FP, Francke U: Absence of H-Y antigen in an XY female with campomelic dysplasia. Hum Genet 1981; 57:23.

128. Brosnan PC, Lewandowski RC, Toguri AG, et al: A familial syndrome of the 46,XY gonadal dysgenesis with anomalies of ectodermal and mesodermal structures. J Pediatr 1981; 97:586.

129. Greenberg F, Gresik MW, Carpenter RJ, et al: The Gardner-Silengo-Wachtel or genito-palato-cardiac syndrome: Male pseudohermaphroditism with micrognathia, cleft palate, and conotruncal cardiac defects. Am J Med Genet 1987; 26:59.

130. Teebi AS, Miller S, Ostrer H, et al: Spastic paraplegia, optic atrophy, microcephaly with normal intelligence, and XY sex reversal: A new autosomal recessive syndrome? J Med Genet 1998; 35:759.

131. Riddick DH, Hammond CB: Long-term steroid therapy in patients with adrenogenital syndrome. Obstet Gynecol 1975; 45:15.

132. White PC, Dupont J, New MI, et al: A mutation in CYP11B1 (Arg-448—His) associated with steroid 11 beta-hydroxylase deficiency in Jews of Moroccan origin. Clin Invest 1991; 87:1664.

133. Naiki Y, Kawamoto T, Mitsuuchi Y, et al: A nonsense mutation (TGG [Trp116]→TAG [Stop]) in CYP11B1 causes steroid 11 beta-hydroxylase deficiency. Clin Endocrin Metab 1993; 77:1677.

134. Skinner CA, Rumsby G: Steroid 11 beta-hydroxylase deficiency caused by a five base pair duplication in the CYP11B1 gene. Hum Mol Genet 1994; 3:377.

135. Bongiovanni AM: Further studies of congenital adrenal hyperplasia due to 3β-hydroxysteroid dehydrogenase deficiency. *In* Vallet HL, Porter IH (eds): Genetic Mechanisms of Sexual Development. New York: Academic Press, 1979, p 189.

136. Rheaume R, Simard J, Morel Y, et al: Congenital adrenal hyperplasia due to point mutation in the type II 3β-hydroxysteroid dehydrogenase gene. Nat Genet 1992; 1:239.

137. Cheng SD, Gasperini R, Muller U: Molecular analysis of aberrations of Xp and Yq. Hum Genet 1992; 88:379.

138. Simard J, Rheaume E, Sanchez R, et al: Molecular basis of congenital adrenal hyperplasia due to 3β-HSD deficiency. Mol Endocrinol 1993; 7:716.

139. Sanchez R, Rheaume D, Laflamme N, et al: Detection and functional characterization of the novel missense mutation Y254D in type II 3β-HSD gene of a female patient with nonsalt-losing 3β-HSD deficiency. J Clin Endocrinol Metab 1994; 78:561.

140. Araki S, Chikazawa K, Sekisuchi I, et al: Arrest of follicular development in a patient with 17 alphahydroxylase deficiency: Folliculogenesis in association with a lack of estrogen synthesis in the ovaries. Fertil Steril 1987; 47:169.

141. Rabinovici J, Blankenstein J, Goldman B, et al: In vitro

fertilization and primary embryonic cleavage are possible in 17 alpha-hydroxylase deficiency despite extremely low intrafollicular 17 beta-estradiol. J Clin Endocrinol Metab 1989; 68:693.

142. Carson SA, Simpson JL: Virilization of female fetuses following maternal ingestion of progestinal and androgenic steroids. *In* Mahesh VB, Greenblatt RB (eds): Hirsutism and Virilization. Littleton, Mass: PSG Publishing, 1994, p 177.

143. Grumbach MM, Ducharme JR, Moloshak RE: On fetal masculinizing action of certain oral progestins. J Clin Endocrinol Metab 1959; 19:1369.

144. Simpson JL, Carson SA: Genetic and nongenetic causes of spontaneous abortion. *In* Sciarra JJ (ed): Gynecology and Obstetrics, vol. III. Philadelphia: Lippincott-Raven, 1998.

145. Verhoeven ATM, Mastboom JL, Van Leusden HAIM, et al: Virilization in pregnancy coexisting with an (ovarian) mucinous cystadenoma: A case report and review of virilizing ovarian tumors in pregnancy. Obstet Gynecol Surv 1973; 28:597.

146. Jones HW, Park IJ: A classification of special problems in sex differentiation. Birth Defects 1971; 7(6):113.

147. Park IJ, Jones HW, Melham RE: Nonadrenal familial female hermaphroditism. Am J Obstet Gynecol 1971; 112:930.

148. Lubinsky MS: Female pseudohermaphroditism and associated anomalies. Am J Med Genet 1980; 6:123.

149. Simpson JL, Kaufman R: Fetal effects of progestogens and diethylstilbestrol. *In* Fraser S, Jansen RPS, Lobo RA, Whitehead MI (eds): Estrogens and Progestogens in Clinical Practice. London: Churchill Livingstone, 1998, pp 533–553.

150. Chang HJ, Clark RD, Bachman H: The phenotype of 45,X/46,XY mosaicism: An analysis of 92 prenatally diagnosed cases. Am J Hum Genet 1990; 46:156.

151. McDonough PG, Tho PT: The spectrum of 45X/46,XY gonadal dysgenesis and its implications (a study of 19 patients). Pediatr Adolesc Gynecol 1983; 1:1.

152. Rosenberg C, Frota-Pessoa O, Vianna-Morgante AM, et al: Phenotypic spectrum of 45,X/46,XY individuals. Am J Med Genet 1987; 27:553.

153. Verp MS, Simpson JL: Abnormal sexual differentiation and neoplasia. Cancer Genet Cytogenet 1987; 25:191.

154. Boscze P, Szamel I, Molnar F, et al: Non-neoplastic gonadal testosterone secretion as a cause of vaginal cell maturation in streak gonad syndrome. Gynecol Invest 1986; 22:153.

155. Lukusa T, Fryns JP, Van den Berge H: Gonadoblastoma and Y-chromosome fluorescence. Clin Genet 1986; 29:311.

156. Hsu LYF: Prenatal diagnosis of chromosome abnormalities through amniocentesis. *In* Milunsky A (ed): Genetic Disorders and the Fetus, 3rd ed. Baltimore: Johns Hopkins Press, 1986, p 155.

157. Frydman M, Kauschansky A, Zamir R, et al: Familial lipoid adrenal hyperplasia: Genetic marker data and an approach to prenatal diagnosis. Am J Med Genet 1986; 25:319.

158. Chung BC, Matteson KJ, Voutilainen R, et al: Human cholesterol side-chain cleavage enzyme P450scc:cDNA cloning assignment of the gene to chromosome 15 and expression in the placenta. Proc Natl Acad Sci USA 1986; 83:8962.

159. Lin D, Gitelman SE, Saenger P, et al: Normal genes for the cholesterol side chain cleavage enzyme, P450scc, in congenital lipoid adrenal hyperplasia. J Clin Invest 1991; 88:1955.

160. Bose HS, Sugawara T, Strauss JF 3rd, et al: The pathophysiology and genetics of congenital lipoid adrenal hyperplasia. International Congenital Lipoid Adrenal Hyperplasia Consortium. N Engl J Med 1996; 335:1870.

161. Perrone L, Criscuolo T, Sinisi AA: Male pseudohermaphroditism due to 3β-hydroxysteroid dehydrogenase-isomerase deficiency associated with atrial septal defect. Acta Endocrinol (Copenh) 1985; 110:532.

162. Heremans GFP, Moolenaar AJ, Van Gelderen HM: Female phenotype in a male child due to 17α-hydroxylase deficiency. Arch Dis Child 1976; 51:721.

163. Nebert DW, Nelson DR, Adesnik M, et al: The P_{450} superfamily: Updated listing of all genes and recommended nomenclature for the chromosomal loci. DNA 1989; 8:1.

164. Biason-Lauber A, Leiberman E, Zachmann M: A single amino acid substitution in the putative redox partner-binding site of P450c17 as cause of isolated 17,20-lyase deficiency. J Clin Endocrinol Metab 1997; 82:3807.

165. Geller DH, Auchus RJ, Mendonca BB, et al: The genetic and functional basis of isolated 17,20-lyase deficiency. Nature Genet 1997; 17:201.

166. Zachmann M, Vollmin JA, Hamilton W, et al: Steroid 17,20-desmolase deficiency: A new cause of male pseudohermaphroditism. Clin Endocrinol 1972; 1:369.

167. Yanase T, Kagimoto M, Suzuki S, et al: Deletion of a phenylalanine in the N-terminal region of human cytochrome P_{450}(17 alpha) results in partial combined 17 alpha-hydroxylase/17,20-lyase deficiency. J Biol Chem 1989; 264:18076.

168. Kagimoto K, Waterman MR, Kagimoto M, et al: Identification of a common molecular basis for combined 17 alpha-hydroxylase/17,20-lyase deficiency in two Mennonite families. Hum Genet 1989; 82:285.

169. Rumsby G, Skinner C, Lee HA, et al: Combined 17 alpha-hydroxylase/17,20-lyase deficiency caused by heterozygous stop codons in the cytochrome P_{450} 17 alpha-hydroxylase gene. Clin Endocrinol (Oxf) 1993; 39:483.

170. Balducci R, Toscano V, Wright F, et al: Familial male pseudohermaphroditism with gynaecomastia due to 17 β-hydroxysteroid dehydrogenase deficiency. A report of 3 cases. Clin Endocrinol 1985; 23:439.

171. Imperato-McGinley J, Peterson RE, Stoller R, et al: Male pseudohermaphroditism secondary to a 17α-hydroxysteroid dehydrogenase deficiency: Gender role with puberty. J Clin Endocrinol Metab 1979; 49:391.

172. Caufriez A: Male pseudohermaphroditism due to 17-ketoreductase deficiency: Report of a case without gynecomastia and without vaginal pouch. Am J Obstet Gynecol 1986; 154:148.

173. Geissler W, Favis D, Wu L, et al: Male pseudohermaphroditism caused by mutations of testicular 17β-hydroxysteroid dehydrogenase 3. Nat Genet 1994; 7:34.

174. Andersson S, Geissler W, Ling W, et al: Molecular genetics and pathophysiology of β-hydroxysteroid dehydrogenase 3 deficiency. J Clin Endocrinol Metab 1996; 81:130.

175. Ulloa-Aguirre A, Mendez PJ, Chavez A, et al: Incomplete regression of Müllerian ducts in the androgen insensitivity syndrome. Fertil Steril 1990; 53:1024.

176. Morris JM, Mahesh VB: Further observations on the syndrome "testicular feminization." Am J Obstet Gynecol 1963; 87:731.

177. Gottlieb B, Trifiro M, Lumbroso R, et al: The androgen receptor gene mutations database. Nucleic Acids Res 1996; 24(1):151.

178. Gottlieb B, Lehvaslaiho H, Beitel LK, et al: The androgen receptor gene mutations database. Nucleic Acids Res 1998; 26:234.

179. Quigley CA, Friedman KJ, Johnson A, et al: Complete deletion of the androgen receptor gene: Definition of the null phenotype of the androgen insensitivity syndrome and determination of carrier status. J Clin Endocrinol Metab 1992; 74(4):927.

180. McPhaul MJ, Marcelli M, Zoppi S, et al: Genetic basis of endocrine disease. 4. The spectrum of mutations in the androgen receptor gene that causes androgen resistance. J Clin Endocrinol Metab 1993; 76(1):17.

181. Park IJ, Jones HW: Familial male hermaphroditism with ambiguous external genitalia. Am J Obstet Gynecol 1970; 108:1197.

182. Griffin JE, Punyashthiki K, Wilson JD: Dihydrotestosterone binding by culture human fibroblasts. Comparison of cells from control subjects and from patients with hereditary pseudohermaphroditism due to androgen resistance. J Clin Invest 1976; 57:1342.

183. Pinsky L, Kaufman M: Genetics of steroid receptors and their disorders. Adv Hum Genet 1985; 16:299.

184. Pinsky L, Kaufman M, Levitzsky LL: Partial androgen resistance due to a distinctive qualitative defect of the androgen receptor. Am J Med Genet 1987; 27:459.

185. Simpson JL, New M, Peterson RE, et al: Pseudovaginal perineoscrotal hypospadias (PPSH) in sibs. Birth Defects 1971; 7(6):140.

186. Opitz JM, Simpson JL, Sarto GE, et al: Pseudovaginal perineoscrotal hypospadias. Clin Genet 1972; 3:1.

187. Imperato-McGinley J, Guerrero L, Gautier T, et al: Steroid 5α-reductase deficiency: An inherited form of male pseudohermaphroditism. Science 1974; 186:1213.

188. Walsh C, Madden JD, Harrod MJ, et al: Familial incomplete male pseudohermaphroditism, type 2. N Engl J Med 1974; 291:944.

189. Peterson RE, Imperato-McGinley J, Gautier T, et al: Male pseudohermaphroditism due to steroid 5α-reductase deficiency. Am J Med 1977; 62:170.

190. Wilson JD, Griffin JE, Russell DW: Steroid 5α-reductase 2 deficiency. Endocrinol Rev 1993; 14:577.

191. Green S, Zachmann M, Mannella B: Comparison of two tests to recognize or exclude 5α-reductase deficiency in prepubertal children. Acta Endocrinol (Copenh) 1987; 114:113.

192. Imperato-McGinley J, Gautier T, Pichardo M, et al: The diagnosis of 5 alpha-reductase in infancy. J Clin Endocrinol Metab 1986; 63:1313.

193. Labrie F, Sugimoto Y, Luu-The V, et al: Structure of human type II 5 alpha-reductase gene. Endocrinology 1992; 131:1571.

194. Andersson S, Berman DM, Jenkins EP, et al: Deletion of steroid 5 alpha-reductase 2 gene in male pseudohermaphroditism. Nature 1991; 354:159.

195. Thigpen AE, Davis DL, Milatovich A, et al: Molecular genetics of steroid 5 α-reductase deficiency. J Clin Invest 1992; 90:799.

196. Simpson ER, Michael MD, Agarwal VR, et al: Cytochromes P450 11: Expression of the CYP19 (aromatase) gene: An unusual case of alternative promoter usage. FASEB 1997; 11:29.

197. Ito Y, Fisher CR, Conte FA, et al: Molecular basis of aromatase deficiency in an adult female with sexual infantilism and polycystic ovaries. Proc Natl Acad Sci USA 1993; 90:11673.

198. Shozu M, Akasofu K, Harada T, et al: A new cause of female pseudohermaphroditism: Placental aromatase deficiency. J Clin Endocrinol Metab 1991; 72:560.

199. Mullis PE, Yoshimura N, Kuhlmann B, et al: Aromatase deficiency in a female who is compound heterozygote for two new point mutations in the P_{450} arom gene: Impact of estrogens on hypergonadotropic hypogonadism, multicystic ovaries, and bone densitometry in childhood. Clin Endocrinol Metab 1997; 82:1739.

200. Lubahn DB, Moyer JS, Golding TS, et al: Alteration of reproductive function but not prenatal sexual development after insertional disruption of the mouse estrogen receptor gene. Proc Natl Acad Sci USA 1993; 90(23):11162.

201. Smith EP, Boyd J, Frank GR, et al: Estrogen resistance caused by a mutation in the estrogen-receptor gene in a man. N Engl J Med 1994; 331(16):1056.

202. Sarto GE, Opitz JM: The XY gonadal agenesis syndrome. J Med Genet 1973; 10:288.

203. Kwok C, Tyler-Smith C, Mendonca B, et al: Mutation analysis of the 2 kb 5′ to SRY in XY females and XY intersex subjects. J Med Genet 1996; 33:465.

204. Schwartz M, Imperato-McGinley J, Peterson RE, et al: Male pseudohermaphroditism secondary to an abnormality in Leydig cell differentiation. J Clin Endocrinol Metab 1981; 53:123.

205. Brown DM, Markland C, Dehner LP: Leydig cell hypoplasia: A case of male pseudohermaphroditism. J Clin Endocrinol Metab 1976, 46:1.

206. Lee PA, Rock JA, Brown TR, et al: Leydig cell hypofunction resulting in male pseudohermaphroditism. Fertil Steril 1981; 37:675.

207. Perez-Palacios G, Scaglia HE, Kofman-Afaro S: Inherited male pseudohermaphroditism due to gonadotrophin unresponsiveness. Acta Endocrinol (Copenh) 1982; 98:148.

208. Saldanha PH, Arnhold IJP, Mendonca BB, et al: A clinico-genetic investigation of Leydig cell hypoplasia. Am J Med Genet 1987; 26:337.

209. Kremer H, Kraaij R, Toledo SP, et al: Male pseudohermaphroditism due to a homozygous missense mutation of the luteinizing hormone receptor gene. Nat Genet 1995; 9(2):160.

210. Salameh W, Shoukair M, Keswani A, et al: Evidence for a deletion in the LH receptor gene in a case of Leydig cell aplasia. In 77th Annual Meeting of Endocrine Society, June 14–17, Washington, DC. 1995; Abstract P2–150:328.

211. Simpson JL: True hermaphroditism. Etiology and phenotypic considerations. Birth Defects 1978; 14(6C):9.

212. Van Niekerk WA, Retief AE: The gonads of human true hermaphrodites. Hum Genet 1981; 58:117.

213. Aaronsen I: True hermaphroditism. A review of 41 cases with observations on testicular history and function. Br J Urol 1985; 57:775.

214. Tegenkamp TR, Brazzell JW, Tegenkamp I, et al: Pregnancy without benefit of reconstructive surgery in a bisexually active true hermaphrodite. Am J Obstet Gynecol 1979; 135:427.

215. Minowada S, Fukutani K, Hara M, et al: Childbirth in a true hermaphrodite. Eur Urol 1984; 10:414.

216. Van Niekerk WA: True Hermaphroditism. New York: Harper & Row, 1974.

217. Raspa RW, Subramanian AP, Romas NA: True hermaphroditism presents as intermittent hematuria and groin pain. Urology 1986; 28:133.

218. Ramsay M, Bernstein R, Zwane E, et al: XX true hermaphroditism in South African blacks: An enigma of primary sexual differentiation. Am J Hum Genet 1988; 43:4.

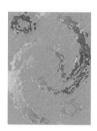

Chapter 8

Abnormal Sexual Differentiation and Hypogonadism: Management and Therapy

SELMA FELDMAN WITCHEL AND PETER A. LEE

Sexual differentiation, or the development of internal and external genitalia, is a complex process dependent on chromosomal constitution in the presence of a gender-appropriate hormonal milieu. Genetic sex, determined at fertilization, directs differentiation of the bipotential genital structures. With a 46,XY chromosomal composition, the bipotential gonad differentiates into a testis by 6 to 7 weeks of gestation. When the chromosomes are 46,XX, ovarian differentiation occurs later, at 9 to 10 weeks of gestation.

Investigations of humans with discrepancies between phenotypic and genetic sex led to identification of the genetic locus responsible for testicular differentiation on the short arm of the Y chromosome, the sex-determining region Y (SRY) gene.[1] The finding of mutations in the SRY gene in 46,XY human females and the creation of a sex-reversed female mouse transgenic only for the mouse Sry gene confirmed that this locus is responsible for testicular differentiation. Subsequently, other genes such as SOX9, WT1, SF-1, and DSS have been shown to play a role in sexual differentiation, because mutations in these genes are often associated with anomalous internal or external genital development.

In addition to genetic factors, the ambient hormonal milieu influences internal and external genital development. Testosterone and dihydrotestosterone induce male internal and external genital development. Müllerian inhibitory hormone (MIH) secreted by the testes induces regression of the müllerian structures. In the absence of stimulation by androgen and MIH, the "default" program of female genital differentiation ensues.

Genital ambiguity, or discordance between phenotype and genetic sex, indicates an abnormality in the process of sexual differentiation. Aneuploidy or abnormalities affecting the sex chromosomes can affect sexual differentiation. Mutations in certain autosomal genes can lead to aberrant sexual differentiation. An atypical or inappropriate hormonal milieu can influence genital differentiation. For example, exposure of a 46,XX female fetus to increased androgen concentrations during gestation induces virilization of the external genitalia. For a 46,XY male fetus, subnormal androgen concentrations or inadequate androgen action in utero impairs to various degrees external genital differentiation. In this chapter we focus on disorders of sexual differentiation that influence achievement of normal reproductive competence.

GONADAL DYSGENESIS

The term *gonadal dysgenesis* describes conditions in which gonadal differentiation is abnormal. A spectrum of aberrant gonadal differentiation—ranging from streak gonads to dysgenic testis—can be seen on histologic examination. In the past, gonadal dysgenesis was categorized as *pure*, *partial*, or *mixed*. As the molecular etiologies of gonadal dysgenesis are elucidated, classification is shifting to specific genetic defects.

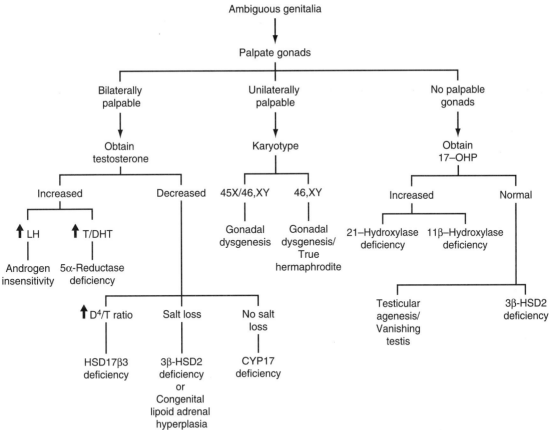

Figure 8–1. The diagnostic approach to the infant presenting with ambiguous genitalia. The possible diagnoses and laboratory studies are suggested based on the presence of the gonads (17OHP = 17-hydroxyprogesterone; LH = luteinizing hormone; 3β-HSD2 = 3β-hydroxysteroid dehydrogenase; CYP17 = 17-hydroxylase; T/DHT = testosterone/dihydroxytestosterone; D⁴/T ratio = Δ4 androstenedione/testosterone; HSD17β3 = 3β-hydroxysteroid dehydrogenase).

DISORDERS INVOLVING SEX CHROMOSOMES

Turner Syndrome

Turner syndrome affects approximately 1 of every 2000 to 2500 liveborn females (Table 8–1). It was first described by Ullrich in 1930 and further by Turner in 1938 to include short stature, webbed neck, low posterior hairline, cubitus valgus, and failure of pubertal development.[2] Other stigmata include high-arched palate, multiple nevi, hypoplastic nails, congenital heart disease, and renal anomalies. The risks for developing autoimmune disorders and hypertension unrelated to congenital renal anomalies are increased. Subsequently, this phenotype was determined to be associated with abnormalities of the X chromosome. The spectrum of X chromosome abnormalities includes monosomies, partial deletions, and structural rearrangements.[3] Mosaic karyotypes, in which the cell line carrying the

aberrant X chromosome co-exists with other cell lines are common. Indeed, it has been speculated that mosaicism in critical cell lines is vital for live birth.[4]

The diagnosis can often be made at birth as a result of the infant's dysmorphic features, particularly peripheral lymphedema. Intrauterine growth retardation with low birth weight is common. With prenatal ultrasound and fetal chromosome analysis, the diagnosis may be made before birth. For girls whose condition eludes diagnosis in the neonatal period, short stature and delayed puberty are the most common reasons for referral and diagnosis.[5]

OVARIAN FAILURE

Initial ovarian differentiation in utero apparently proceeds normally, but follicular atresia is accelerated. By the time of gonadarche, most follicles have disappeared, leaving streak gonads. In the immediate neonatal period, luteinizing

Table 8–1. Features of Turner Syndrome

Short stature
Endocrine abnormalities
   Delayed puberty
   Ovarian failure
   Hypergonadotropic hypogonadism
   Thyroid disorders
   Impaired glucose tolerance
   Diabetes mellitus
   Infertility
Cardiac abnormalities
   Coarctation of the aorta
   Partial anomalous pulmonary venous return
   Bicuspid aortic valves
   Mitral valve prolapse
   Hypertension
   Aortic dissection
Renal anomalies
   Horseshoe kidney
   Duplicated renal collecting system
   Malrotation
   Abnormalities of the renal vascular system
Inflammatory bowel disease
   Crohn disease
   Ulcerative colitis
Ears
   Chronic otitis media
   Cholesteatoma
Lymphatic abnormalities
   Cystic hygroma
   Puffy hands and feet
   Webbed neck
Skeletal abnormalities
   Shortening of the fourth metacarpal
   Shortening of the fourth metatarsal
   Widening of the head of the distal phalanges
   Madelung deformity
   Cubitus valgus
   Schmorl nodes
   Scheuermann disease
   Scoliosis
   Osteoporosis
Genetic
   Presence of Y chromosome material
   Risk of gonadoblastoma or dysgerminoma
Developmental
   Impaired visuospatial skills
   Difficulties with social interactions
Cutaneous
   Increased number of nevi

(LH) and follicle-stimulating hormone (FSH) levels are often elevated. During childhood, when the hypothalamic-pituitary-gonadal (HPG) axis is quiescent, gonadotropin concentrations in girls with Turner syndrome are indistinguishable from those of normal girls. With the reactivation of the HPG axis, the streak gonad does not produce sufficient estradiol, so that negative feedback inhibition fails and gonadotropin concentrations rise. Uterine and vaginal differentiation are normal.

Loci on both the short and long arms of the X chromosome are involved in ovarian function. Women with deletions limited to distal Xq (proximal to Xq13.3-q21.3 or distal to Xq26-28) may develop premature ovarian failure in the absence of other features of Turner syndrome.[6] In rare instances, spontaneous pubertal development or pregnancy occurs. Even within a single family, ovarian function can vary.[7]

SHORT STATURE

Short stature is often the reason for the initial evaluation of a girl with Turner syndrome. X chromosome monosomy and terminal deletions of Xp are invariably associated with short stature.[8] Growth hormone responses to provocative stimulation and physiologic evaluations are variable but tend to be normal.[9] During the prepubertal years, growth hormone and insulin-like growth factor I (IGF-I) concentrations are comparable to those in normal children. Mean 24-hour growth hormone concentrations were similar in girls with Turner syndrome and age-matched girls before 9 years of age but lower in the girls with Turner syndrome after 9 years of age.[10, 11]

OTHER FEATURES

The prevalence of congenital heart disease is greater among girls with Turner syndrome than in the general population. In one series of 136 girls with Turner syndrome confirmed on the basis of short stature or gonadal failure, bicuspid aortic valve was the most common cardiac anomaly (14.7%). Other common anomalies included aortic valve disease, coarctation of the aorta, and partial anomalous pulmonary venous drainage.[12] Aortic dilatation, which can be associated with cystic medial necrosis and acute aortic dissection, is a potentially disastrous complication.[13] Routine reevaluation for this devastating complication is recommended for adolescents and adult women with Turner syndrome. Patients with recognized valvular abnormalities should be given standard subacute bacterial endocarditis prophylaxis.

Skeletal anomalies can occur in Turner syndrome. Shortening of the fourth metacarpal, secondary to premature epiphyseal fusion, is common. Shortening of the fourth metatarsal sometimes also occurs. The "drumstick" shape of the distal phalanges is due to widening of their heads. Madelung deformity is due to impaired distal radial growth, premature fusion of the distal radial growth plate, and shortening of the ulna. Cubitus valgus or increased carrying angle of the elbow is extremely frequent. Characteristic knee findings include projection and enlargement of the metaphyseal portion of the medial aspect of the tibial condyle, which is associated with enlargement of the medial condyle.[14]

In the spine, abnormalities of the cartilaginous end plates (Schmorl nodes) and of the epiphyseal rings (Scheuermann disease) may be found. Typically, Scheuermann disease is not associated with significant pain. In the past, scoliosis in girls with Turner syndrome has not been severe or progressive, but increased use of growth hormone could affect the natural history of scoliosis.

Skeletal demineralization associated with slow bone turnover is another characteristic of Turner syndrome. Markers of bone turnover such as serum osteocalcin and procollagen III amino-terminal extension peptide concentrations are typically low.[15] No consistent differences in bone histology have been identified between Turner syndrome patients and normal humans. The incidence of wrist fractures was reported to be increased in untreated girls aged 9 to 13.[16] Fractures, especially at sites typical for osteoporosis, were increased in adult women with Turner syndrome.[17] Gonadal failure with estrogen deficiency impairs shift to endosteal cortical bone growth and loss of estrogen-mediated acceleration in trabecular bone deposition.[18] Preliminary data suggest that growth hormone treatment was associated with improved bone mineralization.[19, 20] Thus, growth hormone therapy during the prepubertal years and early to mid-pubertal years, in conjunction with estrogen and progesterone therapy throughout adulthood appears to promote bone accretion and achievement of normal peak bone mass. Healthy lifestyle interventions such as adequate calcium intake and weight-bearing activity may help to prevent osteoporosis.[21]

Typical facial features include high-arched palate, micrognathia, and a downward droop of the lateral corners of the eyes. Chronic or recurrent otitis media may persist into adolescence. Hearing loss and cholesteatoma may develop.[22, 23] Girls with Turner syndrome often have increased numbers of nevi. Some girls tend to form keloids, an important consideration for surgical procedures.

Congenital renal anomalies, particularly horseshoe kidneys, duplicated collecting systems, malrotation, or anomalies of the renal vascular system are associated with Turner syndrome.[24] Renal ultrasonography should be performed to assess for these congenital urinary tract defects.[25] Because of the increased risk of hypertension,

blood pressure needs to be monitored. Hypertension can be secondary to coarctation of the aorta or renal disease or of unknown cause. Gastrointestinal disorders such as inflammatory bowel disease and celiac disease can be associated with Turner syndrome.[26, 27] The development of inflammatory bowel disease can retard growth.[28]

Metabolic abnormalities consisting of carbohydrate intolerance and type 2 diabetes mellitus are prevalent in adult women with Turner syndrome,[29] who were found to have impaired glucose tolerance and decreased first-phase insulin response.[30] Using the euglycemic insulin clamp technique, insulin resistance was detected in a small group of affected girls naïve to growth hormone treatment.[31] The natural history of Turner syndrome in adults shows increased prevalences of fractures, both type 1 and type 2 diabetes mellitus, hypertension, and heart disease.[32]

PHENOTYPE-GENOTYPE CORRELATION

In mapping genetic loci responsible for the phenotypic features of Turner syndrome, it is relevant to look for genes whose haploinsufficiency could result in a phenotype. In other words, genes mapped to the pseudoautosomal region with homologues on the Y chromosome or genes not subject to X inactivation are the most likely candidate genes. Comparison of subjects with partial monosomy for the short arm of the X chromosome revealed that loci at Xp11.2-p22.1 affect growth, ovarian function, and palate development, but not lymphedema, congenital heart disease, or webbed neck.[33] Although monosomy for the maternal X chromosome is more common, there appear to be no "parent-of-origin" effects on the physical features of Turner syndrome.[34] Congenital heart disease is more common in patients with ring X chromosomes (33%) and 45,X monosomy (29%) than in those with other structural anomalies.[12]

Cell lines containing all or portions of Y chromosome material can be found in girls with Turner syndrome. In some instances, the Y chromosome material can be identified on cytogenetic analysis. More sensitive techniques involving polymerase chain reaction (PCR) amplification may be necessary to detect evidence of Y chromosome material.[35] The principal concern is the increased risk for gonadoblastoma (see later).

PSYCHOSOCIAL DEVELOPMENT

Earlier literature implied that girls with Turner syndrome are "retarded." It is crucial that this inaccurate information be dealt with promptly, because the majority of girls with Turner syndrome show verbal and nonverbal IQs within the normal range. The verbal intelligence and school performance of affected girls are generally comparable to their unaffected sisters.

Yet, girls with Turner syndrome often have difficulties with certain areas of cognitive functioning. The specific areas include visuospatial performance and mathematical achievement.[36] Geometry, hand-eye coordination, map reading, estimating distances of objects, and playing sports with fast-moving balls may be more difficult for some girls. Impaired social and behavioral function (defined as difficulty with peer relationships, immaturity, and difficulties in recognizing social and nonverbal cues) have been observed.[37–39] Indeed, maintaining relationships with peers can be a lifelong problem. Compared to unaffected sisters, girls with Turner syndrome have more difficulty with adaptive social skills and attention. Although girls with Turner syndrome are within the norms for these areas, differences from their sisters suggest that distinct neurobiologic components are related to numerical or structural alterations of the X chromosome.[40] That monosomy for the maternal X chromosome is associated with greater social, cognitive, and behavioral difficulties as compared with monosomy for the paternal X chromosome indicates a role for imprinting on phenotype.[41]

Situations that are likely to lead to failure should be avoided. For example, cubitus valgus and wrist deformity may make playing the violin difficult. Parents, educators, and physicians should focus on positive attributes. These girls should be encouraged to participate in sports in which height is not important such as ice skating, swimming, and diving. Clothing manufacturers offer petite sizes to provide sophisticated clothing for adolescents and adult women with Turner syndrome.

Delaying puberty to maximize growth potential can have adverse effects on the patient's self-esteem, as one affected woman eloquently stated:

> Without breasts and other secondary sexual development, the boys did not "notice" me in usual junior high school fashion. Perhaps I would not have worried so much about that, for I sensed that I was not ready for predating boy-girl relationships, had it not also tended to isolate me from girlfriends. Few of them were dating regularly, but all were claiming boyfriends and sharing

their interests in dating in intimate sessions. Because they, too, responded to my youthful appearance, I was largely excluded from much of the normal friendships and socialization of early adolescence. I was confused and angry.[42]

DIFFERENTIAL DIAGNOSIS

The typical presenting features of girls with Turner syndrome are short stature and delayed puberty. Over the first few years of life, growth velocity and stature may be within normal limits. Subsequently, growth velocity declines and girls referred in late childhood or early teens are short for chronologic age and for corrected mid-parental height.[43] Subnormal growth velocity may also be the presenting symptom for hypothyroidism, growth hormone deficiency, hypercortisolism, inflammatory bowel disease, and chronic renal disease. Girls with Noonan syndrome may show physical features reminiscent of Turner syndrome, such as short stature, webbed neck, cubitus valgus, and midfacial hypoplasia, although right-sided congenital heart disease, greater prevalence of developmental delay, and a normal karyotype distinguish Noonan syndrome.[44] Autosomal-dominant inheritance with variable expression has been recognized for Noonan syndrome with mapping of a gene associated with the syndrome to the long arm of chromosome 12.[45] Short stature, especially when the parents are short, may be judged a familial attribute. Hence, since the manifestations of Turner syndrome may be limited to short stature, all short girls should be evaluated for it.

The diagnosis of Turner syndrome is based on chromosome analysis. Usually a peripheral blood karyotype is sufficient. In some mosaic patients, analysis of fibroblasts obtained through a skin biopsy may be necessary. Buccal smears can be helpful but do not provide sufficient detail about the specific karyotype.

MANAGEMENT

Comprehensive education of the patient and her family is a priority in the management of a girl with Turner syndrome (Table 8–2). Surveys of affected middle-aged women indicate the need to provide full disclosure about Turner syndrome.[46] Telling a young girl that nothing is wrong when she visits a "special doctor" on a regular basis does not fool her. Such denial may only convince her that she must have a terrible disease. Withholding the diagnosis may intensify

Table 8–2. Health Supervision and Treatment Recommendations for Turner Syndrome

Growth
    Monitor at regular intervals
    Consider growth hormone treatment
Cardiac abnormalities
    Evaluation by pediatric cardiologist
    Echocardiogram
    Appropriate therapy for cardiac lesions
    Prophylaxis for subacute bacterial endocarditis
    Monitor for aortic root dilatation and risk for dissection
    Monitor blood pressure
Renal anomalies
    Renal ultrasonography
    Monitor for urinary tract infections
Ears
    Monitor for otitis media
    Treat otitis media (antibiotics, tympanotomy tubes)
    Monitor for cholesteatoma
    Monitor for hearing loss
Endocrine
    Monitor thyroid function
    Document hypergonadotropic hypogonadism
    Urinalysis to assess for glycosuria
    Oral glucose tolerance test, if necessary
    Hormone replacement therapy to initiate and maintain
        secondary sexual characteristics
    Discuss reproductive options
Genetic
    Review karyotype with family and discuss risk of
        recurrence
    Consider obtaining molecular assay for Y chromosomal
        material
Skeletal
    Observe for scoliosis and other skeletal anomalies
    Hormone replacement therapy to prevent osteoporosis
Educational
    Evaluate and support for spatial perception difficulties
    Evaluate and support for difficulties with social
        interactions
    Support groups for parents and girls with Turner
        syndrome

the negative impact of short stature or delayed puberty on her self-esteem. Reproductive options should be presented in a positive light; the girl can have a family by adoption or through assisted reproductive interventions.

Growth hormone therapy, used frequently to ameliorate the short stature of Turner syndrome, has become an accepted treatment. The average adult height for untreated women with Turner syndrome is 144 cm. Although much individual variation occurs, adult stature near 150 cm is conceivable with early initiation of growth hormone treatment. Growth hormone therapy (0.375 mg/kg/week) improves growth velocity and enhances adult stature: final height is at least 5 cm greater than anticipated from the projected adult height before treatment. Factors that improve height gain include younger age at institution of therapy, frequency and duration of ther-

apy, and delayed skeletal maturation.[47, 48] In another series, growth hormone, alone or in conjunction with oxandrolone (0.0625 mg/kg/day), increased final height, importantly without major side effects apart from a single subject with obesity and hypothyroidism who developed slipped capital femoral epiphysis almost 2 years after starting growth hormone therapy.[49] Growth hormone therapy showed no major or persistent effect on lipoprotein(a) in girls with Turner syndrome.[50] Optimal outcome for adult height occurs when growth hormone therapy is started as soon as growth begins to slow. Hormone replacement therapy is usually necessary to promote pubertal development and menses. Attention needs to be focused on providing hormone replacement therapy throughout adulthood to prevent osteoporosis.[51] Recent studies have indicated the beneficial effects of estrogen in reducing coronary artery disease and preventing dementia and osteoporosis. In one small series of girls with Turner syndrome, combined estrogen and growth hormone therapy increased short-term calcium deposition in bone.[52]

Approximately 5% to 10% of patients with Turner syndrome show spontaneous pubertal development and 2% to 5% become pregnant. Miscarriages tend to be common in pregnancies, however. Oocyte donation is an option to treat infertility.[53]

45,X/46,XY Mosaicism

Individuals with 45,X/46,XY karyotype may be recognized at birth because of genital ambiguity. External genital differentiation ranges from apparently normal female to apparently normal male.[54, 55] Affected infants can show many features typical of Turner syndrome, such as short stature, renal anomalies, webbed neck, and low posterior hairline. Karyotypes are typically 45,X/46,XY, but additional cell lines may occur (i.e., 45,X/46,XX/46,XY). In a series of 45,X/46,XY infants ascertained prior to birth, many showed normal male external genital development without any correlation between the mosaicism percentage and the appearance of the gonads or genitalia.[56] While there is often a streak gonad on one side and a dysgenetic testis on the other side, the spectrum of gonadal differentiation ranges from bilateral streak gonads to bilateral dysgenetic testes.

The degree of masculinization reflects testicular function, which may ultimately depend on the dominant cell type in the undifferentiated gonad.[57] Individuals with dysgenetic testis often have deficient MIH secretion in utero leading to regression of wolffian structures and the presence of müllerian structures. Asymmetry of internal and external genital structures is a valuable clinical clue to this diagnosis in a child with ambiguous genitalia. Although testosterone secretion in utero may have been inadequate for normal virilization, the dysgenetic testis can secrete sufficient testosterone at puberty to induce significant virilization. Genitography, ultrasonography, and magnetic resonance imaging can help to characterize the internal genital structures.[58]

The presence of a dysgenetic testis increases the risk for the development of gonadoblastomas, mixed-tissue tumors composed of admixed nests of germ cells and sex cord cells.[59] It has been suggested that gonadoblastomas are carcinomas in situ from which invasive germ cell tumors, seminomas, embryonal carcinomas, teratomas, choriocarcinomas, and dysgerminomas can develop.[60, 61] Expression of carcinoma in situ markers and presence of aneuploid germ cells in gonadoblastomas provide evidence to support this hypothesis.[62] Malignant degeneration of germ cell elements may occur with subsequent metastatic disease. Breast development may indicate the presence of a gonadal estrogen-secreting tumor rather than normal ovarian function.[63] Calcification within the neoplastic tissue can occur. Generally, surgical excision is curative for gonadoblastoma, though additional treatment may be indicated when invasive elements are present.[64] Although such tumors develop more often during late adolescence or young adulthood, they have been reported in infants.[65]

46,XY Females

Failure of testicular differentiation results in gonads that typically are streaks of fibrous tissue that do not secrete steroid hormones and do not contain obvious germ cells. Female external genitalia result because the infant was not exposed to testosterone in utero. When MIH secretion is also deficient, fallopian tubes and uterus develop. The most common presenting features are delayed puberty or poorly developed secondary sexual characteristics with primary amenorrhea. Stature can be normal or tall. Gonadotropin concentrations are elevated. As in the 45,X/46,XY patient with dysgenetic testicular material, the risk for gonadoblastoma is increased. Gonadal dysgenesis can be categorized as *complete* in which the internal genitalia consist of streak gonads and müllerian structures or *partial* in which dysgenetic testes with a mix of wolffian and mülle-

rian structures are present. Whereas the majority of patients with 46,XY gonadal dysgenesis show no other congenital anomalies, a 46,XY patient with gonadal dysgenesis, mental retardation, and multiple pterygium syndrome has been described.[66]

In approximately 15% to 20% of 46,XY females, mutations have been identified in the *SRY* gene.[67] The majority of the reported mutations cluster in the HMG-box domain, a region believed to bind or interact with DNA. Mutations affecting the regulatory regions of the *SRY* gene appear to be rare.[68] Since the majority of 46,XY females show no mutations in the *SRY* gene, mutations in other genes must also lead to 46,XY gonadal dysgenesis.[69]

46,XX Males

Typical clinical manifestations in the 46,XX male include normal male sexual differentiation with development of hypogonadism, azoospermia, and gynecomastia at puberty. Occasionally, external genitalia may be ambiguous. Most XX males show evidence of the *SRY* gene by PCR amplification. In the majority of cases, the mechanism appears to be transfer of the *SRY* gene through unequal interchange between the homologous regions of the short arms of the sex chromosomes during paternal meiotic division.[70] Three 46,XX males were identified prenatally because of discrepancies between the karyotype and ultrasound appearance of the external genitalia. One pregnancy was terminated for presumed congenital adrenal hyperplasia.[71, 72]

Dose-Sensitive Sex Reversal

Another gene mapped to Xp21 and known as *DAX-1, DSS,* or *AHC,* is important for sexual differentiation and reproductive competence. The protein shows homology to orphan nuclear receptors and appears to function as a transcription factor. Loss of function mutations are associated with X-linked adrenal hypoplasia and hypogonadotropic hypogonadism. Typically, affected males present in the neonatal period with adrenal insufficiency or in the teen years with delayed puberty secondary to hypogonadotropic hypogonadism.[73, 74] Occasionally, X-linked adrenal hypoplasia may be part of a contiguous gene deletion syndrome that includes Duchenne muscular dystrophy and glycerol kinase deficiency.[75] Since internal and external male genital development is normal, *AHC* does not appear to be required for testicular differentiation. Sexual differentiation, pubertal development, and fertility are normal in heterozygous females. Because no women homozygous for loss of function mutations have been recognized, the functional significance of this gene in females remains to be characterized.

Duplication of a critical portion of this locus is associated with male-to-female sex reversal despite normal SRY genes. Among patients studied, gonadal differentiation has ranged from dysgenetic testis to streak gonads. External genital development has been reported to be normal female or ambiguous with internal genital development reflecting an assortment of müllerian- and wolffian-derived structures.[76] Studies of transgenic mice suggest that AHC is important for maintenance of testicular function (rather than promoting ovarian differentiation).[77]

True Hermaphroditism

True hermaphroditism is defined as the presence of both ovarian tissues with follicles and testicular tissues with tubules. Gonads can be ovary, testis, or ovotestis. The most common karyotype is 46,XX. External genital development ranges from normal female to genital ambiguity. Additional findings can include hypospadias, cryptorchidism, and inguinal hernias, which may contain a gonad or uterus. Often, the ovarian component shows normal function. Spontaneous female pubertal development can occur with good potential for fertility.[78] That true hermaphroditism and XX males can occur in the same family without evidence of the SRY gene supports speculation that autosomal genes are involved in testis determination.[79]

AUTOSOMAL ABNORMALITIES

Campomelic Dwarfism

Campomelic dwarfism is an autosomal-dominant osteochondrodysplasia characterized by bowing of femur and tibia, Robin malformation, hypoplastic scapulas, and bilateral clubfeet. Death in the neonatal period due to respiratory failure is common. Approximately two thirds of affected 46,XY fetuses demonstrate male-to-female sex reversal. Hence, external genital development in affected 46,XY fetuses extends from normal female to normal male.[80] The molecular basis of this disorder has been determined to be mutations in the SOX9 gene located at chromosome 17q24.3-q25.1.[81, 82] The phenotype does not

correlate well with the specific genetic mutation in affected individuals, and mutations in the SOX9 gene appear to be an extremely rare cause of 46,XY gonadal dysgenesis.[83]

WT1

Wilms tumor with aniridia, genitourinary abnormalities, hemihypertrophy, and mental retardation (known as WAGR syndrome) was noted to be associated with heterozygous deletions of chromosome 11p13, an observation that led to the identification of the WT1 gene.[84] Gonadoblastoma can develop. Development of transgenic mice demonstrated the importance of WT1 to renal and gonadal development. Examination of the homozygous knockout mice that died in midgestation showed cardiac anomalies as well as absence of kidneys and gonads.[85] The WT1 gene consists of 10 exons and encodes a protein that acts as a transcription factor and as a tumor suppressor. Alternative splicing at two different sites can generate four distinct proteins, with or without exon 5 and with or without the addition of three amino acids (lysine, threonine, serine) between the third and fourth zinc finger domains. One recognized consequence of the alternative splicing at exon 9 is different DNA-binding specificity.[86]

Denys-Drash syndrome is characterized by nephropathy, Wilms tumor, and abnormal genital differentiation.[87, 88] Proteinuria manifests at an early age with progression to nephrotic syndrome and renal failure. The typical histopathology shows diffuse or focal mesangial sclerosis with mesangial cell expansion. The gonads and genitalia of affected 46,XY persons can be streak gonads or dysgenetic testes. Derivatives of both müllerian and wolffian ducts can be present. External genitalia range from normal female to ambiguous. Molecular basis is usually heterozygosity for a missense mutation. It has been suggested that, in combination in the developing testis, SF-I and WT1 induce MIH production.[89] In the presence of a mutant WT1, less MIH may be produced, leading to incomplete regression of müllerian structures.

Frasier syndrome is characterized by focal glomerular sclerosis, gonadal dysgenesis, and 46,XY karyotype. To date, only a single patient with Frasier syndrome has been reported to have Wilms tumor.[90] The molecular basis has been identified to be mutations in intron 9 of WT1, which disrupt splicing and lead to decreased amounts of the +KTS isoform.[91–93] The rarity of Wilms tumor in patients with Frasier syndrome, along with the predominance of the −KTS isoform, suggests that it functions as a tumor suppressor.

Chromosome 9p

Deletions of the distal short arm of chromosome 9 have been detected in 46,XY females with gonadal dysgenesis.[94] Among males with 9p deletions, approximately a third have abnormal external genital differentiation.[95] Two genes, *DMRT1* and *DMRT2*, have been identified at 9p24.3 that appear to be involved in testis development.[96] It remains to be determined whether the mechanism leading to gonadal dysgenesis involves haploinsufficiency or unmasking of a mutated allele due to loss of the normal allele.

Smith-Lemli-Opitz Syndrome

Clinical features of Smith-Lemli-Opitz syndrome include microcephaly, mental retardation, syndactyly, and genital ambiguity in affected 46,XY individuals.[97] Inheritance mode is autosomal-recessive. Affected persons have elevated serum 7-dehydrocholesterol and low serum cholesterol concentrations. Mutations in the sterol δ-7 reductase gene were identified in patients with this disorder.[98]

46,XX Gonadal Dysgenesis

Pure gonadal dysgenesis with a 46,XX karyotype is also characterized by delayed puberty with poor breast development, sparse sexual hair, and primary amenorrhea.[99] Perrault syndrome is characterized by ovarian dysgenesis and sensorineural deafness. Inheritance is autosomal-recessive.[100, 101] In the absence of mutations on the X chromosomes, it can be speculated that XX gonadal dysgenesis represents mutations in autosomal genes involved in ovarian differentiation.

HORMONAL DISORDERS

DISORDERS OF CORTISOL BIOSYNTHESIS

The congenital adrenal hyperplasias (Table 8–3) are autosomal-recessive disorders in which mutations in a steroidogenic enzyme impair cortisol biosynthesis. The loss of negative feedback inhibition leads to increased secretion of adrenocorticotropin (ACTH). The clinical and laboratory features depend on which specific enzyme gene is affected.

21-HYDROXYLASE DEFICIENCY

Decreased 21-hydroxylase activity is the most common cause of congenital adrenal hyperplasia and is one of the most common inherited disorders. Incidence for the classic forms is reported to range from 1 in 5000 to 1 in 15,000, depending on geographic region and inclusion criteria. The incidence for the nonclassic disease may be as high as 1 in 27.[102] The clinical features range from classic salt-losing disease associated with salt loss and prenatal virilization of affected females, to simple virilizing forms associated with prenatal virilization of affected females and postnatal virilization of affected males, to the late-onset forms and cryptic forms.

In this disorder, mutations in the 21-hydroxylase *(CYP21)* gene generate defective protein products that cannot adequately convert 17-hydroxyprogesterone into 11-deoxycortisol and progesterone into deoxycorticosterone. Accumulation of precursors results in overproduction of the adrenal androgens, dehydroepiandrosterone (DHEA) and androstenedione, which are peripherally converted to testosterone. In affected 46,XX fetuses, the excessive androgens induce virilization of the external genitalia, ranging from an almost normal-looking scrotum and phallus, to posterior labial fusion in the absence of clitorimegaly, to normal female external genitalia. Most important, no matter how well-developed the scrotum and phallus seem, the external genitalia appear to be symmetric and gonads are not palpable. Despite various degrees of virilization of the external genitalia, the internal genitalia, including ovaries, fallopian tubes, uterus, and upper vagina, are normal. Owing to genital abnormalities, most affected girls are identified in the neonatal period. Girls with minimal virilization of the external genitalia may present in childhood with clitorimegaly, premature pubic hair, tall stature, accelerated growth rate, and advanced skeletal maturation. With appropriate medical management, it can be anticipated that affected girls, including those with impressive virilization of the external genitalia, will have normal pubertal development and potential for fertility. Symptoms of the mildest form, known as *late-onset* or *nonclassic*, may not develop until puberty. Presenting complaints include hirsutism, oligomenorrhea or amenorrhea, acne, and infertility.

Affected 46,XY infants appear normal at birth and often at the time of hospital discharge. When

Table 8–3. Clinical Features of Disorders Associated with Decreased Steroidogenesis or Steroid Activity

Enzyme	Karyotype	Neonatal	Puberty	Salt Loss
CYP21				
Severe	46,XX	Virilization	PP, HA	+
Moderate		± Virilization	PP, HA	−
Mild		Normal	HA	−
Severe	46,XY	Normal	PP	+
Moderate		Normal	PP	−
Mild		Normal	Normal	−
HSD3β2				
Severe	46,XX	Virilization	PP, HA	+
Moderate		± Virilization	PP, HA	−
Mild		Normal	HA	−
Severe	46,XY	↓ Masc	PP	+
Moderate		± ↓ Masc	PP	−
Mild		Normal	Normal	−
CYP11β1				
Severe	46,XX	Virilization	PP, HA	−
Moderate		± Virilization	PP, HA	−
Mild		Normal	HA	−
Severe	46,XY	Normal	PP	−
Moderate		Normal	PP	−
Mild		Normal	Normal	−
CYP17				
	46,XX	Normal	Delayed/absent	−
	46,XY	↓ Masc	Delayed/absent	−
StAR				
	46,XX	Normal	Normal/absent	+
	46,XY	↓ Masc	Absent	+
HSD17β3				
	46,XX	Normal	Normal	−
	46,XY	↓ Masc	Virilization	−
SRD5A2				
	46,XX	Normal	Normal	−
	46,XY	↓ Masc	Virilization	−
LHR (loss of function)				
	46,XX	Normal	Normal, HA	−
	46,XY	↓ Masc	Absent	−
AR	46,XX	Normal	Normal	−
	46,XY	↓ Masc	Variable	−

+, yes; −, no; ±, sometimes; ↓, undervirilization.

mineralocorticoid deficiency is present, affected males typically present within the first 2 to 3 weeks of life with weight loss, poor feeding, vomiting, and dehydration. Laboratory studies show hyponatremia and hyperkalemia. In unrecognized cases, hypotension develops, and patients sometimes die. Boys may present in childhood with phallic enlargement, premature pubic hair, tall stature, and advanced skeletal maturation. One key feature on physical examination is that testicular volume is prepubertal or significantly less than that anticipated from the stage of phallic and pubic hair development.

The 21-hydroxylase gene is located on chromosome 6, very close to a highly homologous nonfunctional pseudogene (*CYP21P*). The majority of mutations associated with 21-hydroxylase deficiency represent gene conversion events in which *CYP21* has acquired deleterious sequences

from *CYP21P*. Six mutations account for the majority of affected alleles. These mutations include large gene deletions or gene conversion events, the intron 2 splicing mutation, I172N, V281L, Q318X, and R356W. In general, phenotype correlates with genotype. Yet, the clinical features associated with the intron 2 splicing mutation and I172N may vary significantly. Comparison of the clinical features among affected children with the identical genotype (large deletion on one allele and I172N on the identical extended haplotype on the other allele) showed much variation in both the extent of prenatal virilization and severity of mineralocorticoid deficiency.[103] Typically, P30L, V281L, and P453S are associated with "nonclassic" 21-hydroxylase deficiency. Multiple mutations can occur on a single allele, and such mutations act synergistically to impair 21-hydroxylase activity.[104]

Diagnostic laboratory features are elevated serum 17-hydroxyprogesterone concentration and urinary 17-ketosteroid excretion (Table 8–4). Correlation of 17-hydroxyprogesterone concentration with molecular genotype in infants detected through a newborn-screening program showed nonextracted 17-hydroxyprogesterone concentrations to range from 2500 to 80,000 ng/dl.[105] In older children and adolescents, ACTH stimulation tests (0.25 mg IV or IM cosyntropin with hormone determinations at 0 and at 30 or 60 minutes) may be needed to confirm the diagnosis. Molecular genotype analysis is increasingly available.

Newborn screening for 21-hydroxylase deficiency, now more widely available, uses filter paper screening for whole blood 17-hydroxyprogesterone concentration. The cutoff level for most screening programs does not detect those who have a nonclassic form. It is important to mention that preterm or stressed infants often have elevated steroid values that may cross-react in the radioimmunoassay for 17-hydroxyprogesterone. Such infants do not have congenital adrenal hyperplasia and do not require glucocorticoid replacement. The dilemma is to accurately distinguish false-positive results from mild cases.

Prenatal treatment for 21-hydroxylase deficiency remains a controversial subject. If prenatal treatment is elected, dexamethasone therapy administered to the mother must be instituted at the time of her first missed menstrual period, because virilization of the external genitalia takes place early in gestation. Either chorionic villus sampling or amniocentesis in conjunction with molecular genotype analysis is necessary to determine whether the fetus is an affected female. If the fetus is male or is not affected, dexamethasone can be discontinued. Limitations of prenatal therapy include potential unknown consequences of high-dose steroid therapy, the need to treat all at-risk pregnancies, and the recognition of the need for therapy only after a propositus has been identified.

3β-HYDROXYSTEROID DEHYDROGENASE DEFICIENCY

The enzyme 3β-hydroxysteroid dehydrogenase type 2, is expressed almost exclusively in the adrenal glands and gonads, where it predominantly converts 17-hydroxypregnenolone to 17-hydroxyprogesterone. Conversion of DHEA to androstenedione is less efficient in humans. Decreased activity of 3β-hydroxysteroid dehydrogenase leads to genital ambiguity in both sexes (see Table 8–3). In the 46,XX fetus, increased DHEA production occurs with increased peripheral conversion to testosterone and masculinization of the external genitalia. In the 46,XY fetus, impaired enzyme activity interferes with testosterone biosynthesis, the result being insufficient testosterone for normal virilization of the external genitalia. Glucocorticoid and mineralocorticoid deficiencies coexist. Diagnostic laboratory studies are elevated concentrations of 17-hydroxypregnenolone and DHEA with increased 17-hydroxypregnenolone to 17-hydroxyprogesterone ratios (see Table 8–4). Heterozygotes typically show normal responses to ACTH stimulation. Classic 3β-hydroxysteroid dehydrogenase deficiency is due to mutations in the 3β-hydroxysteroid dehydrogenase type 2 (HSD3β2) gene.[106–108]

11β-HYDROXYLASE DEFICIENCY

This enzyme converts 11-deoxycortisol to cortisol. The clinical features are very similar to those of 21-hydroxylase deficiency (see Table

Table 8–4. Typical Laboratory Findings of Genetic Disorders

Gene	Findings
CYP21	Increased 17-hydroxyprogesterone, progesterone, and androstenedione
	Hyponatremia, hyperkalemia, and increased plasma renin activity in salt-losing forms
3βHSD2	Increased 17-hydroxypregnenolone and dehydroepiandrosterone
	Increased 17-hydroxypregnenolone-17-hydroxyprogesterone ratio
	Hyponatremia, hyperkalemia, and increased plasma renin activity in salt-losing forms
CYP11β1	Increased 11-desoxycortisol and androstenedione
	Increased 11-desoxycortisol-cortisol ratio
	Variable hypernatremia, hypokalemia, and suppressed renin activity
CYP17	Increased progesterone, deoxycorticosterone
	Variable hypernatremia, hypokalemia, and suppressed renin activity
StAR	All steroids are low
	Hyponatremia, hyperkalemia, and increased plasma renin activity
17βHSD3	Increased androstenedione and low testosterone
	Increased androstenedione-testosterone ratio
S5AR2	Increased testosterone-dihydrotestosterone ratio
LHR	Increased luteinizing hormone and low testosterone
AR	Increased luteinizing hormone and testosterone
	Normal to increased follicle-stimulating hormone

8–3). Although this form of congenital adrenal hyperplasia is typically associated with hypertension, salt loss may occur in the immediate neonatal period or in treated patients with adrenal suppression.[109] Diagnostic laboratory studies show elevated 11-deoxycortisol concentrations and increased 11-deoxycortisol-cortisol ratios (see Table 8–4). This disorder is secondary to mutations in the 11β-hydroxylase gene, *CYP11β1*.

17α-HYDROXYLASE/17,20-LYASE DEFICIENCY

The enzyme 17α-hydroxylase/17,20-lyase converts pregnenolone to 17-hydroxypregnenolone and then to DHEA. Decreased activity interferes with glucocorticoid and sex steroid biosynthesis (see Table 8–3). Affected 46,XX persons show normal female internal and external genital differentiation. Typically, they present with delayed puberty or poorly developed secondary sexual characteristics and primary amenorrhea. For affected 46,XY individuals, external genital development ranges from normal female to ambiguous because of testosterone deficiency. Indeed, 46,XY individuals with female external genitalia may not be diagnosed until their pubertal development is delayed. Normal testicular production of MIH leads to regression of müllerian duct–derived structures. Increased secretion of deoxycorticosterone and corticosterone is common and may be associated with some degree of hypertension and hypokalemia.

This disorder is secondary to mutations in the 17α-hydroxylase/17,20-lyase gene (*CYP17*). The majority of mutations cause complete inhibition of both enzyme activities.[110] Identification of patients whose 17,20-lyase activity is preferentially affected indicates that the two enzyme activities are regulated independently. Investigation of two such mutations, R347H and R358Q, provides evidence of impaired interaction of CYP17 with oxidoreductase, a protein that donates electrons to microsomal cytochrome P_{450} enzymes, and with cytochrome b_5. The net result is disrupted electron transfer and preferential loss of 17,20-lyase activity.[111]

CONGENITAL LIPOID ADRENAL HYPERPLASIA

Another disorder is characterized by inability to synthesize any adrenal or gonadal steroid hormones (see Table 8–3). Impaired fetal testicular testosterone synthesis results in undervirilization of internal and external genitalia in affected 46,XY fetuses. Thus, both 46,XX and 46,XY infants show female external genital development. Without early diagnosis and treatment, adrenal insufficiency with hyponatremia, hyperkalemia, and cardiovascular collapse is evident early in infancy and the infant dies.[112] Hypergonadotropic hypogonadism is evident in adolescence.

This disorder is due to mutations in the steroid acute regulatory protein (*StAR*) gene.[113] The StAR protein is responsible for the rate-limiting step of acute steroidogenesis, namely the transport of cholesterol into mitochondria. Mutations in *StAR* affect steroidogenesis in two ways. First, StAR-dependent steroidogenesis is impaired. Second, the accumulation of intracellular cholesterol esters is toxic to the adrenal or gonadal cell and destroys any residual StAR-independent steroidogenesis. This model was confirmed by spontaneous pubertal development in an affected 46,XX patient.[114] Carcinoma in situ was described in an intraabdominal testis removed from a 15-year-old 46,XY patient who was raised as a girl and had intermittently followed her hormone replacement regimen.[115] In the early stages of congenital lipoid adrenal hyperplasia, hyperplastic steroidogenic cells with florid lipid deposits are noted that subsequently evolve into small glands with minimal or no lipid deposition.

Management

Treatment involves glucocorticoid (and, if necessary, mineralocorticoid) replacement therapy. The goal of therapy is to decrease adrenal androgen secretion while avoiding side effects secondary to oversuppression, such as reduced growth velocity. For children, oral hydrocortisone is commonly used because it provides the best approximation of physiologic dosing. Physiologic replacement therapy is based on reported daily cortisol production rates of 7 to 12 mg/m²/day in children and adults.[116, 117] For most patients, an oral cortisol dose between 12 and 20 mg/m²/day is sufficient to suppress adrenal androgen oversecretion and maintain normal growth and development. Neonates typically require larger doses (i.e., 25 to 30 mg/m²/day). Adequacy of replacement therapy can be assessed by the lack of progressive virilization, normal growth velocity, appropriate skeletal maturation, normal serum adrenal androgen concentrations for age and stage of maturation, and urinary 17-ketosteroid excretion. Androstenedione is typically more useful, since the level does not fluctuate as markedly as than of 17-hydroxyprogesterone in relation to timing of medication. A more useful measure of oversuppression is the 17-hydroxyprogesterone concentration. For older adolescents or adults, prednisone or dexamethasone can be used.

The usual mineralocorticoid replacement regimen consists of oral fludrocortisone (Florinef). The typical dose is 0.1 mg in a single daily dose; however, neonates and infants may require as much as 0.3 mg daily because of their greater aldosterone production. Occasionally, additional oral sodium chloride is required to prevent hyponatremia. Plasma renin activity serves as an index of the adequacy of mineralocorticoid replacement, although renin activity does not reliably indicate whether the dose is excessive. In older children, a dietary history of salt intake and salt craving provides a clinical parameter of the sufficiency of the replacement regimen. Blood pressure should be monitored.

Increased glucocorticoid dosage is necessary at times of physiologic stress such as fever higher than 101° F, persistent vomiting or diarrhea, major trauma, or a surgical procedure. Three times the usual daily glucocorticoid dose is generally adequate, but higher doses may be necessary for surgical procedures. All families should have—and know how to use—a fast-acting injectable hydrocortisone preparation (e.g., Solu-Cortef) for emergencies. Recommended doses are 25 mg in infants, 50 mg for children younger than 4 years, and 100 mg for all others.

For elective surgery, triple the usual dose can be taken the evening before the procedure. During the procedure, hydrocortisone can be administered by continuous intravenous infusion, along with the usual fluids. Because of the short half-life of intravenous hydrocortisone, continuous infusion is favored over a bolus. When oral mineralocorticoid replacement is not tolerated, intravenous saline may be necessary because parental deoxycorticosterone is generally unavailable. Persons with 11β-hydroxylase deficiency who are taking suppressive glucocorticoid therapy may require mineralocorticoid replacement when under physiologic stress, especially from gastrointestinal illnesses.

Despite apparently adequate glucocorticoid replacement therapy, some women with congenital adrenal hyperplasia develop oligomenorrhea or amenorrhea. These women often benefit from taking oral contraceptives in addition to glucocorticoid therapy. Spironolactone may also help to block androgen action. Because spironolactone use is associated with irregular menstrual bleeding and because of the risk for undervirilization

of a male fetus, oral contraceptives should be used concurrently.

DISORDERS OF TESTOSTERONE BIOSYNTHESIS OR ACTION

In this section we discuss disorders of deficient testosterone synthesis or action. All are inherited disorders whose specific clinical features vary according to the severity of the genetic alteration. Although the most extreme or characteristic phenotype is described, it is important to remember that there is a broad range of phenotypes, from female external genital differentiation to mild hypogonadism in phenotypic males (see Table 8–3).

Leydig Cell Hypoplasia

In Leydig cell hypoplasia, Leydig cell differentiation and testosterone biosynthesis are impaired. The testosterone deficiency leads to failure to stabilize the wolffian ducts and undervirilization of the external genitalia. Because MIH secretion is normal, no uterus develops. This autosomal-recessive disorder is due to loss of function mutations in the LH receptor (*LHR*) gene.[118] Phenotypes in affected 46,XY persons range from female external genitalia to micropenis. Genetic females are asymptomatic until puberty, when they develop oligomenorrhea or amenorrhea, enlarged cystic ovaries, and infertility.[119] Serum LH concentrations and ratios of LH to FSH are elevated and testosterone concentrations low.

17β-Hydroxysteroid Dehydrogenase Deficiency

In this autosomal-recessive disorder, impaired conversion of androstenedione to testosterone results in testosterone deficiency (see Table 8–4). Distinguishing features include perineoscrotal hypospadias with bilateral cryptorchidism at birth and progressive virilization at puberty. In utero, müllerian hormone secretion is sufficient so that a blind vaginal pouch develops in the absence of a uterus or fallopian tubes. And, despite testosterone deficiency in utero, wolffian duct derivatives such as epididymis, vasa deferentia, seminal vesicles, and ejaculatory ducts typically are present. At puberty, clitoromegaly, deepening of the voice, male-pattern sexual hair, and increased muscle mass develop. Presumably, this virilization is due to LH stimulation of testicular androstenedione secretion with peripheral conversion of the androstenedione to testosterone. In some societies, affected persons switch gender identity from female to male during puberty. Laboratory studies demonstrate elevated basal and human chorionic gonadotropin (hCG)-stimulated androstenedione-testosterone ratios.

Several different enzymes show 17β-hydroxysteroid dehydrogenase activity. These enzymes differ in tissue expression, substrate preferences, and co-factors.[120] The specific isozyme expressed in the testis is coded by the type 3 17β-hydroxysteroid dehydrogenase (*HSD17β3*) gene. This disorder is due to loss of function mutations of *HSD17β3*.[121, 122] Women genotyped as being either homozygous or compound heterozygous carriers of *HSD17β3* mutations are asymptomatic.[123]

5α-Reductase Deficiency

Conversion of testosterone to dihydrotestosterone (DHT) in androgen target tissues is impaired in this autosomal-recessive disorder. The clinical features are similar to those of 17β-hydroxysteroid dehydrogenase deficiency in that the external genitalia appear female at birth with perineoscrotal hypospadias. Progressive virilization takes place at the time of puberty. Facial hair is sparse, and male-pattern baldness is rare. This disorder was initially characterized among a consanguineous population in the Dominican Republic, where affected persons are known as "guevedoces" or "penis at 12."[124] Gender identity often changes from female to male as the child virilizes. Laboratory studies document increased basal and hCG-stimulated testosterone-DHT ratios. Analysis of urinary metabolites shows that ratios of etiocholanolone to androsterone and tetrahydrocortisol to 5α-tetrahydrocortisol are increased. This disorder is due to loss of function mutations in the 5α-reductase type 2 (*SRD5A2*) gene.[125]

Androgen Insensitivity

Androgen insensitivity is an X-linked disorder associated with complete or partial resistance to androgen action at the androgen receptor (see Table 8–3).[126–128] Often, the family history contains an affected maternal relative. The disorder is due to mutations in the androgen receptor, which is located on the proximal long arm of the X chromosome. Abnormalities of the androgen

receptor can be classified as receptor-negative (i.e., the ligand fails to bind to the receptor) or receptor-positive (i.e., androgen or DHT can bind to the receptor but the ligand-receptor complex cannot adequately influence gene transcription). In infants, adolescents, and adults, LH and testosterone concentrations are elevated, whereas FSH concentrations may be normal or elevated (see Table 8–4). When androgen resistance is associated with secondary 5α-reductase deficiency the testosterone-DHT ratio increases.[129]

In a state of complete androgen insensitivity, deficient androgen action and normal secretion of MIH results in regression of both wolffian and müllerian duct–derived structures. Affected persons show female external genital development and no internal genital ducts. Presenting features include labial masses, inguinal hernias, and primary amenorrhea. When present, the vagina is a short blind pouch. The testes may be intraabdominal or located within the inguinal canal or the labia majora. At puberty, loss of negative feedback inhibition leads to increased LH and testosterone secretion. Conversion of testosterone to estradiol frequently stimulates spontaneous breast development. Typically, axillary and pubic hair are sparse.

In partial androgen insensitivity syndromes, some response to androgen occurs. The spectrum of clinical manifestations ranges from genital ambiguity to hypogonadism in phenotypic males. Some patients with partial androgen insensitivity assigned female sex of rearing develop virilization with the onset of puberty. *Reifenstein, Gilbert-Dreyfus*, and *Lubs* are eponyms for partial androgen insensitivity syndromes. Phenotypic heterogeneity—in other words different phenotypes with the identical mutation—can occur even within a single family.[130] During the first few months of life, LH and testosterone values are elevated. For partial androgen insensitivity, a trial of testosterone therapy may be indicated to assess the clinical response to androgen. Differential diagnosis includes Denys-Drash, Frasier, and Smith-Lemli-Opitz syndromes. In contrast to these disorders associated with dysgenetic gonads, testicular histology is normal in the androgen insensitivity syndromes and the testis readily responds to hCG stimulation with abundant testosterone secretion.

The androgen receptor protein consists of ligand-binding, DNA-binding, and transactivation domains. Unliganded receptors are localized predominantly to the cytoplasm. Androgens diffuse into target cells where they can bind directly to the androgen receptor or can undergo conversion by 5α-reductase to DHT, which then binds to the androgen receptor. Androgen binding alters the conformation of the ligand-binding domain and is accompanied by receptor phosphorylation. The ligand-receptor complex then moves into the nucleus, where it binds to androgen response elements (ARE) on chromatin and causes changes in gene expression.[131] Mutations associated with androgen insensitivity may impair ligand binding, may alter the kinetics of the ligand-receptor interaction, or may generate transcriptionally inactive proteins.[132, 133] The majority of mutations described to date are point mutations.[134]

Recent interest has focused on a trinucleotide repeat region in exon 1. This variable-length CAG repeat codes for a polyglutamine tract. Expansion of this trinucleotide repeat is associated with spinal bulbar muscle atrophy and mild androgen insensitivity.[135]

Vanishing Testis Syndrome

Humans with well-developed male external genital development and bilateral congenital anorchia are considered to have the vanishing testes syndrome. Such individuals had testes that secreted testosterone at the appropriate time of gestation to elicit normal male sexual differentiation. Affected patients show hypergonadotropic hypogonadism and no significant testosterone response to hCG stimulation. This disorder has been attributed to vascular insufficiency affecting the developing testis. Review of the anatomic and histologic findings in a large series of boys supports the hypothesis that the vanishing testis syndrome is due to testicular torsion, probably late in gestation, and recommends laparoscopic evaluation to assess for residual testicular tissue because of the potential for malignant degeneration.[136, 137]

MANAGEMENT

Often, the initial and most critical management decisions for a patient with inadequate testosterone synthesis or action is to determine gender of rearing. Children with complete androgen insensitivity show normal female external genitalia and have no clinical response to a trial of hCG or testosterone treatment. Since those with complete androgen insensitivity will not respond to testosterone therapy, female sex of rearing is usually assigned. Each case requires individual consideration of the genotypic sex, extent of

erectile tissue, and response to testosterone therapy.[138] Early recognition, diagnosis, and testosterone treatment when indicated is the best treatment for 17β-hydroxysteroid dehydrogenase and 5α-reductase deficiencies. Sex steroid treatment in androgen insensitivity syndromes may be important to prevent decreased bone density.[139]

DISORDERS OF MÜLLERIAN INHIBITORY HORMONE

Persistent müllerian duct syndrome is characterized by müllerian duct–derived structures in association with normal male genital differentiation. Bilateral inguinal hernias early in life are the typical presentation. Often, one hernia sac contains both testes along with müllerian structures (hernia uteri inguinale). This disorder is due to mutations in MIH or its receptor.[140, 141] Usually, testicular function, including spermatogenesis, is normal.

MANAGEMENT: SEX OF REARING

From the first prenatal ultrasound examination until the moment of birth, parents are eager and excited to know the sex of their infant. Genital ambiguity raises major medical, psychosocial, and genetic concerns. Whereas to the clinician, genital ambiguity is a developmental anomaly, for the anxious parents, their extended family, and their friends it is a social emergency. Compounding the difficulties are cultural attitudes about sexual dimorphism, pre-existing expectations for this child, and feelings of guilt and dejection for having given birth to a child with a birth defect, especially a defect that is so emotionally charged. The initial goal of medical management is to determine the most appropriate sex of rearing, and the sex of rearing that may be possible prior to determination of a definitive diagnosis.

It is helpful to inform the parents that their child's genitalia were incompletely formed. This incomplete development represents a visible birth defect. Explanations (which often need to be repeated) of normal fetal sexual differentiation, emphasizing the embryonic bipotentiality of genital structures, can help parents to understand what has happened and provide the rationale for specific diagnostic studies. Demonstration of the precise genital abnormalities on physical examination is very helpful and may increase the parents' level of comfort with their infant. Importantly, the infant should be referred to as *your baby* or *your child*, not *it, he,* or *she*. Parents often obsess on what they "heard" or overheard from healthcare professionals. Such words, especially carelessly spoken ones, can have lasting negative impact. Naming of the infant and birth registration should be postponed until the diagnostic evaluation has enabled selection of the more appropriate sex of rearing.

The first step of the diagnostic evaluation is a careful and thorough physical examination. Important findings include palpable gonads, symmetry of genital appearance, extent of phallic and labioscrotal development, position of urethral meatus, status of müllerian duct–derived structures, and the presence of other anomalies. These physical features indicate the fetal hormonal milieu and do not identify the genetic sex. A family history is valuable to discover other affected individuals, information helpful in diagnosis and management.

Diagnostic studies include a karyotype to ascertain the genetic sex and an imaging study to establish the status of müllerian-derived structures. Although basal steroid hormone concentrations are often diagnostic (see Table 8–4), ACTH or hCG stimulation may be necessary for some infants. Measurement of gonadotropin, glucose, and electrolyte concentrations may also be indicated. Measurement of serum MIH indicates Sertoli cell function. In infants with ambiguous genitalia, low testosterone and low MIH concentrations are consistent with gonadal dysgenesis. Low testosterone with normal or elevated MIH concentrations are associated with defects in testosterone biosynthesis, including Leydig cell hypoplasia.[142] Genotype analyses are increasingly available and are helpful to confirm the molecular basis of the disorder and to help to predict risk of recurrence. In cases of gonadal dysgenesis or an intraabdominal gonad in the presence of Y chromosome material, removal of intraabdominal gonads can be considered to eliminate risk of gonadal neoplasia or malignancy.[143]

The virilized 46,XX infant with 21-hydroxylase deficiency congenital adrenal hyperplasia typically presents with genital ambiguity in the absence of palpable gonads. Abdominal ultrasonography shows a normal uterus and enlarged adrenal glands. Ovaries are present but may be difficult to visualize. Random 17-hydroxyprogesterone, progesterone, and androstenedione concentrations are markedly elevated. At birth, serum electrolyte concentrations are normal. Over the first 5 to 10 days of life, hyperkalemia and hyponatremia develop in the untreated child. Because of the potential for spontaneous female pubertal development and normal fertility with hormone replacement therapy, female sex of rearing, with appropriate genital reconstructive surgery, is usually appropriate. To minimize vaginal scarring, vaginoplasty and dilatation are often delayed until late adolescence, closer to the time when the girl will engage in sexual intercourse.

Symmetric external genitalia and bilateral palpable testes suggest a defect in testosterone biosynthesis or activity. Androgen insensitivity syndromes are characterized by elevated LH and testosterone concentrations in the neonatal period. When the diagnosis of partial androgen insensitivity is suspected because of genital ambiguity, 46,XY karyotype, and typical hormone profile, the clinical response to exogenous testosterone therapy can be used to help to choose sex of rearing. The amount of phallic growth after one or more monthly testosterone injections (25 mg testosterone enanthate per month for 1 to 3 months) provides a clinical assessment of androgen sensitivity. If the response is judged to be satisfactory, male sex of rearing is appropriate. For infants with partial androgen insensitivity and a meager response to exogenous androgen stimulation, female sex of rearing should be considered. Molecular confirmation of mutations in the androgen receptor can be obtained. At this writing, such studies are generally offered only by research laboratories. Nevertheless, results of molecular genetic analysis typically are not available for timely gender assignment but may be helpful for genetic counseling purposes.

Consideration of sex of rearing involves many factors and needs to be individualized for each patient. As much as possible, parents need to be included in discussions and decision making. Recent reports confirm that sex reversal is not a trivial matter.[144, 145] Issues of genital appearance, sexual functioning, and potential for fertility need to be considered. Traditionally, decisions were based on the adequacy of external genital development for adult sexual function. Increasingly, the role of the prenatal and postnatal hormonal milieus of the brain in molding gender identity, sexually dimorphic behavior, and sexual preferences is being pondered.[146] Those who suggest that gender assignment and reconstructive surgery be delayed fail to address the real life issues of how the child will be raised and dressed and which restroom the child will use in kindergarten.[147, 148] Biologic (i.e., prenatal and postnatal hormonal milieu) external genital development, surgical procedures, and social factors (i.e., parents' acceptance of the child and the diagnosis) all influence gender identity.[149] Age at presentation is another factor in decision making, because sex reversal becomes more difficult as the child gets older. Thus, supporting the child in the gender identity already adopted may be the better option if diagnosis is made after 12 to 18 months of age. Once the sex of rearing is determined, however, gender identity should be unequivocal. The infant is either a boy or a girl.

HORMONE REPLACEMENT IN HYPOGONADAL FEMALES

Customarily, sex hormone replacement therapy is recommended for females with hypogonadism. For short stature, especially in association with Turner syndrome, consideration should be given to growth hormone therapy before the institution of sex steroid replacement (see Turner Syndrome). Although low-dose estrogen may speed growth, it also promotes skeletal maturation and epiphyseal fusion.

Estrogen therapy is used to initiate or advance development of secondary sexual characteristics, especially breasts, uterus, and vagina. Current evidence indicates that estrogen therapy is cardioprotective. Preliminary data suggest that estrogen also exerts a positive influence on cognitive function. The three major types of estrogen preparations are (1) physiologic replacements such as 17β-estradiol, available as a transdermal patch; (2) synthetic preparations such as ethinyl estradiol; and (3) conjugated natural estrogens such as Premarin (Table 8–5). The transdermal estradiol patch has largely supplanted topical (vaginal), injectable, and implantable estrogen preparations. Another advantage of the patch is that estrogen delivery is more physiologic with fewer fluctuations in serum concentrations. Because the transdermal patch appears to provide efficacious prophylaxis against osteoporosis and to produce favorable lipoprotein profiles in postmenopausal women, it can be considered as an alternative to oral preparations for young hypogonadal women. The 1:1 estrone-estradiol ratio

is preserved with transdermal estradiol, as it is not with other estrogen preparations. The liver converts oral estrogens to estrone, which increases the estrone-estradiol ratio. Serum estradiol concentrations can readily be determined and the dose adjusted, if necessary. While many adolescents prefer transdermal patches to oral medications, some are bothered by local skin irritation from the adhesive and the visible sign of "being different."

When a uterus is present, cyclic progestin therapy protects against the eventual induction of endometrial hyperplasia or carcinoma secondary to unopposed estrogen treatment.[150, 151] Progesterone can be administered orally, rectally, vaginally, or transdermally. Progestins affect breast maturation, mood, and libido. Androgenicity and impact on endometrium and lipoproteins vary among specific progestins.[152]

The decision when to initiate therapy needs to be individualized according to the underlying diagnosis and the patient's eagerness to experience puberty with her girlfriends. Delayed puberty may exacerbate feelings of being different from peers and negatively affect self-esteem. Low-dose estrogen therapy can be initiated and doses gradually increased to maximize long bone growth and minimize potential side effects such as nausea and breast tenderness. Breast development can usually be induced with ethinyl estradiol, 5 to 10 μg per day; conjugated equine estrogen, 0.3 mg per day; or transdermal estradiol biweekly, 0.05 mg. Once vaginal bleeding occurs or after 6 to 12 months of unopposed estrogen, cyclic estrogen-progestin therapy can be instituted.

Cyclic regimens include continuation of the initial estrogen treatment, oral or transdermal, with the addition of 5 to 10 mg of medroxyprogesterone for 10 to 14 days per month. For example, unopposed estrogen can be started on the first day of the month and continued until day 25. The progestin can be administered on days 15 to 25 of the month. Both hormones can be discontinued on day 26 and menses will occur on days 28 to 31. Oral contraceptives can also be used, their advantage being the simplicity of taking one pill per day. Since girls with Turner syndrome are at increased risk for diabetes mellitus, it is wise to choose an oral contraceptive formulation that contains a norethindrone-type progestin rather than a levonorgestrel type.[153]

Although these regimens are generally tolerated well, occasional patients complain of side effects, which limit compliance. For example, a 14-year-old girl with Turner syndrome who is 58 inches tall and weighs 95 pounds may be

Table 8–5. Common Commercially Available Estrogen Preparations

	Route	Dosage (mg/day)
Estradiol	Oral	1, 2°
Estradiol	Transdermal	0.05, 0.10
Ethinyl estradiol	Oral	0.005, 0.010, 0.020
Estropipate (estrone)	Oral	0.625, 1.25, 2.5, 5.0
Conjugated equine estrogens	Oral	0.3, 0.625, 0.9, 1.25, 2.5

°Minimum dose thought to prevent osteoporosis.

"overdosed" with standard low-dose contraceptives containing 35 μg ethinyl estradiol. If persistent breast tenderness is a problem, changing to a contraceptive preparation containing 20 mg ethinyl estradiol (e.g., Loestrin 1/20, Alesse) may help. For girls who might spontaneously become pregnant, oral contraceptives provide hormone replacement and contraception simultaneously. In general, the clinician who prescribes hormone replacement therapy should be familiar with several different preparations. Recalling the precautions suggested for the 50-μg oral contraceptives of the past, mothers are likely to inquire about long-term risks and benefits of hormone replacement therapy. Apart from increased risk for venous thromboembolic events, there are minimal health risks, and potential health benefits, from oral contraceptives in nonsmokers.[154, 155]

FERTILITY IN HYPOGONADAL FEMALES

The development of techniques for in vitro fertilization has expanded the reproductive options for women with irreversible hypogonadism. Currently, the minimum requirements for becoming pregnant are a uterus and willingness to receive donor oocytes. Donor oocytes can be obtained from anonymous volunteers undergoing elective tubal ligation, women using assisted reproductive techniques, or relatives or other anonymous donors willing to submit to controlled ovarian hyperstimulation and follicular retrieval.[156] Higher pregnancy rates have been achieved more recently, probably owing to different hormone replacement regimens, improved culture techniques, and greater clinical experience with in vitro fertilization. Because at least two women with Turner syndrome developed aortic dissection during pregnancy, the cardiovascular system should be evaluated before oocyte donation.[157] Indeed, the predilection for women with Turner syndrome to develop impaired glucose tolerance, thyroid disorders, and cephalopelvic disproportion has prompted the suggestion that only a single embryo be transferred.[158] Discussion of the relative merits of options to obtain donor oocytes and specific technical details are beyond the scope of this chapter.

REFERENCES

1. Sinclair AH, Berta P, Palmer MS, et al: A gene from the human sex-determining region encodes a protein with homology to a conserved DNA-binding motif. Nature 1990; 346:240.
2. Turner HH: A syndrome of infantilism, congenital webbed neck, and cubitus valgus. Endocrinology 1938; 23:566.
3. Ford CE, Jones KW, Polani PE, et al: A sex chromosome anomaly in a case of gonadal dysgenesis (Turner's syndrome). Lancet 1959; 1:711.
4. Held KR, Kerber S, Kaminsky S, et al: Mosaicism in 45,X Turner syndrome: Does survival in early pregnancy depend on the presence of two sex chromosomes? Hum Genet 1992; 88:288.
5. Committee on Genetics: Health supervision for children with Turner syndrome. Pediatrics 1995; 96:1166.
6. Krauss CM, Turksoy RN, Atkins L, et al: Familial premature ovarian failure due to an interstitial deletion of the long arm of the X chromosome. N Engl J Med 1987; 317:125.
7. Zinn AR, Ouyang B, Ross JL, et al: Del(X)(p21.2) in mother and two daughters with variable ovarian function. Clin Genet 1997; 52:235.
8. Ogata T, Matsuo N: Turner syndrome and female sex chromosome aberrations: Deduction of the principal factors involved in the development of clinical features. Hum Genet 1995; 95:607.
9. Ranke MB, Blum WF, Haug F, et al: Growth hormone, somatomedin levels and growth regulation in Turner's syndrome. Acta Endocrinol 1987; 116:305.
10. Ross JL, Long LM, Loriaux DL, et al: Growth hormone secretory dynamics in Turner syndrome. J Pediatr 1985; 106:202.
11. Albertsson-Wikland K, Rosberg S: Dynamics of growth hormone secretion in girls with Turner syndrome. In Rosenfeld RG, Grumbach MM (eds): Turner Syndrome. New York: Marcel Dekker, 1990, pp 233–246.
12. Prandstraller D, Mazzanti L, Picchio FM, et al: Turner's syndrome: Cardiologic profile according to the different chromosomal patterns and long-term clinical follow-up of 135 nonpreselected patients. Pediatr Cardiol 1999; 20:108.
13. Lin AE, Lippe B, Rosenfeld RG: Further delineation of aortic dilatation, dissection, and rupture in patients with Turner syndrome. Pediatrics 1998; 102:e12.
14. Beals RK: Orthopedic aspects of the XO (Turner's) syndrome. Clin Orthop 1973; 97:19.
15. Bergmann P, Valsamis J, Van Perborgh J, et al: Comparative study of the changes in insulin-like growth factor-I, procollagen-III N-terminal extension peptide, bone gla-protein, and bone mineral content in children with Turner's syndrome treated with recombinant growth hormone. J Clin Endocrinol Metab 1990; 71:1461.
16. Ross JL, Long LM, Feuillan P, et al: Normal bone density of the wrist and spine and increased wrist fractures in girls with Turner's syndrome. J Clin Endocrinol Metab 1991; 73:355.
17. Davies M, Gulekli B, Jacobs H: Osteoporosis in Turner's syndrome and other forms of primary amenorrhea. Clin Endocrinol 1995; 43:741.
18. Rubin K, Schirduan V, Gendreau P, et al: Predictors of axial and peripheral bone mineral density in healthy children and adolescents, with special attention to the role of puberty. J Pediatr 1993; 123:863.
19. Rubin K, Schirduan V, Kennedy D, et al: Effects of rhGH alone or in combination with estrogen on bone accretion in Turner's syndrome. J Bone Miner Res 1990; 5:S252.
20. Lanes R, Gunczler P, Paoli M, et al: Bone mineral density of prepubertal age girls with Turner's syndrome while on growth hormone therapy. Horm Res 1995; 44:168.
21. Rubin K: Turner syndrome and osteoporosis: mechanisms and prognosis. Pediatrics 1998; 102:481.

22. Watkin PM: Otological disease in Turner's syndrome. J Laryngol Otol 1989; 103:731.

23. Sculerati N, Ledesma-Medina J, Finegold DN, et al: Otitis media and hearing loss in Turner syndrome. Arch Otolaryngol Head Neck Surg 1990; 116:704.

24. Matthies F, Macdiarmid WD, Rallison ML, et al: Renal anomalies in Turner syndrome. Clin Pediatr 1971; 10:561.

25. Lippe B, Geffner ME, Dietrich RB, et al: Renal malformations in patients with Turner syndrome: Imaging in 141 patients. Pediatrics 1988; 82:852.

26. Bonamico M, Bottaro G, Pasquino AM, et al: Celiac disease and Turner syndrome. J Pediatr Gastroenterol Nutr 1998; 26:496.

27. Arulanantham K, Kramer MS, Gryboski JD: The association of inflammatory bowel disease and X chromosomal abnormality. Pediatrics 1980; 66:63.

28. Manzione NC, Kram M, Kram E, et al: Turner's syndrome and inflammatory bowel disease: A case report with immunologic studies. Am J Gastroenterol 1988; 83:1294.

29. Nielsen J, Johansen K, Yale H: The frequency of diabetes mellitus in patients with Turner's syndrome and pure gonadal dysgenesis. Acta Endocrinol 1969; 62:251.

30. Gravholt CH, Naeraa RW, Nyholm B, et al: Glucose metabolism, lipid metabolism, and cardiovascular risk factors in adult Turner's syndrome. Diabetes Care 1998; 21:1062.

31. Caprio S. Boulware S, Diamond M, et al: Insulin resistance: An early metabolic defect of Turner's syndrome. J Clin Endocrinol Metab 1991; 72:832.

32. Gravholt CH, Juul S, Naeraa RW, et al: Morbidity in Turner syndrome. J Clin Epidemiol 1998; 51:147.

33. Zinn AR, Tonk VS, Chen Z, et al: Evidence of a Turner syndrome locus or loci at Xp11.2-p22.1. Am J Hum Genet 1998; 63:1757.

34. Mathur A, Stekol L, Schatz D, et al: The parental origin of the single X chromosome: Lack of correlation with parental age or clinical phenotype. Am J Hum Genet 1991; 48:682.

35. Kocova M, Siegel SF, Wenger SL, et al: Detection of Y chromosomal sequences in Turner syndrome by Southern blot analysis of amplified DNA. Lancet 1993; 342:140.

36. Mazzocco MMM: A process approach to describing mathematics difficulties in girls with Turner syndrome. Pediatrics 1998; 102:492.

37. McCauley E, Ito J, Kay T: Psychosocial functioning in girls with Turner's syndrome and short stature: Social skills, behavior problems, and self-concept. J Am Acad Child Adolesc Psychiatry 1986; 25:105.

38. McCauley E, Kay T, Ito J, et al: The Turner syndrome: Cognitive deficits, affective discrimination, and behavior problems. Child Develop 1987; 58:464.

39. Siegel PT, Clopper R, Stabler B: The psychological consequences of Turner syndrome and review of the National Cooperative Growth Study Psychological Substudy. Pediatrics 1998; 102:488.

40. Mazzocco MMM, Baumgardner T, Freund LS, et al: Social functioning among girls with fragile X or Turner syndrome and their sisters. J Autism Dev Disord 1998; 28:509.

41. Skuse D, Elgar K, Morris E: Quality of life in Turner syndrome is related to chromosomal constitution: Implications for genetic counselling and management. Acta Paediatr Suppl 1999; 428:110.

42. Orten JL: Coming up short: The physical, cognitive, and social effects of Turner's syndrome. Health Soc Work 1990; 15:100.

43. Massa GG, Vanderschueren-Lodeweyckx M: Age and height at diagnosis in Turner syndrome: Influence of parental height. Pediatrics 1991; 88:1148.

44. Mendez HMM, Opitz JM: Noonan syndrome: A review. Am J Med Genet 1985; 21:493.

45. Jamieson CR, van der Burgt I, Brady AF, et al: Mapping a gene for Noonan syndrome to the long arm of chromosome 12. Nat Genet 1994; 8:357.

46. Sylven L, Hagenfeldt K, Brondum-Nielsen K, et al: Middle-aged women with Turner's syndrome. Medical status, hormonal treatment, and social life. Acta Endocrinol 1991; 125:359.

47. Betts PR, Butler GE, Donaldson MDC, et al: A decade of growth hormone treatment in girls with Turner syndrome in the UK. Arch Dis Child 1999; 80:221.

48. Plotnick L. Attie KM, Blethen SL, et al: Growth hormone treatment of girls with Turner syndrome: The National Cooperative Growth Study Experience. Pediatrics 1998; 102:479.

49. Rosenfeld RG, Attie KM, Frane J, et al: Growth hormone therapy of Turner's syndrome: Beneficial effect on adult height. J Pediatr 1998; 132:319.

50. Querfeld U, Dopper S, Gradehand A, et al: Long-term treatment with growth hormone has no persisting effect on lipoprotein(a) in patients with Turner's syndrome. J Clin Endocrinol Metab 1999; 84:967.

51. Garden AS, Diver MJ, Fraser WD: Undiagnosed morbidity in adult women with Turner's syndrome. Clin Endocrinol 1996; 45:589.

52. Beckett PR, Copeland KC, Flannery TK, et al: Combination growth hormone and estrogen increase bone mineralization in girls with Turner syndrome. Pediatr Res 1999; 45:709.

53. Hovatta O: Pregnancies in women with Turner's syndrome. Ann Med 1999; 31:106.

54. Aranoff GS, Morishima A: XO/XY mosaicism in delayed puberty. J Adolesc Health Care 1988; 9:501.

55. Wallace TM, Levin HS: Mixed gonadal dysgenesis. Arch Pathol Lab Med 1990; 114:679.

56. Chang HJ, Clark RD, Bachman H: The phenotype of 45,X/46,XY mosaicism: An analysis of 92 prenatally diagnosed cases. Am J Hum Genet 1990; 46:156.

57. Kocova M, Siegel SF, Wenger SL, et al: Detection of Y chromosome sequences in a 45,X/46,XXq- patient by Southern blot analysis of PCR-amplified DNA and fluorescent in situ hybridization (FISH). Am J Med Genet 1995; 55:483.

58. Choi HK, Cho K-S, Lee HW, et al: MR imaging of intersexuality. Radiographics 1998; 18:83.

59. Rutgers JL: Advances in the pathology of intersex conditions. Hum Pathol 1991; 22:884.

60. Sully RE: Gonadoblastoma. A review of 73 cases. Cancer 1970; 25:1340.

61. Müller J, Skakkebaek NE, Ritzén M, et al: Carcinoma in situ of the testis in children with 45,X/46,XY gonadal dysgenesis. J Pediatr 1985; 106:431.

62. Jorgensen N, Muller J, Jaubert F, et al: Heterogeneity of gonadoblastoma germ cells: Similarities with immature germ cells, spermatogonia, and testicular carcinoma in situ cells. Histopathology 1997; 30:177.

63. Scully RE: Gonadal pathology of genetically determined diseases. In Kraus FT, Damjanov I, Kaufman N (eds): Pathology of Reproductive Failure. Baltimore: Williams & Wilkins, 1991, pp 257–285.

64. Chapman WHH, Plymyer MR, Dresner ML: Gonadoblastoma in an anatomically normal man: A case report and review of the literature. J Urol 1990; 144:1472.

65. Olsen MM, Caldamone AA, Jackson CL, et al: Gonadoblastoma in infancy: Indications for early gonadec-

tomy in 46,XY gonadal dysgenesis. J Pediatr Surg 1988; 23:270.

66. Angle B, Hersh JH, Yen F, et al: XY gonadal dysgenesis associated with a multiple pterygium syndrome phenotype. Am J Med Genet 1997; 68:7.

67. Lim HN, Freestone SH, Romero D, et al: Candidate genes in complete and partial XY sex reversal: Mutation analysis of *SRY*, *SRY*-related genes and *FTZ-F1*. Mol Cell Endocrinol 1998; 140:51.

68. Veita R, Ion A, Barbaux S, et al: Mutations and sequence variants in the testis-determining region of the Y chromosome in individuals with a 46,XY female phenotype. Hum Genet 1997; 99:648.

69. Scherer G, Held M, Erdel M, et al: Three novel SRY mutations in XY gonadal dysgenesis and the enigma of XY gonadal dysgenesis cases without SRY mutations. Cytogenet Cell Genet 1998; 80:188.

70. Magenis RE, Casanova M, Fellous M, et al: Further cytologic evidence for Xp-Yp translocation in XX males using in situ hybridization with Y-derived probe. Hum Genet 1987; 75:228.

71. Ginsberg NA, Cadkin A, Strom C, et al: Prenatal diagnosis of 46,XX male fetuses. Am J Obstet Gynecol 1999; 180:1006.

72. Margarit E, Soler A, Carrio A, et al: Molecular, cytogenic, and clinical characterization of six XX males including one prenatal diagnosis. J Med Genet 1998; 35:727.

73. Reutens AT, Achermann JC, Ito M, et al: Clinical and functional effects of mutations in the *DAX-1* gene in patients with adrenal hypoplasia congenita. J Clin Endocrinol Metab 1999; 84:504.

74. Habiby RL, Boepple P, Nachtigall L, et al: Adrenal hypoplasia congenita with hypogonadotropic hypogonadism. J Clin Invest 1996; 96:1055.

75. Bartley JA, Miller DK, Hayford JT, et al: Concordance of X-linked glycerol kinase deficiency with X-linked congenital adrenal hypoplasia. Lancet 1982; 2:733.

76. Bardoni B, Zanaria E, Guioli S, et al: A dosage sensitive locus at chromosome Xp21 is involved in male to female sex reversal. Nat Genet 1994; 7:497.

77. Yu RN, Ito M, Saunders TL, et al: Role of *Ahch* in gonadal development and gametogenesis. Nat Genet 1998; 20:353.

78. Damiani D, Fellous M, McElreavey K, et al: True hermaphroditism: Clinical aspects and molecular studies. Eur J Endocrinol 1997; 136:201.

79. Slaney SF, Chalmers IJ, Affara NA, et al: An autosomal or X linked mutation results in true hermaphrodites and 46,XX males in the same family. J Med Genet 1998; 35:17.

80. Wagner T, Wirth J, Meyer J, et al: Autosomal sex reversal and campomelic dysplasia are caused by mutations in and around the *SRY*-related gene *SOX9*. Cell 1994; 79:1111.

81. Foster JW, Dominguez-Steglich D, Guioli S, et al: Campomelic dwarfism and autosomal sex reversal caused by mutations in an SRY-related gene. Nature 1994; 372:525.

82. Tommerup N, Schempp W, Meinecke P, et al: Assignment of an autosomal sex reversal locus (*SRA1*) and campomelic dysplasia (*CMPD1*) to 17q24.3-q25.1. Nat Genet 1993; 4:170.

83. Meyer J, Südbeck P, Held M, et al: Mutational analysis of the *SOX9* gene in campomelic dwarfism and autosomal sex reversal: Lack of genotype/phenotype correlations. Hum Mol Genet 1997; 6:91.

84. Bruening W, Bardeesy N, Silverman BL, et al: Germline intronic and exonic mutations in the Wilms tumour gene (WT1) affecting urogenital development. Nat Genet 1992; 1:144.

85. Kriedberg JA, Sariola H, Loring JM, et al: WT1 is required for early kidney development. Cell 1993; 74:679.

86. Reddy JC, Licht JD: The WT1 Wilms' tumor suppressor gene: How much do we really know? Biochem Biophys Acta 1996; 1287:1.

87. Denys P, Malraux P, van den Berghe H, et al: Association d'un syndrome anatomopathologique de pseudohermaphrodisme masculin, d'une tumeure de Wilms, d'une nephropathie parenchymateuse et d'un mosaicisme XX/XY. Arch Fran Pediat 1967; 24:729.

88. Drash AL, Sherman F, Hartmann WH, et al: A syndrome of pseudohermaphroditism, Wilms' tumor, hypertension, and degenerative renal disease. J Pediatr 1970; 76:585.

89. Nachtigal MW, Hirokawa Y, Enyeart-Van Houten DL, et al: Wilms' tumor 1 and Dax-1 modulate the orphan nuclear receptor SF-I in sex-specific gene expression. Cell 1998; 93:445.

90. Barbosa AS, Hadjiathansiou CG, Theodoris C, et al: The same mutation affecting the splicing of WT1 gene is present on Frasier syndrome patients with or without Wilms' tumor. Hum Mutat 1999; 13:146.

91. Barbaux S, Niaudet P, Gubler MC, et al: Donor splice-site mutations in WT1 are responsible for Frasier syndrome. Nat Genet 1997; 17:467.

92. Kikuchi H, Takata A, Akasaka Y, et al: Do intronic mutations affecting splicing of WT1 exon 9 cause Frasier syndrome? J Med Genet 1997; 35:45.

93. Klamt B, Koziell F, Poulat F, et al: Frasier syndrome is caused by a defective alternative splicing of WT1 leading to an altered ratio of WT1+/− KTS splice isoforms. Hum Mol Genet 1998; 7:709.

94. Bennett CP, Docherty Z, Robb SA, et al: Deletion 9p and sex reversal. J Med Genet 1993; 30:518.

95. Huret JL, Leonard C, Forestier B, et al: Eleven new cases of del(9p) and features of 80 cases. J Med Genet 1988; 25:741.

96. Raymond CS, Parker ED, Kettlewell JR, et al: A region of chromosome 9p required for testis development contains two genes related to known sexual regulators. Hum Mol Genet 1999; 8:989.

97. Greene C, Pitts W, Rosenfeld R, et al: Smith-Lemli-Opitz syndrome in two 46,XY infants with female external genitalia. Clin Genet 1984; 25:366.

98. Wassif CA, Maslen C, Kachilele-Linjewile S, et al: Mutations in the human sterol-delta7-reductase gene at 11q12–13 cause Smith-Lemli-Opitz syndrome. Am J Hum Genet 1998; 63:55.

99. de S Nazareth HR, Farah LMS, Cunha AJB, et al: Pure gonadal dysgenesis (type XX). Hum Genet 1977; 37:117.

100. Perrault M, Klotz B, Housset E: Deux cas de syndrome de Turner avec surdi-mutute dans une même fratrie. Bull Mem Soc Med Hôp Paris 1951; 16:79.

101. Nishi Y, Hamamoto K, Kajiyama M, et al: The Perrault syndrome: Clinical report and review. Am J Med Genet 1988; 21:623.

102. Speiser PW, Dupont B, Rubinstein P, et al: High frequency of nonclassical steroid 21-hydroxylase deficiency. Am J Hum Genet 1985; 37:650.

103. Jääskelainen J, Levo A, Voutilainen R, et al: Population-wide evaluation of disease manifestation in relation to molecular genotype in steroid 21-hydroxylase (CYP21) deficiency: Good correlation in a well defined population. J Clin Endocrinol Metab 1997; 82:3293.

104. Nikoshkov A, Lajic S, Holst M, et al: Synergistic effect of partially inactivating mutations in steroid 21-hydroxylase deficiency. J Clin Endocrinol Metab 1997; 82:194.

105. Witchel SF, Nayak S, Suda-Hartman M, et al: Newborn screening for 21-hydroxylase deficiency: Results of *CYP21* molecular genetic analysis. J Pediatrics 1997; 131:328.

106. Rhéaume E, Simard J, Morel Y, et al: Congenital adrenal hyperplasia due to point mutations in the type II 3β-hydroxysteroid dehydrogenase gene. Nat Genet 1992; 1:239.

107. Simard J, Rhéaume E, Sanchez R, et al: Molecular basis of congenital adrenal hyperplasia due to 3β-hydroxysteroid dehydrogenase deficiency. Mol Endocrinol 1993; 7:716.

108. Zhang L, Sakkal-Alkaddour H, Chang YT, et al: A new compound heterozygous frameshift mutation in the type II 3β-hydroxysteroid dehydrogenase (*3β-HSD*) gene causes salt-wasting 3β-HSD deficiency congenital adrenal hyperplasia. J Clin Endocrinol Metab 1996; 81:291.

109. Zadik Z, Kahana L, Kaufman H, et al: Salt loss in hypertensive form of congenital adrenal hyperplasia (11β-hydroxylation deficiency). J Clin Endocrinol Metab 1984; 58:384.

110. Yanase T, Simpson ER, Waterman MR: 17α-Hydroxylase/17,20-lyase deficiency: From clinical investigation to molecular definition. Endocrinol Rev 1995; 12:91.

111. Geller DH, Auchus RJ, Miller WL: $P_{450}c17$ mutations R347H and R358Q selectively disrupt 17,20-lyase activity by disrupting interactions with P_{450} oxidoreductase and cytochrome b_5. Mol Endocrinol 1999; 13:167.

112. Miller WL, Strauss JF III: Molecular pathology and mechanism of action of the steroidogenic acute regulatory protein, StAR. J Steroid Biochem Mol Biol 1999; 69:131.

113. Lin D, Sugawara T, Strauss JF III, et al: Role of steroidogenic acute regulatory protein in adrenal and gonadal steroidogenesis. Science 1995; 267:1828.

114. Bose HS, Pescovitz OH, Miller WL: Spontaneous feminization in a 46,XX female patient with congenital lipoid adrenal hyperplasia due to a homozygous frameshift mutation in the steroidogenic acute regulatory protein. J Clin Endocrinol Metab 1997; 82:1511.

115. Korsch E, Peter M, Hiort O, et al: Gonadal histology with testicular carcinoma in situ in a 15-year-old 46,XY female patient with a premature termination in the steroidogenic acute regulatory protein causing congenital lipoid adrenal hyperplasia. J Clin Endocrinol Metab 1999; 84:1628.

116. Kenny FM, Preeyasombat C, Migeon CJ: Cortisol production rate in childhood. II. Normal infants, children, and adults. Pediatrics 1966; 37:34.

117. Linder BL, Esteban NV, Yergey AL, et al: Cortisol production rate in childhood and adolescence. J Pediatrics 1990; 117:892.

118. Kremer H, Kraaij R, Toledo SP, et al: Male pseudohermaphroditism due to a homozygous missense mutation of the luteinizing hormone receptor gene. Nat Genet 1995; 9:160.

119. Arnhold IJ, Latronico AC, Batista MC, et al: Menstrual disorders and infertility caused by inactivating mutations of the luteinizing hormone receptor gene. Fertil Steril 1999; 71:597.

120. Zhang Y, Word RA, Fesmire S, et al: Human ovarian expression of 17β-hydroxysteroid dehydrogenase types 1, 2, and 3. J Clin Endocrinol Metab 1996; 81:3594.

121. Geissler WM, Davis DL, Wu L, et al: Male pseudohermaphroditism caused by mutations of testicular 17β-hydroxysteroid dehydrogenase 3. Nat Genet 1994; 7:34.

122. Andersson S, Geissler WM, Wu L, et al: Molecular genetics and pathophysiology of 17-beta-hydroxysteroid dehydrogenase deficiency. J Clin Endocrinol Metab 1996; 81:130.

123. Mendonca BB, Arnhold IJ, Bloise W, et al: 17β-Hydroxysteroid dehydrogenase 3 deficiency in women. J Clin Endocrinol Metab 1999; 84:802.

124. Imperato-McGinley J, Guerrero L, Gautier T, et al: Steroid 5α-reductase deficiency in man: An inherited form of male pseudohermaphroditism. Science 1974; 186:1213.

125. Thigpen AE, Davis DL, Milatovich A, et al: Molecular genetics of 5α-reductase 2 deficiency. J Clin Invest 1992; 90:799.

126. Quigley CA, De Bellis A, Marschke KB, et al: Androgen receptor defects: Historical, clinical, and molecular perspectives. Endocrinol Rev 1995; 16:271.

127. Viner RM, Teoh Y, Williams DM, et al: Androgen insensitivity syndrome: A survey of diagnostic procedures and management in the UK. Arch Dis Child 1997; 77:305.

128. McPhaul MJ: Molecular defects of the androgen receptor. J Steroid Biochem Mol Biol 1999; 69:315.

129. Imperato-McGinley J, Peterson RE, Gautier T, et al: Hormonal evaluation of a large kindred with complete androgen insensitivity: Evidence for secondary 5α-reductase deficiency. J Clin Endocrinol Metab 1982; 54:931.

130. Rodien P, Mebarki F, Mowszowicz I, et al: Different phenotypes in a family with androgen insensitivity caused by the same M708I point mutation in the androgen receptor gene. J Clin Endocrinol Metab 1996; 81:2994.

131. Brinkmann AO, Blok LJ, de Ruiter PE, et al: Mechanisms of androgen receptor activation and function. J Steroid Biochem Mol Biol 1999; 69:307.

132. Shkolny DL, Beitel LK, Ginsberg J, et al: Discordant measure of androgen-binding kinetics in two mutant androgen receptors causing mild or partial androgen insensitivity, respectively. J Clin Endocrinol Metab 1999; 84:805.

133. Zhu Y-S, Cai L-Q, Cordero JJ, et al: A novel mutation in the CAG triplet repeat region of exon 1 of androgen receptor gene causes complete androgen insensitivity in a large kindred. J Clin Endocrinol Metab 1999; 84:1590.

134. Gottlieb B, Lehvaslaiho H, Beitel LK, et al: The androgen receptor gene mutations database. Nucleic Acids Res 1998; 26:234.

135. La Spada AR, Wilson EM, Lubahn DB, et al: Androgen receptor gene mutations in X-linked spinal and bulbar muscular atrophy. Nature 1991; 352:77.

136. Merry C, Sweeney B, Puri P: The vanishing testis: Anatomical and histological findings. Eur Urol 1997; 31:65.

137. de Vries JDM: Editorial comment. Eur Urol 1997; 31:65.

138. Bin-Abbas B, Conte F, Grumbach MM, et al: Congenital hypogonadotropic hypogonadism and micropenis: Effect of testosterone treatment on adult penile size—why sex reversal is not indicated. J Pediatrics 1999; 134:579.

139. Mizunuma H, Soda M, Okano H, et al: Changes in bone mineral density after orchidectomy and hormone replacement therapy in individuals with androgen insensitivity syndrome. Hum Reprod 1998; 13:2816.

140. Imbeaud S, Belville C, Messika-Zeitoun L, et al: A 27 base-pair deletion of the anti-müllerian type II receptor is the most common cause of the persistent müllerian duct syndrome. Hum Mol Genet 1996; 5:1269.

141. Knebelmann B, Boussin L, Guerrier D, et al: Anti-müllerian hormone Bruxelles: A nonsense mutation associated with the persistent müllerian duct syndrome. Proc Natl Acad Sci 1991; 88:3767.

142. Rey RA, Belville C, Nihoul-Fekete, et al: Evaluation of

gonadal function in 107 intersex patients by means of serum antimüllerian hormone measurement. J Clin Endocrinol Metab 1999; 84:627.

143. Borer JG, Nitti VW, Glassberg KI: Mixed gonadal dysgenesis and dysgenetic male pseudohermaphroditism. J Urol 1995; 153:1267.

144. Diamond M, Sigmundson HK: Sex reassignment at birth: Long-term review and clinical implications. Arch Pediatr Adolesc Med 1997; 151:298.

145. Bradley SJ, Oliver G, Chernick AB, et al: Experiment of nurture: Ablatio penis at 2 months, sex reassignment at 7 months, and psychosexual follow-up in young adulthood. Pediatrics 1998; 102:132A.

146. Reiner W: To be male or female—that is the question. Arch Pediatr Adolesc Med 1997; 151:224.

147. Kessler SJ: Lessons from the Intersexed. New Brunswick, NJ: Rutgers University Press, 1998.

148. Glassberg KI: Editorial: Gender assignment and the pediatric urologist. J Urol 1999; 161:1308.

149. Slijper FM, Drop SL, Molenaar JC, et al: Long-term psychological evaluation of intersex children. Arch Sex Behav 1998; 27:125.

150. Nachtigall LE, Nachtigall RH, Nachtigall RD, et al: Estrogen replacement therapy II. A prospective study in the relationship to carcinoma and cardiovascular and metabolic problems. Obstet Gynecol 1979; 54:74.

151. Whitehead MI, Townsend PT, Pryse-Davies J, et al: Effects of estrogen and progestins on the biochemistry and morphology of the postmenopausal endometrium. N Engl J Med 1981; 305:1599.

152. Carr BR: Uniqueness of oral contraceptive progestins. Contraception 1998; 58:23S.

153. Mishell DR Jr: Family Planning. In Mishell DR, Jr, Stenchever MA, Droegemueller W, Herbst AL (eds): Comprehensive Gynecology, 3rd ed. St Louis: Mosby–Year Book, 1997, pp 283–352.

154. Mishell DR Jr: Cardiovascular risks: Perception versus reality. Contraception 1999; 59:21S.

155. Westhoff CL: Breast cancer risk: Perception versus reality. Contraception 1999; 59:25S.

156. Frydman R, Bydlowski M, Letur-Konirsch H, et al: A protocol for satisfying the ethical issues raised by oocyte donation: The free, anonymous, and fertile donors. Fertil Steril 1990; 53:666.

157. Nagel TC, Tesch LG: Art and high risk patients. Fertil Steril 1997; 68:748.

158. Houvatta O: Pregnancies in women with Turner's syndrome. Ann Med 1999; 31:106.

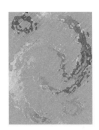

Chapter 9
Nutrition, Growth, and Development

GILBERT B. FORBES

The importance of proper nutrition cannot be overstated, as ultimately the functioning of all physiochemical processes is dependent on an adequate supply of dietary nutrients. Although there is some latitude in the amounts needed, a minimum requirement for each nutrient does exist, and excessive amounts of some nutrients can be harmful. The body can function for a time without food, albeit at less than full capacity, but a more or less continuous supply of nutrients is needed to provide those ingredients that cannot be manufactured within: essential amino acids, vitamins, minerals, and energy. In some respects human beings are more at risk than other mammals, some of which can synthesize certain vitamins or, with the help of intestinal bacteria, can thrive without a dietary supply of essential amino acids. Hibernating animals conserve energy by reducing metabolic rate.

Growth is one of the prime indicators of nutritional adequacy; indeed, growth rate can serve as a bioassay of nutritional status. For many years this has been the standard practice of nutritionists, who have used the growth rates of animals to test the adequacy of various diets. For instance, the observation, many years ago, that highly purified diets did not provide normal growth in rats led to a search for the missing ingredients, resulting in the discovery of some vitamins. The biologic value of various dietary proteins was also established using this technique.

Growth requires energy plus an adequate supply of all essential nutrients; thus, there is no single dietary "growth factor." The effect of a deficiency of one essential nutrient, or of dietary energy, cannot be rectified by giving the others in excess. In children in underdeveloped areas of the world, growth faltering is known to occur with diets low in vitamin A, zinc, vitamin D, or

protein, as well as with diets low in dietary energy. Even chloride deficiency can cause growth failure. In developed countries, diets usually provide sufficient essential nutrients because of the wide variety of foods available, the plentiful supplies of milk, and the fact that a number of foods are fortified with vitamins and minerals. The one exception is iron, for it is known that some adolescents are deficient in this element. Thus, in growth-deficient individuals, the energy content of the diet is most frequently at fault.

Figure 9–1 illustrates the importance of growth rate as an indicator of nutrient deficiency (in this case, vitamin A). Growth rate is exceeded in sensitivity only by female reproductive performance; thus it reflects more subtle deficiency states than can be detected by other techniques.[1]

The great sensitivity of the growth rate to a reduction in energy intake means that growth per se is an integral, inescapable part of adolescent life. Insufficient food has a negative impact on the entire adolescent functional unit (i.e., metabolic rate, activity level, physical performance, and sexual maturation) and on growth rate. If energy intake is inadequate, growth will suffer along with other body functions.

The growing body also responds to energy surfeit. Deliberate overfeeding of adults and adolescents results in weight gain. About two thirds of this gain is fat, and about one third is lean. Of interest is the finding that the weight increment per unit of excess food consumed is the same for women as it is for men.[2] Obese children, who can achieve such a state only via a positive energy balance, are apt to be taller and to have a larger lean weight and larger bones than their thinner peers. Longitudinal studies of children who became obese during childhood show that most of them had had an increase in height percentile status once they had become obese; this change in height status occurred either coincident with the increase in weight or sometime thereafter, but never before.[3] The longitudinal data reported

The research was supported by National Institutes of Health grant HD 18454.

139

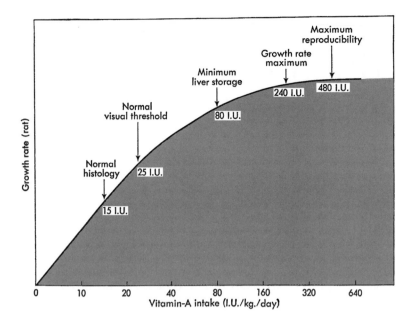

Figure 9–1. Growth rate of rats as a function of vitamin A intake: comparison with other criteria. (From Bessey OA: Evaluation of nutritive status by chemical and other methods. *In* Scheinberg IH [ed]: Infant Metabolism. New York: Macmillan, 1956.)

by Buckler[4] clearly show the effect of subcutaneous fat stores—and hence the magnitude of energy balance—on the stature of adolescent girls (Fig. 9–2).

The plane of nutrition also has an effect on sexual maturation. Girls who have early menarche tend to be heavier and taller at menarche than their premenarchal age-matched peers, and those with late menarche tend to be lighter than their postmenarchal age-matched peers, though stature is comparable. Thus, early maturers have an elevated body mass index (BMI; kg/m^2), and late maturers have a smaller BMI than their age-matched peers. A plot of the data provided by Zacharias and colleagues[5] shows a progressive drop in BMI with age at menarche, in distinct contrast to the progressive increase in BMI that occurs normally at this time of life (Fig. 9–3). Buckler's[4] longitudinal data show that girls who mature early have a greater adolescent growth spurt than those who mature later (Fig. 9–4). Thus, girls who have delayed puberty will appear thin, even undernourished, in comparison to their normally developed age peers. It is possible, of course, that for some delayed development was actually due to poor nutrition.

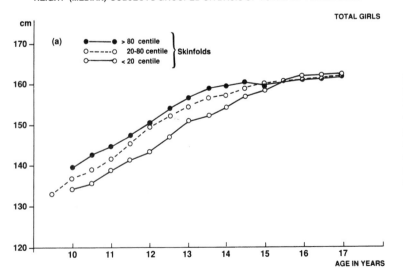

HEIGHT (MEDIAN) SUBJECTS GROUPED ON BASIS OF TOTAL OF 4 SKIN FOLDS

Figure 9–2. Influence of adiposity, as estimated from thickness of skin plus subcutaneous fat, on the height of girls. (Longitudinal data from Buckler JMH: A Longitudinal Study of Adolescent Growth. London: Springer-Verlag, 1990, p 168.)

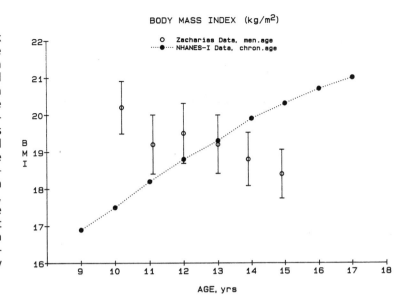

Figure 9–3. Body mass index (BMI) as a function of age in normal girls (●···●). 50th percentile values compiled by Cronk and Roche[18] from data obtained during the National Health and Nutrition Survey. Vertical bars show means and standard errors of BMI at menarche for girls of different menarchal age (men.age). (Data from Zacharias L, Rand WM, Wurtman RJ: A prospective study of sexual development and growth in American girls: The statistics of menarche. Obstet Gynecol Surv 1976; 31:325.)

It should be noted that there is wide variation in menarchal weight; of the 600 subjects studied by Zacharias' group, the heaviest girl was 2½ times the weight of the lightest girl at time of menarche; the coefficient of variation was 15%. Using data from several surveys, Garn and La-Velle[6] documented the fact that a body weight less than the proclaimed "critical value" of 47 kg is not necessarily an impediment to menarche or conception.

Two lines of evidence support the concept that nutrition has an effect on sexual maturation in humans. Obese girls tend to have early menarche, and Stark and colleagues[7] have shown that

early maturing girls are already overweight by age 7 years. Girls living in underdeveloped countries tend to have later menarche. Thus, overnutrition speeds up the maturation process, and undernutrition slows it. Of interest is the demonstration of compromised ovarian function in young women who lose even a little weight.[8]

Underfed animals experience delayed puberty. Young female rats who are underfed have reduced levels of pituitary gonadotropin-releasing hormone (GnRH) and fewer GnRH receptors, so that gonadotropin production or release is subnormal, and vaginal opening does not occur. This situation is promptly reversed by adequate

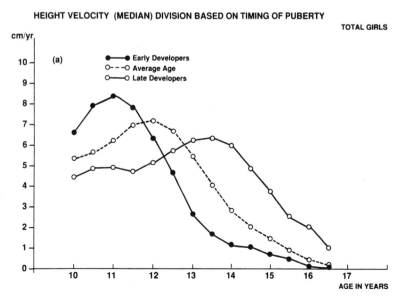

Figure 9–4. Height velocity profiles for early-maturing, average-maturing, and late-maturing girls. (Longitudinal data from Buckler JMH: A Longitudinal Study of Adolescent Growth. London: Springer-Verlag, 1990, p 207.)

food: normal hormonal function is restored, and sexual maturation takes place.[9]

It has been demonstrated that undernutrition diminishes the production of somatomedins, important facilitators of growth produced in the liver by the action of growth hormone. Reduced plasma levels of somatomedins have been recorded in infants with kwashiorkor, and even brief periods of undernutrition in adults produce striking reductions in plasma levels of somatomedins, which are promptly restored by adequate food intake.[10] Deliberate overfeeding is accompanied by a small increase in levels of somatomedins.[11] Thus, nutrition can affect hormones as well as somatic growth.

Several changes have occurred in the growth of children and adolescents since the 19th century. Secular increases in height and weight have been noted in all industrialized societies for which reliable data are available. Female adolescents today are taller and heavier than their age-matched peers of a century ago, and puberty (as judged by menarchal age) is occurring earlier. These changes accompanied the rise of modern nutritional science, and most observers endorse the hypothesis that improved nutrition is responsible for such changes. Two additional factors may have played a role, however: the decline in chronic infection, and the phenomenon of hybrid vigor.

All of this information must be viewed in the context of heredity. At all ages past infancy, there is a reasonable correlation between the heights of children and the heights of their parents. Studies of twins and adoptees show that inheritance is a major factor in weight, stature, BMI, lean weight, and body fat.[12–14]

ASSESSMENT OF GROWTH IN HEIGHT AND WEIGHT

The most commonly used height and weight charts are those based on data collected by the National Committee on Health Statistics on thousands of white children in the United States (Fig. 9–5). Percentile plots are preferred over means and standard deviations because fre-

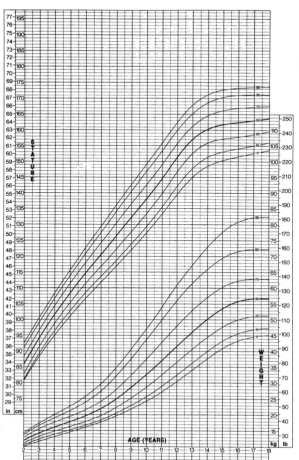

NCHS percentiles for stature and weight for age, girls, 2 to 18 years.

Figure 9–5. Height and weight of girls, based on data from the National Center for Health Statistics. (From Moore WH, Jeffries JE: *In* Johnson TR, Moore WM, Jeffries JE [eds]: Children are Different. Columbus, OH: Ross Laboratories, 1978. Used and reprinted with permission of Ross Laboratories, Columbus, OH 43216, from NCHS Growth Charts, © 1982, Ross Laboratories.)

quency distributions are often skewed. Although black children and adolescents tend to be a bit taller and Hispanics and Orientals somewhat shorter than whites, these charts have proven satisfactory.° Every effort should be made to make an accurate measurement of height and weight and to record age to the nearest month. The best instrument for measuring heights is the Holtain stadiometer,† which consists of a fixed vertical member attached to the wall on which rides a movable headboard maintained in a horizontal position, a direct reading dial, and a footboard with a heel plate. Unfortunately, however, this instrument is expensive. A satisfactory substitute is a meter stick attached to the wall next to a bare floor, with a movable headboard positioned perpendicular to the wall. The sliding-stick devices attached to platform scales are not accurate and should not be used.

The subject must remove his or her shoes and stand erect next to the measuring device in the nonlordotic position, with the eyes and ears forming a horizontal plane; some observers prefer to give a gentle upward tug on the chin. It should be remembered that people are often 1 to 2 cm shorter in the late afternoon than in the early morning. Weight should be determined with the subject dressed in light indoor clothing and the shoes off.

Older children and adolescents may want to know how tall they will be when fully grown; this is especially true of undergrown boys and tall girls. There are two common techniques for making such estimates. The simplest is to average the parents' heights, and then add 6.5 cm for boys and subtract 6.5 cm for girls. Another method is to obtain a radiograph of the wrist and enter bone age and present stature into the prediction tables provided by Bayley and Pinneau.[16]

CHANGES IN BODY COMPOSITION DURING GROWTH

A number of organ systems comprise body weight. Modern technology has made it possible to estimate several components of the body in a relatively noninvasive manner. The growth of these components during adolescence differs somewhat from the growth of the body as a whole.

METHODS FOR ESTIMATING BODY COMPOSITION

The weight of body fluids (plasma volume, total red cell mass, extracellular fluid volume, total body water) is estimated by the principle of isotopic dilution.

Lean body mass (LBM) or, as some prefer, fat-free mass, can be estimated in several ways, based on the fact that neither electrolytes nor water is bound by neutral fat, and by the fact that LBM has a different density than fat. A measurement of total body water or total body potassium can thus yield an estimate of LBM; body fat is the difference between weight and LBM. Measurement of body density yields an estimate of the percentages of body fat and LBM. Urine creatinine excretion is used as an index of muscle mass.

Estimates of skeletal mass are made from the size and density of various bones, using the degree of attenuation of monoenergetic gamma rays; this process is referred to as *single-* or *dual-photon absorptiometry*. The cross-sectional area of the second metacarpal cortex, as read from a plain radiograph, has also been used for this purpose. Computed tomography (CT) and magnetic resonance imaging (MRI) can define the size and shape of various organs and determine muscle mass and body fat.

A new technique is bioelectrical impedance. A weak alternating current is passed between the hand and the foot or between the feet. The measured resistance is said to be a function of lean weight. This technique has the advantage of being quick and easy to use. A problem is the lack of a theoretical basis for it.

Although it is not very precise, anthropometry is an inexpensive and easily used technique for estimating body fat. The two most commonly used techniques are the measurement of skinfold (actually fatfold) thickness, and various body circumferences.

Because human skin is only 0.5 to 2 mm thick, the subcutaneous fat layer accounts for the bulk of the skinfold thickness. The measurement is made by grasping the skin plus subcutaneous tissue between the thumb and forefinger, shaking it gently to exclude underlying muscle, and stretching it just far enough to permit the jaws of a spring-activated caliper to pinch the tissue. Because the jaws of the caliper compress the

---

°Tanner and Davies[15] have devised some charts that portray growth velocity as a function of age for average adolescents, and for early and late maturers. These charts are available from Serono Laboratories, Inc., 280 Pond St., Randolph, MA 02368.

†Holtain Ltd., Crosswell, Crymmych, Pembrokeshire, U.K.

tissue, the caliper reading diminishes for a few seconds; then, the dial is read.

The most frequent site for measurement is over the triceps muscle at a point halfway between shoulder and elbow; other sites are over the biceps, at the inferior tip of the scapula, and at the iliac crest. Individuals with moderately firm subcutaneous tissue and those with very firm tissue that is not easily deformable present something of a problem. In persons who have recently lost weight, the subcutaneous tissue is often flabby; in very obese subjects, the tissue thickness may exceed the maximum jaw width (40 mm) of the caliper.

The ratio of abdomen circumference to hip circumference can be used as an index of body fat distribution. There is some evidence to suggest that adults with high ratios have large accumulations of intraabdominal fat and are somewhat more prone to cardiovascular disease and stroke. Forbes[17] described the changes in this ratio during the adolescent and adult years in normal individuals. It is noteworthy that sex differences first appear during adolescence, girls having a lower ratio than boys.

The cross-sectional area of arm muscle and bone, and that of fat can be calculated from measurements of arm circumference and skinfold thickness* (many authors use the term *arm muscle area*, which is incorrect). Although this technique yields reliable results in thin subjects, it may overestimate arm muscle and bone area and thus underestimate arm fat area in obese ones.

Finally, it should not be forgotten that the use of relative weight—either percentage weight for height or BMI—while far from perfect, can be useful in evaluating large numbers of individuals. Those with high values almost always have increased body fat, especially girls and women. A nomogram for determining BMI from weight and height is shown in Figure 9–6. This index is age dependent, as shown in Figure 9–3, which depicts the 50th percentile for white children and adolescents who participated in the 1971–1974 National Health and Nutrition Survey.[6] Values for adolescent black females tend to be a little higher (by 1% to 4%) than those for whites. Values for Dutch children and for French children are comparable to those shown in the figure.

Table 9–1 lists the various percentile values

---

*Arm muscle + bone area is $(C - \pi SF)^2/4$, and arm fat area is $\frac{SF}{4}(2C - \pi SF)$, where C is arm circumference and SF is skinfold thickness.

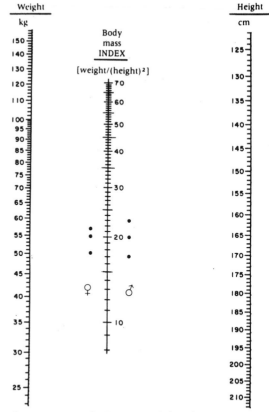

Figure 9–6. By laying a straightedge connecting weight and height, the BMI can be read. The three dots on the left side of the BMI line represent 50th percentile values for females aged 20 *(top)*, 15 *(middle)*, and 10 years *(bottom)*; those on the right side are for males of similar age.

for BMI in girls, compiled by Cronk and Roche.[18] It is evident that the distributions at all ages shown are strongly skewed toward higher values. In evaluating data on BMI, it should be kept in mind that body weight is the sum of lean and fat; thus, individuals with a large body frame may have a generous BMI without having excess body fat.

SUBCUTANEOUS FAT

The region over the triceps muscle is most commonly used for measuring the thickness of skin plus subcutaneous tissue. Measurements at other sites usually yield different values, indicating that the subcutaneous fat mantle does not have a uniform thickness. Indeed, CT and MRI show that a large fraction of total subcutaneous fat in women is located in the hips and thighs. However, the triceps site is easily accessible, and

Table 9–1. Body Mass Index (kg/m²) for Girls

Age (yr)	Percentile						
	5th	*10th*	*25th*	*50th*	*75th*	*90th*	*95th*
6	12.8	13.5	14.0	15.0	16.0	16.9	17.3
7	13.1	13.8	14.5	15.6	16.8	18.4	19.2
8	13.5	14.2	15.1	16.2	17.7	19.9	21.1
9	13.9	14.6	15.6	16.9	18.7	21.3	23.0
10	14.4	15.1	16.2	17.5	19.6	22.7	24.8
11	14.9	15.5	16.7	18.2	20.4	23.8	26.3
12	15.3	16.0	17.3	18.8	21.2	24.8	27.7
13	15.8	16.4	17.8	19.3	21.9	25.6	28.8
14	16.2	16.8	18.2	19.9	22.5	26.1	29.6
15	16.6	17.2	18.6	20.3	23.0	26.5	30.2
16	16.9	17.5	18.9	20.7	23.5	26.7	30.6
17	17.1	17.8	19.2	21.0	23.8	26.9	30.9
18–20	17.6	18.4	19.7	21.6	24.3	27.2	31.2
21–23	17.7	18.5	19.8	21.8	24.4	27.7	31.5

the triceps skinfold thickness does bear a relationship to total body fat content.

Figure 9–7 shows the changes in triceps skinfold thickness during adolescence in white girls who participated in the 1971–1974 National Health and Nutrition Survey. It is apparent that the frequency distributions are strongly skewed toward higher values.

Menarche is an event of considerable physiologic and hormonal significance. It has been known for many years that the peak of the height velocity curve occurs just before menarche and that there is a temporal association with changes in basal oxygen consumption, pulse rate, and blood pressure. In addition, data show that the perimenarchal years are accompanied by an array of changes in body composition, skeletal size, distribution of body fat, muscle strength, and urinary hydroxyproline excretion. Indeed, the increase in LBM at this time of life is as great as the increase in body fat.[19]

LEAN BODY MASS AND BODY FAT

Figure 9–8 shows the time course for body weight, LBM, and body fat (average values) for boys and girls. The developing sex difference in LBM during adolescence is clearly evident. By the end of the second decade of life, the male LBM is roughly equal to female body weight; the male-female ratio for LBM is about 1.44:1,

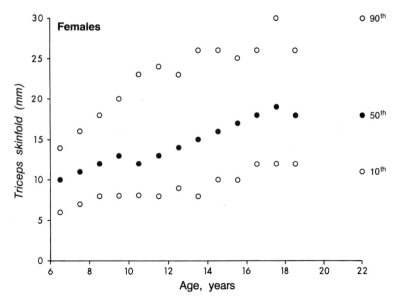

Figure 9–7. Triceps skinfold thickness for females—90th, 50th, and 10th percentiles. (Data from Cronk CE, Roche AF: Race- and sex-specific reference data for triceps and subscapular skinfolds and weight/stature². Am J Clin Nutr 1982; 35:351.)

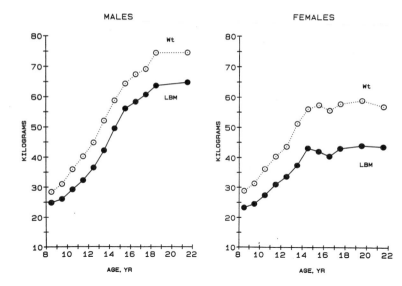

Figure 9–8. Growth of weight and lean body mass (LBM) for girls and boys (mean values); body fat is the difference between weight and LBM. Authors' data based on potassium 40 counting in 551 white females and 559 white males. (From McAnarney ER, Kreipe RE, Orr DP, Comerci GD: Textbook of Adolescent Medicine. Philadelphia: WB Saunders, 1992.)

in contrast to 1.25:1 for body weight. This is one reason boys are stronger than girls and require more energy.

LBM has physiologic and nutritional importance. It constitutes the active metabolic mass of the body, as body fat is relatively inert. There is little or no sex difference in basal metabolic rate when LBM is used as a reference point; total energy expenditure, blood volume, and maximum oxygen consumption are all functions of LBM. Accretion rates of various body constituents are more closely related to LBM than to weight (with its variable fat component).

LBM is a function of height at all ages, and the same is true for total body calcium in adults; thus, tall children should have an athletic advantage over those who are shorter. The variability in LBM for subjects of a given age and sex is less than that for weight, and, thus, body fat variability accounts for a large proportion of the variation in body weight.

Table 9–2 lists average values for a number of body measurements and body constituents for 10-year-olds and 20-year-olds, together with estimates of daily accretion rates for nitrogen, calcium, and iron over the entire decade. At the

Table 9–2. Body Measurements and Constituents at Selected Ages

	Age 10 (M/F)	Age 20 (M/F)	Daily Accretion av Entire Decade (M/F)
Body weight (kg)°	33/34	71/57	
Lean body mass (kg)°	27/26	62/43	
Total body nitrogen (gm)†	840/780	1980/1290	0.31/0.14
Total body calcium (gm)‡	330/290	1100/710§	0.21/0.12
Total body iron (mg)‖	1480/1430	3560/2270	0.57/0.23
Blood volume (ml)‖	2450/2400	5350/3950	
Arm muscle + bone area (cm²)¶	24.4/22.6	59.0/34.0	
Urine creatinine (mg/24 hr)	730/700	1990/1300	
Metacarpal cortex (cm²)#	0.27/0.26	0.56/0.42	

°Authors' data (Fig. 9–8).

†To convert to grams of protein, multiply by 6.25.

‡Data from Christian et al. (1975), extrapolated from photon density measurements of forearm bones; referenced in Forbes GB: Human Body Composition: Growth, Aging, Nutrition, and Activity. New York: Springer-Verlag, 1987.

§Values obtained by neutron activation (S. Cohn et al., 1971, 1980) are 1100 gm for males and 830 gm for females; referenced in Forbes GB: Human Body Composition: Growth, Aging, Nutrition, and Activity. New York: Springer-Verlag, 1987.

‖Data compiled by Hawkins (1964); referenced in Forbes GB: Human Body Composition: Growth, Aging, Nutrition, and Activity. New York: Springer-Verlag, 1987.

¶Midarm cross-sectional area, calculated from skinfold thickness and arm circumference. Data compiled by Frisancho (1981); referenced in Forbes GB: Human Body Composition: Growth, Aging, Nutrition, and Activity. New York: Springer-Verlag, 1987.

#Midshaft cross-sectional area, second metacarpal. Data from Garn et al. (1976); referenced in Forbes GB: Human Body Composition: Growth, Aging, Nutrition, and Activity. New York: Springer-Verlag, 1987.

peak of the adolescent growth spurt, these accretion values will be two to three times greater. At the beginning of the decade there is little, if any, sex difference in any of these values, but it can be seen that the accretion rates (i.e., the amounts added to the body as a result of growth) are considerably greater in boys. By age 20 years, the male-female ratios for the various measurements are in the range of 1.3:1 to 1.7:1, in contrast to a weight ratio of only 1.25:1 and a height ratio of 1.08:1. On average, boys acquire about twice as much nitrogen, calcium, and iron and much more muscle mass, as reflected by arm muscle plus bone cross-sectional area and the daily excretion of creatinine. It should be remembered that these are accretion rates, not dietary requirements, which must take into consideration gastrointestinal absorption and urinary, fecal, and cutaneous losses.

COMPOSITION OF WEIGHT GAIN AND WEIGHT LOSS

Generally speaking, a significant loss of weight, which is the result of nutritional deficit, involves losing both LBM and fat. The relative contributions of these two body components to the total weight loss depend on the initial body fat content and on the magnitude of the energy deficit. Thin persons tend to lose relatively more lean tissue, and obese people lose relatively more fat.[20] Very low energy diets result in considerable erosion of the LBM, despite adequate protein intake, whereas diets providing more than 1000 kcal/day are less hazardous in this respect. Exercise tends to mitigate the effect of low energy intake, but only to a degree; weight loss of more than a few kilograms will still be accompanied by some loss of LBM. Careful studies have shown that an energy deficit, the result of exercise, produces about the same degree of weight loss and negative nitrogen balance as a comparable deficit produced by eating less food. Athletes should be told to eat properly, and girls who aspire to a very thin figure run the risk of subnormal lean weight and thinner bones.

Weight gain, the result of nutritional surfeit, also involves both LBM and fat. The fact that obese persons usually have a somewhat larger LBM than thin individuals favors the hypothesis that obesity is indeed a nutritional disease, the result of a positive energy balance. There is even some evidence for increased skeletal size and slightly higher blood hemoglobin levels. Indeed, obese persons need to eat more than thin ones to stay in energy balance: data on free-living adults and adolescents engaged in light physical activity show that an extra 16 to 20 kcal/day is needed to sustain each additional kilogram of body weight.[2, 21] Data from dietary histories that purport to show otherwise must be regarded with great skepticism.

There are two exceptions to the general rule that LBM and fat increase and decrease together. The first relates to the effect of anabolic agents: androgenic anabolic steroids given in significant amounts and for long enough cause an increase in LBM (including muscle) and a decrease in body fat; the same is true of human growth hormone. This is the reason athletes take steroids and risk undesirable side effects in an effort to enhance athletic performance. The second exception is Prader-Willi syndrome, in which LBM is decreased in the presence of an excess of body fat.[22] Body composition changes in these patients mimic those seen in animals with experimental hypothalamic obesity.

EXERCISE

A regular program of exercise over a period of several weeks can produce a modest increase (1 to 3 kg) in LBM and a decrease in body fat; however, weight loss of more than a few kilograms usually causes some loss of LBM, even with adequate exercise.[23] Excessive exercise can lead to fatigue and even some loss of appetite; the latter, of course, will lead to weight loss.

The fact that the dominant arm of professional tennis players has larger muscle and bone mass testifies to the phenomenon of local muscle hypertrophy in response to vigorous use over prolonged periods. The large muscle bulk of some body builders is sometimes hailed as a result of exercise and muscle training, but without special tests to measure serum testosterone and gonadotropins, it is difficult to rule out the effects of unreported use of androgenic anabolic steroids. Certainly, the generous deltoid muscles of some runners may provide circumstantial evidence of steroid use.

Many athletes, boys and girls alike, have a larger LBM and less body fat than nonathletes. It is not known whether this is the result of training or is principally hereditary. Eating a great deal can augment the LBM, but body fat increases at the same time.

Successful athletes constitute a special group. A study of female participants in the 1972 and 1976 Olympic Games showed that almost all of the finalists in the various events were taller than average for American women aged 18 to 24 years (exceptions were gymnasts, coxswains, and participants in equestrian jumping); the mean difference was 7 cm. With the exception of discus throwers and shot putters, however, average BMI values were close to the 50th percentiles shown in Table 9–1 and Figure 9–3.[24] This must mean that the smaller body fat burden of the female athlete is counterbalanced by a somewhat larger LBM.

SPECIAL SITUATIONS

Nutrition is a most important determinant of growth.[25] Suboptimal nutrition slows the rate of growth and sexual maturation, and excess calories speed up both processes. It has been established that significant changes in body weight incident to nutritional factors involve both the lean and the fat components of the body: both components decrease with undernutrition and increase with overnutrition.[25]

Adolescents vary considerably in body size. All other things being equal, larger teenagers need more to eat than those who are small. Basal metabolic rate is known to be a function of body size when expressed in absolute terms (i.e., kilocalories per unit time). Studies of adolescent girls using advanced techniques have shown that total energy expenditure is related to body size; the slope of the regression line for adolescent girls is 20 kcal/day per kilogram body weight.[21] Obviously, obese girls must eat more than their thin peers to maintain their greater body weight. There are three situations in adolescence for which nutritional surveillance and advice are particularly important.

The first is pregnancy, which involves rapid weight gain, almost all of it in the second and third trimesters. The average gain is 75 gm/day. Assuming an energy expenditure of 8 kcal/gm gain, the extra energy need is about 600 kcal daily, or about 25% of the average nonpregnant female intake. Extra iron and calcium are needed to support the increased maternal blood volume and the demands of the fetal skeleton. Underweight and poorly nourished girls deserve special consideration.

Second, athletes have a higher energy expenditure than the average adolescent and therefore need more food if they are not to lose weight. With the possible exception of iron, there is no need for extra nutrients other than calories. Hot weather increases the need for water and, when sweating is profuse and prolonged, for salt.

The third group are those who follow fad diets, which may be deficient in one or more essential nutrients. Growth faltering can occur with diets low in cholesterol and saturated fat if attention is not given to energy intake.

A word should be said about the nutritional benefits of exercise. Exercise demands more food but not necessarily more essential nutrients. Assuming a well-balanced diet, the result will be a greater intake of such nutrients and thus less likelihood of a specific deficiency. Support for the long-term benefits comes from a study showing that even modest exercise programs can reduce the risk of non–insulin-dependent diabetes mellitus.[26]

REFERENCES

1. Bessey OA: Evaluation of nutritive status by chemical and other methods. *In* Scheinberg IH (ed): Infant Metabolism. New York: Macmillan, 1956, p 284.
2. Forbes GB: Human Body Composition: Growth, Aging, Nutrition, and Activity. New York: Springer-Verlag, 1987.
3. Forbes GB: Nutrition and growth. J Pediatr 1977; 91:40.
4. Buckler JMH: A Longitudinal Study of Adolescent Growth. London: Springer-Verlag, 1990.
5. Zacharias L, Rand WM, Wurtman RJ: A prospective study of sexual development and growth in American girls: The statistics of menarche. Obstet Gynecol Surv 1976; 31:325.
6. Garn SM, La Velle M: Reproductive histories of low-weight girls and women. Am J Clin Nutr 1983; 37:862.
7. Stark O, Peckham CS, Moynihan C: Weight and age at menarche. Arch Dis Child 1989; 64:383.
8. Lager C, Ellison PT: Effect of moderate weight loss on ovarian function assessed by salivary progesterone measurements. Am J Hum Biol 1990; 2:303.
9. Delemarre-van de Waal HA, Plant TM, van Rees GB, et al (eds): Control of the Onset of Puberty. III. New York: Excerpta Medica, 1989.
10. Clemmons DR, Klibanski A, Underwood LE, et al: Reduction of plasma immunoactive somatomedin-C during fasting in humans. J Clin Endocrinol Metab 1981; 53:1247.
11. Forbes GB, Brown MR, Welle SL, Underwood LE: Hormonal response to overfeeding. Am J Clin Nutr 1989; 49:608.
12. Bouchard C, Savard R, Despres J-P, et al: Body composition in adopted and biological siblings. Hum Biol 1985; 57:61.
13. Stunkard AJ, Sorensen TIA, Hanis C, et al: An adoption study of human obesity. N Engl J Med 1986; 314:193.
14. Forbes GB, Sauer EP, Weitkamp LR: Lean body mass in twins. Metabolism 1995; 44:1442.
15. Tanner JM, Davies PSW: Clinical longitudinal standards for height and height velocity for North American children. J Pediatr 1985; 107:317.
16. Bayley N, Pinneau SR: Tables for predicting adult height from skeletal age: Revised for use with the Greulich-Pyle hand standards. J Pediatr 1952; 40:432.
17. Forbes GB: The abdomen:hip ratio. Normative data and observations on selected patients. Int J Obesity 1990; 14:149.
18. Cronk CE, Roche AF: Race- and sex-specific reference data for triceps and subscapular skinfolds and weight/stature². Am J Clin Nutr 1982; 35:351.

19. Forbes GB: Body size and composition of perimenarchal girls. Am J Dis Child 1992; 146:63.
20. Forbes GB: Lean body mass-body fat interrelationships in humans. Nutr Rev 1987; 45:225.
21. Bandini LG, Schoeller DA, Dietz WH: Energy expenditure in obese and nonobese adolescents. Pediatr Res 1990; 27:198.
22. Schoeller DA, Levitsky LL, Bandini LG, et al: Energy expenditure and body composition in Prader-Willi syndrome. Metabolism 1988; 37:115.
23. Forbes GB: Exercise and body composition. J Appl Physiol 1991; 70(3):994.
24. Khosla T: Sport for tall. Br Med J 1983; 287:736.
25. Phillips LS: Nutrition, metabolism, and growth. In: Daughaday WH (ed): Endocrine Control of Growth. New York: Elsevier, 1981.
26. Helmsick SP, Ragland DR, Leung RW, Paffenbarger RS: Physical activity and reduced occurrence of noninsulin-dependent diabetes mellitus. N Engl J Med 1991; 325:147.

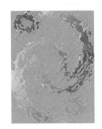

Chapter 10

Effects of the Thyroid on Gonadal and Reproductive Function During Childhood and Adolescence

Thomas P. Foley, Jr.

The interrelationships between hypothalamic-pituitary-gonadal (HPG) axis and thyroid function have been known for nearly two centuries. The alterations in thyroid function tests in pregnant women and those who take oral contraceptives are familiar to physicians, even though errors in interpretation are not infrequent. Specific thyroid diseases alter normal reproductive function, particularly in females, at puberty and during adult life.[1, 2] The most common causes of acquired abnormalities of thyroid function in areas of the world where dietary iodine intake is sufficient are autoimmune thyroid diseases (ATDs), Graves disease and autoimmune (Hashimoto) thyroiditis. Autoimmune diseases, including ATDs, are much more common in adolescent and adult women than in men.[3]

HYPOTHALAMIC-PITUITARY-THYROID REGULATION: THYROID HORMONE

The regulation of thyroid hormone secretion and action is less complex than that of the HPG system, particularly in females (Fig. 10–1). There are two sources for the iodothyronines in serum: (1) Thyroxine (T_4) and, in much smaller amounts, the triiodothyronines (T_3 and reverse T_3) are synthesized and secreted directly by the thyroid gland. (2) The monodeiodination of T_4 generates the most potent iodothyronines, 3,3',5-L-triiodothyronine (T_3) and the biologically inactive stereoisomer reverse rT_3 (rT_3, known chemically as 3,3', 5'-L-triiodothyronine).[4] These hormones circulate bound to three distinct proteins: thyroxine-binding globulin (TBG), transthyretin (TTR), and albumin. TBG has the greatest binding affinity for the iodothyronines, and albumin has the greatest binding capacity; however, the biologically active hormones that mediate the action of thyroid hormones at the cellular level exist in the unbound, or free, form. The concentrations of free T_4 and free T_3 directly correlate with the biologic status of thyroid hormone function and can be directly measured using methods that are generally available in commercial laboratories.[5]

Thyroid-stimulating hormone (TSH), a pituitary glycoprotein, regulates thyroid hormone synthesis and secretion and, in part, thyroid gland growth.[6] Thyroid growth also is controlled by local growth factors such as insulin-like growth factor 1 (IGF-1) and epidermal growth factor (EGF).[5] The synthesis and release of TSH is regulated in part by stimulation of the hypothalamic hormone, thyrotropin-releasing hormone (TRH), and in part by the pituitary intracellular concentration of T_3. The latter is derived from circulating free T_3 concentrations and by the intrapituitary conversion of T_4 to T_3. This enzymatic reaction is very important in the regulation of TSH synthesis and release. When the availability of T_4 for conversion to T_3 is decreased in the pituitary gland, TSH synthesis and secretion increase in an effort to restore free T_4 concentrations to normal.[7] Therefore, T_4 concentrations are very important in the regulation of TSH secretion, even though their biologic potency at the cellular level is minimal as compared with that of T_3. The earliest sign of thyroid gland

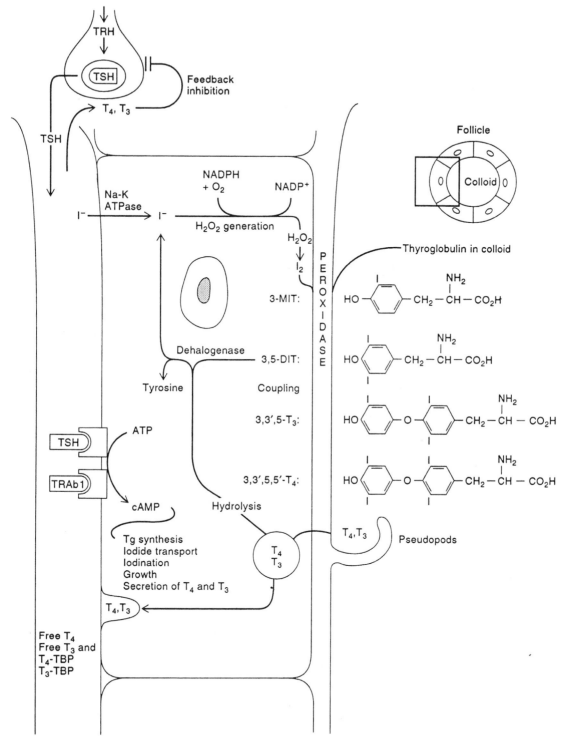

Figure 10–1. A schematic representation of the synthesis and secretion of thyroid hormones by the thyroid gland. Dietary sources of iodide are absorbed into the circulation, and, under the influence of TSH stimulation, iodide is concentrated by the thyroid, immediately oxidized to iodine, and incorporated into tyrosyl residues on thyroglobulin. Mono- and diiodotyrosyl residues are coupled to form tetraiodothyronine (T_4) or triiodothyronine (T_3). T_4 and T_3 are released by proteolysis and secreted into the circulation on stimulation by TSH.

failure is a decrease in T_4 secretion. Initially, however, the concentration of circulating free T_4 usually remains within the normal range. The decrease in the free T_4 concentration is recognized by the pituitary, and the first detectable abnormalities in thyroid function in response to thyroid gland failure are increases in pituitary TSH content, release of TSH into the circulation, and the concentration of TSH in serum.

The gonadotropins follicle-stimulating hormone (FSH) and luteinizing hormone (LH), TSH, and human chorionic gonadotropin (hCG) are glycoproteins that share identical alpha subunits within a species.[6] The beta subunits mediate the biologic response only when the alpha and beta subunits are combined to form the intact hormone and when postranslational glycosylation is completed. There are sequence homologies between the beta subunits of TSH, LH, and hCG and the peripheral receptors such that in high concentrations these hormones may display biologic properties of their related glycoproteins. These activities contribute in part to the increased thyroid gland function in the presence of increased concentrations of hCG and the precocious onset of puberty that is observed in children with severe primary hypothyroidism, or myxedema.

The deiodination of T_4 to T_3 and rT_3 in peripheral tissues is regulated by the nutritional and metabolic needs of the organism and may be altered in certain pathophysiologic conditions.[4] During nutritional deprivation, particularly when carbohydrate intake is reduced, there is preferential deiodination of T_4 to rT_3. Similarly, during acute, serious illnesses, there is preferential deiodination of T_4 to rT_3; this is known as the *nonthyroidal illness (NTI) syndrome*, or the *euthyroid sick syndrome*. In addition, total T_4 may be decreased, but free T_4 levels remain normal to high normal when measured by definitive methods such as equilibrium or direct dialysis. Maintenance of high normal free T_4 concentrations in the NTI syndrome is the likely mechanism whereby TSH secretion remains in the normal range even in the presence of a low T_3 concentration. These metabolic alterations are thought to be a mechanism in which the organism adapts to a decreasing need for a highly catabolic hormone, T_3, by producing the biologically inactive stereoisomer rT_3. Therefore, when a patient with the NTI syndrome is tested, the results are usually a low total T_3 value, an elevated rT_3, normal or decreased total T_4, normal or high-normal free T_4, and normal, measurable TSH. In advanced-stage NTI syndrome, free T_4 concentrations may decline even though serum TSH values remain normal or low, indicating that a state of hypothalamic hypothyroidism had developed.

The metabolic effects of thyroid hormone are mediated by T_3 at the cellular level.[8] This action is very similar to that of the steroid hormones, in that T_3 binds to a thyroid hormone response element that is bound to the DNA receptor that controls transcription and translation and thus regulates protein synthesis. There is also evidence to suggest that T_3 directly stimulates oxidative phosphorylation in the mitochondria, an action separate and distinct from its effect on protein synthesis.

There are important physiologic and pathophysiologic relationships between thyroid function and gonadal function.[1, 2] Estrogen in higher concentrations in serum during pregnancy and during oral contraceptive therapy stimulates hepatic synthesis and secretion of TBG. This effect of estrogen alters thyroid function tests but does not change the thyroid status of the patient. In the presence of an increased concentration of TBG, total T_4 increases but free T_4 and TSH remain normal. When indirect measurements of free T_4 are made using the resin uptake test with radiolabeled T_3 (RT_3U) in the presence of estrogen, the effect of increased TBG will be to increase the total T_4 and decrease the RT_3U. The estimated free T_4 (EFT) or free T_4 index (FTI) is calculated by the product of the total T_4 and RT_3U. The high T_4 and low RT_3U values will give a product that is normal, reflecting a normal free T_4 concentration in this circumstance.

When a newborn's TBG is very low or unmeasurable, the total T_4 is low but the free T_4 by direct dialysis is normal.[9] In laboratories that still perform the RT_3U, it is elevated, but the product, FTI, should be normal; however, in the absence of TBG, the FTI may be artifactually low. Since familial TBG deficiency usually is inherited as an X-linked trait, the female is the heterozygote and has a slightly decreased or moderately low level of total T_4. The free T_4 is normal.[9] When the RT_3U test is performed, the value is increased and the calculated FTI is normal. This disorder is relatively common and may lead to inappropriate treatment with T_4 when women are tested for thyroid hormone abnormalities during an infertility evaluation, except when free T_4 is measured, and it is normal.

There are other drugs that either alter the binding of thyroid hormones to thyroid hormone–binding proteins or interfere with binding (Table 10–1). Anabolic steroids and androgens decrease TBG synthesis, secretion, and serum concentrations. Certain anticonvulsant medications, particularly phenytoin (Dilantin), compete

Table 10–1. Clinical Conditions and Drugs That Interfere with Iodothyronine Binding to Thyroid-Binding Proteins

Decreased concentrations of thyroid-binding globulin

    Acromegaly, active
    Androgenic steroids
    L-asparaginase
    Familial deficiency thyroid-binding globulin
    Glucocorticoids
    Nephrotic syndrome
    Severe illness
    Thyrotoxicosis

Inhibitors of binding

    Drugs
        5-Fluorouracil
        Halofenate
        Mitotane
        Phenylbutazone
        Phenytoin
        Salicylate

Increased concentration of thyroid-binding globulin

    Acute intermittent porphyria
    Drugs
        Clofibrate
        Heroin
        Methadone
        Perphenazine
    Estrogens, endogenous and exogenous
        Contraceptives
        Neonate
        Pregnancy
    Familial excess of thyroid-binding globulin
    Hepatitis, infectious or chronic active
    Hypothyroidism

Familial abnormalities of albumin and transthyretin

Iodothyronine antibodies (anti-T_4 and anti-T_3)

with T_4 for binding to TBG. The thyroid function tests show normal TBG levels and decreased total T_4 values, and in some instances there are artifactual abnormalities in the RT_3U test. In these cases, direct measurement of free T_4 using equilibrium or direct dialysis methods may be the only reliable way to assess the free T_4 concentration and differentiate alterations in T_4 binding from hypothalamic or pituitary hypothyroidism.[9] These measurements of free T_4 are available from commercial laboratories that have expertise in endocrine testing and they are important to use when there are discrepancies in the expected results of thyroid function tests or when certain therapeutic or clinical conditions are present. Such conditions include the NTI syndrome, when alterations in thyroid function may result in an incorrect diagnosis of hypothalamic or pituitary hypo- or hyperthyroidism.

    Results of other tests of thyroid function differ between men and women and are altered during contraceptive therapy or pregnancy.[1, 2] The TSH and prolactin responses to TRH are greater in women than in men. This effect is particularly evident when estrogen concentrations in preovulatory women are greater than those of women in the luteal phase of the cycle or those of men. During pregnancy, associated changes in thyroid function include increases in thyroid size, in total production of thyroid hormone, in secretory activity of the thyroid by histologic evaluation, and in the uptake of radioactive iodine.

THYROTOXICOSIS AND THE REPRODUCTIVE SYSTEM

    There is a long history of the association of thyrotoxicosis and abnormalities in HPG regulation. The first report of thyrotoxicosis, by Parry in 1825, described menstrual abnormalities in two women as follows:

She nursed for a year the child of her first lying-in, during which time she did not menstruate. Subsequently to that period she had five times miscarried; and for the last four months her menses had been irregular as to intervals, and defective in quantity and colour.[10]

    This woman had been seen in 1786 with tachycardia, exophthalmos, and goiter. In another case the description read "menses, since the commencement of the malady, defective." In 1940, von Basedow reported the occurrence of amenorrhea as a common symptom in postmenarchal women.[11]

    Menarche may occur at an earlier than normal age if hyperthyroidism develops in a prepubertal girl, presumably as a result of the effects of excessive thyroid hormones on mild advancement of skeletal maturation, which is an indication of an advance in biologic maturation.[1] Onset of menses may be delayed in prepubertal thyrotoxic girls, however, an effect that is analogous to amenorrhea in adult women. Oligomenorrhea, anovulation, and menometrorrhagia also have been reported, although the last condition is more often associated with hypothyroidism. These changes would be expected to return to normal when a euthyroid state is achieved during therapy.[1]

PATHOGENESIS

    Autoimmune thyrotoxicosis (Graves disease or Parry disease) is the most common cause of thyrotoxicosis (Table 10–2). The disease is caused

Table 10–2. Causes of Thyrotoxicosis Pathogenesis

Juvenile Hyperthyroidism	Juvenile Hypothyroidism
Autoimmune (Graves disease)	Chronic autoimmune thyroiditis
Autonomous hyperfunctioning nodular disease	Lymphocytic thyroiditis with thyromegaly
Toxic adenoma	Hashimoto thyroiditis (struma lymphomatosis) with
McCune-Albright syndrome	thyromegaly
Hyperfunctioning thyroid carcinoma (rare)	Fibrous variant with atrophy
Thyroid-stimulating hormone–mediated hyperthyroidism	Congenital hypothyroidism, late-onset, mild disease
Thyroid-stimulating hormone–secreting pituitary adenoma	Ectopic thyroid dysgenesis
Pituitary resistance to thyroid hormone	Dyshormonogenesis
Toxic thyroiditis	Peripheral resistance to thyroid hormone
Thyrotoxic phase of subacute thyroiditis	Endemic goiter
Thyrotoxic presentation of autoimmune thyroiditis	Iodine deficiency
Ingestion of thyroid hormone	Environmental goitrogen
Iodide-induced hyperthyroidism (Jodbasedow)	Drugs
Tumor-secreting thyroid stimulators (rare)	Lithium
Hydatidiform mole	Antithyroid drugs
Choriocarcinoma	Iodide excess in association with other thyroid disease
	Thyroid irradiation
	Thyroidectomy

by an abnormality in the immune system that results in the production of immunoglobulin G (IgG), usually subclass 1, that stimulates the TSH receptor.[12] Thyroid hormones do not modulate the stimulatory response of the thyroid to these antibodies, known as *TSH receptor antibodies* (TRAb), and unregulated oversecretion of T_4 and T_3 causes most of the clinical symptoms of the disease. These symptoms are found in any disease associated with thyrotoxicosis and are not specific for Graves disease. Specific antibodies, either the same antibody clone or an antibody distinct from the thyroid-stimulating antibody, are reported to cause the exophthalmos and other ocular signs in of autoimmune thyrotoxicosis.[13] Exophthalmos is a clinical sign specifically associated with Graves disease, and its presence is diagnostic.

Thyrotoxicosis of other causes is very uncommon or rare during adolescence—TSH-mediated hyperthyroidism from either pituitary TSH-secreting adenomas or the syndrome of resistance

to thyroid hormone with thyrotoxicosis; overdosing with exogenous thyroid hormones; toxic thyroiditis from the release of preformed thyroid hormones after a viral (subacute thyroiditis) or autoimmune (Hashimoto disease) insult to the thyroid; autonomous hyperfunction of the thyroid, from a thyroid adenoma, the McCune-Albright syndrome, or, very rarely, thyroid carcinoma; iodide-induced hyperthyroidism (jodbasedow disease); and tumor-secreting thyroid stimulators that are rarely seen in women with hydatidiform mole or choriocarcinoma.[14] In these latter diseases, high levels of hCG stimulate the thyroid to increase secretion of thyroid hormones and cause hyperthyroidism.

CLINICAL SYMPTOMS AND SIGNS

During childhood and adolescence, the symptoms and signs of thyrotoxicosis are similar to those in adults (Table 10–3). Children and ado-

Table 10–3. Thyrotoxicosis

Clinical Symptoms and Signs	Initial Clinical Evaluation
Thyromegaly	T_3, T_4, free T_4, thyroid-stimulating hormone
Tachycardia	Complete blood and differential counts
Nervousness and insomnia	Thyroid-stimulating hormone–receptor antibody
Increased pulse pressure and palpitations	Radionuclide image (*only* in presence of nodule[s])
Proptosis	Radioiodide uptake (*only* when the diagnosis and cause are
Increased appetite, often with weight loss	not known conclusively)
Tremor, restlessness	
Heat intolerance	
Deteriorating school performance	
Enuresis	

lescents often exhibit deteriorating academic performance; abnormal sleeping habits (enuresis, difficulty falling asleep, and restless sleep); and the expected symptoms of muscle weakness, fatigue, heat intolerance, excessive perspiration, increased appetite with loss in weight or stable weight, nervousness, irritability, and emotional lability. Thyromegaly is almost always present in a child or young adult when hyperthyroidism (excess thyroid hormone secretion from the thyroid gland) is the cause of thyrotoxicosis. Except when a thyroid nodule secretes thyroid hormone, the gland is diffusely enlarged, soft to firm, nontender, smooth, and usually symmetrically enlarged (Fig. 10–2).[14] Tachycardia with increased pulse pressure is expected; proptosis from exophthalmos usually is mild to moderate in severity during childhood and adolescence and occurs

less often and is less severe than in adults (see Fig. 10–2). Other eye signs seen in children and adolescents are generally limited to stare, eyelid lag, and retraction, although periorbital edema and conjunctival injection and edema are occasionally observed.

DIAGNOSTIC EVALUATION

A patient who presents with the classic symptoms and signs of Graves disease—diffuse thyromegaly, exophthalmos, and tachycardia—requires minimal diagnostic procedures before therapy.[14] Thyroid function tests should include measurement of serum free T_4 and TSH using a sensitive assay that discriminates normal from low values, a complete blood count with differen-

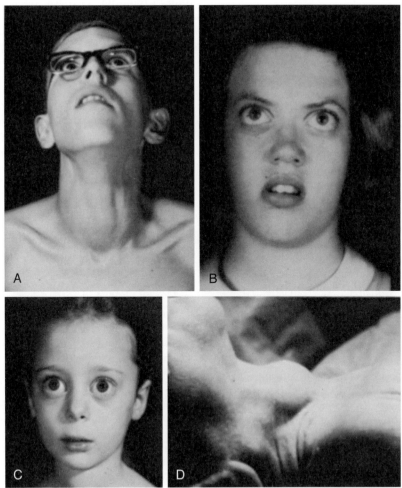

Figure 10–2. Manifestations of autoimmune thyrotoxicosis (Graves disease). *A*, Diffuse thyromegaly, in an adolescent. *B*, Diffuse thyromegaly in an adolescent with exophthalmos. *C*, Exophthalmos and diffuse thyromegaly in a young girl. *D*, Diffuse thyromegaly secondary to congenital transient Graves disease in a neonate.

tial, and preferably (although not necessarily) measurement of TRAb by a TSH receptor–binding inhibitory immunoglobulin (TBII) method to document an autoimmune origin (Table 10–3).

When the origin of thyrotoxicosis is less obvious, other diagnostic tests may be necessary to exclude other causes.[15] Such tests include measurement of serum T_3 whenever a thyroid nodule is present or the free T_4 is normal or only slightly elevated; measurement of radioiodide uptake at 4 to 6 hours and 24 hours after the tracer dose to differentiate hyperthyroid causes of thyrotoxicosis from other causes; a radioiodine scan and/or ultrasonography of the thyroid if nodular thyroid disease is present; and pituitary magnetic resonance imaging (MRI) and determination of the serum alpha subunit if serum TSH is inappropriately normal or elevated in the presence of elevated concentrations of free T_4 and T_3.[16]

Thyroglobulin and thyroid peroxidase antibody titers in serum may be useful to detect autoimmune thyroiditis (Hashimoto disease); either as a cause of transient, toxic thyroiditis with thyrotoxicosis or as a disease intercurrent with autoimmune thyrotoxicosis (Graves disease).

MANAGEMENT

The initial therapy for thyrotoxicosis is directed toward control of the exaggerated adrenergic responsiveness of moderate or severe thyrotoxicosis and the excessive thyroid hormone synthesis and secretion.[15, 17] Usually, symptoms can be controlled by beta-adrenergic blocking agents such as propranolol in doses for adolescents as low as 10 to 20 mg every 6 to 8 hours, assuming no contraindications to their use (e.g., asthma, congestive heart failure). After 2 to 3 weeks, as euthyroidism develops in response to antithyroid therapy the dose of propranolol can be tapered and discontinued over 1 or 2 weeks.[18]

Antithyroid medications—methimazole (MTZ) and propylthiouracil (PTU)—are prescribed in three divided doses totaling 0.5 to 1.0 mg/kg per day for MTZ or 5 to 10 mg/kg per day for PTU.[15, 19] Once euthyroidism is achieved, the maintenance dose of MTZ and possibly of PTU can be prescribed once daily[20, 21]; PTU therapy may need to continue in either two or three divided doses. When the thyroid is blocked and the total and free T_4 and T_3 values decrease into the hypothyroid range, the serum TSH may remain suppressed below normal for several weeks as a result of the effect of prolonged hypothalamic-pituitary suppression from chroni-

cally elevated T_4 and T_3 concentrations. Once serum TSH values become elevated, there are two options for maintenance therapy: (1) the addition of T_4 therapy in a once daily dose of 1 μg/kg while maintaining the blocking doses of the antithyroid drug (known as *combined therapy*); or (2) a decremental "tapering" of the antithyroid dose.[15] The advantage of combined therapy is less frequent patient monitoring to ensure the optimal dose for the antithyroid medication and the ability to suppress thyroid gland function and expression of the antigen, the TSH receptor. Continuation of T_4 therapy after remission and discontinuation of antithyroid therapy may, but likely does not, reduce the risk of subsequent recurrence of thyrotoxicosis.[22]

The most effective and safest mode of definitive therapy for autoimmune thyrotoxicosis is radioiodide ablation.[15, 23, 24] Permanent hypothyroidism requiring T_4 replacement therapy is the goal of radioiodide therapy and often is the preferred initial treatment for adults, particularly in North America. The risk for subsequent development of benign or malignant tumors of the thyroid after radioiodine ablative therapy does not differ from the risk reported in the general population, possibly because thyroid tissue is destroyed rather than partially damaged. This therapy is acceptable for adolescents and adults.[24] There is very limited experience with radioiodide ablative therapy in young children, even though theoretically the risk for thyroid tumors would be low if the gland were completely destroyed. The risk for thyroid carcinoma after exposure to radioactive iodine from the Chernobyl accident was greatest in the youngest children, especially those exposed in utero.[23] Because radioiodine readily crosses the placenta and ablates the fetal thyroid after 11 to 12 weeks of gestation, it is contraindicated during pregnancy. A screening test for pregnancy is mandatory before radioiodine therapy is initiated in female patients between the time of menarche and menopause.[25]

The current indications for surgical therapy for thyrotoxicosis are limited.[17] The presence of a toxic thyroid nodule and a nodule within the thyroid gland of patients with Graves disease, which may be indicative of thyroid carcinoma, is an indication for definitive surgical therapy. Subtotal thyroidectomy may be indicated for treatment of Graves disease during pregnancy when antithyroid drugs, given in lower doses to reduce the risk of hypothyroidism to the fetus, are not successful in maintaining a mild hyperthyroid or euthyroid state. Definitive surgical therapy is also indicated when one or two courses of radioiodide therapy have failed or there are other contraindications to radioiodide exposure.

HYPOTHYROIDISM AND THE REPRODUCTIVE SYSTEM

Hypothyroidism may have a profound effect on growth and sexual maturation of children and adolescents.[26] With severe primary hypothyroidism, there may be complete cessation of growth and a long delay in skeletal maturation. In most cases, pituitary or hypothalamic hypothyroidism is associated with other pituitary hormone deficiencies and causes growth retardation, particularly when associated with growth hormone deficiency.[27] Even with panhypopituitarism, however, some growth is observed. Congenital hypothyroidism does not cause abnormalities of the reproductive system unless compliance with therapy is poor.

Hypothyroidism during the prepubertal years usually delays the onset of puberty; when it develops during puberty, it halts sexual maturation.[26, 27] Hypothyroidism—primary, secondary (pituitary), or tertiary (hypothalamic)—is an important cause of delayed puberty, is associated with slowing of growth, and is reversed by T_4 therapy. Patients with primary hypothyroidism may have an enlarged sella turcica as a result of the hyperplasia of thyrotrophs (TSH-secreting cells in the pituitary) in response to the marked increase in TSH secretion. This abnormality usually is differentiated by MRI from hypothalamic and pituitary tumors, which cause deficiencies in the secretion of TRH and/or TSH.

Infrequently, hypothyroidism that develops during childhood is associated with isosexual precocity and precocious menstruation in females[26, 28, 29] and with testicular enlargement in males.[30] Gonadal stimulation from pubertal levels of gonadotropins is evidenced by breast development in girls and testicular enlargement in boys; however, there is no evidence of precocious adrenarche, as pubic and axillary hair are absent. The hypothetical explanation for sexual precocity is based on the common alpha subunits; partial sequence homology of the beta subunits and weak cross-reacting bioactivity of the pituitary glycoproteins (LH, FSH, TSH hCG); and stimulation of the FSH receptor by very high levels of TSH.[30, 31]

CAUSES: PRIMARY, PITUITARY, AND HYPOTHALAMIC

The most common cause of acquired primary hypothyroidism is chronic autoimmune thyroiditis.[27] There are three common variants: lymphocytic thyroiditis of childhood and adolescence with thyromegaly, but usually not severe hypothyroidism; Hashimoto thyroiditis with thyromegaly, also known as *struma lymphomatosa*; and a chronic fibrous variant.[27, 32] These diseases present as growth deceleration and/or thyromegaly.

Other causes of primary hypothyroidism include late-onset, mild congenital hypothyroidism; sporadic thyroid dysgenesis with ectopic tissue; familial thyroid dyshormonogenesis with thyromegaly; or the very rare disease known as *peripheral resistance to thyroid hormone* (see Table 10–2).[27] Nearly all cases of congenital primary hypothyroidism are detected by newborn screening and rarely present during childhood except in areas where screening is unavailable or is inadequate or when the condition is missed by the screening program. The most common cause of primary hypothyroidism is endemic goiter and cretinism caused by iodine deficiency, or selenium deficiency, or environmental goitrogens. With the increased use of ionizing radiation to treat cervical, cranial, and thyroid tumors and Graves disease, the number of patients with radiation-induced primary hypothyroidism is increasing. During the early recovery phase of toxic thyroiditis from subacute or viral thyroiditis, primary hypothyroidism develops for several weeks, until the thyroid gland recovers. Certain medications are known to block thyroid hormone synthesis (PTU, MTZ) or thyroid hormone release (iodides, lithium) and to cause primary hypothyroidism usually with goiter.[27]

The pituitary and hypothalamic forms of hypothyroidism usually are caused by space-occupying lesions in and between the hypothalamus and pituitary or by the effects of radiation therapy for tumors in this region.[33] Isolated TRH or TSH deficiency has been reported as both a familial and a sporadic disease.[34] Other causes, usually associated with other pituitary hormone deficiencies, include congenital midline malformations of the central nervous system, trauma, infections, and inflammatory processes.

Clinical Symptoms and Signs

During childhood and adolescence, the most characteristic clinical signs of hypothyroidism are deceleration of growth, thyromegaly, and abnormal sexual development (Fig. 10–3).[26, 27] Nonspecific symptoms such as lethargy, easy fatigability, weight gain (although usually not obesity), weakness, cold intolerance, constipation, and dry skin may be present (Table 10–4). Because these

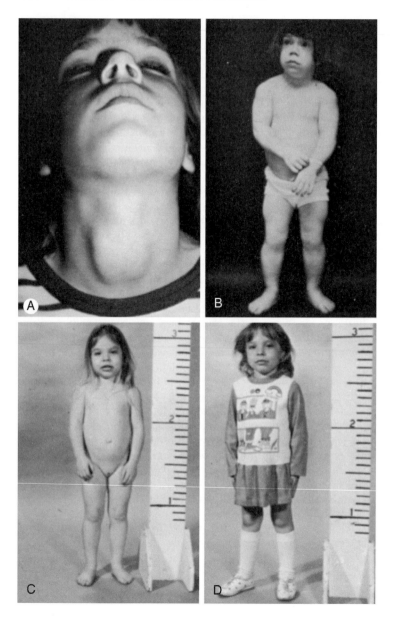

Figure 10–3. Manifestations of autoimmune (Hashimoto) thyroiditis. *A,* In a young adolescent with diffuse thyromegaly, the right lobe is larger than the left. *B,* Primary hypothyroidism and the Kocher-Debré-Sémélaigne syndrome (muscular hypertrophy in a person with chronic primary juvenile hypothyroidism) in a young boy. *C,* Advanced primary hypothyroidism, growth retardation, and myxedema secondary to the fibrous variant of autoimmune (Hashimoto) thyroiditis in a young girl; *D,* The patient after 2 months' treatment with L-thyroxine.

Table 10–4. Hypothyroidism

Clinical Symptoms and Signs	Initial Evaluation
Deceleration of linear growth	Growth curve
Delayed skeletal maturation	Thyroid-stimulating hormone
Delayed pubertal development; rarely, precocious puberty	T_4, free T_4
Delayed dental development and tooth eruption	Bone age
Myopathy, weakness, fatigue, muscular hypertrophy	Thyroid antibodies
Pale, dry, sallow skin	Thyroperoxidase (thyroid microsomal) antibody,
Galactorrhea	thyroglobulin antibody
Constipation	Thyroid-stimulating hormone
Cold intolerance	Radioiodide uptake (*only* when diagnosis and cause are
Pseutotumor cerebri	indeterminate)

symptoms develop very gradually, the child or parent often is not aware of them until T_4 therapy is initiated and symptoms subside. Other signs include delayed dental maturation and tooth eruption, coarse hair and hair loss, galactorrhea, and a sallow appearance to the skin (see Fig. 10–3). These symptoms and signs are seen infrequently in hypothalamic and pituitary hypothyroidism because of the mild degree of hypothyroidism.[33, 34]

Diagnostic Evaluation

The diagnosis of primary hypothyroidism is confirmed by the elevation of serum TSH, usually a value greater than 20 mU/L.[27] Patients with growth retardation and the symptoms and signs of hypothyroidism have very low levels of T_4 and free T_4, but serum T_3 values may remain within the normal range until the classic presentation of myxedema develops. The diagnosis of autoimmune thyroiditis can be established by detecting thyroid antibodies (thyroglobulin and thyroid peroxidase antibodies) or TSH receptor–blocking antibodies in serum (Table 10–4). Pituitary and hypothalamic hypothyroidism are confirmed by a low free T_4 value with a normal, indetectable or (on rare occasions in hypothalamic hypothyroidism) mildly elevated serum TSH value that is less than 20 mU/L.[35] The latter effect occurs because the biologic activity of TSH is impaired in hypothalamic hypothyroidism as a result of reduced or abnormal glycosylation of the molecule; TSH can be measured by immunoassays, however, because the antibodies in the assay are directed against the peptide portion of the molecule that is secreted in response to the low circulating level of free T_4.[6, 36] No other evaluation or tests are usually required for diagnosis.

Management

Hypothyroidism is usually one of the easier diseases to manage, and the cost of therapy is low.[27] The synthetic preparations of L-thyroxine should be used, particularly in children. In older children and adolescents, a dose of 1 to 3 μg/kg per day (approximately 100 μg/m²/day) generally produces a clinical and biochemical euthyroid state. To avoid interference in absorption by certain foods, T_4 should be taken at least 30 minutes before a meal or at bedtime.[27] A patient who forgets a dose should take a double dose the next day. Once normal serum levels of T_4 and TSH are achieved, thyroid function tests need be

monitored only annually, unless patient compliance or reliability of T_4 preparations is in question.

CLINICAL PRESENTATIONS AND THE ROLE OF THYROID HORMONES IN PATHOGENESIS

PUBERTAL DELAY

In the evaluation of a child with pubertal delay, both primary hypothyroidism and hypothalamic-pituitary disease (with or without hypothyroidism) must be excluded.[26] For the diagnosis of autoimmune thyroiditis with primary hypothyroidism, serum TSH (elevated), free T_4 (low), and thyroid peroxidase and thyroglobulin antibodies (positive in a titer greater than 1:4 or a detectable concentration [in units per ml] in children) are the initial, and usually definitive, diagnostic tests. An elevated TSH level without an abnormally low T_4 level is considered compensated primary hypothyroidism and would not be expected to account for pubertal delay. Because hypothalamic-pituitary hypothyroidism after age 8 years is nearly always associated with other hypothalamic or pituitary hormone abnormalities, pubertal delay in such cases during adolescence is associated with gonadotropin deficiency. Confirmation of the diagnosis of hypothalamic or pituitary hypothyroidism requires a low serum free T_4 level (preferably determined by a definitive test such as direct or equilibrium dialysis)[9] and a low, normal, or mildly elevated TSH level (not greater than 20 mU/l).[35] MRI of the hypothalamic-pituitary area is necessary to distinguish a space-occupying lesion from idiopathic hypothalamic-pituitary hypothyroidism.[33] A TRH test is required to differentiate hypothalamic from primary pituitary disease as a cause of central hypothyroidism.[33, 36] Failure to demonstrate a rise in TSH after TRH in the presence of a low free T_4 value supports the diagnosis of primary pituitary TSH deficiency. The prolactin (PRL) response to TRH would be normal or exaggerated unless the pituitary gland were completely destroyed, in which case there would be no TSH or PRL response.

PRECOCIOUS PUBERTY

Early breast development or testicular enlargement without adrenarche is a rare presentation of advanced primary hypothyroidism. The usual cause is autoimmune thyroiditis, but it can be any disease associated with chronic primary hypothyroidism duration, usually with symptoms and signs of myxedema and onset during childhood. The initial thyroid evaluation is the same as that described for primary hypothyroidism and pubertal delay (i.e., measurement of serum TSH, free T_4, and thyroid antibodies).

HYPERPROLACTINEMIA

Primary and hypothalamic hypothyroidism can both be associated with hyperprolactinemia, and pubertal or young adult patients may present with amenorrhea and galactorrhea.[26] In early stages of disease with mild hypothyroidism, the basal PRL level may be normal, but the PRL response to TRH may be exaggerated, as the TSH response is. Young adults who present with either an unexplained elevated PRL level or galactorrhea should be screened for hypothyroidism (i.e., with measurement of serum TSH and free T_4).

GROWTH ABERRATIONS

Mild accelerations in growth may occur with thyrotoxicosis, but such patients will have obvious clinical disease by the time growth acceleration is observed. In hypothyroidism, however, the first and only sign of the disease may be a deceleration in growth velocity. These patients must be screened for hypothyroidism (i.e., with measurement of serum TSH and free T_4).

RAPID PUBERTAL ADVANCE DURING TREATMENT OF HYPOTHYROIDISM

Patients with chronic primary hypothyroidism associated with growth deceleration and retarded skeletal maturation who present during late childhood or early adolescence may experience both rapid growth acceleration and pubertal advance when euthyroidism is restored with appropriate doses of T_4.[37] The onset of puberty may occur before growth has caught up to the growth percentile achieved before the hypothyroidism developed. Furthermore, because the pubertal response may proceed more rapidly than the growth response, the patient may reach adult height, with epiphyseal fusion, before catch-up growth is completed and thus fail to attain the genetically predetermined height, the *target*

height.[37] This problem is demonstrated in the growth chart (Fig. 10–3). The patient grew at the 50th percentile before hypothyroidism developed around age 6 years; however, after therapy and completion of pubertal development, her height was only at the 25th percentile. Short adult stature is more likely to occur in children whose hypothyroidism in more severe and prolonged and who begin treatment in the early teenage years.

REFERENCES

1. Longcope C: The male and female reproductive systems in thyrotoxicosis. In Braverman LE, Utiger RD (eds): Werner and Ingbar's The Thyroid, 7th ed. Philadelphia: Lippincott-Raven, 1996, Part IV, pp. 671–677.
2. Longcope C: The male and female reproductive systems in hypothyroidism. In Braverman LE, Utiger RD (eds): Werner and Ingbar's The Thyroid, 7th ed. Philadelphia: Lippincott-Raven, 1996, Part V, pp. 849–852.
3. Foley TP Jr: Disorders of the thyroid in children. In Sperling MA (ed): Clinical Pediatric and Adolescent Endocrinology. Philadelphia: W.B. Saunders, 1996, pp 171–194.
4. Leonard JL, Koehrle J: Intracellular pathways of iodothyronine metabolism. In Braverman LE, Utiger RD (eds): Werner and Ingbar's The Thyroid, 7th ed. Philadelphia: Lippincott-Raven, 1996, Part I, pp. 125–161.
5. Vassart G, Dumont JE, Refetoff S: Thyroid disorders. In Scriver CR, Beaudet AL, Sly WS, Valle D (eds): The Metabolic and Molecular Bases of Inherited Disease, 7th ed. New York: McGraw-Hill, 1995, Part 13, pp. 2883.
6. Scanlon MF, Toft AD: Regulation of thyrotropin secretion. In Braverman LE, Utiger RD (eds): Werner and Ingbar's The Thyroid, 7th ed. Philadelphia: Lippincott-Raven, 1996, Part I, pp. 220–240.
7. Larsen PR, Silva JE, Kaplan MM: Relationships between circulating and intracellular thyroid hormones: Physiological and clinical implications. Endocrine Rev 1981; 2:87–102.
8. Oppenheimer JH, Schwartz HL, Strait KA: The molecular basis of thyroid hormone actions. In Braverman LE, Utiger RD (eds.): Werner and Ingbar's The Thyroid, 7th ed. Philadelphia: Lippincott-Raven, 1996, Part I, pp. 162–184.
9. Nelson JC, Weiss RM, Wilcox RB: Underestimates of serum free thyroxine (T4) concentrations by free T_4 immunoassays. J Clin Endocrinol Metab 1994; 79:76–9.
10. Parry CH: Elements of Pathology and Therapeutics. 1825; 2:111–128.
11. von Basedow CA: Exophthalmos durch Hypertrophie des Zellgewebes in der Augenhöhle. Wochenschr Heilk 1840; 6:197–204; 220–228.
12. Weetman AP, Yateman ME, Ealey PA, et al: Thyroid-stimulating antibody activity between different immunoglobulin G subclasses. J Clin Invest 1990; 86:723–727.
13. Hiromatsu Y, Fukazawa H, Wall JR: Cytotoxic mechanisms in autoimmune thyroid disorders and thyroid-associated ophthalmopathy. Endocrinol Metab Clin North Am 1987; 16:269–286.
14. La Franchi S, Mandel SH: Graves' disease in the neonatal period and childhood. In Braverman LE, Utiger RD (eds): Werner and Ingbar's The Thyroid, 7th ed. Philadelphia: Lippincott-Raven, 1996, Part VIII, pp. 1000–1008.

15. Dallas JS, Foley TP Jr: Hyperthyroidism. *In* Lifshitz F (ed): Pediatric Endocrinology: A Clinical Guide, 3rd ed. New York: Marcel Dekker, 1995, pp 401–414.
16. Weintraub BD, Gershengorn MC, Kourides IA, et al: Inappropriate secretion of thyroid stimulating hormone. Ann Intern Med 1981; 95:339.
17. Solomon B, Glinoer D, Lagasse R, et al: Current trends in the management of Graves' disease. J Clin Endocrinol Metab 1990; 70:1518–1524.
18. Levey GS: The heart and hyperthyroidism. Use of beta-adrenergic blocking drugs. Med Clin North Am 1975; 59:1193–1201.
19. Cooper DS: Antithyroid drugs. N Engl J Med 1984; 311:1353.
20. Jansson R, Dahlberg PA, Johansson H, et al: Intrathyroidal concentrations of methimazole in patients with Graves' disease. J Clin Endocrinol Metab 1983; 57:129–132.
21. Okuno A, Yano K, Inyaku F, et al: Pharmacokinetics of methimazole in children and adolescents with Graves disease. Studies on plasma and intrathyroidal concentrations. Acta Endocrinol (Copenh) 1987; 115:112–118.
22. Hashizume K, Ichikawa K, Sakurai A, et al: Administration of thyroxine in treated Graves' disease. N Engl J Med 1991; 324:947–953.
23. Foley TP Jr, Charron M: Radioiodine treatment of juvenile Graves disease. Exp Clin Endocrinol Diabetes 1997; 105 (Suppl 4):61–65.
24. Rivkees SA, Sklar C, Freemark M: The management of Graves' disease in children, with special emphasis on radioiodine treatment. J Clin Endocrinol Metab 1998; 83:3767–3776.
25. Stoffer SS, Hamburger JI: Inadvertent ^{131}I therapy for hyperthyroidism in the first trimester of pregnancy. J Nucl Med 1976; 17:146–149.
26. Styne DM: Thyroid dysfunction: An adolescent gynecologic perspective. Curr Opin Obstet Gynecol 1995; 7:367–370.
27. Foley TP Jr: Acquired hypothyroidism in infants, children and adolescents. *In* Braverman LE, Utiger RD (eds): Werner and Ingbar's The Thyroid, 8th ed. Philadelphia: Lippincott-Raven, 2000, Part C, pp 983–988.
28. Hubble D: Endocrine relations. Lancet 1:1, 1955.
29. Van Wyk J, Grumbach MM: Syndrome of precocious menstruation and galactorrhea in juvenile hypothyroidism: An example of hormonal overlap pituitary feedback. J Pediatr 1960; 57:416.
30. Franks RC, Stempfel RS: Juvenile hypothyroidism and precocious testicular maturation. J Clin Endocrinol Metab 1963; 23:805.
31. Anasti JN, Flack MR, Froehlich J, et al: A potential novel mechanism for precocious puberty in juvenile hypothyroidism. J Clin Endocrinol Metab 1995; 80:276.
32. Foley TP, Schubert WK, Marnell RT, et al: Chronic lymphocytic thyroiditis and juvenile myxedema in uniovular twins. J Pediatr 72:201–207, 1968.
33. Arslanian S, Foley TP Jr, Lee PA: Endocrine and systemic manifestation of brain tumors in children. *In* Deutsch M (ed): Management of Childhood Brain Tumors. Boston: Kluwer Academic, 1990, pp. 137–173.
34. Foley TP Jr: Congenital hypothyroidism. *In* Braverman LE, Utiger RD (eds): Werner and Ingbar's The Thyroid, 8th ed. Philadelphia: Lippincott-Raven, 2000, Chapter 82, Part B, pp 977–983.
35. Illig R, Krawczynska H, Torresani T, et al: Elevated plasma TSH and hypothyroidism in children with hypothalamic hypopituitarism. J Clin Endocrinol Metab 41:722–728, 1975.
36. Martino E, Bartalena L, Faglia G, Pinchera A: Central hypothyroidism. *In* Ingbar SH, Braverman LE, Utiger RD (eds): Werner and Ingbar's The Thyroid, 7th ed. Philadelphia: Lippincott-Raven 1996, Part V, pp. 779–791.
37. Rivkees SA, Bode HH, Crawford JD: Long-term growth in juvenile acquired hypothyroidism: the failure to achieve normal adult stature. N Engl J Med 1988; 318:599–602.

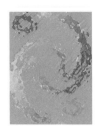

Chapter 11
Molecular Biology and Genetics Aspects

STEPHEN S. WACHTEL AND LEE P. SHULMAN

The clinical applications of molecular biology have increased considerably in the past decade. Genetics is no longer the singular bailiwick of geneticists; molecular methods have become useful diagnostic tools in most clinical specialties, including diverse ones such as infectious disease, pathology, and clinical immunology. This has enabled more accurate diagnosis and has improved delineation of disease and monitoring of treatment. In addition, molecular biology has entered the arena of adolescent and pediatric gynecology. Professionals who provide gynecologic care to adolescent and pediatric patients thus should be aware of the novel molecular technologies available for the diagnosis and management of problems they are likely to encounter.

We address a number of the molecular biologic methods available to clinicians—methods for identification of specific DNA sequences by Southern blotting and hybridization, DNA sequence analysis, genetic fingerprinting, and amplification of specific DNA sequences by the polymerase chain reaction (PCR). We review application of these methods to two problems frequently encountered in the adolescent and pediatric population: sexual assault and abnormal sexual development. The format is introductory and readily accessible to nonspecialist readers. A more comprehensive description of laboratory methods is beyond the scope of this chapter. Interested readers are encouraged to review the technical literature cited throughout the text.

MOLECULAR BIOLOGY: RECOMBINANT DNA METHODS

RESTRICTION ENZYMES

The fleas we know have other fleas,
Upon their backs to bite 'em,
And these in turn have other fleas,
And so ad infinitum.

The validity of this little rhyme has yet to be ascertained, but we do know that bacterial cells are hosts for viruses called *bacteriophages*, or simply *phages*—minute particles that exist in the mysterious and obscure reaches between the realms of life and nonlife. Whether they are alive or not, bacterial viruses are, in a real sense, parasites of bacterial cells. In general, the individual phage particle consists of a duplex molecule of DNA surrounded by a protein coat. The phage attaches to the cell wall of the bacterium and injects its DNA into the cell. As a consequence of that injection, the protein- and DNA-synthesizing programs of the bacterial cell are subverted: *viral* proteins and DNA chains are produced, not those of the bacterium. These components are assembled into new virus particles inside the bacterium, so that the infected cell is now little more than a shell containing a hundred or so virus particles. The cell virtually explodes, thereby releasing the nascent viruses into the surrounding milieu.

Students of medicine know that the entire "life cycle" of the virus lasts about 20 minutes and that, given the proper host and environment, billions of viruses can be produced within a couple of hours. Yet bacterial cells are not without their defenses. Among the armamentarium of proteins produced by bacteria are enzymes that cut viral DNA into harmless segment. These enzymes recognize very short base sequences that are common in viral DNA but rare in bacterial DNA. An example is *Eco*RI (for *Escherichia coli* restriction enzyme one), which cuts DNA wherever it encounters this sequence:

--- GAATTC ---
--- CTTAAG ---

The cut is made as follows:

--- G • AATTC ---
--- CTTAA • G ---

Bacterial enzymes that cut DNA in this way are called *restriction enzymes* because they restrict the ability of viruses to infect and reproduce. Many different restriction enzymes have been identified in a variety of bacteria. The sequence of bases that the restriction enzyme cuts is called a *restriction site* or *recognition sequence*. The fragments resulting from digestion of DNA with a particular restriction enzyme are called *restriction fragments*.

Restriction enzymes are valuable tools for molecular biology, because they allow geneticists to dissect, analyze, and reassemble DNA in a predictable and controlled fashion. For example, by using several alternative restriction enzymes with a given sample of DNA, it is possible to produce a *restriction map* that shows a linear sequence of restriction sites and restriction fragments in the sample under study (differences in restriction maps among individuals are called *restriction fragment length polymorphisms (RFLPs)*. As another example, geneticists can use restriction enzymes to remove a sequence of bases between two restriction sites in one piece of DNA and insert it into another piece of DNA that contains the same restriction sites. The product of this kind of manipulation is called *recombinant DNA*.

The techniques of recombinant DNA allow human DNA sequences to be placed into bacterial (plasmid) or viral DNA, and this enables large-scale replication of the human sequences, for, when the bacterial or viral DNA is replicated, the human DNA is also replicated. Given the short life cycle of bacteria and bacterial viruses, it is thus possible to generate millions of copies of a desired sequence. This is called *cloning* or, more precisely, *molecular cloning*. The target DNA can be removed from the recombinant molecule by applying the same restriction enzyme used to insert it. Cloning allows comprehensive analysis of DNA—determination of the exact sequence of nucleotide bases, for example—and thereby elucidation of the precise order of amino acids in the corresponding protein.[1]

PROBES

The human genome contains about 10^9 base pairs (bp) of DNA. Thus, the DNA in a single gene (usually about 300–2000 bp) represents only a tiny fraction of the total. To identify a particular gene, we thus require a specific *probe*, a sequence of DNA able to react with the target

sequence. The probe may correspond to the entire gene or to certain sequences within it.

One way to obtain a probe is to identify a target messenger RNA (mRNA) by separating it from newly synthesized protein, for example, and to synthesize DNA by use of the mRNA as a template. The enzyme that catalyzes this reaction is called *reverse transcriptase*. The initial product of the reaction is a hybrid molecule consisting of one strand of mRNA and one strand of complementary DNA (cDNA). When the reaction is complete, the mRNA is degraded with alkali, and the single-stranded cDNA is converted, by the enzyme *DNA polymerase*, into double-stranded cDNA, which can be cloned and used as a probe.[2]

There are alternative ways to develop probes. For instance, enriched populations of Y chromosomes (or any other chromosomes) can be obtained by flow cytometry. If the Y chromosomal DNA is digested with restriction enzymes, the result is a series of Y-specific DNA fragments. Some of these can be used as probes to evaluate children with ambiguous genitalia, as the presence of a Y-chromosome or a portion thereof may be responsible for some cases of sexual ambiguity in children. In addition, Y-specific probes are valuable for evaluating XX males. Because sex reversal in XX males usually is due to Y-X crossovers involving transfer of the testis-determining gene *(TDF)*, and, because the Y-X crossovers may involve more or less Y material, those probes that are closer to *TDF* would be expected to be found in a greater proportion of XX males than would those that are farther distal. This has enabled construction of maps depicting the relative positions of a number of Y probes and has led to the discovery of the ZFY gene, an early candidate for the human *TDF*, and, more recently, to the discovery of *SRY*, the actual testis-determining gene.

IDENTIFICATION OF SPECIFIC SEQUENCES

Southern Blotting

For the sake of illustration, say that a young woman whose presenting complaints are amenorrhea, eunuchoid habitus, and short stature is found to have a karyotype of 46,X + marker. The marker chromosome is small and could be part of the short arm of the X or the Y. Keeping in mind that females who possess Y fragments are at increased risk for gonadal malignancy,[3] we wish to determine the nature of the marker chromosome. Let us assume that we have a probe—call it Y-1—that represents a DNA segment proximal to the Y centromere. By the following method called *Southern blotting,*[4] we can then determine whether the marker is Y-derived.

A sample of DNA is first extracted from blood of the patient. The DNA is then fractionated by digestion with restriction enzyme; e.g., the *Eco*RI restriction enzyme. Wherever the enzyme encounters its recognition site (— GAATTC —) it will cut (— G / AATTC —), and the result will be a series of fragments of varying sizes. Next, the DNA fragments are placed in a gel matrix and exposed to an electric field in which they migrate according to size, the smaller fragments faster than the larger ones. The fragments can, accordingly, be classified by the number of pairs of DNA bases that they contain. It is convenient to describe the size of such fragments in terms of the thousands of base pairs that they contain. These are referred to as *kilobase pairs* or *kilobases* (kb). A particular fragment might contain 5.5 kb, for instance, or 6.8 kb.

When the migration *(electrophoresis)* is completed, the DNA fragments are denatured and transferred *(blotted)* onto a nitrocellulose or nylon matrix and thereby immobilized. By this method, the DNA fragments can be removed from the gel and transferred in exactly the same positions that they occupied in the gel.

Copies of the probe, Y-1, are placed onto the filter under conditions that favor *hybridization*—the reaction of sequences in the probe with complementary sequences in the target DNA, which is denatured before transfer (so probe and target DNA both are single-stranded). The hybridization reaction is visualized by the use of radiolabeled or chemiluminescent probes. The result is a band, or a series of bands on the filter or photographic plate, identifing the fragment to which the probe has bound. The size of the fragment is determined by comparing the position of the band with markers of known size (Fig. 11–1).

In the test being described, DNA from the patient would be compared with samples of DNA from normal male and female controls. Given that the probe is Y chromosome–specific, we should expect to find at least a single hybridization band in the male DNA, and absence of that band in the female DNA. Presence of the band in the patient would signal the presence of at least that part of the Y chromosome that corresponds to the probe. Using alternative probes from across the Y, one could determine the approximate amount of Y material in the marker chromosome.

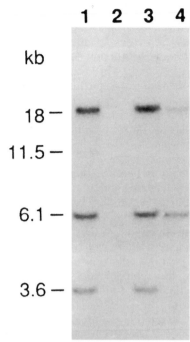

Figure 11–1. Southern blot. Autoradiograph of genomic DNA hybridized with ^{32}P-labeled probe pT5.1.1.PH, which identifies Y chromosome–specific sequences in the mouse. Lanes contain mouse DNA as follows: 1, normal XY male; 2 normal XX female; 3, sex-reversed XX male with Y-X crossover; 4, sex-reversed XX male carrying deleted Y-X crossover. The sizes of the fragments identified by the probe can be estimated by comparison with the kilobase (kb) markers at left. (From Mitchell MJ, Bishop CE: A structural analysis of the Sxr region of the mouse Y chromosome. Genomics 1992; 12:26.)

When a probe represents part or all of a specific gene, it is possible to determine whether that gene is present in a genome. In certain cases, by the application of small *(oligonucleotide)* probes, geneticists can use Southern blotting techniques to identify particular mutations within genes.

Northern Blotting

Northern blotting technique is essentially similar to that described for Southern blotting, except that mRNA, rather than DNA, is probed. As a result, the geneticist obtains a measure of transcription (expression) of the target gene. Say, for example, that a sequence has been identified as a candidate for a gene involved in ovarian development. By northern blotting it may be ascertained whether the gene is transcribed in ovary or lung or kidney, and it may be shown whether the gene is transcribed in the gonadal ridge about the time of ovarian differentiation. That is how northern blotting was used to evaluate the candidacy of *SRY*, the testis-determining gene. An RNA transcript hybridizing with the *SRY* probe (pY53.3) was identified in testis but not in male lung or kidney,[5] and a corresponding transcript was identified in the gonadal ridge of the fetal mouse just before emergence of the seminiferous tubules.[6]

Dot Blots and Slot Blots

For rapid screening of desired sequences in DNA and RNA, the samples to be analyzed are digested and denatured (as in Southern or Northern blotting), but then the extracted DNA or RNA is applied directly to a nitrocellulose or other matrix, without electrophoresis. By application of a particular probe, the investigator can then determine whether the corresponding sequence is present in the sample, without reference to the size of the fragments that may be recognized by the probe (this information is not available in the absence of electrophoresis). The difference between slot blots and dot blots lies in the shape of the recess or template in the apparatus used to capture the DNA or RNA under study. The slot is a thin rectangle, whereas the dot is a small circle. In both cases, the formats facilitate consistent loading of samples. The amount of sample hybridizing with a particular probe can be quantified by densitometry.

Stringency

Stringency refers to the conditions of the hybridization reaction that determine the stability of the resulting DNA duplex. A stringency of 80% means that 80% of the base pairs in a duplex are matched. It is possible to vary the stringency of hybridization—in Southern blots, for example—by changing the temperature and salt concentration when the filter is washed. At higher stringency (higher temperature, lower salt concentration), a greater degree of base pair matching is required between probe and target DNA for hybridization to occur (that is, for the probe to recognize the target sequence). By varying temperature and salt concentration, the geneticist can apply the probe to the identification of sequences related to, but not identical with, the target sequence.

Consider this example. The gene for the plate-

let-activating factor receptor (PAFR) was cloned several years ago in guinea pig DNA, but not yet in human DNA. Given the likelihood of strong evolutionary conservation (the PAFR belongs to the G protein–coupled receptor superfamily), the guinea pig probe was used to isolate a corresponding human sequence by screening a human cDNA library at reduced stringencies. Fragments with which the probe hybridized could be cloned and the desired human sequence identified by testing for function or by partial sequence analysis (see below).

DNA SEQUENCING

It may be said that one of the chief goals of the geneticist is to determine the nucleotide sequence of genes, for this allows comparison of normal (wild-type) and mutant genes and thus correlation of discrete lesions (e.g., nucleotide base substitutions, deletions, etc.) with particular disorders. Moreover, knowledge of DNA sequence facilitates the generation of restriction maps, identification of segments that encode proteins, and comparison with known sequences—a useful means of obtaining information about novel sequences and their products.

Current methods enable the geneticist to decipher routinely the sequence of a gene or a particular DNA fragment. Initially, two methods were employed in this regard: the method of Maxam and Gilbert,[7] which involved chemical modification and cleavage of specific nucleotides, followed by electrophoresis of the resulting fragments in high-resolution acrylamide gels, and the dideoxy chain termination method of Sanger et al,[8] which involved synthesis of small fragments of DNA in a way that curtailed elongation of each fragment at a position corresponding to a particular base; this was also followed by electrophoresis in acrylamide.

According to the method of Sanger et al,[8] which was the more widely used, a series of $2',3'$-dideoxynucleotides was first prepared, representing each of the four bases (ddATP, ddTTP, ddCTP, ddGTP). Because each of these bases possessed a normal $5'$-triphosphate, each could be taken up into the growing DNA chain by DNA polymerase. But once incorporated, a dideoxynucleotide (ddNTP) blocked chain growth because it would not form a bond with the deoxynucleotide (dNTP) next in line, and elongation of that fragment was terminated. For sequencing, four polymerase reactions were performed, each involving one of the four nucleotide bases (which had been labeled). When the ddNTPs

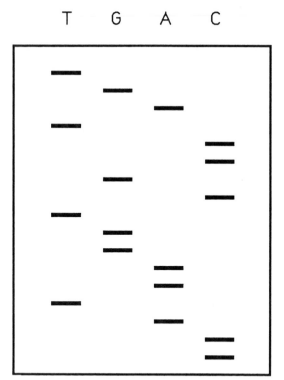

Figure 11–2. DNA sequencing. Graphic representation of autoradiograph depicting nucleotide bands in a sequencing gel. The order of nucleotides in the segment analyzed is C-C-A-T-A-A-G-G-T-C-G-C-C-T-A-G-T.

were mixed with "normal" bases (dNTPs) in the correct ratio, some of the polymerizing reactions were terminated while most others continued. The result was a series of DNA fragments, each one a single base longer than the preceding one and each terminating at a particular base (A,T,C,G). The fragments were then separated by electrophoresis in an acrylamide gel. The pattern of migration, which corresponded exactly to the particular sequence of nucleotides in the segment of DNA under study, was visualized by autoradiography or chemiluminescence (Fig. 11–2). By this method, it was possible to determine the sequence of about 250-300 bases at a time. For larger segments, 250-300 bp were read in alternative fragments, and the overlapping sequences were combined to give the complete sequence.

The Sanger reaction has been automated. The electrophoresis step, identification of the particular band pattern, and analysis of bands is now regularly performed by commercially available machines. According to one method, fluorescent label is incorporated into the four bases, which can be run and read in a single lane because they

fluoresce at different wavelengths. The readout consists of a series of four peaks, each representing one of the four nucleotide bases. An additional method for dideoxy sequencing involves an application of thermal cycling that resembles the polymerase chain reaction (PCR; see later). Several kits are available for routine application of this method.

DNA FINGERPRINTING

The human genome contains long repetitive DNA sequences, known as *satellites*. They are so called because they are representative of small shoulders, or satellites, off the main peak in cesium chloride density ultracentrifugation profiles of DNA (Fig. 11–3). Satellite DNA typically occurs in the heterochromatic regions of the chromosomes, which are usually genetically inert; the DNA in these regions is sometimes called *junk DNA*. Within these regions, the G:C and A:T

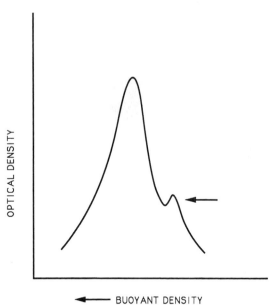

Figure 11–3. Satellite DNA. The buoyant density of double-stranded DNA—a function of G-C content—may be determined by centrifugation through a cesium chloride density gradient. The main peak depicted in the figure includes 90% of the DNA in the genome. This is centered around a value of 1.70 gm–cm^{-3}, corresponding to an average G-C content of 42%, which is typical of mammals. The small peak at the right *(arrow)*, represents 10% of the genome. This is a satellite DNA with a G-C content of 30% and a buoyant density of 1.69 gm–cm^{-3}. Satellites may have densities larger or smaller than those represented by the main peak.

base pairs are distributed unequally, and thus, satellite DNA has a density that is different from the density of the main body of DNA.

A number of polymorphic *minisatellites* have been identified in human DNA. These consist of tandem repeats of a core sequence containing, say, 10 to 15 bp, as in the (AGGGCTGGAGG)n sequence described by Jeffreys et al.[9] This particular type of satellite DNA is also known as *variable numbers of tandem repeats* (VNTRs), as these repeated sequences are characterized by hypervariable numbers of these sequences throughout the genome. The great variability in the number of repeated sequences is probably generated by unequal crossing over, which yields a composite of specific VNTRs that differ from individual to individual; in other words, a *DNA fingerprint*. Southern blotting and hybridization with probes comprising multiple repeats of the core sequence can be used to detect several distinct sequences simultaneously, thereby en-

abling identification of individuals for family, demographic, and linkage studies. Evidently, these sequences are inherited in mendelian fashion; they exhibit germline and somatic stability.

DNA fingerprinting has been used to identify individuals and to determine genetic relationships in many species, including dog, cat, house sparrow, lesser snow goose, and various sea turtles and whales. An example of DNA fingerprinting in the sea turtle is given in Figure 11–4. In humans, DNA fingerprinting has been applied to paternity testing and forensic medicine. In an immigration case in England, DNA fingerprinting enabled positive identification of a Ghanian boy who wanted to live with his mother.[10]

The validity of DNA fingerprint analysis has been questioned, particularly in criminal cases involving sexual assault. The major problem is that the methods for identification of DNA samples may yield inconclusive or even spurious data. In an editorial on the subject of genetic

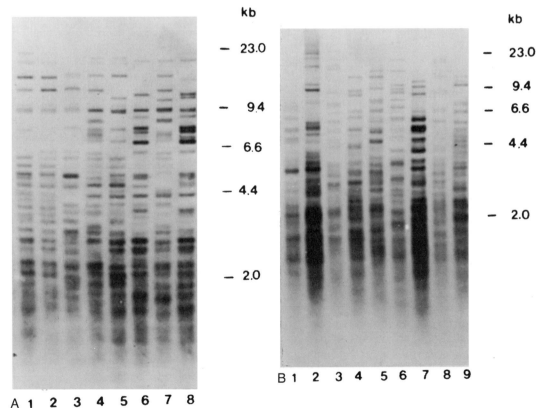

Figure 11–4. DNA fingerprinting. Variable hybridization patterns obtained in two freshwater turtles by use of the Bkm probe (GATA) after digestion of DNA with the restriction enzyme *Bst*N1: *(a) Trionyx spiniferous* (spiny soft shell) and *(b) Trachemys scripta* (red-eared slider). Each of the numbered lanes contains the "fingerprint" of a particular animal. The size of the individual fragments (or bands) can be approximated by reference to the kilobase (kb) markers to the right of each Southern blot. (From Demas S, Wachtel S: DNA fingerprinting in reptiles: Bkm hybridization patterns in Crocodilia and Chelonia. Genome 1991; 34:472.)

fingerprinting, Lander[11] pointed out that artifacts can be generated by forensic DNA samples, which are likely to be degraded or contaminated. Citing the work by Budowle et al,[12] he noted, moreover, that, when fresh DNA from the victim's blood was compared with forensic samples from the vaginal epithelium in 111 cases of rape, corresponding fragments differed by as much as 5% molecular weight and that, during electrophoresis, forensic samples exhibited a tendency to migrate faster than freshly extracted sample did. In addition, it was indicated that little has been published on laboratory-to-laboratory variations in fingerprint analysis (or even variations within a laboratory) and that the problem of "band shifting" due to contamination, degradation, or differences in sample concentration, remains to be solved.

Despite these caveats, DNA fingerprinting is being used more and more often in criminal and civil cases. This has particular applications in cases of sexual abuse. In particular, restriction fragment length polymorphisms (RFLPs) are now widely employed for comparing forensic DNA samples with samples provided by criminal suspects. RFLPs are highly polymorphic in the human population, and a group of five or more may be tested in alternative samples with little likelihood of a random match. Depending on the population frequencies of the individual RFLPs, the probability of randomly matching a group of five RFLPs in a blood sample with the RFLPs in a semen sample taken in a rape case may be on the order of 10^{-5} to 10^{-6}, or even less.

The PCR is also being applied for DNA fingerprinting. In this case, particular forensic sequences are amplified and compared with corresponding sequences from a suspect (see later).

POLYMERASE CHAIN REACTION (PCR)

The ability to amplify a particular segment of DNA—to produce billions or even trillions of copies of a single DNA molecule—has sparked a revolution in molecular biology. DNA amplification by the PCR was first described by Saiki et al[13] of the Cetus Corporation. The method has since found a broad range of applications in medicine, genetics, and evolutionary biology.[14]

The PCR consists of three basic steps: (1) denaturation of double-stranded DNA, (2) attachment of oligonucleotide primers that delineate a target sequence, and (3) synthesis of new DNA that corresponds to the target sequence. Usually, each step is carried out at a particular

temperature; for example, denaturation at 94–98° C, primer attachment (*annealing*) at 37–65°C and replication at 72°C. The target sequence is amplified by running the PCR through several, say 20–40, cycles; this results in an exponential increase in the number of target sequences, because the products generated in cycle n can serve as templates in the next cycle $(n + 1)$.

Although large fragments of DNA can be amplified in the PCR, most reactions are limited to segments of no more than 400 bp. As an example, say that we wish to amplify a 300-bp segment in a particular gene. We must have the nucleotide sequences of the regions that immediately flank the target sequence. Then we can produce the oligonucleotide primers that will delineate the sequence to be amplified. The primers are single-stranded DNA molecules of about 18–24 bp. Once annealed to the target sequence, they initiate replication and control the direction of synthesis (Fig. 11–5). The reaction is catalyzed by the heat-stable enzyme *Taq* polymerase, obtained from the thermophilic bacterium, *Thermus aquaticus*. Use of *Taq* polymerase enables the entire reaction to be carried out in a single tube in a temperature-cycling apparatus.

The potential applications of PCR in the Pediatric adolescent population are numerous. A brief summary of some of them follows (for a more detailed description of the applications of PCR, see Erlich[14]).

Diagnosis

In the aforementioned female patient with the 46,X,+mar karyotype, the origin of the marker chromosome was identified by Southern blotting. But this could be done more easily by PCR with oligonucleotide primers delineating Y chromosome–specific sequences. As another example, the products of PCR amplification can be tested for single base changes with oligonucleotide probes, as in the original report by Saiki and associates,[13] where the authors describe a method for diagnosis of sickle cell anemia by detection of polymorphism within the β-globin gene.

Oncology

Mutations within the *ras* oncogene, common in certain tumors, can likewise be diagnosed by PCR in combination with short DNA probes used to hybridize with the amplified fragments.

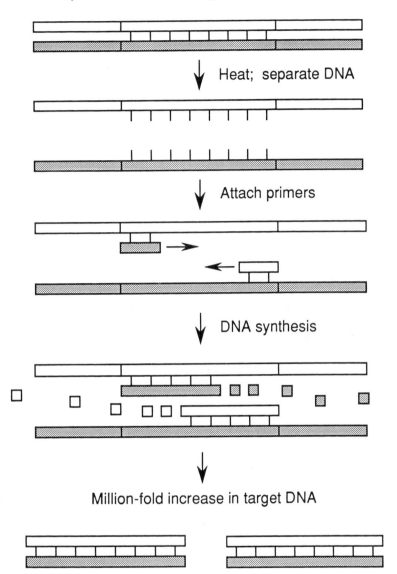

Figure 11–5. Polymerase chain reaction (PCR). The weak bonds that unite the individual DNA strands are broken by heating, and the strands are separated. Then the single-stranded primers are attached. The primers delineate the sequence to be replicated and determine the orientation of DNA synthesis. Replication is accomplished in the presence of heat-resistant Taq polymerase (the small squares represent the incoming nucleotides). The process may be repeated through numerous cycles, generating millions or billions of copies of a desired sequence. See text for a detailed description of the method.

Heat; separate DNA

Attach primers

DNA synthesis

Million-fold increase in target DNA

Forensics

PCR has enabled evaluation of minute quantities of degraded DNA in samples that could not be used for standard DNA fingerprint analysis. The alternative method, involving Southern blotting, calls for quantities of intact high-molecular-weight DNA greater than those needed for the PCR.

Genetics

By reverse transcription, it is also possible to amplify DNA from mRNA templates. This enables study, not only of the presence of a gene but also of its expression.

FORENSIC APPLICATIONS OF RECOMBINANT DNA TECHNOLOGY: SEXUAL ASSAULT

The methods described here have generated considerable enthusiasm in forensic medicine. As noted above, recombinant DNA techniques can provide data on identification of individuals and can be applied for the evaluation of tissue specimens not previously amenable to forensic analysis. DNA analysis is now widely used to determine parentage, to identify people physically involved in homicide, sexual assault, and other crimes, and to identify the victims of kidnapping, murder, or natural disasters. Molecular methods do not necessarily require fresh blood or tissue samples. They can be used to analyze blood or tissue samples that have been exposed to the environment for varying periods.

Gynecologists who specialize in treating pediatric and adolescent patients are frequently called upon to assess young victims of sexual assault. In addition to his or her central role in the emotional and physical care of these patients, the gynecologist must help government authorities to identify the responsible parties. Thus, gynecologists must be aware of the methods currently used for inclusion or exclusion of those suspected of sexual assault. In this section, we review the application of recombinant DNA methods to the evaluation of sexual assault, in particular, and the applications and limitations of these methods in various legal jurisdictions.

FORENSIC DNA FINGERPRINTING

DNA fingerprinting can be used to identify the source of seminal fluid and other tissues recovered from sexual assault victims. It can also be used to detect more than one assailant. If the sexual assault occurred soon after consensual sexual intercourse with a different partner, DNA fingerprinting could distinguish between tissue from the partner and that of an assailant. Despite the power of DNA fingerprinting in identifying sexual assailants, the data produced by such analyses have limitations. Problems range from improper preparation of specimens to faulty interpretation of data.[15] These problems have limited universal acceptance of DNA fingerprinting in cases of sexual assault.[16]

DNA Extraction

For forensic analysis, DNA can be obtained from any nucleated cell. However, the quality of analysis correlates with the quality of the specimen from which the DNA is extracted. Extraction of high-quality DNA is related to the size and age of the specimen and to the environmental conditions where it was collected, and eventually stored.[17] For example, a 72-hour-old dried semen specimen does not usually yield DNA of the same quality as a specimen obtained from the vaginal vault 6 hours after ejaculation. A general rule is that a specimen produced recently and not exposed to extremes of heat or cold yields higher-quality DNA than an older specimen that has been exposed to the environment. Universal standards for tissue volume and environmental conditions have yet to be determined.

DNA Storage and Transport

Though desirable, immediate extraction of DNA from a specimen at a crime scene is not always possible. Appropriate conditions for storage of various tissues amenable to forensic DNA analysis are listed in Table 11–1. Which storage condition to use depends on the specific tissue, the type of analysis to be performed, and how long the sample or extracted DNA will be stored or transported. DNA is relatively stable and, once extracted, can be shipped at room temperature or, if frozen, kept indefinitely. Repeated freezing and thawing results in degradation and is not recommended. DNA can also be stored in chloroform (optimal concentration 5 μl/ml) for long periods.

VARIABLE NUMBER OF TANDEM REPEATS

What method is used to identify persons involved in sexual assault depends on the quality and quantity of the specimen available and what type of information is being sought. When a recently ejaculated seminal specimen is recovered, DNA fingerprinting utilizing probes of VNTRs may be used. As noted above, VNTRs are characterized by repetitive sequences in specific regions of the human genome and are polymorphic in different persons: (i.e., the number and location of these sequences differ from person to person).[18-21] Thus, analysis of VNTRs in DNA extracted from seminal fluid recovered from the vaginal vault of an assault victim can be used to differentiate the victim's own DNA and the DNA of consensual sexual partners from that of the purported assailant.

Once extracted from the seminal specimen, the DNA is exposed to restriction enzymes, sub-

Table 11–1. Storage of Tissue or Extracted DNA

Tissue	Storage Requirements
Unextracted tissue	Room temperature
	4°C
	−25° to −195°C
	Fixed in alcohol or saline
Extracted DNA	Room temperature
	4°C
	Chloroform (5 μl/ml)
	Frozen (kept indefinitely)
Tissue lysate	Unextracted tissue placed in a solution of 100 mmol *Tris*-HCl, 40 mmol ethylenediamine tetraacetic acid, 0.2% sodium dodecylsulfate (pH 8.0)

jected to gel electrophoresis, and blotted onto a nitrocellulose filter (see section on molecular biology, earlier). Hybridization using either multilocus or single-locus VNTR probes may then be performed; which probes to use depends on the type of information required. Multilocus VNTR probes produce a complex banding pattern for each individual (see Fig. 11–4) and are used for paternity determination and to resolve questions of relatedness. Single-locus probes produce a maximum of two bands, which represent the two alleles at a given gene locus. Several single-locus probe analyses can be performed to provide data on several genetic loci and can usually include or exclude a sexual assailant suspect. The sensitivity and specificity of VNTR analysis depends on the clarity of the DNA-banding pattern, which is directly related to the quality of the DNA and to the quality control program implemented by each laboratory.[16]

SINGLE-LOCUS POLYMORPHISM

Unfortunately, recently ejaculated seminal specimens are not always recoverable from a crime scene. In some cases, victims do not seek medical treatment until several days after the assault; in other cases, the assailant does not ejaculate in the vagina or does not ejaculate at all. In these cases, degraded seminal specimens, fingernail scrapings, or hair samples may provide the only recoverable DNA from the assailant. In these cases the amount of DNA is often small and not amenable to multilocus or single-locus VNTR analysis, but single-locus polymorphism probes can be used to exclude sexual assailant suspects.[22]

Single-locus polymorphism probes identify deletions, additions, or inversions at specific sites in the genome, the presence or absence of which may differ between individuals.[23] These probes may be applied to small or degraded DNA specimens, and Southern blot and dot blot techniques both may be used in the analyses. The dot blot technique, similar to Southern blot but without the electrophoresis, is especially useful because it depends simply on hybridization of a probe and a DNA sample. Thus, dot blots provide data sooner and are less costly than Southern blots. Despite the advantages of single-locus polymorphism probe analysis, the technique is not very specific and may require multiple probes to include or exclude suspects.[22]

STATISTICAL ANALYSIS

The principal question addressed by those who use molecular methods in cases of sexual assault is whether DNA obtained at the crime scene is the same as the DNA of a suspect. Statistical analysis thus is used to estimate the probability that DNA obtained at the crime scene is or is not that of a particular suspect. The analyst takes into account not only the frequency in the general population of the studied allele(s) but also the probability that the alleles analyzed are sufficient to include or exclude suspects. Selection of specific statistical methods thus depends on what data are available and what information is being sought. Statistical tests used in forensic medicine have been reviewed by Kirby.[16]

LEGAL CONSIDERATIONS

Despite the relatively wide acceptance of DNA analysis by civil and criminal courts, the limitations previously mentioned have served to prevent universal admissibility of molecular biology results into criminal and civil legal proceedings. DNA forensic technology is relatively new[9] and the data generated by DNA techniques are considered novel and are not always accepted as evidence. For novel scientific data to be admitted as evidence in a court of law, they usually must pass two "tests"—the Frye test and the relevancy test. The Frye test[24] is based on the case *Frye v. United States*,[25] in which the District of Columbia Court of Appeals decided, ". . . the thing from which the deduction is made must be sufficiently established to have gained general acceptance in the particular field to which it belongs." The Frye test thus is meant to assure that only data resulting from reliable scientific tests are admitted as evidence. Once data from a novel scientific diagnostic test are admitted as evidence in a certain legal jurisdiction, similar data can in the future be admitted *in that particular jurisdiction* without the need to demonstrate further the reliability of the method. Without universal standards and guidelines, data from DNA analyses resulting from different DNA techniques or generated by different laboratories may be required to "pass" another Frye test within a certain legal jurisdiction that may have already admitted, as evidence, similar DNA analyses performed in a different laboratory.

The relevancy test asserts that novel scientific data are similar to other expert testimony,[26] allowing the data to be admitted but also allowing them to be ". . . attacked by cross-examination and refutation."[27] The relevancy approach neither accepts nor refutes the Frye test; rather, it permits judges more latitude in accepting such evidence. The relevancy approach has been promulgated by some Federal jurisdictions. The Third Circuit Court of Appeals held, ". . . some scientific evidence can assist the trier of fact in reaching an accurate determination of facts in issue even though the principles underlying the evidence have not become generally accepted in the field to which they belong." Such rulings permit parties to attempt refutation of the findings of DNA analysis based on demonstration of one or several of the aforementioned limitations.

As more legal jurisdictions accept molecular biology methods as commonplace, data generated by DNA analysis will be utilized more easily in criminal and civil cases, although such data may not be considered "relevant" if discrepancies in the analysis or its interpretation are demonstrated in court. Only strict, universal quality control standards for all aspects of DNA analysis,[17] like those currently in place for forensic blood protein tests, will serve to ensure that information generated by DNA analysis will truly be representative of the individuals involved and thus properly utilized to assess innocence or guilt.

MOLECULAR GENETICS IN THE STUDY OF SEXUAL DIFFERENTIATION

Pediatric and adolescent gynecologists are frequently called upon to evaluate abnormal sexual differentiation and genital tract anomalies. Although sexual differentiation involves a complex interaction of genetic, hormonal, and environmental influences, genetics plays an increasing role in the diagnosis of sexual ambiguity and genital tract anomalies. In this section, we review recent advances in the molecular genetics of sexual differentiation.

NORMAL SEX DIFFERENTIATION: THE SRY GENE

It is well-known that the Y chromosome determines sex (the embryo becomes a male in the presence of the Y and a female in its absence), but it is not known how this is accomplished. During the last quarter century, several Y-situated genes and sequences were candidates for the testis-determining gene *(TDF)*—among them, the *HYS* gene, which governs expression of the serologic H-Y ("male") antigen; the Bkm minisatellite, a tetranucleotide originally recovered from the sex-determining W chromosome

of the banded krait (a snake); the *ZFY* gene, which encodes a zinc finger protein; and the *SRY* gene, which encodes a protein with a conservative DNA-binding motif.

Among those sequences,[28] the *SRY* gene was shown to be the long sought testis determinant. It is highly conservative: *SRY*-like sequences are found in a broad spectrum of vertebrate species, including representatives of five major classes.[5, 29] The *SRY* gene contains a conservative motif of 80 amino acids that have "striking" homology to part of the Mc mating-type protein of the fission yeast *Schizosaccharomyces pombe*, and to a DNA-binding motif found in the nuclear high-mobility group proteins, HMG1 and HMG2. The mouse homolog *(Sry)* is located in the smallest region of the mouse Y chromosome known to induce the testis and is deleted in a line of XY females. It is expressed in the gonadal ridge of the mouse embryo precisely at the time of testicular development, and its transcription is curtailed after formation of the seminiferous tubules. It is expressed in the somatic cells of the gonad, not in the germ cells (presence of germ cells is not a prerequisite of testicular differentiation). Also, microinsertion of a 14-kb segment of DNA containing *Sry* evoked development of testes in at least some transgenic XX mice.[30] Further evidence of a testis-determining role for *SRY* was provided in cases of sex reversal in humans. For example, mutations and deletions of *SRY* were found in certain women with XY gonadal dysgenesis (characterized by failure of testicular differentiation, presence of streak gonads, and primary amenorrhea).

Some 80% of women with XY gonadal dysgenesis have *SRY* genes that are indistinguishable from those of normal males, at least with respect to the conservative region. This finding, together with other data that we now summarize, provides evidence of roles for other genes in testicular organogenesis and insight into the nature of primary (gonadal) sex determination. Thus, absence of *SRY* in certain XX males[31] argues for unregulated expression of "downstream" X-linked or autosomal testis-determining genes, and presence of apparently intact *SRY* genes in (most) women with XY gonadal dysgenesis argues for mutation in those same genes. Indeed, X-linked and autosomal transmission is indicated in familial cases of XY gonadal dysgenesis, and X-chromosome rearrangements have been correlated with failure of testicular development in persons with Gardner-Silengo-Wachtel (genitopalatocardiac) syndrome.

AUTOSOMAL GENES IN XY GONADAL DYSGENESIS

According to the scheme advanced by Wolf et al,[32] the structural genes for testicular differentiation are on an autosome, are repressed by genes in the noninactivated part of the X, and are derepressed by a gene on the Y. It follows that some forms of XY gonadal dysgenesis are due to failure of the autosomal genes and are transmitted as autosomal recessive traits. After excluding kindreds with likely X-linked inheritance, Simpson et al[33] evaluated segregation ratios in 24 families. Among those were twelve with a single case of XY gonadal dysgenesis, six with two cases, and six with three cases. Although X-linked recessive and male-limited autosomal dominant transmission could not be ruled out, the frequency of affected relatives was no different from the frequency that would be expected were the condition inherited as an autosomal recessive trait limited to XY embryos. Moreover, autosomal genes would seem likely in the etiology of XY gonadal dysgeneis because the majority of cases seem to arise sporadically.

In fact, two autosomal sex-reversing genes have now been suggested, one on chromosome 17 and one on chromosome 9. Some infants with campomelic dysplasia are XY females. Study of de novo reciprocal translocations in three such cases enabled assignment of the autosomal sex-reversal locus *SRA1* to 17q24.3—q25.1.[33–35] As for the corresponding locus on chromosome 9, partial monosomy for the short arm of chromosome 9 in at least seven cases of XY sex reversal has allowed assignment of another sex-determining locus in 9p24.1—pter.[36, 37]

X-LINKED GENES IN XY GONADAL DYSGENESIS

Several cases of XY gonadal dysgenesis can be attributed directly to failure of X-linked genes. Among the familial cases surveyed by Simpson et al,[33] X-linked recessive inheritance was demonstrated in four.[38] The last family, described by Mann et al,[39] included three affected sisters, an affected maternal second cousin, and a maternal aunt. The maternal grandmother of the affected siblings had a sister who was infertile and presumed to be an XY female. The maternal great grandmother had three infertile sisters, each presumed to be an affected XY female.

As noted above, rearrangements of the X chromosome have been detected in cases of the Gardner-Silengo-Wachtel syndrome, which in-

volves sex reversal in XY female infants with multiple congenital abnormalities.[40] For example, Bernstein et al[41] described an anomalous additional band in the short arm of the X chromosome in a profoundly retarded girl whose somatic features included ventricular septal defect, cleft palate, asymmetry of skull and facies, etc. The initial karyotype, 46,Xp+Y, represented a duplication of part of the short arm [46,dup(X)(p21-pter)Y].

When the child died at 5 years of age, necropsy disclosed hypoplastic uterus and tubes. Ovaries could not be detected macroscopically, but histologic examination of the uterine adnexa revealed a small focus of ovarian stroma with scattered degenerative follicles. There was no sign of testicular architecture. The external genitalia were those of a normal female. When amniocentesis revealed the abnormal 46,Xp+Y karyotype in fetal cells during a later pregnancy, the parents elected to abort the fetus at 20 weeks of gestation. The fetus, a phenotypic female, exhibited the various abnormalities observed in the proband, but the fetal gonads were normal ovaries with numerous follicles and germ cells.

Similar findings have been reported by Stern et al[42] in a single infant and by Scherer et al[43] in sisters. More recently, Arn et al[44] described maternal half siblings with ambiguous external genitalia and a small duplication in the segment Xp21.2–p22.11. On that basis, a "new" gene, *SRVX (sex reversal X)*, was assigned to the segment. Soon after, Bardoni et al[45] narrowed the locus of the gene (which they called *DSS* for *dosage-sensitive sex reversal*) to a 160-kb segment in Xp21 overlapping the *adrenal hypoplasia* locus. Further study of the region revealed a candidate gene for *DSS* called *DAX-1 (DSS-AHC critical region on the X chromosome, gene 1)*.[46] Although duplication at the *DSS (DAX-1)* locus can block male development in an XY embryo, the relevant gene is not a regular part of the male-determining cascade because absence of *DSS* does not interfere with testicular differentiation.

GENETICS OF TESTICULAR DIFFERENTIATION: SUMMARY

In aggregate, these data indicate the existence of at least three genes in a differentiative pathway that culminates in organization of the fetal testis. One of the genes, *SRY*, is situated on the Y chromosome; two are autosomal. A simple scheme would have the primary switch on the Y chromosome. Accordingly, *SRY* would encode a protein that binds to and activates another gene or group of genes. In fact, the SRY protein recognizes and binds a short sequence in the *MIS* (*müllerian-inhibiting substance*) gene, thereby bending the sequence and activating transcription of *MIS*.[47]

Failure or deletion of any of the genes in the testis-determining pathway would result in the formation of an XY ovary, which would degenerate to be replaced by a streak gonad (XY gonadal dysgenesis). Translocation of the *SRY* gene to an X, or activation of the downstream autosomal genes in the absence of the Y, would result in an XX testis.

When duplicated, a fourth gene, *DSS*, situated on the X chromosome, can block normal differentiation of the testis. This gene may have a role in ovarian differentiation.[45–47] A candidate for *DSS* has been described. Called *DAX-1*, it overlaps *AHC* and resembles genes in the nuclear hormone receptor family. Like *SRY*, it encodes a protein that regulates transcription. A representative scheme for sex determination in the human is shown in Figure 11–6.

OVARY-DETERMINING GENES

It seems reasonable to assume that ovarian differentiation is also under genetic control, but,

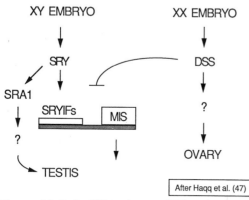

Figure 11–6. In XY embryos, SRY activates autosomal genes such as *SRA1* and other yet to be named genes in chromosome 9p. This leads ultimately to development of the testis. In addition, SRY produces a factor or factors (SRYIF) that bind the müllerian inhibition substance (MIS) gene; this leads to production by testicular Sertoli cells of MIS. The X-linked DSS gene (*DAX-1*) may play a role in differentiation of the ovary.[45–47] When duplicated in XY embryos, DSS blocks normal differentiation of the testis, causing the syndrome of XY gonadal dysgenesis.[47] (After Haqq CM, King C-Y, Ukiyama E. et al: Molecular basis of mammalian sexual determination. Science 1994; 266:1494.)

except for the possible involvement of *DSS*, the genes responsible for development of the female gonad have not been identified. Human embryos with the 45,X karyotype (indicating loss of a second sex chromosome) develop the characteristic features of Turner syndrome—short stature, epicanthal folds, high-arched palate, low nuchal hairline, webbed neck, shieldlike chest, coarctation of the aorta, ventricular septal defect, etc. As in cases of 46,XY gonadal dysgenesis, the gonads commence development as ovaries, but, in the absence of the second X chromosome, the ovaries degenerate and are replaced at around the time of birth or shortly thereafter by streak gonads, which have no endocrine activity. This indicates occurrence of noninactivated X-linked genes that are critical for the maintenance of the ovary.[48]

Besides X-linked genes, certain autosomal genes may be required for maintenance of the ovary, because autosomal inheritance is indicated in certain forms of gonadal dysgenesis in females with a "normal" 46,XX karyotype. In some families, one sibling may exhibit gonadal dysgenesis and another, primary amenorrhea with extreme ovarian hypoplasia. In other cases, XX gonadal dysgenesis may occur in subjects with severe somatic anomalies. An example is Perrault syndrome, in which XX gonadal dysgenesis and neurosensory deafness are combined.[48]

GENETIC CONTRIBUTIONS TO NORMAL AND ABNORMAL FEMALE GENITAL TRACT DEVELOPMENT

Normal development of the female reproductive tract involving proper differentiation of the müllerian ducts and the urogenital sinus depends on complex interaction between genetic, hormonal, and environmental factors. Disruption of this interaction can result in a wide spectrum of genital tract abnormalities, including imperforate hymen, vaginal septa, vaginal atresia, incomplete müllerian fusion, and müllerian aplasia. These may be isolated anomalies or associated with others. Moreover, several mendelian disorders include abnormalities of the female reproductive tract as a component of their phenotypic expression.

Müllerian tract abnormalities may result in gynecologic problems in pediatric and adolescent patients requiring assessment, diagnosis, and treatment. Here, we review the genetic factors that contribute to müllerian or wolffian duct anomalies in young girls; diagnosis and management of müllerian duct abnormalities are reviewed in Chapter 7.

EMBRYOLOGY

There are two pairs of primordial genital ducts in the human embryo, the wolffian, or *mesonephric*, ducts and the müllerian, or *paramesonephric*, ducts. One pair persists in each sex, and one pair regresses. The wolffian ducts drain the mesonephric kidneys, which disappear at 11 to 12 weeks of fetal development. In XY embryos, under the influence of androgens secreted by the newly differentiated testis, the wolffian ducts form the epididymis, ductus deferens, and ejaculatory duct.[49] In the absence of androgens or in androgen-insensitive embryos, the wolffian ducts fail to differentiate and instead regress, leaving behind only small remnants. Unlike müllerian duct regression, which requires the MIS, wolffian duct regression does not require a specific substance. Rather, it occurs in the absence of androgens.

The müllerian ducts develop as invaginations on the lateral surface of the wolffian ducts. The superior portions of the müllerian ducts remain separate and eventually form the fallopian tubes. The inferior portions become the Y-shaped uterovaginal primordium, consisting of a uterine segment and a vaginal segment.[50]

The external genitalia arise from a common, undifferentiated primordium. At 4 weeks of fetal development, a genital tubercle with lateral labioscrotal and urogenital folds appears at the cranial end of the cloacal membrane. The genital tubercle elongates to become a phallus, equally long in males and females. In the absence of dihydrotestosterone (DHT, a 5α-reductase metabolite of testosterone), the growth of the phallus slows considerably and the genital tubercle forms the clitoris, the urogenital folds do not fuse (they form the labia minora[51]) and the labioscrotal folds become the labia majora. The vaginal vestibule, into which the urethra, vagina, and vestibular ducts open, arises from the cavernous tissue derived from walls of the urogenital sinus.[50]

CLINICAL PRESENTATION AND EVALUATION

Genital abnormalities cause significant psychological and emotional duress for affected children and their families. Intensive diagnostic testing is often necessary. Symptomatic abnormalities frequently require surgical repair. Although most female genital abnormalities are sporadic, an important part of the diagnostic evaluation of affected girls and women should be a detailed family history, as familial clustering of particular abnormalities or associated ones is useful in formulating a correct diagnosis and in assessing risk for other family members and offspring of affected persons.

Most patients with müllerian and urogenital sinus anomalies undergo normal secondary sexual development and present because of amenorrhea or abnormal menses. This is because müllerian and urogenital anomalies are end-organ abnormalities and, therefore, not often associated with mutations of the primary sex-determining genes. Thus, these patients usually have normal levels of sex steroids and regulatory hormones. However, genital tract abnormalities that are a result of sex chromosome abnormalities may be associated with gonadal dysgenesis.

Most forms of isolated müllerian duct and urogenital sinus abnormalities are inherited in polygenic/multifactorial fashion (mendelian forms of isolated müllerian duct abnormalities are discussed below). In addition, some müllerian duct abnormalities may be a component of a mendelian multiple malformation syndrome. Next, we discuss the genetics of specific müllerian duct abnormalities (those that occur only sporadically are not included).

SPECIFIC FEMALE GENITAL TRACT ABNORMALITIES

Fusion of the Labia Minora

In girls, agglutination of the labia minora usually follows genital infection or trauma resulting from sexual abuse. Congenital fusion of the labia minora is a rare occurrence that has been reported in siblings and in several families.[52, 53]

Imperforate Hymen

The hymen usually ruptures spontaneously during the prenatal period, permitting outflow of mucus during the prepubescent period and menstruum at menarche. When the hymen is imperforate, accumulation of mucus (hydrocolpos) and blood (hematocolpos) within the vagina or blood within the uterus (hematometra) occurs. Although affected siblings have been described,[54] most cases are isolated events.

Transverse Vaginal Septa

Transverse vaginal septa are believed to arise from a failure in fusion and/or canalization of the urogenital sinus and/or müllerian duct derivatives. Two observations support this statement: (1) septa usually occur at predicted sites of fusion of the müllerian and urogenital sinus derivatives, and (2) cranial surfaces of septa are lined with columnar (müllerian) epithelium, whereas caudal surfaces are lined by squamous (urogenital sinus) epithelium.[55] Although transverse vaginal septa usually occur sporadically, McKusick et al[56, 56a] (MIM#236700)* have described an autosomal recessive disorder in the Amish population in which affected females have transverse vaginal septa in addition to ophthalmic (congenital cataracts) and orthopedic (severe scoliosis, unilateral absence of the leg) abnormalities. Kaufman et al[57] reported another autosomal recessive disorder (MIM#236700)* in which affected patients have not only transverse vaginal septa but also congenital heart disease and postaxial polydactyly. This disorder has not been reported among the Amish.

Longitudinal Vaginal Septa

Vaginal septa also occur in the longitudinal axis, either in a coronal or sagittal orientation. Unlike transverse septa, longitudinal septa probably do not arise from fusion or canalization abnormalties but rather from abnormal mesodermal proliferation or persistence of epithelium during canalization.[55] Like transverse septa, most longitudinal septa occur sporadically in the population. However, Edwards and Gale[58] described an autosomal dominant syndrome (MIM#114150) characterized by longitudinal vaginal septa, urinary tract anomalies, and hand abnormalities (camptobrachydactyly). Johanson and Blizzard[59] described an autosomal recessive disorder (MIM#243800) involving longitudinal vaginal septa, aplastic nasal ala, microcephaly, deafness, hypothyroidism, skeletal dysplasia, and gastrointestinal malabsorption.

Vaginal Atresia

Vaginal atresia occurs when the urogenital sinus fails to contribute to the inferior portion of

---

*MIM# refers to the reference number describing the appropriate mendelian disorder found in McKusick VL: Mendelian Inheritance in Man. Baltimore: Johns Hopkins University Press 1991.

the vagina. The lower portion of the vagina is thus replaced by fibrous tissue, above which well-developed müllerian structures are usually found. Like both types of vaginal septa, most cases occur sporadically. Nonetheless, vaginal atresia may be part of an autosomal recessive syndrome consisting of renal, genital, and middle ear anomalies (MIM#267400). Winter and colleagues[60] and Turner[61] have described families whose female siblings exhibited vaginal atresia, anomalies of the ossicles of the middle ear, and varying degrees of renal dysgenesis.

Müllerian Aplasia

Müllerian aplasia, often called *Mayer-Rokitansky-Kuster-Hauser* syndrome, is the congenital absence or hypoplasia of the fallopian tubes, uterine corpus, uterine cervix, and proximal vagina.[62–65] Müllerian aplasia must be distinguished from vaginal atresia, a condition in which the distal vagina is replaced by fibrous tissue but normal müllerian structures lie superior to the vaginal aplasia (Fig. 11–7). Because ovarian function is usually unaffected, girls with müllerian aplasia undergo normal secondary sexual development but lack uterine enlargement and menarche. The blind-ending vagina is shortened to 1–2 cm and is derived totally from invagination of the urogenital sinus.[55] In addition to abnormality of the müllerian duct derivatives, a large percentage of patients with müllerian aplasia exhibit urologic and skeletal abnormalities. Duncan et al[66] suggested that the aforementioned müllerian, renal, and cervicospinal abnormalities be grouped in a distinctive, nonrandom association known as MURCS (*m*üllerian, *r*enal, *c*ervicospinal).

Most patients with müllerian aplasia have a 46,XX karyotype, but some exhibit sex chromosome mosaicism (45,X/46,XX; 46,XX/47,XXX)[67] or deletions in the short arm of a G-group autosome.[68] Although familial aggregates of müllerian aplasia have been described,[69, 70] the mode of inheritance is still unclear. Lischke[71] reviewed three families in which monozygotic twins were discordant, making autosomal recessive inheritance unlikely. Shokeir[72] proposed sex-limited (female) autosomal dominant inheritance based on his study of 16 families in Saskatchewan. Yet Carson et al[73] found no other affected relatives among the families of 23 probands, an observation that suggests multifactorial/polygenic inheritance. These discrepant results could be explained by genetic heterogeneity (i.e., expression of a different gene or group of genes could result in similar phenotypes). The MURCS anomalad

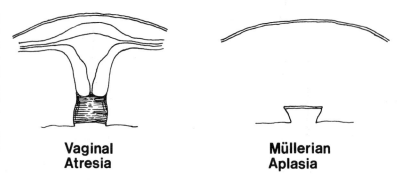

Figure 11–7. Müllerian aplasia. Diagrammatic comparison of vaginal atresia and müllerian aplasia. Vaginal abnormality is a cardinal feature of both disorders. (From Shulman LP, Elias S: Developmental abnormalities of the female reproductive tract: Pathogenesis and nosology. Adolesc Pediatr Gynecol 1988; 1:230.)

Vaginal Atresia

Müllerian Aplasia

usually occurs sporadically. Greene and coworkers[74] reported a family in which the MURCS anomalad was identified in several female members.

Incomplete Müllerian Fusion

Incomplete müllerian fusion results in a spectrum of anomalies that includes unicornuate uterus, arcuate uterus, subseptate uterus, septate uterus, uterus bicornis unicollis (bicornuate uterus), uterus bicornis bicollis, and the didelphic uterus (completely separate hemiuteri, each of which leads to a separate cervix and vagina) (Fig. 11–8). Most retrospective surveys estimate the prevalence of incomplete fusion at around 0.1%,[75, 76] but obstetricians who have explored uteri immediately after delivery have reported a

prevalence of 2% to 3%.[77, 78] Among the latter studies, a relatively large percentage of affected patients exhibited an arcuate or subseptate uterus, anomalies oftentimes difficult to detect except in the immediate postpartum period.

Although familial aggregates of incomplete müllerian fusion have been described,[79] the only formal genetic analysis was reported by Elias et al,[80] who sought to determine the frequency with which symptomatic müllerian fusion anomalies occurred in relatives of a small but genetically unbiased sample of 24 probands. Only one of 37 (2.7%) female siblings older than 16 appeared to have a symptomatic uterine anomaly; none of 24 mothers, 45 maternal aunts, or 50 paternal aunts were affected. This low frequency of affected relatives is more consistent with polygenic/multifactorial causes than with other genetic causes.

Incomplete müllerian fusion can also be a

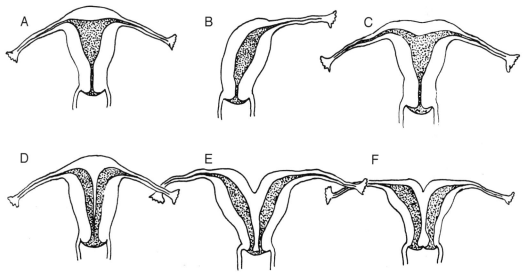

Figure 11–8. Incomplete müllerian fusion. Diagrammatic representation of the spectrum of anomalies of müllerian fusion: *A*, normal uterus; *B*, uterus unicornis (unicornate uterus); *C*, uterus arcuatus (arcuate uterus); *D*, uterus septus (septate uterus); *E*, uterus bicornis unicollis (bicornuate uterus); *F*, uterus didelphys (didelphic uterus). (From Shulman LP, Elias S: Developmental abnormalities of the female reproductive tract: Pathogenesis and nosology. Adolesc Pediatr Gynecol 1988; 1:230.)

component of a multiple malformation syndrome. Fraser syndrome (MIM#219000) is an autosomal recessive disorder characterized by cryptophthalmos, middle and outer ear malformations, hypertelorism, laryngeal stenosis, and syndactyly. Affected females may also have a bicornuate uterus.[81] The hand-foot-genital (HFG) syndrome (MIM #140000) is an autosomal dominant disorder in which patients exhibit skeletal abnormalities of the hands and feet (small feet, short great toes, abnormal thumbs, clinodactyly), hypospadias and displaced urethral meatus in affected males, and incomplete müllerian fusion anomalies, urinary incontinence, and malposition of ureteral orifices in affected females.[82] Like other dominantly inherited disorders, HFG syndrome demonstrates considerable variation in expression among affected family members.

Persistence of Müllerian Structures in Males

Persistence of uterus and fallopian tubes in males is due to absence or mutation of the MIS or its receptor. Affected males usually present with inguinal hernias, cryptorchidism, and/or infertility. Diagnosis is frequently made at the time of surgical intervention, when rudimentary or developed müllerian duct derivatives are discovered. Nilson[83] reported the first case in 1939; subsequently, familial aggregates were reported.[84, 85] Study of the familial aggregates revealed recessive inheritance, although it is not clear whether it is autosomal or X-linked.[86]

REFERENCES

1. Watson JD, Tooze J, Kurtz DT: Recombinant DNA. New York: WH Freeman, 1983.
2. Berger SL, Kimmel AR: Guide to Molecular Cloning Techniques. San Diego: Academic, 1987.
3. Simpson JL, Golbus MS, Martin AO, Sarto GE: Genetics in Obstetrics and Gynecology. New York: Grune & Stratton, 1982.
4. Southern EM: Detection of specific sequences among DNA fragments separated by gel electrophoresis. J Molec Biol 1975; 98:503.
5. Sinclair AH, Berta P, Palmer MS, et al: A gene from the human sex-determining region encodes a protein with homology to a conserved DNA-binding motif. Nature 1990; 346:244.
6. Koopman P, Münsterberg A, Blanche C, et al: Expression of a candidate sex-determining gene during mouse testis differentiation. Nature 1990; 348:450.
7. Maxam A, Gilbert W: A new method for sequencing DNA. Proc Nat Acad Sci USA 1977; 74:560.
8. Sanger F, Nicklen S, Coulson AR: DNA sequencing with chain-terminating inhibitors. Proc Nat Acad Sci USA 1977; 74:5463.
9. Jeffreys AJ, Brookfield JFY, Semenoff R: Positive identification of an immigration test-case using human DNA fingerprints. Nature 1985; 317:818.
10. Jeffreys AJ, Wilson V, Thein SL: Individual-specific 'fingerprints' of human DNA. Nature 1985; 316:76.
11. Lander ES: Research on DNA typing catching up with courtroom application (Invited editorial). Am J Hum Genet 1991; 48:819.
12. Budowle B, Giusti AM, Waye JS, et al: Fixed-bin analysis for statistical evaluation of continuous distributions of allelic data from VNTR loci for use in forensic comparisons. Am J Hum Genet 1991; 48:841.
13. Saiki RK, Scharf S, Faloona F, et al: Enzymatic amplification of β-globin sequences and restriction site analysis for diagnosis of sickle cell anemia. Science 1985; 37:170.
14. Erlich HA: PCR Technology. Principles and Applications for DNA Amplification. New York: Stockton, 1989.
15. King M-C: An application of DNA sequencing to a human rights problem. In Friedmann T (ed): Molecular Genetic Medicine. San Diego: Academic, 1991, pp 117–134.
16. Kirby LT: DNA Fingerprinting: An Introduction. New York: Stockton, 1990.
17. Mudd JL, Hartmann JM, Kuo MC, et al: Guidelines for a quality assurance program for DNA restriction fragment length polymorphism analysis. Crime Lab Digest 1989; 16:41.
18. Chandley AC, Mitchell AR: Hypervariable minisatellite regions are sites for crossing-over at meiosis in man. Cytogenet Cell Genet 1988; 48:152.
19. Jeffreys AJ: Highly variable minisatellites and DNA fingerprints. Biochem Soc Trans 1987; 15:309.
20. Jeffreys AJ, Royle NJ, Wilson V, et al: Spontaneous mutation rates to new length alleles at tandem-repetitive hypervariable loci in human DNA. Nature 1988; 332:278.
21. Royle NJ, Clarkson RE, Wong Z, et al: Clustering of hypervariable minisatellites in the proterminal regions of human autosomes. Genomics 1988; 3:352.
22. Zumwalt RE: Application of molecular techniques to forensic pathology. In Fenoglio-Preiser CM, Willman CL (eds): Molecular Diagnostics in Pathology. Baltimore: Williams & Wilkins, 1991, pp 339–354.
23. Schumm JW, Knowlton R, Braman J, et al: Identification of more than 500 RFLPs by screening random genomic clones. Am J Hum Genet 1988; 42:143.
24. Levin R: DNA typing on the witness stand. Science 1989; 244:1033.
25. Frye v. United States. 293 F. 1013 (D.C. Cir 1923).
26. Comment. DNA Identification Tests and the Courts, 63 Wash L Rev 1988; 903, 905, n. 2.
27. United States v. Baller, 519 F. 2d463, 466 (4th Cir, 1975).
28. Wachtel SS, Tiersch TR: The search for the male-determining gene. In Wachtel SS (ed): Molecular Genetics of Sex Determination. San Diego: Academic, 1994, pp 1–22.
29. Tiersch TR, Mitchell MJ, Wachtel SS: Studies on the phylogenetic conservation of the SRY gene. Hum Genet 1991; 87:571.
30. Koopman P, Gubbay J, Vivian N, et al: Male development of chromosomally female mice transgenic for Sry. Nature 1991; 351:117.
31. Ferguson-Smith MA, North MA, Affara NA, et al: The secret of sex. Lancet 1990; 336:809.
32. Wolf U, Fraccaro M, Mayerová A, et al: A gene controlling H-Y antigen on the X chromosome. Hum Genet 1980; 54:149.
33. Simpson JL, Blagadowidow N, Martin AO: XY gonadal dysgenesis: Genetic heterogeneity based upon clinical observations, H-Y antigen status and segregation analysis. Hum Genet 1981; 58:91.

34. Tommerup N, Schempp W, Meinecke P, et al: Assignment of an autosomoal sex reversal locus *(SRA1)* and campomelic dysplasia *(CMPD1)* to 17q24.3–q25.1. Nature Genet 1993; 4:170.

35. Wagner T, Wirth J, Meyer J, et al: Autosomal sex reversal and campomelic dysplasia are caused by mutations in and around the SRY-related gene *SOX9*. Cell 1994; 79:1111.

36. MacDonald MT, Flejter W, Sheldon S, et al: XY sex reversal and gonadal dysgenesis due to 9p24 monosomy. Am J Med Genet 1997; 73:321.

37. Veitia R, Nunes M, Brauner R, et al: Deletions of distal 9p associated with 46,XY male to female sex reversal: Definition of the breakpoints at 9p23.3–p24.1. Genomics 1997; 41:271.

38. Wachtel SS, Simpson JL: XY sex reversal in the human. *In* Wachtel SS (ed): Molecular Genetics of Sex Determination. San Diego: Academic, 1994, pp 287–309.

39. Mann JL, Corkery JJ, Fisher HJW, et al: The X-linked recessive form of XY gonadal dysgenesis with a high incidence of gonadal germ cell tumors: Clinical and genetic studies. J Med Genet 1983; 20:264.

40. Greenberg F, Greesick MV, Carpenter RJ, et al: The Gardner-Silengo-Wachtel syndrome: Male pseudohermaphroditism with micrognathia, cleft palate, and conotruncal cardiac defect. Am J Hum Genet 1987; 26:59.

41. Bernstein R, Koo GC, Wachtel SS: Abnormality of the X chromosome in human 46,XY female siblings with dysgenetic ovaries. Science 1980; 207:768.

42. Stern HJ, Garrity AM, Saal HM, et al: Duplication of Xp21 and sex reversal: Insight into the mechanism of sex determination. Am J Hum Genet 1990; 47(Suppl):A41.

43. Scherer G, Schempp W, Baccichetti C, et al: Duplication of an Xp segment that includes the ZFX locus causes sex inversion in man. Hum Genet 1989; 81:291.

44. Arn P, Chen H, Tuck-Muller CM, et al: SRVX, a sex-reversing locus in Xp21.2–p22.11. Hum Genet 1994; 93:389.

45. Bardoni B, Zanaria E, Guiloi S, et al: A dosage sensitive locus at chromosome Xp21 is involved in male to female sex reversal. Nature Genet 1994; 7:497.

46. Zanaria E, Muscatelli F, Bardoni B, et al: An unusual member of the nuclear hormone receptor superfamily responsible for X-linked adrenal hypoplasia congenita. Nature 1994; 372:635.

47. Haqq CM, King C-Y, Ukiyama E, et al: Molecular basis of mammalian sexual determination: Activation of müllerian inhibiting substance gene expression by SRY. Science 1994; 266:1494.

48. Fisher E, Scambler P: Human haploinsufficiency — one for sorrow, two for joy. Nature Genet 1994; 7:5.

49. Gyllensten L: Contributions to embryology of the urinary bladder: Development of definitive relationships between openings of the wolffian ducts and the ureters. Acta Anat 1949; 7:305.

50. Bulmer D: The development of the human vagina. J Anat 1957; 91:490.

51. Jirasek JE: Atlas of Human Prenatal Morphogenesis. Boston: Martinus-Nijhoff, 1983, pp 64–68.

52. Sueiro MB, Piloto R: Aderencia incompleta dos pequinos labios com caracter familiar. Gaz Med Port 1963; 16:513.

53. Willman SP, Carr BR, Klein VR: Familial fusion of the labia minora (Abstract). Proc Greenwood Genet Center 1988; 7:140.

54. McIlroy DM, Ward IV: Three cases of imperforate hymen occurring in one family. Proc R Soc Med 1930; 23:633.

55. Simpson JL: Gynecologic disorders. *In* King RA, Rotter JI, Motulsky AG (eds): The Genetic Basis of Common Disease. Oxford: Oxford University Press, (in press).

56. McCusick VA, Weilbaecher RG, Gragg GW: Recessive inheritance of a congenital malformation syndrome. JAMA 1968; 204:111.

56a. McKusick VL: Mendelian Inheritance in Man. Baltimore: Johns Hopkins University Press, 1991.

57. Kaufman RL, Hartmann AF, McAlister WH: Family studies in congenital heart disease II: A syndrome of hydrometrocolpos, postaxial polydactyly and congenital heart disease. Birth Defects 1972; 8:85.

58. Edwards JA, Gale RP: Camptobrachydactyly: A new autosomal dominant trait with two probable homozygotes. Am J Hum Genet 1972; 24:464.

59. Johanson A, Blizzard R: A syndrome of congenital aplasia of the alae nasi, deafness, hypothyroidism, dwarfism, absent permanent teeth and malabsorption. J Pediatr 79; 982:1971.

60. Winter JSD, Kohn G, Mcllman WJ, et al: A familial syndrome of renal, genital and middle ear anomalies. J Pediatr 1968; 72:88.

61. Turner G: A second family with renal, vaginal and middle ear anomalies. J Pediatr 1970; 76:641.

62. Mayer G: Über Verdoppelungen des Uterus und ihre Arten, nebst Bemerkungen über Hasenscharte und Wolfsrachen. J Chir Auger 1829; 13:525.

63. Küster H: Uterus bipartitus solidus rudimentarius cum vagina solida. Z Geb Gyn 1910; 67:692.

64. Rokitansky H: Über die sogenannten Verdoppelungen des Uterus. Med J Öst Staat 1938; 26:39.

65. Hauser GA, Schreiner WE: Das Mayer-Rokitansky-Kuster syndrome. Schweiz Med Wochenschr 1961; 91:381.

66. Duncan PA, Shapiro LR, Klein RM: The MURCS association. Am J Obstet Gynecol 1987; 156:1554.

67. Stott RB, Cameron JS, Ogg CS, et al: XO/XX mosaicism in the Rokitansky-Kuster-Hauser syndrome. Lancet 1971; ii:1380.

68. Linquette M, Gasnault JP, Dupont-Lecompte J, et al: Le syndrome de Rokitansky-Kuster-Hauser et les syndromes voisins d'aplasie uterovaginale. Rev Fr Endocrinol Clin 1968; 9:41.

69. Anger D, Hemet J, Ensel J: Forme familial du syndrome de Rokitansky-Kuster-Hauser. Bull Fed Gynecol Obstet Franc 1966; 18:229.

70. Jones HW, Mermut S: Familial occurrence of congenital absence of the vagina. Am J Obstet Gynecol 1972; 114:1100.

71. Lischke JH, Curtis CH, Lamb EJ, et al: Discordance of vaginal agenesis in monozygotic twins. Obstet Gynecol 1973; 41:920.

72. Shokeir MHK: Aplasia of the müllerian system: Evidence for probable sex-limited autosomal dominant inheritance. Birth Defects 1978; 14:147.

73. Carson SA, Simpson JL, Malinak LR, et al: Heritable aspects of uterine anomalies. II. Genetic analysis of müllerian aplasia. Fertil Steril 1983; 40:86.

74. Greene RA, Bloch MJ, Huff DS, et al: MURCS association with additional congenital anomalies. Hum Pathol 1986; 17:88.

75. Simpson JL: Genetic aspects of gynecologic disorders occurring in 46,XX individuals. Clin Obstet Gynecol 1972; 15:157.

76. Semens JP: Congenital anomalies of female genital tract. Functional classification based on review of 56 personal cases and 500 reported cases. Obstet Gynecol 1962; 68:371.

77. Hay D: Uterus unicollis and its relationship to pregnancy. J Obstet Gynecol Br Emp 1961; 82:330.

78. Greiss FC, Manzy CH: Genital anomalies in women. An evaluation of diagnosis, incidence and obstetric performance. Am J Obstet Gynecol 1961; 82:330.

79. Verp MS, Simpson JL, Elias S, et al: Heritable aspects of uterine anomalies. I. Three familial aggregates with müllerian fusion anomalies. Fertil Steril 1983; 40:80.

80. Elias S, Simpson JL, Carson SA, et al: Genetic studies in incomplete müllerian fusion. Obstet Gynecol 1984; 63:276.

81. Fraser GR: Our genetical 'load.' A review of some aspects of genetical variation. Hum Genet 1962; 25:387.

82. Elias S, Simpson JL, Feingold M, et al: The hand-foot-uterus syndrome: A rare autosomal dominant disorder. Fertil Steril 1978; 9:239.

83. Nilson O: Hernia uteri inguinalis beim manne. Acta Chir Scand 1939; 83:231.

84. Sloan WR, Walsh CR: Familial persistent müllerian duct syndrome. J Urol 1976; 115:459.

85. Brook CGD, Wagner H, Zachmann M, et al: Familial occurrence of persistent müllerian structures in otherwise normal males. Br Med J 1973; 1:771.

86. Imperato-McGinley J, Peterson RE: Male pseudohermaphroditism: The complexities of male phenotypic development. Am J Med 1976; 61:251.

87. Mitchell MJ, Bishop CE: A structural analysis of the Sxr region of the mouse Y chromosome. Genomics 1992;12:26.

88. Demas S, Wachtel S: DNA fingerprinting in reptiles: Bkm hybridization patterns in Crocodilia and Chelonia. Genome 1991; 34:472.

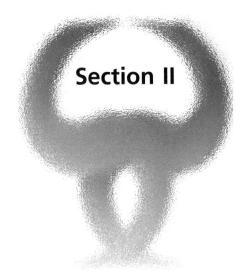

Section II

Medical Problems

ASSOCIATE EDITOR: DAVID MURAM

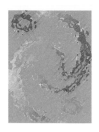

Chapter 12

Genital Examination of Prepubertal and Peripubertal Females

Susan F. Pokorny

The information in this chapter will not be put to its best use if the physician cannot adequately examine the child's reproductive organs, but the physician examining a young child should keep in mind that experiences related to the genitourinary and rectal area play a key role in a child's psychological development. Thus, the physician should consider the appropriateness of the examination, in terms of both the timing and the type of information sought with the examination. The full pelvic examination sequence applied to reproductive-aged women is never used in a prepubertal child, but there is no physical reason why, with proper physician skill and patient preparation, a speculum examination cannot be performed on a virginal adolescent.

APPROPRIATENESS OF THE EXAMINATION

EDUCATIONAL EXAMINATIONS

Prevailing thought in American culture is that the female genital system should be kept out of sight and out of mind until some magic moment when a woman should be knowledgeable about "womanly things."[1] This does not allow children to develop the cognitive skills they need to acknowledge early signs or symptoms of genital disorders, nor does it help them to ward off the coercive, clandestine advances of sexual molesters or abusers. With this in mind, it seems appropriate that all pediatric primary care providers include a detailed educational genital examination in each annual physical examination.

The child should be allowed to leave on undergarments until it is time for the genital examination, as this conveys the message that the genitals are a special area of the body. When it comes

time for the genital examination, the physician might say something like, "Now I'm going to check a special part of your body to see that everything is growing well." The examination can then be carried out, as described later in this chapter, and information obtained from the examination shared with both child and parent. Because children and young adolescents are concrete thinkers, it is *during the course of the examination* that the most meaningful information can be imparted.

During or immediately after the examination, it is important that the physician point out to the child that the examination was sanctioned by the parent or guardian, who was present. The physician might use this moment to explain to the child that no one else should attempt to examine or touch her genital area, and should that happen, she should inform a parent or guardian. Because children are concrete thinkers, they need this type of explicit instruction.[2]

By addressing issues referable to the genital area in an open and comfortable fashion, very often the physician is also providing the parent with vocabulary and communication skills that will sustain future parent-child dialogues about the child's reproductive system.

DIAGNOSTIC EXAMINATIONS

When a child is brought for a specific genital complaint, the physician starts with a patient history and then conducts a physical examination. Because genital symptoms are frequently presented in colloquialisms and anatomically incorrect terms, the physician will have to rely most on the physical examination for the diagnosis of most pediatric gynecologic disorders.

The physician planning a diagnostic genital

examination must look for features in the history that dictate what information should be obtained from the examination and the sequence in which such information is to be obtained. For example, not every 4-year-old girl with vaginal discharge needs to undergo vaginoscopy, but many do, particularly when the discharge is copious, bloody, or persistent. On the other hand, there is no reason to put a 4-year-old child with lichen sclerosus through a vaginal examination when the diagnosis can be made with external procedures.

Genital examination of the prepubertal child relies on obtaining the patient's compliance by promising to do her no physical harm. Occasionally, there is not enough time for the physician to develop rapport with the child and, thereby, her trust. For example, in cases of a penetrating perineal injury or a recent sexual assault, it is imperative that an examination be performed immediately, regardless of the child's compliance. In these situations, the physician should consider the appropriateness of an examination under anesthesia or heavy sedation. On the other hand, if the genital complaint is chronic or the injury clearly superficial, the physician can consider allowing a diagnostic examination to evolve over several sessions (i.e., sequential examinations).

The timing between sequential examinations will also be dictated by certain aspects of the history. A history of bleeding at any time during the course of the illness that cannot be explained on the first examination dictates more urgent follow-up for further studies.[3] In contrast, the spacing of follow-up examinations for chronic vulvitis might be more leisurely, allowing time for removal of environmental contact irritants and for therapeutic trials of medications.

Because girls have low levels of circulating sex steroid hormones as compared with reproductive-aged women, it is important to remember that the vast majority of pediatric gynecology complaints will be related to growth, inflammation, lesions, or reactions of the skin and mucosa of the external genitalia or, to a lesser degree, of the mucosa of the vaginal canal. The cervix, uterus, and fallopian tubes are so hormonally inert and undeveloped that they are typically evaluated only when a neoplasm grows to a pathologically obvious size; colposcopy of the cervix and hysterosalpingography cannot be performed in children because of the small size of these structures. Likewise, the ovaries are not routinely evaluated unless signs and symptoms of a neoplastic or endocrine disorder are apparent.

The physician must decide which cases warrant only an external examination and which require visual inspection of the vaginal canal. If there is a history of bleeding and no cause has been found or there is persistent or recurrent infection, vaginoscopy is mandatory to rule out a foreign object or neoplasm.

PERFORMING AN ADEQUATE GENITAL EXAMINATION

GETTING THE CHILD TO COMPLY

Giving the child a sense of control over the examination and making a commitment not to cause discomfort sets the stage for obtaining as much information as possible and giving age-appropriate educational guidance (Table 12–1). If the child is being seen because of a genital complaint, it is advisable to have some idea of the area of the family's concern before contact with the patient. If too much time is spent obtaining a report of all the historical details of the complaint, the child will become restless and anxious. This history can be obtained most expeditiously by having the parent complete a questionnaire before the patient meets the physician. This questionnaire should include the following: the length of time the problem has existed; the pivotal issues, signs, or symptoms; the presence or absence of common environmental irritants; past treatments and diagnoses; skin and/or allergic conditions of the patient and/or family

Table 12–1. Suggestions for Genital Examinations of Young and Adolescent Girls

Obtain the patient's cooperation.
  This is necessary to create teachable moments and to afford adequate examinations.
Get the patient to comply.
  She must have control over the examination.
  She must be promised no physical pain.
  She must know what information is being sought.
Special measures in the prepubertal female's examination:
  Inform the child that the genital examination is sanctioned.
  Involve the child with a hand-held mirror and a magnification device.
  Position the child with her feet in the stirrups, on the examiner's lap, or sitting on a parent's lap. Drape her legs over the parent's thighs.
  Attempt to examine in both the supine and knee-chest positions.
  Be knowledgeable about the various spread methods to reveal the vestibule.
  Use instruments only when necessary.
Special aspects of the peripubertal genital examination:
  Understand the impact of estrogen.
  Take advantage of the stimulus phenomenon.
  Choose a speculum of proper width after the introitus is evaluated.

members; and recently prescribed medications not related to the complaint, particularly antibiotics. Occasionally, the physician will have to address earlier genital trauma in the child's history to elucidate a confusing array of symptoms and concerns. By keeping an open, nonjudgmental attitude the physician can detect caretaker practices that might be contributing to the child's signs and symptoms.[4]

The questionnaire allows the physician to move more rapidly to the examination itself and to concentrate on developing rapport with the child. The patient is much more likely to comply with the examination when the physician is able to explain succinctly to the child why the examination must be done and that it will not hurt her. A simple way of doing this is to say something like, "I understand your mother has some worries about your girl parts. Why don't we just look, and I'll tell you what I see."

Compliance for a genital examination in a premenarcheal child is greatly facilitated by the use of a hand-held mirror. The mirror can be held by the patient, a nurse, or the patient's parent so that the patient can see her external genitalia while the examination is being performed.

Before she removes her clothes, the patient can be shown the mirror and how it will allow her to see her genitalia. While the patient is sitting on the edge of the examination table or on her parent's lap, the physician or nurse can demonstrate how the patient can see her shoes or feet in the mirror. Once the patient knows how to do this, it is simple to slightly adjust the mirror so that she can see her external genital area. This can be described as a "trick to look around corners."

Once the child knows how the mirror will allow her to observe the examination, it is easy to get her to remove her clothing. A comment from the examiner about not being able to see through underpants is usually an adequate clue, and the patient will typically quickly remove her underclothing so that the examination can proceed.

Other methods have been described to reduce anxiety and gain the patient's cooperation. Muram and colleagues showed that videocolposcopy was well accepted by patients and significantly reduced their apprehension.[5] In another study, patients were randomized to one of three distraction techniques used during the genital examination: passive play (being read to), active play (singing, blowing bubbles), or viewing a movie through video eyeglasses. The study showed that levels of physical distress were lowest among children who used video glasses and highest among those randomly assigned to passive play (p = .02). Children randomized to video glasses also expressed higher levels of satisfaction than those randomized to active (p = .001) or passive (p = .05) play.[6]

When the child is to remove her underclothing, she should be offered a drape. Most young children will not request a drape and will not know how to use it without instructions. Nevertheless, by draping the child's lower body for the genital examination, the physician is again indicating to the child that the genital area is a special part of the body and that the physician has respect for any modesty the patient might have. The physician does not want to be so matter of fact about the examination that the child might stop in the waiting room to show everyone else the parts of her anatomy that the physician has just shown her. Draping symbolizes to the child that the physician-directed genital examination is a special situation.

POSITIONING THE CHILD FOR THE EXAMINATION

The ideal position for good visualization of the child's external genitalia is the supine position with the buttocks on the end of a gynecologic examination table. Her head should be elevated so that constant communication may be maintained with the examiner, who is positioned at the end of the table. The examiner should be comfortably seated and have adequate light. The child's feet can be placed in the gynecologic table stirrups or in the examiner's lap.

The child can also sit on her parent's lap with her legs spread open and draped across the parent's thighs. Ideally, the parent should sit, semireclined, on the end of the gynecologic table, with both feet in the stirrups. There are several advantages to this position: the parent can hold the mirror so that both he or she and the child can see the child's external genital area; the parent's arms enwrap and reassure the child; and the elevated position of the child makes the examination much easier.

After as much visual information as possible has been obtained from the supine frog-leg position, the child should be encouraged to assume the prone knee-chest position, preferably with her back slightly swayed. Although this is a more anxiety-provoking position and the child cannot watch the examination with the hand-held mirror, by retracting the perineal tissues laterally and superiorly a different, and sometimes more thorough, view of the hymen can be gained (Figs. 12–1, 12–2). The main advantage to this position, if the child cooperates and relaxes her abdominal muscles, is that more of the vaginal canal can be visualized than in the supine frog-leg position. Occasionally, with a well-focused light and when discharge or inflammation is minimal, the cervix can be identified at the vaginal apex.

THE NONCOMPLIANT CHILD

Occasionally a child is so traumatized by previous examinations or by sexual abuse that, even though all of the steps just prescribed are followed, she will not allow an external genital examination. At this point, if the examiner makes a particularly strong appeal to the child's "need to know that everything down there is okay," it is surprising how many eventually comply with the examination.

If the examiner has the impression that a child who was previously traumatized is being

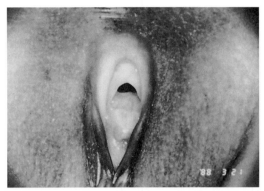

Figure 12–2. The same child shown in Figure 12–1 but in the knee-chest position. (From Pokorny SF: Pediatric gynecology. *In* Stenchever MA [Ed]: Office Gynecology. St. Louis: Mosby–Year Book, 1992, pp 106–135.)

manipulative, the child should be told that she may leave but that she cannot be assured that "everything is okay." The examiner might even leave the room to see other patients and give the victimized child time to reconsider and perhaps agree to the examination. Invariably, these children will position themselves to allow an external examination. A child who is extremely frightened should be allowed to use her own hands to spread the labia laterally so that the vaginal introitus can be visualized.

To force a genital examination on any child is saying, symbolically, that older and stronger persons have the right of access to that part of her body. Given the prevalence of abuse of children, this is not the message that should be communicated. An examination forced on a previously traumatized child might cause more psychological harm. Furthermore, no matter how many people restrain the child, the examination will be inadequate, as the perineum must be somewhat relaxed for adequate visualization of the hymen.

Sedation of an anxious, fearful child for a genital examination is frequently inadequate or requires a degree of sedation that is dangerous in most outpatient settings. Like a forced examination, an examination with inadequate sedation symbolizes to the child that older, stronger people have the right of access to the child's genital area without her permission, and opportunities to teach her otherwise are missed. When a pathologic condition is strongly suspected, an examination under anesthesia is usually warranted. When such a condition is unlikely or of minimal clinical consequence, it is advisable to continue to work sequentially with the patient on an out-

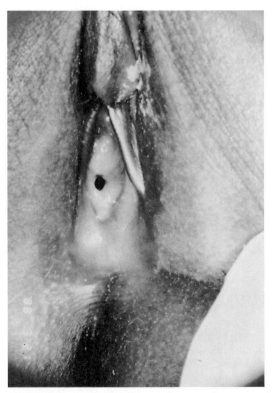

Figure 12–1. Appearance of normal external genitalia of a prepubertal female in the supine position using the lateral spread technique. (From Pokorny SF: Pediatric gynecology. *In* Stenchever MA [Ed]: Office Gynecology. St. Louis: Mosby–Year Book, 1992, pp 106–135.)

patient basis until an adequate examination can be completed.

Clearly, a noncompliant child taxes the patience of the examiner and everyone else involved. Nevertheless, the cultural message conveyed by, and the long-term therapeutic benefits obtained from, allowing the child to control the pace of the examination far outweigh the information obtained from a forced genital examination.

MAGNIFICATION AND DOCUMENTATION

The physician should not begin a genital examination of a prepubertal child without having available some means to magnify the tissue. The genital structures are small, and minute details are frequently needed to make a correct diagnosis and choose the proper therapeutic intervention. An otoscope with the truncated ear canal piece removed, a hand-held map-reading magnifying glass, operative microscopic eye loupes, a dermatologist's circular magnifying light, a colposcope, and a cervicoscope have all been used as magnifiers. The cost of the instrument, its easy use and mobility, and the setting for its use must all be considered. The colposcope and cervicoscope have photographic capabilities that are useful for documenting structures and lesions and that other instruments do not afford, but they are expensive and cumbersome to use.

The advantages of magnification—and the discipline required to document what is observed—enhance the visual acumen of the examiner. Physicians should approach the examination with the idea that they will be seeing normal genital structures that have the potential for individual, physiologic, and acquired variations.

All adequate genital examinations of the prepubertal child should be documented in the child's medical record with a detailed, labeled sketch of the external genitalia (Figs. 12–3, 12–4). This detailed sketch becomes part of a database from which to investigate future genital complaints.

A simple way to sketch findings is to start with a diamond-shaped space representing the vestibule of the child in the supine position; the clitoris would be positioned at 12:00 o'clock, the patient's left side at 3:00 o'clock, the posterior fourchette at 6:00 o'clock, and the patient's right side at 9:00 o'clock. The urethra and vaginal opening can be placed within the diamond space and lesions or other details placed accordingly.

This explicit detailed documentation of find-

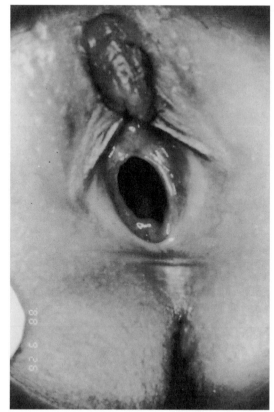

Figure 12–3. Vulva of a child showing a disruption of the hymen's posterior rim at the 6 o'clock position, associated with a small bump at the 7 o'clock position.

ings is extremely important for very young, preverbal children and for mentally or verbally handicapped children who cannot, should there ever be a need, make an "outcry" about sexual abuse. Documentation of baseline genital findings at a given point in time is invaluable should a future examination produce evidence of unexplained genital trauma.

VISUALIZING THE VESTIBULE

Usually, the small structures of the vestibule cannot be adequately evaluated unless the adjacent labia majora are spread laterally and posteriorly. By placing the index finger from each hand or the index and middle finger or thumb and index finger from one hand on both labia majora, lateral to the vestibule, and slightly posterior to the vaginal orifice, the examiner can usually spread the tissues laterally and posteriorly enough so that the vestibular structures can be

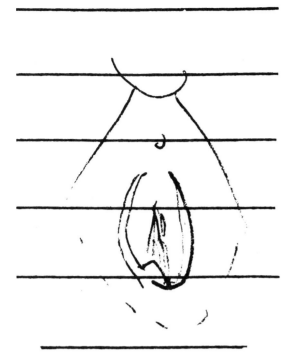

Figure 12–4. Example of how the vulva of a prepubertal child can be sketched in the medical record for documentation of minute details. This is a sketch from the medical record of the child in Figure 12–3.

adequately visualized. This is called the *supine lateral spread method* (Fig. 12–5).

If that attempt is inadequate, each labium major should be grasped gently in the same location used for the two-fingered method just described but using both hands. Gentle traction is placed on the labia, pulling toward the examiner and slightly posteriorly and laterally. While doing this, the examiner should continue to reassure the patient, being careful to not "pinch" the grasped labia. At the point of maximal traction, if the child is instructed to take a deep breath, the change in intraabdominal pressure so created will invariably allow the vestibular tissues to fan out so that the hymen and vaginal opening can be readily visualized. This is called the *supine lateral traction method*.

PHYSICAL FINDINGS

ANATOMIC STRUCTURES

The physical findings of the external genital examination should be recorded in standard, anatomically correct terms (Fig. 12–6). The *vulva* encompasses the mons, the labia majora, and

the vestibule; the *vestibule* is the externalized mucosal surface demarcated by the clitoris, the labia minora, Hart's line, and the posterior fourchette; the *perineal body* is the bridge of tissue between the vestibule and the rectum; the *perineum* encompasses all structures from the anterior mons or pubic symphysis, the lateral border of the labia majora or ischial tuberosities, and the posterior perirectal area or coccyx; *introitus* refers to a mouth or an opening, in this case, that to the vagina.

The most obvious landmark of the perineum of the prepubertal female is the clitoris. Because of extreme variability in both clitoral size and the subcutaneous adipose tissue of the mons pubis, the clitoris occasionally seems quite strikingly large. Once the clitoral complex is identified, the next most prominent structures are the labia minora. These raised, thin mounds form the lateral anterior margins of the vestibule and course toward the midline to meet under the clitoral complex. A thin, sharp apex of the labia minora is compatible with the atrophic state of most prepubertal females.

The vestibule is lined with glabrous epithelium. The vestibular sulcus between the vaginal orifice and the posterior fourchette, the fossa navicularis, can be deep, forming a considerable pocket, or shallow and almost nonexistent. The fossa navicularis and the lateral vestibular sulci are densely vascular; the density of capillaries in these areas makes them persistently erythematous.

The urethra is in the anterior vestibule. It might be a minute, pinpoint orifice, cleftlike, or

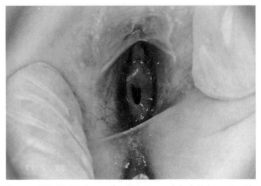

Figure 12–5. Vulva of a 3-year-old child; note the density of capillaries on the vestibular sulcus. (Erythema of the atrophic mucosa can be confused with inflammation.) Also note the bands and crypts of the minor vestibular glands in the periurethral sulcus. (From Pokorny SF: Physical examination of the reproductive systems of female children and adolescents. Curr Probl Obstet Gynecol Fertil 1990;13:202–213.)

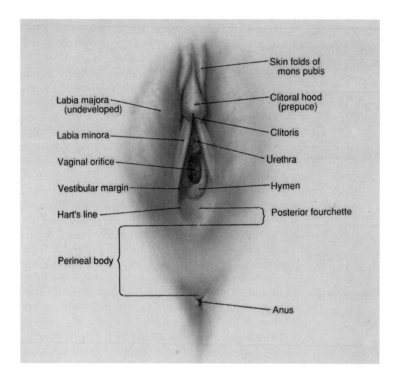

Labia majora (undeveloped)

Labia minora

Vaginal orifice

Vestibular margin

Hart's line

Perineal body

Skin folds of mons pubis

Clitoral hood (prepuce)

Clitoris

Urethra

Hymen

Posterior fourchette

Anus

Figure 12–6. External genitalia of the prepubertal female. The goal of the external genital examination is to identify all of these structures.

surrounded by a marked and variable amount of mucosa. At times it appears quite patulous. In the periurethral area, bands of tissue or deep crypts are frequently noted. The great variability in the appearance of these structures is caused by the minor vestibular glands.

Posterior to the urethra, with the child in the supine position, is the opening into the vagina. The vaginal orifice, or introitus, is surrounded by a collar of tissue called the *hymen*. Lateral and circumferential to the vaginal orifice is a sulcus in the vestibule. Crypts occur in this sulcus and are quite variable in their appearance. Again, these are the major vestibular glands; they are less apparent and not as common as those in the periurethral area.

In children with vulvovaginitis or marked estrogen depletion of the tissues, spreading the labial tissues laterally to visualize the vestibular structures sometimes creates a fissure in the superficial tissue of the posterior fourchette. Such lesions heal rapidly with warm tub-baths and removal of irritants.

ESTROGEN STATUS

Understanding the estrogen status of a young female is essential to determining how the genital examination is best performed. This determination is also important to arrive at an appropriate diagnosis and a treatment plan. Although

estrogen stimulation drops rapidly after birth (with separation from the maternal circulation), the newborn infant's gonadotropin level remains elevated for some time and the effect of estrogen on the vulvar tissues persists well into the third year of life. Capillaries cannot be seen in the estrogenized mucosa, which has a moist, whitish pink color.

From the toddler years until the peripubertal years (age 9 or 10), estrogen effect is minimal and the vulvovaginal mucosa is extremely thin and atrophic. "Road map" capillary beds should be visible. In areas where these capillaries are dense (i.e., the sulcus of the vestibule and very often the periurethral area), the tissue is erythematous and can be mistaken for inflammation. When inflammation is causing the erythema, tissue redness is more generalized and the mucosa thickened and edematous, to the extent of obscuring the capillary beds so easily seen in normal atrophic prepubertal mucosa.

THE HYMEN: VARIATIONS, CONFIGURATIONS, AND ALTERATIONS

Most hymenal membranes have a distinct orifice. In some cases the orifice is so small as to justify the term *microperforation* (Fig. 12–7). Another, more common, variation is the septate hymen (Fig. 12–8), marked by two distinct ori-

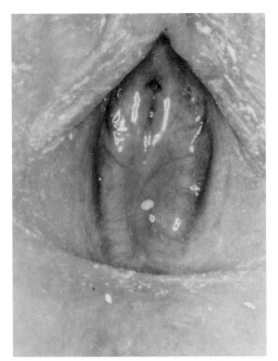

Figure 12–7. A seemingly imperforate hymen in a prepubertal female. A small probe was passed into the vagina via a microperforate opening in the suburethral area. (From Pokorny SF, Pokorny WJ: Pediatric gynecology. *In* Ashcraft KW, Holder TM [Eds]: Pediatric Surgery, 2nd ed. Philadelphia: WB Saunders, 1993, p 975.)

dinally septate vagina, which is often associated with müllerian duplication anomalies.

It is not uncommon, with sequential examinations, for a seemingly imperforate hymen ultimately to be discovered to be a microperforate hymen. Gentle probing with a small catheter or feeding tube in the suburethral area usually reveals a passage into the vagina. This usually requires no surgical intervention, since drainage is not impeded, and, under estrogen stimulation at puberty, many of these microperforations enlarge.

When an imperforate hymen is detected at birth because of a small hydrocolpos that does not extend above the pelvic brim, hymenotomy can be performed in the newborn nursery. The infant is held in the dorsal lithotomy position by assistants; local anesthetic is applied; a cruciform incision is made in the bulging membrane; and the redundant margins are excised. Because of the profusely "estrogenized" mucosa of the neonate, hemostasis is rarely a problem and can usually be managed by silver nitrate cauterization.

If imperforate hymen is suspected (Fig. 12–9) and the child shows no retention of secretions fices with an intervening bridge of tissue that usually runs in the anteroposterior direction but can also run from side to side or diagonally. It is important to distinguish a septate hymen, which has no association with upper reproductive tract müllerian duplication anomalies, from a longitu-

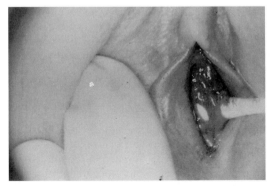

Figure 12–8. Septate hymen with a probe demonstrating that this is not a duplicate vagina. (From Pokorny SF: Pediatric gynecology. *In* Stenchever MA [Ed]: Office Gynecology. St. Louis: Mosby–Year Book, 1992, pp 106–135.)

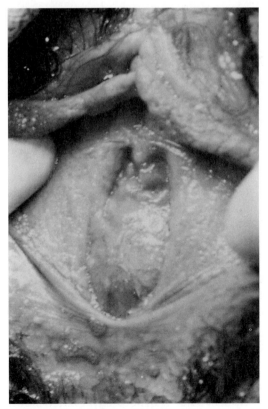

Figure 12–9. A bulging imperforate hymen with a hematocolpos in a 13-year-old girl.

(i.e., a hydromucocolpos), which can be easily detected on rectal examination, surgery should be postponed until estrogen production is noted at puberty—but before significant hematocolpos develops.

Frequently, periurethral cysts in neonates are confused with a small hydromucocolpos and bulging imperforate hymen (Fig. 12–10). If the physician carefully probes the suburethral area, the anteriorly positioned vaginal introitus will be found. The probe or feeding tube can then be slid posteriorly, past the cyst and into the vagina, proving the patency of the latter. The hymen may be stretched thin over the 2- to 4-cm, yellowish suburethral cyst (Fig. 12–11). Such cysts spontaneously resolve over the first month of life or so and do not require excision or drainage unless they become infected or produce symptoms.

In reviews of 265 prepubertal hymens and 333 newborn hymens, respectively, Pokorny and Kozinetz[7] and Mor, Merlob, and Reisner[8] found incidences of 3.8% and 3% for hymen variants

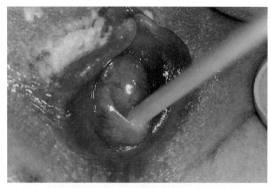

Figure 12–11. Photograph of the same patient shown in Figure 12–10 illustrates that the hymen was stretched thin over the yellowish periurethral cyst, which resolved spontaneously over several months. (From Pokorny SF, Pokorny WJ: Pediatric gynecology. *In* Ashcraft KW, Holder TM [Eds]: Pediatric Surgery, 2nd ed. Philadelphia: WB Saunders, 1993, p 975.)

(septation, microperforation, imperforation), respectively.

HYMENAL CONFIGURATIONS

In addition to the congenital variants just described, the physician should be aware that hymens of prepubertal girls exhibit many variations in how they surround the vaginal orifice. These are called *hymenal configurations* (Fig. 12–12).[9] If the hymen is thought of as a skirt or collar of tissue surrounding the mouth of the vagina, the various configurations can be better conceptualized.

In most girls, the hymenal collar completely surrounds the vaginal orifice. If the opening in the membrane is not in the center, almost always it is displaced toward the urethra. This type of hymen is considered to be *annular* or *circumferential* (see Fig. 12–5).[9–11] If the orifice is so far anterior that there is no room for development of a hymenal rim in the suburethral area, there will be no hymenal tissue from 10:00 or 11:00 o'clock to 1:00 or 2:00 o'clock. This hymenal configuration is called a *crescent* or *posterior rim*.[9–11] Depending on how high the collar of tissue is, this might be a "high" (Fig. 12–13) or a "low" (Fig. 12–14) posterior rim.

In other children, the hymen seems to be more redundant, and, not infrequently, it has scallops on its free margin. This configuration is definitely more common in the estrogenized state (Fig. 12–15), but aspects of it—especially the scallops on the margins of a redundant hymen—are sometimes observed in prepubertal

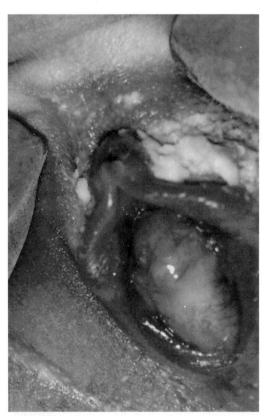

Figure 12–10. A periurethral cyst in a newborn that gives the appearance of an imperforate hymen and a small hydromucocolpos. (From Pokorny SF: Pediatric gynecology. *In* Stenchever MA [Ed]: Office Gynecology St. Louis: Mosby–Year Book, 1992, p 119.)

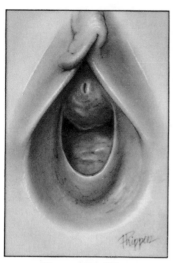
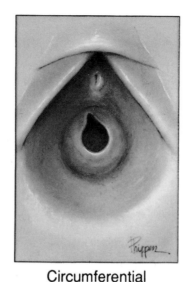
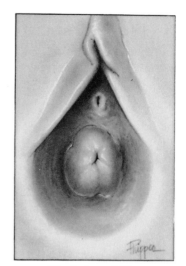

Posterior Rim

Circumferential
Smooth Rim

Fimbriated Rim

Figure 12–12. Various hymen configurations. (From Pokorny SF: Configuration of the prepubertal hymen. Am J Obstet Gynecol 1987; 157:950–956.)

children. This configuration has been called *fimbriated* or *denticular*.[9–11]

The diameter of the hymenal orifice can be influenced by the hymen's configuration, by the method of spreading the vulvar tissues, and by the degree of perineal muscle relaxation when the measurements are taken. Two other factors that influence orifice diameter (because they thicken the hymenal tissue and thus make the orifice smaller) are inflammation and estrogenization of the tissue.

Occasionally, a physician examines a child who seems to have no hymenal tissue at all; any that can be visualized is only nubbins of tissue randomly arranged around the mouth of the vagina (Fig. 12–16). All females are born with a hymen, and falls and severe blows to the adjacent perineal or vulvar tissues do not result in the finding of no hymenal tissue.[12] In adult patients, hymenal caruncles develop after the stretch trauma of vaginal childbirth. Likewise, hymenal remnants or caruncles are evidence of significant stretch trauma to a prepubertal child's vaginal introitus and are the most consistent residual physical findings of severe childhood sexual abuse involving vaginal penetration. Thus, hymenal caruncles in a prepubertal child should not be ignored by the clinician and should be reported to proper authorities for investigation of sexual abuse.

Evaluation of the prepubertal hymen should proceed by steps as the examiner seeks information: Is this a hymen variant such as imperforate, microperforate, or septate hymen? How is the hymen configured around the vaginal introitus (general variations)? Are there any breaks or bumps in it (minute variations)?

The hymen's contour is most variable in the suburethral area, but the majority of hymens have a smooth free margin from 3:00 o'clock to 9:00 o'clock and no irregularities, mounds, or indentations. When such variations are noted, it is imperative that they be described in *anatomically descriptive* terms, *not* "action descriptive" terms such as *ruptured*, *virginal*, or *marital* (Fig. 12–17).

Many annular hymens have a cleft or an indentation in the collar in the suburethral hymen from 10:00 o'clock to 2:00 o'clock (see Fig. 12–5). Not infrequently, the crescent hymen has symmetric scallops, flaps, or wings of tissue, of the same color and thickness as the remainder of the hymen, positioned bilaterally on the hymen margins from 9:00 o'clock to 3:00 o'clock. The scallops that grace the free margins of the fimbriated hymen are uniform in their arrangement. Occasionally, they form a "stellate" orifice, but, because this term describes an orifice and not a hymen, its use should be discouraged. When evaluating scalloped hymen contours, it is important to document the integrity of the hymenal tissue collar and to confirm that the scallop indentations do not represent breaks that extend through the collar of tissue down to the vaginal wall (Fig. 12–18).

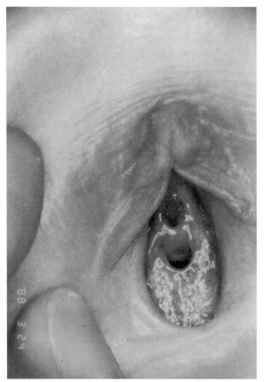

Figure 12–13. Hymen with a high posterior rim. Note that there is no hymenal tissue in the suburethral area.

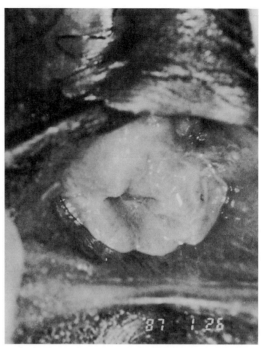

Figure 12–15. Fimbriated or denticular redundant hymen with scallops along its rim. (From Pokorny SF: Configuration of the prepubertal hymen. Am J Obstet Gynecol 1987; 157:950–956.)

Hymenal tags are not uncommon in newborns and seem to be related to estrogen stimulation. In the newborn, they are small (1 to 3 mm), isolated exophytic mucosal lesions, and the majority resolve. Occasionally, one persists, most likely secondary to end organ–related heightened sensitivity to low levels of estrogen. In older children, these tags typically are isolated, asymmetric mounds of tissue. In thickness and color

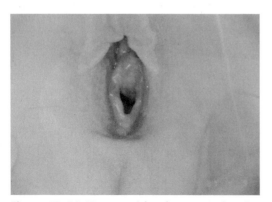

Figure 12–14. Hymen with a low posterior rim.

they resemble that of the hymenal collar. Occasionally, they outgrow their blood supply, become more polypoid, and create an inflammatory, and occasionally bloody, discharge. When the latter alterations occur, it is difficult to distinguish the tags from a pedunculated, friable condyloma acuminatum. In such cases, excisional biopsy is warranted (Fig. 12–19).

Some mounds of tissue on the hymen margin at 6:00 o'clock most likely represent remnants of a septate hymen (Fig. 12–20). Other bumps on the hymen margin are thought to be acquired. Some are situated on the rim of the hymen on one side or the other, usually from 3:00 o'clock to 9:00 o'clock on the posterior hymenal margin, and, like the retracted septal remnant described earlier, are thicker than the hymen itself and in many cases are discolored (i.e., more erythematous than the hymen; Fig. 12–21). Biopsy studies have proven that many of these consist of inflammatory granulation tissue or are histologically suggestive of human papillomavirus. It is not clear whether inflammation alone can cause these isolated hymenal bumps to form or whether a traumatic event must occur.[8]

Symmetric bumps on the hymen may repre-

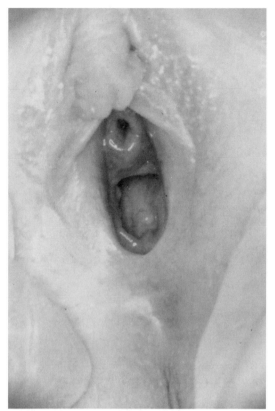

Figure 12–16. Remnants-only hymen in a 7½-year-old girl several years after multiple episodes of penile-vaginal penetration. (From Pokorny SF: Pediatric vulvovaginitis. *In* Kaufman R, Fredrich EG, Gardner HL: Benign Disease of the Vulva and Vagina. Chicago: Year Book Medical, 1989, p 58.)

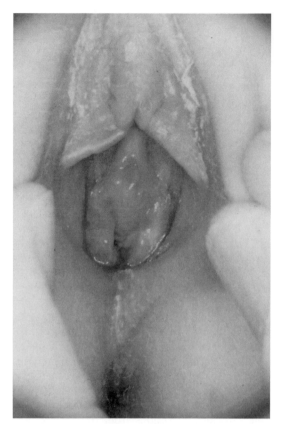

Figure 12–17. Hymen with a break at the 6 o'clock position.

sent retractions of a traumatic hymenal laceration at the 6:00 o'clock position (Figs. 12–22, 12–23). Interpretation of bumps and breaks on the hymen is controversial, but, in a reported series of 265 prepubertal hymens, such bumps and breaks were three times more likely to be associated with sexual abuse than with other pediatric gynecologic conditions.[8]

More recent studies examined the normal anatomic features of the prepubertal genitalia.[13–15] The investigators observed a significant decrease in the amount of hymenal tissue during the first year of life, and some girls with an annular hymen at birth had a crescentic hymen at age 1 year. No notches were seen on the inferior aspect of the hymen. External ridges observed at birth usually resolved by age 3 years. Many of the tags that were seen at birth were not observed at age 3 years.

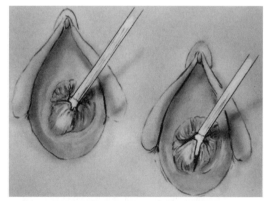

Figure 12–18. Fimbriated redundant hymens occasionally need to be examined with a small probe or swab to determine whether an indentation extends to the base of the hymen collar. This figure shows a tear at the 6 o'clock position. (From Pokorny SF: Physical examination of the reproductive systems of female children and adolescents. Curr Probl Obstet Gynecol Fertil 1990; 13:202–213.)

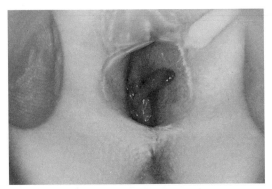

Figure 12–19. Hymenal polyp.

INSTRUMENTATION OF THE VAGINA

VAGINAL ASPIRATOR

Although the estrogen effect on the mucosa of prepubertal children varies from child to child, the majority of children who are past the stage of toilet training have very atrophic genital mucosa. Such mucosa is very sensitive to touch and can easily be lacerated by inflexible instruments. Furthermore, cotton-tipped swabs, which are often used to collect secretions from the vagina, are abrasive and painful.

A soft rubber catheter is excellent for flushing the vagina with fluid, but it is not ideal for collecting undiluted vaginal secretions. Because the vagina is a closed space, when vaginal fluid is aspirated into the catheter, invariably, the cathe-

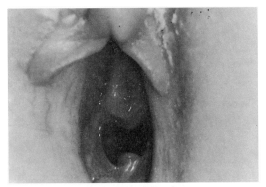

Figure 12–20. Vestibule of a 5-year-old child. Note the patulous urethra. A biopsy of a mound of tissue on the hymen margin at the 6 o'clock position demonstrated fibroelastic tissue, compatible with hymenal septal remnant. (From Pokorny SF: Physical examination of the reproductive systems of female children and adolescents. Curr Probl Obstet Gynecol Fertil 1990; 13:202–213.)

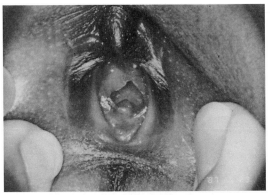

Figure 12–21. Vulva of a 4-year-old child. A biopsy of a mound of erythematous tissue at the 6 o'clock position on hymen rim revealed chronic inflammation. (From Pokorny SF: Physical examination of the reproductive systems of female children and adolescents. Curr Probl Obstet Gynecol Fertil 1990; 13:202–213.)

ter tip is sucked against the vaginal wall, and the yield is a variable, but usually disappointingly small, amount of vaginal aspirant.

An atraumatic method for obtaining vaginal aspirant fluid uses a makeshift catheter within a catheter (Fig. 12–24).[16] Using aseptic technique, the proximal 4 inches of a butterfly intravenous tube is passed into the distal 4½ inches of a soft No. 12 urinary bladder catheter. A 1-ml tuberculin syringe with 0.5 to 1.0 ml of aspirating fluid is attached to the hub of the butterfly tubing. The entire amount of vaginal wash solution can be flushed into the vagina and aspirated back into the syringe; this can be done several times to produce a good admixture of secretions from the upper vagina. The aspirant can be used for wet mounts, Gram stain, culture, and as forensic material.

Because young girls are not aware of the vaginal canal, frequently, it is frightening for them to watch the catheter slide into the canal. Thus, if at all possible, they should be discouraged from watching this procedure with the hand-held mirror.

Most children will comply with the vaginal wash procedure (see earlier) if they are shown that no needles are attached to the catheter apparatus. Sometimes, squirting a few drops of the flushing fluid onto their hand or allowing them to touch and feel a sample catheter is reassuring. The procedure is performed with the child in the supine frog-legged position. The examiner should explain what will happen in terms the child can understand (e.g., "I am going to wash out your girl parts and you will feel it, but it will

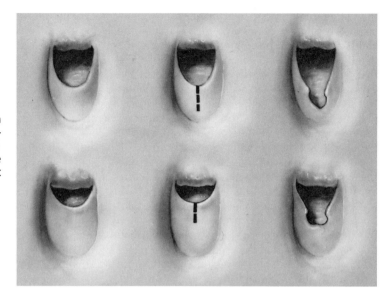

Figure 12–22. Posterior rim breaks. (From Pokorny SF, Kozinetz CA: Configuration and other anatomic detail of the prepubertal hymen. Adolesc Pediatr Gynecol 1998; 1:99.)

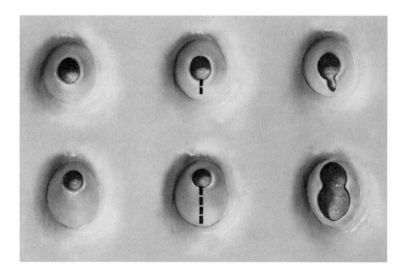

Figure 12–23. Circumferential breaks. (From Pokorny SF, Kozinetz CA: Configuration and other anatomic detail of the prepubertal hymen. Adolesc Pediatr Gynecol 1988; 1:99.)

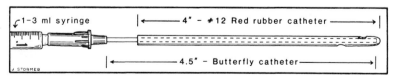

Figure 12–24. Catheter-in-catheter aspirator used to obtain secretions from the prepubertal vagina. (From Pokorny SF, Stormer J: Atraumatic removal of secretions from the prepubertal vagina. Am J Obstet Gynecol 1987; 156:581–582.)

not hurt."). Then, using one hand to spread the labia so that the vaginal introitus is visualized, the catheter apparatus, held in the other hand, is quickly slipped at least 2 to 3 cm into the child's vagina. The examiner should brace the hand against the child's mons pubis or thigh, so that, should the child move suddenly when the catheter is inserted into the vagina, the catheter will stay in place. Once the child is again assured that the catheter is not hurting her, the examiner can inject and aspirate the fluid in and out of the vagina a few times to get a good admixture of vaginal secretions, aspirate the fluid back into the syringe, and then quickly remove the entire apparatus.

Occasionally, topical anesthetics are helpful for pediatric gynecologic procedures (e.g., when the vaginal canal needs to be vigorously flushed to remove a foreign object (such as a toilet paper wad) or in preparation for vaginoscopy. Because local anesthetic might interfere with the results, it is not routinely used when vaginal aspirant is needed for cultures or forensic material.

Viscous xylocaine (2% jelly) can be applied with a cotton ball or dripped directly on the vestibule. Once it has taken effect, a urinary bladder catheter is placed into the child's vagina. With her buttocks over the drain basin on the end of the gynecologic examination table, aseptic solution (e.g., bladder irrigant with povidone-iodine) is flushed into her vagina.

OTHER INSTRUMENTS

To adequately visualize the vaginal canal of a prepubertal child, the instrument of choice must be narrow in diameter and have irrigating capability. Instillation of the irrigation fluid expands the vaginal canal and flushes out discharge and debris, so that the entire vaginal canal and cervix can easily be visualized. Hysteroscopes and pediatric cystoscopes are ideal for this task.

All bivalved instruments, even nasal specula, cause damage to the atrophic tissues of the prepubertal child's vagina, and rarely can they be opened wide enough to provide the same—and necessary—degree of visualization described earlier. The large otoscope and the Cameron-Miller vaginoscope, although the latter was designed specifically for children, also afford inferior visualization of the vaginal canal as compared with an endoscope in a fluid-expanded vaginal canal. *Pediatric speculum* is a misnomer. Such instruments are too short (less than 8 cm) to allow the examiner to see the vaginal apex of a peripubertal

child and too wide for the vaginal introitus of a small child, where they can cause serious injury.

Any inflexible instrument has the potential to injure an unanesthetized prepubertal child's vulva should the child move while the instrument is in the vagina. When the vaginal canal must be visualized and it is thought that the child will comply with the examination, the instrument of choice is a flexible fiberoptic endoscope with irrigating capability.

Viscous xylocaine can be placed on the vestibule. The fiberoptic endoscope with infusing irrigating fluid can then be inserted gently into the vaginal canal. Once the scope is in the canal, the labia can be squeezed together gently, to allow the irrigating fluid to expand the vagina.

Ideally, for this procedure the child should sit, semireclined, with her buttocks slightly over the end of the gynecology table and her feet in the stirrups. The drain basin of the table should be positioned so that the irrigating fluid drains into it.

Promising the child that she will be allowed to look into the scope once the examiner is finished helps to obtain her cooperation. Most fiberoptic endoscopes are long enough to allow the intravaginal part to be steadied and the eyepiece handed to the patient, so that she, too, may look.

SPECIAL ASPECTS OF THE PERIPUBERTAL GENITAL EXAMINATION

It is appropriate to consider the use of a speculum for genital examination of estrogenized

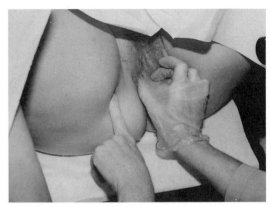

Figure 12–25. Extinction of stimulus phenomenon being applied to obtain patient compliance for her first pelvic examination. Note the nonexamining finger being pressed into the patient's perineum in preparation for placement of the examiner's finger into the patient's vaginal introitus.

peripubertal girls. Estrogen has a profound impact on introital tissues: It imparts a degree of pliability and distention not found in "nonestrogenized" prepubertal introitus. For example, a speculum of a size that can be used in a peripubertal girl, just a year or so earlier, would have lacerated her vulvar tissues.

The examiner should first attempt to place the examining index finger *through* the vaginal introitus before inserting the speculum. This practice has several advantages: It allows detection of hymenal variants. It is necessary for teaching the patient to relax. It allows the examiner to determine what width of speculum blade will afford the most comfort *and* the best visibility.

Applying the "extinction of stimuli" phenomenon is valuable for a young female's first pelvic examination. This neurologic phenomenon makes it possible to use a primary distracting stimulus to lessen, defuse, and extinguish a second stimulus. The procedure consists of describing, one by one, the sensations she will experience as the examining (index) finger enters the vaginal introitus.

In essence, the examiner presses a nonexamining finger into the patient's perineum, close to the pantyline, before touching the introitus with the examining finger. The examination should not proceed until the patient acknowledges that the pressure sensation she is feeling is not painful. She should report an awareness of a pressure sensation (Fig. 12–25).

The patient is then forewarned that she will feel the same type of pressure sensation as the examining finger slowly enters the vaginal introi-

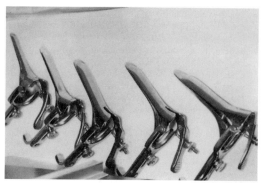

Figure 12–27. The physician should have a variety of speculum widths (0.8 to 3.0 cm) to choose from when performing a girl's first pelvic examination. (From Pokorny SF: Physical examination of the reproductive systems of female children and adolescents. Curr Probl Obstet Gynecol Fertil 1990; 13:202–213.)

tus. The more anxious the patient is, and the tighter the introital tissues feel, the more pressure the nonexamining (distracting) finger should apply to the perineum to defuse and extinguish the sensation the patient is feeling at the introitus (Fig. 12–26).

Once the examining finger is through the introitus, it should remain there. At this point, the patient can be instructed how to relax the perineal body by allowing her knees to drop outward. Once this is accomplished, a speculum of the proper width can easily be chosen (Fig. 12–27).

REFERENCES

 1. Cassell C: Swept Away. Why Women Fear Their Own Sexuality. New York: Simon and Schuster, 1984.
 2. Jenny C, Sutherland SE, Sandahl BB: Developmental approach to preventing the sexual abuse of children. Pediatrics 1986; 78:1034.
 3. Cowan BD, Morrison JC: Management of abnormal genital bleeding in girls and women. N Engl J Med 1991; 324(24):1710–1715.
 4. Herman-Giddens ME, Berson NL: Harmful genital care practices in children. JAMA 1989; 261:577.
 5. Muram D, Jones CE: The use of video-colposcopy in the gynecologic examination of children and adolescents. Adolesc Pediatr Gynecol 1993; 6:154–156.
 6. Berenson AB, Wiemann CM, Rickert VI: Use of video eyeglasses to decrease anxiety among children undergoing genital examinations. Am J Obstet Gynecol 1998; 178(6):1341–1345.
 7. Pokorny SF, Kozinetz CA: Configuration and other anatomic details of the prepubertal hymen. Adolesc Pediatr Gynecol 1988; 1:97.
 8. Mor N, Merlob P, Reisner SH: Types of hymen in the newborn infant. Eur J Obstet Gynecol Reprod Biol 1986; 22:225.

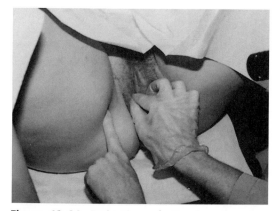

Figure 12–26. Extinction of stimulus phenomenon being demonstrated for a patient's first pelvic examination. Note that the nonexamining finger continues to be pressed into the patient's perineum while the examiner's other index finger probes the introitus.

9. Pokorny SF: Configuration of the prepubertal hymen. Am J Obstet Gynecol 1987; 157:950–956.

10. Emans SJ, Woods ER, Flagg NT, et al: Genital findings in sexually abused symptomatic and asymptomatic girls. Pediatrics 1987; 79:778.

11. Enos W, Conrath T, Byer J: Forensic evaluation of the sexually abused child. Pediatrics 1986; 78:385–398.

12. Pokorny SF, Pokorny WJ, Kramer W. Acute genital injury in the prepubertal female. Am J Obstet Gynecol 1992; 166(5):1461–1466.

13. Berenson AB:A longitudinal study of hymenal morphol-

ogy in the first 3 years of life. Pediatrics. 1995; 95(4):490–496.

14. Berenson AB: Appearance of the hymen at birth and one year of age: A longitudinal study. Pediatrics. 1993; 91(4):820–825.

15. Berenson AB, Heger AH, Hayes JM, et al: Appearance of the hymen in prepubertal girls. Pediatrics 1992; 89(3):387–394.

16. Pokorny SF, Stormer J:Atraumatic removal of secretions from the prepubertal vagina. Am J Obstet Gynecol 1987; 156(3):581–582.

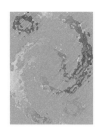

Chapter 13

Vulvovaginitis in Children and Adolescents

FREDERICK J. RAU AND DAVID MURAM

Vulvovaginal inflammation, the most common reproductive system disorder of girls, accounts for 40% to 85% of visits to pediatric gynecology services.[1-3] Symptoms of vulvovaginitis in this age group commonly arouse parental anxiety because of the perceived rarity of vulvovaginitis in children or the fear of childhood sexual abuse. In addition, concern over lack of appropriate supervision and hygiene in day care or other settings may be appropriate. The majority of children with vulvovaginitis have an easily treated, nonspecific disorder, but a small percentage have infections that are associated with a systemic illness or child abuse.

RECOGNIZING VULVOVAGINITIS IN A CHILD

DEFINITION

In prepubertal children, vulvovaginitis is defined as inflammation of the vulva or vagina in response to any of a variety of stimuli. The pattern of inflammation and the causes are very different in younger persons as compared with adolescents and adults. For example, typically pediatric vulvovaginitis has no specific pathogens that can be identified as being clearly foreign to normal vaginal flora. Instead, overgrowth of resident bacteria in relation to those on the vulvovaginal epithelium produces a set of signs and symptoms commonly seen in clinical practice.

HISTORY AND ONSET OF SYMPTOMS: WHEN TO INTERVENE

As parents and caregivers know, a female child occasionally complains of vulvar discomfort or itching. Persistent symptoms noted by the child or observed by the caretaker increase concern. Clinical features most common with childhood vulvovaginitis include vulvar pruritus and pain, vulvar dysuria, and evidence of vulvovaginal inflammation (manifested as vaginal discharge, erythema, edema, odor, or vaginal spotting or bleeding; Table 13–1).[1, 4]

The child or parent may notice a single predominant sign or symptom, or a combination of any (or all) may be seen. Conservative treatments may be attempted at home—baths with or without added soothing compounds, going without underwear, bland ointments. If the child's complaints persist or if examination of the child's vulva or underwear reveals signs of discharge or inflammation, medical attention will be sought. Certain aspects of the child's history are helpful in identifying contributing factors. For example, a young, preverbal child may be seen rubbing or scratching her vulva, and that may be the only sign that vulvovaginitis might be present. The girl may be uncomfortable with diaper changing, urination, or defecation. Persistent urinary frequency, urgency, or vulvar dysuria may be present in a child of any age. If a discharge is present, helpful clues to the degree of bacterial superin-

Table 13–1. Clinical Features of Vulvovaginitis in Children

Feature	Prevalence (%)
Vaginal discharge	53–88
Erythema	33
Pruritus	32
Vulvar dysuria	12–15
Vaginal bleeding/spotting	1–9
Odor	8
Pain	1–4

Table 13–2. Factors That Can Contribute to Childhood Vulvovaginitis

Behavioral factors
   Inadequate front-to-back wiping
   Inattention to perineal hygiene at home or day program
   Over vigorous vulvar cleansing
   Bubble baths, deodorant soaps
   Sandbox play
   Masturbation
Physiologic factors
   Family respiratory or gastrointestinal illness
   Diabetes mellitus or immunodeficiency state
   Limited antibodies in vaginal secretions
   Anestrogenic vaginal epithelium, neutral pH
   Eczema, seborrhea, other dermatologic condition
   Sexual abuse
Anatomic factors
   Confining clothing
   Decreased labial fat pads
   Small labia minora
   Thin, delicate, vulvar skin
   Vulva anatomically close to anus

fection are its color, duration, and odor. For example, a green discharge and a significant odor are more likely to indicate significant aerobic and anaerobic contamination, and may even indicate a predominant organism. The duration of vulvar inflammatory symptoms such as itching, burning, pain, and vulvar dysuria should be reviewed, as they can persist long after the discharge resolves. Other aspects of a child's history relevant to vulvovaginitis are reviewed in Table 13–2. The history need not be exhaustive. If the child appears anxious or apprehensive, other history questions may be asked during the examination.

WHAT TYPE OF EXAMINATION?

The appropriate examination for office evaluation of childhood vaginitis usually involves a "mini" inspection of the vulva and lower vagina.[5] It is important to communicate to the referring clinician and parents that you will not be doing a pelvic examination in the manner traditional for adult women. Nasal and "pediatric" duckbill speculums have little (if any) place in the evaluation of prepubertal children with vulvovaginitis, as they cause intense pain owing to the relatively nondistensible prepubertal hymen and vagina and do not provide additional information. Nonthreatening methods of putting the parents at ease and bonding with the child should be used. Inspection of the vulva and perianal area for erythema, edema, excoriations, discharge or blood, or any other vulvar lesions should be done first. Magnification using a coloposcope is occa-

sionally helpful, especially if childhood sexual abuse is in question. The labial traction method affords visualization of the inner labia, clitoris, urethra, hymenal contour, and distal vagina. In some patients with persistent or recurrent infections, a foreign body in the vagina is the cause. The most common foreign body is wadded-up fragments of toilet paper, but a variety of objects have been found. The knee-chest position can improve visualization of the middle and upper vagina.[6] The perineal body and anus should be inspected for hygiene, excoriations, trauma, and skin changes. It is helpful to use a mirror or to show the parent the findings of interest. Review of vulvar anatomy and affirmation of findings that were noted at home help the family to contribute to the treatment and follow-up plans.

USE OF MICROSCOPIC EXAMINATION AND CULTURES

As in evaluation of adult vaginitis, examination of vaginal secretions in children with symptoms of vulvovaginitis can be helpful in arriving at a preliminary diagnosis and formulating a treatment plan during the initial office visit. The benefit of routine vaginal cultures in children thought to be at low risk for childhood sexual abuse is, however, less clear, especially when little or no vaginal discharge is seen despite erythema and edema. A variety of methods have been suggested to retrieve vaginal secretions, in a relatively atraumatic way, when obtaining a specimen is deemed necessary Table 13–3.

Nasopharyngeal Calgiswabs and cotton-tipped applicators are readily available to clinicians. The applicator is moistened with nonbacteriostatic saline and is gently passed through the hymenal orifice into the distal vagina. Care must be taken to avoid touching the hymenal edge when collecting the specimens. If the child is very apprehensive, the applicator can be rested vertically at the hymenal orifice. The labia majora are then gently pressed together in the midline and the child is encouraged to cough. Muram has de-

Table 13–3. Methods of Collecting Vaginal Secretions from Children

Intravaginal nasopharyngeal Calgiswab or male urethral swab dipped in nonbacteriostatic saline
Adult-size cotton swab outside the hymenal orifice
Catheter-within-a-catheter technique
Vulvovaginal irrigation with warm saline
Pediatric feeding tube attached to a syringe

scribed a method in which warm saline is gently sprayed toward the distal vagina to increase the yield of intravaginal secretions.[7] Two or three cotton applicators are then placed vertically just outside the hymen, and the child is instructed to cough to express the intravaginal specimen. A variety of aspiration methods, such as the catheter-within-a-catheter method,[8] pediatric feeding tubes, or eye-dropper techniques, are described in greater detail in Chapter 12.

Examination of the specimen under the microscope can assess for *Candida* spores or hyphae and leukocytes and can rule out the remote possibility of trichomoniasis. A decision must be made whether to perform bacterial or yeast cultures. At this time, opinions differ on the usefulness of vaginal cultures in children with vulvovaginitis.[9–12] Many authors feel that they are not necessary, because most patients who are likely to have nonspecific vulvovaginitis have it in association with inadequate perineal hygiene.[10] When a vaginal discharge persists despite conservative measures, when vaginal bleeding has been noted, or if childhood sexual abuse is an issue, vaginal cultures to isolate a predominant organism and identify sexually transmitted diseases can be helpful.[13] In a large percentage of children with vulvovaginitis, no specific pathogen (nonspecific vaginitis) can be identified. Alteration of normal bacterial populations in the prepubertal vagina and the vaginal and vulvar inflammatory response are responsible for the symptoms.

A variety of studies have examined the vaginal flora in populations of children with and without symptoms Table 13–4.[4, 9, 14–18] These studies indicate that the isolated organisms in children with and without symptoms of vulvovaginitis can vary significantly, depending upon the population studied. At baseline, a wide variety of aerobic, anaerobic, and, occasionally, fungal, organisms can be found in asymptomatic children.[9, 16–18] Predominant organisms in asymptomatic children include *Staphylococcus epidermidis*, diphtheroids, lactobacilli, α-hemolytic and nonhemolytic streptococci, *Escherichia coli*, peptococci, peptostreptococci, and *Clostridia* and *Bacteroides* species. *Candida* was cultured very rarely (fewer than 5%) in asymptomatic girls (in contrast to postpubertal subjects). The bacterial population does appear to change significantly in symptomatic patients. For example, an early study by Emans and Goldstein found that 53% of their patients with vulvovaginitis had normal vaginal flora, *E. coli*, or other gram-negative organisms, whereas 47% had a "specific" identified cause.[6] The predominant organisms were *E. coli* and group A streptococci. Zeiguer and colleagues found a specific pathogen in 58.5% of girls with vaginitis.[4] In this Argentinian study, a large percentage of cultures were positive for *Chlamydia trachomatis* and *Neisseria gonorrhoeae*. No anaerobic data were reported; however, Gerstner and colleagues obtained vaginal cultures through a vaginoscope from a group of symptomatic and asymptomatic girls. Both groups had a wide variety of aerobic and anaerobic organisms; however, the symptomatic group had a higher prevalence of anaerobes such as *Peptococcus*, *Peptostreptococcus*, and *Bacteroides*.[18] *Candida* species were also found in a larger percentage of girls in the symptomatic group; lactobacilli were found less frequently. These findings may be somewhat altered by previous antibiotic therapy for other conditions. The overlap in bacterial flora between symptomatic and asymptomatic girls is striking. This overlap suggests that, in some children, other factors, such as bacterial content in the vaginal fluid or the inflammatory response of the vulvovaginal epithelium, play a crucial role in the clinical presentation and response to therapy. These findings may be somewhat altered by previous antibiotic therapy.

CLASSIFICATION AND THERAPY OF CHILDHOOD VULVOVAGINITIS

PHYSIOLOGIC DISCHARGE

A vaginal discharge in a child during the newborn period and during early pubertal development is usually considered normal. In the newborn period, maternal estrogens passed in utero to the child can cause mucous secretion by the endocervical glands that is manifested as a clear white discharge. Additionally, in some children the discharge may contain blood owing to endometrial shedding. With the onset of estrogen secretion from the ovaries at pubarche, a similar, thick, mucoid discharge is often seen. This physiologic secretion is not associated with an odor or symptoms of vulvovaginal inflammation; however, when the discharge dries on the skin it sometimes causes local irritation or even secondary infection. Reassurance and explanation in distinguishing normal secretions from those that might indicate vaginitis is helpful to the adolescent and her family.

TYPES OF CHILDHOOD VULVOVAGINOPATHIES

Based on the clinical history, examination, wet-mount, and KOH examination, and cultures,

Table 13–4. The Types of Microbes Identified in Children with Vulvovaginitis

Investigators	Normal Flora or No Growth (%)	Normal Flora and at Least 1 or More Bacteria (1 Isolate) (%)	Predominant Aerobic Organism(s)	Predominant Anaerobic Organism(s)	Candida (%)	Sexually Transmitted Organism(s) (%)	Other
Emans and Goldstein[6]	26	40	Escherichia coli, group A streptococci	No data	8	11	
Paradise[28]	47	39	E. coli	Bacteroides spp.	0	11	Shigella
Gerstner[18]	0	100	Enterococci, E. coli, Staphylococcus epidermidis	Peptococcus, Eubacterium, Peptostreptococcus, Bacteroides	25	0	Fewer lactobacilli in symptomatic children
Pierce and Hart[14]	45	55	E. coli, Haemophilus influenzae, streptococci	?	3.5	0	
Zeiguer[4]	45	55	Haemophilus spp, Ureaplasma urealyticum	?	1.5	19–29	32% had pinworms
Jones[16]	76	24	Streptococcus pyogenes, H. influenzae	No data	0	0	High prevalence of Haemophilus spp.

childhood vulvovaginitis can be classified into nonspecific (50% to 80%) and specific (20% to 50%). Fewer than 5% of patients will have vaginitis caused by an organism thought to be sexually transmitted (see Chapter 21). The history is commonly helpful in identifying factors that would make a specific type of vaginitis more likely, such as a recent upper respiratory tract or gastrointestinal infection, or concerns about childhood sexual abuse. If the culture data are not available, the initial therapy must be based on history, examination, and wet-mount findings. Very often, the initial presentation and findings suggest nonspecific vaginitis, and a treatment plan can be based on this assumption.

BEHAVIORAL INTERVENTION AND MEDICATION THERAPY

A number of principles have been suggested for behavioral modification for children with vulvovaginitis. These can be described as attempts at "improvement of perineal hygiene." Behavioral interventions for children and caretakers attempt to eliminate practices that render children susceptible to vaginitis (see Table 13–2). The goals of these interventions are to keep the vulva cool, dry, and less irritated. Subsequent disruption of the "itch and scratch cycle" will provide immediate and long-term relief. Suggested interventions include these:

- Frequent sitz/tub baths with warm water only
- Urinating with knees, thighs, and labia apart to prevent urine reflux into vagina
- Front-to-back perineal wiping after a bowel movement
- Use of unscented toilet tissue
- Avoidance of vulvar exposure to harsh soaps (i.e., bubble baths, shampoo, deodorant soaps)
- Cotton underwear to absorb vaginal discharge
- Avoid tight pants and leotards
- Mild unscented soap for face and body washing (limit exposure)
- Pat vulva dry or dry with hair dryer on low setting
- Avoid exposure to potential sources of bacteria (e.g., sandboxes, pets)

Nonspecific Vulvovaginitis

Therapy of acute, nonspecific vulvovaginitis in children should focus on improving perineal hygiene, as described above, and relieving symptoms. Tub/sitz baths with plain warm water, colloidal oatmeal, or Domeboro solution can be very soothing to an acutely inflamed vulva. Witch hazel pads can also be soothing. After patting the vulva dry, low-potency topical steroid (hydrocortisone, 1% or 2.5%, or triamcinolone, 0.025%) will relieve itching and inflammation in children with significant pruritus. The clinician has the option of monitoring the child's response to improved hygiene for 2 to 3 days or to prescribe a course of antibiotics. There are no data to suggest which children might benefit from such treatment. Most clinicians base their clinical decision on the duration of symptoms, severity of inflammation, and results of previous attempts at therapy. In a referral-type practice, conservative or behavioral measures have usually been attempted; thus antibiotics are commonly used—with excellent short-term results. Based on culture data,[4, 6, 9, 18] several antibiotics are appropriate choices for nonspecific vulvovaginitis. These include amoxicillin, amoxicillin/clavulanic acid, or a cephalosporin such as cefaclor, cephalexin, or cefixime. Erythromycin or trimethoprim/sulfamethoxazole may be used for penicillin-allergic children. A 7- to 10-day course is usually prescribed. If the history indicates previous antibiotic use for another infection (e.g., otitis media, bronchitis/sinusitis), disturbed bacterial homeostasis should be anticipated and likely vulvovaginal denudation that is contributing to the child's symptoms. In this situation, a course of topically applied estrogen cream bid for 7 to 14 days will promote healing and decrease the chronic inflammation. This approach is especially helpful in chronic nonspecific vulvovaginitis without a significant discharge or in patients with denudation of mucosal surfaces.

Recurrent nonspecific vulvovaginitis is a very frustrating problem for the child, family, and clinician. A variety of strategies have been suggested that utilize an individualized, trial and error approach.[10] Failure of initial medical therapy to alter the child's symptoms should alert the physician to the possibility that the vaginal discharge may be caused by other disorders (e.g., foreign body, ectopic ureter, or even a neoplasm). Diagnostic vaginoscopy is indicated, as either an in office or an operating room procedure (see later). If a discharge recurs after *successful* treatment with oral antibiotics and the diagnostic vaginoscopy findings are normal, a suppressive dose of the same antibiotic at bedtime for 2 months is frequently very effective. Perineal hygiene, culture results, and the possibility of a foreign body must be reevaluated. If vulvar inflammatory symptoms persist after antibiotics and steroid cream, a course of estrogen cream, twice daily for 1 to 3 weeks, promotes growth of the epithelial layer and can disrupt the inflammatory cycle.

Intermittent vulvar pain along with intense itching (clinically, *transient vulvitis*) is a puzzling variant of vulvovaginitis. Minimal signs of inflammation (if any) persist, but frightening (usually nocturnal) episodes of pain cause great distress for the child and her family. No therapy is clearly effective, but an individualized approach using estrogen cream, antihistamines at bedtime, lidocaine gel, and reassurance can be offered.

Specific-Organism Vulvovaginitis

RESPIRATORY PATHOGENS

Respiratory pathogens of vulvovaginitis in children include group A β-hemolytic streptococci, *Streptococcus pneumoniae*, *Haemophilus influenzae*, *Moraxella catarrhalis*, and *Neisseria meningitidis*. The history usually suggests a pharyngeal or respiratory tract illness, and the culture results indicate the pathogen. Group A β-hemolytic streptococci are the most frequent cause of vaginitis-associated vaginal bleeding in children.[19] Q-tip culturing or vaginoscopy can be used to reveal significant inflammation of the atrophic vaginal epithelium. The mechanism is usually autoinoculation from respiratory secretions, or possibly via a hematogenous route. A nonspecific discharge and intense vulvitis are seen initially, but streptococcal infections can cause perianal cellulitis and vulvar abscesses.[20–22] Treatment of group A "strep" infection is amoxicillin, 40 mg/kg per day, in three doses for 10 days. Erythromycin ethylsuccinate, 30 to 50 mg/kg per day in four doses, or cefixime, 8 mg/kg per day, in one or two doses are alternatives. A recent review identified *H. influenzae* as the second most common pathogen of vulvovaginitis in a series of 104 pediatric patients.[23] Therapeutic options for *Haemophilus* organisms are amoxicillin clavulanate, 20 to 40 mg/kg per day, divided in two doses; erythromycin-sulfisoxazole, 50 mg/kg per day; trimethoprim-sulfamethoxazole (TMP/SMX), 8 mg/kg per day; or cefaclor, 20 to 40 mg/kg per day, in divided doses.

GASTROINTESTINAL PATHOGENS

While *E. coli* is commonly associated with nonspecific vulvovaginitis, two gastrointestinal pathogens, *Shigella* spp. and *Yersinia enterocolitica* have been identified as rare but specific organisms in symptomatic children. Recurrent

vaginal discharge and bleeding should alert the clinician to the possibility of *Shigella* vulvovaginitis. In a review of 38 patients with *Shigella* vaginitis, 47% had bleeding associated with their vaginal discharge. A relatively small number of children had vulvar inflammatory symptoms such as pain, pruritus, or dysuria.[24] The lower genital tract is inoculated from a preexisting gastrointestinal infection. Cultures of the stool may not always prove positive, and other contact persons should be cultured. Treatment is 6 to 10 mg TMP and 30 to 50 mg SMX/kg per day PO or IV every 12 hours for 5 days. Tetracycline, and ampicillin are also effective against sensitive strains.

A second gastrointestinal pathogen, *Y. enterocolitica*, has been identified as a cause of vulvovaginitis in children. This case report traced a child's *Y. enterocolitica* vulvovaginitis to contaminated tofu.[25] A gastrointestinal illness initially was seen, followed by typical acute vulvovaginitis. Treatment is also TMP/SMX in doses similar to those for *Shigella*.

PINWORMS

Pinworms are 1 cm long, thin, white worms that make their way from the anus to the vagina. In addition to classic perianal pruritus, *Enterobius vermicularis* can also cause symptoms of vulvovaginal pruritus, which is difficult to distinguish from vulvovaginitis. Fecal bacteria may also be carried by the pinworms, leading to bacterial superinfection of the vulva. If nocturnal pruritus is evident, a flashlight examination at night may identify the worms. Alternatively, a morning "Scotch Tape" test can identify the eggs. Treatment is mebendazole, one 100-mg dose repeated 2 weeks later.

CANDIDA INFECTIONS

Despite the temptation to assign the cause of vaginal irritation and redness to "yeast," *Candida* is rarely the cause of vulvovaginitis in children. In most studies, symptomatic children have demonstrated positive cultures for *Candida* in no more than 8%.[4, 6, 9, 14, 16] *Candida* vulvovaginitis is clinically recognized by vulvar erythema and edema associated with whitish plaques of the involved surfaces. Satellite lesions may be seen. KOH prep can assist in identifying spores and hyphae. Biggy culture medium is necessary to grow the organism. A true *Candida* infection in children is commonly preceded by a course of antibiotics. Estrogenic effects of early puberty place young adolescents at much higher risk for a *Candida* infection. If laboratory confirmation of *Candida* is made in a prepubertal child, inquiry should be made to exclude antibiotic use, diabetes mellitus, or an immune deficiency state.

External antifungal creams—anecdotally—have a high failure rate owing to persistent intravaginal organisms. Treatment of *Candida* vulvovaginitis in children and younger adolescents is problematic owing to the difficulty of administering intravaginal medication. One technique that has been helpful is a variation of the catheter-within-a-catheter method described by Pokorny.[8] First, a 10-ml syringe is filled with a dose of antifungal cream. A No. 16 IV catheter (no needle) is attached and placed into a shortened No. 10 urethral catheter. The urethral catheter is placed into the vaginal fornix, and the dose of cream is injected with the syringe. A single dose usually suffices for complete resolution of symptoms, but repeat doses occasionally are necessary—at the office or at home. Topical corticosteroid creams are important for immediate symptom relief. The safety and efficacy of oral antifungal agents such as fluconazole have not been determined in children.

TRICHOMONIASIS

Trichomonas vaginalis is a protozoan and a relatively common cause of vaginitis in adolescents and adult women. Although usually thought of as clearly a sexually transmitted pathogen, neonatal and early childhood trichomoniasis associated with perinatal transmission has been described.[26] A very young child presents with a profuse white-yellow discharge and significant vulvar erythema and edema. Motile or nonmotile trichomonads can easily be seen on a saline mount. Childhood sexual abuse should obviously be considered, but nonsexual transmission is possible. Recommended treatment is oral metronidazole, 15 mg/kg per day, in three doses.

VAGINAL FOREIGN BODIES AND VAGINOSCOPY

A common concern among caretakers and clinicians who see children with vulvovaginitis is the possibility of a vaginal foreign body. Anecdotal tales abound of buttons, ointment tube tops, pen tops, bobby pins, dice, crayons, and other objects in a child's vagina, but the most common foreign object is balled-up wads of toilet paper that are trapped in the lower third of the vagina. In one series, approximately 79% of all "foreign bodies" were found to be toilet tissue.[27] The child may rub herself, or a caretaker may wipe her vulva so that fragments of tissue make their way into the vagina. The classic sign of a vaginal foreign body is a foul-smelling vaginal discharge, which may be blood-tinged owing to the intense or chronic inflammatory response. Vaginal cultures show common organisms of nonspecific vaginitis. A common scenario that may alert the clinician is failure of discharge and inflammation to resolve after conscientious perineal hygiene and medical therapy. In one study, 4% of girls who presented with genital symptoms were found to have a vaginal foreign body. The presence of vaginal bleeding raised the probability of a foreign body to approximately 18% when discharge was present and 50% when no discharge was present.[28] Although the most common cause of vaginal bleeding is vulvovaginitis, continued vaginal bleeding or spotting after medical therapy should prompt vaginal and cervical visualization by vaginoscopy.

When a foreign body is suspected, several options are available for further evaluation. Using the labial traction method of vulvovaginal examination, the physician can occasionally see—and retrieve—a foreign body situated at the posterior vaginal wall. The knee-chest position is superior for mid- and upper vaginal visualization. If toilet tissue is seen or suspected, in-office vaginal lavage with warm saline or water can remove some or all of the fragments. A cooperative child, and topical lidocaine gel applied to the hymen, are helpful. There are limitations to the efficacy of office lavage; if the object is heavy, or embedded in the vaginal epithelium, or has a certain shape, lavage will not be successful. When visualization of the vagina and cervix is necessary, a slender (3-mm), flexible hysteroscope with warm saline irrigation is an excellent method of in-office vaginoscopy. However, with an anxious child or a reluctant parent, vaginoscopy under a short-acting anesthetic using a pediatric arthroscope or cystoscope can provide prompt resolution for a difficult clinical problem. In addition to evaluation for a foreign body, vaginoscopy is indicated for suspicion of significant trauma, neoplasm, congenital anomaly, and persistent or recurrent vulvovaginitis.[19] An undiagnosed foreign body can remain in a child for years and intermittently cause symptoms due to erosion and tissue necrosis.[29]

VULVAR DERMATITIS

Vulvar dermatitis is a frequent cause of vulvitis without associated vaginitis. In young children, diaper dermatitis is related to the mixed irritative effects of urine and stool. *Candida* is commonly associated with diaper dermatitis. Seborrhea and atopic dermatitis are common in children.[19] Vulvar involvement of both conditions causes subacute vulvar inflammation and pruritus. In addition, thin, fine vulvar fissures are common. Frequent fissure locations include superior to the clitoris in the midline, within the interlabial groove, and in the perineal and perianal regions. These and other vulvar disorders are discussed in Chapter 14.

VULVOVAGINITIS DUE TO SYSTEMIC ILLNESSES

A number of childhood illnesses cause associated vulvovaginitis, which can be severe. Viral illnesses such as varicella, measles, and rubella can involve the vulva and vagina in association with the acute infection. In *varicella*, vesicular lesions may develop on the vulvar and vaginal epithelium in conjunction with other mucous membranes. Rupture of the vesicles rapidly forms 2- to 3-mm ulcerative lesions.[30] In children with measles, Koplik's spots (small, irregular, bright red spots with a tiny bluish-white speck in the center) are seen in the labial mucosa early on in the rash development.[30] These lesions coalesce to form diffuse red patches with bluish white elevations. Complete resolution occurs. The pink-red maculopapular exanthem of rubella commonly involves the vulvar skin. Bacterial illnesses such as diphtheria can cause ulcerative vulvovaginitis. The lesions typically are deep, rounded, "punched out" ulcerations, which can coalesce and form a reservoir of organisms.[30] Other systemic illnesses such as leukemia and erythema multiforme produce ulcerative, necrotic lesions of the vagina, vulva, and urethra. Crohn's disease can produce ulcerative vulvar lesions commonly associated with perianal involvement. In addition to therapy of the primary disorder, oral metronidazole and topical corticosteroids are helpful for resolution and prevention of chronic vulvar or perineal fistulas. Behçet's syndrome may produce painful, recurrent ulcers of the vulva in children. Other systemic signs of Behçet's syndrome, such as uveitis, cutaneous vasculitis, arthritis, or meningoencephalitis, are usually seen. Topical corticosteroids and analgesics are necessary for relief of symptoms, but vulvar scarification can be seen.[31] Kawasaki syndrome can produce erythematous, raised, pruritic plaques or a maculopapular rash that can affect the vulvar and perineal areas.

VULVOVAGINITIS IN ADOLESCENTS

Adolescence is often associated with unique gynecologic concerns. Pubertal hormone changes promote alteration of the vaginal flora from that of a child to that of an adult. As a result, infectious processes are different and more prevalent. It has been noted that the signs and symptoms of vulvovaginitis (e.g., vaginal discharge and pruritus) were second only to menstrual disorders as the presenting complaint in more than 2000 visits by adolescent girls to a gynecology clinic.[1]

The sequelae of these infections include more serious disorders of the upper genital tract (e.g., salpingo-oophoritis with resultant infertility). Other lesions of concern, including premature rupture of membranes and asymptomatic cervicitis, may be noted in this patient population. Finally, the epidemic of human papillomavirus (HPV) infections has been linked to increased risk of developing cervical cancer.

Evaluation of an adolescent who presents with signs and symptoms of vulvovaginitis must take into consideration the pubertal status, current or recent sexual involvement (voluntary or associated with assault), and contraceptive method (if any), as these may affect management. The possibility of sexually transmitted infection is a significant concern to these patients; thus, the clinical setting provides the opportunity to educate the patient and facilitate compliance with recommended therapy. Sexual activity among adolescents predisposes them to exposure to a host of pathogens. Because sexually transmitted diseases are discussed in Chapters 21 and 22, the present discussion is limited to the evaluation and management of the common causes of vulvovaginitis in adolescents.

Vulvar and vaginal inflammation can result from a wide variety of causes. In postpubertal adolescents, especially those who are sexually active, it usually begins as a primary vaginitis; the associated discharge may incite a secondary vulvitis. In many patients, it may be impossible to identify accurately the anatomic origin of the presenting symptoms, and other information is needed to determine whether the upper genital tract is affected. Sexual activity increases the risk of vulvovaginal infections and sexually transmitted diseases in adolescents. In young females with symptoms suggestive of vulvovaginitis, it is very helpful to seek these risk factors, as they may suggest a pathogen.

Lactobacilli help to control the vaginal microflora and maintain its steady state. Lactic acid, produced during *Lactobacillus* metabolism and by vaginal epithelial cells, promotes low vaginal pH. Lactobacilli continue to thrive in this environment. They also possess many antagonistic properties, and some strains produce metabolites (such as H_2O_2) that help to maintain this dominance.[32] Changes in pH or glycogen status affect the lactobacilli in a way that permits other organisms to predominate. Antibiotics, douches, alkaline secretions during menses, alkaline soaps, and poorly controlled diabetes mellitus are among the more common causes of such changes in microflora. Variations in dominance and population levels of each bacterial species are noted throughout the cycle, as the vaginal pH varies from neutral to acidic. Some researchers suggest that frequent and unprotected intercourse may also alter pH status because of the strong alkalinity of seminal fluid and vaginal lubricating secretions.[32]

Once the normal vaginal flora is replaced by a pathogen, the vaginal mucosa becomes irritated and inflamed, often with an associated increase in production of vaginal secretions, discharge, and changes in odor or color. The color may range from yellow-white to greenish brown, especially if it is associated with bleeding. Pruritus and vulvar irritating symptoms are common. These include burning, dyspareunia, vulvar dysuria, and ill-defined discomfort of the genitalia. Pelvic pain, abnormal uterine bleeding, and other signs of pelvic inflammatory disease may be evident if an ascending infection is present. The differential diagnosis of vaginal discharge is outlined in Table 13–5.

Evaluation of the discharge with respect to magnitude, color, character, odor, and pH is important. Mixing of vaginal secretions with a 10% solution of potassium hydroxide (KOH) facilitates the identification of *Candida*. Liberation of a

distinctive fishy odor immediately after the addition of KOH is one of the diagnostic features of bacterial vaginosis. This odor is attributable to volatile amines in the vaginal fluid, presumably the products of anaerobic bacterial metabolism. Microscopic evaluation of a wet-mount preparation is a significant part of the office evaluation. Specific culture may be required to isolate a specific pathogen (e.g., *Chlamydia*, *N. gonorrhoeae*).

HORMONAL CHANGES

After puberty, the vaginal ecosystem resembles that of the adult, with an epithelial lining, enzymes, substrates, microflora, and secretions. Vaginal secretions are composed of the products of vaginal transudation, endocervical mucous secretions, endometrial and tubal fluids, exfoliated cells, and fluid from sebaceous, sweat, and Bartholin's glands. The vaginal flora is dependent on pH and glycogen-glucose availability for bacterial metabolism. Under the influence of endogenous estrogens, the vaginal mucosa proliferates, thickens, and accumulates glycogen. Fermentation of glycogen results in a decrease in the pH to levels of 4.0 to 4.5. This environment favors acidogenic, glycogen-metabolizing bacteria, predominantly lactobacilli.[33] Other such bacteria include acidogenic corynebacteria, Enterobacteriaceae spp., and *Bacteroides fragilis*. Various staphylococci, streptococci, diphtheroids, *Candida albicans*, and other species of anaerobic bacteria have also been reported.

Discharge-Producing Hormonal Alterations

Some 6 to 12 months before menarche, physiologic vaginal secretions increase in production, resulting in a physiologic discharge (leukorrhea). In general, this discharge is clear or yellow-white, mucoid, and not irritating. It is frequently copious, but not malodorous. Staining of underclothing may result from the drying of secretions, with a resultant change to a yellow-brown color. Dried secretions may also cause vulvar pruritus, although the vulva is not inflamed.[34] Evaluation of the discharge by microscopy notes normal flora with an absence of leukocytes and pathogenic bacteria. The pH of the secretions is below 4.5. Good perineal hygiene should be encouraged, and the patient should be reassured that this is not indicative of a disease.

Table 13–5. Common Causes of Vaginal Discharge

Physiologic
  Hormonal changes
  Cervical ectopy
Inflammatory
  Foreign body
  Bacterial
  Nonspecific vulvovaginitis
  Bacterial vaginosis
  Candida
  Trichomonas
Sexually transmitted diseases
  Gonorrhea
  Chlamydia
  Salpingo-oophoritis (pelvic inflammatory disease)
  Condyloma accuminata

Cervical Ectopy

Ectopy represents the presence of the one cell–thick columnar epithelium extending from the endocervix out onto the visible ectocervix. Ectopy is normally found during early adolescence and gradually recedes as squamous metaplasia replaces the ectopic columnar epithelium. Oral contraceptive use favors the persistence or reappearance of ectopy. In ectopy, the cervical os may contain clear or slightly cloudy mucus. Colposcopy shows that the epithelium is intact and not ulcerated. Cauterization to eliminate ectopy is not warranted.

Ectopy may make the cervix more susceptible to infection with *N. gonorrhoeae* or *C. trachomatis* by exposing a larger area of susceptible columnar epithelium. Moreover, ectopy may increase susceptibility to human immunodeficiency virus (HIV) infection. If cervicitis supervenes, the area of ectopy may become edematous and fragile, and bleed in response to gentle swabbing.

Risk Factors

Sexual activity increases the risk of vulvovaginal infections and sexually transmitted diseases in adolescents. Oral contraceptives and douches, as well as the alteration of immune mechanisms by chemotherapeutic agents such as antibiotics or systemic illness such as diabetes mellitus have the potential to increase the risk of vulvovaginitis. Certain sexual practices; obesity; the wearing of tight, noncotton underclothing; and poor perineal hygiene can also play a role in the development of vulvovaginitis in the adolescent female. When evaluating young females with symptoms suggestive of vulvovaginitis, it is very helpful to identify these risk factors, as they may suggest the possible pathogen.

Clinical Features

The presenting symptoms may differ according to the organism. Once the normal vaginal flora is replaced by a pathogen, the vaginal mucosa becomes irritated and inflamed, often with a resulting increase in production of vaginal secretions and discharge and a change in odor or color. Adolescents with vulvovaginitis may note these changes. The color ranges from yellow or white to greenish brown, especially if the discharge is associated with bleeding. Pruritus and vulvar irritation symptoms are common. These include burning, dyspareunia, vulvar dysuria, or ill-defined discomfort of the genitalia. Pelvic pain, abnormal uterine bleeding, and other signs of pelvic inflammatory disease may be evident if an ascending infection is present.

APPROACH TO THE ADOLESCENT PATIENT

Conveying the belief that her problem is significant helps greatly in establishing a trusting relationship with the adolescent patient. Confidentiality is of utmost importance to adolescents, and the nature of the physician-patient relationship should be clearly stated. This is especially true when sexual activity is a concern. The clinician must also be aware that adolescents often use common gynecologic symptoms as a prelude to the discussion of more pressing concerns, such as possible pregnancy, contraceptive needs, or fear of a sexually transmitted illness. Sensitive listening and "reading between the lines" are in order in this setting.

Patient History

It is important to note the characteristics of the discharge and associated vulvar inflammation. Additional information should include pubertal status, menstrual history, the use of menstrual hygiene products, and medications. Timing of the onset of symptoms with respect to the menstrual cycle, sexual activity, or the use of medications should also be noted. Inquiry should be made, if applicable, into the number of sexual partners, any recent change in partners, and a history of dyspareunia, dysuria, or orogenital sexual activity.[35] Open-ended questions such as "Do you have a boyfriend?" and "Is it serious?" are useful in establishing communication early on. With time, more direct questions can be asked.

The presence of the parent or guardian usually limits discussion of sexuality. Talking with the adolescent in private yields a more accurate history. In some cases, the vulvovaginal symptoms may embarrass a young teenager, who may have difficulty revealing pertinent historical data and may be very reluctant to be examined. Supportive and nonthreatening discussion is critically important.

Physical Examination

For younger adolescents, vulvovaginitis often occasions their first pelvic examination. This setting provides an excellent opportunity to discuss pubertal changes, reproductive health, and the importance of routine gynecologic care. Discussion and reassurance regarding the pelvic examination and its importance are extremely helpful in creating a positive experience. Adult stirrups may be successfully used for most teenage patients.

The initial phase of the genital examination consists of an inspection of the vulva for distribution of pubic hair and signs of inflammation or vulvar skin disease, discharge, or trauma. After emphasizing normal findings or confirming visualization of potentially abnormal areas, the labia are gently separated, and the hymen and vestibule are inspected. The degree of estrogenization and caliber of the orifice are noted.

Decisions about how the discharge is sampled and whether a speculum is used are based primarily on the degree of relaxation, the size of the hymenal opening, and previous sexual activity. If an adolescent is not sexually active and has a small hymenal orifice, vaginal cultures or saline and potassium hydroxide wet-mounts can be obtained without the use of a speculum using an intravaginal saline-soaked, cotton-tipped swab. This may be especially appropriate if the girl has not used tampons in the past. If the patient has successfully used tampons, the Huffman-Graves speculum may be used to visualize the cervix and collect the appropriate specimens. In a sexually active adolescent, the cervix should be sampled for *N. gonorrhoeae* and *Chlamydia*. A Pap smear is important in sexually active teenagers to screen for HPV and other manifestations of cervical inflammation or dysplasia. A rectoabdominal or vaginoabdominal examination is required to de-

tect uterine or adnexal tenderness or, at times, the presence of a pelvic mass.

CAUSES AND MANAGEMENT

In adolescents, mixed infections are common. Evaluation of the discharge with respect to volume, color, character, odor, and pH is important. Microscopic evaluation of a wet-mount preparation is a significant part of the office evaluation. A specific culture may be required to determine whether a chlamydial or gonorrheal infection is present. The most common causes of vulvovaginitis are bacterial vaginosis, trichomoniasis, and candidiasis (Table 13–6).

BACTERIAL VAGINOSIS

Overgrowth of aerobic and anaerobic vaginal bacterial flora upsets the normal predominance of lactobacilli and results in bacterial vaginosis, the most common cause of vulvovaginitis in the reproductive age group.[36] Bacterial vaginosis accounts for approximately one third of all cases of vulvovaginitis in women.[37] It occurs when the normal vaginal flora is replaced by *Gardnerella vaginalis* (a gram-negative rod), *Mycoplasma hominis*, *Bacteroides* spp., or *Mobiluncus* spp. (a curved gram-negative rod).

Bacterial vaginosis is not currently considered a sexually transmitted disease, as its prevalence has been found to be similar in sexually active and in virginal females.[38] Many of the sexual partners of females with bacterial vaginosis have been found to be colonized with the same organ-

Table 13–6. Clinical Features of Vulvovaginitis

	Candidiasis	*Gardnerella vaginalis*	Trichomoniasis
Signs and symptoms	Pruritus Vulvovaginitis erythema White curdlike discharge	Vulvitis (rare) Gray-white "amine-like" discharge	Pruritus Vaginal erythema
Vaginal smear	Filaments and spores (10% potassium hydroxide)	Epithelial cells with bacteria "clue cells" Gram-negative rods Positive whiff test Fish odor with potassium hydroxide	Motile, flagellated organisms (saline)
pH	Acidic with nitrazine paper	5.0–5.5	6.5–7.5
Treatment	Clotrimazole Miconazole Nystatin Gentian violet or boric acid	Metronidazole Ampicillin	Metronidazole

Douching is not usually recommended for the adolescent.
From Sanfilippo JS: Adolescent girls with vaginal discharge. Pediatr Ann 1986; 15(7):509–519.

ism, however, and symptoms often follow unprotected intercourse. Some women may be more susceptible to acquiring bacterial vaginosis. Eschenbach and coworkers observed that women with bacterial vaginosis lack the H_2O_2-producing strains of lactobacilli that usually inhibit growth of the pathogens.[39]

Clinical Features

Although many women remain asymptomatic, the common presenting symptom of bacterial vaginosis is vaginal discharge with a foul odor—often a thin, homogeneous, gray discharge with a fishy odor. The organism, a surface parasite, is unable to invade the vaginal wall, and, therefore, acute inflammatory reaction is rare. Bacterial vaginosis has been associated with upper genital tract disorders (e.g., endomyometritis, chorioamnionitis, and pelvic inflammatory disease). *Mobiluncus* spp. have been associated with vaginal bleeding.[40]

On examination, discharge is usually noted at the introitus and may also be adherent to the vaginal walls. The mucosal surface often appears normal, without signs of acute inflammation. The vaginal pH is above 4.5, and on mixture of the fluid with a 10% potassium hydroxide solution, a fishy odor may be noticed (the "whiff" test). Metabolism of *G. vaginalis* produces amines. This positive whiff test is caused by the alkalinization of amines produced by the organism. Microscopic evaluation of a saline wet-mount preparation shows stippled vaginal epithelial cells, the borders of which appear obscured by the adherent bacteria. This typical appearance is called the "clue cell," and when 20% or more of the vaginal

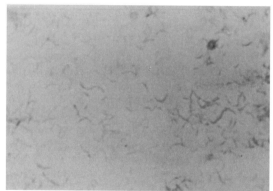

Figure 13–2. Typical comma-shaped cell seen in bacterial vaginosis caused by the curved rod-shaped *Mobiluncus* species. (From Mårdh P-A: The vaginal ecosystem. Am J Obstet Gynecol 1991; 165:1165–1166.)

epithelial cells show these features, some investigators consider it to be diagnostic for bacterial vaginosis (Fig. 13–1).[41] Few, if any, leukocytes are noted. The corkscrew movement pattern of the highly motile *Mobiluncus* bacterial rods may be another diagnostic feature seen on wet-mount slides (Fig. 13–2).[42] A Gram stain of the vaginal fluid reveals mixed flora with relatively few lactobacilli.[43]

Routine cultures generally are not helpful, and the diagnosis of bacterial vaginosis is confirmed on the basis of the presence of the clinical and wet-mount observations (Table 13–7).[44] The sensitivity and specificity of the wet-mount examination are given next.

Diagnosis

Wet Prep Alone
Sensitivity: 98%
Specificity: 94%

Wet Prep with KOH
Specificity: 99%

Treatment

The current treatment of bacterial vaginosis consists of an oral 7-day course of metronidazole (750 mg once daily).[45] With this regimen, an 80% to 90% cure rate has been reported. A single

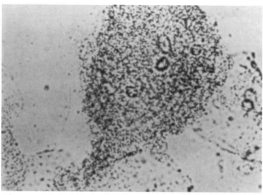

Figure 13–1. Typical "clue cell" of bacterial vaginosis. Note *Gardnerella vaginalis* attached to vaginal epithelial cell. (Courtesy of Dr. David Muram.)

Table 13–7. Clinical and Wet-Mount Criteria in Bacterial Vaginosis

A homogeneous, adherent discharge
Positive whiff test
"Clue" cells
pH > 4.5

2-gm dose has been suggested to improve patient compliance, but it has been associated with a significant failure rate.[41] Clindamycin, either oral or intravaginal, is an alternative treatment.[46] It is not clear whether an asymptomatic patient should be treated, although, in light of the potential for an ascending infection, it may well be necessary to treat asymptomatic women. Sexual partners are often not treated unless bacterial vaginosis recurs.[47]

TRICHOMONIASIS

T. vaginalis, a motile protozoan, is a common cause of vulvovaginitis in adolescent females, (15% to 20% of all cases of vulvovaginitis).[41] Although the organism is known to survive for several hours in wet towels or chlorinated water reservoirs,[48] it is transmitted primarily through sexual contact.

Clinical Features

The presenting complaint is usually a vaginal discharge. Because *T. vaginalis* also infects the urethra and Skene's glands, dysuria and vulvar pruritus are often present. Rarely, dyspareunia is a symptom of trichomoniasis. The discharge ranges from scant to profuse; is usually malodorous; and may be yellow, green, or gray. The trichomonads produce carbon dioxide, which may cause the discharge to appear frothy.

On examination, vulvar and vaginal erythema are common. Punctate hemorrhages of the vagina and cervix ("strawberry cervix") are visible in about 20% of cases.[35] Colposcopic evaluation may enhance detection of this abnormality (in about 45% of cases).[41] Such cervical involvement may result in postcoital bleeding, which may alter the color of the discharge.

Growth of the organism is optimal at a pH of 5.5 to 6.0; the vaginal pH in patients with trichomoniasis is generally above 5.0. Diagnosis is based on microscopic examination of the wet-mount preparation. Motile, flagellated, tear-shaped organisms are seen (Fig. 13–3), although, often, a number of seemingly lifeless ones can be observed. Many leukocytes are also identified. Unlike in bacterial vaginosis, lactobacilli may be present. Occasionally, trichomonads are noted on routine urinalysis. The Pap smear detects the trichomonads in about 60% of cases but is an unreliable test because of a high false-positive rate.[49] Gram stains are of little value.[41] Cultures are very sensitive but are rarely required to confirm the diagnosis.

Treatment

Treatment may consist of antibiotic therapy and local vulvar care. Systemic therapy is preferred to adequately treat the urethral and periurethral reservoirs. Metronidazole remains the medication of choice. The oral 7-day regimen of 250 mg three times per day has a cure rate of 95%[50]; the one-time dose of 2 gm has a cure rate of 88%.[41] Single-dose therapy facilitates patient

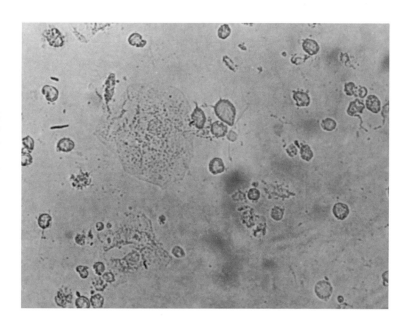

Figure 13–3. A wet mount showing motile trichomonads in the center and nonviable forms mixed with white blood cells in the periphery. (From Friedrich EG Jr: Vulvar Disease, 2nd ed. Philadelphia: WB Saunders, 1983.)

compliance and can even be administered in an office setting. Sexual partners should be treated simultaneously with the single-dose regimen. Metronidazole-resistant strains have been identified,[51] and infections with such strains may require treatment with higher doses for longer periods of time or, alternatively, a combination of oral and vaginal therapy. Monif suggests routine use of condoms and postcoital douching with an acidic solution as preventive therapy.[35]

CANDIDA *VULVOVAGINITIS*

Candida vulvovaginitis is fairly common in adolescents. Although prevalence estimates for this group are not readily available, it probably accounts for about 25% of all vulvovaginitis cases. Asymptomatic colonization may be present in as many as 20% of healthy women.[41]

C. albicans accounts for some 85% to 90% of all yeast organisms isolated from the human vagina.[41] Other *Candida* species (e.g., *Candida tropicalis*, *Torulopsis glabrata* [also known as *Candida glabrata*], and *Candida parapsilosis*) are becoming more prevalent as agents of vulvovaginitis. This increase probably reflects an increase in their resistance to conventional antifungal therapy. This results in an increased prevalence of treatment failures and recurrent *Candida* infections.[52] Although penile colonization has been observed in 20% of the male partners of women with recurrent *Candida* infections,[53] *Candida* vulvovaginitis is not considered a sexually transmitted disease.

Candida infection often follows disturbances in the normal vaginal ecosystem (e.g., diabetes mellitus, pregnancy, broad-spectrum antibiotic therapy, or another immunosuppressive state). The clinical observation that *Candida* vulvovaginitis most frequently appears in the luteal phase of the menstrual cycle is supported by the idea that modulation of the immune system may be influenced by the woman's hormone status.[54] Combination oral contraceptives containing estrogen predispose patients to *Candida* vulvovaginitis in a similar manner. A recent course of antibiotics can alter the microbiologic flora of the pubertal vagina, making *Candida* more likely to overgrow. Diabetes mellitus can predispose to *Candida* infections, and glucose screening—up to and including a glucose tolerance test—may be appropriate, although the latter has not been found to be cost-effective as routine screening.[41] Transmission by close contact (e.g., bedclothes) appears to be less likely. Increased body moisture associated with tight or restrictive clothing is a predisposing factor. Fashion consciousness among adolescents may increase the importance of this last factor as a cause for vulvovaginitis.

Clinical Features

The presenting complaint in *Candida* vulvovaginitis is usually severe vulvar pruritus. Secondary vulvar dysuria and dypareunia may also be present. There may be a small amount of white or yellow curdlike discharge that tends not to have an odor. The non–*C. albicans* species rarely cause dyspareunia or dysuria and therefore are associated with less discomfort than *C. albicans*.

Examination reveals diffuse erythema and hyperemia of the vulva. Inflammation may extend inferiorly to the perianal region or laterally toward the inner thighs. Excoriation and desquamated areas may be seen. White plaques or satellite *Candida* lesions may be identified. The dermatologic appearance can sometimes be confused with lichen sclerosus. The pH of the discharge is below 4.5.

The diagnosis is made by examination of the fungal hyphae and buds with a saline or potassium hydroxide wet-mount preparation (Fig. 13–4). Leukocytes and epithelial cells are usually present. Hyphae and pseudohyphae are noted on Gram stain. Culture may be obtained if the diagnosis is in doubt.

Treatment

Predisposing factors should be assessed and, if possible, corrected. Control of serum glucose,

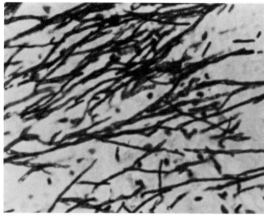

Figure 13–4. *Candida albicans* growing as hyphae and pseudohyphae within infected tissue (original magnification × 320). (From Monif GRG: Infectious Disease in Obstetrics and Gynecology. Hagerstown, MD: Harper & Row, 1974.)

use of oral contraceptives containing low-dose estrogen, avoidance of perfumed vaginal hygiene products, completion of antibiotic therapy, or a change to cotton undergarments (preferably less tight fitting ones) may be necessary.

Intravaginal therapy with antimycotic preparations (creams, suppositories, or tablets) for 3 to 7 days is the standard regimen. Traditional therapy consists of any of the imidazoles (miconazole, clotrimazole). The triazoles (e.g., terconazole) provide broad-spectrum coverage of C. albicans as well as non–C. albicans species.[52] In adolescent females, a shorter course of therapy promotes patient compliance, as deference to the desires of sexual partners may be a factor.

The topical and oral azoles (imidazoles and triazoles) currently available are associated with high cure rates (85% to 90%) in most patients with infrequent episodes of vulvovaginal candidiasis. However, C. glabrata and C. tropicalis have been shown to be less sensitive than C. albicans to standard imidazole antifungal agents such as miconazole and clotrimazole.[55–57]

Topical agents are the standard first-line therapy for vulvovaginitis. They have been shown to be safe and relatively free of untoward effects, the most common of which are headache and abdominal cramps (0.2% for both), and local burning, itching, or discomfort (0.9% to 6.0%).[58]

The availability of effective oral medications for the eradication of vulvovaginal candidiasis is important for adolescents, who may be reluctant to use intravaginal medication. Furthermore, shorter-course therapies are preferred by patients and help to ensure compliance, which has been shown to decline with longer treatment. Single-day therapies are available, require minimal effort, and have been shown to be as effective as short-course (3- to 7-day) regimens for acute episodes of vulvovaginal candidiasis.[59–61] Gastrointestinal symptoms and headache are the most frequently reported side effects with oral antifungal agents. Because data on teratogenicity are limited, oral agents should be avoided in pregnant adolescents and those contemplating pregnancy. Treatment of the male partner is not routinely recommended.

Recurrent Candida Vulvovaginitis

Recurrent or chronic Candida vulvovaginitis has become a problem. Whether because of the presence and persistence of vaginal yeast species or inconstant—and incomplete—therapy (associated with patient noncompliance) has been debated. More frequent use of broad-spectrum an-

tibiotic therapy has also been implicated. Defective T-cell function in immunodeficiency states allows the organisms to persist.[62] Over-the-counter availability of imidazoles may allow for subsequent selection of non–C. albicans species. Use of the triazoles in initial therapy may prevent this situation. However, in cases of recurrence, prophylactic postmenstrual therapy with intravaginal clotrimazole (500 mg each month)[63] or suppresive therapy with low-dose oral ketoconazole (100 mg daily for up to 6 months) has been found to be beneficial. Treatment of sexual partners has not been shown to be useful.

VULVOVAGINITIS OF UNUSUAL CAUSES

A foreign body within the vagina can produce persistent discharge with secondary vulvar irritation that will not respond to medical therapy. In adolescents, the most common vaginal foreign body is a forgotten tampon, usually found high in the proximal vagina, where it may have been "resting" for days or weeks. The discharge is usually dark brown, purulent, and malodorous. On removal of the tampon, symptoms abate. Vaginal ulcerations may appear if several weeks have elapsed before discovery and removal of the object.[48]

Chemical or allergic vulvovaginitis is more common in adolescents who use exogenous chemicals such as feminine hygiene sprays, douches, and deodorant tampons or creams, all of which can produce vaginal irritation.[43] Severe vulvar pruritus, burning, and discomfort are common. It is important to obtain a thorough history of possible allergens or irritants so that the diagnosis of Candida vulvovaginitis is not established incorrectly.[41]

REFERENCES

1. Koumantakis EE, Hassan EA, Deligeoroglou EK, Creatsas GK: Vulvovaginitis during childhood and adolescence. J Pediatr Adolesc Gynecol 1997; 10(1):39–43.
2. Grunberger W, Fisch LF: Pediatric gynecological outpatient department. A report on 600 patients. Wien Klin Wochenschr 1982; 94:614–618.
3. Pierce AM, Hart CA: Vulvovaginitis: Causes and management. Arch Dis Child 1991; 67:509–511.
4. Zeiguer NJ, Muchinik GR, et al: Vulvovaginitis in Argentinian children: Evaluation of determinant pathogens. Adolesc Pediatr Gynecol 1993; 6:25–31.
5. Gidwani GP: Approach to evaluation of premenarchal child with a gynecologic problem. Clin Obstet Gynecol 1987; 3:643.
6. Emans SJ, Goldstein DP: The gynecologic examination

of the prepubertal child with vulvovaginitis: Use of the knee-chest position. Pediatrics 1980; 65:758.

7. Muram D: Personal communication, 1993.
8. Pokorny SF, Storner LVN: Atraumatic removal of secretions from the prepubertal vagina. Am J Obstet Gynecol 1987; 156:581.
9. Paradise JE, et al: Vulvovaginitis in premenarchal girls: Clinical features and diagnostic evaluation. Pediatrics 1982; 70:193.
10. Emans SJ, Laufer MR, Goldstein DP: Pediatric and Adolescent Gynecology, 4th ed. Philadelphia: Lippincott-Raven, 1998, p 84.
11. Pokorny SF: Pediatric vulvovaginitis. *In* Kaufman RH, Faro S (eds): Benign Diseases of the Vulva and Vagina, 4th ed. St. Louis: Mosby, 1994, pp 56–57.
12. Bacon J: Pediatric vulvovaginitis. *In* Goldfarb A (ed): Clinical Problems in Pediatric and Adolescent Gynecology. New York: Chapman & Hall, 1996, p 24.
13. Muram D, Speck PM, Dockter M: Child sexual abuse examination: Is there a need for routine screening for *N. gonorrhoeae*? Adolesc Pediatr Gynecol 1996, 9:79–80.
14. Pierce AM, Hart CA: Vulvovaginitis: Causes and management. Arch Dis Child 1991; 67:509–511.
15. Koumantakis EE, Hassan EA, et al: Vulvovaginitis during childhood and adolescence. J Pediatr Adolesc Gynecol 1997; 10:39–43.
16. Jones R: Childhood vulvovaginitis and vaginal discharge in general practice. Family Pract 1996; 13:369–372.
17. Hammerschlag MR, et al: Anaerobic microflora of the vagina in children Am J Obstet Gynecol 1978; 131:853.
18. Gerstner GJ, et al: Vaginal organisms in prepubertal children with and without vulvovaginitis: A vaginoscopic study. Arch Gynecol 1982; 231:247.
19. Altchek A: Nonendocrine vaginal bleeding. *In* Lifshitz F, (ed): Pediatric Endocrinology, 3rd ed. New York: Marcel Dekker, 1996, p 207.
20. Spear RM, Rothbaum RJ, et al: Perianal streptococcal cellulitis. J Pediatr 1985; 107:557.
21. Kokx NP, Comstock JA, Facklam RR: Streptococcal perianal disease in children. Pediatrics 1987; 80:659–663.
22. Zeiguer NJ, et al: Vulvar abscesses caused by *Streptococcus pneumoniae*. Pediatr Infect Dis J 1992; 11:1335.
23. Cox RA: *Haemophilus influenzae*: An underrated cause of vulvovaginitis in young girls. J Clin Pathol 1997; 50:765–768.
24. Murphy TV, Nelson JD: *Shigella* vaginitis: Report of 38 patients and review of the literature. Pediatrics 1979; 63:511.
25. Watkins S, Quan L: Vulvovaginitis caused by *Yersinia enterocolitica*. Pediatr Infect Dis 1984; 3(5):444.
26. Danesh IS, Stephen JM, Gorbach J: Neonatal *Trichomonas vaginalis* infection. J Emerg Med 1995; 13(1):51–54.
27. Henderson P, Scott R: Foreign body vaginitis caused by toilet tissue. Am J Dis Child 1966; 111:529.
28. Paradise JE, Willis ED: Probability of vaginal foreign body in girls with genital complaints. Am J Dis Child 1985; 139:472–476.
29. Le SQ, Chantilis SJ, Carr BR: A typical presentation of a vaginal foreign body. Obstet Gynecol 1996; 88(4):736.
30. Katz A, Gershon AA, Hotez PJ (eds): Krugman's Infectious Diseases of Children, 10th ed. St. Louis: Mosby-Year Book, 1998.
31. Fivozinsky KB, Laufer MR: Vulvar disorders in prepubertal girls: A literature review. J Reprod Med 1998; 43:763–773.
32. Redondo-Lopez V, Cook RL, Sobel JD: Emerging role of lactobacilli in the control and maintenance of the vaginal bacterial microflora. Rev Infect Dis 1990; 12(5):856–872.

33. Friedrich EG: Vaginitis. Am J Obstet Gynecol 1985; 152:247–251.
34. Sanfilippo JS: Adolescent girls with vaginal discharge. Pediatr Ann 1986; 15(7):509–519.
35. Monif GRG: Infectious Vulvovaginitis. Keystone Heights, Fl: Rose Printing, 1985.
36. Kent HL: Epidemiology of vaginitis. Am J Obstet Gynecol 1991; 165:1168–1176.
37. Sobel J: The diagnosis and management of bacterial vaginosis. STD Bull 1992; 11(3):3–11.
38. Bump R, Bueshing WJ: Bacterial vaginosis in virginal and sexually active adolescent females: Evidence against exclusive sexual transmission. Am J Obstet Gynecol 1988; 158(4):935–939.
39. Eschenbach DA, Davick PR, Williams BL, et al: Prevalence of hydrogen peroxide–producing lactobacillus species in normal women and women with bacterial vaginosis. J Clin Microbiol 1989; 27(2):251–256.
40. Larsson PB, Bergman BB: Is there a causal connection between motile, curved rods, *Mobiluncus* species and bleeding complications? Am J Obstet Gynecol 1986; 154:107–108.
41. Sobel JD: Vaginal infections in adult women. Med Clin North Am 1990; 74(6):1573–1602.
42. Mårdh P-A: The vaginal ecosystem. Am J Obstet Gynecol 1991; 165:1163–1168.
43. Gerstner GJ, Grunberger W, Boschitsch E, Rotter M: Vaginal organisms in prepubertal children with children with and without vulvovaginitis. A vaginoscopic study. Arch Gynecol 1982; 231:247–252.
44. Amsel R, Toten PA, Spiegel CA, et al: Nonspecific vaginitis: Diagnostic criteria and microbial and epidemiologic associations. Am J Med 1983; 74:14–22.
45. Centers for Disease Control: 1989 sexually transmitted diseases treatment guidelines. MMWR 1989; 38(no. S-8):36.
46. Hillier S, Krohn MA, Watts H, et al: Microbiologic efficacy of intravaginal clindamycin cream for the treatment of bacterial vaginosis. Obstet Gynecol 1990; 76(3):407–413.
47. Thomason JL, Gelbart SM, Scaglione NJ: Bacterial vaginosis: Current review with indications for asymptomatic therapy. Am J Obstet Gynecol 1991; 165:1210–1217.
48. Altchek A: Vulvovaginitis, vulvar skin disease, and pelvic inflammatory disease. Pediatr Clin North Am 1981; 28(2):397–431.
49. Krieger JN, Tam MR, Stevens CE, et al: Diagnosis of trichomoniasis: Comparison of conventional wet-mount examination with cytologic studies, cultures and monoclonal antibody staining of direct specimens. JAMA 1988; 259:1223–1227.
50. Lossick JG, Kent HL: Trichomoniasis: Trends in diagnosis and management. Am J Obstet Gynecol 1991; 165:1217–1222.
51. Grossman JH III, Galask PG: Persistent vaginitis caused by metronidazole-resistant *Trichomonas*. Obstet Gynecol 1990; 76(3):521–522.
52. Horowitz BJ: Mycotic vulvovaginitis: A broad overview. Am J Obstet Gynecol 1991; 165:1188–1192.
53. Horowitz BJ, Edelstein SW, Lippman L: Sexual transmission of *Candida*. Obstet Gynecol 1987; 69:883–886.
54. Kalo-Klein A: *Candida albicans*: Cellular immune system interaction during different stages of the menstrual cycle. Am J Obstet Gynecol 1989; 161:1132–1136.
55. Horowitz BJ, Edelstein SW, Lippman L: *Candida tropicalis* vulvovaginitis. Obstet Gynecol 1985; 66:229–232.
56. Takada M, Kubota T, Hogaki M, et al: Attributes of microorganisms that contribute to recurrence and intractability of vaginal mycosis. Nippon Sanka Fujinka Gakkai Zasshi 1986; 38:1125–1134.

57. Odds FC: Resistance of yeasts to azole-derivative antifungals. J Antimicrob Chemother 31:463–471, 1993.)

58. Tobin MJ: Vulvovaginal candidiasis: Topical vs. oral therapy. Am Fam Phys 1995; 51:1715–1720.

59. Stein GE, Gurwith D, Mummaw N, Gurwith M: Single-dose ticonazole compared with 3-day clotrimazole treatment in vulvovaginal candidiasis. Antimicrob Agents Chemother 1986; 29:969–971.

60. Sobel JD, Brooker D, Stein GE, et al: Single oral dose fluconazole compared with conventional clotrimazole topical therapy of *Candida* vaginitis. Fluconazole Vagini-tis Study Group. Am J Obstet Gynecol 1995; 172(4 Pt 1):1263.

61. Kaplan B, Rabinerson D, Gibor Y: Single-dose systemic oral fluconazole for the treatment of vaginal candidiasis. Int J Gynaecol Obstet. 1997; 57(3):281.

62. Ashman RB, Papadimitriou JM: What's new in the mechanisms of host resistance to *Candida albicans* infection? Pathol Res Pract 1990; 186:527–534.

63. Roth AC, Milsom I, Forrsman L, Wahlen P: Intermittent prophylactic treatment of recurrent vaginal candidiasis by postmenstrual application of a 500 mg clotrimazole vaginal tablet. Genitourin Med 1990; 66:357–360.

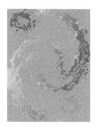

Chapter 14

Dermatologic Conditions of the Vulva

C. MARJORIE RIDLEY

To describe all dermatologic conditions of the vulva is outside the scope of this text. The clinical features, diagnosis, and management of those conditions that are common and of those that are less so but nevertheless important, will be discussed. There are several sources for the reader who wishes to explore further the subject of skin disease in general or vulvar disease in particular.[1, 2]

The patient may present, not to a dermatologist, but to a clinician unfamiliar with dermatologic problems, for instance to a gynecologist or a pediatrician or to a physician in genitourinary medicine who deals mainly with sexually transmitted disease. Interdisciplinary clinics obviously have value, and the growth of interest in pediatric dermatology as a separate specialty has also been a significant help.

An accepted classification of the conditions is essential. The current recommendations of the International Society for the Study of Vulvovaginal Disease (Table 14–1) is to be superseded shortly by a more logical system, whereby all the conditions will be listed in a simple morphologic and descriptive fashion such as would be met with in appropriate texts,[2] and, for example, the term *squamous cell hyperplasia*, which has no clinical meaning, will be dropped.

The appearance of vulvar lesions is affected by the warmth and moisture in the region; bullae rupture, and scaly areas become moist and macerated. Throughout life, the vulvar skin responds differently from that in other parts of the body, for example as regards absorptive capacity, transepidermal water evaporation, water-holding capacity of the stratum corneum, and susceptibility to irritants.[3]

HISTORY AND EXAMINATION

Wherever possible, a history should be obtained from the patient as well as from the par-

Table 14–1. International Society for the Study of Vulvovaginal Disease

Classification of Nonneoplastic Epithelial Disorders of Vulvar Skin and Mucosa 1987

Lichen sclerosus
Squamous cell hyperplasia
Other dermatoses
Mixed epithelial disorders may occur. In such cases it is recommended that both conditions be reported. For example, lichen sclerosus with associated squamous cell hyperplasia should be reported as lichen sclerosus and squamous cell hyperplasia. Squamous cell hyperplasia with associated vulvar intraepithelial neoplasia (formerly hyperplastic dystrophy with atypia) should be diagnosed as vulvar intraepithelial neoplasia.
Squamous cell hyperplasia is used for those instances in which the hyperplasia is not attributable to another cause. Specific lesions or dermatoses involving the vulva (for example, psoriasis, lichen planus, lichen simplex chronicus, *Candida* infection, condyloma acuminatum) may include squamous cell hyperplasia, but should be diagnosed specifically and excluded from this category.

Adapted from Ridley CM, Frankman O, Jones ISC, et al: New nomenclature for vulvar disease. Report of the Committee. Am J Obstet Gynecol 1989; 160:769. With permission of Mosby–Year Book, Inc.

ent. It is important to ensure that adolescents be given the opportunity to speak in private. An adequate and systematic physical examination is essential. This aspect is dealt with in detail in Chapter 12. It is usually satisfactorily achieved with the patient lying on her back with the legs abducted. A very small child can be examined lying on the knees of a parent or guardian. The labia minora spontaneously separate, and the vestibule can be clearly visualized. This position also usually allows the perineum and perineal area to be evaluated; otherwise, the left lateral or knee-chest position is employed. A mounted illuminated magnifying mirror is useful for observation of detail. The normal appearances must be appreciated; they vary throughout neonatal life, infancy, childhood, and adolescence. The findings should be noted on a diagram. A photograph is often useful. Details of how to conduct an internal examination and to take specimens to investigate for infection are presented in Chapter 12. When there is suspicion of sexual abuse, the examination and investigation must be carried out by an experienced physician who is aware of the criteria and of what procedures to follow. It is often necessary to examine the rest of the skin, including the mouth, hair and scalp, and nails. When the diagnosis is not clear but is unlikely to be of serious import, sensible symptomatic management is justifiable. It is important, however, in this situation, to reevaluate until a diagnosis has been reached or until the problem has resolved.

BIOPSY

When a biopsy is indicated, it is usually feasible to carry it out as an outpatient procedure. A cooperative parent can be of help during the procedure, but it is better to exclude those who are likely to be upset by it. For adolescents, a eutectic mixture of prilocaine and lidocaine (Emla cream) is applied; adduction of the thighs promotes the anesthetic effect, which usually takes about 10 minutes to develop. In children, this cream can cause methemoglobinemia and the preparation is not advised for them.[4] Lidocaine solution 1% is introduced through a fine-gauge needle or a dental cartridge. A disposable punch gives a good specimen for most purposes, with diameters of 3, 4, or 6 mm being used according to circumstances. The core of tissue can be snipped off at the base with sharp scissors, inflicting minimal distortion of the specimen. Larger defects may require an absorbable suture, whereas smaller ones require only pressure or light cautery to achieve hemostasis. Specimens for electron microscopy or immunofluorescence are rinsed in normal saline and then placed directly into special media or are quick-frozen.

VULVAR DISORDERS

In practice, there is to some extent a spectrum of disease across all age groups, but here these conditions are considered under the headings of (1) those associated largely with neonates and infants and (2) those more likely to be seen in older girls or adolescents.

DISORDERS IN THE NEONATE AND INFANT

Infants born prematurely tend to have immature skin that is imperfectly keratinized and easily damaged, losing heat and water rapidly.[5] The normal neonate has anatomically mature skin, but a number of functional deficiencies (e.g., inadequate eccrine sweating) commonly lead to skin changes. Sebaceous secretion is sometimes excessive and the child is susceptible to infection. Maternally induced hormonal changes are evident in the edema and erythema, which can last as long as a few weeks after birth, and often there is a vaginal discharge. The hymen may be thickened and pinkish until the age of about 4 years. A hymenal polyp is sometimes seen in a newborn as a polypoid structure, which represents a thickening of the hymen and looks like a tag[6] (Fig. 14–1). It is said to occur in 6% of newborns within the first 48 hours of life and tends to disappear within a few days.

Perianal Dermatitis

Perianal dermatitis has been described in neonates, especially ones who have been fed cow's milk formula. The skin is red and eroded; diaper rash may or may not be associated. Treatment consists of careful cleansing, bland lubricants, and protective agents such petroleum jelly.

Miliaria

Miliaria related to obstruction of the eccrine sweat duct is common in neonates, and to some extent in infants, perhaps in relation not only to obstruction of the duct but also to overheating.

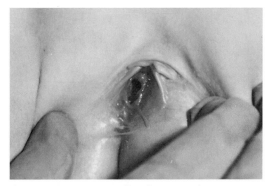

Figure 14–1. Hymenal polyp noted on gynecologic examination of a newborn.

The anogenital area is a common site. *Miliaria crystallina* refers to lesions caused by obstruction in the stratum corneum and *miliaria rubra* to those related to a deeper obstruction. The latter is the usual form. Groups of papulovesicles or pustules develop on a red background and last for a few days. Secondary infection may occur. Lesions must be differentiated from toxic erythema of the newborn, whose lesions are typically pustular and contain eosinophils. The condition responds to scrupulous hygiene and bland emollients such as aqueous cream.

Intertrigo

Intertrigo is common and develops as a result of friction, obesity, and moisture. Miliaria and secondary infection are often associated. Attention to hygiene, bland emollients, and perhaps a mild topical corticosteroid is effective treatment.

Impetigo

Impetigo is a risk in the first week or so of life. It is usually caused by *Staphylococcus aureus*, commonly phage group II, especially type 71, which may be acquired from the mother, another relative, or staff. Bullae that rapidly become crusted affect the genital area and elsewhere, and complications ensue if treatment with systemic antibiotics is not properly and rapidly prescribed. Outbreaks occur when the source is not promptly identified and treated.

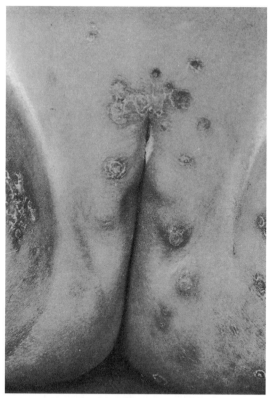

Figure 14–3. Note diaper rash, with eroded papules. (From Ridley M, Oriel JD, Robinson AJ: A Colour Atlas of Diseases of the Vulva. London: Chapman and Hall, 1992.)

Diaper Rash

Diaper rash is common and usually develops after the first weeks of life. It can be persistent (Fig. 14–2).

IRRITANT DERMATITIS

Irritant dermatitis is the commonest form of diaper rash. It is caused by friction and wetting, is aggravated by the effects of fecal contamination, urine of pH above 8 (which increases the activity of fecal proteases), and secondary infection with *Candida* and bacteria. It occurs more frequently in bottle-fed infants. The erythema has a glazed appearance and is sharply demarcated; the flexural areas are usually spared. Sometimes papules with eroded, shallow, ulcerated summits develop (Fig. 14–3). The rash usually clears uneventfully when diapers are no longer worn.

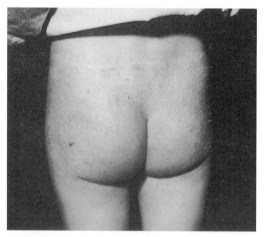

Figure 14–2. Diaper dermatitis. Note the clear demarcation of the diaper area with the irritation.

SEBORRHEIC DERMATITIS

Diaper seborrheic dermatitis is not related to the condition reported in adults (see Fig. 14–3). It is often associated with lesions elsewhere, particularly on the scalp. The diaper area is diffusely red. In differentiating it from atopic dermatitis, the nature of the lesions on other parts of the body and the relative absence of itching in the seborrheic type can be helpful, but it is often impossible to distinguish them completely except with the passage of time.

DIAPER PSORIASIS

Diaper psoriasis is probably not related to the psoriasis seen in older children and adults, the subjects not having the HLA patterns associated with that condition. Nevertheless, a few subjects do seem to be significantly likely to develop psoriasis later. The patches are strikingly scaly and well-defined, and there are often lesions elsewhere (Fig. 14–4).

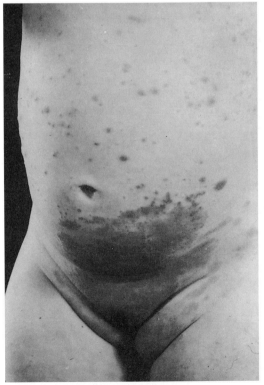

Figure 14–4. Diaper psoriasis showing well-defined lesions of the diaper area of the trunk. (From Ridley M, Oriel JD, Robinson AJ: A Colour Atlas of Diseases of the Vulva. London: Chapman and Hall, 1992.)

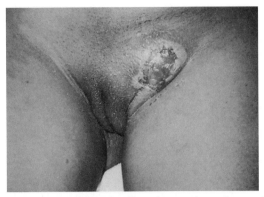

Figure 14–5. Infantile gluteal granuloma located in the left inguinal area.

DIFFERENTIAL DIAGNOSIS

The differential diagnosis of all these diaper rashes includes Langerhans cell histiocytosis, acrodermatitis enteropathica, and syphilis, all of which are rare and all likely to produce morphologically identifiable lesions in other areas.

Management calls for cleansing with a bland preparation such as emulsifying ointment and application of a protective agent such as petroleum jelly. A mild topical corticosteroid will be useful, often combined with an antifungal or antibacterial agent, but potent ones can lead to muscle wasting and systemic absorption. Whether or not the diaper is of the disposable or nondisposable type matters less than that it be changed frequently, which is all-important.

INFANTILE GLUTEAL GRANULOMA. A rare condition in which oval, livid, eroded nodules appear, often on a background of a resolving irritant diaper rash, is gluteal granuloma.[7] The histology is granulomatous. It may be related to occlusion and potent topical corticosteroids. It responds to reduction in the strength of the corticoseroid application and to simple measures, but may leave scarring (Fig. 14–5).

ACRODERMATITIS ENTEROPATHICA. Acrodermatitis enteropothica, a rare condition that is the result of zinc deficiency, can be inherited as a recessive defect of zinc absorption or acquired, for example, as a consequence of prematurity, drug effects (penicillamine, chelating agents), or total parenteral nutrition. The histologic picture is nonspecific. The lesions affect the face and anogenital area; they are bright red, often eroded, well-defined, and resistant to conventional treatments for diaper rash or eczema (Fig. 14–6). If treatment is long deferred, hair will be lost. Serum zinc levels are usually low but can be unreliable, and clinical diagnosis is paramount.

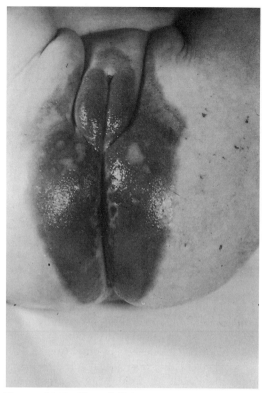

Figure 14–6. Zinc deficiency. Note red, eroded areas. (From Ridley M, Oriel JD, Robinson AJ: A Colour Atlas of Diseases of the Vulva. London: Chapman and Hall, 1992.)

Treatment with oral zinc—temporary or long-term according to the cause—is effective.

LANGERHANS CELL HISTIOCYTOSIS. The diaper area is involved, as are other parts of the body, in the so-called Letterer-Siwe form of histiocytosis (Fig. 14–7). The lesions are yellowish, often purpuric papules. The histologic picture is diagnostic: typical large cells contain lobulated nuclei and, on electron microscopy, Birbeck granules, together with histiocytes, eosinophils, and giant cells. The prognosis depends on the presence and extent of systemic involvement, and this factor also dictates treatment.

Labial Adhesions. Estrogen deficiency and inflammation have been postulated as causes. Adhesions were present in 1.4% of infants in one reported series (Fig. 14–8).[8] In another study of 50 children, as a rule, the adhesions appeared before age 2 years, but none before age 2 months.[9] Fusion, when almost complete, leaves only a pinhole meatus, situated anteriorly. A line of demarcation is always to be found between the clitoral hood and the labia minora,[10] a finding that helps to distinguish it from ambiguous genitalia. Other lesions in the differential diagnosis include lichen sclerosus (usually with associated texture changes, papules, loss of pigment, and obliteration of contours), scarring related to trauma such as sexual abuse or circumcision procedures, and rare conditions such as cicatricial pemphigoid.

Resolution is often spontaneous; in one series of 10 children it occurred in five patients within 6 months, in nine in 12 months, and in all by 18 months.[11] Where there are problems with pooling of urine or infection,[12] gentle manual separation by the mother using an application of an emollient or an estrogen cream is effective, though recurrences are frequent. Estrogen cream is capable of being absorbed, and it should not be used for more than about 2 weeks at a time. Surgical separation is very rarely, if ever, justified.

CONDITIONS OF OLDER CHILDREN AND ADOLESCENTS

Infestations and Infections

ECTOPARASITES

PEDICULOSIS. Pediculosis pubis may be encountered in adolescents and diagnosed by

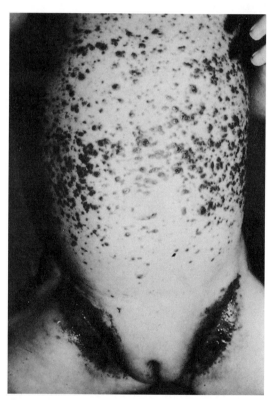

Figure 14–7. Langerhans cell histiocytosis, showing papules on the trunk and diaper area. (From Ridley M, Oriel JD, Robinson AJ: A Colour Atlas of Diseases of the Vulva. London: Chapman and Hall, 1992.)

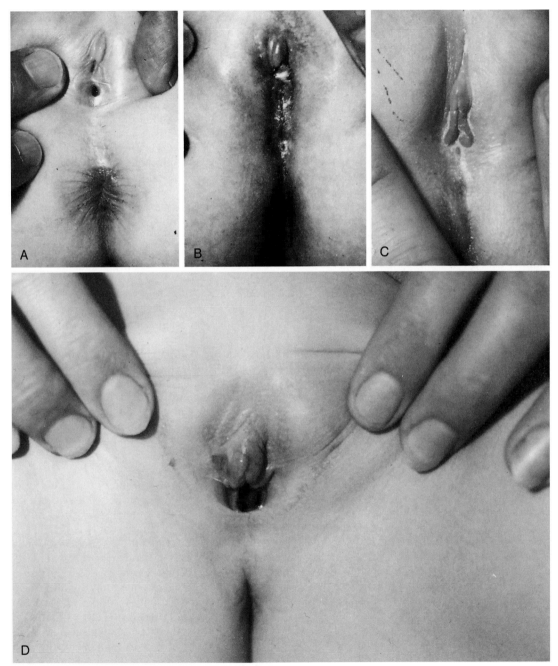

Figure 14–8. Labial adhesions. *A–C,* Small vaginal opening with complete closure of the vagina secondary to adhesions. *D,* Intact hymen and introitus with lateral displacement of the adherent area.

seeing nits and lice on the pubic hair. It is treated with aqueous solutions of malathion or carbaryl applied and left for 12 hours.

SCABIES. Scabies may occur at any age, but lesions of the vulva are extremely rare.

OXYURIASIS. *Enterobius* infestations (threadworm, whipworm) are common. These worms live in the large bowel and move out of the anus to lay eggs at night. Larvae hatch and reenter the canal, beginning the cycle a new. Pruritus ani is the usual symptom. Sometimes, however, the worms enter the vagina and pruritus vulvae ensues. Applying transparent adhesive tape to the perianal area in the morning before washing is a convenient way to isolate the ova, which can then be identified under the microscope. Piperazine salts should be administered to the whole family as well as to the patient. Hand washing and nail scrubbing after defecation and before meals are important in preventing reinfection. *Ascaris* and *Trichuris* infestations have occasionally been found in children.

FUNGAL INFECTIONS

CANDIDA. *Candida* is a common complication of diaper rash. *Candida* vulvovaginitis is rare in children but occurs in adolescents as in adults. Treatment is with imidazoles. Vulvar lesions of mucocutaneous candidiasis, a rare condition associated with immunosuppression, are marked by large plaques of *Candida*-infected tissue that are resistant to treatment.[13]

PITYRIASIS VERSICOLOR. A superficial infection caused by the yeastlike *Pityrosporon orbiculare*, pityriasis versicolor is usually manifested as scaly macules on the trunk that in postpubertal patients are brownish on pale skin and whitish on dark skin. Lesions of the face and in the genital area have been reported in West Indian infants of African extraction.[14] The diagnosis is made by visualizing spores and hyphae in a skin scraping to which is added a drop of 10% potassium hydroxide. Treatment with a topical imidazole, for example, clotrimazole, is effective.

BACTERIAL INFECTIONS

Mixed bacterial infections may be associated with poor hygiene, with maceration resulting from vaginal discharge, or with excoriation of any sort. Staphylococci are responsible for folliculitis in the pubic area. An underlying cause, such as diabetes, trauma following depilation procedures, or pediculosis, should always be sought. Oral

antibiotics may be required, in conjunction with local measures such as mupirocin ointment and antiseptic washes, for example, povidone-iodine. Staphylococcal infections of Bartholin's gland and duct are rare before adulthood. Staphylococci are also responsible for bullous impetigo in children and in babies, and sometimes, in conjunction with streptococci, for nonbullous forms.

Streptococci alone sometimes cause nonbullous impetigo. Treatment of all forms of impetigo is with antibiotics usually, unless the eruption is particularly severe, topically applied. Streptococcal cellulitis tends to occur, and to recur, in tissue that for any reason is chronically edematous. Penicillin V or erythromycin is effective in treatment and suppression and often must be taken for months, or even years. The organisms also occasionally cause a distinctive streptococcal dermatitis without true cellulitis.[15] This dermatitis is of three types; in one, the perianal skin is pink, moist, and tender; in another it is slightly red with fissures; and in the third it is beefy red with scaling and crusts. The organism, always a beta-hemolytic *Streptococcus* species, comes from the gastrointestinal tract or by way of the hands, throat, or skin. Such lesions may complicate underlying skin disease, for instance lichen sclerosus, or arise on apparently normal skin. Penicillin V or erythromycin is effective treatment, and topical antiseptics such as povidone-iodine are useful in preventing recurrence. Syphilis and gonorrhea are discussed in Chapters 21 and 22.

VIRAL INFECTIONS

All viral infections are more florid, and often atypical in presentation, in patients who are immunosuppressed, for example, with the human immunodeficiency virus.

VARICELLA-ZOSTER VIRUS. Varicella-zoster virus may affect the vulva as part of the generalized rash of varicella (chicken pox). Zoster is rare in young subjects; involvement of the 3rd sacral dermatome produces vulvar lesions.

HERPESVIRUS HOMINIS (HERPES SIMPLEX) AND HUMAN PAPILLOMAVIRUS. Vulvar features of viral infection by herpesvirus hominis and human papillomavirus are discussed in detail in Chapters 21 and 22. It suffices to point out that, while nonsexual transmission of genital herpesvirus is possible in a child, such lesions should arouse strong suspicion of sexual abuse. The position in regard to the human papillomavirus is somewhat different. Although sexual abuse always comes to mind in a child with anogenital warts, there is no doubt that they can transmitted by nonsexual contact, from the patient herself or from others or vertically, during passage through the birth canal. The incubation period can be as long as a year. Moreover, both types usually associated with genital warts, and those where that is not the case, may be involved. Typing of the virus may yield information on the site from which the warts are derived but it neither proves nor rules out sexual transmission.[16, 17]

MOLLUSCUM CONTAGIOSUM. Molluscum exists in two types but appears not to be site-specific.[18] The lesions are firm papules with an umbilicated center from which whitish material extrudes or can be extracted. Rarely do they present diagnostic difficulty. Curetted material can be examined as a wet-mount film or sent for histologic examination if there is any doubt. Treatment via local destruction, for example, piercing with a pointed applicator or cryotherapy, is effective but painful, and thus is a problem in children. Many dermatologists prefer to persuade the parents to await natural remission. Children usually have extragenital lesions, but some have anogenital ones. Whether investigation into the possibility of sexual abuse is undertaken depends on the circumstances. Adolescents sometimes have sexually transmitted anogenital molluscum.

VULVAR MANIFESTATIONS OF SYSTEMIC DISEASE

Acrodermatitis enteropathica and Langerhans cell histiocytosis were discussed earlier.

CROHN'S DISEASE

A condition of unknown cause, Crohn's disease can affect both children and adolescents.[19] Cutaneous lesions, usually oral and anogenital, may antedate intestinal signs and symptoms. The oral mucosa is sometimes thickened in a cobblestone pattern. The vulva is edematous with lymphangiectases, sinuses, abscesses, and tags

(Fig. 14–9). The bowel lesions are characterized histologically by noncaseating granulomas, but lesions of the skin are often nonpecific, showing only edema and lymphatic dilatation. The lymphangiectases are easily mistaken for warts,[20] and hidradenitis is also included in the differential diagnosis. Topical corticosteroids are helpful to some extent, and treatment of the intestinal lesions, for example, with metronidazole, often produces improvement of the skin lesions.

BEHÇET'S SYNDROME

A serious and multisystem disease likely to be of viral origin, the syndrome should be diagnosed only if accepted criteria are fulfilled; that is, recurrent oral ulceration accompanied by at least two of the following findings (Table 14–2): recurrent genital ulcers, eye lesions, cutaneous lesions (e.g., erythema nodosum, pyoderma and sterile pustules), and a positive anergy test.[21] The onset is sometimes in adolescence. Vulvar ulcers are painful, shallow, and persistent lesions that often cause scarring and tend to involve the labia minora. The histologic findings may be nonspecific or show thrombosed arterioles. Treatment includes topical antibiotics, corticosteroids, and anesthetic agents, as well as oral steroids, colchicine, immunosuppressives, and even thalidomide. The prognosis depends on the extent and nature of systemic involvement.

APHTHOUS ULCERS

Minor aphthous oral ulcers usually occur alone, but the major variant, often familial and tending to cause scarring, is sometimes accompanied by vulvar ulceration of similar type (Fig. 14–10). The cause is uncertain and the histologic findings nonspecific. Treatment is usually topical and much the same as that for the ulcers of Behçet's syndrome.

Table 14–2. Recurrent Ulcers of the Vulva

Lesion	Cause	Incidence	Family History	Other Sites	Histologic Findings	Scarring
Behçet's syndrome	Unknown, possibly viral	Very rare	Negative	Essential for diagnosis	Nonspecific	Common
Aphthous ulcer (major type)	Unknown, some cases genetic	Less rare	May be positive	Mouth	Nonspecific	Common
Other genital ulcers	Unknown, some cases probably viral	Rare	Negative	None	Nonspecific	Rare

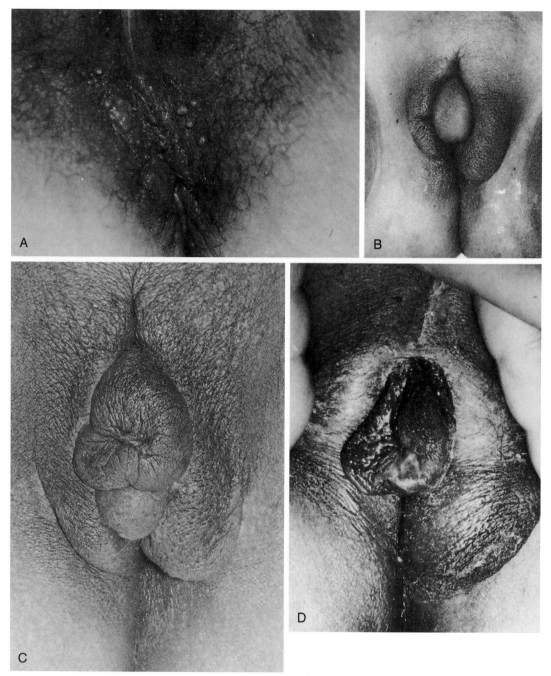

Figure 14–9. *A*, Perianal lesions of lymphangiectasia, suggestive of Crohn's disease. *B–D*, Vulvar involvement of Crohn's disease. (*A* from Ridley M, Oriel JD, Robinson AJ: A Colour Atlas of Diseases of the Vulva. London, Chapman and Hall, 1992.)

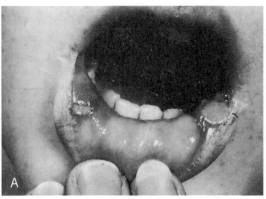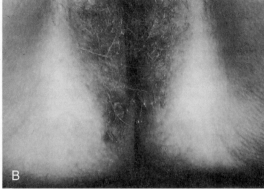

Figure 14–10. *A*, Aphthous ulcers of the mouth, and *B*, Vulvar area. (From Ridley CM: The Vulva. Edinburgh: Churchill Livingstone, 1988.)

OTHER NONINFECTIVE ULCERS OF UNCERTAIN ORIGIN

Many other names, such as *Lipschutz* and *Sutton*, have been attached to a variety of ulcers, often nonrecurrent ones. Some have no doubt been aphthous. Some are associated with leukemia, some with pityriasis lichenoides, and some with infectious mononucleosis.[22–24] Mononucleosis may be the main, but not the only, cause of ulcers of acute onset and fever in young girls. The histologic findings are nonspecific and the treatment symptomatic.

GENETIC DISORDERS

DARIER'S DISEASE (KERATOSIS FOLLICULARIS)

Darier's disease is inherited as an autosomal dominant trait. Its lesions appear late in childhood and gradually spread. The flexures are especially vulnerable. Horny papules coalesce, becoming macerated and infected. Patients are prone to bacterial and viral infections, and the vulva is often a site of severe outbreaks. The histologic findings are diagnostic, showing hyperkeratosis, parakeratosis, acanthosis, and acantholyic cells, which keratinize to form abnormal cells, the so-called *corps ronds*. Topical treatment with corticosteroids, antibacterials, antiseptics, and retinoic acid is of some benefit. Severe cases can be improved dramatically by an oral retinoid, acitretin, but side effects and teratogenic potential limit its use. Genetic counseling should be offered.

EPIDERMOLYSIS BULLOSA

A genetically determined mucocutaneous condition, epidermolysis bullosa has many different forms that are distinguished on clinical, genetic, and electron microscopic grounds. Lesions are likely to be present at birth or from an early age. When mucosal surfaces are involved, there may be scarring, depending on whether the bulla forms below the lamina lucida or within it. The labia, vagina, vestibule, and anal areas may all be affected (Fig. 14–11). No specific treatment is available; genetic counseling is important.

BENIGN FAMILIAL CHRONIC PEMPHIGUS (HAILEY-HAILEY DISEASE)

A rare condition, Hailey-Hailey disease is genetically determined by a dominant gene. Le-

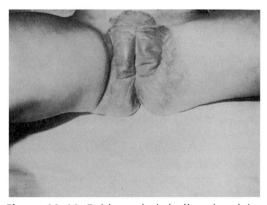

Figure 14–11. Epidermolysis bullosa involving the vulvar area.

sions appear in adolescence in some subjects, though often much later. They affect flexural areas, including the anogenital region. They are mostly associated with keratinized skin, but vaginal involvement has been reported.[25] The skin appears moist, red, and fissured, with or without visible blistering. Lesions are exacerbated by fungal *(Candida)*, bacterial, or viral infection and by allergic contact dermatitis. On histologic examination, the extensive acantholysis is easily confused with Darier's disease; *corps ronds*, however, are not present and the clinical appearance is usually sufficiently distinctive. The mainstays of treatment are topical corticosteroids and antibacterial agents, both occasionally also given systemically. A variety of drugs, including cyclosporine, have been used in difficult cases, with variable results, and surgical procedures, including grafting, are sometimes necessary.

DISORDERS OF SKIN APPENDAGES

DISORDERS OF HAIR

Folliculitis

Folliculitis, usually a result of depilatory preparations, is not uncommon and was discussed earlier.

Alopecia Areata

A condition of unknown cause but associated with autoimmune disease, alopecia is not uncommon, and in adolescents, patches may affect the pubic hair, usually in combination with lesions elsewhere. They are round and smooth. On histologic examination, early-stage lesions show some inflammation centered on the hair bulb, and later the follicles appear to be smaller and higher in the dermis than normal. There is no effective treatment, but the prognosis for spontaneous regrowth is often good.

Hidradenitis Suppurativa

Hidradenitis is now thought to be an affection of the follicular epithelium.[26] Its cause is unknown, but it rarely develops before puberty. The breasts, axillae, and particularly the anogenital area are involved. Painful, reddened nodules turn into abscesses, often with sinuses and fistu-

las. During quiescent periods, small bridged scars with comedones are seen. In severe cases the whole area is involved in a painful, unsightly mass. The differential diagnosis includes chronic infections such as granuloma inguinale and lymphogranuloma venereum, but the condition that most commonly causes difficulty is Crohn's disease. Oral antiandrogens[27] and long-term antibiotic therapy, as well as topical measures, have a limited role. Oral retinoids such as acitretin have been used, with varying effect, but the drug has side effects and is teratogenic. Surgery is often the best option. Minor procedures, small excisions, or extensive procedures with grafting may be necessary, depending on the severity of the condition.[28]

DISORDERS OF SWEAT GLANDS: FOX-FORDYCE DISEASE

Miliaria is discussed earlier.

A rare condition, of unknown cause, Fox-Fordyce disease is characterized by close-set, itchy papules of the breasts, axillae, and pubic area. They appear after puberty and tend to improve during pregnancy. Obstruction of the apocrine sweat glands leads to inflammation. Treatment is unsatisfactory, but alternatives include oral contraceptives, ultraviolet irradiation, and topical corticosteroids or retinoic acid.

DISORDERS OF PIGMENTATION

Hyperpigmentation

Hyperpigmentation may arise as a result of deposition of hemosiderin or melanin. Hemosiderin is found in many cases of lichen sclerosus and lichen planus. Melanin is responsible for the pigmentation in such lesions as seborrheic warts, lentigines, moles, and vulvar intraepithelial neoplasia. It is also responsible for the postinflammatory pigmentation that is a common sequela of lichen planus and that in dark-skinned persons may follow any inflammatory process.

Acanthosis Nigricans

In childhood and adolescence, this rare pigmented condition in the flexures may be hereditary. It is associated with insulin resistance. There is rarely ever cause for anxiety about associated malignancy, as there is in adults. The skin is dark, velvety, and thickened, and on histologic examination shows hyperkeratosis, acanthosis, and papillomatosis. The lesions must be differentiated from the diffuse darkening of these areas common in obese patients, particularly in dark-skinned ones.

Hypopigmentation

In dark-skinned persons, hypopigmentation may follow any inflammatory condition (Fig. 14–12).

Vitiligo

Vitiligo is of unknown cause but is associated with autoimmune disease. The loss of pigment is complete; melanocytes may be reduced in number, absent, or nonfunctional. It may affect the anogenital area at any age. The principal differential diagnosis is lichen sclerosus, although in the latter the examiner can usually detect a change of texture. The two lesions are quite likely to coexist,

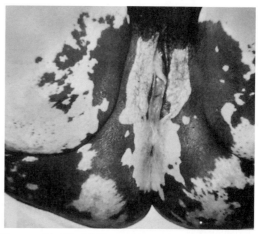

Figure 14–13. Vitiligo. Note the depigmented areas of the vulva.

however. The pigmentation is unlikely to return, and there is no effective treatment that is feasible in the genital area (Fig. 14–13).

BULLOUS (BLISTERING) DISEASES

A simple classification of bullous disease is presented in Table 14–3.

Bullous Diseases not of Immune-Mediated Causes

Impetigo, epidermolysis bullosa, and familial benign chronic pemphigus (Hailey-Hailey disease) were discussed earlier.

Stevens-Johnson Syndrome

The Stevens-Johnson syndrome is a variant of erythema multiforme with mucosal involvement; other skin manifestations may be conspicuous or absent. It is often precipitated by drugs or by herpesvirus hominis infection. The oral, ocular, and genital mucosae are attacked. The bullae rupture to leave painful denuded surfaces; acral targetlike lesions may coexist; and systemic disturbance is considerable. Scarring may be a sequela; introital adenosis is a rare complication.[29, 30] The bullae are subepidermal, and vascular changes and epidermal necrosis are associated. The main elements in the differential diagnosis are toxic epidermal necrolysis (TEN) and staphylococcal scalded skin syndrome

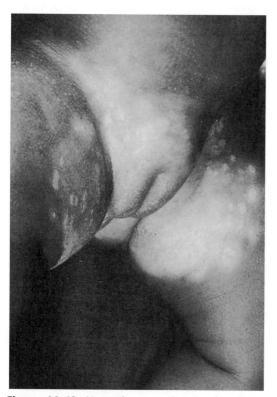

Figure 14–12. Hypopigmentation in the diaper area after resolution of diaper rash in a dark-skinned child. (From Ridley CM: The Vulva. Edinburgh: Churchill Livingstone, 1988.)

Table 14–3. Bullous Diseases

Disease	Cause	Site of Bullae	Immunofluorescence	Treatment
Epidermolysis bullosa	Genetic	Variable	Negative	Symptomatic
Benign familial chronic pemphigus	Genetic	Intraepidermal, acantholytic	Negative	Antibiotics, corticosteroids
Stevens-Johnson syndrome	Idiopathic, drugs, or herpes hominis (herpes simplex) virus	Subepidermal, with necrosis and vasculitic changes	Negative	Symptomatic (intensive care)
Toxic epidermal necrolysis	Drug or cause unknown	Subepidermal, marked necrosis	Negative	Symptomatic (intensive care)
Staphylococcal scalded skin syndrome	Bacterial	Intraepidermal, superficial	Negative	Antibiotics
Impetigo (bullous type)	Bacterial (staphylococci)	Intraepidermal	Negative	Antibiotics
Pemphigus vulgaris	Immune-mediated	Intraepidermal, acantholytic	+ IgG, intraepidermal	Immunosuppressives and many other drugs
Linear IgA disease	Immune-mediated	Subepidermal	+ IgA at basement membrane zone	Sulfapyridine and many other drugs
Cicatricial pemphigoid°	Immune-mediated	Subepidermal	+ IgG at basement membrane zone	Immunosuppressives and many other drugs
Bullous pemphigoid°	Immune-mediated	Subepidermal	+ IgG at basement membrane zone	Immunosuppressives and many other drugs

°In these two conditions immunofluorescence may not always be positive, in which case they can be distinguished only clinically, that is, by the scarring associated with cicatricial pemphigoid.

(SSSS). When the eruption is precipitated by a herpetic infection, long-term acyclovir prevents recurrences. Any medication that might be implicated must be withdrawn. The use of systemic steroids remains controversial. Cyclosporine may be used. In severe cases, treatment in a burn unit is essential.

Toxic Epidermal Necrolysis and Staphylococcal Scalded Skin Syndrome

TEN and SSSS are not always clinically distinctive. SSSS usually affects children and is provoked by a staphylococcal exotoxin, usually of phage type 2. TEN is precipitated by medications, but not by herpetic infection. The skin peels off over large areas, but the target lesions of erythema multiforme are absent, and mucosal surfaces are severely affected. The patient is very ill with fever, pain, secondary infection, and systemic involvement. In SSSS, there is an intraepidermal split below the granular cell layer, whereas in TEN the whole epidermis is necrotic with a subepidermal bulla and basal layer de-

struction. Thus, scarring, ocular and genital, is a sequela of TEN but not of SSSS. Distinguishing correctly between TEN and SSSS is vital, as the treatments are different, and histologic examination may be required. Stevens-Johnson syndrome may be difficult to distinguish unless skin lesions typical of erythema multiforme are present.

Management of SSSS is antibiotics. That of TEN is the same as treatment for Stevens-Johnson syndrome.

IMMUNOBULLOUS DISEASES

Some immune-mediated bullous disorders have a predilection for the vulvar area (Fig. 14–14).[31] They affect keratinized skin and mucosa, and often involve the eyes and mouth. Their pathogenesis lies in the development of antibodies against basement membrane and epidermal tissue. A blister is the result of interaction between the antibodies and the target cells, which are those that promote adhesion to the underlying dermis and to each other. Immunofluorescence, either direct (on the skin) or indirect (to detect circulating antibodies in the blood), is an

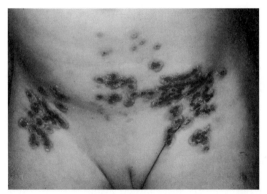

Figure 14–14. Chronic bullous disease of childhood (linear IgA disease). Note the clustered lesions on the lower trunk. (From Ridley CM: The Vulva. Edinburgh: Churchill Livingstone, 1988.)

essential technique for differentiation. Because clinically based nomenclature is giving way to more precise characterization in terms of the target cells, new names are often encountered.

Pemphigus Vulgaris

Pemphigus is rare in young subjects but has been reported on occasion in conjunction with a specific tumor.[32] Both mucosa and keratinized skin are involved. The vagina may be affected. When lesions are widespread, the patient is very ill and denuded surfaces ooze profusely. The bulla is intraepidermal with marked acantholysis, and immunoglobulin G (IgG) is deposited between the cells.

Chronic Bullous Disease of Childhood (Linear IgA Disease)

Linear IgA disease is characterized by tense bullae, often in clusters, on the keratinized skin of the genital area and elsewhere (see Fig. 14–14). It tends to improve at puberty, but may leave scars. The bullae are subepidermal and there is a band of IgA at the basement membrane zone.

Cicatricial Pemphigoid and Bullous Pemphigoid

Tense bullae affect the genital area and may involve the vaginal, oral, and ocular mucosa (the latter particularly in the case of cicatricial pem-

phigoid). On clinical findings, however, these diseases are distinguished by the fact that only the cicatricial form is associated with scarring. They are identical in showing subepidermal bullae and deposition of IgG at the basement membrane zone, although, in both, results of immunofluorescence testing are somewhat capricious. Both are rare in the young but have been reported, *with* genital involvement, in children.[31]

DIFFERENTIAL DIAGNOSIS

The differential diagnosis of immunobullous disorders contains, mainly, all such lesions and then lichen sclerosus and lichen planus. In children, sexual abuse occasionally must be considered as a differential diagnosis. The chief difficulty is that the clinical and histologic changes are not always specific where vulvar lesions are concerned and immunofluorescence tests are not always consistent. Lesions elsewhere are often more easily recognized.

MANAGEMENT

A detailed account of management for these diseases is outside the scope of this chapter. Generally speaking, topical bland preparations and corticosteroids are employed, but they help only those who are mildly affected. More often, management must address widespread disease and the use of potentially dangerous drugs, such as steroids, dapsone, sulfapyridine, sulfamethoxypyridine, minocycline, nicotinamide, azathioprine, and cyclosporine. The patient should be under the supervision of an experienced dermatologist who will cooperate, as appropriate, with the gynecologist and ophthalmologist.[2]

INFLAMMATORY DISORDERS

PSORIASIS

Psoriasis often affects the flexures, and anogenital lesions are not uncommon (Fig. 14–15). The usual scaling is often lost at this site, but the bright erythema and the sharp outline make diagnosis easy. Histologic examination shows parakeratosis, acanthosis, elongation of rete ridges, a thinner or absent granular layer, and perivascular inflammation; collections of neutrophils are sometimes seen in the horny layer. The lesions are responsive to bland emollients and topical

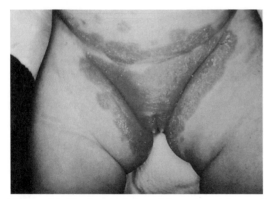

Figure 14–15. Psoriasis involving the vulvovaginal area.

corticosteroids, which can be safe and potent at the onset provided that the patient is carefully monitored. Tar, dithranol, and calcipotriol should not be used in the genital area.

SEBORRHEIC DERMATITIS

The lesions of seborrheic dermatitis are common in flexures and are less bright and less well-defined than those of psoriasis. The two can, nevertheless, be difficult to distinguish, clinically and histologically. Indeed, they can be intercurrent or change from one to the other.

ECZEMA

Even when it is severe elsewhere, atopic eczema rarely affects the vulva, except with diaper rash of infancy. Eczema at that site is more likely to be an irritant or allergic reaction complicating some other condition. Contact allergic dermatitis is confirmed by patch testing and appears to be more common when the anal area is involved by the rash.[33] Care must be taken to distinguish relevant positive findings from irrelevant ones. Relevant substances are commonly preservatives, local anesthetics, or other medicaments. The skin is erythematous and readily becomes thickened and excoriated. The histologic picture is that of spongiosis, parakeratosis, and acanthosis with dermal inflammation. The principal lesion in the differential diagnosis is psoriasis. The sharp outline of psoriatic lesions—and, often, the presence of typical lesions elsewhere—is helpful. The disease is managed with soothing preparations such as potassium permanganate solution, 1:10,000, followed by bland emollients or a topical corticosteroid ointment, and treatment of any secondary

infection. Combinations of a corticosteroid and an antifungal or antibacterial agent such as miconazole are useful.

LICHENIFICATION

Lichenification is the term given to thickening of the skin which is associated with itching lesions, particularly those of eczema and psoriasis. The skin looks pale in color and its markings are increased. Histologically, it is characterized by hyperkeratosis and marked acanthosis. To break the vicious cycle of scratching and itching, the topical steroid must be potent, and at night a mild anxiolytic and sedative, such as hydroxyzine, is helpful.

LICHEN SCLEROSUS

Lichen sclerosus affects all areas of the body, at all ages and in persons of both sexes.[34, 35] Anogenital lesions in girls are not uncommon and present several features of considerable importance. The cause is not known with certainty but is known to be linked to autoimmune disease.[36] Infectious agents, particularly *Borrelia burgdorferi*, have been suspected but the association appears to be unlikely.[37, 38] Recently, evidence of significant linking with class 2 HLA has been reported.[39]

The lesions of lichen sclerosus are ivory-colored, flat-topped papules that coalesce into plaques (Fig. 14–16); atrophy, purpura, and ecchymosis are common, as is the Koebner phenomenon (that is, the appearance of lesions in response to trauma). Extragenital lesions sometimes occur. Lesions on the vulva may involve the labia minora, the clitoris, and the surrounding tissue of the genitocrural folds, as well as the labia majora when they have developed, and they can extend into the perianal area in a figure-of-eight pattern. Nevertheless, many patients have sparse manifestations. Soreness and itching are variable. Perianal lesions sometimes lead to constipation, which is treated inappropriately when the underlying condition is not recognized. Histologic examination usually shows a thin epidermis with an underlying hyalinized zone, and, below that, a band of inflammatory cells. At other times, the epidermis may appear hyperkeratotic with pointed and forked rete ridges.

The differential diagnosis includes labial adhesions, where the only change is fusion; vitiligo, where there is only loss of pigment; and, most

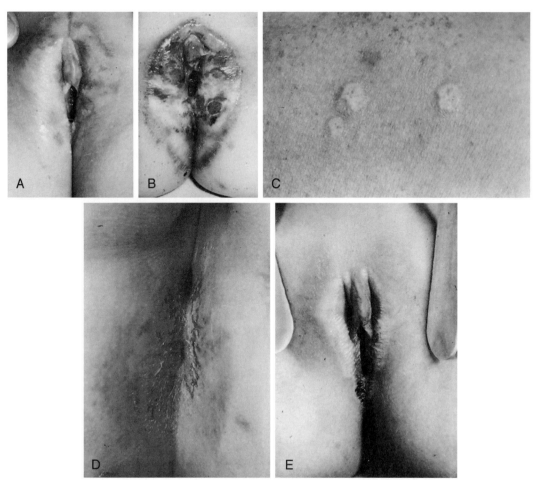

Figure 14–16. Lichen sclerosus. *A*, Areas of pallor. *B*, Vulvar lesions with secondary ulcerations. *C*, Ivory papules on the trunk. *D*, Perianal secondary infection. *E*, Intense purpura that bleeds with minimal trauma.

important, sexual abuse. It has been postulated that the trauma of abuse could provoke the appearance of lichen sclerosus, an example of the Koebner phenomenon,[40] but this idea is not generally accepted. Sexual abuse and lichen sclerosus can, of course, coexist, and each clinical case must be assessed and investigated as necessary and on its own merits.

For management, bland emollients, for example, aqueous cream for washing and after washing, are important, as is scrupulous hygiene and treatment of secondary infection. There is no place for testosterone or estrogen cream. Mild topical corticosteroids can suppress symptoms, but it is now generally accepted that a very potent corticosteroid, clobetasol propionate 0.05%, is dramatically effective in children, as it is in adults. It not only relieves symptoms but apparently arrests the disease process, halting tissue destruction and, in mildly affected children, ef-

facing all trace of the disease.[41] Concerns about safety seem to be unfounded; the minute amounts required do not carry the risk of local or systemic side effects. Obviously, careful supervision is necessary, instruction being given on a safe amount to be used in a given time. After a reducing regimen has controlled the condition, maintenance is achieved by occasional use, an approach probably more effective than resorting to a milder preparation.

The prognosis is good in so far as most cases improve around puberty. Some girls have a recurrence in adolescence or as adults.[42] With this new approach, however, the natural history of lichen sclerosus may be much modified. Parents can certainly be assured that intercourse and pregnancy will be possible. With lichen sclerosus, there is a small but definitely increased risk of squamous cell carcinoma, and though this eventuality is almost entirely confined to older women, it has been reported in adolescents.[43] Again, it is not yet known whether this risk will be modified by the new treatment regimens.

LICHEN PLANUS

Lichen planus, which has clinical and histologic similarities with lichen sclerosus, is rare in young people—at any anatomic site. However, a vulvar example of its rare form, *lichen planus pemphigoides*, was reported in a child,[44] and, in the erosive vulvovaginal-gingival form, it is sometimes seen in adolescents.[45] In this latter manifestation, lesions affect the vulva with painful erosions and destruction of architecture; the vagina with erosions that may lead to synechiae and stenosis; and the mouth with an erosive gingivitis, and, sometimes, buccal and labial lesions. Histologic examination shows hyperkeratosis, an increased granular layer, acanthosis with a saw-toothed, irregular appearance, basal cell liquefaction, and a bandlike dermal infiltrate in close apposition to the dermis.

The clinical course is usually chronic and treatment is unsatisfactory. The patient may present to a gynecologist, who is not familiar with her disease. Unfortunately, surgical intervention without the judicious use of dilators and potent topical corticosteroids can be detrimental. Systemic steroids, retinoids, cyclosporine, and other potent medications are sometimes prescribed, and it is imperative that the patient be under the care of a multidisciplinary team, including a dermatologist. In anogenital lichen planus, generally, there is risk of squamous cell carcinoma, but it has rarely (if ever) been reported in this particular form of the disease.

CYSTS AND TUMORS[46]

Unless the diagnosis is beyond doubt, any mass of the vulva should be excised or biopsy samples taken for study.

CYSTS

Congenital cysts may be discovered at any age. When in the vestibule, they are primarily mucinous and, when more lateral, principally mesonephric. Other cysts, such as sebaceous and epidermal cysts, and cysts of Bartholin's gland duct, are unlikely to be seen before adult life.

TUMORS

Nonepithelial Tumors[47]

Some malignant nonepithelial tumors can involve the vagina of infant girls and present as a vulvar mass.

NEUROFIBROMATOSIS TYPE 2

Lesions of neurofibromatosis may appear on the vulva in a child or adolescent—alone, or as part of more widespread manifestations of the disease. They may be nodular or more diffuse. Clitoral involvement has sometimes been mistaken for ambiguous genitalia.[48] Such lesions tend to be reported selectively, and the true incidence is unknown. Malignant change is possible, but rare. Histologic examination shows Schwann cells, thick bundles of collagen, and mucoid material. The tumors can be excised; the diffuse masses, less easily.

HEMANGIOMA

A hemangioma may be a hamartoma rather than a true neoplasm (Fig. 14–17). That most commonly seen on the vulva is the cavernous hemangioma, or strawberry mark, a large mass, often ulcerated or secondarily infected. On histologic examination, there are large vascular channels lined with a single layer of endothelial cells. Infection is treated with topical agents, and hemorrhage is rarely a problem (except in the rare Kasabach-Merritt syndrome, when the tumor leads to thrombocytopenia for which systemic steroids are given). The prognosis is good: natural resolution leaves areas of lax and shrivelled skin, which, if unsightly, can be treated by plastic surgery.

LYMPHANGIOMA

Lymphangiomas present as soft masses, often in the labia majora, or as the tiny, frogspawn-like vesicles of lymphangioma circumscriptum. The latter lesions tend to occur in young adults, and hemorrhage into the vesicles can mimic angiokeratomas, which, however, are unlikely to be seen in this age group. Lymphatic spaces are lined by endothelial cells that contain lymphocytes and erythrocytes. Excision is unsatisfactory, as underlying lymphatic spaces often communicate. The carbon dioxide laser has been helpful.[49]

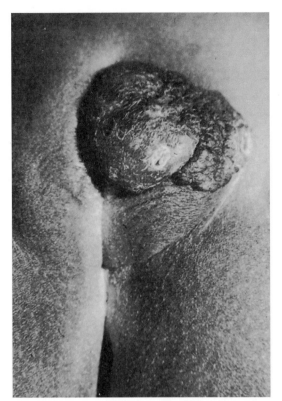

Figure 14–17. Strawberry-type hemangioma on the vulva.

LIPOMA

Lipomas can develop at any age. They usually affect the labia majora, and have no unusual features, appearing as soft, rounded masses of mature adipose cells.

Epithelial Tumors[50]

VULVAR INTRAEPITHELIAL NEOPLASIA

A subject of great importance, vulvar intraepithelial neoplasia (VIN) is currently under intensive study. The brief account that follows is, of necessity, not comprehensive.

VIN is currently classified as differentiated and undifferentiated types. The former is found almost always in older women, a complication as a rule of lichen sclerosus, and will not be discussed further here. The latter, undifferentiated type, however, is closely associated with human papillomavirus types 16 and 18 and is found in younger age groups. It is customary, at present, though not altogether satisfactory, to speak of the full-thickness undifferentiated type as VIN3,

and to discount those of lesser extent. At least two cases of this type have been reported in girls.[51, 52] One was in a 3-year-old victim of sexual abuse; the lesion regressed after biopsy. The second was in a girl aged 2 without evidence of sexual abuse; papillomavirus types 16 and 18 were found, and that lesion responded to cryotherapy.

Today, VIN3 is not uncommon in adolescents. The appearances are variable, consisting of solitary or, more often, flat or raised patches that can be warty or smooth, and reddish, pale, or brown in color. Biopsy, often repeated and multiple, is needed to check for the presence of invasive carcinoma, which sometimes supervenes; predisposing factors are smoking and immunosuppression. As cervical intraepithelial neoplasia is often associated, and potentially more serious, the cervix, too, must be kept under observation. Histologic examination shows full-thickness atypia, with a pattern of either close-set abnormal cells or a more disorderly arrangement of such cells with koilocytes; the two appearances may coexist. Treatment is unsatisfactory. In a young and otherwise healthy patient, careful observation is an option, although remission is rare. When there are symptoms or adverse factors, excision must be done with care, to avoid, whenever possible, unacceptable tissue loss. The alternatives, such as cryotherapy or 5-fluorouracil, unfortunately produce poor results. Laser treatment is painful. Moreover, it is ineffective in hairy areas where the VIN extends into the follicles.

SQUAMOUS CELL CARCINOMA

Squamous cell carcinoma is rare in adolescents but has been reported with lichen sclerosus.[43]

MELANOCYTIC LESIONS

LENTIGINES. Lentigines may be single or multiple. They are brown and macular. The LAMB syndrome (*l*entigines, *a*trial myxoma, *m*ucocutaneous myxomas, and *b*lue nevi) has been reported in a girl of 13 who had vulvar lentigines.[53] Histologically, there is increased pigmentation and increased numbers of melanocytes in the basal layer, with some melanophages in the underlying dermis.

MOLES. Intraepidermal, compound, and junctional nevi are quite common at the vulva. Ideally, they should be excised, since the patient may find them difficult to observe and malignant melanoma of the vulva has a poor prognosis. Some unusual compound nevi in young women can easily be mistaken for malignant melanoma; nests of odd shaped cells are found in the dermis.[54] A true vulvar malignant melanoma was reported in a girl aged 14 years who, presumably coincidentally, had lichen sclerosus.[55] A juvenile mole, or Spitz nevus, may occur at this site. It is a brown nodule and benign and has a distinctive histologic appearance of spindle and epithelioid nevus cells in the epidermis, sometimes with giant cells.

ADNEXAL NEOPLASMS. The only adnexal neoplasm likely to be encountered in children or adolescents is syringoma, a benign tumor of eccrine origin. Many cases have been reported in young adults, usually in association with lesions elsewhere, and they have also been reported in children.[56] They are small skin-colored papules. The histologic appearance is of comma-shaped ducts surrounded by fibrous tissue and lined with epithelial cells.

REFERENCES

1. Champion RH, Burton JL, Burns DA, Breathnach SM, et al (eds): Rook, Wilkinson, Ebling Textbook of Dermatology, 6th ed. Oxford: Blackwell Scientific, 1998.
2. Ridley CM, Neill SM (eds): The Vulva, 2nd ed. Oxford: Blackwell Scientific, 1999.
3. Oriba HA, Elsner P, Maibach HI: Vulvar physiology. Semin Dermatol 1989; 8:2.
4. Frayling IM, Addison GM, Chattergee K, Meakin G: Methaemoglobinaemia in children treated with prilocaine-lignocaine cream. Br Med J 1990; 301:153.
5. Immature skin. Lancet 1989; ii (8672):1138.
6. Borglin NE, Selander P: Hymenal polyps in newborn infants. Acta Paediatr (Suppl) 1962; 135:28.
7. Bluestein J, Furner EB, Phillips D: Granuloma gluteale infantum: Case report and review of the literature. Pediatr Dermatol 1990; 7:196.
8. Christensen EH, Oster J: Adhesions of labia minora (synechia vulvae) in childhood. Acta Paediatr Scand 1971; 60:709.
9. Capraro VJ, Greenberg H: Adhesions of the labia minora: A study of 50 patients. Obstet Gynecol 1972; 39:65.
10. Pokorny SF: Prepubertal vulvovaginopathies. Obstet Gynecol Clin North Am 1992; 19:39.
11. Jenkinson SD, Mackinnon AE: Spontaneous separation of fused labia minora in prepubertal girls. Br Med J 1984; 289:160.
12. Finlay HVL: Adhesions of the labia minora in childhood. Proc R Soc Med 1965; 58:929.
13. Odds FC: *Candida* and Candidosis, 2nd ed. London: Bailliere Tindall, 1988.
14. Jeliffe DB, Jacobson FW: The clinical picture of tinea versicolor in Negro infants. J Trop Hyg 1954; 57:290.
15. Krol AL: Perianal streptococcal dermatitis. Pediatr Dermatol 1990; 7:97.
16. Padel AF, Venning VA, Evans MF, et al: Human papillomaviruses in anogenital warts in children: Typing by in situ hybridisation. Br Med J 1990; 300:1491.
17. Handley JM, Maw RD, Bingham EA, et al: Anogenital warts in children. Clin Exp Dermatol 1993; 18:241.
18. Porter CD, Blake NW, Archard LC, et al: Molluscum contagiosum virus types in genital and non-genital lesions. Br J Dermatol 1989; 120:37.
19. Lally MR, Orenstein SR, Cohen BA: Crohn's disease of the vulva in an 8-year-old girl. Pediatr Dermatol 1988; 5:103.
20. Handfield-Jones SE, Prendiville WJ, Norman S: Vulvar lymphangiectasia. Genitourin Med 1989; 65:335.
21. Wechsler B, Davatchi F, Mizushima Y, et al: Criteria for diagnosis of Behçet's disease. Lancet 1990; 335:1078.
22. Muram D, Gold SS: Vulvar ulcerations in girls with myelocytic leukemia. South Med J 1993; 86:293.
23. Burke DA, Adams RM, Arundell FD: Febrile ulceronecrotic Mucha-Habermann's disease. Arch Dermatol 1969; 100:200.
24. Lampert A, Assier-Bonnet H, Chevallier B, et al: Lipschutz's genital ulceration: A manifestation of Epstein-Barr virus primary infection. Br J Dermatol 1996; 135:663.
25. Vaclavinkova V, Neumann E: Vaginal involvement in familial benign chronic pemphigus (morbus Hailey-Hailey). Acta Derm Venereol 1982; 62:80.
26. Yu CCW, Cook MG: Hidradenitis suppurativa: A disease of follicular epithelium rather than apocrine glands. Br J Dermatol 1990; 122:763.
27. Mortimer PS, Dawber RPR, Gales MA, Moore RA: A double-blind controlled cross-over trial of cyproterone acetate in females with hidradenitis suppurativa. Br J Dermatol 1990; 122:263.
28. Banerjee AK: Surgical treatment of hidradenitis. Br J Surg 1992; 79:863.
29. Wilson EEB, Malinak LR: Vulvovaginal sequelae of Stevens-Johnson syndrome and their management. Obstet Gynecol 1988; 71:478.
30. Bonafe JL, Thibaut I, Hoff J: Introital adenosis associated with the Stevens-Johnson syndrome. Clin Exp Dermatol 1990; 15:356.
31. Marren P, Wojnarowska F, Venning V, et al: Vulvar involvement in autoimmune bullous diseases. J Reprod Med 1993; 38:101.
32. Coulson IH, Cook MG, Bruton J, Penfold C: Atypical pemphigus vulgaris associated with angiofollicular lymph node hyperplasia (Castleman's disease). Clin Exp Dermatol 1986; 11:656.
33. Goldsmith PC, Rycroft RJG, White I, et al: Contact sensitivity in women with anogenital dermatoses. Contact Dermatol 1997; 36:174.
34. Meffert JJ, Davis BM, Grimwood RE: Lichen sclerosus. J Am Acad Dermatol 1995; 32:393.
35. Meyrick Thomas RH, Ridley CM, McGibbon DH, Black MM: Lichen sclerosus in women. J R Soc Med 1996; 89:694.
36. Meyrick Thomas RH, Ridley CM, McGibbon DH, Black MM: Lichen sclerosus and autoimmunity—a study of 350 women. Br J Dermatol 1988; 118:41.
37. Aberer E, Stanek G: Histological evidence for spirochetal origin of morphea and lichen sclerosus et atrophicans. Am J Dermatopathol 1987; 9:374.
38. Farrell AM, Millard PR, Schomberg KH, Wojnarowska F: An infective aetiology for lichen sclerosus: Myth or reality? Br J Dermatol 1997; 137 (Suppl 30): 25.
39. Marren P, Yell J, Charnock FM, et al: The association between lichen sclerosus and antigens of the HLA system. Br J Dermatol 1995; 132:197.
40. Warrington SA, de San Lazaro C: Lichen sclerosus et atrophicus and sexual abuse. Arch Dis Child 1996; 75:512.

41. Fischer G, Rogers M; Treatment of childhood vulvar lichen sclerosus with a potent topical corticosteroid. Pediatr Dermatol 1997; 14:235.

42. Ridley CM: Genital lichen sclerosus (lichen sclerosus et atrophicus) in childhood and adolescence. J R Soc Med 1993; 86:69.

43. Pelisse M: Lichen sclerosus. Ann Dermatol Venereol 1987; 114:411.

44. Hernando LB, Sebastian FV, Sanchez H, et al: Lichen planus pemphigoides in a 10-year-old girl. J Am Acad Dermatol 1992; 26; 124.

45. Pelisse M: The vulvo-vaginal-gingival syndrome: A new form of erosive lichen planus. Int J Dermatol 1989; 28:381.

46. Fox H, Buckley CH: Tumour-like lesions and cysts of the vulva. In Ridley CM, Neill SM (eds): The Vulva, 2nd ed. Oxford: Blackwell Scientific, 1999.

47. Fox H, Buckley CH: Non-epithelial tumours of the vulva. In Ridley CM, Neill SM (eds): The Vulva, 2nd ed. Oxford: Blackwell Scientific, 1999.

48. Friedrich EG, Wilkinson EJ: Vulvar surgery for neurofibromatosis. Obstet Gynecol 1985; 65:135.

49. Bailin P, Kantor GK, Wheeland RG: Carbon dioxide laser vaporization of lymphangioma circumscriptum. J Am Acad Dermatol 1986; 14:257.

50. Fox H, Buckley CH: Epithelial tumours of the vulva. In Ridley CM, Neill SM (eds): The Vulva, 2nd ed. Oxford: Blackwell Scientific, 1999.

51. Halasz C, Silvers D, Crum CP: Bowenoid papulosis in a 3-year-old girl. J Am Acad Dermatol 1986; 14:326.

52. Weitzner JM, Fields KW, Robinson MJ: Pediatric Bowenoid papulosis: Risks and management. Pediatr Dermatol 1989; 6:303.

53. Rhodes AR, Silverman RA, Harrist TJ, Perez-Atayde AR: Mucocutaneous lentigines cardiomucocutaneous myxomas and multiple blue nevi: The LAMB syndrome. J Am Acad Dermatol 1984; 10:72.

54. Friedman RJ, Ackerman AB: Difficulties in the diagnosis of melanocytic nevi on the vulva of premenopausal women. In Ackerman AB (ed): Pathology of Malignant Melanoma. Chicago: Year Book, 1981, p 119.

55. Friedman RJ, Kopf AW, Jones WB: Malignant melanoma in association with lichen sclerosus on the vulva of a 14-year-old girl. Am J Dermatopathol 1984; 6:253.

56. Scherbenske JM, Lupton GP, Hames WD, Kirkle DB: Vulvar syringomas occuring in a 9-year-old child (Correspondence) J Am Acad Dermatol 1988; 19:575.

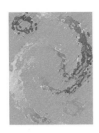

Chapter 15

Vaginal Bleeding in Childhood and Menstrual Disorders in Adolescence

CLAIRE TEMPLEMAN, S. PAIGE HERTWECK,
DAVID MURAM, AND JOSEPH S. SANFILIPPO

Bleeding in an adolescent girl is clinically significant when it is prolonged or blood loss is excessive. In comparison, vaginal bleeding in early childhood, regardless of its duration and quantity, is always clinically important. Such bleeding may be caused by local vulvar or vaginal lesions or may arise from the endometrium as a manifestation of precocious puberty. In adolescent girls, excessive or irregular bleeding from the vagina is one of the most common disorders of menstrual function. Most of these girls suffer from dysfunctional uterine bleeding. Determining the cause of vaginal bleeding in children and adolescents can be a challenge to the clinician.

BLEEDING GENERATED BY VULVAR AND VAGINAL DISORDERS

A detailed history and careful inspection of the external genitalia reveal the cause of bleeding in many girls with vulvar lesions.[1, 2] To rule out local vaginal lesions (e.g., tumors, foreign bodies), vaginoscopy and examination under anesthesia are the mainstays of evaluation. In infants and children, the hymenal orifice normally admits 0.5-cm vaginoscopy. An instrument 0.8 cm in diameter can be used to examine most older premenarchal girls. The more common vulvar and vaginal disorders that cause bleeding in children are listed in Table 15–1.

The illustrations in this chapter are courtesy of the North American Society for Pediatric and Adolescent Gynecology.

VULVOVAGINITIS

Vulvovaginitis is the most common gynecologic disorder in children. Young girls are susceptible to infections because perineal hygiene is often less than adequate and contamination by stool or debris is common. In addition, the vaginal mucosa is thin and atrophic and, therefore, less resistant to infections. The symptoms of vulvovaginitis vary from minor discomfort to relatively intense perineal pruritus or a sensation of burning accompanied by a foul-smelling discharge. The irritating discharge inflames the vulva and often causes the child to scratch the affected area to the point of bleeding. Acute vulvovaginitis may denude the thin vulvar or vaginal mucosa, but bleeding usually is minimal, and, as a rule, the discharge is little more than blood staining. Inspection of the vagina reveals an area of redness and soreness that may be minimal or may extend laterally to the thighs and posteriorly to the anus (Fig. 15–1). Vaginoscopy is necessary to exclude a foreign body or tumor in a girl who has recurrent vaginal infections or a foul-smelling, bloody discharge.[2]

Table 15–1. Causes of Vulvar and Vaginal Bleeding in Children

Vulvovaginitis
Foreign body
Urethral prolapse
Vulvar skin disorders
Trauma
Sarcoma botryoides
Adenocarcinoma of the cervix or vagina

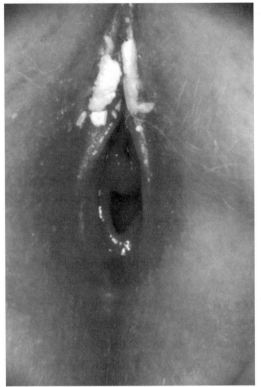

Figure 15–1. Vulvitis in a prepubertal girl. Vulvar erythema present. (See Color Fig. 15–1.)

Infection with group A beta-hemolytic streptococci (Fig. 15–2) or *Shigella* species may result in bloody vaginal discharge in prepubertal females.[3] Wet-mount specimens and cultures often confirm the diagnosis.[2–5] In general, broad-spectrum antibiotics (e.g., ampicillin) are very useful. In all instances, proper instruction in vulvar hygiene should be given to both the parent and the child. When infection is severe and mucosal damage extensive, a short course of topical estrogen cream, one fingertip applied twice daily for 7 to 10 days, is prescribed to promote healing of vulvar and vaginal tissues. When irritation is intense, hydrocortisone cream, 0.5% to 1.0%, may be necessary to alleviate the pruritus. A complete discussion of vulvovaginitis can be found in Chapter 13.

FOREIGN BODIES

Foreign bodies in the vagina induce an intense inflammatory reaction and result in a blood-stained, foul-smelling discharge (Fig. 15–3). Usually, the child does not recall inserting the foreign object or will not admit to it. The foreign body most commonly found consists of rolled pieces of toilet paper that appear as amorphous conglomerates of grayish material. They are found most frequently on the posterior vaginal wall. Because many foreign bodies are not radiopaque, radiographs are of little value. Vaginoscopy may be necessary to remove objects from the vagina and to exclude other causes for the bleeding. Often, a foreign body in the lower third of the vagina can be removed by washing it out with warm saline. Unfortunately, recurrences are quite common.[2, 4, 5]

URETHRAL PROLAPSE

Occasionally, vulvar bleeding is the result of urethral prolapse (Fig. 15–4). The urethral mucosa protrudes through the meatus and forms a hemorrhagic, characteristic, donut-shaped annular mass that bleeds quite easily.[7] Prolapse is diagnosed when the urethral orifice is identified in the center of the mass, which is separate from the vagina. When the lesion is small and urination is unobstructed, a short course of therapy with estrogen cream is beneficial. Although

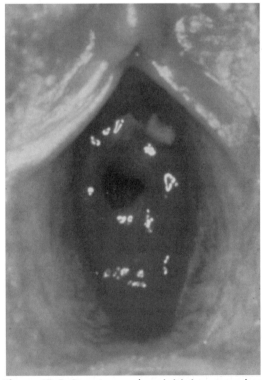

Figure 15–2. Streptococcal vaginitis in a prepubertal girl. Note the purulent material near the urethra. Gross erythema of the hymen obscures the normal vascular pattern. (See Color Fig. 15–2.)

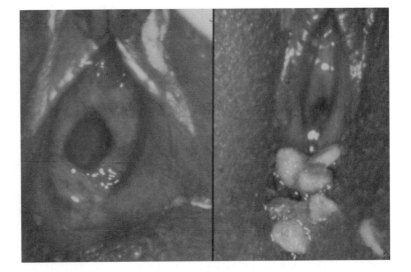

Figure 15–3. The cause of vaginal discharge and bleeding was, initially, puzzling. After vaginal irrigation, it was revealed to be small pieces of toilet paper. (See Color Fig. 15–3.)

this form of treatment may lead to resolution of the prolapse, the recurrence rate, especially with large prolapses, has been reported to reach 67%.[7] Resection of the prolapsed tissue and insertion of an indwelling catheter for 24 hours may be necessary when urinary retention is present or the lesion is large and necrotic.[2, 6, 8]

LICHEN SCLEROSUS

Lichen sclerosus, a destructive inflammatory condition of the skin (Fig. 15–5) that is common in postmenopausal women, occasionally affects young children. Symptoms are vulvar irritation, dysuria, and pruritus. Examination of the vulva reveals flat, ivory-colored papules that may coalesce into plaques. The clitoris, posterior fourchette, and anorectal area frequently are affected. The lesions do not extend laterally beyond the middle of the labia majora or spread into the vagina, and they tend to bruise easily, forming bloody blisters that are susceptible to secondary infection. On histologic examination, the skin shows flattening of the rete pegs, hyalinization of the subdermal tissues, and keratinization. Histologic confirmation is not usually indicated in children.

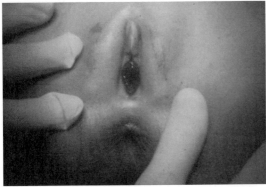

Figure 15–4. Urethral prolapse in a prepubertal girl. (See Color Fig. 15–4.)

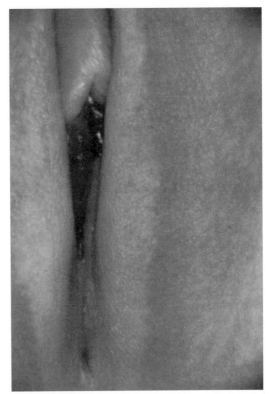

Figure 15–5. Lichen sclerosus in a young girl. Note the pale labia majora and ecchymosis of the labia minora. (See Color Fig. 15–5.)

In mild cases, symptomatic treatment is recommended—attention to hygiene, avoidance of irritants and excessive bathing with harsh soaps, and use of a protective emollient such as A and D Ointment. Hydroxyzine hydrochloride (Atarax) may be given 1 hour before bedtime to decrease nocturnal itching. In unsuccessful or in more severe cases, topical hydrocortisone, ointment or cream, 0.5–1%, applied three to four times daily for 1 to 4 weeks plus liberal use of emollients, is successful. Some physicians prefer to use more potent steroids, e.g., clobetasol 0.05%, although some of these medications are not recommended for use in children under 12 years of age. A recent randomized study comparing clobetasol propionate with, respectively, 2% testosterone propionate, 2% progesterone, and a placebo revealed that improvement in symptoms, gross aspects, and histologic features was seen only in the clobetasol-treated patients.[10] After the clobetasol regimen, regular use of emollients has been useful, although, owing to the chronic nature of this disorder, a second course of steroids is sometimes necessary.

GENITAL TRAUMA

The external genitalia of children, as compared with those of adults, are not as well-protected against injury. Fortunately, most such injuries are minor. Commonly, the trauma is caused by a blunt blow to the vulva, although infrequently the injury results from a fall on a sharp object, which sometimes penetrates the perineal body or vagina. Although most injuries are accidental, a significant number of genital tract injuries in children are caused by physical or sexual abuse. Therefore, it is extremely important for the examining physician to determine how the child sustained the injury. In the case of sexual abuse, the victimized child must be removed from an unsafe environment.[11]

A blunt injury may cause blood vessels beneath the perineal skin to rupture. Blood accumulates under the skin and forms a hematoma, a rounded, tense, and tender swelling whose size depends on the amount of bleeding (Fig. 15–6). Usually, a contusion to the vulva does not require treatment. A small vulvar hematoma often can be controlled by pressure with an ice pack, but a large hematoma, or one that continues to increase in size, should be incised, the clotted blood removed, and the bleeding points ligated. A prophylactic broad-spectrum antibiotic is advisable. The vulva should be kept clean and dry.[6]

Most vaginal injuries occur when an object penetrates the vagina through the hymenal open-

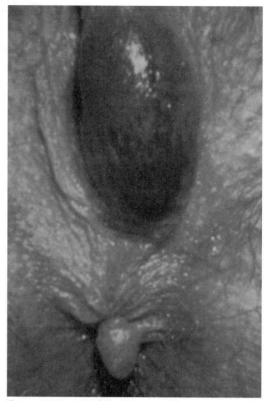

Figure 15–6. Straddle injury to the vulva resulted when this girl fell on the middle bar of a boys' bicycle. The hymen was spared in this case. (See Color Fig. 15–6.)

ing. Hymenal injuries rarely involve the hymen alone; often, the thin vaginal mucosa is lacerated along with the hymen. Usually, there is very little bleeding from a hymenal injury, but any such bleeding is indicative of vaginal penetration, and thus the possibility of additional vaginal injuries exists. In such cases, a detailed examination is necessary to exclude injuries to the upper vagina. When a vaginal laceration extends to the vaginal vault, laparotomy may be indicated to rule out extension of the tear into the broad ligament or the peritoneal cavity. Bladder and bowel integrity must be confirmed by catheterization and rectal palpation.[2, 4, 11]

GENITAL TUMORS

Benign tumors of the vulva, particularly hemangiomas, sometimes cause vulvar bleeding. Capillary hemangiomas cause only minimal bleeding, if any. They usually disappear as the child grows older and thus require no treatment except for reassurance to the parent. In contrast, cavernous hemangiomas are composed of vessels of considerable size, and injury to them may cause serious hemorrhage. Thus, they are best treated surgically, by either excision or occlusion of the feeding vessels.[4]

Although uncommon, genital tumors must be considered whenever a girl is found to have a chronic genital ulcer, a traumatic swelling of the external genitalia, tissue protruding from the vagina, or a foul-smelling, bloody discharge. Embryonal carcinoma of the vagina, or rhabdomyosarcoma (sarcoma botryoides), is most common in children (Fig. 15–7), but, when it involves the cervix, its incidence peaks during adolescence. Characteristically, the tumors arise in the submucosal tissue of the anterior vagina and then spread rapidly beneath an intact vaginal epithelium. Next, the vaginal mucosa bulges into a series of polypoid growths that may protrude through the vaginal orifice. The diagnosis is confirmed by histologic examination of a biopsy specimen. Although, in the past, radical pelvic exenteration was the treatment—and survival 15%—today, the combination of (1) intensive chemotherapy followed by (2) limited surgical resection that preserves the bladder and rectum, and (3) postoperative irradiation results in survival rates higher than 85%.[13] A combination chemotherapy regimen of vincristine, *d*-actinomycin, and cyclophosphamide has been used with success. When the tumor is amenable to surgical removal after chemotherapy, radical hysterectomy (preserving the ovaries) and vaginectomy are performed. Exenteration is not recommended. When, after chemotherapy, the tumor is still unresectable, radiotherapy helps to shrink the tumor and control its growth (see Chapters 33 and 36).[13]

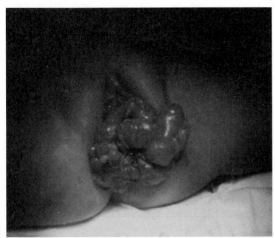

Figure 15–7. Lesions of sarcoma botryoides (vulvovaginal rhabdomyosarcoma) protrude from the vagina of a 3-year-old girl. (See Color Fig. 15–7.)

RARE CAUSES OF BLEEDING IN PREPUBERTAL GIRLS

Rarely, prepubertal vaginal bleeding has an anatomic or endocrine-mediated cause. In an 8-month-old girl, a sliding inguinal hernia containing the uterus, fallopian tube, and ovary was reported to be associated with vaginal bleeding that resolved once the hernia was repaired.[14]

Primary hypothyroidism that presents as precocious puberty and heavy vaginal bleeding has been described.[15] In these cases bilaterally enlarged, multicystic ovaries, and retarded bone age are often observed. The postulated mechanism behind such a clinical picture assumes that follicle- and thyroid-stimulating hormones, (FSH, TSH) may act through the same receptor and therefore that, in some patients, TSH elevation stimulates the gonadal FSH receptor. Resolution of the precocious puberty, vaginal bleeding, and hypothyroidism can be achieved by treatment with L-thyroxine.

Treatment of congenital adrenal hyperplasia in female infants has been associated with vaginal bleeding.[16] The authors postulate that during intrauterine life exposure to elevated androgen levels prevents down-regulation of the ovarian gonadotropin receptors. When, in the postnatal period, androgens are suppressed with glucocorticoid treatment, gonadotropin levels rise markedly and cause a transient, augmented end-organ response.

ENDOMETRIAL SHEDDING

Bleeding that arises from the endometrium per se is usually endometrial shedding and, in the pediatric age group, is often associated with sexual precocity. Precocious puberty is the onset of sexual maturation at any age that is more than 2 SD earlier than the norm. At present, the appearance of secondary sexual characteristics before 8 years of age or onset of menarche before age 10 is considered precocious,[17–19] although more recent data of 17,000 girls across the United States aged 3 to 12 years record breast or pubic hair development at 7 to 8 years in 6.7% of white and 27.2% of African Americans.[20] Occasionally, for reasons that remain unclear, only one sign of pubertal development is present (e.g., premature thelarche or premature menarche). Such manifestations sometimes are caused by a transient elevation in the circulating levels of estrogen or by extreme sensitivity of the target tissue to very low (prepubertal) levels of sex hormones. Such isolated development may be the first sign of precocious puberty, however, and re-evaluation at regular intervals is therefore indicated.

PHYSIOLOGIC ENDOMETRIAL SHEDDING (Table 15–2)

During the first few weeks of life, a newborn female responds physiologically to stimulation of placentally acquired maternal estrogens. The effects may be seen for perhaps a month, but rarely longer. The most obvious effect, breast budding, occurs in nearly all infants born at term. Vaginal discharge is quite common, as the cervical glands secrete a considerable amount of mucus, which combines with exfoliated vaginal cells. Occasionally, after birth and subsequently with declining estrogen levels, the stimulated endometrial lining is shed and vaginal bleeding occurs. Such bleeding ceases within the first 7 to 10 days of life. Further evaluation is required if bleeding first appear or persists after 10 days of age.[2, 4, 5]

DYSFUNCTIONAL UTERINE BLEEDING

Dysfunctional uterine bleeding (DUB) is defined as excessive, prolonged, or unpatterned bleeding from the uterine endometrium that is not related to anatomic lesions of the uterus.[21] The most common cause of DUB is anovulation secondary to a disturbance of the normal hypothalamic-pituitary-ovarian axis. Anovulation accounts for more than 75% of all cases of DUB.[22]

Table 15–2. Causes of Endometrial Shedding in Children

Physiologic
  Neonatal withdrawal bleeding
Early sexual development (incomplete form)
  Premature menarche
Early sexual development (complete forms)
  Immature hypothalamic-pituitary-ovarian axis
    Exposure to estrogens
      In the food chain
      Through medications
    Endogenous estrogen production
      Functional ovarian cysts
      Ovarian neoplasms
      Other hormone-producing neoplasms
  Mature hypothalamic-pituitary-ovarian axis
    Idiopathic precocious puberty
    Central nervous system lesions
    McCune-Albright syndrome

Table 15–3. Menstrual Abnormalities

Polymenorrhea: Frequent irregular bleeding at intervals of less than 18 days
Oligomenorrhea: Infrequent irregular bleeding at intervals of more than 45 days
Metrorrhagia: Bleeding between regular periods
Menorrhagia: Excessive uterine bleeding occurring regularly (synonymous with *hypermenorrhea*)
Hypomenorrhea: Decreased menstrual flow at regular intervals
Menometrorrhagia: Frequent, irregular, excessive, and prolonged uterine bleeding

---

Some have advocated that DUB should perhaps be renamed *anovulatory uterine bleeding*.

The normal menstrual cycle usually consists of a mean interval of 28 days and a mean duration of 4 days (± 2 to 3 days).[23] Normal menstrual flow is approximately 30 ml per cycle[24] and the upper normal limit 60 to 80 ml.[25] Bleeding at intervals of 21 days or less that lasts at least 7 days or 80 ml total volume is considered abnormal. Definitions of various menstrual abnormalities are listed in Table 15–3.

Approximately 10% to 15% of all gynecologic patients have DUB, but it is more common in adolescents.[22] The cause involves the slow maturation of the hypothalamic-pituitary-ovarian axis, especially for the first 18 months after menarche in adolescent girls, and thus cycles are usually anovulatory. Although menarche occurs, on average, at 12.8 years of age in the United States, it can take as long as 5 years for regular ovulatory cycles to ensue.[26] McDonough and Ganett observed anovulation in 55% to 82% of cycles in adolescents between the time of menarche and 2 years after menarche, in 30% to 45% of the cycles from 2 to 4 years after menarche, and in no more than 20% of cycles from 4 to 5 years after menarche.[27] Jones reported abnormal bleeding in more than 500 adolescent females who were followed for 5 years, 75% of whom were anovulatory. Thus, there is a relatively strong association between anovulation and DUB in adolescents.[28]

Normal ovulation involves regular cyclic production, first of estradiol (to initiate ovarian follicular growth and endometrial proliferation) and then of ovulation (to produce a significant increase in progesterone, which stabilizes the endometrium). Without ovulation and subsequent progesterone production, a state of unopposed estrogen occurs. This causes dilatation of the spiral arterial supply in the endometrium and resultant endometrial proliferation and associated abnormal height without proper structural support. The result is spontaneous superficial breakage with random asynchronous bleeding.[24] Eventually, increased estrogen has a negative effect on the hypothalamus and pituitary gland, causing reductions in gonadotropin-releasing hormone (GnRH), FSH, and luteinizing hormone (LH), and in estrogen as well. This results in vasoconstriction and collapse of the thickened, hyperplastic endometrial lining, with heavy, and often prolonged, bleeding.[29]

Although anovulation is the most common finding associated with DUB, a number of ovulatory patients have intermenstrual bleeding. The mechanism of this particular disorder is unclear. In addition, conditions of prolonged progesterone excretion after ovulation, as a result of a persistent corpus luteum cyst (Halban syndrome), can result in 6 to 8 weeks of amenorrhea followed by irregular menstrual flow.[30]

Diagnosis

DUB is a diagnosis of exclusion. Initial attempts to identify anovulation as the cause of irregular bleeding should be directed at ruling out organic lesions in the reproductive tract and coagulation disorders. Organic disorders that can cause symptoms resembling those of simple anovulatory bleeding include benign intrauterine neoplasms, reproductive tract malignancies, bleeding with early pregnancy (as in threatened abortion), ectopic pregnancy, and hydatidiform mole. Associated blood dyscrasias include thrombocytopenic purpura, von Willebrand disease (vWD), platelet dysfunctions, and platelet storage pool diseases (Table 15–4).

Despite the many possibilities, the usual diagnosis in an adolescent patient remains anovulation. Although the most common cause of anovulation in adolescents is immaturity of the hypothalamic-pituitary-ovarian axis, any hypothalamic dysfunction associated with stress, strenuous exercise or weight loss, or systemic disease also can affect ovulation. In particular, congenital adrenal hyperplasia, Cushing syndrome, hepatic dysfunction, adrenal insufficiency, and thyroid dysfunction can interfere with the process.[21] In some cases, the interaction is not well understood, but the hormonal derangement associated with adrenal dysfunction interacts with the central regulating mechanisms of ovulation, and it is thought that thyroid abnormalities and liver dysfunction result in derangement of the metabolic clearance rate of estrogen.[22]

It had been accepted for a long time that the

Table 15–4. Differential Diagnosis of Dysfunctional Uterine Bleeding

Pregnancy complications
  Abortion
  Ectopic pregnancy
  Trophoblastic disease
Benign and malignant neoplasms of the genital tract
  Cervical polyp
  Vaginal adenosis
  Vaginal carcinoma
  Cervical carcinoma
  Granulosa-theca cell tumors
  Endometriosis
  Leiomyoma
Genital tract infection
  Vaginitis
  Cervicitis
  Vaginal foreign body
  Intrauterine contraceptive device
  Salpingo-oophoritis
Endocrinopathies
  Polycystic ovarian disease
  Hyperprolactinemia
  Hypothyroidism
  Hyperthyroidism
Exogenous drugs or hormones
Trauma
Coagulation disorders
  Idiopathic thrombocytopenic purpura
  Von Willebrand disease
Chronic systemic illness
  Liver cirrhosis
  Renal failure

second most common cause of abnormal uterine bleeding in adolescents is coagulopathy. Claessens and Cowell,[31] who reviewed 59 patients admitted over a 9-year period to a children's hospital for acute menorrhagia found that 19% (11 patients) of all such admissions were attributable to a primary coagulation disorder: idiopathic thrombocytopenic purpura (ITP; four cases), vWD (three cases), Glanzmann disease, a primary qualitative platelet disorder (two cases), Fanconi anemia, and thalassemia major. Forty-four percent of these patients required transfusions. The authors concluded that one in four patients with severe menorrhagia and one in five who require hospitalization have a coagulation disorder.

In contrast, Falcone and coworkers[32] reviewed 61 patients with a primary diagnosis of DUB who were admitted to three pediatric hospitals over a 10-year period. The mean age at presentation was 13.8 years. Of the 61 patients, only two (3%) were found to have a newly diagnosed hematologic disorder (ITP and acute promyelocytic leukemia, respectively) but 29% (18 patients) had a history of a significant medical problem, and for three of these patients it was a hematologic disease. Almost all patients (92%) responded to intravenous or oral estrogen. Forty percent required a blood transfusion.

Smith and coworkers[33] reviewed 46 hospital admissions for menorrhagia in 37 adolescents over a 15-year period. The average age at admission was 15.9 years. For the 46 admissions, the causes of menorrhagia were anovulation, hematologic disease (15 patients, but newly diagnosed in only one), and chemotherapy related to infections. The most common hematologic disorder was vWD (five cases), followed by thrombocytopenia (four cases), and Fanconi anemia, chronic ITP, and aplastic anemia in three, two, and one case, respectively. Hormone treatment was successful in controlling the bleeding in 83% of cases (38 patients); dilation and curettage was necessary for eight patients owing to failed medical treatment or suspected uterine disease. Blood transfusion was required by 63% of patients.

Judging from the literature, the incidence of newly diagnosed hematologic disease in adolescents admitted with menorrhagia is low, 2.7% and 3% in series by Smith and Falcone, respectively. For patients with an existing hematologic disease, however, the risk of admission for menorrhagia may be as high as 33%.[33] Treatment of these patients is successful in more than 80% of cases when an estrogen preparation (either intravenous or oral) is combined with resuscitation via blood transfusion.

The most common hematologic disorder in adolescents is thrombocytopenic purpura.[26] Platelets and fibrin participate directly in the hemostasis achieved in a bleeding menstrual endometrium. Therefore, deficiencies in these constituents, like those of thrombocytopenia and vWD, cause the associated increased blood loss with menses.[24] Similarly, there have been case reports of menorrhagia in persons with platelet storage pool disease, a defect that prevents platelet aggregation.[34]

Von Willebrand disease is the most common inherited bleeding disorder; it is heterogeneous and estimated to occur in about 0.1% of the population.[35] Reductions in the plasma concentrations of vWF, or a selective impairment of its activity, decrease platelet adhesion and cause clinical bleeding. There are three major types of vWD. All forms, with the exception of type 3 disease, are inherited as autosomal dominant traits. Affected patients are heterozygous with one normal and one abnormal vWF allele. Patients with type 3 disease have a recessive form. They are usually the offspring of two parents with mild type 1 disease. The clinical symptoms vary by the degree of impairment. In cases with

mild impairment, bleeding occurs only after surgery or trauma. More severely affected patients have spontaneous bleeding episodes (e.g., epistaxis, genitourinary bleeding). Some patients with type 3 disease have severe mucosal bleeding and occasionally develop hemarthroses like those of hemophiliacs. The laboratory findings are variable, but the diagnosis can be established according to the following criteria: (1) prolonged bleeding time, (2) reduction in plasma vWF concentration, (3) reduction in biologic activity, and (4) reduced factor VIII activity.

Evaluation

An evaluation for abnormal bleeding begins with a detailed gynecologic history, which should include age at menarche, frequency and duration of menses, last and previous menstrual periods, and a sexual history. Medications should also be carefully recorded, as they, too, can be associated with anovulatory bleeding. Medications that tend to increase the cytochrome P_{450} mechanism in the liver (e.g., seizure medications) also increase the metabolism of steroid hormones and thus may result in DUB. A careful systems review should be obtained, with particular emphasis on evaluation of bleeding disorders (easy bruisability, epistaxis, gingival bleeding) and endocrinopathies (hirsutism, galactorrhea, thyroid dysfunction). The physical examination is an opportunity to assess Tanner staging and look for signs of endocrine abnormalities. A pelvic examination must investigate the possibility of pregnancy, a foreign body, or an anatomic source of bleeding.

Essential laboratory tests include a complete blood cell count with platelet evaluation, a blood smear, a serum pregnancy test, and a coagulation profile, including prothrombin time and partial thromboplastin time. In severe cases, a vWF assessment and a bleeding time should be ordered. These coagulation tests should be completed before transfusion or hormonal treatment. Endocrine evaluation should be complemented by thyroid function studies. Usually, thyroxine (T_4) and TSH levels are sufficient.

Treatment

Management of DUB depends in large part on the presenting signs and symptoms, examination findings, and the hemoglobin and hematocrit levels (Table 15–5). Irregular vaginal bleeding may be controlled with oral contraceptives. In general, a 30- to 35-μg ethinyl estradiol prepara-

Table 15–5. Management of Dysfunctional Uterine Bleeding

Hemoglobin Value (gm/100 ml)	Management
>12	Reassurance
	Menstrual calendar
	Iron supplements
	Periodic reevaluation
10–12	Reassurance and explanation
	Menstrual calendar
	Iron supplements
	Cyclic progestin therapy or oral contraceptives
	Reevaluation in 6 months
<10	Explanation
No active bleeding	Evaluation for coagulation defect
	Transfusion/iron supplements
	Oral contraceptives
	Reevaluation in 6–12 months
Acute hemorrhage	Evaluation for coagulation defect
	Transfusion
	Fluid replacement therapy
	Hormonal hemostasis (intravenous conjugated estrogen)
	Intensive progestin therapy
	Dilation and curettage (when hormonal hemostasis fails)
	Oral contraceptives for 6–12 months

tion is adequate. For the short term, it may be necessary to increase the dose of ethinyl estradiol to 50 µg if the original dose proves ineffective. Oral contraceptives reduce menstrual blood flow by at least 60% in patients with a normal uterus.[38] Failure to control hypermenorrhea with cyclic estrogen-progestin therapy implies the possibility of an anatomic cause such as a myoma, polyp, or bleeding diathesis.

In many cases of anovulatory bleeding, it is feasible to substitute only the missing progestin. Progesterones and progestins are antiestrogenic when given in pharmacologic doses.[39] Progesterone induces the enzyme 17-hydroxysteroid dehydrogenase in endometrial cells. This enzyme complex converts estradiol to estrone. Progestins diminish the estrogenic effect on target cells by inhibiting augmentation of estrogen cytosol receptors, which ordinarily modulate estrogen action. These influences account for the antimitotic antigrowth impact of progestins on the endometrium. In the treatment of oligomenorrhea, with withdrawal, flow can be initiated by a progestational agent such as medroxyprogesterone acetate (10 mg daily, 10 to 14 days per month). If this regimen fails to induce bleeding, further evaluation is necessary. For the treatment of

menometrorrhagia or polymenorrhea, progestins are prescribed for 10 to 14 days to induce stromal stability, which is followed by a withdrawal flow.

During an acute anovulatory bleeding episode, the bleeding may be controlled with a 50-µg estrogen-progestin oral contraceptive. Therapy consists of one pill taken four times daily for 1 to 5 days. If this dosage does not cause menstrual flow to cease, a diagnosis other than anovulation must be considered, including myomas or polyps. If the flow diminishes significantly or abates predictably, the oral contraceptive should be tapered down to one dose per day for the remainder of the 21-day cycle, after which withdrawal flow occurs. When oral contraceptives containing 0.05 mg ethinyl estradiol are used to induce amenorrhea in patients before bone marrow transplantation, the possibility of developing intrahepatic cholestasis must be considered. Jaundice as a result of this complication was recently reported in two such patients, which resolved after oral contraceptives were discontinued. The mechanism for such a complication is thought to be competition between glucuronide conjugates and estrogen metabolites for a transport protein in the bile canaliculi.

Intermittent vaginal bleeding frequently is associated with lower circulating estrogen levels and resultant breakthrough bleeding. Progestins do not control this type of bleeding, which is common in adolescents who have long been anovulatory and whose persistent desquamation has left little residual endometrial tissue. Therefore, estrogen therapy must be administered before progestin. For acute or heavy uterine bleeding, intravenous conjugated estrogens (15 to 25 mg) may be administered and repeated in 6 to 12 hours.[40] After the bleeding ceases, the patient may be prescribed either cyclic combination estrogen-progestin oral contraceptives or cyclic progestins. For patients whose bleeding is less dramatic, estrogen oral contraceptives or oral conjugated estrogens (1.25 mg orally for 7 to 10 days) may be prescribed.

Physicians frequently encounter irregular bleeding in patients who have taken oral contraceptives or medroxyprogesterone acetate (Depo-Provera). Irregular bleeding occurs in the first part of the cycle and may be secondary to decreased estrogen input that results in an unstable, atrophic endometrial lining. Such irregular bleeding also occurs in 25% of patients taking medroxyprogesterone for similar reasons. Cyclic estrogen in the form of conjugated estrogens (2.5 mg daily for 7 days during the cycle) should control this problem. Bleeding of new onset or a change in bleeding pattern in sexually active patients taking Depo-Provera should prompt an evaluation for sexually transmitted disease.

Antiprostaglandins act on the endometrial vasculature. The concentrations of prostaglandins E (PGE) and $F_{2\alpha}$ ($PGF_{2\alpha}$) in the endometrium increase progressively during the menstrual cycle. The prostaglandin synthetase inhibitors appear to decrease menstrual blood loss,[41] perhaps by altering the balance between the platelet-proaggregating vasoconstrictors thromboxane A_2 and B_2 and the antiaggregating vasodilator prostacyclin. Whatever the exact mechanism, prostaglandin inhibitors diminish menstrual blood loss in adolescents and the bleeding associated with chronic endomyometritis (e.g., that associated with an intrauterine contraceptive device). These compounds may be prescribed in conjunction with cyclic hormone therapy. Typically, they are initiated at the first sign of menses or with the first cramping episode at the time of menses and are taken throughout the menstrual cycle. Antifibrinolytic agents such as aminohexanoic acid (Amicar) have been found in a randomized controlled trial to decrease blood loss in patients with primary menorrhagia by 40% to 50%.[43] Its place in the management of menorrhagia is as second-line therapy when organic lesions have been ruled out and when estrogen preparations are ineffective or contraindicated.[42] The side effects of this medication are dose-dependent and affect mainly the gastrointestinal tract (nausea, vomiting, abdominal pain, diarrhea).[43] The other potential adverse effect is thrombus formation; however, no studies have yet addressed this question specifically.

Failure to respond to medical therapy usually occurs when progestins are used to control bleeding in patients with hypoestrogenic or desquamated endometrium. Dilation and curettage is the last line of therapy for anovulatory irregular bleeding in adolescents and is rarely necessary, except when a patient known to have a bleeding diathesis does not respond to hormone treatment. If bleeding persists, the physician should suspect an anatomic abnormality that was not identified during the dilation and curettage. Further diagnostic evaluation (e.g., sonohysterography or hysteroscopy) should be considered.

In the rare situations when hormone therapy is contraindicated or bleeding is excessive and uncontrollable, GnRH analogues have been recommended, not only to decrease menorrhagia but also to produce amenorrhea.[44] McLauchlen and coworkers reported that, in four patients with menorrhagia, after 12 weeks of intranasal GnRH analogue (buserelin) treatment, total menstrual blood loss had decreased significantly by the second and third posttreatment cycle.[44]

The long-term prognosis for adolescents with irregular bleeding can be described as guarded at best. About 5% continue to have severe episodes of anovulatory bleeding and merit endocrine evaluation. The importance of continued follow-up is illustrated by the results of a 25-year prospective evaluation of adolescents with DUB. Of 291 patients, 60% continued bleeding for 2 years after initial onset. Persistent problems were noted in 50% of patients after 4 years and in 30% after 10 years.[45] Except for those with blood dyscrasias, patients who had normal menses before irregular bleeding commenced have a more favorable prognosis.

REFERENCES

1. Emans SJH, Goldstein DP: Pediatric and Adolescent Gynecology, 3rd ed. Boston: Little, Brown, 1990.
2. Muram D: Pediatric and adolescent gynecology. *In* Pernol ML, Benson RC (eds): Current Gynecologic and Obstetric Diagnosis and Treatment. Norwalk, Conn: Appleton & Lange, 1991, pp 629–656.
3. Davis TC: Chronic vulvovaginitis in children due to *Shigella flexneri*. Pediatrics 1975; 56:41.
4. Huffman JW, Dewhurst CJ, Capraro VJ: The Gynecology of Childhood and Adolescence, 2nd ed. Philadelphia: WB Saunders, 1981.
5. Huffman JW: Premenarchal vulvovaginitis. Clin Obstet Gynecol 1977; 20:581.
6. Muram D, Massouda D: Vaginal bleeding in children. Contemp Obstet Gynecol 1985; 27:41–52.
7. Capraro VJ, Bayonet-Rivera NP, Magosas I: Vulvar tumor in children due to prolapse of urethral mucosa. Am J Obstet Gynecol 1970; 108:572.
8. Desai SR, Cohen RC: Urethral prolapse in a premenarchal girl: Case report and literature review. Aust NZ J Surg 1997; 67:660–667.
9. Mercer LJ, Mueller CM, Hajj SN: Medical treatment of urethral prolapse. Adolesc Pediatr Gynecol 1988; 1:182–184.
10. Bracco GL, Carli P, Sonni L, et al: Clinical and histologic effects of topical treatments of vulval lichen sclerosus: A critical evaluation. J Reprod Med 1993; 38:37.
11. Muram D: Detecting and managing sexual abuse in children. Contemp Obstet Gynecol 1988; 31:34–48.
12. Muram D: Genital tract trauma in pre-pubertal children. Pediatr Ann 1986; 15:616–620.
13. Julian JC, Mergueriapa PA, Shortliffe LM: Pediatric genitourinary tumors. Curr Opin Oncol 1995; 7:265.
14. Zitsman JL, Cirincione E, Margossian H: Vaginal bleeding in an infant secondary to sliding inguinal hernia. Obstet Gynecol 1997; 89:840–842.
15. Gordon CM, Austin DJ, Radovick S, et al: Primary hypothyroidism presenting as severe vaginal bleeding in a prepubertal girl. J Pediatr Adolesc Gynecol 1997; 10:35–38.
16. Uli N, Chin D, David R, et al: Menstrual bleeding in a female infant with congenital adrenal hyperplasia: Altered maturation of the hypothalamic pituitary ovarian axis. J Clin Endocrinol Metab 1997; 82:3298–3302.

17. Dewhurst J: Practical Pediatric and Adolescent Gynecology. New York: Marcel Dekker, 1980.
18. Dewhurst J: Female Puberty and Its Abnormalities. Edinburgh: Churchill Livingstone, 1984.
19. Zacharias L, Rand WM, Wurtman RJ: A prospective study of sexual development and growth in American girls: The statistics of menarche. Obstet Gynecol Surv 1976; 31:325.
20. Herman-Giddens ME, Slora EJ, Wasserman RC, et al: Secondary sexual characteristics and menses in young girls seen in office practice: A study from the Pediatric Research Office Settings Network. Pediatrics 1997; 99:505.
21. American College of Obstetricians and Gynecologists: Dysfunctional Uterine Bleeding. ACOG Technical Bulletin, No. 134. Washington, DC: 1989.
22. Sanfilippo J, Yussman M: Gynecologic problems of adolescence. In Lavery J, Sanfilippo J (eds): Pediatric and Adolescent Obstetrics and Gynecology. New York: Springer-Verlag, 1985, p 61.
23. Mishell DR: Abnormal uterine bleeding. In Mishell DR, Stenchever MA, Droegemuller W, et al (eds): Comprehensive Gynecology, 3rd ed. St Louis: CV Mosby, 1997, p 1025.
24. Speroff L, Glass R, Kase N: Dysfunctional uterine bleeding. In Clinical Gynecologic Endocrinology and Infertility, 4th ed. Baltimore: Williams & Wilkins, 1994, p 531.
25. Hallberg L, Hogdahl AM, Nilsson L, et al: Menstrual blood loss—a population study: Variations at different ages and attempts to define normality. Acta Obstet Gynecol Scand 1966; 45:320.
26. Gidwani GP: Vaginal bleeding in adolescents. J Reprod Med 1984; 29:419.
27. McDonough PG, Ganett P: Dysfunctional uterine bleeding in the adolescent. In Barrom BN, Belisle BS (eds): Adolescent Gynecology and Sexuality. New York: Masson, 1982.
28. Jones GS: Endocrine problems in the adolescent. Md State Med J 1967; 16:45.
29. Spellacy WN: Abnormal bleeding. Clin Obstet Gynecol 1983; 26:702.
30. Dunnihoo D: Abnormal uterine bleeding. In Fundamentals of Gynecology and Obstetrics. Philadelphia: JB Lippincott, 1990, p 543.
31. Claessens EA, Cowell CA: Acute adolescent menorrhagia. Am J Obstet Gynecol 1981; 139:277.
32. Falcone T, Desjardins C, Bourque J, et al: Dysfunctional uterine bleeding in adolescents. J Reprod Med 1994; 39:761–764.
33. Smith YR, Quint EH, Hertzberg BS: Menorrhagia in adolescents requiring hospitalization. J Pediatr Adolesc Gynecol 1998; 11:12–15.
34. Walker RW, Gustavson LP: Platelet storage pool disease in women. J Adolesc Health 1983; 3:264.
35. Rodeghiero F, Castaman G, Dini E: Epidemiological investigation of the prevalence of von Willebrand's disease. Blood 1987; 69:454–459.
36. Ewenstein B: Bleeding disorders: Clinical evaluation in women with bleeding disorders—the role of the OB/GYN. Highlights of a multi-disciplinary roundtable discussion. Armour Pharmaceutical Company Educational Publications, 1995, pp 4–9.
37. Sham RL, Francis CW: Evaluation of mild bleeding disorders and easy bruising. Blood Rev 1994; 8:98–104.
38. Nilsson L, Ribrybo G: Treatment of menorrhagia. Am J Obstet Gynecol 1971; 110:712.
39. Gurpide E, Gusberg SB, Tseng L: Estradiol binding and metabolism in human endometrial hyperplasia and adenocarcinoma. J Steroid Biochem Mol Biol 1976; 7:891.
40. DeVore GR, Owens O, Kase N: Use of intravenous premarin in the treatment of dysfunctional uterine bleeding—double-blind, randomized control study. Obstet Gynecol 1982; 59:285.
41. Anderson AB, Hynes PJ, Guillebaud J, et al: Reduction of menstrual blood loss by prostaglandin-synthetase inhibitors. Lancet 1976; 1:774.
42. Bonnar J, Sheppard BL: Treatment of menorrhagia during menstruation: A randomized controlled trial of ethamsylate, mefenamic acid and tranexamic acid. BMJ 1996; 313:579–582.
43. Mannucci PM: Hemostatic drugs. N Engl J Med 1998; 339:245–250.
44. McLauchlen RI, Healy DL, Burger HG: Clinical aspects of LH/RH analogs in gynecology: A review. Br J Obstet Gynaecol 1986; 93:431.
45. Southam AL, Richart RM: The prognosis for adolescents with menstrual abnormalities. Am J Obstet Gynecol 1966; 94:637.

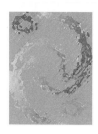

Chapter 16

Dysmenorrhea and Pelvic Pain

GITA P. GIDWANI AND MARSHA KAY

Pelvic pain and dysmenorrhea are frequent complaints seen by practitioners who treat adolescent females. In this chapter we discuss the causes of acute and chronic pelvic pain (CPP) and the management of the patient with CPP and dysmenorrhea.

The differential diagnosis of pelvic pain can be a clinical challenge, owing to stress and coping mechanisms of the young adult. Her family may exaggerate the intensity of the symptoms. In patients with recurrent abdominal pain (RAP) who have a negative clinical evaluation, an acute surgical emergency may arise, and the healthcare team must be able to ask the appropriate questions on the telephone to "triage" the acute episodes in patients with CPP.

Pelvic pain can arise from numerous causes. An approach to diagnosis and treatment in adolescents with acute and chronic pelvic pain and dysmenorrhea is presented.

ACUTE PELVIC PAIN

The gynecologist may find that adolescents (in contrast to adults) present to the emergency department with acute pain secondary to dysmenorrhea. On the other hand, an adolescent with obstructive müllerian symptoms may complain of chronic pelvic pain. Thus, it is important to remember that there is a fine line between pain of different causes. The causes of acute pelvic pain in the female reproductive tract may be related to complications of spontaneous abortion or tubal pregnancy; torsion, rupture, or hemorrhage of an ovarian cyst; or infection of the pelvic organs (Table 16–1). Pelvic inflammatory disease (PID) is extremely important to consider in the differential diagnosis of acute abdominal pain. It has been identified as the gynecologic disorder that most often leads to hospitalization of reproductive-aged women in the United States.[1] An adolescent presenting with acute pelvic pain should undergo a pelvic and rectal examination. Otherwise, a number of diagnostic possibilities may be missed.

Nonreproductive causes (e.g., appendicitis, volvulus of the bowel, intestinal obstruction, perforation of the bowel, mesenteric adenitis) will produce acute peritoneal irritation and may require immediate surgical intervention. Urinary tract lesions (e.g., acute cystitis, acute pyelonephritis, ureteral calculus) may present with acute pain. Other causes of acute pelvic pain include bone and joint infections of the sacrum, ileum, or hip; slipped femoral epiphysis; and intraabdominal abscess.

Steps in taking an adequate history must include questions about sexual activity and missed

Table 16–1. Causes of Acute Pelvic Pain in Adolescent Females

Gynecologic causes
　Pregnancy complications (e.g., incomplete or threatened abortion, tubal pregnancy)
　Infections (e.g., postabortal endometritis or acute pelvic inflammatory disease)
　Ovarian cyst—rupture, torsion, or hemorrhage
　Obstructive anomalies of the müllerian duct system (e.g., hematocolpos, complete transverse vaginal septum)
Nongynecologic causes
　Gastrointestinal causes
　　Acute appendicitis
　　Volvulus
　　Meckel's diverticulitis
　　Intestinal obstruction
　　Mesenteric adenitis
　　Regional enteritis
　　Ulcerative colitis
　　Pancreatitis
　Urinary tract causes
　　Acute cystitis
　　Acute pyelonephritis
　　Ureteral calculus
　Other causes
　　Bone and joint infections of the sacrum, ileum, or hip
　　Slipped femoral epiphysis
　　Intraabdominal abscess

or abnormal menses. It is very important that these points be addressed when the parent is elsewhere, as it is difficult for a frightened adolescent to give a history of sexual activity or missed periods if her parents do not know that she is sexually active. In general, one must always consider the possibility of pregnancy in the adolescent. At this stage, measurement of vital signs and abdominal examination for signs of peritoneal irritation or to rule out a palpable mass or tenderness must be attempted. A regular pelvic examination is very helpful at this time.

A narrow vaginal speculum (e.g., a small Pedersen) must be available for examination of young girls. Cultures for gonococcal and *Chlamydia* infections are obtained as necessary. The size of the uterus, the presence or absence of tenderness of the cervix and adnexa, and the presence or absence of an adnexal mass are important findings of the examination.

The basic laboratory work must include a pregnancy test, complete blood count, urinalysis with cultures and determination of the erythrocyte sedimentation rate, as indicated. Pelvic ultrasonography may be very useful to identify free fluid, suspected pregnancy, or leaking, torsion, or hemorrhage of an ovarian cyst. Ovarian cysts measuring 2 to 3 cm are usually purely physiologic. To diagnose partial or complete torsion of the ovary, attention must be paid to the patient's symptoms, rather than to the ultrasound. A child or adolescent experiencing waves of acute pelvic pain, with or without nausea, may be experiencing complete or intermittent torsion of the ovary or fallopian tube. For unclear reasons girls in the 7- to 10-year age group are especially prone to ovarian torsion, an event that is more common on the right side. Because ultrasound and Doppler studies for ovarian torsion have not achieved 100% sensitivity, a high level of clinical suspicion is paramount. At the present time ovarian torsion can be undone and the ovary saved, so early diagnosis is of the utmost importance.[2, 3]

Management depends on how definitively the clinical examination reveals the diagnosis. If the diagnosis is not clear, surgical intervention is necessary. Laparoscopy is being used increasingly for treatment of ectopic pregnancy and for diagnosis and treatment of hemoperitoneum secondary to a ruptured corpus luteum cyst. Subacute conditions (e.g., urinary tract infections, PID, gastroenteritis, mesenteric adenitis) can be treated medically, and occasionally further tests (e.g., urography) may be necessary to detect urinary calculi.

Patients whose diagnosis is in doubt present a clinical dilemma. Examples include those with clinical evidence of PID who are not responding to usual therapy; patients with a ruptured ovarian cyst or incomplete torsion of an ovarian cyst; and patients with questionable appendicitis. In these individuals, according to Goldstein,[4] laparoscopic examination and definitive treatment prevent long periods of inpatient observation and pain and avoid surgical catastrophes like ruptured appendix. The patient can also be discharged quickly after the laparoscopy and can resume scholastic and athletic activities within 48 to 72 hours.

According to data from Boston Children's Hospital collected between 1980 and 1986, 47% of 121 laparoscopies performed on such patients had complications related to ovarian cyst(s); 11% had appendicitis; and in 17%, no abnormality was found.[4]

Whitworth and colleagues,[5] in a study of women patients, suggested that diagnostic laparoscopy should be considered even when appendicitis is suspected.[5] The surgical risk involved in the procedure under general anesthesia is low, and as surgeons become more adept at removing the appendix through the laparoscope, this will clearly be the procedure of choice in most acute cases.

DYSMENORRHEA

Dysmenorrhea is equated with difficult menstrual flow. Primary *dysmenorrhea* is painful menstruation in the absence of gross disease of the pelvic organs. *Secondary dysmenorrhea* describes painful menstrual periods in women who have gross pathologic conditions of the pelvic organs (e.g., endometriosis, salpingitis, congenital anomalies of the müllerian system).

INCIDENCE

Andersch and Milsom[6] noted that dysmenorrhea was reported by 72% of an urban population of women. The scoring system they used may be of assistance in planning additional questionnaire studies (Table 16–2). Table 16–3 describes the prevalence and severity of dysmenorrhea. It should be noted that 15.4% of the responders said that their menstrual cycle limited daily activity; however 27.6% had no dysmenorrhea. There is a significant correlation between the severity of dysmenorrhea, duration of menstruation, and the quantity of menstrual flow as assessed by the respondents. There was a significant difference in the prevalence and severity of dysmenorrhea

Table 16–2. Verbal Multidimensional Scoring System for Assessment of Dysmenorrhea

Grade	Working Ability	Systemic Symptoms	Analgesics
Grade 0: Menstruation is not painful, and daily activity is unaffected.	Unaffected	None	Not required
Grade 1: Menstruation is painful but seldom inhibits normal activity; analgesics are seldom required; mild pain.	Rarely affected	None	Rarely required
Grade 2: Daily activity affected; analgesics required and give sufficient relief so that absence from work or school is unusual; moderate pain.	Moderately affected	Few	Required
Grade 3: Activity clearly inhibited; poor effect of analgesics; vegetative symptoms (e.g., headache, fatigue, nausea, vomiting, and diarrhea); severe pain.	Clearly inhibited	Apparent	Poor effect

From Andersch B, Milsom I: An epidemiologic study of young women with dysmenorrhea. Am J Obstet Gynecol 1982; 144:655.

between nulliparous women and women whose pregnancy had been terminated by induced or spontaneous abortion. The prevalence and severity of dysmenorrhea in parous women were significantly lower. In this study, a total of 50.9% of the respondents had missed time from work or school. Only 31% of those women had been evaluated.

In another epidemiologic study, data were collected from the approximately 7000 adolescents, 2699 of them menarchal. The prevalence of dysmenorrhea was striking: 59.7% reported discomfort or pain in connection with menstrual periods.[7] Of those who reported pain, 14% described it as severe, 37% as moderate, and 49% as mild. The prevalence of dysmenorrhea increased with chronologic age, from 39% for 12-year-olds to 72% for 17-year-olds. Dysmenorrhea also increased with sexual maturity, from 38% of those at Tanner stage III to 66% at Tanner stage V, and from 31% at gynecologic age 1 to 78% at gynecologic age 5.

Of the total sample, 14% frequently missed school because of menstrual pain, and of those

Table 16–3. Dysmenorrhea Prevalence and Severity

	Number of Patients	Percentage
Grade 0	162	27.6
Grade 1	201	34.3
Grade 2	133	22.7
Grade 3	90	15.4

From Andersch B, Milsom I: An epidemiologic study of young women with dysmenorrhea. Am J Obstet Gynecol 1982; 144:655.

with severe dysmenorrhea, 50% reported missing school. Although black adolescents reported no increased *incidence* of dysmenorrhea, they were absent from school more frequently than whites *because* of dysmenorrhea, even when socioeconomic status was taken into account. Only 14.5% of the adolescents with dysmenorrhea had ever sought help for this problem. Interestingly, 30% of parents were not aware of their daughter's dysmenorrhea.[7]

Since a lot of nonprescription medications have been introduced, adolescents may be using such medications for the management of discomfort. To determine how adolescents use medication to manage menstrual discomfort, a survey was done by Campbell and coworkers[8] in a public high school, where it was found that 93% of the 386 adolescents had experienced menstrual discomfort during the last three menstruations. Overall, 70% of them had used over-the-counter (OTC) medication to manage the discomfort, and 17% had used prescription medication. After evaluating the data, they concluded that adolescents frequently suffer from menstrual discomfort and use OTC medication to manage the discomfort, but they may not be using them correctly.

In a similar study by Chambers and colleagues,[9] from Halifax, Nova Scotia, 651 junior high school students proceeded to self-administer medications for pain, but a number of them did misuse OTC medications (e.g., taking aspirin too often). This fact underscores the importance of providing adolescents with correct information about these medications. Chambers and colleagues found that, in the preceding 3 months, 58.3% to 75.9% of adolescents reported taking an OTC medication for pain without first checking with an adult.

HISTORY AND PATHOGENESIS

The discovery of prostaglandins by Pickles[10] and intrauterine studies by Ackerland and colleagues[11] proved that menstrual pain was not a myth but a condition that could be treated with certain agents, namely, nonsteroidal antiinflammatory drugs (NSAIDs).[12]

PROSTAGLANDINS AND THEIR PHARMACOLOGY

The precursor for the synthesis of prostaglandins is arachidonic acid, an essential fatty acid derived from dietary sources and stored primarily in cell plasma membranes. Any type of thermal,

mechanical, or chemical stimulus is thought to cause release of arachidonic acid from its depots, a process that leads to the synthesis of prostaglandins. In the uterus, these prostaglandins are formed by two different enzyme systems: the cyclooxygenase pathway, which results in formation of prostaglandins, and the lipoxygenase pathway, which produces a series of monohydroxy acids and leukotriene products (Figs. 16–1, 16–2).[13]

The cyclooxygenase pathway of arachidonic acid metabolism has been well studied. This pathway produces the classic prostaglandins PGE_2, PGD_2, and $PGF_{2\alpha}$ as well as thromboxanes and prostacyclin. All of these products have potent and diverse physiologic activities, many of them opposing (e.g., vasoconstriction and vasodilatation; smooth muscle contraction and relaxation). It is the cyclooxygenase enzyme system that becomes compromised when patients are treated with NSAIDs.

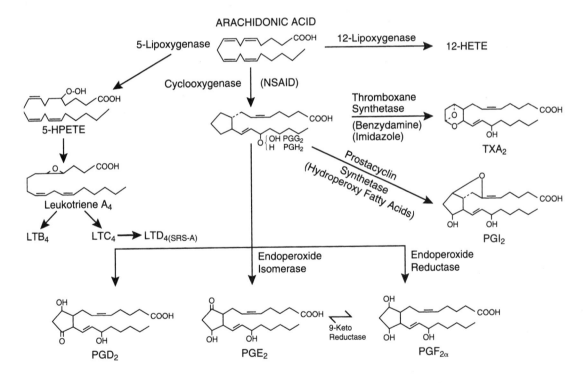

5 HPTE — 5 hydroxyperoxyeicosatetraenoic acid
12 HETE — 12 hydroxyeicosatetric acid
LTB_4 — leukotriene B_4
LTC_4 — leukotriene C_4
PGI_2 — prostacyclin
TXA_2 — thromboxane A_2

Figure 16–1. Metabolism of arachidonic acid. (From Dawood MY, McGuire JL, Demers LM [eds]: Premenstrual Syndrome and Dysmenorrhea. Munich: Urban & Schwarzenberg, 1985. © 1985, Williams & Wilkins Co., Baltimore.)

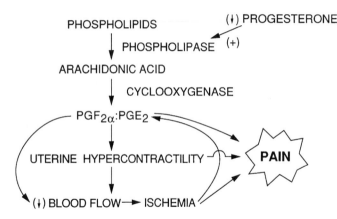

Figure 16–2. Prostaglandins in dysmen-orrhea. (From Dawood MY, McGuire JL, Demers LM [eds]: Premenstrual Syndrome and Dysmenorrhea. Munich: Urban & Schwarzenberg, 1985. © 1985, Williams & Wilkins, Baltimore.)

The second pathway by which arachidonic acid is converted to prostaglandins is the lipoxygenase pathway. In this synthetic process, the leukotrienes, extremely potent smooth muscle–stimulating substances, are the end product. Several forms of lipoxygenase systems exist in the cells. The 5-lipoxygenase and 12-lipoxygenase compounds, the two most prevalent in tissues and cells, catalyze the oxidation of arachidonic acid to one of two monohydric acids: 5-hydroperoxyeicosatetraenoic acid (5-HPETE) or 12-hydroperoxyeicosatetraenoic acid (12-HPETE). Ultimately, 5-HPETE gives rise to the leukotrienes, which can affect uterine activity. Currently it is believed that in the 30% to 40% of patients with dysmenorrhea who do not respond to cyclooxygenase inhibitors, the contribution of the lipoxygenase pathway may produce symptoms of dysmenorrhea.

It is important to note that prostaglandins are not stored, and de novo synthesis is the reason they are found in tissues and biologic fluids when menstruation starts. These substances are rapidly bioinactivated, and the enzymes involved in the biodegradation of $PGF_{2\alpha}$ and PGE_2 are widely distributed throughout the body. A major increase in prostaglandin release generally occurs within the first 36 to 48 hours after the onset of menses (Fig. 16–2). This increase in uterine prostaglandins coincides with the loss of hormonal support of the endometrial lining. The source of prostaglandins is believed to be the human endometrium, which can synthesize both $PGF_{2\alpha}$ and PGE_2.[14–16]

DIAGNOSIS

Primary Dysmenorrhea

It is imperative to differentiate primary dysmenorrhea (that not related to organic causes)

from secondary dysmenorrhea (that related to some organic cause). Primary dysmenorrhea occurs 6 to 12 months after menarche, when ovulatory cycles have been established. The onset of symptoms dates back to menarche or shortly thereafter. A thorough history, pelvic examination, and rectal examination will rule out any major abnormality, such as müllerian anomaly or PID in a sexually active teenager. The organic causes that are responsible for dysmenorrhea are included in Table 16–4.[17] A family history of endometriosis must alert the physician to the possibilty of endometriosis in a teenager.[18] Dyspareunia, infertility, and irregular, heavy periods with dysmenorrhea suggest organic disease.[19, 20]

TREATMENT

The general measures include reassurance and educational counseling. Mild analgesics and a simple explanation to allay anxiety after an adequate evaluation will help the patient to cope with mild symptoms. Narcotic analgesics should not be prescribed routinely because of the high risk of abuse.

Nonsteroidal Antiinflammatory Drugs

Prostaglandin synthetase inhibitors have had a profound impact on the treatment of primary

Table 16–4. Causes of Secondary Dysmenorrhea

Endometriosis
Pelvic inflammatory disease
Adenomyosis
Uterine polyps, uterine myomas
Congenital obstructive müllerian malformations
Cervical stricture or stenosis
Ovarian cysts
Pelvic adhesions

Table 16–5. Prostaglandin Synthetase Inhibitors

Carboxylic acids (type I)
  Salicylic acid esters (e.g., aspirin, diflunisal [Dolobid])
  Acetic acids (e.g., indomethacin [Indocin], sulindac
    [Clinoril], tolmetin [Tolectin], diclofenac [Voltaren])
  Propionic acids (e.g., ibuprofen [Motrin, Advil, Nuprin,
    Rufin], fenoprofen [Nalfon], naproxen [Naprosyn],
    naproxen sodium [Anaprox], ketoprofen [Orudis],
    suprofen [Suprol], flurbiprofen [Ansaid])
  Fenamic acids (e.g., mefenamic acid [Ponstel],
    meclofenamate, tolfenamic acid, flufenamic acid)
Enolic acids (type II)
  Pyrazolones (e.g., phenylbutazone)
  Oxicans (e.g., piroxicam [Feldene])

dysmenorrhea. They are considered NSAIDs in large part because they reduce the edema and erythema associated with inflammation. They are antithrombotic agents (i.e., inhibit the aggregatory response of these blood elements), potent antipyretics, and extremely potent analgesics. The two classes—carboxylic acids (type I) and enolic acids (type II)—are shown in Table 16–5. The type I prostaglandin synthetase inhibitors inhibit cyclooxygenase enzymes and therefore block the conversion of arachidonic acid to cyclic endoperoxides. Type II inhibitors tend to decrease isomerase and reductase enzyme activity and therefore prevent the conversion of cyclic endoperoxide to prostaglandins. Because cyclic endoperoxides have more potent uterotonic effects than prostaglandins, it is preferable to use type I inhibitors to treat dysmenorrhea.[16]

The doses of various NSAIDs are included in Table 16–6, and their side effects are shown in Table 16–7. Although all NSAIDs have the common property of inhibiting prostaglandin synthesis, any given NSAID may have different tissue sources. For this reason they sometimes exhibit different pharmacologic properties in the laboratory and in clinical practice. Thus, aspirin is a good antipyretic but lacks effective antiinflammatory action and may increase menstrual flow; thus, it is less often used in the treatment of dysmenorrhea. The varying severity of their side effects also affects the frequency of use. For example, indomethacin provides excellent relief of pain but has a number of side effects and thus is not usually prescribed.

Table 16–6. Clinical Trials of NSAIDs in Dysmenorrhea

Class	Number of Patients	Regimen	Pain Relief (% of Patients)
Salicylates			
Aspirin	92 (1978–1980)	500–650 mg qid	Slight to no effect
Acetic acids			
Indomethacin	278 (1975–1979)	25–50 mg tid	71–100
Diclofenac sodium	35 (1981)	25 mg tid	69
Propionic acids			
Naproxen (NA)	224 (1977–1983)	200–285 mg qid	61–90
Ibuprofen	245 (1974–1983)	400 mg tid	56–100
Ketoprofen	23 (1979)	50 mg tid	90
Suprofen	610 (1983)	200 mg qid	63–84
Fenamates			
Flufenamic acid	90 (1974–1979)	125–200 mg tid	77–100
Mefenamic acid	138 (1977–1983)	250–500 mg tid	59–95
Meclofenamate	18	Single dose	71
Butaphenes			
Phenylbutazone	NA	NA	NA
Oxyphenbutazone	NA	NA	NA
Oxicans			
Piroxicam (Feldene)	68	20–40 mg	90

NA, No information available.
Modified from Dawood MY, McGuire JL, Demers LM (eds): Premenstrual Syndrome and Dysmenorrhea. Munich: Urban & Schwarzenberg, 1985. © 1985, Baltimore: Williams & Wilkins, 1985.

Table 16–7. Side Effects of Nonsteroidal Antiinflammatory Drugs

Gastrointestinal
  Indigestion
  Nausea
  Constipation
  Vomiting
  Diarrhea
Central nervous system
  Headache
  Dizziness
  Vision and hearing disturbances
  Irritability
  Drowsiness
Other
  Allergic reactions (e.g., skin rash)
  Bronchospasm
  Hematologic disease
  Renal dysfunction (e.g., fluid retention)

Modified from Dawood MY, McGuire JL, Demers LM (eds): Premenstrual Syndrome and Dysmenorrhea. Munich: Urban & Schwarzenberg, 1985. © 1985, Williams & Wilkins Co., Baltimore.

Ibuprofen and naproxen have been widely used in clinical practice. A trial of mefenamic acid (Ponstel) is useful when propionic acids are ineffective. Fenamates are potent inhibitors of prostaglandins and can antagonize the action of prostaglandins already synthesized. NSAIDs have definite advantages over oral contraceptives, as, generally, they are administered for only 2 or 3 days. Their success has confirmed that prostaglandins are a major cause of dysmenorrhea. In adolescents, a trial of 6 months, with necessary adjustments in dose and compound, usually proves effective.[21–23]

NSAIDs reduce not only uterine hypercontractility but also other side effects of dysmenorrhea (e.g., dizziness, nausea, vomiting). NSAIDs' high rate of success has made them the first line of treatment for dysmenorrhea. The failure of NSAIDs in some patients suggests that other mediators (e.g., leukotrienes) may contribute to this disorder.

Oral Contraceptives

Oral contraceptives have been known to prevent menstrual cramps. In an adolescent who is sexually active, an oral contraceptive has the dual functions of preventing pregnancy and treating dysmenorrhea. In clinical practice, a trial of 2 to 3 months of oral contraceptives for the control of dysmenorrhea will demonstrate whether the patient will respond.

If the patient does not respond to NSAIDs or oral contraceptives, an aggressive evaluation,

including diagnostic laparoscopy, should be performed to rule out an organic cause. Multiple studies, including Davis and coworkers[24] have shown that, when dysmenorrhea responds neither to NSAIDs nor to oral contraceptives, endometriosis is likely the reason. Thus, Davis and colleagues reported that, in 49 patients with severe dysmenorrhea all examined by laparoscopy, 36 had histologically proven endometriosis.

Other Treatment Measures

In some patients NSAIDs produce undesirable side effects and, so, are contraindicated. For them, an alternative is Trimodal hydrochloride tablets.[25] Trimodal has central-acting analgesic properties and is indicated for moderate to severe pain. It is composed of codeine, 10 mg oxycodone, prescribed as 50- mg pills. Dosage is 50 to 100 mg every 6 hours, not to exceed eight pills in 24 hours. Other methods (e.g., transcutaneous electrical nerve stimulation [TENS]) have been used. A study by Kaplan and colleagues[26] showed that, of 102 nulliparous women with dysmenorrhea, 58 (56.9%) reported complete relief from TENS and 31 (30.4%) moderate relief. These patients stopped using analgesic methods during the trial. Acupuncture has also been found to be successful in managing the pain of chronic primary dysmenorrhea; 90.9% showed improvement after acupuncture.[27] Calcium channel blockers have been shown to reduce intrauterine pressure and are effective for dysmenorrhea. Other symptoms (i.e., nausea, vomiting, and diarrhea) were not relieved, however, an observation that suggests that the effect of the medication was restricted to smooth muscle relaxation. Because the side effects associated with calcium channel blockers were severe, they have limited clinical utility. Further research to develop lipoxygenase inhibitors and leukotriene antagonists, in combination with cyclooxygenase inhibitors, may increase the success rate of medical therapy to 100%.

Nitroglycerin for management of pain of primary dysmenorrhea has been reported in a multicenter pilot study; transdermal nitroglycerin produced excellent pain relief in 90% of patients. Headaches were reported by 20% of the patients. A randomized, placebo-controlled study is under way to confirm the findings.[28]

A longitudinal study of risk factors for duration and severity of menstrual cramps in a cohort of college women was published by Harlow's group.[29] Among the 165 women aged 17 to 19 years matriculating at a local university whose menstrual pain lasted 5 days, the pain was modified by weight, smoking, and alcohol consumption. It was found that being overweight was an important risk factor and that frequent alcohol consumption reduced the probability of having menstrual cramps but increased duration and severity when they did occur. Smokers' cramps tended to last longer. Thus, it is wise for us to counsel adolescents with dysmenorrhea about the importance of a healthy lifestyle—avoiding alcohol, quitting smoking, and achieving ideal weight.

Durant and associates,[30] found that girls who were under great stress experienced more severe symptoms during the first month of therapy for dysmenorrhea as compared with the control population. As therapy continued, however, life stresses ceased to have a significant influence. Clinicians should encourage patients to eat a proper diet, limit intake of caffeine and chocolate, stop smoking, keep an ideal weight, and seek professional help for extraordinary stresses in their lives. It is important to understand that having control over pain enables people to deal more effectively with other stressors. Thus, a very aggressive approach to the control of dysmenorrhea is paramount. If it is relieved by oral contraceptives, many physicians prescribe these for 6 to 9 months and discontinue treatment during the summer. It is important to bring these patients back for follow-up and to continue monitoring them while prescribing oral contraceptives and antiprostaglandins to help them to cope.

DIAGNOSIS AND TREATMENT OF PELVIC PAIN OF OTHER CAUSES (Table 16–8)

MITTELSCHMERZ

Mittelschmerz is pain at the time of ovulation. The pain, which may be described as severe or colicky or as a dull ache, is sometimes accompanied by a clear discharge, and sometimes even vaginal bleeding. Pain ususaly lasts 6 to 7 hours but may persist as long as 48 to 72 hours. This condition is very easily diagnosed by comparing the dates of pain with the dates of menstruation or by keeping a formal basal body temperature chart to demonstrate that the pain is cyclic and related to ovulation. Spillage of fluid from the ruptured ovarian follicle may be seen on ultrasound. An NSAID, or sometimes simply acetaminophen, relieves symptoms in most cases.

Table 16–8. Causes of Recurrent Abdominal Pain in Adolescent Females

Gynecologic causes
  Dysmenorrhea
  Mittelschmerz
  Pelvic inflammatory disease
  Endometriosis
  Müllerian obstructive anomalies
  Ovarian cysts
Nongynecologic causes
  Lactose malabsorption
  Chronic constipation
  Giardiasis
  Crohn's disease
  Irritable bowel syndrome
  Unusual causes
    Meckel's diverticulum
    Midgut malrotation
    Schönlein-Henoch purpura
    Acute intermittent porphyria
    Ureteropelvic junction obstruction
  Abdominal wall trigger points
  Psychogenic causes

PELVIC INFLAMMATORY DISEASE

PID has been noted with increasing frequency in young girls. Gonococci and chlamydiae are primarily responsible. Symptoms are lower abdominal pain, vaginal discharge, and dysuria. The clinician must have a high index of suspicion for PID so that appropriate cultures can be obtained from the cervix.

Adolescents with lower abdominal pain who are suspected to have PID must be examined by pelvic laparoscopy when either of these indications develops.

1. Recurrence of PID when the diagnosis was established without positive cervical cultures or other objective signs and symptoms.
2. Persistence of significant pelvic pain and symptoms after 4 to 7 days of aggressive treatment for culture-proven PID.

Westrom and coworkers objectively measured the accuracy of laparoscopic diagnosis of PID. Rome and colleagues demonstrated in inpatients with indeterminate PID that routine use of laparoscopy was a valuable diagnostic adjunct. Laparoscopy is definitely useful for accurately diagnosing PID.[31, 32]

Because undiagnosed PID eventually results in infertility, the cost and risk-benefit ratio for laparoscopy must be weighed when an adolescent is affected. Conversely, adolescents should not be given a diagnosis of "chronic PID" without adequate documentation. This subject is discussed further in Chapter 39.

ENDOMETRIOSIS

Endometriosis in the adolescent can cause chronic pelvic pain.[17]

Adequate medical treatment after laparoscopic confirmation of the diagnosis will help to relieve chronic pelvic pain. Multiple studies have shown that the oral contraceptives Depo-Provera and Lupron can be effective in the long-term treatment of these patients. Because presacral neurectomy and laparoscopic uterine nerve ablation are unproven treatments, they must not be used for adolescents with endometriosis.[33–35]

MÜLLERIAN OBSTRUCTIVE ANOMALIES

Müllerian obstructive anomalies may go long undetected in an adolescent whose complaint is acute or chronic recurrent pain. Obstructive anomalies may be missed unless they are ruled out by a pelvic examination. Goldstein and associates showed that müllerian anomalies had been missed for a long time in patients with CPP and were discovered only on laparoscopic examination. See Chapter 39 for further discussion.

OVARIAN CYSTS

A multifollicular ovary with preovulatory follicles measuring 2 cm is common in adolescents. Functional cysts of the ovary are cysts of the ovarian follicle, corpus, or theca luteum, are smaller than 3 cm, and are not neoplastic. Unfortunately, widespread use of pelvic sonography has resulted in patients being told that they have a "cyst," and this conjures up visions of neoplasm or cancer of the ovary. The following principles are useful in the management of ovarian masses in adolescents:

1. When a palpable mass feels fixed or solid, it should be treated surgically. Tumor markers, α-fetoprotein, β-HCG, serum lactate dehydrogenase (LDH), and CA-125 tests should be done preoperatively.
2. Abdominal plain film should be considered for young patients with masses larger than 5 cm. Benign, mature teratomas are the most common ovarian tumor of young women. Some 40% of the tumors contain teeth, a finding that clinches the diagnosis. Occasionally, a phlebolith or a calcified or malignant tumor is mistaken for calcium.
3. A 5- to 7-cm cystic mass that is mobile can be managed conservatively with 6 weeks' ob-

servation. The patient is instructed to go to a hospital emergency department if acute pain develops. Previous studies have shown that about three fourths of these cysts disappear without further treatment.

4. Although oral contraceptives have been known to decrease ovarian cyst formation, recent studies do not substantiate this. It is also apparent from recent data that if an oral contraceptive is used, the preparation should contain 35 to 50 μg of ethinyl estradiol in a combined pill.[36]
5. Exacerbation of pain during periods of observation of a large cyst should prompt evaluation. Rupture and spillage of fluid or hemorrhage may cause peritoneal irritation. Complete or incomplete ovarian torsion is another serious complication. Currently, we are advocating conservative surgical treatment of adnexal torsion, i.e., untwisting and conserving the ovary, which can be accomplished safely when circulation to the adnexa is not compromised. It is thus very important that we challenge ourselves to detect torsion of the ovary early. Again, in a case of torsion, the decision to use the laparoscope and do a complete cystectomy and oophoropexy will depend on the surgeon's expertise. It is important that when minilaparotomy is attempted, conservative microsurgical techniques, suturing to prevent adhesions, and other "antiadhesion" measures be taken. The primary objective is to conserve the young woman's fertility.

CHRONIC PELVIC PAIN

CPP in adult gynecology patients has been defined as noncyclic pelvic pain of more than 6 months' duration that is not relieved by nonnarcotic analgesics. CPP is a very general term that encompasses pain associated with laparoscopically evident abnormalities (e.g., endometriosis), nonreproductive somatic disease (e.g., irritable bowel syndrome [IBS]), and somatic "psychogenic" disorders. In adult patients, CPP accounts for a significant number of laparoscopies and hysterectomies.[3] The annual direct and indirect costs of this syndrome have been estimated to be $2 billion. Aggressive management of recurrent abdominal pain (RAP) in female adolescents can spare them from becoming adults with CPP.[37]

RECURRENT ABDOMINAL PAIN

In 1958, Apley and Naish[38] reported that 10% to 15% of pediatric and adolescent females pre-

Table 16–9. Recurrent Abdominal Pain: Items in the History

The history must include:
1. Age at menarche
2. Onset of symptoms in relation to menarche
3. Duration of pain
4. Localization of pain: consistent or variable, and severity
5. Cyclic or noncyclic pain, especially in relation to menses
6. Severity of pain, including consistency or variability, with subjective rating scale and functional rating scale
7. Menstrual history
8. Sexual history, including dyspareunia
9. History of sexually transmitted diseases or pelvic inflammatory disease (PID)
10. Careful history of bowel pattern, including history of bloating, nausea, vomiting, and a dietary history in the past 24 hours
11. Urinary tract symptoms
12. General health changes (e.g., weight, fever, joint problems, fatigue, headaches)
13. Symptoms of androgen excess (e.g., acne, oily skin)
14. Family history (e.g., endometriosis, dysmenorrhea, Crohn's disease)

sented with RAP, but only in 1 of 20 patients were they able to identify an organic cause for it. Since 1959, advances in endoscopy have helped to identify an organic cause in a significant percentage of patients. Apley noted that an organic cause must be ruled out before the patient can be considered "functional." Obviously, not all patients fit into the organic or psychogenic category; some are best managed with reassurance and professional consultations, as necessary. Table 16–9 includes some of the features of history taking.

Over the years, various adolescent specialists have outlined principles for management of abdominal pain. Some useful pointers are outlined in Table 16–10. It is important to remember that

Table 16–10. Principles of Treatment of Patients with Recurrent Abdominal Pain

1. Validate the patient's pain.
2. Relieve symptoms.
3. Establish validity of a nonorganic cause.
4. Empower the parent.
5. Use concrete language.
6. Evaluation must be completed at one session so the patient will know that all tests have been done.
7. Psychosocial referral, if necessary, even if an organic cause is found (e.g., minimal endometriosis, pelvic inflammatory disease, or other pelvic disease).
8. Frequent visits must be made after surgery, as patients experience a placebo effect and later will consult another physician if they cannot see the first surgeon.

we must prevent these patients from becoming "chronic pain syndrome patients."[39]

A multidisciplinary approach is absolutely necessary for these patients when the surgeon does not find disease in the pelvis that accounts for the disability and pain. Major operative procedures (e.g., oophorectomy, ovarian cystectomy, cutting of presacral or uterosacral nerves) must be avoided. A number of other methods are available for these patients: practicing relaxation skills, TENS, biofeedback, and applying anesthetic agents for "trigger points." Physiotherapy is also very useful in the rehabilitation of a CPP patient, and she should be encouraged to return to normal activities. Tables 16–9 and 16–10 outline the history and treatment principles for patients with RAP.

Peters and associates[40] in Sweden compared adult women randomly assigned to a standard treatment that included laparoscopy or to an integrated treatment approach that included somatic, psychological, dietary, environmental, and physiotherapeutic modalities. Evaluation of these women 1 year later showed that an integrated approach improved their pelvic pain significantly more often than did the standard approach. Laparoscopy plays an important role in diagnosing reproductive system abnormalities (e.g., endometriosis, PID, or müllerian abnormality may cause the adolescent to have permanent reproductive damage later in adult life.)

For adolescents with CPP, initial laparoscopy and aggressive treatment—surgical and medical—of the condition is in order. Most teenagers respond to this. Repeated surgical procedures must be avoided in teenagers. A consultation from an adolescent specialist should be obtained if the pain recurs.

In a study of RAP in patients referred to Vanderbilt University, Walker and associates drew the following conclusions[41]:
1. Measures of emotional distress are not useful in differentiating pain of organic cause from other pain.
2. Attention to psychosocial dysfunction may promote recovery of patients both with or without organic etiologies for abdominal pain.
3. When a child's family has a high level of "illness behavior," attempts must be made to decrease the family's focus on the child's physical symptoms and the child is encouraged to resume normal activity.
4. The majority of mothers of children with abdominal pain, regardless of cause, believe that one or more of the psychosocial factors contributed to their child's abdominal pain.

Therefore, it is important that we seek the

help of other disciplines in our attempts to help patients with CPP, whether laparoscopy reveals an organic cause or no lesion. This approach is in keeping with the old dictum that medicine is an art and not all science.[42, 43]

PELVIC PAIN OF NONREPRODUCTIVE CAUSES

Gastrointestinal (GI) and urinary tract sources of chronic abdominal pain may be difficult to distinguish from those of gynecologic origin. RAP is thought to affect at least 10% of school-aged children.[44] In the past, the frequency of reports of RAP to physicians was only 10%, but increasing numbers of children and teenagers may be coming to evaluation because of the increasing recognition of the variety of organic causes of RAP in the pediatric age group.[45] Several studies have shown a female predominance.[46]

Nonorganic pain is usually periumbilical and is associated with a family medical history of functional GI problems. The length and severity of attacks may not be helpful in elucidating the cause.[46] Differentiating between GI and reproductive tract causes of chronic abdominal pain is particularly difficult in adolescent females and frequently requires a coordinated approach between the pediatric gastroenterologist and pediatrician or gynecologist.

Lactose Malabsorption

One common cause of GI pain is lactose malabsorption,[47] a disorder that affects between 5% and 20% of the population and is more common in certain ethnic and national groups, including African Americans and Asians. In one study, lactose malabsorption was present in 24% of children aged 6 to 18 years who had RAP.[48] Forty-six percent of African American children in that series were lactose intolerant, as compared with 20% of white children ($p < .02$).[48] Lactose malabsorption is characterized by crampy abdominal pain, excess flatus, diarrhea, and bloating. Most patients seem to benefit from withdrawing lactose from their diet; this benefit however, is not limited to those who are lactose malabsorbers. Patients who are lactose absorbers may also benefit from lactose withdrawal. Failure of response to short-term withdrawal of milk and cheese products from the diet does not rule out lactose intolerance because there are many unsuspected dietary sources of lactose.[48]

Lactose absorption is best evaluated by a breath hydrogen test (BHT). After a standard oral lactose load (usually 2 gm/kg, to a maximum of 50 gm), serial analyses of breath hydrogen samples are performed. An increase of more than 10 (and especially of more than 20) ppm from the baseline confirms lactose malabsorption and suggests that lactose withdrawal or enzyme supplementation would be beneficial.[47] In the series by Webster and coworkers, patients who were taken off lactose completely or who took enzyme supplements did significantly better, over the long-term, than patients who had normal lactose absorption and, presumably, pain of another cause. Patients on a lactose-free diet should receive a calcium supplement. If, despite a negative BHT, lactose malabsorption is still suspected a lactulose BHT can confirm the diagnosis. Lactulose is a nonabsorbable disaccharide, and, after administration of a standard lactulose load, BHT should reveal an increase of at least 10 to 20 ppm. This test is used to identify individuals who cannot produce significant amounts of hydrogen in the colon and therefore do not exhale it in their breath. It helps to eliminate false-negative results. Another cause of a false-negative lactose BHT is recent use of an antibiotic. Patients who require long-term antibiotic therapy and cannot stop taking it for a BHT can be evaluated by serial serum glucose determinations after an oral lactose load. Malabsorption of other carbohydrates, such as fructose, sucrose, and sorbitol, may also result in diarrhea and symptoms similar to those of lactose intolerance. Sucrose malabsorption can be evaluated by comparable oral tolerance tests.

Chronic Constipation

A second cause of chronic abdominal pain that is often confused with pain of reproductive system origin is chronic constipation. The actual incidence of this disorder is difficult to determine, although a significant number of persons are affected. Chronic constipation is marked by a history of infrequent bowel movements or straining with bowel movements. There is significant variation in any person's normal stool frequency, and diet is an important variable. Bowel movements as frequent as three times a day or as infrequent as once every 3 days are considered within normal limits. Some younger children develop overflow incontinence with chronic constipation, and a history of fecal soiling should be elicited. In many cases the constipation is not recognized, and the chief presenting complaint is diarrhea. This diagnosis of constipation is best established by a careful physical examination, including rectal examination. Important confirmatory tests include rectal motility to evaluate the degree of distention in the rectum and to rule out Hirschsprung disease. Biofeedback therapy, in conjunction with rectal motility testing, may help patients to overcome their abdominal pain. Some patients have a condition known as *paradoxical contraction of the puborectalis muscle*, which results in ineffective relaxation during attempts to defecate. Biofeedback training is especially helpful for these patients. In patients with long-standing constipation, it may take a long while for the rectum to return to normal size and for patients to be able to sense when they need to defecate. Some authors have noted a decrease in the frequency of attacks of RAP in response to the addition of dietary fiber; the mechanism is thought to be alteration in colonic transit time.[49] Irregular bowel habits may be a component of some female reproductive disorders, including endometriosis, and the presence of constipation does not exclude other intraabdominal or pelvic disease.[50] Patients with severe constipation may have a palpable lower abdominal mass, which can mimic a uterine lesion, or even pregnancy. An enema usually "delivers" the mass. Manual disimpaction is required occasionally, but usually, pediatric patients should be sedated for this type of procedure.

Giardiasis

The incidences of both symptomatic and asymptomatic *Giardia* infections are very variable. It may be a significant pathogen in young children, especially those who attend day care.[51] Other persons at risk include family members of children attending day care, travelers, immigrants from abroad, swimmers in contaminated water (where animals defecate or the water is otherwise contaminated), campers, and immunodeficient persons.[52] The clinical presentation is very variable and may be characterized by acute enteritis or persistent and relapsing diarrhea. Patients may also exhibit abdominal distention, nonspecific cramping, flatulence, and failure to thrive. Occasionally, they develop urticaria or bronchospasm related to *Giardia*.[52] The diagnosis is best established by stool cultures obtained on three separate occasions and examination for ova and parasites or antigen detection. An endoscopically obtained small bowel biopsy specimen may also yield the diagnosis. Persons who have contact with contaminated water should be considered at risk for this disorder. The treatment is

quinacrine, metronidazole, or furazolidone. Treatment may be repeated, if necessary. Patients with *Giardia* infection are frequently lactose intolerant; the intolerance resolves with adequate therapy unless the patient is genetically predisposed to secondary lactase deficiency.

Crohn's Disease and Ulcerative Colitis

Inflammatory bowel disease (IBD) has a bimodal peak of onset. The first peak occurs in adolescence, and approximately 20% to 30% of cases of IBD are diagnosed in childhood or adolescence.[53] Many patients with IBD have a family history of either ulcerative colitis (UC) or Crohn's disease, especially in first-degree relatives, as studies from the Cleveland Clinic Foundation have demonstrated.[54, 55]

Crohn's disease is a serious cause of abdominal pain that may be missed without serial follow-up of patients, as long-term studies performed at the Mayo Clinic have shown.[56] A 23-year retrospective review of an outpatient population demonstrated that the mean age of onset of Crohn's symptoms in pediatric patients was 11.6 years with a mean diagnostic delay of 9.5 months.[53] Although Crohn's disease is characterized by abdominal pain, diarrhea, weight loss, anorexia, fever, impaired growth, primary or secondary amenorrhea, and joint symptoms, as many as 7% of patients may present with isolated abdominal pain. Failure to gain weight appropriately, on a weight to height basis, poor progression through the Tanner stages, and a decrease in height percentile for age or height velocity on serial measurements are clinical signs suggestive of Crohn's disease.[57]

The presence of Crohn's disease may be suggested by abnormal results on screening laboratory tests, including a complete blood cell count and erythrocyte sedimentation rate. A rectal examination should be performed to check for occult blood in every patient with RAP and for any evidence of perianal disease. Many patients undergo surgery for abdominal pain or suspected acute or "chronic" appendicitis before the correct diagnosis of Crohn's disease is made. Patients with Crohn's disease most often have involvement of the terminal ileum, but any portion of the alimentary tract from the mouth to the anus may be involved. Diagnostic clues on physical examination include recurrent mouth sores, joint pains, clubbing of the fingers, recurrent rashes of the anterior lower extremities with or without nodules, perianal disease, and a family history.[57]

Table 16–11. Physical Examination and Laboratory Findings Suggestive of Inflammatory Bowel Disease

	Crohn's Disease	Ulcerative Colitis
Physical examination		
Growth failure	Present	Present but less common
Weight loss	Present	Present
Clubbing	Present	Present
Arthritis, especially large joints	Present	Present
Skin manifestations	Present	Present
Erythema nodosum (EN)		
pyoderma gangrenosum (PG)		(EN > PG)
Stomatitis, aphthous ulcers	Present	Not characteristic
Ocular disease; iritis, uveitis	Present	Present
Hepatic disease: hepatitis, sclerosing cholangitis	Present	Present
Fistulas	Perianal, enterocutaneous, enterocolic, enteroenteral enterovesical, enterovaginal	Absent
Renal disease: stones	Present	Less common
Laboratory findings		
Anemia	Present	Present
Thrombocytosis	Present	Present
Hypoalbuminemia	Present	Present
Increased sedimentation rate	Present	Present
Liver function test abnormalities	Sometimes present	Sometimes present

Patients who complain of nocturnal bowel movements, fecal urgency and tenesmus, heme-positive stools, and abdominal pain that is relieved by passage of a loose or soft stool should be evaluated for IBD. The diagnosis is usually established by colonoscopy with biopsy or esophagogastroduodenoscopy (EGD).[58] Upper GI (UGI) x-ray examination with small bowel follow-through (SBFT) can be suggestive, especially if terminal ileal narrowing or a fistula is demonstrated, but care should be taken to avoid misinterpreting lymphonodular hyperplasia of the terminal ileum, which is a normal finding in children and adolescents with terminal ileal Crohn's disease.[58]

The symptoms of ulcerative colitis (UC) are less frequently misinterpreted than those of Crohn's disease, because the presentation tends to be more dramatic—rectal bleeding, protracted diarrhea, significant weight loss—and, therefore, patients seek medical attention earlier. The majority of patients have a less fulminant presentation, however and sometimes have constitutional symptoms such as weight loss and growth failure.[59] Like Crohn's disease, there is often a considerable delay in the diagnosis of ulcerative colitis. Findings on physical examination are similar to those of Crohn's disease, except that perianal disease is absent and disease is limited to the colon (Table 16–11). Laboratory findings are also similar, except for a higher rate of positive tests for antineutrophilic cytoplasmic antibody

(ANCA) in patients with UC (Table 16–12).[60] Treatment options are similar to those for Crohn's, although surgical options are significantly different; thus, whenever possible, it is important to establish the correct diagnosis before surgery.[57] Some 10% to 15% of newly diagnosed pediatric patients have "indeterminate colitis", an appellation that means that Crohn's disease of the colon cannot be initially distinguished from UC.[59] With long-term follow-up, a substantial fraction of these patients ultimately are determined to have Crohn's disease. Although both UC and Crohn's disease are associated with increased risk of GI tract malignancy, the risk is significantly higher for patients with UC, and strategies are in place for dysplasia screening and colectomy, should dysplasia be detected. IBD should not be confused with irritable bowel syndrome (IBS).

Celiac Disease

Celiac disease is an inherited form of gluten intolerance characterized by small bowel villus atrophy in response to gliadin. The disease is most common in persons of Northern European descent. Patients with gluten-sensitive enteropathy are intolerant of wheat, rye, barley, and oats but can eat rice and maize. The condition frequently presents in infancy after the introduction of gluten into the diet, but it may not appear

Table 16–12. Evaluation of Common Causes of Recurrent Abdominal Pain

Suspected Diagnosis	Diagnostic Test(s) of Choice
Acid peptic disease	EGD with biopsy, pH probe
Eosinophilic gastroenteritis	Antral biopsy
Helicobacter pylori	Antral biopsy, culture, breath test
Celiac disease	Antigliadin and anti-endomysial antibodies EGD with small bowel biopsy
Constipation	Rectal examination, KUB, rectal motility
Giardia lamblia infection	Stool O&P × 3, or stool antigen detection EGD with small bowel biopsy
Inflammatory bowel disease	CBC, ESR, Albumin
Crohn's disease	UGI-SBFT, EGD, colonoscopy with biopsy
Ulcerative colitis	Colonoscopy with biopsy
Lactose intolerance	Lactose breath hydrogen test
Pancreatitis	Serum amylase and lipase, abdominal ultrasound, computed tomography if recurrent, ERCP

O&P = ova and parasites; CBC = complete blood count; ESR = erythrocyte sedimentation rate; ERCP = endoscopic retrograde cholangiopancreatography.

until adolescence or early adulthood. Failure to thrive, diarrhea, irritability, fat malabsorption, and abdominal bloating are the signs. Older patients may have less dramatic symptoms—nonspecific abdominal pain, cramping, bloating, diarrhea, and fatigue.[61] Osteomalacia, iron deficiency anemia, folate deficiency, and hypoalbuminemia may be present.[58] Diagnosis is suggested by positive antigliadin antibodies (IgG, IgA) and anti-endomysial antibodies but should be confirmed by EGD and small bowel biopsy because of the possibility of false-positive antibody results. Complete gluten withdrawal from the diet restores the villi to their normal appearance. Life-long avoidance of dietary gluten is necessary because of the significantly increased risk of small bowel lymphoma in undiagnosed patients with celiac disease or patients who do not comply with the diet. First-degree relatives of affected patients appear to have approximately a 10% risk (70% to 75% for monozygotic twins) of celiac disease and, so, should be screened.[62]

Irritable Bowel Syndrome

IBS may be a cause of RAP in older adolescents or young adults.[62] It is especially prevalent in patients who present to a gynecologist for evaluation.[63] Patients characteristically have altered bowel habits alternating between constipation and diarrhea. Other signs are looser stools and more frequent bowel movements and symptoms including abdominal pain, a sense of incomplete evacuation, straining, and bloating. IBS affects 14% of high school students and 6% of middle school students.[64] IBS symptoms are no more frequent in high school girls than boys, but are more common in patients who test positive for anxiety trait and depression or who regularly have headaches.[64] Dietary therapy that includes addition of fiber may provide symptomatic relief for these patients. It is important to establish that the abdominal distention is not related to menses and that the pain is long standing. IBS must be excluded if there is any evidence of blood on rectal examination, if the patient has a history of bowel resection, or if an organic disease is detected.

Esophagitis, Gastritis, and Duodenitis

In the past, esophagitis, gastritis, and duodenitis were frequently underdiagnosed in children using standard GI radiography. Fiberoptic and video endoscopy and their subsequent application to pediatrics have made it possible to identify these problems in children and adolescents. In a review of children ultimately found to have peptic ulcer disease who had undergone a UGI series before endoscopy, 50% of gastric ulcers and 11% of duodenal ulcers were not detected by x-ray.[65] Endoscopy yielded the diagnosis in 97% of these patients. In one patient with a duodenal ulcer, the endoscope could not be passed to visualize the ulcer because of a deformed duodenal bulb; that ulcer was diagnosed by UGI study.[65] In another review of 22 children with endoscopically confirmed gastric or duodenal ulcers, UGI barium examination was normal in 54% of patients (false-negative), missing 6 of 7 gastric ulcers and 5 of 15 duodenal ulcers.[65a] Endoscopy has a higher diagnostic yield than plain films in patients with mucosal changes such as esophagitis or gastritis without ulceration.[65b] At the Cleveland Clinic Foundation, Balsells and coworkers reported their experience with endoscopy in more than 2000 pediatric patients.[66] Of the 1945 EGDs performed, the most common indication was abdominal pain (31% of patients). Dyspepsia—defined as at least one of these symptoms (abdominal pain, nausea, eructation, heartburn)—was the indication for EGD in 35% of cases.[66] Esophagitis was detected endoscopically in 27% of patients. Acid peptic disease (gastritis, duodenitis, gastric or duodenal erosions) was present in 22% of cases. In patients older than 17 years, acid peptic disease was diagnosed in half of all examinations.[66] Minor complications occurred in 0.36% of patients, and procedure-related major complications occurred in one (0.06%) patient. In that case, the complication was related to a therapeutic esophageal dilation after a severe injury from swallowing a caustic substance.[66] Tam and Saing retrospectively reviewed 533 endoscopies in children over a 13-year period; for 34%, the indication was abdominal pain.[67] The investigators found that 22% of the patients had esophagitis, gastritis, duodenitis, or ulcerative disease. There was no endoscopy-related death in that series.[67] In younger children especially, historical findings alone may not suggest the diagnosis of acid peptic disease because of the child's inability to localize the abdominal pain or identify precipitating or exacerbating factors. Tam and associates reviewed their 18-year experience with peptic ulcer disease, predominantly chronic duodenal ulcers, in children.[68] Forty-six percent of their patients had a history of epigastric pain, and, of these, only 43% (one fourth of the entire study population) had typical "ulcer pain." The location of the pain may lead to diagnostic errors. Five children with perforated duodenal ulcers presented with right lower quadrant pain and were thought preoperatively to have appendicitis.[68] Older adolescents have more typical symptoms of acid peptic disease, including substernal pain and acid regurgitation. The availability of ibuprofen OTC and the increasingly frequent use of this medication for indications such as fever and headache has increased the prevalence of acid peptic disease in our practice. Proton pump inhibitors have proven to be a very effective treatment for moderate to severe acid peptic disease in pediatric patients, and today surgery for this condition is very unusual.

Although its pathologic role in the development of antral gastritis and duodenal ulceration has now been established, the role of *Helicobacter pylori* in the pathogenesis of RAP in children is less clear.[69] *H. pylori* colonization cannot be distinguished from other disorders on the basis of abdominal pain and vomiting.[69] The diagnosis is established by EGD and by Giemsa staining, culture, or rapid urease testing of biopsy specimens.[70] Less invasive breath testing methods have recently become available.[69] Therapy is directed at eradicating the organism—and includes various conbinations of bismuth subsalicylate, proton pump inhibitors, and antibiotics (including amoxicillin, metronidazole, tetracycline, and macrolide antibiotics).[71]

Eosinophilic gastroenteritis may cause RAP in pediatric patients and is frequently difficult to detect. Because any layer of the GI tract may be involved, the clinical presentation varies accordingly. Involvement of the mucosal layer typically produces signs similar to those of IBD or acid peptic disease: pain, weight loss, anemia, and hypoproteinemia. Submucosal and muscle involvement typically affects the gastric antrum and may mimic pyloric stenosis with recurrent vomiting and gastric outlet obstruction.[72, 73] Serosal involvement may result in hypoproteinemia and eosinophilic ascites. Diagnosis is usually confirmed by EGD with mucosal biopsy, but full thickness biopsy is occasionally necessary. Therapy consists of cromolyn sodium (a mast cell stabilizer), inhibition of gastric acid production, and intermittent doses of corticosteroids. It is not unusual for affected patients to have undergone several endoscopies before the correct diagnosis is established.

Pancreatitis

Pediatric and adolescent patients with pancreatitis typically have severe acute attacks of mid-epigastric abdominal pain, which sometimes radiates to the back. The pain may also be harder to localize and may appear to originate from the lower chest or lower abdomen. Often, severe nausea and vomiting are associated with the pain, and sometimes a low-grade fever.[74] Children with pancreatitis typically assume a position with the trunk flexed and the knees drawn up. Exquisite abdominal tenderness is usually present. Bluish discoloration around the flanks or umbilicus indicates very severe disease.[74] Risk factors for pediatric patients include gallstones of any cause, hyperlipidemia, medications and toxins (including alcohol), metabolic disease, trauma, structural abnormalities, mutations of the cystic fibrosis gene, and hereditary pancreatitis.[75] A significant fraction of cases are idiopathic.[75] With subsequent attacks, the severity of the abdominal pain may decrease. This makes the diagnosis more difficult if not initially suspected.[76] The diagnosis is suggested by serum amylase and lipase determinations,[75] and confirmed by kidney/ureter/bladder (KUB) films, abdominal ultrasound, computed tomography, and magnetic resonance imaging.[75] On KUB, pancreatic calcification may be seen in patients with long-standing disease. A normal KUB does not rule out pancreatitis. Endoscopic retrograde cholangiopancreatography may be helpful in patients with recurrent attacks when anatomic abnormalities are suspected and in some cases is therapeutic for biliary or pancreatic duct obstruction. Antioxidant therapy may be appropriate in patients with hereditary pancreatitis.[77]

Uncommon Nonreproductive Causes of Abdominal Pain

Chronic or recurrent abdominal pain may have an uncommon cause unrelated to the reproductive system, including anatomic and other abnormalities.

MECKEL'S DIVERTICULUM

Meckel's diverticulum is the most common congenital anomaly of the intestinal tract (prevalance 0.3% to 3%). Patients with complications related to Meckel's diverticulum are usually younger than 2 years. Approximately 55% of patients with Meckel's diverticulum have abnormal mucosa in the diverticulum, with gastric mucosa present in 80% to 85% of cases.[78-81] Complications of Meckel's diverticulum include bleeding (detected by technetium scan with pentagastrin stimulation), obstruction caused by intussusception or volvulus, diverticulitis, and perforation. Pain may be secondary to ulceration of the normal intestinal mucosa adjacent to the diverticulum. Onset of abdominal pain due to Meckel's diverticulum typically is abrupt. The majority of patients with Meckel's diverticulum are asymptomatic, and their condition is discovered incidentally or at autopsy.

MIDGUT MALROTATION

Another unusual cause of abdominal pain that may present with intermittent cramping or vomiting is midgut malrotation.[82] This condition may also present with acute volvulus, especially in the newborn period. In a retrospective review from Texas Children's Hospital the mean age of 16 children older than 6 weeks whose midgut malrotation was treated surgically was 4 years (range up to 15 years). Approximately half of them presented with chronic abdominal pain or vomiting. A clue to the presence of malrotation was visible peristalsis. In nonacute cases, the pain was characteristically intermittent, and symptoms had been present for an average of 6 months. Symptoms were often related to partial duodenal obstruction with Ladd bands, and symptoms resolved postoperatively. Proper evaluation for suspected malrotation includes a UGI series with small bowel follow through (SBFT). Volvulus due to midgut malrotation has also been reported in adults; the consequences of volvulus can be severe and life threatening.

SCHÖNLEIN-HENOCH PURPURA

Schönlein-Henoch purpura is characterized by purpura, arthritis, and abdominal pain, with or without glomerulonephritis.[83] Two thirds of patients have abdominal pain, which may be severe or colicky. As many as 10% of patients may undergo exploratory laparotomy before the diagnosis is established. Fifty percent of patients have heme-positive stools, and 30%, melanotic stools. The abdominal pain of Schönlein-Henoch purpura may develop before the characteristic rash does. The disease may also be complicated by intussusception or massive GI bleeding, and early diagnosis is imperative. Older children seem to have more severe disease than toddlers. Abdominal radiography may reveal characteristic thumbprinting of the colon. Corticosteroid therapy has been prescribed for this disorder, with mixed results, but it appears to shorten the duration of the abdominal pain.[84]

ACUTE INTERMITTENT PORPHYRIA

Acute intermittent porphyria is an autosomal dominant disorder more common in females. Onset is typically in late puberty or early adulthood; the cause is diminished uroporphyrin synthetase activity. Precipitating factors (found in 75% of patients) include use of barbiturates or sulfonamides, premenstrual segment of the cycle, infection, fasting, and alcohol consumption. Acute intermittent porphyria is characterized by recurrent attacks of neurologic, abdominal, and psychological symptoms. The attacks may last several days, and asymptomatic periods intervene. Patients also experience constipation and associated vomiting. From some, a history of pain or paraesthesias in the extremities may be elicited, and as many as 20% of patients may have tonic-clonic seizures related to the disorder. If the condition is not identified, death may occur from respiratory paralysis or cardiac arrhythmia secondary to "sympathetic overdrive." No treatment is available; management consists of avoiding the precipitating factors. A correct diagnosis is important to reduce long-term morbidity.[85]

ABDOMINAL EPILEPSY

Some authors have described abdominal epilepsy as a very rare cause of RAP. Characteristically, the pain is paroxysmal, abrupt in onset, located in the middle to upper abdomen, and associated with autonomic phenomena and mental status changes.[86] Patients have postictal symptoms after the attack and then are able to resume normal activity. The characteristic electroencephalographic finding is a spiked wave pattern with a temporal lobe focus. The existence of this disorder is disputed, and its actual prevalence in pediatric patients is difficult to determine. A response to anticonvulsant medication is necessary for the diagnosis to be considered correct.[87]

URETEROPELVIC JUNCTION (UPJ) OBSTRUCTION

Although UPJ obstruction is an uncommon cause of RAP (confirmed in fewer than 1% of patients evaluated for this disorder), abdominal pain as an isolated finding is not an uncommon presentation and may occur in as many as 70% of patients older than 1 year. The abdominal pain is nonspecific and may radiate to the groins, upper quadrants, and flanks. Only a small percentage of affected patients have associated gross hematuria. The problem is usually unilateral, the left side being affected more often than the right, but it is bilateral in as many as 20% of patients. The condition is caused by intrinsic anomalies at the UPJ, including aberrant vessels, fibrous bands, and kinks. The diagnosis is readily established by intravenous pyelography, and a high index of suspicion is required.[88]

PSYCHOGENIC DISORDERS

Some preliminary evidence suggests that recurrent and chronic abdominal pain may also be the result of a psychogenic disorder and may represent an altered response to the normal stresses of everyday life. Some studies have found that children with RAP are likely to have a history of manifesting stress as GI tract disorders (e.g., preschool stomach aches),[89] but no evidence suggests an increased incidence of psychosis in these children or a disrupted social environment. Their family histories do, however, indicate a high incidence of functional GI tract disorders.

ABDOMINAL WALL TRIGGER POINTS

Slocumb, in a study of 122 CPP patients, found that the single most common site of pain is the abdominal wall.[90] Needle localization was used to identify sources of pain in the fat and fascial planes above the aponeurosis in these patients. The tender points generated most of pain for 90% of patients in this series. Tension of the rectus muscle, produced either by elevating both legs or by lifting the head and shoulder, exacerbated the abdominal wall pain, because the tender points were pressed against the firm rectus muscles.[91]

Diagnosis and treatment of focal tender points in the abdominal wall by infiltration of local anesthetic (e.g., 1% procaine or 0.25% bupivacaine) has been shown to block this pain. Slocumb found that pain relief lasted for days or months. This therapeutic modality has also been combined with antidepressants and nonsteroidal antiinflammatory agents, and psychological counseling whenever necessary. During the examination the physician should try to elicit any abdominal trigger points in patients with chronic pain. The workup of patients with chronic pain can be accomplished in steps.

PATIENT HISTORY

The examiner should begin by asking the patient to describe the pain, localizing it, and then asking about factors that aggravate pain. If the pain is related to endometriosis, at least in the early stages, a cluster of symptoms, seems to appear around the time of menses or at the time of ovulation.

A careful history of bowel function will reveal symptoms suggestive of irritable bowel syndrome. Manning and coworkers administered a questionnaire of 156 different symptoms to 109 selected patients.[92] Four symptoms—distention, relief of pain with bowel movement, loose and frequent bowel movements with onset of pain and mucus, and a sense of incomplete evacuation—were common in those who had IBS. A rectal examination and guaiac test are recommended. If the guaiac study is positive or perianal disease is found, especially in conjunction with an elevated erythrocyte sedimentation rate, the possibility of IBD must be considered. Hard stool in the rectal vault suggests constipation as a possible cause of pain.

The physician should also try to elicit any history of bulimia and anorexia nervosa. Anorexia nervosa can easily be detected when the patient's body weight is at least 25% below expected weight, she has intense fear of gaining weight and a distorted body image, and she has missed at least three consecutive menstrual periods. Patients with bulimia, on the other hand, may be very outgoing, sociable, sexually active, have normal periods, and be very secretive about her bingeing. Associated findings include recurrent bouts of depression, low self-esteem, and substance abuse. The bingeing and purging put these patients at risk for chronic constipation and laxative dependence, dental erosion and caries, esophagitis, and electrolyte abnormalities. Denial of symptoms—by the patient and sometimes by the family—is typical. The diagnosis can be established only if the physician suspects an eating disorder and tries to elicit a compatible history, which may not be forthcoming until the second or third visit.

It is important to elicit any history of lactose intolerance, constipation, drinking of large amounts of carbonated drinks or iced tea, or gum chewing. A musculoskeletal examination, which may involve a straight leg–raising test and compression of different trigger points, must also be done.

Most important in the evaluation of chronic abdominal or pelvic pain is that the workup proceed in a stepwise and directed manner. Initial screening examinations should include a complete blood cell count with differential, determination of erythrocyte sedimentation rate, liver function tests, urinalysis with culture, amylase determination, plain film abdominal radiography, stool cultures for ova and parasites, stool guaiac test, measurements of height and weight recorded on growth charts, and a gynecologic examination. Secondary evaluation may include BHT, determination of lead level, porphyrin determination, intravenous pyelography, UGI series with SBFT, and barium enema, EGD, or colonoscopy (see Table 16–12).

An ultrasound examination of the pelvis is very often used to evaluate these patients. Ultrasound ordinarily identifies any major müllerian abnormalities but not endometriosis or PID unless these are accompanied by a large ovarian abscess or endometrioma. On the other hand, an ovarian cyst 1 to 2 cm in diameter in such a patient can lead the examiner to think that the cyst is causing the pain; however, the cyst may not account for the symptoms. It is thus important that physicians be selective about choosing the proper diagnostic tests. Laparoscopic examination and other GI endoscopic procedures are necessary for a number of these patients.

MANAGEMENT

Often, these patients are angry and frustrated because they have seen many physicians, have had numerous tests, and usually have missed a considerable amount of scholastic and extracurricular activities. Parents and teachers can become overprotective. Physicians should avoid recommending home tutoring or giving special considerations such as notes to excuse the patient from physical fitness activities. It is best to complete the evaluation as quickly as possible and in a deliberate stepwise manner. The physician must place the adolescent in proper perspective—her emotional development in relation to her chronologic age. For example, a 16-year-old who is dependent on her mother will need to be followed until late adolescence. Every attempt must be made to rule out organic causes with noninvasive tests and, if necessary, by endoscopic examination of the GI tract and liberal use of the laparoscope.

When the condition has an organic cause an adolescent should never be told, "The pain is in your head" or "You'll grow out of it" and then be referred for psychiatric evaluation. Similarly, when the history includes sexual or physical abuse or a triggering event is noted (e.g., the death of a parent or friend) a search still must be undertaken to rule out organic causes that may have been causing the pain. After the workup has been completed, patients can be managed according to the specific cause.

In adolescents, depression can also be associated with abdominal pain. Formal psychiatric treatment with antidepressants may be necessary. Depending on the diagnosis, methods of pain reduction may include biofeedback, stress management, and self-hypnosis. These are used effectively by neurologists and other specialists to manage chronic degenerative disease of the back and migraine headaches. Psychogenic abdominal pain is truly a diagnosis of exclusion.

Long-term follow-up and availability of the physician for any type of emergency is a necessity for patients with abdominal pain. The goal of the healthcare team is to determine the cause of pain and allow the adolescent to resume normal activities. Recurrent pelvic pain is a pervasive problem in pediatric and adolescent patients and demands aggressive evaluation, often with a multidisciplinary approach, to find the cause and institute appropriate treatment.

REFERENCES

1. Velebil P, Wingo PA, Xia Z, et al: Rate of hospitalization for gynecologic disorders among women of reproductive age in the United States. Obstet Gynecol 1995; 86:764.
2. Shaler E, Pelez D: Laparoscopic treatment of adnexal torsion. Surg Gynecol Obstet 1993; 176:448.

3. Fleischer AC, Stein SM, Cullinan JA, Warner MA: Color Doppler sonography of adnexal torsion. J Ultrasound Med 1995; 14:523.
4. Goldstein DP: Acute and chronic pelvic pain. Pediatr Clin North Am 1989; 36:573.
5. Whitworth CM, Whitworth PA, et al: Value of diagnostic laparoscopy in young women with possible appendicitis. Surg Gynecol Obstet 1988; 167(3):187–190.
6. Andersch B, Milsom I: An epidemiologic study of young women with dysmenorrhea. Am J Obstet Gynecol 1982: 144:655.
7. Klein J, Litt J: Epidemiology of adolescent dysmenorrhea. Pediatrics 1981; 68(5):661.
8. Campbell MA, McGrath PJ: Use of medication by adolescents for the management of menstrual discomfort. Arch Pediatr Adolesc Med 1997; 151(9):905–913.
9. Chambers CT, Reid GJ, et al: Self-administration of over-the-counter medication for pain among adolescents. Arch Pediatr Adolesc Med 1997; 151(5):449–455.
10. Pickles VR: Prostaglandins and dysmenorrhea—historical survey. Acta Obstet Gynecol Scand 1979; 87(Suppl 58):7.
11. Ackerland M, Anderson KF, et al: Effects of terbutaline on myometrial activity, uterine blood flow and lower abdominal pain in women with primary dysmenorrhea. Br J Obstet Gynaecol 1976; 38:673–678.
12. Gidwani G: Dysmenorrhea—myths and facts. Cleve Clin Q 1983; 50:567.
13. Schwartz A, Zor U, et al: Primary dysmenorrhea: Alleviation by an inhibitor of prostaglandin synthesis and action. Obstet Gynecol 1974; 44:709–712.
14. Dawood MY, McGuire JL, et al: Premenstrual Syndrome and Dysmenorrhea. Baltimore-Munich: Urban & Schwarzenberg, 1985.
15. Jacobsen J, Cavalli-Bjorkman K, et al: Prostaglandin synthetase inhibitors and dysmenorrhea—a survey and personal clinical experience. Acta Obstet Gynecol Scand 1979; 87(Suppl 1): 73.
16. Dawood MY: Dysmenorrhea and prostaglandins: Pharmacological and therapeutic considerations. Drugs 1981; 22:42.
17. Gidwani GP: Treating endometriosis in the adolescent. Contemp OB/GYN 1989; 33:75.
18. Malinak LR, Buttram VC, et al: Heritable aspects of endometriosis. Am J Obstet Gynecol 1980; 137:332–337.
19. Laufer MR: Endometriosis in adolescents. Curr Opin Pediatr 1992, 4:582–589.
20. Reese KA, Reddy S, Rock JA: Endometriosis in an adolescent population—The Emory Experience. J Pediatr Adolesc Gynecol 1996; 9:125–128.
21. Chan WY, Fuchs F, et al: Effects of naproxen sodium on menstrual prostaglandins and primary dysmenorrhea. Obstet Gynecol 1983; 61:285.
22. Jacobsen J, Lundstrom V, et al: Naproxen in treatment of OC-resistant primary dysmenorrhea. Acta Obstet Gynecol Scand 1983; 113 (Suppl):87.
23. Smith RP, Powell JR: Simultaneous objective and subjective evaluation of meclofenamate sodium in the treatment of primary dysmenorrhea. Am J Obstet Gynecol 1987; 157(3):611.
24. Davis GD, Thillet E, Lindemann J: Clinical characteristics of adolescent endometriosis. J Adolesc Health 1993; 14(5):362–368.
25. Emans SJ, Laufer M, Goldstein DP: Dysmenorrhea, Tramadol, pelvic pain and PMS. In Callaghan P (ed): Pediatric and Adolescent Gynecology. Philadelphia: Lippincott-Raven, 1998, p 374.
26. Kaplan B, Rabinerson D, et al: Clinical evaluation of a new model of a transcutaneous electrical nerve stimulation device for the management of primary dysmenorrhea. Gynecol Obstet Invest 1997; 44(4):255–259.
27. Helms JM: Acupuncture for the management of primary dysmenorrhea. Obstet Gynecol 1987; 69(1):51–56.
28. The Transdermal Nitroglycerin/Dysmenorrhea Study Group: Transdermal nitroglycerin in the management of pain associated with primary dysmenorrhea: A multinational pilot study. J Int Med Res 1997; 25:41–44.
29. Harlow SD, Park M: A longitudinal study of risk factors for the occurrence, duration and severity of menstrual cramps in a cohort of college women (published erratum appears in Br J Obstet Gynaecol 1997; 104[3]:386). Br J Obstet Gynaecol 1996;103(11):1134–1142.
30. Durant RH, Jay MS, et al: Factors influencing adolescents for dysmenorrhea. Am J Dis Child 1985; 139:489.
31. Westrom L, Joesoef R, Reynolds G, et al: PID and fertility: A cohort study of 1844 women with laparoscopically verified disease and 657 control women with normal laparoscopic results. Sex Transm Dis 1992; 19:185.
32. Rome ES, Moszczenski SA, Craighill MC, et al: An inpatient clinical pathway for pelvic inflammatory disease. Clin Perform Qual Health Care 1995; 3:185–196.
33. Vercellini P, Trespidi L, et al: Endometriosis and pelvic pain: Relation to disease stage and localization. Fertil Steril 1996; 65(2):299–304.
34. Crosignani PG, De Cecco L, et al: A three-year clinical investigation into efficacy, cycle control and tolerability of a new low-dose monophasic oral contraceptive containing gestodene. Gynecol Endocrinol 1996; 10(1):33–39.
35. Vercellini P, Trespidi L, et al: A gonadotropin-releasing hormone agonist versus a low-dose oral contraceptive for pelvic pain associated with endometriosis. Fertil Steril 1993; 60:75–79.
36. Steinkaupf MP, Hammond KR, Blackwell RE: Hormonal treatment of functional ovarian cysts—a randomized prospective study. Fertil Steril 1990; 54:775–777.
37. Reiter RC: Chronic pelvic pain. In Pitkin RM, Scott JR (eds): Clinical Obstetrics and Gynecology. Philadelphia: Lippincott-Raven, 1990, p 117.
38. Apley J, Naish N: Recurrent abdominal pain: A field survey of disease in childhood. Arch Dis Child 1958; 33:165.
39. Steege JF, Metzger DA, et al: Chronic Pelvic Pain, An Integrated Approach. Philadelphia: WB Saunders, 1998, p 9.
40. Peters AAW, VanDorst E, Jellis B, et al: A randomized clinical trial to compare two different approaches in women with chronic pelvic pain. Obstet Gynecol 1991; 77:740.
41. Walker LS, Green JW, et al: Psychosocial factors in pediatric abdominal pain: Implications for assessment and treatment. Clin Psychologist 1993; 46(4):206.
42. Gidwani GP: Chronic pelvic pain: Steps to take before and after operataive intervention. In Pokorny SF (ed): Pediatric and Adolescent Gynecology. Chapman & Hall, 1996, pp. 41–53.
43. Pokorny SF: Pediatric and Adolescent Gynecology. Chapman & Hall, 1996.
44. Wyllie R, Kay M: Causes of recurrent abdominal pain (Editorial). Clin Pediatr (Phila) 1993; 32:369–371.
45. Pineiro-Carrero VM, Andres JM, Davis RH, Mathias JR: Abnormal gastroduodenal motility in children and adolescents with recurrent functional abdominal pain. Pediatrics 1988; 113(5):820–825.
46. Poole SR: Recurrent abdominal pain in childhood and adolescence. Am Fam Physician 1984; 30(2):131–137.
47. Blumenthal I, Kelleher J, Littlewood JM: Recurrent abdominal pain and lactose intolerance in childhood. Br Med J Clin Res Ed 1981; 282(6281):2013–2014.

48. Webster RB, DiPalma JA, Gremse DA: Lactose maldigestion and recurrent abdominal pain in children. Dig Dis Sci 1995; 40(7):1506–1510.

49. Feldman W, McGrath P, Hodgson C, et al:. The use of dietary fiber in the management of simple, childhood, idiopathic, recurrent, abdominal pain. Results in a prospective, double-blind, randomized, controlled trial. Am J Dis Child 1985; 139(12):1216–1218.

50. Gidwani G: Endometriosis more common than you think. Contemp Pediatr 1989; 6:99–110.

51. Ish-Horowicz M, Korman SH, Shapiro M, et al: Asymptomatic giardiasis in children. Pediatr Infect Dis J 1989; 8(11):773–779.

52. Korman S, Deckelbaum R: Giardiasis in children—diagnosis and treatment. Resident Staff Physician 1989; 35:61–65.

53. Bousvaros A: Inflammatory bowel disease. Int Semin Paediatr Gastroenterol Nutr 1997; 6:1.

54. Farmer RG, Michener WM, Mortimer EA: Studies of family history among patients with inflammatory bowel disease. Clin Gastroenterol 1980; 9(2):271–277.

55. Michener WM, Caulfield M, Farmer RG, et al: Genetic counselling and family history in IBD: 30 years experience at the Cleveland Clinic. Can J Gastroenterol 1990; 4:350–354.

56. Castile RG, Telander RL, Cooney DR, et al: Crohn's disease in children: Assessment of the progression of disease, growth, and prognosis. J Pediatr Surg 1980; 15(4):462–469.

57. Wyllie R, Sarigol S: The treatment of inflammatory bowel disease in children. Clin Pediatr 1998; 37:421–426.

58. Wyllie R, Kay MH: Colonoscopy and therapeutic intervention in infants and children. Gastrointest Endosc Clin North Am 1994; 4:143–160.

59. Issenman RM: Inflammatory bowel disease: Presentation and clinical features. Int Semin Paediatr Gastroenterol Nutr 1997; 6:2–6.

60. Proujansky R, Fawcett PT, Gibney KM, et al: Examination of anti-neutrophil cytoplasmic antibodies in childhood inflammatory bowel disease. J Pediatr Gastroenterol Nutr 1993; 17:193–197.

61. Goggins M, Kelleher D: Celiac disease and other nutrient related injuries to the gastrointestinal tract (Review; 175 refs). Am J Gastroenterol 1994; 89(8 Suppl):S2–17.

62. Hyams JS, Treem WR, Justinich CJ, et al: Characterization of symptoms in children with recurrent abdominal pain: Resemblance to irritable bowel syndrome. J Pediatr Gastroenterol Nutr 1995; 20:209–214.

63. Hogston P: Irritable bowel syndrome as a cause of chronic pain in women attending a gynaecology clinic. Br Med J Clin Res Ed 1987; 294(6577):934–935.

64. Hyams JS, Burke G, Davis PM, et al: Abdominal pain and irritable bowel syndrome in adolescents: A community-based study. J Pediatrics 1996; 129:220–226.

65. Nord KS, Rossi TM, Lebenthal E: Peptic ulcer in children: The predominance of gastric ulcers. Am J Gastroenterol 1981; 75(2):153–157.

65a. Drumm B, Rhoads JM, Stringer DA, et al: Peptic ulcer disease in children: Etiology, clinical findings and clinical course. Pediatrics 1988; 82:410–414.

65b. Newman J. Radiographic and endoscopic evaluation of the upper GI tract. Radiol Technol 1998; 69:214–226.

66. Balsells F, Wyllie R, Steffen R, Kay M: Use of conscious sedation for esophagogastroduodenoscopy in children, adolescents and young adults. A 12 year review. Gastrointest Endosc 1995; 41:333.

67. Tam PK, Saing H: Pediatric upper gastrointestinal endos-

copy: A 13-year experience. J Pediatr Surg 1989; 24(5):443–447.

68. Tam PK, Saing H, Lau JT: Diagnosis of peptic ulcer in children: The past and present. J Pediatr Surg 1986; 21(1):15–16.

69. Wyllie R: *Helicobacter pylori* disease in childhood (Editorial). Clin Pediatr (Phila) 1995; 34:463–465.

70. Laine L, Lewin D, Naritoku W, et al: Prospective comparison of commercially available rapid urease tests for the diagnosis of *Helicobacter pylori*. Gastrointest Endosc 1996; 44(5):523–526.

71. Falk GW: *H.pylori* 1997: Testing and treatment options (Review; 19 refs). Cleve Clin J Med 1997; 64(4):187–192.

72. Steffen RM, Wyllie R, Petras RE, et al: The spectrum of eosinophilic gastroenteritis. Report of six pediatric cases and review of the literature. Clin Pediatr (Phila) 1991; 30:404–411.

73. Kay MH, Wyllie R, Steffen RM: The endoscopic appearance of eosinophilic gastroenteritis in infancy. Am J Gastroenterol 1995; 90:1361–1362.

74. Weizman Z: Acute pancreatitis. *In* Wyllie R, Hyams JS (eds): Pediatric Gastrointestinal Disease: Pathophysiology Diagnosis Management, 1st ed. Philadelphia: WB Saunders, 1993, pp 873–879.

75. Mathew P, Wyllie R, Caulfield M, et al: Chronic pancreatitis in late childhood and adolescence. Clin Pediatr (Phila) 1994; 33:88–94.

76. Wyllie R: Hereditary pancreatitis (Editorial; Comment). Am J Gastroenterol 1997; 92(7):1079–1080.

77. Mathew P, Wyllie R, Van Lente F, et al: Antioxidants in hereditary pancreatitis. Am J Gastroenterol 1996; 91:1558–1562.

78. Diamond RH, Rothstein RD, Alavi A: The role of cimetidine-enhanced technetium 99m pertechnetate imaging for visualizing Meckel's diverticulum. J Nucl Med 1991; 32:1422–1424.

79. Wyllie R: Intestinal duplications, Meckel diverticulum, and other remnants of the omphalomesenteric duct. *In* Behrman RE, Kleigman RM, Arvin AM (eds): Nelson: Textbook of Pediatrics, 15th ed. Phildelphia: WB Saunders, 1996, pp 1067–1069.

80. Rossi P, Gourtsoyiannis N, Bezzi M, et al: Meckel's diverticulum: Imaging diagnosis (see Comments). (Review; 55 refs). AJR Am J Roentgenol 1996; 166(3):567–573.

81. Arnold JF, Pellicane JV: Meckel's diverticulum: A ten-year experience. Am Surgeon 1997; 63(4):354–355.

82. Brandt ML, Pokorny WJ, McGill CW, Harberg FJ: Late presentations of midgut malrotation in children. Am J Surgery 1985; 150(6):767–771.

83. Goldman LP, Lindenberg RL: Henoch-Schoenlein purpura. Gastrointestinal manifestations with endoscopic correlation. Am J Gastroenterol 1981; 75(5):357–360.

84. Rosenblum ND, Winter HS: Steroid effects on the course of abdominal pain in children with Henoch-Schönlein purpura. Pediatrics 1987; 79:1018–1021.

85. Pattison CW, Haynes IG: Acute intermittent porphyria. A non-surgical cause of abdominal pain. Practitioner 1984; 228(1390):420–421.

86. Peppercorn MA, Herzog AG: The spectrum of abdominal epilepsy in adults. Am J Gastroenterol 1989; 84(10):1294–1296.

87. Singhi PD, Kaur S: Abdominal epilepsy misdiagnosed as psychogenic pain. Postgrad Med J 1988; 64(750):281–282.

88. Byrne WJ, Arnold WC, Stannard MW, Redman JF: Ureteropelvic junction obstruction presenting with recurrent abdominal pain: Diagnosis by ultrasound. Pediatrics 1985; 76(6):934–937.

89. McGrath PJ, Goodman JT, Firestone P, et al: Recurrent abdominal pain: A psychogenic disorder? Arch Dis Child 1983; 58:888–890.
90. Slocumb JC: Neurological factors in chronic pelvic pain: Trigger points and the abdominal pelvic pain syndrome. Am J Obstet Gynecol 1984; 149(5):536–543.
91. Thomson WH, Dawes RF, Carter SS: Abdominal wall tenderness: A useful sign in chronic abdominal pain. Br J Surg 1991; 78(2):223–225.
92. Manning AP, Thompson WG, Heaton KW, Morris AF: Towards positive diagnosis of the irritable bowel. Br Med J 1978; 2(6138):653–654.

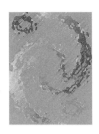

Chapter 17

Androgens and the Adolescent Girl

Robert L. Rosenfield and José F. Cara

Androgen production during puberty is necessary for the regulation of the maturational changes that characterize adolescence. In adolescent girls, androgens serve primarily as hormonal precursors for the biosynthesis of estrogens. When androgen production is excessive, normal sexual maturation may be altered and a variety of clinical signs and symptoms ensue, including premature pubarche, hirsutism or hirsutism equivalents such as excessive acne, and anovulatory menstrual irregularities. Appropriate recognition, evaluation, and treatment of hyperandrogenic disorders is important if normal sexual function is to be restored. Here, we will discuss current concepts of androgen physiology, review advances in our understanding of the causes of hyperandrogenic disorders, and provide recommendations for the diagnosis and treatment of hyperandrogenism in childhood and adolescence.

ANDROGENS: PHYSIOLOGIC AND PATHOPHYSIOLOGIC ACTIVITY

BIOSYNTHESIS

Steroid hormone biosynthesis involves the sequential enzymatic processing of cholesterol to form one of five possible types of end-products, namely progestins, mineralocorticoids, glucocorticoids, androgens, and estrogen (Fig. 17–1).[1, 2] Relatively few enzymes in the steroid biosynthetic cascade are required for steroid hormone biosynthesis by the adrenal glands and gonads, because many can perform more than one sequential reaction.

The biosynthesis of androgens is regulated by the trophic hormones adrenocorticotropin (ACTH) in the adrenal cortex and luteinizing hormone (LH) in the gonads. They regulate the rate-determining step for the secretion of all steroid hormones,[1] the conversion of cholesterol to

pregnenolone. This is a 2-step process involving cytochrome P450scc (Fig. 17–2), an enzyme mediator of the chemical reactions involved in cholesterol side chain cleavage, and the steroidogenic acute regulatory protein, which transports cholesterol into the inner mitochondrial membrane.[2] Cytochrome P450c17 is rate limiting for the formation of cortisol and sex hormones, and its level of expression is absolutely dependent on trophic hormone stimulation. This one enzyme possesses both 17-hydroxylase and 17,20-lyase activities. The first of these two sequential activities is necessary to form cortisol, and both are necessary to form the 17-ketosteroids dehydroepiandrosterone (DHEA) and androstenedione, which are in turn the precursors of all potent sex steroids. P450c17 mediates conversion of pregnenolone by a two-step chemical reaction involving 17-hydroxylation (to 17-hydroxypregnenolone) followed by 17,20-lyase activity (to DHEA). Progesterone undergoes parallel reactions to androstenedione: P450c17 carries out 17-hydroxylation to 17-hydroxyprogesterone, and this in turn is converted into androstenedione by 17,20-lyase activity. The P450c17 gene product does not efficiently form androstenedione from 17-hydroxyprogesterone, but there is some evidence for the existence of a P450c17-independent pathway, so the quantitative importance of this path in the intact follicle is not known. The 17,20-lyase activity of P450c17 is regulated differently from its 17-hydroxylase activity; phosphorylation of enzyme serine residues and electron transfer enzymes selectively up-regulate the lyase activity. The enzymes Δ^5-isomerase-3β-hydroxysteroid dehydrogenase (3β-HSD) and 17β-HSD are non–P450 steroidogenic enzymes that convert pregnenolone to progesterone and DHEA to androstenedione. Androstenedione is the major precursor for both testosterone and estrogen formation in the gonads; it is converted by 17β-HSD to form testosterone or aromatized

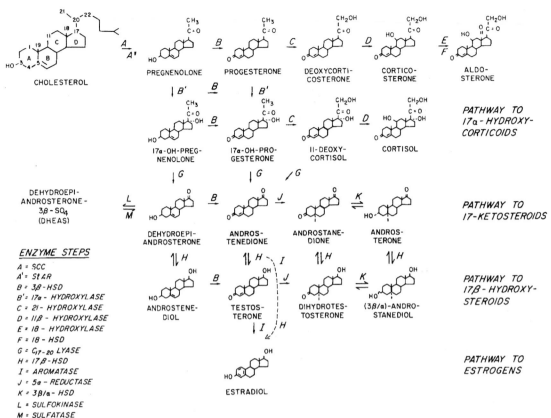

Figure 17–1. Pathways of steroid hormone biosynthesis from cholesterol. Relevant carbon atoms of cholesterol are designated by conventional numbers and rings by letters. The flow of hormonogenesis is generally downward and to the right. The top line shows the pathway to progestins and mineralocorticoids, the second line the pathway to glucocorticoids, the third line the pathway to 17-ketosteroids, and the fourth line to androgens. The bottom and dotted lines indicate the pathways to estrogen (the long dotted line involves the 17-ketoestrogen estrone [not shown] as an intermediate). HSD, hydroxysteroid dehydrogenase; SCC, site chain cleavage; StAR, steroidogenic acute regulatory protein. (Modified with permission from Rosenfield RL: The ovary and female sexual maturation. *In* Kaplan, SA (ed): Clinical Pediatric Endocrinology, Vol 2. Philadelphia: WB Saunders, 1989, p 259.)

by aromatase (cytochrome P450arom) to form estrone.

Only the adrenal cortex and gonads actively secrete steroids. In normal women, the ovaries and adrenal glands normally contribute about equally to testosterone production.[3, 4] Approximately half of the total testosterone originates from direct secretion, and half is derived from peripheral conversion of secreted 17-ketosteroids. Other tissues, including liver, adipose tissue, and skin, contain some of these enzymes, which allows for the further processing of steroids synthesized in the adrenals and gonads.

REGULATION OF SECRETION

Androgens are secreted by both the adrenal glands and ovaries in response to their respective

tropic hormones, ACTH and LH.[2] Since they are in a sense byproducts of estradiol and cortisol secretion by the ovaries and adrenal glands, respectively, androgen levels in females are not under specific hormonal control; there is no direct negative feedback control by the pituitary gland, as there is for cortisol and estradiol secretion. Hence, there is no hormonal regulatory mechanism to control androgen levels. Rather, intraglandular paracrine and autocrine mechanisms seem to play a major role in the regulation of androgen secretion by these glands.

Adrenal Glands

Adrenal 17-ketosteroid secretion gradually begins during middle childhood as a result of adrenarche, an incomplete aspect of puberty in

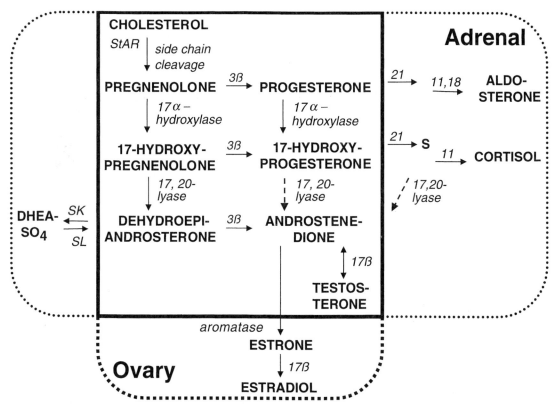

Figure 17–2. Outline of the major steroid biosynthetic pathways involved in androgen production. The area enclosed by the solid line contains the core steroidogenic pathway utilized by both the gonads and adrenal glands. The areas enclosed by the dotted lines contain the steroidogenic pathways utilized specifically by the ovaries and adrenal glands, as indicated. The Δ^5 path is on the left-hand side of 3β and the Δ^4 path in the right-hand columns. S, 11-deoxycortisol. The enzymes are italicized: *3β*, Δ^5-3β-hydroxysteroid dehydrogenase (HSD); *21*, 21-hydroxylase; *11,18*, 11β-hydroxylase/ 18-hydroxylase-dehydrogenase; *17β*, 17β-HSD; SCC, side chain cleavage; *StAR*, steroidogenic acute regulatory protein. (Modified with permission from Ehrmann DA, Rosenfield RL: An endocrinologic approach to hirsutism. J Clin Endocrinol Metab 1990; 71:1–4. © The Endocrine Society.)

which maturational changes permit the adrenal cortex to secrete 17-ketosteroids.[2] Although young children secrete as much cortisol in proportion to body size as adults, they form hardly any 17-ketosteroids. During adrenarche, there is a change in the pattern of the adrenal secretory response to ACTH, with striking increases in 17-hydroxypregnenolone and DHEA production (Fig. 17–3).[5] As a result, DHEA sulfate (DHEAS, the sulfated derivative of DHEA) becomes the predominant androgen secreted by the adrenal glands.

These adrenarchal changes seem to be related to the development of the zona reticularis of the adrenal cortex.[2] This zone has low 3β-HSD activity and possesses the sulfokinase activity to sulfate the DHEA that accumulates. DHEA synthesis increases because of a combination of the low 3β-HSD activity and an apparent increase in the 17,20-lyase activity of P450c17. This zone has

been postulated to originate from cells of the fetal adrenocortical zone that have failed to undergo involution. Its development as a continuous zone begins at about age 6 years and correlates with the DHEAS production. DHEAS production rises steadily from this point in time to peak at about age 18 years (Fig. 17–4).[6]

The nature of the factor or factors responsible for bringing about the adrenarchal changes in the adrenal glands has been the subject of considerable controversy.[2, 7] A pituitary source of the putative adrenarche factor has been postulated, since DHEA and DHEAS are depressed out of proportion to cortisol in hypopituitarism or by low glucocorticoid doses.[8] Several substances have been implicated as the pituitary hormone that brings about the adrenarchal change, including "cortical androgen stimulating hormone" and proopiomelanocortin-related peptides. The fact that adrenarche represents a change in the ste-

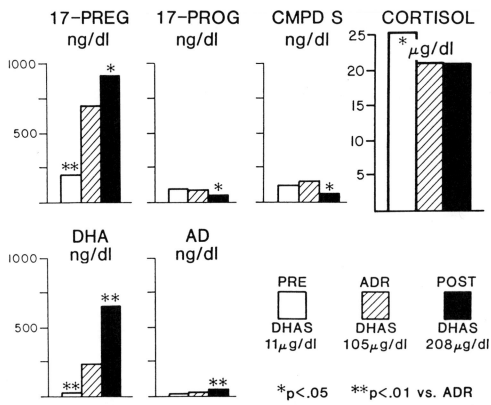

Figure 17–3. Changing pattern of adrenal steroidogenic response to ACTH stimulation with maturation. Shown are the plasma steroid levels 30 minutes after a 10-µg/m² intravenous bolus of ACTH in prepubertal children (PRE), children with precocious adrenarche (ADR), and follicular-phase adult females (ADULT). The layout is organized according to the biosynthetic pathway (see Figs. 17–1, 17–2). Note that children with precocious adrenarche have 17-hydroxypregnenolone (17-PREG) and dehydroepiandrosterone (DHEA) responses intermediate between those of prepubertal children and adults. 17-PROG, 17-hydroxyprogesterone; CMPD S, 11-deoxycortisol; AD, androstenedione. (Reproduced with permission from Rosenfield RL: The ovary and female sexual maturation. *In* Kaplan SA (ed): Clinical Pediatric Endocrinology, Vol 2. Philadelphia: WB Saunders, 1989, p 259.)

roidogenic response pattern of the adrenal gland to ACTH suggests that potential adrenarche factor(s) may control the growth and differentiation of the zona reticularis or regulate steroidogenic enzyme activity. Intraadrenal factors, such as estradiol, have also been postulated as potential adrenarchal factors[9] and may function as modulators of adrenal steroidogenic enzyme activity.

Insulin and insulin-like growth factors (IGFs) may modulate the response of adrenal steroids to ACTH.[2] Insulin infusion has recently been reported to modestly potentiate the 17-ketosteroid response to ACTH in a pattern compatible with increases in 17-hydroxylase and 17,20-lyase activities, the former more prominently. Insulin excess might explain the enhanced responsiveness of 17-ketosteroids to ACTH in simple obesity. Recent in vitro studies have directly shown that insulin and IGFs up-regulate adrenal

17-hydroxylase, 17,20-lyase, and 3β-HSD activity. It is becoming clear that other factors are involved in the intraadrenal modulation of the response to ACTH. For example, interleukin 6 is strongly expressed in the zona reticularis of the adrenal cortex and is capable of stimulating DHEA secretion.

In most children, adrenarchal androgen production becomes clinically apparent (as pubarche, the appearance of pubic hair) at about the same time as true pubertal development (also called *gonadarche*). Because the control mechanisms that initiate adrenarche are different from those responsible for initiating puberty, adrenarche is sometimes not chronologically related to true puberty. Adrenarche and gonadarche are dissociated in a variety of clinical conditions, including idiopathic premature puberty, gonadal dysgenesis, isolated gonadotropin deficiency, and

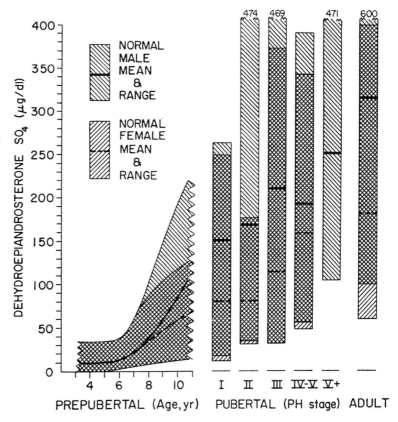

Figure 17–4. Normal range of plasma dehydroepian-drosterone sulfate (SO_4) in relation to age and pubertal stage. (Reproduced with permission from Rosenfield RL, Rich BH, Lucky AW: Adrenarche as a cause of benign pseudopuberty in boys. J Pediatr 1982; 101:1005.)

constitutional delay of puberty.[10] Whereas neither adrenal androgens nor corticoids are stimulated by gonadotropins, DHEAS production is depressed moderately in hypogonadism for reasons that are not clear.

The Ovary

Because of the pubertal increase in gonadotropin secretion, ovarian androgen and estrogen secretion increase during puberty. The combined action of LH on theca-interstitial (thecal) cells and of follicle-stimulating hormone (FSH) on ovarian granulosa cells, respectively, is necessary for the development and maintenance of normal ovarian function.[2] Androgenic precursors (especially androstenedione) are produced by theca cells under LH stimulation. These are aromatized to estrogen by FSH-stimulated granulosa cell aromatase activity. Androgens seem to stimulate the differentiation of small follicles yet limit the number of follicles that are allowed to mature further and so may be involved in the selection of a single follicle for ovulation. As the

dominant follicle emerges, increased amounts of both androstenedione and estradiol are secreted, the ratio favoring estradiol in healthy preovulatory follicles.

Androgens can be viewed as a necessary evil in the ovary.[2] On one hand, they are obligate intermediates in the biosynthesis of estradiol. On the other, intraovarian androgen excess hinders the development of a preovulatory follicle, committing follicles to atresia.[11] Atretic follicles are predominantly androgenic ones because they are relatively deficient in aromatase activity. Consequently, androgen-induced follicular atresia seems to predispose to further androgen production, producing a vicious cycle of hyperandrogenism. Therefore, it seems critical for the function of the ovary that the intraovarian androgen concentration be kept to a minimum. How ovarian androgen secretion is minimized while the formation of estrogen is optimized is not known. Since there is no long-loop feedback (via the pituitary) for specifically regulating ovarian androgen secretion, another mechanism must exist. We have postulated that, normally, androgen excess is prevented primarily by the down-regulation process, whereby excessive or protracted LH stimulation leads to intraovarian desensitization of the responses to LH at the level of P450c17.[12]

A number of hormones and growth factors seem to be involved in the intraovarian modulation of P450c17 steroidogenic responsiveness to LH.[12] Desensitization to LH is mediated in part by ovarian steroids. It appears likely that estrogen inhibits this response by a short-loop (paracrine) negative feedback mechanism. Androgens, on the other hand, may well be inhibitory by an autocrine mechanism. These inhibiting modulators seem to be counterbalanced by hormones and growth factors that amplify P450c17 activities, including insulin, IGF-I,[13, 14] and inhibin, plus numerous other small peptides.[2, 12]

BLOOD LEVELS AND TRANSPORT

The total plasma concentrations of androgens and intermediates in their biosynthesis are shown in Table 17–1.[15] Plasma levels of DHEAS normally reflect adrenal androgen production, whereas plasma testosterone and androstenedione levels are accounted for by both ovarian and adrenal androgen secretion. Plasma 17-hydroxyprogesterone, like testosterone and androstenedione, may arise from either the adrenal glands or ovaries. Of the circulating androgens, testosterone is the most important, biologically and clinically, because of its relatively high plasma concentration and potency at the target organ level.

More than 96% of the plasma testosterone and structurally related 17β-hydroxysteroids circulate in plasma bound to carrier proteins; only a small fraction remains free.[16, 17] Sex hormone–binding globulin (SHBG) and albumin are the principal sex steroid–binding proteins in plasma. Although there has been interest in the possibility that albumin-bound testosterone is bioactive, only the free steroid is bioavailable.[18, 19] Because of its high binding affinity, SHBG concentration

is the major determinant of the fraction of 17β-hydroxysteroids binding to plasma albumin and of the fraction that remains free and biologically active in blood.

SHBG is a glycoprotein synthesized in the liver.[17] Isoelectric focusing studies have shown heterogeneity of the circulating forms, but the clinical significance of this finding is not known. It has structural homology to a noncirculating androgen-binding protein synthesized in the Sertoli cell of the testis.[20] Its synthesis is modulated by a number of physiologic and pathologic states that ultimately affect its plasma concentration: SHBG levels are increased by estrogens and thyroid hormone excess; plasma concentrations are decreased by androgen, glucocorticoid, growth hormone, and most importantly insulin.[21] Because SHBG levels are often decreased in hyperandrogenic states and obesity, serum free testosterone levels are often elevated in women whose total testosterone levels are normal. Consequently, the plasma free testosterone concentration is more often elevated in women with hirsutism or acne than is the plasma total testosterone concentration, reflecting the truly elevated plasma concentration of bioavailable androgen.[22]

MECHANISMS OF ACTION

Androgens exert their effects by binding to the androgen receptor of target tissues (Fig. 17–5).[23, 24] The biologic activity of testosterone is dependent in large part on its being converted to dihydrotestosterone (DHT). DHT is formed by 5α-reductase activity, primarily in target tissues and liver. In skin, 5α-reductase activity resides primarily in sebaceous and sweat glands and in dermis, rather than in hair follicles. Plasma 3α-androstanediol glucuronide, a metabolite of DHT, has been touted as a marker of hypersensitivity of the hair follicle to androgen.[25] However, the extent to which this metabolite arises from hepatic or skin 5α-reductase activity is controversial.[26]

Table 17–1. Typical Normal Ranges for Plasma Androgens and Intermediates*

	17-Hydroxy-pregnenolone (ng/dl)	17-Hydroxy-progesterone (ng/dl)	11-Deoxy-cortisol (ng/dl)	Cortisol (μg/dl)	DHEA (ng/dl)	Andro-stenedione (ng/dl)	Testosterone (ng/dl)
Prepubertal, 2–8 yr	<25–235	<25–65	<25–160	5–25	<25–120	<25–50	<15
Adrenarchal†	<25–355	<25–95	<25–120	5–25	100–420	30–75	10–45
Adult female	40–360	30–130‡	30–220	5–25	100–1000	55–200	20–75

*Normal range may differ slightly among laboratories.
†Children with premature adrenarche.
‡17-Hydroxyprogesterone increases in the preovulatory phase to peak as high as 360 ng/dl in the luteal phase of the cycle.
From Rosenfield RL. Hyperandrogenism in peripubertal girls. Pediatr Clin North Am 1990; 37:1333.

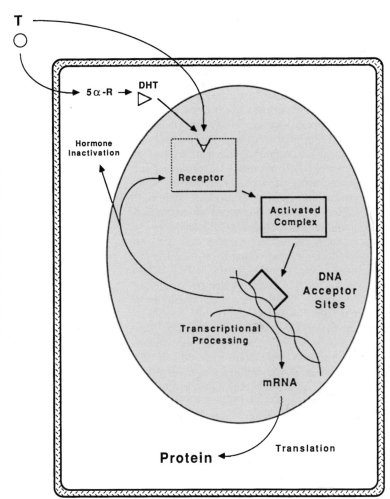

Figure 17–5. Mechanism of action of testosterone on target cells. Testosterone (T) binds to its intracellular receptor directly or after its prior conversion to dihydrotestosterone (DHT). The resulting activated receptor complex binds to its specific hormone response element on DNA, stimulating transcription and translation of specific genes. 5α-R, 5α-reductase.

DHT has greater biologic potency than testosterone owing to its higher affinity for and slower dissociation from the androgen receptor.[27]

The androgen receptor has been cloned and the gene determined to be located on the long arm of the X chromosome; it is subject to X inactivation.[27] It is homologous with other receptors of the nuclear receptor superfamily, which includes receptors for other steroids.[28, 29] Androgen binding to the androgen receptor leads to an activated ligand-receptor complex that binds to the androgen receptor response element on nuclear DNA, stimulating transcription of target genes and leading to increased protein synthesis. As in other androgen target tissues, androgen receptors have been demonstrated in the pilosebaceous unit.[24] Genetic mutations in the androgen receptor can lead to quantitative or qualitative losses of androgen receptor function, producing the various syndromes of androgen resistance;[30] however, excess activity of the androgen receptor itself has not been incriminated as a cause of hirsutism.

PILOSEBACEOUS RESPONSE TO ANDROGENS AND ANDROGEN EXCESS

Hair can be categorized as vellus hair or terminal hair.[23, 24] Vellus hair is fine, soft, and not pigmented, and terminal hair is long, coarse, and pigmented. Virtually all hair follicles are associated with sebaceous glands to form pilosebaceous units (PSUs). The growth of the hair follicle of PSUs is controlled by an induction factor(s) still to be characterized that is elaborated by the dermal papilla. In target areas, androgens cause the prepubertal pilosebaceous unit to differentiate into either a sexual hair follicle (in which the vellus hair transforms into a terminal hair) or into a sebaceous gland (in which the sebaceous component proliferates and the hair remains vellus). Androgens are thus necessary for sexual hair and sebaceous gland development. Antiandrogens reverse this process, causing pilosebaceous units to revert toward the prepubertal state. Male-pattern sexual hair (for example, mustache and beard) develops in sites where relatively high levels of androgen are necessary for pilosebaceous unit differentiation. The greater density of terminal hairs in the androgen-sensitive areas of men (compared with women) is accounted for by a greater proportion of pilosebaceous units with terminal rather than vellus hairs. Male-pattern baldness is largely the result of conversion of terminal hair into sebaceous follicles.

Hirsutism is defined as excessive male-pattern hair growth in women.[23] Hirsutism must be distinguished from hypertrichosis, which is the proper term for the excessive growth of androgen-independent hair that is vellus, prominent in nonsexual areas, and most commonly familial or caused by metabolic disorders (for example, thyroid disturbances, anorexia nervosa) or medications (for example, phenytoin, minoxidil, or cyclosporine). In adult Caucasian women, hirsutism can be defined as a total score of 8 or more on the scale of Ferriman and Gallwey (Fig. 17–6). Thus, it is normal for women to have a few sexual

hairs in most "male" areas (such as the mustache and beard areas).

The cutaneous manifestations of androgen excess include hirsutism, acne, and balding;[31] however, these are variably expressed manifestations of hyperandrogenism. Some patients have hirsutism or acne alone, others both, and still others neither. Balding in a diffuse pattern can be the sole symptom.[32]

An increase in the plasma free testosterone concentration underlies half of all cases of mild hirsutism and a third of the cases of persistent, mild acne in adolescents (Table 17–2).[31] Moderately severe hirsutism or cystic acne is even more likely to be hyperandrogenic.[31, 33] However, it must be noted that the amount of sexual hair and sebaceous gland development seems to depend as much on the factors that determine sensitivity of the PSUs to androgens as on the plasma androgen level itself. At one end of the normal spectrum are women whose PSUs seem hypersensitive to normal blood free androgen levels; this seems to account for "idiopathic" hirsutism and acne. At the other end of the spectrum are women whose PSUs are relatively insensitive to androgen; this seems to account for "cryptic" hyperandrogenemia (hyperandrogenism without skin manifestations).

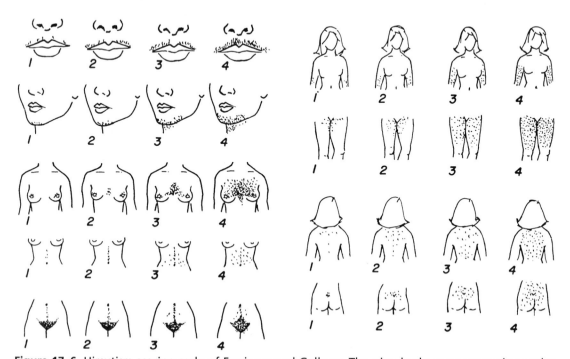

Figure 17–6. Hirsutism scoring scale of Ferriman and Gallwey. The nine body areas possessing androgen-sensitive pilosebaceous units are graded from 0 (no terminal hair) to 4 (frankly virile) and totaled. (Reproduced with permission from Ehrmann DA, Rosenfield RL: An endocrinologic approach to hirsutism. J Clin Endocrinol Metab 1990; 71:1–4. © The Endocrine Society.)

Table 17–2. Clinical Scoring System for Acne Vulgaris*

Score	Class	Lesions
	Microcomedones	Comedones, <2 mm diameter
1	Minor	Comedones, 2 mm or greater (<10)
2	Mild	Comedones (10–20; pustular or nonpustular)
3	Moderate	Comedones (>20) or pustules (<20)
4	Severe	Pustules (>20)
5	Cystic	Inflammatory lesions >5 mm

*Face and trunk may be graded separately.
From Rosenfield RL. Hyperandrogenism in peripubertal girls. Pediatr Clin North Am 1990; 37:1333.

HYPERANDROGENIC DISORDERS

Hyperandrogenemia should be suspected when development of sexual hair is premature or excessive. Skin manifestations, alternatively, may consist of acne or diffuse alopecia or may not be present at all. Androgen excess is often associated with menstrual irregularity, but a third of cases are eumenorrheic. Androgen excess is often associated with obesity, particularly of an android distribution (waist to hip ratio over 0.85), and acanthosis nigricans (a consequence of undue insulin resistance). A high index of suspicion is therefore warranted when a patient presents with any single one of these signs.

The term *polycystic ovary syndrome* (PCOS) has come to be used loosely for the unexplained chronic hyperandrogenism that accounts for most cases that present at or beyond adolescence.[34] Hyperandrogenism arises from abnormal adrenal or ovarian function in most cases but occasionally from abnormalities in the peripheral formation of androgen. Functional abnormalities (Table 17–3) are much more common than tumors.

ADRENAL DISORDERS

Premature Pubarche and Premature Adrenarche

Normally, the first manifestation of the adrenal and gonadal contributions to androgen production is pubarche, the appearance of pubic hair. Presexual pubic hair (Tanner II) appears in girls at age 11.2 ± 1.1 (mean $\pm$ SD) years, and sexual pubic hair (Tanner III) appears at $11.9 \pm$

1.1 years of age.[6, 35] Pubarche typically follows the onset of breast development, which begins at the age of 10.8 ± 1.0 years of age.[36]

Premature pubarche refers to the appearance of sexual hairs before 8.5 years of age. Premature pubarche requires the presence of adrenarche. It is often considered to be synonymous with *premature adrenarche*.[6, 35] This term implies that children with early pubarche have undergone normal adrenarche prematurely, which is probably true in many cases. In some children, however, premature pubarche represents inordinate sensitivity of sexual hair follicles to normal adrenal androgen levels. In others, premature adrenarche may be an early manifestation of exaggerated adrenarche, which is discussed in the next section.

The best hormonal indicator of adrenarche is a plasma level of DHEAS greater than 40 µg/dl (see Fig. 17–4). In children with premature adrenarche, plasma testosterone levels also rise into the early pubertal range, approximating 20 ng/dl. Clinically, the androgen excess is so subtle that the only other sign of increased androgen production may be a few microcomedones. Typically, there is no other evidence of virilization: no clitoromegaly, no growth spurt, and no discordant advancement of bone age. In more than 90% of children with premature adrenarche, the responses of steroid intermediates to ACTH are

Table 17–3. Causes of Female Hyperandrogenism

Functional adrenal hyperandrogenism
  Premature pubarche and premature adrenarche
  Primary functional adrenal hyperandrogenism/exaggerated adrenarche
  Congenital adrenal hyperplasia
  Prolactin or growth hormone excess
  Dexamethasone-resistant FAH
    Cushing disease
    Cortisol resistance
    Apparent cortisone reductase deficiency
Functional gonadal hyperandrogenism
  Primary polycystic ovary syndrome due to functional ovarian hyperandrogenism
  Secondary polycystic ovary syndrome
    Adrenal virilizing disorders and rests
    Ovarian steroidogenic blocks
    Syndromes of severe insulin resistance
  Hermaphroditism
  Chorionic gonadotropin–related
Peripheral androgen overproduction
  Obesity
  Idiopathic hyperandrogenism
Tumoral hyperandrogenism
Androgenic drugs

Modified from Rosenfield RL: Current concepts of polycystic ovary syndrome. Ballière's Clin Obstet Gynecol 1997; 11:307.

between the prepubertal and adult ranges (see Fig. 17–3). The predominant steroids are the Δ^5-3β-steroids, 17-hydroxypregnenolone, and DHEA. Recent data suggest that premature adrenarche may predispose to the subsequent development of polycystic ovary syndrome during adolescence, which is discussed later.[37] This is particularly true of those who have the higher androgen levels and probably will subsequently prove to have exaggerated adrenarche.

The distinction of premature adrenarche from mild (nonclassic) virilizing congenital adrenal hyperplasia (CAH) has been a matter of considerable controversy. On one hand, in some clinics as many as 40% of children who present with premature pubarche have been diagnosed as having nonclassic CAH due to 21-hydroxylase deficiency.[38, 39] This high incidence is clearly skewed by the presence of patients of ethnic groups that have a high incidence of CAH, such as Ashkenazi Jews and Hispanics, in these clinics. On the other, much of the dispute centers around the distinction of mild 3β-HSD deficiency from premature adrenarche based on the responses of steroid intermediates to ACTH stimulation. Some investigators had designated Δ^5-steroid responses greater than those of Tanner stage II or III controls as indicating 3β-HSD deficiency, thus concluding that 3β-HSD deficiency is a common cause of premature adrenarche,[38] but it is now clear from molecular genetic studies that 3β-HSD deficiency is rarely the cause of premature pubarche.[40] Table 17–4 shows the typical ranges of steroid intermediate responses to ACTH in normal and prematurely adrenarchal subjects.

Primary Functional Adrenal Hyperandrogenism and Exaggerated Adrenarche

Functional adrenal hyperandrogenism (FAH), glucocorticoid-suppressible ACTH-dependent 17-ketosteroid excess, is found in approximately half of hyperandrogenic females and PCOS patients.[2, 12] The vast majority of FAH is "primary" (idiopathic), because fewer than 10% of cases of adrenal hyperandrogenism can be incontrovertibly attributed to any well-established pathophysiologic cause. This entity was originally termed *exaggerated adrenarche*, a concept that fit with the observation that fully half of all women with 17-ketosteroid hyperresponsiveness to ACTH have a pattern of steroid intermediates that resembles an exaggeration of adrenarche. Typically, they have moderately excessive 17-hydroxypregnenolone and DHEA responses to ACTH together with modest androstenedione hyperresponsiveness. Occasionally, they have mild abnormalities of 17-hydroxyprogesterone or 11-deoxycortisol in response to ACTH. Alternatively, this entity has been considered by others to represent nonclassic forms of CAH; however, molecular genetic studies and combined ovarian and adrenal function testing have shown that enzyme mutations are rare.

Currently, several lines of evidence support the concept that primary FAH is due to dysregulation of adrenal steroidogenesis rather than an exaggeration of the adrenarchal process:

1. The 17-ketosteroid hyperresponsiveness to ACTH can be interpreted as overactivity of 17-hydroxylase/17,20-lyase in the adrenal cortex, and in two thirds of cases there is apparent overactivity of these steps in the ovaries.

2. The adrenal overproduction of 17-ketosteroids is associated with increased levels of the adrenarche marker DHEAS in only a small minority of cases (approximately 20%).

3. There is evidence of widespread but variable dysregulation of a number of aspects of corticosteroid secretion and metabolism, such as a tendency for hypercortisolism and evidence of increased 11β-hydroxysteroid dehydrogenase activity. In addition, evidence is accumulating that hyperinsulinemia is related to adrenal dysregulation, as it is to ovarian dysregulation.

Table 17–4. Typical Normal Range of Steroid Levels Post-ACTH*

	17-Hydroxy-pregnenolone (ng/dl)	17-Hydroxy-progesterone (ng/dl)	11-Deoxy-cortisol (ng/dl)	Cortisol (μg/dl)	DHEA (ng/dl)	Andro-stenedione (ng/dl)
Prepubertal, 2 yr	130–340	80–180	<25–350	13–50	45–120	<25–80
Adrenarchal†	240–1100	40–190	40–300	13–50	285–495	55–140
Adult female	150–1070	35–130‡	40–200	13–50	225–1470	55–185

*30 min post-ACTH 10 μg/m² as intravenous bolus. Values 60 min after 250 μg ACTH are similar.
†Children with typical premature adrenarche.
‡17-Hydroxyprogesterone increases in the preovulatory phase to peak as high as 360 ng/dl in the luteal phase of the cycle.
From Rosenfeld RL. Hyperandrogenism in peripubertal girls. Pediatr Clin North Am 1990; 37:1333.

Primary FAH occurs as an isolated abnormality in approximately one quarter of hyperandrogenic women (that is, those who have no evidence of ovarian hyperandrogenism). Although the menstrual cycle is normal in two thirds of these patients, in the remainder it is associated with anovulatory signs, so it may present as an adrenal variant of PCOS, which is discussed later.[41, 42] Primary FAH is also found in half of patients with classic and nonclassic PCOS.

Congenital Adrenal Hyperplasia

CAH results from an autosomal-recessive defect in the activity of any one of the steroidogenic enzymes necessary for the synthesis of corticosteroid hormones by the adrenal gland (see Figs. 17–1 and 17–2).[43, 44] Because of the enzyme defect, the adrenal gland cannot efficiently secrete glucocorticoids (especially cortisol) or mineralocorticoids (primarily aldosterone). There is a lack of negative feedback inhibition of ACTH or of renin-angiotensin secretion, respectively, which markedly increases the secretion of these trophic hormones and leads to compensatory hyperplasia of the adrenal cortex. The result is defective synthesis of end product, on one hand, and accumulation of steroid precursors immediately before the enzyme defect, on the other. The clinical presentation depends on the severity of the enzyme deficiency. In cases in which the enzyme deficiency is mild, secretion of end product is sometimes restored to normal, but only at the expense of the accumulation of precursors before the defective enzyme step. In these cases, the disorder may not become clinically apparent until childhood or adolescence.

Each enzyme deficiency produces a characteristic clinical syndrome and biochemical abnormality, depending on which of the adrenal end products is deficient and which precursors accumulate. Several clinical syndromes resulting from deficient adrenal enzyme activity have been described, including sex hormone deficiency CAH, isolated mineralocorticoid deficiency CAH, and virilizing CAH.[43–46]

Virilizing CAH is the result of a deficiency of 21-hydroxylase, 3β-HSD, or 11β-hydroxylase. In virilizing CAH, inefficient cortisol synthesis is associated with the accumulation of androgenic precursors that produce excessive virilization of female infants with genital ambiguity in the newborn period or hyperandrogenism later in childhood. These disorders may be associated with altered mineralocorticoid production, mineralo-

corticoid deficiency with salt wasting in the case of 21-hydroxylase and 3β-HSD deficiency, or salt retention with hypertension in the case of 11β-hydroxylase deficiency.

Virilizing CAH due to 21-hydroxylase deficiency is a common inherited condition that can be manifested as excessive virilization either early in life or later in childhood and adolescence. It accounts for more than 90% of the cases of CAH and has an overall incidence in the general population of about 1 in 12,000. Several distinctive clinical syndromes have been described, the result of a spectrum of variations in the severity of the enzyme defect. Classic 21-hydroxylase deficiency is the result of a severe enzyme deficiency that presents in the newborn period with variable signs and symptoms of excessive virilization and adrenal insufficiency. It leads to ambiguous genital development in female infants and can be associated with mineralocorticoid deficiency (salt-wasting CAH) or in many cases normal mineralocorticoid function (simple virilizing CAH). Because the genital development of males is not affected, boys usually present with either adrenal insufficiency and salt wasting shortly after birth (when associated with mineralocorticoid deficiency) or with signs of androgen excess later in childhood (in simple virilizing CAH).

CAH also has a "nonclassic" presentation, manifesting in its late-onset, or attenuated, form as premature pubarche or presenting with peri- or postpubertal onset of hirsutism, acne, or amenorrhea. Such nonclassic cases account for about 5% of adult hirsutism in the general population[12] and approximately 10% in adolescents. Some cases are entirely "silent"; they are discovered serendipitously in family studies and have no clinical manifestations. These nonclassic forms of 21-hydroxylase deficiency CAH have been shown to be due to distinct 21-hydroxylase mutations that cause only mild enzyme deficiencies.[47] Studies of the molecular biology of 21-hydroxylase deficiency have provided important tools for its diagnosis. The gene for 21-hydroxylase (P450c21) is located on chromosome 6 and is closely linked to the human major histocompatibility complex (MHC or HLA), residing between HLA-B and HLA-DR. DNA probes are now available to detect the most common mutations. This has made rapid prenatal diagnosis possible for most affected families and afforded the potential for therapy in utero. This is accomplished by administering dexamethasone to the mother as soon as pregnancy is recognized to prevent the genital abnormalities produced in severe cases.[47, 48]

Utilizing ACTH response patterns, HLA typ-

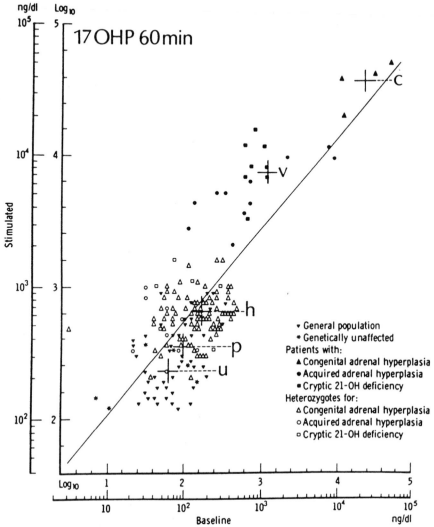

Figure 17–7. Patterns of response to ACTH stimulation among normals and subjects with various degrees of 21-hydroxylase deficiency. The graph shows the baseline and ACTH-stimulated levels of 17-hydroxyprogesterone in unaffected individuals (u), the general population (p), heterozygotes for 21-hydroxylase deficiency (h), nonclassical variants homozygous for 21-hydroxylase deficiency (v), and classical 21-hydroxylase–deficient patients (c). The data include males and females regardless of phase of menstrual cycle or age. ACTH was administered intravenously as a 250-μg bolus. (Reproduced with permission from New MI, Lorenzen F, Lerner AJ, et al: Genotyping steroid 21-hydroxylase deficiency: Hormonal reference data. J Clin Endocrinol Metab 1983; 57:320. © The Endocrine Society.)

ing, and molecular genetic techniques, New and her colleagues developed normative data that have permitted the accurate diagnosis of the different 21-hydroxylase deficiency syndromes (Fig. 17–7).[47] These investigators have shown that the rapid 17-hydroxyprogesterone response to an intravenous bolus of ACTH identifies both nonclassic and classic virilizing CAH better than baseline steroid levels. The degree of clinical severity correlates with the degree of 21-hydroxylase deficiency demonstrated by the ACTH test. Importantly, the response to an ACTH bolus also

usually identifies carriers of the gene abnormality.

Severe 3β-HSD deficiency leads to defective cortisol and mineralocorticoid synthesis, and adrenal insufficiency develops in the newborn period. Because of deficient synthesis of Δ⁴-steroids (including androgens), affected male infants classically have insufficient virilization and sexual ambiguity. Affected infant girls, on the other hand, are often virilized because of the very high levels of the weakly androgenic DHEA and its more androgenic metabolites.[49] When the enzyme deficiency is mild, virilization later in childhood or adolescence may be the first sign of accumulation of these androgenic precursors.[40, 50] The controversy about the distinction of mild 3β-HSD deficiency from simple premature adrenarche was discussed earlier.

Typically, 11β-hydroxylase deficiency presents with genital ambiguity in females and subsequent incomplete sexual precocity in association with hypertension. Atypical cases marked by late-onset hirsutism without hypertension have been reported but are rare.[51, 52]

Other Adrenal Disorders

Glucocorticoid-suppressible hyperandrogenism occurs in hyperprolactinemia and acromegaly. Hyperprolactinemia may mimic PCOS. It may present with hirsutism or acne. Although menstrual disturbance and galactorrhea are typical, they are not always present.[53] Polycystic ovaries and LH hyperresponsiveness may be associated with prolactinoma.[54, 55] DHEA and DHEAS levels are elevated, as is the plasma free testosterone, in part because of a direct effect of hyperprolactinemia on adrenal cortical function. Acromegaly may also be associated with PCOS, either because of a direct effect of the elevated IGF-I levels on steroidogenesis or because of adrenal androgenic hyperfunction.[56]

Adrenal hyperandrogenism can have a number of other causes, which are relatively rare. Resistance to dexamethasone suppression is caused by Cushing syndrome, cortisol resistance, or excessively rapid cortisol metabolism. In Cushing syndrome, levels of androstenedione are typically relatively more elevated than those of DHEA.[57] Cortisol resistance may cause premature pubarche or late-onset hirsutism.[58] In these patients, functional abnormality of the glucocorticoid receptor leads to compensatory hypersecretion of ACTH and hypercortisolemia without other clinical or biochemical findings of Cushing syndrome. The clinical findings are due to overproduction of nonglucocorticoid adrenal steroids, and hypertension with hypokalemia may be associated with the syndrome. Congenitally rapid cortisol metabolism due to apparent 11β-hydroxysteroid dehydrogenase deficiency may resemble mild cortisol resistance.[59]

Adrenal tumors can lead to virilization.[60] They are more common in the first decade of life, and approximately half are benign. Malignant adrenal tumors are more common in toddlers and younger children, and both carcinomas and adenomas can be bilateral. They may be associated with hemihypertrophy, Beckwith-Weidemann syndrome, or another syndrome that predisposes to neoplasia or malformations of the genitourinary system.[61] Furthermore, the sites of virilizing adrenal tumors can be most unusual; a case with associated glucocorticoid excess has even been reported that developed within an adrenal rest tumor of the ovary.[62]

An adrenal tumor must be suspected when a child exhibits rapidly progressive virilization. There is often pubic hair development, clitoral enlargement, acne, and accelerated growth and skeletal maturation. When associated with Cushing syndrome, the excessive glucocorticoid production blunts the growth spurt typical of prepubertal virilization.[63] Occasionally, these tumors develop in utero and produce clitoral hypertrophy and labial fusion in the newborn.

Adrenal tumors characteristically produce DHEAS values greater than 600 μg/dl.[60] However, the pattern of steroid secretion may be atypical. Some adrenal tumors secrete only testosterone and have a degree of gonadotropin dependency.[64] Occasionally, dexamethasone suppression is required to distinguish a congenital tumor from CAH.

OVARIAN DISORDERS

The most frequently encountered cause of peripubertal androgen excess is primary functional ovarian hyperandrogenism (FOH), which accounts for most cases of PCOS (see Table 17–3). Our experience in adults and adolescents indicates that approximately two thirds of hyperandrogenic females have a PCOS-type of FOH indicative of dysregulation of androgen secretion (see later). This is not necessarily associated with the ultrasonographic and gonadotropic abnormalities classically associated with PCOS. As described in some detail later, FOH is characterized by subnormal suppression of plasma androgens after suppression of adrenocortical function by dexamethasone and by an elevated 17-hydroxyprogesterone response to a gonadotropin-releasing hormone (GnRH) agonist or human chorionic gonadotropin challenge test.

Primary Polycystic Ovary Syndrome Due to Functional Ovarian Hyperandrogenism

The classic form of PCOS was described in 1935 by Stein and Leventhal as a syndrome of amenorrhea, hirsutism, and obesity associated with bilateral polycystic ovaries.[65] It was subsequently discovered that these patients typically had elevated LH levels and an increased ratio of serum LH to FSH.[66, 67] The clinical and ovarian morphologic appearance of this disorder has long been appreciated to be very variable,[68] and hyperandrogenism is now known to be a constant feature of the syndrome.[69] This observation led to a common clinical definition of the syndrome as "otherwise unexplained chronic hyperandrogenic anovulation,"[70, 71] even though it is now known that anovulation is not always a feature of the syndrome.[34]

It is now clear that FOH underlies the vast majority of classic PCOS cases (that is, those whose chronic hyperandrogenism syndrome is associated with the characteristic ultrasonographic ovarian or gonadotropin abnormalities).[12, 34] Classic PCOS accounts for only half of FOH, however. Half of FOH patients have nonclassic PCOS, that is, they have a PCOS-type of ovarian dysfunction without the ultrasound or gonadotropin abnormalities that characterize the classic syndrome.[34, 72] Two thirds of FOH patients have anovulatory symptoms: The spectrum of menstrual patterns includes amenorrhea, oligoamenorrhea, dysfunctional uterine bleeding, and regular ovulatory cycles. Obesity is not necessarily present, and when it is, it alters the syndrome's manifestations, aggravating the inherent insulin resistance and attenuating LH pulse amplitude.[73]

The clinical and endocrine picture of PCOS/FOH is similar to that in adults.[74, 75] Patients have various menstrual disturbances, PSU disorders, or obesity-related symptoms for the most part. Patients occasionally present because of primary amenorrhea. Noteworthy is the fact that some have suggestive symptoms dating back to mid-childhood, including premature pubarche[37] and true precocious puberty.[76] Rapid weight gain with the onset of puberty is frequently the chief complaint and is sometimes associated with unusually tall stature and prognathism (pseudoacromegaly).[77] Acanthosis nigricans can be the presenting complaint rather than the associated obesity.[78] Acne and hirsutism are common but do not necessarily concern the patient. With a high index of suspicion, the diagnosis can be established in early puberty, before menarche, as early as about age 10 years.

The overall incidence of ovarian hyperandrogenism seems to be similar in adolescents and adults. Among 43 volunteers aged 10 to 16 years, two were hyperandrogenic (5%), and the one who consented to further testing had FOH (2.5%).[22] The incidence of polycystic ovaries on laparoscopy is 1.4% and on autopsy 3.5%. This

evidence is consistent with the long-standing impression that in most cases the menstrual pattern in PCOS has been abnormal since adolescence.[79]

There is considerable interest in the possibility that PCOS/FOH is caused by congenital disorders that first appear during puberty. The model of a complex genetic trait is the most attractive, in which a number of predisposing genetic traits converge to cause the syndrome to surface.[34] It has been proposed that one of these is a "polycystic ovary–premature male-pattern baldness gene," since one study suggested that these are the female and male phenotypes of an autosomal-dominant trait.[80] Insulin resistance, an important element in the syndrome (discussed later), seems to be another predisposing trait. PCOS/FOH has a relationship to adult-type diabetes mellitus. Approximately one third of our patients have a parent with diabetes mellitus,[81] and PCOS/FOH patients have a high incidence of diabetes-like defects in both insulin secretion and insulin sensitivity.[82] Intrauterine growth retardation has been cited as a predisposing factor for premature pubarche–related FOH and insulin resistance.[83] An environmental condition may be the determinant that causes a predisposing congenital trait to be manifested. Prime among candidate environmental factors are obesity and puberty itself, both conditions of insulin resistance. Insulin resistance is greater in normal, healthy adolescents than in either prepubertal or sexually mature persons, quite likely owing to a sex hormone–dependent increase in growth hormone secretion.[84] Indeed, it has been postulated that PCOS/FOH represents a state of "hyperpuberty" in which both the insulin resistance and LH excess of puberty are exaggerated.[85] In accord with this theory, adolescents with classic PCOS are more insulin resistant than normal adolescents.[86]

Normal puberty resembles PCOS/FOH in a number of ways. It is characterized not only by insulin resistance and increasing LH and androgen levels but by relative infertility and frequently multicystic or polycystic ovarian morphology. About half of menstrual cycles are anovulatory in the first two postmenarcheal years.[87] Adolescents with irregular menstrual cycles were found to have higher levels of serum LH and plasma total testosterone, free testosterone, or androstenedione than adolescents with regular menstrual cycles.[87–89] The testosterone levels were above the normal adult range in 12% to 35% of these anovulatory girls independent of hirsutism, acne, or obesity. The limited data suggest that the LH and androgen levels of these adolescents fall when they develop ovulatory cycles but are persistently high in those who do not.[90, 91] The persistently anovulatory group tends to develop larger, more polycystic ovaries over time.[92] The morphology of the normal adolescent ovary has long been considered polycystic,[93] and histologic examination typically has shown thecal luteinization.[79, 94] From ultrasound imaging, it appears that about one quarter of normal adolescents develop "multicystic" ovaries (four to ten follicles of 4 to 10 mm diameter in the maximum plane without increased ovarian stroma), which are considered to be a variation of normal,[95] and another quarter develop polycystic ovaries (10 or more follicles and increased ovarian stroma).[96] The distinction between these two conditions is often subjective and problematic.[97, 98] Regression of polycystic ovaries occurs in no more than 20% of cases.[92, 96]

The pathogenesis of PCOS has been a matter of heated debate.[69, 71, 99–101] Part of the controversy surrounds the issue of whether hyperandrogenism in PCOS arises from adrenal or ovarian sources. Because of frequent adrenal 17-ketosteroid hyperresponsiveness to ACTH, some investigators believe that PCOS originates as an adrenal disorder during puberty. According to this school of thought, adrenal hyperandrogenism is central to its pathogenesis via a complex cycle of events in which secretion of androstenedione and its peripheral conversion to estrone initiate the syndrome (Fig. 17–8).[100, 101] Yen and coworkers have suggested that exaggerated adrenarche initiates this process. More specifically, increased secretion of androstenedione by the adrenal gland leads to increased concentrations of estrogen, primarily estrone, through its peripheral conversion in adipose and other tissues. The elevated androgen levels also decrease SHBG concentrations, increasing further the concentration of estradiol that is free and biologically active. The increase in the plasma concentration of estradiol sensitizes the pituitary to secrete excessive LH, resulting in a high LH-FSH ratio, which leads to excessive stimulation of ovarian thecal androstenedione production and deficient granulosa cell aromatase activity. The resulting increase in ovarian androgens leads to polycystic ovaries while contributing further to the circulating pool of androgens, perpetuating the vicious cycle of hyperandrogenism. We consider this theory, while plausible, to be unlikely for several reasons.[69] Estrone is a weak estrogen and attempts to reproduce gonadotropin secretory abnormalities through exogenous estrone administration have not increased LH concentrations. Furthermore, recent findings suggest that an important element of ovarian dysfunction is independent of elevated LH levels.[2]

A new model has been proposed in which FOH is the common denominator of most PCOS.[12, 15] The androgen secretory disorder is functional because there is no necessary anatomic basis for it. It is gonadotropin dependent because suppression of gonadotropins lowers androgen production. We postulate that PCOS arises from heterogeneous disorders that increase the intraovarian concentration of androgen. Very high concentrations of androgen in the ovary would seem both to stimulate the formation of many small antral follicles ("microcysts") and to arrest the maturation of these follicles, thus preventing the emergence of a dominant follicle and committing an inordinate number of follicles to atresia.[2]

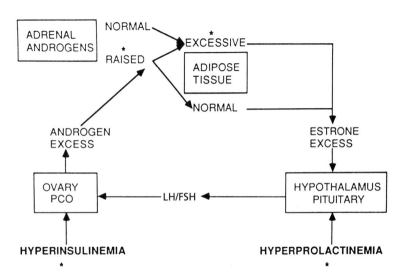

Figure 17–8. Pathophysiology of polycystic ovary syndrome according to the "estrone hypothesis." Adrenal hyperandrogenemia leads to excess estrone that preferentially stimulates pituitary LH secretion and results in secondary ovarian hyperandrogenism. *More than one potential initiating event may occur in a given patient. (Reproduced from McKenna TJ: Pathogenesis and treatment of polycystic ovary syndrome. N Engl J Med 1988; 318:558, with permission of the New England Journal of Medicine.)

At least 80% of primary classic PCOS cases appear to arise from a recently discovered type of abnormality, abnormal regulation (dysregulation) of ovarian androgen secretion. We found that the vast majority of women with classic PCOS have a characteristic pituitary-gonadal response to an acute GnRH agonist challenge test (Fig. 17–9).[12, 102] Their gonadotropin responses often resemble those of males in that they have significantly greater early LH and lesser FSH responses than normal females. They have greater 17-hydroxyprogesterone and, to a lesser extent, greater androgenic responses than those of normal women. Responses of 17-hydroxypregnenolone and DHEA are less consistently elevated, and pregnenolone is not elevated at all in

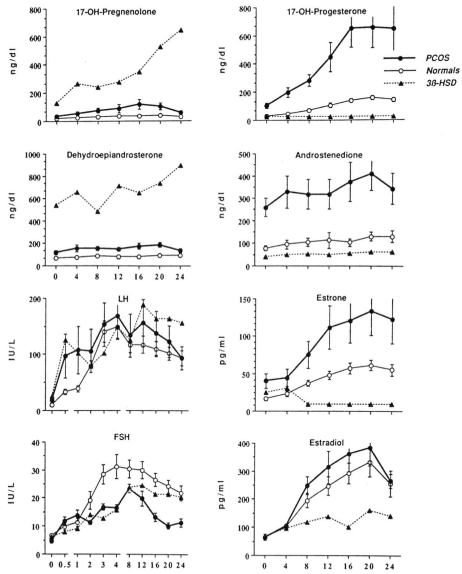

Figure 17–9. Patterns of response to GnRH agonist (nafarelin) testing in patients with functional ovarian hyperandrogenism (PCOS) and a patient with partial 3β-HSD deficiency (3β-HSD) in comparison with normal early follicular phase females (Normals). PCOS patients have significantly greater early (30–60 min) LH and lesser mean FSH responses than normal women. Their 17-hydroxyprogesterone responses (P <.001) and androstenedione responses (P <.05) are significantly increased. Estrogen responses tend to be greater. This steroidogenic pattern is different from that found with an intraovarian steroidogenic block, as exemplified by the patient with 3β-HSD deficiency. (Reproduced with permission from Rosenfield RL: Hyperandrogenism in peripubertal girls. Ped Clin North Am 1990; 37:1333.)

PCOS patients. There is no evidence of a discrete block in the steroidogenic pathway, since the responses of all steroids on the pathway from 17-hydroxyprogesterone to estrone and estradiol are normal or elevated. The elevated responses of 17-hydroxyprogesterone and androstenedione, without evidence of a block in the subsequent steroidogenic steps or consistent abnormalities in the earlier steps in the steroidogenic pathway, suggest increased ovarian 17-hydroxylase and 17,20-lyase activities.

This PCOS-like type of ovarian dysfunction affects more than half of hyperandrogenic patients.[12, 72] It was noteworthy that half of the FOH patients had a nonclassic type of PCOS, one in which the PCOS-type of ovarian dysfunction was not associated with sonographic abnormalities or LH excess. After dexamethasone suppression of adrenal function, the peak response of 17-hydroxyprogesterone to GnRH agonist correlated well with the free testosterone level, and the concordance between the two tests was 85%. Thus, these tests reflect closely related aspects of ovarian dysfunction.

Abnormal regulation of ovarian androgen secretion usually seems to result from escape from desensitization to LH.[2, 12, 15] In addition, we postulate that, in cases of nonclassic PCOS/FOH (that is, those whose LH is not excessive), there is dysregulation of androgen secretion as the result of endocrine, paracrine, or autocrine factors that modulate the ovarian androgen response to LH. Thus, we suspect that abnormal regulation of ovarian steroidogenesis, particularly prominent at the level of P450c17, underlies most cases of PCOS/FOH. This dysregulation prevents the normal coordination of intraovarian androgen with estrogen production that is so important for the proper function of the ovaries.

We have postulated that similar intrinsic abnormalities in the regulation of P450c17 within the adrenal cortex could explain the association with adrenal 17-ketosteroid hyperresponsiveness to ACTH in half the cases of PCOS (see Primary Functional Adrenal Hyperandrogenism and Exaggerated Adrenarche, which is mentioned earlier).[2, 15] Occasionally, isolated primary FAH is associated with a PCOS-like clinical syndrome.[72]

The cause of dysregulation of steroidogenesis is not clear. It is tempting to ascribe classic PCOS to ovarian overstimulation by the LH excess typical of the syndrome, although a primary role for LH excess is arguable.[2] PCOS patients given a fixed dose of the LH analogue human chorionic gonadotropin (hCG) have 17-hydroxyprogesterone and androstenedione hyperresponses. In addition, theca cells from polycystic ovaries secrete

abnormal amounts of steroids in culture, both before and after LH stimulation. Perhaps the most important variable that militates against a primary role of LH excess as a cause of the hyperandrogenism is the desensitization process. Normal thecal cells are very sensitive to the down-regulating effect of LH levels within the physiologic range. Maximal stimulation of 17-hydroxyprogesterone and androstenedione secretion by thecal cells in culture normally occur at LH concentrations approximating the upper portion of the normal range for follicular phase serum LH levels, and a further increase in LH dosage produces no further rise. However, studies both in vivo and in vitro suggest that the steroid responses of PCOS/FOH do not fall along the normal LH-steroid dose-response curve but seem displaced upward and to the left. Thus, the defect in steroidogenesis appears to be the result of escape from normal down-regulation of thecal cell secretion rather than from overstimulation by LH. What, then, elevated LH might have to do with PCOS is not clear, but some evidence suggests that it may be the result of modest androgen excess causing resistance to progesterone.[69, 102a]

The pattern of steroid secretion is similarly abnormal in nonclassic PCOS. This group of patients also has an LH-17–hydroxyprogesterone dose-response curve that is shifted upward and to the left. Thus, we favor the concept that the fundamental defect underlying the androgen excess of PCOS/FOH is ovarian hyperresponsiveness to gonadotropin action because of escape from down-regulation. The ovarian dysfunction seems independent of LH excess, although gonadotropins are permissive. The LH excess may intensify the intrinsic ovarian hyperandrogenic dysfunction.

The cause of the apparent escape of theca cells from down-regulation is unclear. The cause could be extrinsic or intrinsic to the ovaries. It is tempting to link the dysregulation to the insulin excess so common in FOH.[103] Insulin and androgen levels are correlated in PCOS, principally because hyperinsulinemia amplifies the effect of trophic hormones on steroidogenesis,[2, 34] whereas hyperandrogenism seems to contribute only modestly to insulin resistance. The abnormality of thecal function in PCOS resembles the escape from desensitization that occurs when normal cells are treated with insulin or IGF. The ovaries in PCOS behave as if they are responsive to excess insulin or IGFs in a state of resistance to the glucose-metabolic effects of insulin; however, insulin abnormalities are variable, and insulin excess is on average moderate although it can be striking.[104] Therefore, although insulin excess may be a provocative factor, it is rarely the sole cause of the syndrome. Alternatively, it has been proposed that FOH arises from a defect common to both insulin action and ovarian steroid biosynthesis. An increase in phosphorylation of serine residues of the insulin receptor results in resistance to insulin, and serine phosphorylation of P450c17 up-regulates its 17,20-lyase activity.[105]

A major role for defects in the intrinsic intraovarian processes by which thecal and granulosa cell function are coordinated has been postulated. An intrinsic defect in theca cell function in response to LH is a possibility[104, 106, 107] that has gained support from the demonstration of persistent dysfunction of passaged theca cells in culture.[108] Alternatively, the granulosa cell may be the site of the primary defect.[2] IGFs are candidates for being FSH-induceable factors capable of interfering with down-regulation of steroidogenesis, and a defect in the IGF system could account for the altered set point of the granulosa cell response to FSH. Inhibin is another FSH-dependent candidate. Recent clinical studies documented elevated serum inhibin-B levels in PCOS, a finding compatible with the excessive numbers of developing ovarian follicles. Since inhibin stimulates androgen synthesis and androgen in turn stimulates inhibin production, the potential exists for a vicious cycle to develop within the ovary that could cause androgen excess and inhibit follicular development. It is theoretically possible that follicular maturation arrest (resulting in a premature commitment of follicles to atresia) may be the initial event that leads to PCOS; however, it seems certain at least to be contributory. Atretic follicles are relatively androgenic and hypoestrogenic; this imbalance between the production of androgen and estrogen would be expected to perpetuate the cycle of hyperandrogenism and follicular maturation arrest.

Secondary Polycystic Ovary Syndrome

Secondary PCOS arises from frankly virilizing disorders, ovarian steroidogenic blocks, or primary, severe insulin resistance syndromes. Frankly virilizing disorders like poorly controlled virilizing CAH or exogenous androgen administration to transsexual females have been shown to produce the ovarian anatomic changes of Stein-Leventhal syndrome, namely cortical sclerosis, cysts, and hyperthecosis, probably because of the great increase in the intraovarian concentration

of androgen.[12] The frank virilization of classic CAH can also cause FOH. Women with virilizing CAH may have polycystic ovaries and high serum LH levels.[109] Adrenal rests of the ovaries, sometimes associated with CAH, may also mimic PCOS.[110] Ovarian steroidogenic blocks in the pathway to estradiol may, on rare occasions, cause hyperandrogenism, estrogen deficiency, and multicystic ovaries. These can result from congenital defects in the activity of ovarian 3β-HSD,[102] 17β-HSD,[111] or aromatase (see Fig. 17-1).[112, 113] The aromatase mutations reported to date have resulted in congenital virilization with ambiguous genitalia. Virtually every form of extreme insulin resistance, whether due to anti–insulin receptor antibodies, insulin receptor defects, or postreceptor defects, has been reported to be associated with PCOS.[12] The hyperinsulinemia of these insulin resistance syndromes may cause ovarian hyperandrogenism by acting through the IGF-I receptor.[13, 14, 114]

Functional Ovarian Hyperandrogenism of Other Causes

True hermaphroditism is characterized by the presence of *functional* testicular *and* ovarian tissue. This tissue may be separate or it may be combined in a single gonad, in which case it is called an *ovotestis*. True hermaphrodites occasionally present as menstruating, phenotypic females with signs of androgen excess such as clitoromegaly.[115] The diagnosis can be made by the response to gonadotropin stimulation.[116]

Virilization during pregnancy may be due to androgen hypersecretion by a luteoma or hyperreactio luteinalis,[117] which is a condition of benign hyperplastic thecal luteinization of the ovary, solid and cystic, respectively, that regresses spontaneously postpartum. Luteomas do not appear to be associated with excessive levels of hCG; in contrast, hyperreactio luteinalis is almost always associated with hCG excess. Virilization occurs in 10% to 50% of mothers with luteomas and in 25% of those with hyperreactio luteinalis. Fetal virilization is rare, owing to placental aromatization of androgen to estrogen.

PERIPHERAL OVERPRODUCTION OF ANDROGEN

Obesity can cause hyperandrogenemia and amenorrhea, and thus mimic PCOS.[2, 118] Because testosterone formation from androstenedione is increased and SHBG is suppressed, testosterone production is increased and the plasma free testosterone level is high. Estrone formation from androstenedione is also increased, and estradiol metabolism is diverted to active rather than inactive metabolites.[119] Insulin resistance is also characteristic.

Fewer than 10% of our series of hyperandrogenemic women had idiopathic disease (that is, hyperandrogenemia whose source an intensive search failed to conclusively identify as adrenal or ovarian).[69, 120] We suspect that this condition arises from increased peripheral metabolism of inactive steroid precursors to active androgens. We are left with this diagnosis for chronically hyperandrogenic females who demonstrate normal steroid responses to ACTH, GnRH agonist, and dexamethasone testing. Dexamethasone and estrogen-progestin, alone or in combination, suppress plasma free testosterone to normal levels in these cases.

OVARIAN TUMORS

Virilizing ovarian tumors may be malignant or benign and are frequently suspected on the basis of rapidly progressive virilization, testosterone concentrations greater than 200 ng/dl, and characteristic ultrasound or computed tomography findings. The most common virilizing ovarian tumor is Sertoli Leydig cell (arrhenoblastoma), which is occasionally gonadotropin responsive.[121] Ovarian lipid cell tumors are also typically gonadotropin responsive and depend in part on ACTH.[122] Typically, ovarian virilizing tumors secrete mostly androstenedione and thus are characterized by a disproportionate elevation of plasma androstenedione relative to testosterone. Characteristically, mild elevation of urinary 17-ketosteroid excretion results.

DRUGS WITH ANDROGENIC ACTIVITY

Testosterone and anabolic steroids must be considered when a hirsute adolescent, especially an athlete, does not have endogenous hyperandrogenemia.

DIAGNOSIS OF HYPERANDROGENIC STATES

The diagnosis of hyperandrogenism requires a high index of suspicion and a thorough and systematic approach on the part of the physician. A thorough history inquires into the timing and progression of (1) pubarche and breast development and (2) the signs and symptoms of hyperandrogenism, the use of medications, and similar complaints in other family members. Particular attention should be paid to the menstrual history. The physical examination should concentrate on the scoring of hirsutism and acne and assess the extent of virilization and estrogenization. When appropriate, a complete gynecologic examination should be performed and adnexal or adrenal masses carefully sought. The decision to perform a full pelvic examination of a teenager demands judgment. The anatomy of internal organs is now better assessed by abdominal ultrasound than by bimanual or rectal examination. Ancillary diagnostic procedures, such as adrenal computed tomography (CT), should be obtained when indicated by the history and physical examination findings.

Key elements in the history and physical examination may provide important clues to the diagnosis. Onset of virilization in the newborn period with labial fusion and clitoromegaly suggests onset in utero, which is often seen in CAH and less often with congenitally virilizing tumors. Isolated pubic hair development in a young girl suggests precocious adrenarche, whereas more extensive development of pubic or axillary hair, acne, growth spurt, and inordinately advanced bone age suggests a frankly virilizing disorder such as nonclassic CAH. Rapidly progressive virilization, especially that associated with markedly elevated androgen levels or signs of Cushing syndrome, should alert the physician to the possibility of an adrenal or ovarian tumor. PCOS is suggested by peripubertal onset of hirsutism, acne, obesity, or menstrual abnormalities associated with normal estrogenization. Although physiologic anovulation is normal in the perimenarcheal stage of development, a girl who fails to establish a normal menstrual pattern within 2 years after menarche has a 50% chance of experiencing ongoing menstrual disturbances,[123] so this is an indication for PCOS screening.

The laboratory evaluation of hyperandrogenism should include determinations of plasma testosterone and DHEAS.[120] Free testosterone and androstenedione determinations may also be considered. Determinations of urinary 17-hydroxycorticoids and 17-ketosteroids are seldom helpful. The 17-hydroxyprogesterone level is meaningful in the diagnosis of nonclassic CAH only when obtained as an early morning (8 AM) specimen.[124] Baseline plasma testosterone values in the frankly male range (> 350 ng/dl) are pathognomonic for ovarian or adrenal virilizing tumors, whereas levels above 200 ng/dl strongly suggest the presence of such lesions. A very high basal DHEAS level (> 600 μg/dl) suggests an adrenal neoplasm. In such cases, ultrasound, CT, or MRI usually demonstrates the mass and establishes the diagnosis.

Much more commonly, especially in cases of FAH or FOH, the baseline plasma total testosterone value may be normal or only minimally elevated. In most cases, however, free testosterone is elevated or the SHBG level low, a reflection of the hyperandrogenic state. Some authorities believe it is important to measure both total and free testosterone, since normal total testosterone does not rule out all important hyperandrogenic disorders. Because the assay of plasma free testosterone is not standardized among laboratories, some investigators prefer ancillary measurement of plasma androstenedione.

Hyperandrogenemia is a feature of most severe cases of hirsutism or acne and about half of mild cases.[31, 33] Because of the episodic and cyclic secretion of androgens, however, a random value may be misleadingly normal. Clearly, it is both costly and impractical to measure many steroids on multiple occasions; a strategy must be used to derive maximal diagnostic information from limited sampling. When key historical, physical, or laboratory features do not point to a specific diagnosis (such as an ovarian or adrenal tumor) and serum LH, FSH, prolactin, and thyroxine do not yield diagnostic information, we feel that diagnostic screening is usually reasonably accomplished with dexamethasone suppression testing.[120]

Dexamethasone suppression testing is performed by administering a "low" dose (2.0 mg per day) in divided doses by mouth for 4 days (or for 7 days to patients who are very obese or have a relatively high DHEAS level). The pattern of response of plasma free testosterone, DHEAS, and cortisol usually segregates patients diagnostically. Normal suppression of androgens is most specifically indicated by a reduction of plasma free testosterone into the normal range for dexamethasone-suppressed, nonhirsute women. In our laboratory, dexamethasone suppressibility is considered normal in a peri- or postmenarcheal female when plasma free testosterone is less than 8 pg/ml. Normal adrenal suppression is indicated by a reduction in both DHEAS and cortisol to levels below the normal range for adult controls (<70 and <3 μg/dl, respectively, in our laboratory). Failure of cortisol suppression indicates noncompliance with the dexamethasone test regimen, a dexamethasone-resistant form of FAH such as Cushing syndrome, or a virilizing tumor.

The vast majority of patients who respond to dexamethasone with normal suppression of adrenal steroids but subnormal suppression of free testosterone have the common FOH form of PCOS.[69, 120] In practical terms, the diagnosis of PCOS is one of exclusion. Positive ovarian ultrasound findings or an elevated serum LH level or LH-FSH ratio may be a useful corroborating test (classic PCOS), but neither finding is specific for PCOS/FOH. Both may be found in hyperprolactinemic and CAH patients, as discussed above. On the other hand, patients with nonclassic PCOS have ovarian sonograms and LH levels that are normal.

Two ovarian sonographic abnormalities are found in postmenarcheal females with classic PCOS, a polycystic follicular appearance, and excess stroma. A conservative definition of a polycystic appearance that is widely accepted is 10 or more follicular cysts (characteristically smaller than 10 mm in diameter) in the maximal ovarian plane.[125] In the most severe form of PCOS, hyperthecosis, however, cysts are lacking. Stroma is the major determinant of ovarian volume, and an increase in ovarian volume is a more consistent finding in patients with PCOS/FOH than an excessive number of cysts.[12, 126] An ovarian volume of 11 cm^3 or greater[92] or a maximum plane area of 6 cm^2 or greater[126] is excessive.

It is important to keep in mind that polycystic ovaries are not synonymous with PCOS. Twenty percent of normal volunteers have polycystic ovaries.[127] This finding is but one indication of the "nonspecificity" of ultrasonography. It is also important to distinguish a polycystic ovary from a multicystic one. Multicystic changes are common during normal adolescence. Multicystic ovary has been defined as one that contains 6 to 10 follicles in the 4- to 9-mm range in the maximal plane; the critical distinction is that a multifollicular ovary does not show an increase in stroma.[128] This distinction can be problematic, however (see the section on PCOS). In the final analysis, the pelvic ultrasound examination is most important to help rule out a rare virilizing disorder.

Suppression of plasma free testosterone into the normal range after a therapeutic trial of combination estrogen and progestin (i.e., oral contraceptives) is very suggestive of PCOS. Two considerations figure in interpreting the response to this treatment, however. On the one hand, the free testosterone value may not drop to normal as expected. Typically, the reason is a prominent degree of associated primary FAH. In this case, glucocorticoid therapy must be added to suppress androgens to normal. Such a response argues against a tumor as the source of the androgen excess. The physician must also keep in mind that gonadotropin dependence is occasionally associated with a virilizing ovarian[121] or adrenal[64] tumor.

GnRH agonist testing may be useful in confirming the diagnosis of PCOS. A serum 17-hydroxyprogesterone level greater than 200 to 300 ng/dl 24 hours after administration of a 10-μg/kg subcutaneous test dose of the GnRH agonist leuprolide or a 5000 IU intramuscular injection of hCG is characteristic of PCOS.[12, 129, 130]

Normal suppression of androgens after dexamethasone challenge demands that CAH be ruled out. The diagnosis can be confirmed in most cases by measuring steroid intermediates after an intravenous bolus of ACTH, since acute stimulation of adrenocortical steroid production yields a steroid pattern indicative of the nature and severity of the enzyme defect. New and colleagues developed a nomogram based on ACTH testing that delineates the types of steroid response for the classic and nonclassic forms of CAH secondary to 21-hydroxylase deficiency (see Fig. 17–7). A 17-hydroxyprogesterone level is measured 60 minutes after intravenous injection of 250 μg of cosyntropin; the nonclassic type of 21-hydroxylase deficiency CAH has levels over 1200 ng/dl, and the classic type has levels over 12,000 ng/dl.

The diagnosis of the nonclassic forms of 3β-HSD deficiency and 11β-hydroxylase deficiency requires responses of 17-hydroxypregnenolone and 11-deoxycortisol, respectively, that are at least 7 SD above the normal mean (see Table 17–4).[2] Less severe abnormalities of steroid intermediates are best understood as representing primary FAH. No means are available that distinguish FAH-exaggerated adrenarche from premature adrenarche in childhood unless steroid intermediate responses to ACTH exceed the normal range.

At the end of this sequence of testing, very few cases of hyperandrogenemia are left unexplained. "Idiopathic hyperandrogenemia" may be accounted for in some patients by abnormal peripheral androgen metabolism, in which case it is suppressible by dexamethasone, estrogen plus progestin, or a combination of the two. Our experience with GnRH-agonist testing suggests that much hyperandrogenemia that is now considered idiopathic is attributable to nonclassic PCOS/FOH. When androgens are consistently normal in a patient with hirsutism, the diagnosis is truly idiopathic hirsutism, a cosmetic problem due to

apparently increased sensitivity of PSUs to androgen.

TREATMENT OF HYPERANDROGENISM

Treatment of hyperandrogenism in adolescence must be undertaken with an understanding of its pathophysiologic mechanisms and directed at the underlying cause. Surgical extirpation is the treatment of choice for adrenal and ovarian tumors. In the case of adrenal tumor, care must be taken to examine both adrenal glands at the time of surgery, to investigate the possibility of bilateral lesions, and to search for remaining functional adrenal tissue.[60] Coverage with glucocorticoids is important, both at surgery and afterward, if there is glucocorticoid secretion by the tumor. Surgical correction results in normalization of plasma and urinary steroid abnormalities within days. When surgery is not successful or impossible because of metastases, chemotherapy may be attempted, but it generally has limited success.

In classic virilizing CAH, as in all types of CAH, provision of the missing end product, namely glucocorticoid, mineralocorticoid, or both, ameliorates adrenal insufficiency, inhibits trophic hormone stimulation, and suppresses elevated steroid levels. Glucocorticoid replacement is usually accomplished by the administration of hydrocortisone, 10 to 25 mg/m² per day, divided into three doses. Mineralocorticoid replacement, necessary in all salt-losing and non–salt-losing patients with elevated plasma renin activity, is usually achieved with Florinef, 0.05 to 0.2 mg/day. In adolescents and older persons, normalization of ACTH and plasma androgens can usually be achieved with prednisone in doses of 5 to 7.5 mg per day in two doses, the larger fraction to be taken at bedtime. Adequate control is typically associated with 17-hydroxyprogesterone levels approximating high-normal values (200 ng/dl). Failure of menses to normalize in an adolescent suggests incomplete control of progesterone levels or coincident PCOS.[131]

Clinical remission of hyperandrogenic signs and symptoms typically occurs with adequate replacement therapy; however, treatment must be individualized and closely monitored and adjusted, since over- and undertreatment are both associated with adverse effects. In this regard, and especially in younger persons, particular attention must be given to the growth and development pattern and progression of bone age.

Glucocorticoids are also indicated for some

patients with other forms of FAH but are generally less effective.[8] The sequelae of glucocorticoid therapy can be minimized by using a modest bedtime dose (about 5 mg prednisone or 0.25 mg dexamethasone) to selectively reduce adrenal androgen secretion without causing adrenal insufficiency. Long-term use of more than 0.25 mg dexamethasone is likely to cause Cushingoid side effects. Glucocorticoids are not indicated for premature adrenarche, which usually seems to be a normal phenomenon that occurs prematurely, but which requires monitoring as a risk factor for PCOS.

The treatment of FOH, including PCOS, is directed at correcting menstrual irregularities, alleviating symptoms of androgen excess, and, when appropriate, inducing ovulation. No treatment is ideal or universally successful, and therapy must be individualized according to the needs and desires of the individual.

In general, cyclic progestin administration is the method of choice for the treatment of adolescent menstrual irregularities when hirsutism is absent and fertility is not an issue. Medroxyprogesterone acetate (Provera) is used in doses of 10 mg at bedtime daily for 7 days, commencing at intervals of 3 weeks to 2 months. The more frequent dosing is chosen for patients with intractable, dysfunctional uterine bleeding and the less frequent dosing for patients with amenorrhea, as the long intervals permit possibly spontaneous menses. Adolescents who are sexually active need to be warned about the need for barrier contraception while taking cyclic Provera therapy.

For patients whose menses cannot be regulated with progestin alone, oral contraceptives are usually of benefit. An estrogen-progestin combination contraceptive pill that has low androgenic activity is generally recommended (see later). Modest breakthrough bleeding can be managed by doubling the dose each day it occurs.

When progestin or oral contraceptive therapy fails to control dysfunctional uterine bleeding or when bleeding is profuse and rapid and causes significant anemia, conjugated estrogens (Premarin) can be administered in a dose of 10 mg intravenously or a comparable oral dose every 4 hours until bleeding stops. The patient may then be maintained for 3 weeks on oral Premarin, 10 mg daily, and if breakthrough bleeding occurs during this time, the Premarin dose can be increased in 5-mg increments to a maximum of 20 mg per day. An antiemetic should also be prescribed. On the last 5 days of this 3-week regimen, Provera should be added to prevent endometrial hyperplasia and further breakthrough bleeding. If these regimens fail, dilatation and curettage or suction curettage should be performed. If medical management fails, a genital tract tumor must be considered.

When functional hyperandrogenism is associated with hirsutism or acne, treatment should be directed at interrupting one or more of the steps leading to their expression: (1) inhibition of adrenal or ovarian androgen synthesis and secretion, (2) alteration of binding of androgens to SHBG, (3) impairment of the peripheral conversion of androgen precursors to active androgen, and (4) inhibition of androgen action at the target level.[120] Because the maximal effect of pharmacologic agents on hair growth takes 9 to 12 months and is sometimes not totally effective, concomitant local cosmetic measures (bleaching, plucking, waxing, electrolysis) are usually necessary.

In the absence of specific contraindications or associated cardiovascular risk factors, the treatment of choice for hyperandrogenism that produces symptomatic, mild hirsutism in a teenager with PCOS is combination estrogen-progestin therapy. This is a very effective treatment for hyperandrogenic acne. This type of therapy lowers free testosterone levels by reducing serum gonadotropin levels, increasing SHBG levels, and modestly decreasing DHEAS levels. Estrogen-progestin therapy can be expected to arrest hirsutism but may not lead to substantial improvement. Furthermore, the choice of progestin is important: norgestimate and ethynodiol diacetate have the least adrenogenic potential and norethindrone acetate and norgestrel the highest. Chronic GnRH agonist therapy, an alternative means to suppress ovarian androgen production, is indicated only when estrogen-progestin therapy is contraindicated and should be used with sufficient estrogen add-back therapy to prevent osteoporosis.

Moderate or severe hirsutism can be improved by treatment with antiandrogens, a class of hormone antagonists that inhibit the binding of androgens to the androgen receptor. Agents in this category include spironolactone, cyproterone acetate, and flutamide. Spironolactone is most widely used in the United States and is clinically antiandrogenic and progestational in high doses. We recommend starting on 100 mg twice daily. The maximum effect cannot be expected for 9 to 12 months, at which point a lower maintenance dose can be considered. Simultaneous administration of cyclic estrogen-progestin is indicated to ensure a regular menstrual cycle and prevent pseudohermaphroditism in the fetus should the teenager become pregnant. Side effects of spironolactone treatment include initial diuresis, irregular uterine bleeding, hyperkalemia, and postural hypotension, which may limit the long-term use necessary to sustain improvement. A serum chemistry panel should be performed at regular intervals. We recommend this treatment only for adolescents who are very troubled by severe hirsutism.

Cyproterone acetate is a potent progestational and antiandrogenic agent that has proved very successful in the treatment of hirsutism and menstrual irregularity.[132] It is administered in a "reverse cyclic" manner, generally in a dose of 50 mg per day during the first 10 days of a 21-day course of estrogen. It has limited adverse effects but is not currently available in the United States because of its association with breast cancer when administered to beagle pups. Flutamide is a potent nonsteroidal agent with selective antiandrogenic properties, but it is potentially hepatotoxic.

Weight reduction is sometimes successful in reversing hyperandrogenemia and menstrual disorders.[133, 134] The deleterious effects of obesity on hyperandrogenic anovulation are probably mediated by insulin excess. Insulin-lowering treatments may be useful adjuncts to therapy in some cases, but their place in therapy has yet to be well defined. Metformin reduces hepatic glucose production and promotes weight loss. Troglitazone is an insulin-sensitizing agent that does not affect weight.

Women with PCOS are relatively infertile and some may have success in conceiving spontaneously. When pregnancy is an issue, measures should be directed at promoting ovulation. Several medical maneuvers are now available for ovulation induction, including clomiphene citrate, pulsatile GnRH, hMG-hCG, and should these fail, more complex regimens.[135] Women who want to become pregnant may also benefit from the expertise of an experienced reproductive endocrinologist. Such measures are beyond the scope of medical management of most adolescents with FOH, however. There is virtually no place for surgical management of adolescent PCOS except as an incidental procedure when an ovarian tumor is suspected.

REFERENCES

1. Miller W: Molecular biology of steroid hormone synthesis. Endocr Rev 1988; 9:29.
2. Rosenfield RL: Ovarian and adrenal function in polycystic ovary syndrome. Endocrinol Metab Clin North Am 1999; 28:265.
3. Rosenfield RL: The ovary and female maturation. In Sperling M (ed): Pediatric Endocrinology. Philadelphia: WB Saunders, 1996, p 329.
4. Abraham G: Ovarian and adrenal contributions to peripheral androgens during the menstrual cycle. J Clin Endocrinol Metab 1974; 39:340.
5. Rich BH, Rosenfield RL, Lucky AW, et al: Adrenarche: Changing adrenal response to adrenocorticotropin. J Clin Endocrinol Metab 1981; 52:1129.
6. Rosenfield RL: Normal and almost normal variants of precocious puberty: Premature pubarche and premature thelarche revisited. Horm Res 1994; 41:7.
7. Grumbach M, Richards C, Conte F, et al: Clinical disorders of adrenal function and puberty: An assessment of the role of the adrenal cortex in normal and abnormal puberty in man and evidence for an ACTH-like pituitary adrenal androgen stimulating hormone. In James V, Serio M, Giusti C, Martini L (eds): The Endocrine Function of the Human Adrenal Cortex. London: Academic Press, 1978, p 583.
8. Rittmaster R, Givner M: Effect of daily and alternate day low dose prednisone on serum cortisol and adrenal androgens in hirsute women. J Clin Endocrinol Metab 1988; 67:400.
9. Byrne C, Perry Y, Winter J: Kinetic analysis of adrenal 3β-hydroxysteroid dehydrogenase activity during human development. J Clin Endocrinol Metab 1985; 60:934.
10. Sklar C, Kaplan S, Grumbach M: Evidence for dissociation between adrenarche and gonadarche: Studies in patients with idiopathic precocious puberty, gonadal dysgenesis, isolated gonadotropin deficiency, and constitutionally delayed growth and adolescence. J Clin Endocrinol Metab 1980; 51:548.
11. Hoffman F, Meger RC: On the action of intraovarian injection of androgen on follicle and corpus luteum maturation in women. Geburtshilfe Frauenheilklinic 1965; 25:1132.
12. Ehrmann DA, Barnes RB, Rosenfield RL: Polycystic ovary syndrome as a form of functional ovarian hyperandrogenism due to dysregulation of androgen secretion. Endocr Rev 1995; 16:322.
13. Cara JF, Rosenfield RL: Insulin-like growth factor I and insulin potentiate luteinizing hormone–induced androgen synthesis by rat ovarian theca-interstitial cells. Endocrinology 1988; 123:733.
14. Hernandez E, Resnick C, Holtzclaw W, et al: Insulin as a regulator of androgen biosynthesis by cultured rat ovarian cells: Cellular mechanism(s) underlying physiological and pharmacological hormonal actions. Endocrinology 1988; 122:2034.
15. Rosenfield RL, Barnes RB, Cara JF, et al: Dysregulation of cytochrome P450c17α as the cause of polycystic ovary syndrome. Fertil Steril 1990; 53:785.
16. Rosenfield RL, Moll GW Jr: The role of proteins in the distribution of plasma androgens and estradiol. In Molinatti G, Martini L, James V (eds): Androgenization in Women. New York: Raven Press, 1989, p 25.
17. Hammond G: Molecular properties of corticosteroid-binding globulin and sex-steroid–binding proteins. Endocr Rev 1990; 11:65.
18. Moll G Jr, Rosenfield RL: Estradiol inhibition of pituitary luteinizing hormone release is antagonized by serum proteins. J Steroid Biochem 1986; 25:308.
19. Ekins R: Measurement of free hormones in blood. Endocr Rev 1990; 11:5.
20. Gershagen S, Lundwall A, Fernlund P: Characterization of the human sex hormone binding globulin (SHBG) gene and demonstration of two transcripts in both liver and testis. Nucl Acid Res 1989; 17:9245.
21. Nestler JE, Balascini CO, Matt DW, et al: Suppression

of serum insulin by diazoxide reduces serum testosterone levels in obese women with polycystic ovary syndrome. J Clin Endocrinol Metab 1989; 68:1027.

22. Moll G Jr, Rosenfield RL: Plasma free testosterone in the diagnosis of adolescent polycystic ovary syndrome. J Pediatrics 1983; 102:461.

23. Rosenfield RL: Pilosebaceous physiology in relation to hirsutism and acne. Clin Endocrinol Metab 1986; 15:341.

24. Rosenfield RL, Deplewski D: Role of androgens in the developmental biology of the pilosebaceous unit. Am J Med 1995; 98(1A):80S.

25. Lobo R, Paul W, Gentzsschein E, et al: Production of 3α-androstanediol glucuronide in human genital skin. J Clin Endocrinol Metab 1987;65:711.

26. Rittmaster RA: Androgen conjugates: Physiology and clinical significance. Endocr Rev 1993; 14:121.

27. Lubhan DB, Joseph DR, Sullivan PM, et al: Cloning of human androgen receptor – complementary DNA and localization to the X chromosome. Science 1988; 240:327.

28. Forman B, Samuels H: Interactions among a subfamily of nuclear hormone receptors: The regulatory zipper model. Molec Endocrinol 1990; 4:1293.

29. Carson-Jurica MA, Schrader WT, O'Malley BW: Steroid receptor family: Structure and function. Endocrinol Rev 1990; 11:201.

30. Quigley C, De Bellis A, Marchke K, et al: Androgen receptor defects: Historical, clinical, and molecular perspectives. Endocr Rev 1995; 16:271.

31. Reingold SB, Rosenfield RL: The relationship of mild hirsutism or acne in women to androgens. Arch Dermatol 1987; 123:209.

32. Futterweit W, Dunaif A, Yeh H-C, et al: The prevalence of hyperandrogenism in 109 consecutive female patients with diffuse alopecia. J Am Acad Dermatol 1988; 19:831.

33. Marynick SP, Chakmakjian ZH, McCafffree DL, et al: Androgen excess in cystic acne. N Engl J Med 1983; 308:981.

34. Rosenfield RL: Current concepts of polycystic ovary syndrome. Baillière's Clin Obstet Gynaecol 1997; 11:307.

35. Rosenfield RL, Qin K: Normal adrenarche. In Rose BD (ed): UpToDate (CD). Wellesley, Mass: UpToDate, 1998.

36. Rosenfield RL, Barnes RB: Menstrual disorders in adolescence. Endocrinol Metab Clin North Am 1993; 22:491.

37. Ibañez L, Potau N, Virdis R, et al: Postpubertal outcome in girls diagnosed with premature pubarche during childhood: Increased frequency of functional ovarian hyperandrogenism. J Clin Endocrinol Metab 1993; 76:1599.

38. Temeck J, Pang S, Nelson C, et al: Genetic defects of steroidogenesis in premature pubarche. J Clin Endocrinol Metab 1987; 64:609.

39. Oberfield S, Mayes D, Levine L: Adrenal steroidogenic function in a Black and Hispanic population with precocious pubarche. J Clin Endocrinol Metab 1990; 70:76.

40. Pang S: Congenital adrenal hyperplasia. Baillière's Clin Obstet Gynaecol 1997; 11:281.

41. McKenna TJ: Current concepts: Pathogenesis and treatment of polycystic ovary syndrome. N Engl J Med 1988; 318:558.

42. Lobo R: The role of the adrenal in polycystic ovary syndrome. Semin Reprod Endocrinol 1984; 2:251.

43. Miller W, Levine L: Molecular and clinical advances in congenital adrenal hyperplasia. 1987; 111:1.

44. White P, New M, Dupont B: Congenital adrenal hyperplasia. N Engl J Med 1987; 316:1519.

45. Ritzén E: Adrenogenital syndrome. Curr Opin Pediatr 1992; 4:661.

46. Bose H, Sugawara T, Strauss JI, et al: The pathophysiology and genetics of congenital lipoid adrenal hyperplasia. N Engl J Med 1996; 335:1870.

47. New M: Steroid 21-hydroxylase deficiency (congenital adrenal hyperplasia). Am J Med 1995; 98(Suppl A):2S.

48. Svetlana L, Wedell A, Bui T-H, et al: Long-term somatic follow-up of prenatally treated children with congenital adrenal hyperplasia. J Clin Endocrinol Metab 1998; 83:3872.

49. Cara J, Moshang T Jr, Bongiovanni A, et al: Elevated 17-hydroxyprogesterone and testosterone in a newborn with 3β-hydroxysteroid dehydrogenase deficiency. N Engl J Med 1985; 13:618.

50. Rosenfield RL, Rich BH, Wolfsdorf JI, et al: Pubertal presentation of congenital Δ5-β-hydroxysteroid dehydrogenase deficiency. J Clin Endocrinol Metab 1980; 51:345.

51. Zachmann V, Vollman A, New MI, et al: Congenital adrenal hyperplasia due to deficiency of 11β-hydroxylation of 17α-hydroxylated steroids. J Clin Endocrinol Metab 1971; 33:501.

52. Joehrer K, Geley S, Strasser-Wozak E, et al: CYP11B1 mutations causing non-classic adrenal hyperplasia due to 11beta-hydroxylase deficiency. Hum Molec Genet 1997; 6:1829.

53. Glickman SP, Rosenfield RL, Bergenstal RM, et al: Multiple androgenic abnormalities, including elevated free testosterone, in hyperprolactinemic women. J Clin Endocrinol Metab 1982; 55:251.

54. Futterweit W, Krieger DT: Pituitary tumors associated with hyperprolactinemia and polycystic ovary disease. Fertil Steril 1979; 31:608.

55. Monroe S, Levine L, Chang J, et al: Prolactin-secreting pituitary adenomas. J Clin Endocrinol Metab 1981; 52:1171.

56. Lim N, Dingman J: Androgenic adrenal hyperfunction in acromegaly. N Engl J Med 1964; 271:1189.

57. Hauffa BP, Kaplan SL, Grumbach MM: Dissociation between plasma adrenal androgens and cortisol in Cushing's disease and ectopic ACTH-producing tumour: Relation to adrenarche. Lancet 1984; 1:1373.

58. Malchoff CD, Javier EC, Malchoff DM, et al: Primary cortisol resistance presenting as isosexual precocity. J Clin Endocrinol Metab 1990; 700:503.

59. Phillipov G, Palermo M, Shackleton C: Apparent cortisone reductase deficiency: A unique form of hypercortisolism. J Clin Endocrinol Metab 1996; 81:3855.

60. Lee P, Winter R, Green O: Virilizing adrenocortical tumors in childhood: Eight cases and a review of the literature. Pediatrics 1985; 70:129.

61. Fraumeni J, Miller R: Adrenocortical neoplasms with hemihypertrophy, brain tumors and other disorders. J Pediatrics 1967; 70:129.

62. Adeyemi S, Grange A, Giwa-Osagie O, et al: Adrenal rest tumour of the ovary associated with isosexual precocious pseudopuberty and cushingoid features. Eur J Pediatr 1986; 145:2236.

63. Voutilainen R, Leisti S, Perheentupa J: Growth in Cushing syndrome. Eur J Pediatr 1985; 144:141.

64. Werk E, Sholiton L, Kaalejs L: Testosterone-secreting adenoma under gonadotropin control. N Engl J Med 1973; 289:767.

65. Stein IF, Leventhal ML: Amenorrhea associated with bilateral polycystic ovaries. Am J Obstet Gynecol 1935; 29:181.

66. MacArthur JW, Ingersall FM, Worcester J: The urinary excretion of interstitial cell and follicle-stimulating hormone activity by women with diseases of the reproductive system. J Clin Endocrinol Metab 1958; 18:1202.

67. Yen S, Vela P, Rankin J: Inappropriate secretion of follicle-stimulating hormone and luteinizing hormone in polycystic ovarian disease. J Clin Endocrinol Metab 1970; 30:435.

68. Goldzieher J, Axelrod L: Clinical and biochemical features of polycystic ovarian disease. Fertil Steril 1963; 14:631.

69. Barnes RB, Rosenfield RL: The polycystic ovary syndrome: Pathogenesis and treatment. Ann Intern Med 1989; 110:386.

70. Zawadzki J, Dunaif A: Diagnostic criteria for polycystic ovary syndrome: Towards a rational approach. *In* Dunaif A, Givens J, Haseltine F, Merriam G (eds): Polycystic Ovary Syndrome, Current Issues in Endocrinology and Metabolism. Cambridge: Blackwell Scientific, 1992, p 377.

71. Franks S: Polycystic ovary syndrome. N Engl J Med 1995; 333:853.

72. Ehrmann DA, Rosenfield RL, Barnes RB, et al: Detection of functional ovarian hyperandrogenism in women with androgen excess. N Engl J Med 1992; 327:157.

73. Arroyo A, Laughlin GA, Morales AJ, et al: Inappropriate gonadotropin secretion in polycystic ovary syndrome: Influence of adiposity. J Clin Endocrinol Metab 1997; 82:3728.

74. Apter D, Bützow T, Laughlin G, et al: Accelerated 24-hour luteinizing hormone pulsatile activity in adolescent girls with ovarian hyperandrogenism: Relevance to the developmental phase of polycystic ovarian syndrome. J Clin Endocrinol Metab 1994; 79:119.

75. Rosenfield RL: Polycystic ovary syndrome and its presentation at puberty. Frontiers Neuroendocrinol 1996; 17:189.

76. Rosenfield RL: Are adrenal and ovarian functions normal in true precocious puberty? Eur J Endocrinol 1995; 133:399.

77. Flier JS, Moller DE, Moses AC, et al: Insulin-mediated pseudoacromegaly: Clinical and biochemical characterization of a syndrome of selective insulin resistance. J Clin Endocrinol Metab 1993; 76:1533.

78. Dunaif A, Green G, Phelps R, et al: Acanthosis nigricans, insulin action, and hyperandrogenism: Clinical, histological, and biochemical findings. J Clin Endocrinol Metab 1991; 73:590.

79. Merrill JA: The morphology of the prepubertal ovary: Relationship to the polycystic ovary syndrome. South Med J 1963; 56:225.

80. Carey A, Waterworth D, Patel K, et al: Polycystic ovaries and premature male pattern baldness are associated with one allele of the steroid metabolism gene CYP 17. Hum Molec Genet 1994; 3:1873.

81. Ehrmann DA, Barnes RB, Rosenfield RL, et al: Prevalence of impaired glucose tolerance and diabetes in women with polycystic ovary syndrome. Diabetes Care 1999; 22:141.

82. Ehrmann DA: Relation of functional ovarian hyperandrogenism to non–insulin dependent diabetes mellitus. Baillière's Clin Obstet Gynaecol 1997; 11:335.

83. Ibañez L, Potau N, Francois I, et al: Precocious pubarche, hyperinsulinism, and ovarian hyperandrogenism. J Clin Endocrinol Metab 1998; 83:3558.

84. Caprio S, Plewe G, Diamond MP, et al: Increased insulin secretion in puberty: A compensatory response to reductions in insulin sensitivity. J Pediatrics 1989; 114:963.

85. Nobels F, Dewailly D: Puberty and polycystic ovarian syndrome: The insulin/insulin-like growth factor I hypothesis. Fertil Steril 1992; 58:655.

86. Apter D, Bützow G, Laughlin A, et al: Metabolic features of polycystic ovary syndrome are found in adolescent girls with hyperandrogenism. J Clin Endocrinol Metab 1995; 80:2966.

87. Apter D, Vihko R: Serum pregnenolone, progesterone, 17-hydroxyprogesterone, testosterone, and 5α-dihydrotestosterone during female puberty. J Clin Endocrinol Metab 1977; 45:1039.

88. Siegberg R, Nilsson C, Stenman U-H, et al: Endocrinologic features of oligomenorrheic adolescent girls. Fertil Steril 1986; 46:852.

89. Venturoli S, Porcu E, Fabbri R, et al: Menstrual irregularities in adolescents: Hormonal pattern and ovarian morphology. Hormone Res 1986; 24:269.

90. Venturoli S, Porcu E, Fabbri R, et al: Longitudinal evaluation of the different gonadotropin pulsatile patterns in anovulatory cycles of young girls. J Clin Endocrinol Metab 1992; 74:836.

91. Apter D, Vihko R: Endocrine determinants of fertility: Serum androgen concentrations during follow-up of adolescents into the third decade of life. J Clin Endocrinol Metab 1990; 71:970.

92. Venturoli S, Porcu E, Fabbri R, et al: Longitudinal change of sonographic ovarian aspects and endocrine parameters in irregular cycles of adolescence. Pediatr Res 1995; 38:974.

93. Polhemus D: Ovarian maturation and cyst formation in children. Pediatrics 1953; 11:588.

94. Kraus F, Neubecker R: Luteinization of the ovarian theca in infants and children. Am J Clin Pathol 1962; 37:389.

95. Brook C, Jacobs H, Stanhope R: Polycystic ovaries in childhood. Br Med J 1988; 296:878.

96. Bridges NA, Cooke A, Healy MJR, et al: Standards for ovarian volume in childhood and puberty. Fertil Steril 1993; 60:456.

97. Ardaens Y, Robert Y, Lemaitre L, et al: Polycystic ovarian disease: Contribution of vaginal endosonography and reassessment of ultrasonic diagnosis. Fertil Steril 1991; 55:1062.

98. Apter D, Bützow T, Laughlin G: Hyperandrogenism during puberty and adolescence, and its relationship to reproductive function in the adult female. *In*: Frajese G, Steinberger E, Rodriguez-Rigau L (eds): Reproductive Medicine: Serono Symposia. New York: Raven Press, 1993, 93:265.

99. Goldzieher J: Polycystic ovarian disease. Clin Obstet Gynecol 1973; 16:82.

100. Yen S: The polycystic ovary syndrome. Clin Endocrinol 1980; 12:177.

101. McKenna T: Pathogenesis and treatment of polycystic ovary syndrome. N Engl J Med 1988; 318:558.

102. Barnes RB, Rosenfield RL, Burstein S, et al: Pituitary-ovarian responses to nafarelin testing in the polycystic ovary syndrome. N Engl J Med 1989; 320:559.

102a. Eagleson CA, Gingrich MB, Pastor CL, et al: Polycystic ovarian syndrome: Evidence that flutamide restores sensitivity of the gonadotropin-releasing hormone pulse generator to inhibition by estradiol and progesterone. J Clin Endocrinol Metab 2000; 85:4047.

103. Dunaif A: Insulin resistance and the polycystic ovary syndrome: Mechanism and implications for pathogenesis. Endocr Rev 1997; 18:774.

104. Ehrmann DA, Jeppe S, Byrne M, et al: Insulin secretory defects in polycystic ovary syndrome: Relationship to insulin sensitivity and family history of non–insulin-dependent diabetes mellitus. J Clin Invest 1995; 96:520.

105. Zhang L-H, Rodriguez H, Ohno S, et al: Serine phosphorylation of human P450c17 increases 17,20-lyase activity: Implications for adrenarche and the polycystic ovary syndrome. Proc Natl Acad Sci (USA) 1995; 92:10619.

106. Gilling-Smith C, Willis DS, Beard RW, et al: Hypersecretion of androstenedione by isolated theca cells from polycystic ovaries. J Clin Endocrinol Metab 1994; 79:1158.

107. Gilling-Smith C, Story H, Rogers V, et al: Evidence for a primary abnormality of thecal cell steroidogenesis in the polycystic ovary syndrome. Clin Endocrinol 1997; 47:93.

108. Nelson VL, Legro RS, Strauss JF III, McAllister JM: Augmented androgen production is a stable steroidogenic phenotype of propagated theca cells from polycystic ovaries. Mol Endocrinol 1999; 13:946.

109. Dewailly D, Vantyghem-Haudiquet MC, Sainsard C, et al: Clinical and biological phenotypes in late-onset 21-hydroxylase deficiency. J Clin Endocrinol Metab 1986; 63:418.

110. Barnes RB, Rosenfield RL, Ehrmann DA, et al: Ovarian hyperandrogenism as a result of congenital adrenal virilizing disorders: Evidence for perinatal masculinization of neuroendocrine function in women. J Clin Endocrinol Metab 1994; 79:1328.

111. Pang S, Softness B, Sweeney W, et al: Hirsutism, polycystic ovarian disease, and ovarian 17-ketosteroid reductase deficiency. N Engl J Med 1987; 316:1295.

112. Conte F, Grumbach M, Ito Y, et al: A syndrome of female pseudohermaphroditism, hypergonadotropic hypogonadism, and multicystic ovaries associated with missense mutations in the gene encoding aromatase (P450arom). J Clin Endocrinol Metab 1994; 78:1287.

113. Morishima A, Grumbach MM, Simpson ER, et al: Aromatase deficiency in male and female siblings caused by a novel mutation and the physiologic role of estrogens. J Clin Endocrinol Metab 1995; 80:3689.

114. Moller DE, Flier JS: Insulin resistance—mechanisms, syndromes, and implications. N Engl J Med 1991; 325:938.

115. Talerman A, Jarabak J, Amarose AP: Gonadoblastoma and dysgerminoma in a true hermaphrodite with a 46, XX karyotype. Am J Obstet Gynecol 1981; 140:475.

116. Pablo-Mendez J, Schiavon R, Diaz-Cueto L, et al: A reliable endocrine test with human menopausal gonadotropins for diagnosis of true hermaphroditism in early infancy. J Clin Endocrinol Metab 1998; 83:3523.

117. Hensleigh PA, Woodruf JD: Differential maternal-fetal response to androgenizing luteoma or hyperreactio luteinalis. Obstet Gynecol Surv 1978; 33:262.

118. Glass A: Endocrine function in human obesity. Metabolism 1981(30).

119. Lustig R, Bradlow H, Fishman J: Estrogen metabolism in disorders of nutrition and dietary composition. In Pirke K, Wuttke W, Schweiger U (eds): The Menstrual Cycle and Its Disorders. Berlin: Springer-Verlag, 1989, p 119.

120. Ehrmann D, Rosenfield R: An endocrinologic approach to the patient with hirsutism. J Clin Endocrinol Metab 1990; 71:1.

121. Hatch R, Rosenfield RL, Kim MH, et al: Hirsutism: Implications, etiology, and management. Am J Obstet Gynecol 1981; 140:815.

122. Rosenfield RL, Cohen RM, Talerman A: Lipid cell tumor of the ovary in reference to adult-onset congenital adrenal hyperplasia and polycystic ovary syndrome. J Reprod Med 1987; 32:363.

123. Southam A, Richart E: The prognosis for adolescents with menstrual abnormalities. Am J Obstet Gynecol 1966; 94:637.

124. Rosenfield RL, Lucky AW: Acne, hirsutism, and alopecia in adolescent girls. Endo Metab Clin North Am 1993; 22:507.

125. Franks S: Polycystic ovary syndrome: A changing perspective. Clin Endocrinol 1989; 31:87.

126. Robert Y, Dubrulle F, Gaillandre L, et al: Ultrasound assessment of ovarian stroma hypertrophy in hyperandrogenism and ovulation disorders: Visual analysis versus computerized quantification. Fertil Steril 1995; 64:307.

127. Polson D, Adams J, Wadsworth J, et al: Polycystic ovaries—a common finding in normal women. Lancet 1988; 1:870.

128. Adams J, Franks S, Polson DW, et al: Multifollicular ovaries: Clinical and endocrine features and response to pulsatile gonadotropin-releasing hormone. Lancet 1985; 2:1375.

129. Ehrmann D, Schneider D, Sobel B, et al: Troglitazone improves defects in insulin action, insulin secretion, ovarian steroidogenesis, and fibrinolysis in women with polycystic ovary syndrome. J Clin Endocrinol Metab 1997; 82:2108.

130. Ibañez L, Hall J, Potau N, et al: Ovarian 17-hydroxyprogesterone hyperresponsiveness to gonadotropin-releasing hormone (GnRH) agonist challenge in women with polycystic ovary syndrome is not mediated by luteinizing hormone hypersecretion: Evidence from GnRH agonist and human chorionic gonadotropin stimulation testing. J Clin Endocrinol Metab 1996; 81:4103.

131. Rosenfield RL, Bickel S, Razdan AK: Amenorrhea related to progestin excess in congenital adrenal hyperplasia. Obstet Gynecol 1980; 56:208.

132. Kuttenn F, Rigaud C, Wright F, et al: Treatment of hirsutism by oral cyproterone acetate and percutaneous estradiol. J Clin Endocrinol Metab 1980; 51:1107.

133. Kopelman PG, White N, Pilkington F, et al: The effect of weight loss on sex steroid secretion and binding in massively obese women. Clin Endocrinol 1981; 14:113.

134. Bates G, Whitworth N: Effect of body weight reduction on plasma androgens in obese, infertile women. Fertil Steril 1982; 38:406.

135. Barnes R: Diagnosis and therapy of hyperandrogenism. Baillière's Clin Obstet Gynaecol 1997; 11:369.

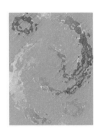

Chapter 18
Adolescent Sexuality
ROBERT T. BROWN

Little is more basic to the nature of human beings than sexuality. The melding of parental gametes assigns us our genotypic sex; then, other physiologic, cultural, and societal factors help to shape our phenotypic expression of that chromosomal throw of the dice. From the earliest moments out of the uterus, the shaping begins. With that first question, "Is it a girl or a boy?" a host of forces begins to direct what kind of woman or man an infant will become. Here, we will examine the contributions of the various factors that shape humans as men and women and will explore the results of that shaping in terms of how adolescents express their sexuality. In addition, we will look at how Americans formally transmit knowledge of sexuality to their children and adolescents by means of education in sex and sexuality.

Human sexuality includes the physical characteristics of and capacities for specific sex behaviors, together with psychosocial values, norms, attitudes, and learning processes that influence these behaviors. It also involves a sense of gender identity and related concepts, behaviors, and attitudes about self and others as men or women in the context of society.[1] Whereas biologic factors such as genotype and hormonal influences on the developing brain affect sexuality from the moment of conception, other extrinsic factors begin to exert their influences at birth. The family's perception of maleness or femaleness, rooted as it is in the norms and expectations of their culture and of society in general, is expressed to the infant from the start. Because we are a species for whom assignment of gender is basic, it may be difficult to discern the various factors that make humans women and men. Therefore, it is instructive to look at an analogous species for whom gender is nonexistent. This can be done only through literature, and the novel in which it is best expressed is *The Left Hand of Darkness* by Ursula LeGuin.[2] In this story, LeGuin introduces a species that is similar to humans but without sex differentiation until individuals go "into heat" to procreate. All children and adolescents are treated equally, and the concept of gender difference is unnecessary and

unknown. All relationships in this society are free of the influence of gender as we know it.

BIOLOGY

Biology determines a person's genotype and the major factors in that genotype's phenotypic expression. If a girl has two X chromosomes but an enzyme defect in her adrenal glands, she may be born with masculinized genitalia. The reaction of her family to this defect will greatly influence this girl's self-concept as a woman. Even if the girl is not fully masculinized, she may have severe acne or hirsuitism, which, undoubtedly, will influence her self-image. Similarly, a girl born without a second X chromosome (i.e., with Turner syndrome) is perceived at birth as undeniably female and may for the rest of her life be treated as a girl, rather than as a woman, because, without pharmacologic assistance, she will not mature.

Because of possible influences of androgens on the fetal brain, a particular girl may be more "boyish" than her peers, or a combination of genetic factors may make her more adept at sports. This physical capability may make her seem more "masculine" and affects how she is perceived by others—and ultimately by herself.

FAMILY

A child's first sense that he or she is a boy or girl—and what exactly that means—is conveyed by the parents early in childhood.[3] As the child develops, he or she witnesses how the mother behaves as a woman, how the father behaves as a man, and how they behave toward each other. These impressions go a long way in helping the child to define what a man or woman should be.[4] These images are colored by the attitudes of other members of the family, such as grandparents and siblings. Absence of one of the parents or of someone who assumes that parental role can make it difficult for a child to understand how women and men behave with each other. Girls "test" how to behave as a woman with their fathers or with another close adult male. Without that input, many girls may go "looking for Daddy" and may engage in considerable risk-taking behavior toward that end.[5] Such behavior may lead to adolescent parenthood or to abusive situations. Inappropriate behavior on the part of a girl's male authority figure may also color her view of sexuality. A girl who has been sexually abused is likely to have very poor self-image. Many such victims attempt suicide or become prostitutes.[6] A girl who is reared in a home where the parents are caring, loving, supportive, and affectionate toward each other, and where the bounds of propriety are observed, as an adult will be able, in all likelihood, to enter into a mature, positive relationship.

CULTURE

Cultural attitudes greatly influence how an adolescent can express sexuality, and they do so in several ways. First, culture assigns men and women specific roles. When these roles are sharply delimited, the choices open to the adolescent for expressing manhood or womanhood are few. On the other hand, cultural ambiguity about sexual behavior leaves adolescents with many options but little guidance. Similarly, the culture dictates how sexual feelings may be expressed. There are four basic types of cultures in this regard: sexually repressive, sexually restrictive, sexually permissive, and sexually supportive.[7] Each type of culture has a distinctive approach to the emergent sexuality of its youth.

A *sexually repressive culture* attempts to suppress sexuality. The Puritans of Colonial New England were an example of such a culture. Sexual play among the young was not allowed and premarital chastity was required. Sexuality was associated with guilt, fear, and anger. Sexual pleasure had little value.

A *sexually restrictive culture* also attempts to limit sexuality. Such cultures are common; the United States, in the first 60 years of the 20th century, is a fairly typical example. In such a culture, there is little sexual play in childhood, and premarital chastity is required of at least one of the sexes. Typically, these cultures are ambivalent about sex and tend to fear it, primarily for the problems that it can cause.

Tolerance of sexuality is characteristic of a *sexually permissive culture* where there are fewer formal prohibitions. Children may participate in sex play as long as it is not overt—as long as

adults do not see it. Sexual activity among adolescents and before marriage is the norm; sex is considered a normal and valued part of life. Although somewhat common in non-European, and some European, cultures, this approach to sexuality appeared in the United States in the early 1960s and lasted to the mid 1980s. Because of the associated problems (AIDS, other sexually transmitted diseases, and adolescent pregnancy) American culture may be reverting to a restrictive attitude toward sexuality.

Sexually supportive cultures have been especially common among the peoples of Oceania. These cultures cultivate sexuality. Sex is seen as indispensable for human happiness, and sexual experimentation is encouraged in the young. Customs and institutions supply sexual information and experience to young people of all ages, and there is no sexual latency period in a child's life.

The United States consists of a mix of cultures and, therefore, has a great variety of attitudes toward and opinions about child and adolescent sexuality. One of the problems American youths sometimes encounter is conflict between the culture in which they were raised and the cultures of others with whom they interact. One of the upshots of our "global village," produced by the media, is the blurring of the distinctions between the mores of many of the cultures in our country. Youths who spend a great deal of time in front of the television may much more readily question the values their natal culture imparts to them.

SOCIETY

In some instances, culture is uniform throughout society, but this is not the case in the United States, where various cultures blend into a harmonious (it is to be hoped) whole while each retains features important to it (a cultural salad bowl rather than a melting pot). With children growing up among so many—and at times disparate—cultures, conflicts between the sexuality values adolescents absorb from the family of origin and those that they confront in society at large are inevitable. Comfort and security with sexuality, as it learned in the home, might enable adolescents to negotiate the conflicting messages they confront as they mature.

For adolescents, one of the predominant sources of information about current societal norms of sexual roles and behaviors is the media, particularly television. The media exert a powerful influence on adolescents by exposing them to an adult world of which they were formerly unaware. Many parents abdicate their responsibility to teach their children about sex and sexuality; increasingly, television, movies, and magazines are the principal sources of information and about "normal" behavior.[8, 9]

No other leisure-time activity is more widely pursued than watching television, especially among children. Adolescents watch less television than children,[10] but what they do watch is heavily laden with messages about sex roles and sexual behaviors. The possible influence of media on adolescents' sexual behavior is discussed later.

The Development of Adolescent Sexuality

It is the *mix* of the influences described earlier that determines how an adolescent will develop as a sexual being, in terms of both self-image and behavior. To understand the sequence, it is necessary to understand basic adolescent development.

Adolescent development is categorized in three primary arenas: organic, cognitive, and psychosocial. *Organic development* is puberty, which is discussed in Chapter 5. *Cognitive development*, as delineated by Piaget, occurs by age-specific stages.[11] Children begin to think in an adult fashion at about the age of 12 years. Piaget calls this type of thinking *formal operational thought*. Full capacity to think in this manner is not attained, however, until at least age 15 or 16 years. Early and middle adolescents (10- to 13-year-olds and 14- to 16-year-olds, respectively) cannot be expected to function in adult fashion most of the time. To understand ideas, they need explicit examples. In the medical setting, for example, history taking must be specific and directive. In the same vein, instructions to a teenager should be very concrete.

Psychosocial development encompasses an adolescent's ability to view himself or herself realistically and to relate to others. A convenient way of understanding this facet of development is to divide it into four tasks that the adolescent must achieve before he or she can be said to have effectively entered adulthood:
1. Effective separation or *independence* from the family of origin
2. A realistic *vocational* goal
3. A mature level of *sexuality*
4. A realistic and positive *self-image*[12]

Sexuality refers to more than just the capacity to participate in physical sexual behavior. It includes the way a person views herself or himself as a woman or a man in our society and how that person relates to other women and men in general, and to one particular person specifically. Sexuality includes the ability of a person to enter into and to maintain an intimate relationship on a basis giving and trust.

Early adolescents express sexuality in ways that may seem humorous to adults but that are painful to the adolescents. Adolescents think a great deal about the opposite sex, but given appropriate adult supervision, rarely do much with their thoughts. Although they have many fantasies about the opposite sex and much contact in school, social contact occurs primarily in situations created by and supervised by adults. School dances are classic situations for the study of early expressions of adolescent sexuality. At junior-high dances, the girls form a mass in the middle of the dance floor that bounces in time to the music, while the boys, averaging a head shorter than the girls, circle around the outside and, now and then, dart toward the middle to "count coup." The girls try to ignore these forays while occasionally sending off "scouting" parties of at least three girls to the bathroom.

As boys and girls grow into middle adolescence, their efforts at relating to those to whom they are romantically inclined center more on group dating and social activities. Teenagers at this stage of development are more secure in their physical self-image and are more prone to spend time with others in their peer group. Normally, any romantic involvement they may have is with a partner who is of similar age and is characterized, not by the giving nature of a mature relationship, but by more selfish motivations. A girl is preoccupied with how her partner matches up to her image of the ideal "catch" and a boy with how far he can go sexually, with this girl. Feelings are intense and all-encompassing to the teenagers, involved. The partner, however, can never really match up to the image that the other has created, so the relationship has a very short life span by adult standards. By late adolescence, the young person usually has grown to the point where he or she can enter into a relationship in a more adult fashion. Such relationships are usually characterized by greater concern of the participants for the feelings and welfare of the other. The capacity for true intimacy has begun to develop, and the adolescents are capable of adult-type relationships. While this internal process is proceeding, it is subject to all the forces that I outlined earlier and to the conditioning the adolescent received as a child.

SEXUAL ACTIVITY

Adolescent sexuality, given all the influences on its development and given the many reasons

Table 18–1. Negative Consequences of Adolescent Sexuality

Premature sexual activity
Pregnancy
Sexually transmitted diseases
Sexual preference
Gender identity issues

why adolescents might want to experiment with this essentially adult behavior, can have many negative consequences. The first potentially negative consequence is participating in sexual intercourse. Other potential negative consequences, many of which stem from premature engagement in sexual activity, are pregnancy, sexually transmitted diseases, forced sex, and problems of gender preference and identity (Table 18–1). In this section the epidemiology of adolescent sexual activity is reviewed.

Before reviewing the data, it is important to consider which factors can influence an adolescent girl's sexual career. We know, for example, that the higher a mother has gone in her education, the later her daughter will begin to have sexual intercourse. We know also that girls who have menarche before age 12 are at greater risk for early onset of sexual activity. Religious affiliation and active religious involvement also help to delay onset of sexual activity, and girls whose families are not intact when they are 14 years

old may begin having sexual intercourse earlier. Other factors that may bear on age of sexual debut include socioeconomic status, whether the mother was a teen parent, degree of goal orientation, abuse of substances, peer pressure, media pressure, poor communication with parents, and poor discipline.[13]

Data on rates of sexual activity and on age of sexual debut are not as accurate as one would like. For example, the national Youth Risk Behavior Survey (YRBS) data from the Centers for Disease Control and Prevention are derived from high school students only, so age peers who are not in school are not included. Our knowledge of the behavior of younger teens and of those not in school must therefore come from other sources. Data from an urban population in Miami, Florida, show first intercourse beginning before age 12 (Table 18–2). YRBS data from 1995 and data from several other sources show that sexual activity increases with increasing age, a finding that is not altogether surprising (Figs. 18–1, 18–2). Here one can also see how many adolescents are using condoms. The Miami study also made the disturbing finding that as many as 24% of adolescents aged 12 to 13 years have already begun to have sexual intercourse.[14] Table 18–3, which combines data from several sources, gives a broader picture of adolescent sexual activity at various ages and in different American populations.[15] What is clear is that, no matter

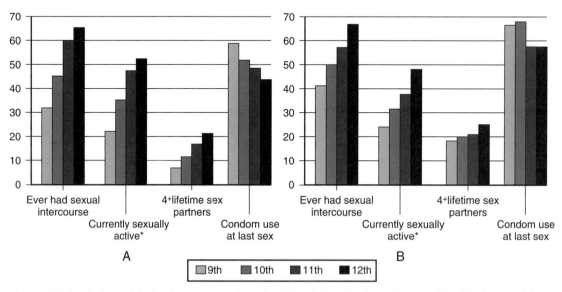

Figure 18–1. *A,* Sexual behavior among female U.S. high school students, 1995 (% by grade). *B,* Sexual behavior among male U.S. high school students, 1995 (% by grade). Asterisk indicates sexual intercourse during 3 months before survey. (Adapted from U.S. Department of Health and Human Services, Centers for Disease Control: Youth risk behavior surveillance—United States 1995. MMWR 1996; 45(SS-4):1.)

Table 18–2. Age of First Intercourse in an Urban Population (*n* = 1602)

Ever Had Intercourse?	59%: Yes
Age at First Intercourse (years old)	Percentage
<12	17
12–13	24
14–15	37
≥16	22
Total	100

Adapted from U.S. Department of Health and Human Services, Centers for Disease Control and Prevention: Sexual behaviors and drug use among youth in dropout-prevention programs—Miami, 1994. MMWR 1994; 43:873.

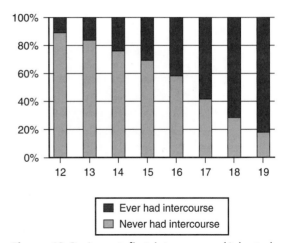

■ Ever had intercourse
□ Never had intercourse

Figure 18–2. Age at first intercourse. (Adapted from Blum RW: The State of Adolescent Health in Minnesota. Minneapolis: University of Minnesota, 1989.)

what their origin or socioeconomic status, many adolescents are sexually active (Fig. 18–3).[16]

Whether early adolescent sexual activity is linked to other adolescent risk behaviors depends on which population is examined. Among the general adolescent population, there is such a link (Fig. 18–4).[16] Among African-American adolescents, however, early sexual activity is not linked to other risk behaviors (Figs. 18–5, 18–6).[17] One other correlation that must be cited is that between early sexual debut in adolescent girls and forced intercourse: the earlier a girl starts her sexual career, the more likely it is that her first sexual experience was rape (Fig. 18–7).[18] Finally, adolescents who do not have sexual intercourse still may participate in sexual activities such as fellatio, cunnilingus, anal intercourse, and masturbation. The rates of these activities are shown in Figure 18–8.[19]

HOMOSEXUALITY

While a significant proportion of adolescents either engage in sexual activity with same sex partners or identify themselves as being gay or lesbian, little mention is made in healthcare texts of their specific developmental issues and healthcare needs.[20–25] Given that this is a pediatric and adolescent *gynecology* text, discussion will be limited to lesbian girls and young women.

Most recent estimates are that some 2% to 4% of adolescent and adult women are lesbians.[23, 25, 26] Many more may have engaged in same-sex sexual activity during their adolescence. Given the potential negative consequences of publicly acknowledging their homosexual orientation, many lesbian adolescents and women reveal themselves only to others in the gay community. The percentage of bisexual women is thought to be much smaller.

Although with regard to healthcare needs of lesbian adolescents, it is important to understand that the developmental issues these young

Table 18–3. Teenage Sexual Activity, % Sexually Active

		Age, (years)					
		13		14		15	
Study	Patients (*n*)	Male	Female	Male	Female	Male	Female
Zelnik & Kantner, 1979	1,717	14	2	35	19	52	44
Harris, 1986	1,000	11	10	35	22	57	53
National Survey of Adolescent Males, 1988	1,880	—	—	33	—	66	—
Blum, 1989	36,284	17	11	29	26	57	45
National Household Survey, 1990	536	6	3	29	37	67	56
National Longitudinal Survey of Youth, 1992	1,825	15	3	35	27	72	66
Youth Risk Behavior Survey, 1993	16,296	—	—	44	32	60	55
Youth Risk Behavior Survey, 1995	10,904	13	5	41	32	60	57

From Strasburger VC, Brown RT: Adolescent Medicine: A Practical Guide, 2nd ed. New York: Lippincott-Raven, 1998, p 153.

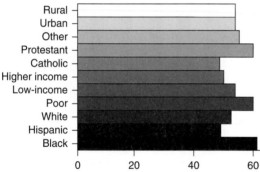

Figure 18–3. Percentage of adolescent women who ever had intercourse—1988. (Adapted from The Alan Guttmacher Institute: Sex and America's Teenagers. New York: Alan Guttmacher Institute, 1994, p 18.)

women face are common to all young women. Lesbian adolescents and young adults are subject to the same challenges that all adolescents face: developing independence, developing a mature sexuality, choosing an appropriate vocational focus, and achieving a realistic and positive self-image.[12] Their sexual orientation superimposes an additional developmental burden that can make traversing adolescence even more of a challenge. Like heterosexual adolescents, lesbian girls must cope with exposure to use of tobacco, drugs, and alcohol. They also are subject, probably even more so than their heterosexual peers, to depression and other psychological morbidity and suicidal ideation and suicide attempts.[27, 28] A contributing factor to apparently increased rates of depression, running away from home, and

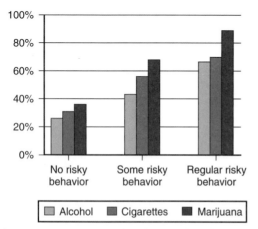

Figure 18–4. Sex and other risk behaviors. (Adapted from The Alan Guttmacher Institute: Sex and America's Teenagers. New York: Alan Guttmacher Institute, 1994, p 27.)

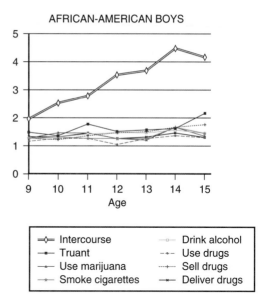

Figure 18–5. High-risk behavior among African American boys. (Adapted from Stanton B, Romer D, Ricardo I, et al: Early initiation of sex and its lack of association with risk behaviors among adolescent African-Americans. Pediatrics 1992; 13–19, with permission.)

suicide attempts is the stress associated with being gay. This stress includes ridicule from peers, the whole issue of "coming out" to family and friends and the public, and the fact of or fear of discrimi-

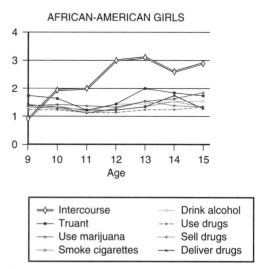

Figure 18–6. High-risk behavior among African American girls. (Adapted from Stanton B, Romer D, Ricardo I, et al: Early initiation of sex and its lack of association with risk behaviors among adolescent African-Americans. Pediatrics 1992; 13–19, with permission)

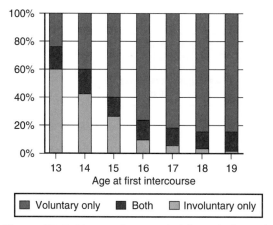

Figure 18–7. Very early sexual debut. (Adapted from The Alan Guttmacher Institute: Sex and America's Teenagers. New York: Alan Guttmacher Institute, 1994, p 28.)

nation in the work place. Figure 18–9 depicts the impact that stigma and prejudice can have on lesbian and gay youths. Stigmatization and prejudice toward lesbians can vary by status within a given racial, ethnic, or functional minority group as well.

The health care of lesbian girls should be no

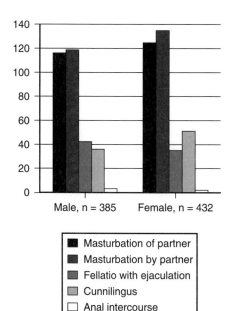

Figure 18–8. Sexual practices by gender of virginal high school adolescents. (Adapted from Schuster MA, Bell RM, Kanouse DE. The sexual practices of adolescent virgins: Genital sexual activities of high school students who have never had vaginal intercourse. Am J Public Health 1996; 86:1570–1576.)

different from that afforded any patient, either in quantity or quality. Any prejudice against gays and lesbians in clinicians should be acknowledged and overcome if the clinician is to provide good care to these patients. When such a prejudice cannot be surmounted, referral must be made to more sympathetic clinicians. Almost every major community in the United States has counselors and support groups for gay and lesbian youths and for their parents and families. The physician who cares for young women should have available phone numbers and addresses of such resources for patients who want to use them.

Lesbian girls are subject to the same health concerns as all other young women. They need anticipatory guidance for risk behaviors, discussion of developmental concerns, periodic physical evaluations, and acute illness care. The fact that they define themselves as lesbian does not mean that they have not had heterosexual relationships; therefore, they need screening for sexually transmitted diseases and Pap smears, just as do their heterosexual peers. Lesbian girls may need more in-depth mental health screening because of the added burden of growing up as "outsiders." Gay and lesbian youths may be more subject to alcohol abuse than their heterosexual peers because of the social importance of bars as safe gathering places for homosexuals. Therefore, the clinician should be familiar with effective drug and alcohol services that are known to be gay-friendly. Lesbians may also need to avail themselves of services from their physician and other health care workers for intervention with their families and for support while they are coming out.

The health care visit for a lesbian girl should be no different, in any way, from that for any young girl. Appropriate safeguards for confidentiality should be provided and communicated to the patient, and history should be sought in terms that assure a lesbian adolescent that revelation of her sexual orientation is accepted without reservation. When questioning about sexual activity, for example, the clinician must be sure to ask whether the patient has been sexually active with either girls or boys. In asking about relationships, the clinician should ask these questions: *Do you have a girlfriend or boyfriend?* and *Have you been, or are you, involved in a romantic relationship with a girl or boy?* When such questions are asked in a nonjudgmental manner, they signal to a girl who is gay or who is grappling with this issue, that it is okay to be open, because the clinician will be accepting. When a girl shows some confusion about her sexual orientation, the

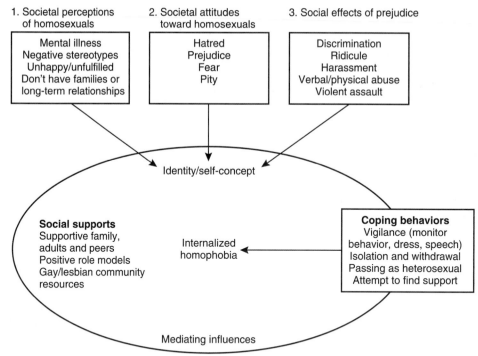

1. Societal perceptions of homosexuals

| Mental illness
Negative stereotypes
Unhappy/unfulfilled
Don't have families or
long-term relationships |

2. Societal attitudes toward homosexuals

| Hatred
Prejudice
Fear
Pity |

3. Social effects of prejudice

| Discrimination
Ridicule
Harassment
Verbal/physical abuse
Violent assault |

Identity/self-concept

Social supports
Supportive family,
adults and peers
Positive role models
Gay/lesbian community
resources

Internalized
homophobia

Coping behaviors
Vigilance (monitor
behavior, dress, speech)
Isolation and withdrawal
Passing as heterosexual
Attempt to find support

Mediating influences

Figure 18–9. Impact of stigma and prejudice (homophobia) on lesbian and gay identity. (Adapted from Ryan C, Futterman D. Experiences, vulnerabilities, and risks. Adolesc Med State Art Rev 1997; 8(2):227, with permission.)

clinician should help to reassure her that it sometimes take many years before a person is sure about this question. Mention should be made that, for any one person, sexual attraction can be either all heterosexual, all homosexual, or any gradation between.

Physical examination should be conducted in the appropriate manner. Although women who are exclusively homosexual have lower incidences of abnormal Pap smears and STDs, one cannot assume that a lesbian young woman has not had a sexual encounter with a man sometime in the past.[29] Indeed, she might be bisexual. Therefore, the physician or other clinician should afford the young woman access to routine pelvic examinations and Pap smears, applying the same criteria to these evaluations that are appropriate for any young woman.

Sexuality Education

The negative consequences of the expression by adolescents of their sexuality, such as adolescent pregnancy and STDs, particularly AIDS, have emphasized as never before the need for sex education. The American public, who overwhelmingly support such education for children and youth, understand this.[30] But, although no one disputes the need for our young people to be better educated in this area, what should constitute such education and where best to provide it are still being debated.

It is a given that sexuality is an essential component of all human beings. Our perceptions of ourselves as men and women color all of our relationships and influence many of our behaviors. With this in mind, it would seem logical that education about topics of sexuality would also take this broad focus. It should include not only the mechanics of sexual behavior but also material designed to help children and adolescents understand themselves as men and women and to help them learn how to express their sexuality in positive ways. Unfortunately, in most instances this is not the case. Traditionally sex education provided by parents has been limited to "the birds and the bees," in religious institutions, to "Don't do it until you're married," and in school, to the biology of reproduction. The other great sex educator in this country, the media (especially television), has dealt with what men and women are and how they behave toward each other, though mostly irresponsibly.[31]

If parents do teach their children and adolescents about sexuality, it is usually a cursory presentation that gives little information about relationships and behavior as men and as women. Instead, mechanical facts are conveyed, along with a dose of guilt.[32] Nevertheless, even though they may never mention the word *sex*, parents, by example, are the primary sexuality educators of their children. Parents want to be the sexuality educators of their children for the most part, but for several reasons they feel not up to the task: their own ignorance; their discomfort in discussing sexual issues; confusion about their personal beliefs, feelings, and attitudes; and potential conflict with their children over those same attitudes, feelings, values, and beliefs.[33] It seems that, were they trained properly in the role, parents could be their children's best source of sexuality education.

Because of parental default in this arena (for whatever reasons), it has devolved on the schools to be the primary providers of formal sex education in the United States. Most states require or otherwise encourage sex and/or AIDS education.[34] At least 60% of American teenagers receive some sex education during their school years.[35] Sex education in the schools definitely increases adolescents' knowledge about sex,[34] and it does not encourage them to initiate sexual activity.[36] Whether it influences behavior is not clear.[37–39]

Although most sex education courses include the essential facts of human reproduction and today most discuss AIDS and the major STDs, until recently fewer delved into contraception, and many made no mention of interpersonal relationships and acceptance of one's own sexuality.[34] One of the problems with sex education in the schools is that certain topics, such as contraception, are taught in high school to students whose initial sexual activity occurred in their elementary and middle school years.[40–42] Thus, these children are starting out with no information or with erroneous information passed to them by their peers. Kids with unreliable knowledge, or no knowledge, develop inappropriate attitudes about sex, and more often engage in high-risk sexual behavior.[42] Sexuality education in the early school years might help to alleviate this problem.

Although schools are increasingly providing sex education, the medium whereby children and adolescents get most of their information—good or bad—is the media, specifically television.[43] More teens feel pressure to have sex from media than from peers or partners.[44] Each year, television programs contain at least 14,000 sexual references, innuendos, and behaviors, few of which involve the use of birth control, self-control, abstinence, or issue of responsibility.[45] Soap operas,

a favorite of teenage girls, contain at least eight episodes of extramarital sex for every one of sex between married spouses. Public service announcements about AIDS are relatively common, but they make no mention about how to prevent AIDS while having sex (i.e., by using condoms). And, still, we have no advertisements for contraceptives on network television.[46]

Whatever the sex education bias of the educator—abstinence or comprehensive instruction and preparation—all agree that education is needed and that it is best provided in the home. When other industrialized countries have just as much teen sexual activity as does the United States, but so much lower rates of adolescent pregnancy and sexually transmitted disease, we have to look long and hard at our system. We then have to try to develop a uniform approach that takes into account the many cultural differences in our society.

Comment must be made about abstinence only and abstinence-preferred education. With funding from the federal government, more and more states are trying to limit all sexuality education to promoting abstinence only.[47] The dangers of this kind of education are, first, that it ignores teens who already are sexually active and who want information about responsible sexual activity, and, second, that it engenders guilt in the half of high school students who are sexually active. There is no clear evidence that it works.[48]

The author would like to thank Harold E. Regan, Jr., M.A., for his assistance in preparing, proofreading, and editing the manuscript.

REFERENCES

1. Chilman CS: Adolescent Sexuality in a Changing American Society—Social and Psychological Perspectives. Bethesda, Md: U.S. Department of Health, Education, and Welfare, Center for Population Research, 1980, p. 3.
2. LeGuin UK: The Left Hand of Darkness. New York: Ace Books, 1969.
3. Moore RE: Normal childhood and early adolescent sexuality: A psychologist's perspective. Semin Adolesc Med 1985; 1:97–100.
4. Strasburger VC: Normal adolescent sexuality: A physician's perspective. Semin Adolesc Med 1985; 1:101–115.
5. Gordon S, Scales P, Everly K: The Sexual Adolescent, 2nd ed. North Scituate, Mass: Duxbury Press, 1979.
6. Hibbard RA, Orr DP: Incest and sexual abuse. Semin Adolesc Med 1985; 1:153–164.
7. Currier RL: Juvenile sexuality in global perspective. In Constantine LL, Martinson FM (eds): Children and Sex, New Findings, New Perspectives. Boston: Little, Brown, 1981, pp 9–19.
8. Strasburger VC, Comstock GA (eds): Adolescents and the Media. Adolesc Med: State Art Rev 1993; 4(3).
9. Strasburger VC, Brown RT: Adolescent Medicine: A

Practical Guide, 2nd ed. New York: Lippincott-Raven, 1998.

10. AC Nielsen Co: Report on television. 1984.
11. Piaget J: The intellectual development of the adolescent. In Caplan G, Lebovici E (eds): Adolescence—Psychosocial Perspectives. New York: Basic Books, 1969.
12. Brown RT: Growth and Development. In Strasburger VC, Brown RT: Adolescent Medicine: A Practical Guide, 2nd ed. New York: Lippincott-Raven, 1998, p 1–22.
13. Braverman PK, Strasburger VC: Adolescent sexual activity. Clin Pediatr 1996; 33(2):100–109.
14. U.S. Department of Health and Human Services, Centers for Disease Control and Prevention: Sexual behaviors and drug use among youth in dropout-prevention programs—Miami, 1994. MMWR 1994; 43:873.
15. Strasburger VC: Adolescent sexuality and health-related problems. In Strasburger VC, Brown RT (eds): Adolescent Medicine: A Practical Guide, 2nd ed. New York: Lippincott-Raven, 1998, p 151–327.
16. The Alan Guttmacher Institute: Sex and America's Teenagers. New York: Alan Guttmacher Institute, 1994 p 19.
17. Stanton B, Romer D, Ricardo I, et al: Early initiation of sex and its lack of association with risk behaviors among adolescent African-Americans. Pediatrics 1993; 92:13–19.
18. Harlap S, Kost K, Forest JD: Preventing Pregnancy, Protecting Health: A New Look at Birth Control Choices in the United States. New York: Alan Guttmacher Institute, 1991.
19. Schuster MA, Bell RM, Kanouse DE: The sexual practices of adolescent virgins: Genital sexual activities of high school students who have never had vaginal intercourse. Am J Public Health 1996; 86:1570–1576.
20. Bidwell RJ: Sexual orientation and gender identity. In Friedman SB, Fisher M, Schonberg SK (eds): Comprehensive Adolescent Health Care. St. Louis, Mo: Quality Medical Publishing, 1992.
21. Kinsey AC, Pomeroy WB, Martin CE: Sexual Behavior in the Human Male. Philadelphia: WB Saunders, 1948.
22. Kinsey AC, Pomeroy WB, Martin CE, Gebbard PH: Sexual Behavior in the Human Female. Philadelphia: WB Saunders, 1953.
23. Laumann EO, Gagnon JH, Michael RT, Michaels S: The Social Organization of Sexuality: Sexual Practices in the United States. Chicago: University of Chicago Press, 1994.
24. Rathus SA, Nevid JS, Fichner-Rathus L: Human Sexuality in a World of Diversity. Boston: Allyn and Bacon, 1993.
25. Sell RL, Wells J, Wypij D: The prevalence of homosexual behavior and attraction in the United States, the United Kingdom and France: Results of national population-based samples. Arch Sex Behav 1995; 24:235.
26. Ryan C, Futterman D: Lesbian and gay adolescents—identity development. Adolesc Med State Art Rev 1997; 8(2):211–23.
27. Ryan C, Futterman D: Adolescent mental health concerns. Adolesc Med State Art Rev 1997; 8(2):263–274.
28. Garofalo R, Wolf RC, Kessel S, et al: The association between health risk behaviors and sexual orientation among a school-based sample of adolescents. Pediatrics 1998; 101(5):895–902.

29. Zenilman J: Sexually transmitted diseases in homosexual adolescents. J Adolesc Health Care 1988; 9(2):129–138.
30. Louis Harris and Associates: Public Attitudes Toward Teenage Pregnancy, Sex Education and Birth Control New York: 1988, p 24.
31. Strasburger VC: Adolescent sexuality and the media. Pediatr Clin North Am 1989; 36:747–773.
32. Kelly GF: Parents as sex educators. In Brown L (ed): Sex Education in the Eighties. New York: Plenum, 1981, p 101–113.
33. Vincent ML, Clearie AF, Schluchter MD: Reducing adolescent pregnancy through school and community-based education. JAMA 1987; 257:3382–3386.
34. The Alan Guttmacher Institute: Risk and Responsibility: Teaching Sex Education in America's Schools Today. New York: 1989.
35. Kenney AM, Guardado S, Brown L: What states and school districts want students to be taught about pregnancy prevention and AIDS. Fam Plann Perspect 1989; 21(2):56–64.
36. Marsiglio W, Mott FL: The impact of sex education on sexual activity and contraceptive use, and premarital pregnancy among American teenagers. Fam Plann Persect 1986; 18:151–162.
37. Anderson JD, Kann L, Holtzman D, et al: HIV/AIDS knowledge and sexual behavior among high school students. Fam Plann Perspect 1990; 22(6):252–255.
38. Scott-Jones D, Turner SL: Sex education, contraceptive and reproductive knowledge, and contraceptive use among black adolescent females. J Adolesc Res 1988; 3:171–187.
39. Laszlo AT, Johnson J (eds): AIDS Education for High-Risk Youth: Assessing the Present, Planning for the Future. Rockville, Md: Community Research Branch, National Institute on Drug Abuse, 1990, pp 41–42.
40. Banks IW, Wilson PI: Appropriate sex education for black teens. Adolescence 1989; 93:233–245.
41. Brooks-Gunn J, Furstenberg FF Jr: Adolescent sexual behavior. Am Psychol 1989; 44:249–257.
42. Melchert T, Burnett KF: Attitudes, knowledge, and sexual behavior of high-risk adolescents: Implications for counseling and sexuality education. J Counsel Develop 1990; 68:293–298.
43. Sprafkin J, Silverman LT: Sex on prime-time. In Schwartz M (ed): TV and Teens. Reading, Mass: Addison-Wesley, 1982, p 130–135.
44. Roper Starch Worldwise, Inc: Teens Talk About Sex: Adolescent Sexuality in the 90s. New York: SIECUS, 1994.
45. Harris L and Associates: Sexual Material on American Network Television During the 1987–1988 Season. New York: Planned Parenthood Federation of America, 1988.
46. Strasburger VC: Adolescents and the Media: Medical and Psychological Impact. Thousand Oaks, Calif: SAGE, 1995.
47. SIECUS Report: Pressure mounts for abstinence-only-until-marriage programs. 1998; 5(2):1–2.
48. Jacobs CD, Wolf EM: School sexuality education and adolescent risk-taking behavior. J School Public Health 1995; 64(3):91–95.

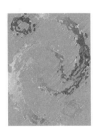

Chapter 19
Adolescent Contraception

RAMONA I. SLUPIK

There are 25 million teenagers in the United States; 4 million are sexually active. More than 1 million females aged 15 to 19 years become pregnant each year, and the vast majority of these pregnancies are unintended.[1] Fifty percent of young women have had sex by age 17.4, and 50% of male teens report having intercourse by age 16.6.[2] By their 18th birthday, 56% of female adolescents and 73% of males have made their sexual debut ("coitarche").[3] Factors that increase the likelihood for early sexual activity in female teens include lower socioeconomic status, living in a single-parent household, engaging in other risky behavior such as using alcohol or drugs, and having peers who are already sexually active. For young men and African-American women, the pace and timing of pubertal development is also a strong predictor (Table 19–1).[3]

The younger the teen is at the time of coitarche, the more likely that the sexual episode was not voluntary. In one study, 74% of young women who had intercourse before age 14 and 60% of those who had sex before age 15 reported being forced into the act.[4] The same factors that influence the likelihood that a teen will engage in sexual intercourse at an early age are also associated with lower contraceptive use. Risk-taking behaviors such as substance abuse and unprotected sex tend to be linked. Teens who engage in risky behavior are more likely to be depressed or less able to handle the stresses of adolescence. Lower socioeconomic status and single parentage are often the sequelae of similar sexual behavior in the parent and thus may be perceived as condoned. Teenagers who live in poor urban neighborhoods, where violence and child neglect are everyday occurrences, may also feel "doomed" to a lifestyle where taking risks is common.

The consequences of early sexual activity without contraception are well-known. These youngsters are more likely to experience an unwanted pregnancy at an earlier age, thus increasing the chances that they will drop out of, and never return to, school. Then their prospects are only low-paying job opportunities and a future as a low-income, single parent. Thus, the cycle often perpetuates itself.

The goals of the healthcare practitioner in the 21st century should be to increase awareness of younger teens and educate them in the sequelae of early sexual activity, particularly unprotected sex. Low-cost confidential contraceptive services, and information on and treatment of sexually transmitted diseases (STDs) must be provided in a private, reassuring, and confidential setting. Healthcare providers should also review the benefits unique to various types of contraception with each adolescent, so that, together, they can select the best method for her and her partner.[5–7]

In the area of sexuality, ignorance and denial remain prominent among our nation's dominant traits. Despite advances in scientific technology and research, the topic of sexual intercourse is taboo in most American households, and few schools have an adequate sex education program.[8] As a result, most United States youths first learn about sex outside the home, and, as a consequence, their attitudes toward birth control are influenced less by parental standards than by their misinformed, misguided peer group. This unwillingness on the part of elders to confront the issue of sex education persists, despite the fact that numerous studies have demonstrated that teenagers armed with basic knowledge of reproductive biology and contraceptive methods are less likely to be sexually promiscuous, be-

Table 19–1. Factors That Increase the Risk of Early Sexual Activity

Low socioeconomic status
Living in a single-parent home
Engaging in risky behavior: cigarettes, alcohol, drugs
Having sexually active peers
In some cases, early or rapid pubertal development

come pregnant, or contract STDs.[3] The home in which sexual behavior is discussed openly and honestly, with parents who are receptive to the special needs of their adolescent, is much less likely to have to endure the heartbreak of a youngster's undesired, out-of-wedlock pregnancy, dropping out of school, or running away.

Factors to keep in mind when choosing a contraceptive method for an adolescent include:

1. Acceptability: Is it a method the patient will continue to use consistently?

2. Effectiveness of method and frequency of intercourse: Does the method lend itself to the "unplanned" coital episode often seen in this age group?

3. Number of partners/STD concerns: Is the patient adequately protected?

4. Cost/access to medical care: Can the patient afford the method for the long term? Motivation/self-discipline of patient and male partner: Will a need to interrupt foreplay result in nonuse of the method?

5. Safety/risk: Will short-term convenience result in long-term drawbacks?

6. Personal religious and/or parental philosophy: Will it influence usage?

The healthcare professional's pragmatic approach to the individual adolescent and her lifestyle will result in a choice that maximizes that method's effectiveness and the girl's continuing use. It is essential to foster a supportive attitude of trust and confidentiality; encouraging follow-up ensures the patient's satisfaction with her chosen method, early detection of side effects or complications, and the chance to switch to another type of contraception when appropriate.

COMBINED ORAL CONTRACEPTIVE PILLS

Oral contraceptives are the method of choice for many United States teenagers.[9] Advantages include its effectiveness rate (92% to 97%, even with an occasional missed or late pill) and the lack of requirement for interruption of foreplay or the cooperation of the male partner. Multiple other noncontraceptive benefits of the pill have often been cited but generally are not appreciated by younger women (Table 19–2).[10, 11] Most notable is the recent approval by the FDA of one oral contraceptive pill (OCP), 35 μg ethinyl estradiol with 180 mg norgestimate for days 1 to 7; 215 mg days 8-14, and 250 mg days 15 to 21 for the treatment of acne, even when contraception is not the primary goal.[12] As acne and hirsu-

Table 19–2. Noncontraceptive Health Benefits of Oral Contraceptives

Increased menstrual cycle regularity
Decreased incidence of dysmenorrhea, menorrhagia, iron-deficiency anemia, dysfunctional bleeding, premenstrual syndrome
Decreased risk of benign breast disease
Decreased risk of pelvic inflammatory disease (and sequelae, including ectopic pregnancy)
Decreased risk of functional ovarian cysts
Decreased risk of acne and hirsutism
Decreased risk of ovarian cancer
Decreased risk of endometrial cancer
Decreased risk of colon cancer
Improved bone density
Decreased risk of rheumatoid arthritis

tism are prevalent in the teenage years, this may prove to be the pill of choice for adolescents with these attendant difficulties. In general, pills containing a low androgenic progestin, such as norgestimate or desogestrel, are preferred, especially for this age group (Table 19–3).

Furthermore, the common use of lower-dose pills (i.e., those that contain no more than 35 μg of ethinyl estradiol) has rendered former contraindications irrelevant. At the present time, compliant teens with homozygous sickle cell disease, mitral valve prolapse without regurgitation, and controlled hypertension or diabetes mellitus (without vascular or renal complications or retinopathy) and without other risk factors such as smoking, may safely use low-dose combined OCPs.[13, 14]

All adolescents should be thoroughly counseled on the first visit to encourage acceptance and minimize the doubts inherent in the selection of any birth control method. Positive presensitization like this is best accomplished by addressing questions before they are asked, such as those about weight gain and breakthrough bleeding. Teens who are reassured that a low-dose oral contraceptive pill will not cause weight gain, and in fact will provide multiple other noncontraceptive benefits, are much more likely to continue to take their pills over the long term.[7, 11, 15] For example, young women who experience relief of severe dysmenorrhea with the pill are eight times more likely to be consistent OCP users.[16]

The major drawback to OCPs is that the girl must be motivated to take a pill every day. Even without perfect compliance, however, the pill is somewhat forgiving: the highest reported accidental pregnancy rates in less than perfect users in the United States are 8% (i.e., 92% effectiveness).[17] Better than average users are cited as

Table 19–3. Oral Contraception Formulations

Brand Name	Manufacturer	Estrogen	Dose (µg)	Cycle Days	Progestin	Dose (mg)	Cycle Days
	*Monophasic°: Estrogen, 20–35 µg ("low-dose")*						
Brevicon	Syntex	EE	35	1–21	NET	0.5	1–21
Demulen	Searle	EE	35	1–21	EDDA	1.0	1–21
Desogen 35	Rugby Organon	EE	30	1–21	DES	0.15	1–21
Levlen	Berlex	EE	30	1–21	LNG	0.15	1–21
Loestrin 1/20	Parke-Davis	EE	20	1–21	NETA	1.0	1–21
Loestrin Fe 1/20†	Parke-Davis	EE	20	1–21	NETA	1.0	1–21
Loestrin 1.5/30	Parke-Davis	EE	30	1–21	NETA	1.5	1–21
Loestrin Fe 1.5/30°	Parke-Davis	EE	30	1–21	NETA	1.5	1–21
Lo/Ovral	Wyeth-Ayerst	EE	30	2–21	NG	0.3	1–21
Modicon	Ortho	EE	35	1–21	NET	0.5	1–21
Nordette	Wyeth-Ayerst	EE	30	1–21	LNG	0.15	1–21
Norinyl 1 + 35	Syntex	EE	35	1–21	NET	1.0	1–21
Ortho-Novum 1/35	Ortho	EE	35	1–21	NET	1.0	1–21
Ovcon 35	Mead-Johnson	EE	35	1–21	NET	0.4	1–21
Marvelon	Wagner-Caileut	EE	35	1–21	NET	0.5	1–21
Mercilon		EE	20	1–21	DES	0.15	1–21
Minulet		EE	30	1–21	GES	0.075	1–21
Ortho-Cept	Ortho	EE	30	1–21	DES	0.15	1–21
	*Monophasic°: Estrogen, 50 µg*						
Demulen 1/50	Searle	EE	50	1–21	EDDA	1.0	1–21
Genora		EE	50	1–21	NET	1.0	1–21
Nalova 1/50	Searle	EE	50	1–21	NET	2.0	1–21
Norethin 1/50	Roberts	EE	50	1–21	NET	1.0	1–21
Norinyl 1/50	Syntex	ME	50	1–21	NET	1.0	1–21
Norlestrin 1/50	Parke-Davis	EE	50	1–21	NETA	1.0	1–21
Norlestrin Fe 1/50†	Parke-Davis	EE	50	1–21	NETA	1.0	1–21
Ortho-Novum 1/50	Ortho	ME	50	1–21	NET	1.0	1–21
Ovcon 50	Mead Johnson	EE	50	1–21	NET	1.0	1–21
Ovral	Wyeth-Ayerst	EE	50	1–21	NG	0.5	1–21
	*Biphasic°*						
Ortho-Novum 10/11	Ortho	EE	35	1–21	NET	0.5	1–10
						1.0	11–21
Ortho-Novum 7/7/7	Ortho	EE	35	1–21	NET	0.5	1–7
						0.75	8–14
						1.0	15–21
	*Triphasic*						
Tri-Levlen	Berlex	EE	30	1–6	LNG	0.5	1–6
			40	7–11		0.075	7–11
			30	12–21		0.125	12–21
Tri-Norinyl	Syntex	EE	35	1–7	NET	0.5	1–7
			35	8–16		1.0	8–16
			35	17–21		0.5	17–21
Triphasil	Wyeth-Ayerst	EE	30	1–6	LNG	0.5	1–6
			40	7–11		0.075	7–11
			30	12–21		0.125	12–21
Tri-Minulet		EE°	30	1–6	LNG	0.05	1–6
			40	7–11		0.075	7–11
			30	12–21		0.125	12–21
Tri-Nova		EE°	30	1–6	LNG	0.05	1–6
			40	7–11		0.075	7–11
			30	12–21		0.125	12–21
Ortho Cyclen	Ortho	EE	35	1–7	NGM	0.180	1–7
				8–15		0.215	8–14
				15–21		0.280	16–21
Mircette	Organon	EE	20	1–21	DSG	0.15	1–21
			10	24–28			
	*Progestin Only*						
Micronor‡	Ortho				NET	0.35	
Nor-Q.D.§	Syntex				NET	0.35	
Ovrette§	Wyeth-Ayerst				NG	0.075	

°All are available in 21- or 28-day pill packages.
†Last seven pills in 28-day pack contain 75 mg ferrous fumarate.
‡Available in 28-day pill package.
§Available in 42-day pill package.
DES, Desogestrel; EDDA, ethynodiol diacetate; EE, ethinyl estradiol; GES, gestodene; LNG, levonorgestrel; ME, mestranol; NET, norethindrone; NETA, norethindrone acetate; NG, norgestrel; NGM, norgestimate.

having a 4% mean pregnancy rate, and perfect-use pregnancy rates are still less than 1%, even with low-dose pills (i.e., not more than 35 μg of ethinyl estradiol).[18]

As always, OCP users should be counseled to take a "belt and suspenders" approach to their sexual activity: using oral contraceptives to prevent pregnancy and a latex condom with spermicide to protect against STDs.[15, 19]

There are a few conditions in which the use of a 50-μg OCP containing estrogen should be considered: namely, long-term use of drugs that induce the liver's cytochrome P_{450} enzyme system and thus speed up estrogen metabolism, thus lowering the circulating estrogen levels and the resultant efficacy of the oral contraceptive. The antiseizure medications phenytoin, phenobarbital, primidone, ethosuximide, and carbamazepine; the antitubercular agent rifampin; and the antifungal griseofulvin are included in this category.[20, 21]

ACNE

Adolescents with acne experience not only its physical effects but also oftentimes they must deal with its psychological aspects. To this concern, oral contraceptives have become an integral part of management of acne. Work published by a number of clinicians has established the efficacy of androgen suppression and clinical improvement of acne. A number of progestins have been evaluated, including work reported by Lucky and co-workers, who noted triphasic preparations with norgestimate and 35 μg of ethinyl estradiol had a significantly greater decrease in mean percent total acne lesions.[21a] Their study design was a prospective randomized clinical trial. Hence, the strength of recommendation was Level I of the Bradford Hill Evidence–based medicine categorizing.[21b] Similar supporting data were provided by Redmond and associates in the obstetrical and gynecological literature.[21c] The Food and Drug Administration has added treatment of acne to the labeling of this oral contraceptive.

Subsequent to these studies, 20 μg preparations have been shown to be efficacious in treating acne. Specifically, levonorgestrel, 100 μg, and ethinyl estradiol, 20 μg, in a double-blind, placebo controlled clinical trial of 350 patients 14 years of age or older, were noted to result in significant (p .05) improvement in total, inflammatory, and noninflammatory lesion scores. The study evaluated patients over a 6-month period.[21d]

PROGESTIN-ONLY PILL

The progestin-only pill available in the United States today, also known as the *mini-pill*, contains either 0.35 mg norethindrone or 0.75 mg norgestrel. Each pack contains 28 active tablets, which are taken one a day, continuously, unlike other OCPs. Its contraceptive mechanism is similar to that of combined OCPs in some respects: altered, thickened cervical mucus and a progestational effect on the endometrium to prevent implantation. Ovulation is suppressed only 60% of the time, however, so the failure rate is higher than those of combined OCPs—about three pregnancies per 100 woman-years in younger women (as compared with 0.3 per 100 woman-years in women older than 40). It is estimated that half of these pregnancies are due to user failure. The patient must be counseled to take the pill at the same time every day, and if she misses the hour by 3 hours or more, she should use a backup method of contraception for 48 hours.[20] Irregular pill taking may also give rise to a higher than usual incidence of breakthrough bleeding.[21]

Despite these inconveniences, the progestin-only pill is still the contraceptive method of choice for young, breastfeeding mothers. The higher prolactin level during lactation enhances the antiovulatory effect and lowers the failure rate.[20] These young women often begin coital activity before the first postpartum visit, when traditionally contraceptive counseling is begun. The progestin-only pill is approved for initiating at 6 weeks postpartum for patients who are breast-feeding full time, and at 3 weeks after delivery for patients who are breast-feeding part-time or supplementing. These U.S. Food and Drug Administration (FDA) and package labeling indications are designed to reduce the rate of unintended pregnancies in young women, who may ovulate as early as 3 to 4 weeks after delivery, a time when most either assume they are unable to conceive or have not yet had a chance to resume their "usual" contraceptive method.

The progestin-only pill is also useful in medical conditions where estrogen is either absolutely or theoretically contraindicated. In contrast to older age groups, these conditions are rare in adolescents, but they include active thrombophlebitis or thromboembolic disease (unless anticoagulation therapy is used); and severe systemic lupus erythematosus (due to the hypothetically increased risk of exacerbation of vascular disease). Additional contraindications to estrogen include uncontrolled diabetes mellitus with vascular complications (e.g., retinal changes, proteinuria) and active liver disease (because of the theoretical risk that an injured liver will be incompetent to metabolize estrogen) the result being hypercoagulability.[22] There may also be an advantage to minimizing or eliminating estrogen altogether when prescribing contraceptives for young women with classic migraine accompanied by focal neurologic complaints, theoretically to minimize the chance of microvascular thrombus formation in vulnerable areas.[23]

EMERGENCY CONTRACEPTION

Emergency contraception (EC) is a postcoital method of pregnancy prevention. The availability of EC reduces the number of unintended pregnancies, and subsequently, the abortion rate. This is a particular problem with teens. EC is designed primarily for use in an isolated emergency. It is also used for adolescents who have intercourse only infrequently but is not recommended for such use, as a consequence is menstrual cycle disturbances and irregular bleedings. Because EC does not prevent all pregnancies, this regimen is no substitute for regular use of oral contraceptives, but EC definitely has a place in family planning and fertility regulation in adolescents.

The most common method used as EC is an altered dose of an ordinary OCP. In 1977, Dr. Yuzpe reported prescribing two tablets of Ovral taken within 72 hours after intercourse, and a second dose 12 hours later. He reported only one pregnancy among 608 women so treated.[24] Many other studies confirmed the efficacy of this method; the failure rate was 1.5% to 2%.[25-29] Despite the efficacy of this method, its use is rather limited.

To stem the tide of unintended pregnancies, some physicians began to evaluate ways to increase the availability and utilization of EC. Some began to question the limiting nature of the Yuzpe regimen.[30] Grou and Rodriguez reviewed the literature looking for evidence supporting the current 72-hour time limit for treatment. From their retrospective data review, they concluded that, theoretically, the time limit could be extended. They recommended large-scale clinical trials to investigate changing the 72-hour time limit.[30]

A 1988 study evaluated the knowledge and use of EC among health professionals in Tower Hamlets.[31] Eighty-five percent of primary care physicians responded, and 91% of them had received requests for postcoital contraception within the previous 6 months. Only a third of general practitioners made information about postcoital contraception available in their offices. Family planning physicians and nurses had the most accurate knowledge to ensure appropriate prescribing and to inform their women patients of this method.

A telephone survey examined the availability of EC at college health centers in the mid-Atlantic United States.[32] Of the 124 completed responses, 43 schools (35%) reported distributing EC. The major reasons the schools listed for not distributing EC pills (81, or 65%) were inadequate staffing, religious convictions, no perceived need, and availability of the same service from a source in the local community.

Similarly, a national survey of adolescent health experts found that the majority of physicians who prescribe EC do so infrequently and that most physicians cited lack of demand for the limited use of EC. Furthermore, fewer than half of these experts regularly counsel patients about EC during routine health visits, and only a few advise virginal teens of its availability.[33]

Another study evaluated the knowledge, attitudes, and EC practices of general practitioners in New South Wales.[34] The authors compared two randomly selected groups of physicians, 100 rural and 100 urban general practitioners (GPs). Rural GPs were more knowledgeable about EC than the urban doctors (95% versus 78%), and more women than men knew about it. More urban GPs frequently prescribed EC (26% versus 6%) and female GPs prescribed it more readily than male GPs (22% versus 12%). There was great variation in the prescribed regimens, especially among rural GPs. Twenty-five percent of urban GPs and 31% of rural GPs did not offer women information about EC, whereas 16% of both groups included such information in any discussion of contraceptive options, and 18% gave information about emergency contraception as a backup to barrier methods. The study highlighted the need to educate both the public and healthcare providers about EC.

The small demand may be due in part to misconceptions about or ignorance of how ECs work. Harper and Ellertson evaluated the knowledge of and perceptions about EC pills among college-aged students.[35] They conducted focus group discussions with the students who had easy access to EC. They found that basic awareness about the method was high, although knowledge of the details of appropriate use, such as the window of opportunity, the level of effectiveness, and the possible side effects was wanting. Approval of the method was widespread among both female and male students. Many of their concerns stemmed from incomplete information about how the regimen works. Students noted how rarely EC pills are discussed and were curious to know more. They asked for routine education in the method and more general discussion.

In a follow-up study, the same authors conducted telephone interviews with 550 undergraduate and graduate students in Princeton, who were selected randomly for participation in the survey.[36] The response rate was 82%. The investigators found that basic awareness and approval of EC were widespread, yet respondents lacked detailed knowledge, which did prompt health-related and ethical misgivings about it. Respondents with accurate information, especially those who knew that the therapy is a large dose of regular OCPs and that side effects were generally minor, were significantly more likely than others to report a favorable attitude. Many students confused the Yuzpe regimen with the abortifacient RU 486. Students reported that discussion of the method is rare, and many wanted to know more about it.

Other investigators attempting to identify barriers to the use of EC examined knowledge about and perceived availability of EC.[37] They interviewed 100 women who sought termination of pregnancy and 100 women who wanted contraceptive advice. Only 7% of women had used EC in the month they conceived. When asked why they had not used EC, 38% said they had not heard of it and 41% did not know where to obtain it. Approximately 50% knew the correct interval for effective use of EC. Sixty-two percent attending the abortion clinics would have used EC if they had had a supply at home, and 57% said they would have used it had it been available over the counter. The discrepancy between the numbers of women who knew of EC (72%) and the numbers who used it to try to prevent pregnancy (7%) indicates that there are barriers to obtaining and using the emergency contraceptive pill.[37]

Wessel and Buscher reported on 150 women who requested EC.[38] Eighty percent of them used another method of contraception and requested EC because they believed their regular method had failed. "Condom accidents" accounted for 70% of the failures. The authors concluded that the intention to prevent an unwanted pregnancy through EC indicates a more responsible attitude toward sexuality and that the popularity of EC may increase.[38]

George and coworkers attempted to assess women's knowledge of EC.[39] They distributed a questionnaire to 1290 women aged 16 to 50 years. More than three quarters of the women had heard of EC; these were mainly women who used contraception, who had relatively more education, or who were not Muslim. Only 53% of barrier method users knew that EC could be used as a backup when other methods failed. Only a fifth of women had heard about it from their GP or another health professional, whereas half had obtained their information from the media. They concluded that healthcare providers should routinely provide information on EC to users of barrier methods of contraception.

In a study by Savonius and coworkers, 200 women who applied for legal abortion within the first trimester of pregnancy were interviewed.[40] Of all of the women interviewed, 93% claimed to have adequate knowledge of contraception. At the time of conception, 11.5% were using safe methods (OCPs 8%; IUDs 3.5%), 63% used less safe methods, and 26% used no contraception. Of the condom users, 76.7% reported that the condom broke or slipped off or that they had not used condoms consistently. EC might have prevented some of these unintended pregnancies.

Some investigators examined the feasibility and effectiveness of telephone follow-up on the use of EC at a college health center.[41] They made 264 telephone calls to 97 women who had received EC and were successful in reaching 65 (67%) of them. The women reported a high rate of compliance with the medical regimen—and very few side effects from EC. A majority said that EC did not affect their ability to pursue daily activities. On weighing the (relatively few) problems after EC distribution against the time, effort, and cost required to reach just over two thirds of the women, the researchers concluded that EC telephone follow-up procedure was neither cost-effective nor particularly useful.

Other products have been shown to be effective EC. Timed-release pellets of levonorgestrel (LNG) were implanted subdermally in mice after the animals had mated and ovulated but before implantation of embryos would have occurred.[42] Mice in some groups were sacrificed on day 14 of gestation, and numbers of fetuses and resorption sites were counted; mice in other groups were allowed to carry to term. Pellets designed to release 5 mg of hormone in 90 days were totally effective in preventing uterine implantation of embryos. Although, when administered on day 2, the 5-mg pellets did not prevent embryos from implanting in all cases, they prevented pregnancies from going to term by causing resorption of the embryos that did implant. When the pellets were implanted on day 3 of the postcoital period, implantation of embryos occurred and fetuses were carried to term. Results of the study indicate that subdermal implants of LNG inserted postcoitally prevent uterine implantation of embryos in mice when the implants are inserted *before day 3* of the postcoital period.

A study investigated the potential postcoital contraceptive mechanisms of the crude extract of Sri Lankan marine red algae, *Gelidiella acerosa*, in rats.[43] The dose was 1000 mg/kg per day and the route of administration oral. The results showed that the crude extract possessed potent postcoital contraceptive activity when administered on days 7 to 8 of pregnancy and, so, had a narrow window of opportunity. The postcoital contraceptive activity was postimplantation, loss or fetal death (89%), between days 9 and 14 of gestation. The extract was not estrogenic, or antiestrogenic, or a stressor but it appeared to be antiprogestational (i.e., it reduced ovarian progesterone output). It has been suggested that the crude extract may reduce ovarian progesterone release, possibly via antiplatelet and PGE_2-depressing activity. Another study showed that a hexane extract of the seeds of *Nigella sativa* L. has similar activity (Table 19–4).[44]

In conclusion, the traditional Yuzpe method of EPC has been thoroughly studied and is regarded as safe and well-tolerated. After a pregnancy test (home or office) to rule out a preexisting gestation, two combined OC tablets containing 50 µg of ethinyl estradiol should be administered as soon as possible, preferably within 72 hours, although this is not an absolute limit. Two more tablets should be taken 12 hours later. The major side effect, nausea, can be avoided by advising the patient to take an antinausea medication (e.g., OTC dimenhydrinate, i.e., Dramamine) 30 minutes before the OC doses. Victims of sexual assault and others at risk for STDs should still visit their healthcare practitioner's office, but they should not put off institution of ECP.

DYSFUNCTIONAL UTERINE BLEEDING

Anovulatory uterine bleeding is common in the perimenarchal years.[44a] It has been ascribed to "immaturity" of the hypothalamic-pituitary-ovarian axis. The diagnosis of dysfunctional uterine bleeding (DUB) is one of exclusion and arrived at once organic etiologies have been ruled out. Management requires assessment to include a pregnancy test, thyroid-stimulating hormone (TSH) level, and, as indicated, prolactin level. Determination of serum follicle-stimulating hormone (FSH) level may be indicated when a diagnosis of ovarian failure is entertained.[44a]

Management has been reported to include use of oral contraceptives (OCP). In work reported by Davis and co-workers, in which a multicenter, randomized, double-blind study involving 201 patients was conducted, triphasic OCPs containing norgestimate and ethinyl estradiol proved efficacious. Specifically, improvement occurred in 65% of the treatment group versus 40% in the placebo group. This was significant (alpha = 0.05; 1-beta = 0.80). The authors concluded that norgestimate with ethinyl estradiol was effective treatment for metrorrhagia, menometrorrhagia, oligomenorrhea, and polymenorrhea-related DUB.[44b]

LONG-ACTING HORMONAL METHODS

DEPO-PROVERA

Depo-Provera, 150 mg of depot medroxyprogesterone acetate (DMPA) injected intramuscularly, is becoming increasingly popular among adolescents as it renders daily compliance, interruption of foreplay, and cooperation of the male partner unnecessary. It is still "user-dependent," however, to the extent that it requires the patient to return to a healthcare professional's clinic for repeat injections every 12 weeks to ensure contraceptive efficacy. Although recommended dosing is every 3 months, its mechanism of action is

Table 19–4. Prescriptive Equivalents for the Yuzpe Method of Emergency Contraception*

Trade Name	Formulation	Number of Pills Taken with Each Dose
Ovral	0.05 mg of ethinyl estradiol 0.50 mg of norgestrel	2
Lo/Ovral	0.03 mg of ethinyl estradiol 0.30 mg of norgestrel	4
Nordette	0.03 mg of ethinyl estradiol 0.15 mg of levonorgestrel	4
Levlen	0.03 mg of ethinyl estradiol 0.15 mg of levonorgestrel	4
Triphasil	(Yellow pills only) 0.03 mg of ethinyl estradiol 0.125 mg of levonorgestrel	4
Tri-Levlen	(Yellow pills only) 0.03 mg of ethinyl estradiol 0.125 mg of levonorgestrel	4

*Treatment consists of two doses taken 12 hours apart. Use of an antiemetic agent before taking the medication will lessen the risk of nausea, a common side effect.
Emergency contraception, ACOG Practice Patterns. No. 3, 1996.

suppression of ovulation, which does not occur for at least 14 weeks after the standard 150-mg injection.[9]

Menstrual cycle irregularities provoke the most concern about DMPA and may be the most common reason for premature discontinuation. Irregular bleeding or spotting occurs in as many as 25% to 50% of users in the first 6 to 12 months of dosing. Over time, however, excessive vaginal bleeding may be largely circumvented by administering the usual 150-mg dose monthly during the first 3 months (i.e., the first three doses); by decreasing menometrorrhagia, long-term compliance is increased.[45] Most DMPA users become amenorrheic. Alternatively, when persistent bleeding or spotting threatens to prompt discontinuation of DMPA, estrogen supplementation (e.g., 1.25 mg conjugated oral estrogen daily or its equivalent) usually reduces or eliminates bleeding. Furthermore, the sooner oligomenorrhea or amenorrhea can be achieved the better. Most teenagers perceive this as an appealing feature of the drug that improves continuation rates by more than 50%.[46] When a patient with amenorrhea presents for repeat injection more than 14 weeks after the previous dose, pregnancy should be ruled out before the next dose is administered.

DMPA offers a unique advantage for certain handicapped adolescents, particularly those with seizure disorders. In addition to the advantages of oligomenorrhea or amenorrhea that a compromised patient or her caretaker would appreciate, injectable DMPA has been shown to raise the seizure threshold and, thus, to lower seizure frequency. DMPA also improves contraceptive efficacy as compared with OCPs that contain estrogen, if they are also taking antiseizure medications that induce hepatic enzymes, notably phenobarbital, phenytoin, and carbamazepine. Increased hepatic metabolism of the estrogen in OCPs in these cases can increase the failure rate.[21] Reliable contraception is also particularly important for socially disenfranchised patients such as these, who may be partially or wholly institutionalized and thus be at greater risk for sexual assault or molestation. For these patients, a method such as DMPA may have multiple benefits. Concern has been expressed about bone demineralization with Depo-Provera.[21] Further prospective studies will provide clinically applicable information about this product.

NORPLANT

Norplant is a sustained-release, progestin (levonorgestrel) contraceptive device, consisting of six thin, flexible Silastic matchstick-sized rods. They are implanted beneath the dermis and are designed to remain in place for up to 5 years. Advantages of the method include ease of continuance and freedom from worry about daily compliance, interruption of foreplay, and cooperation of the male partner.

Side effects associated with Norplant include irregular bleeding or spotting, headaches, and acne.[9, 19] Various methods have been tried to prevent irregular bleeding; the most successful of these has been short-term administration of oral low-dose estrogen (e.g., 1.25 mg conjugated estrogen or 2 mg estradiol for 7 to 10 days).[20]

Because of its extremely efficient contraceptive effect (99%), most adolescents will decide to continue with the Norplant method, particularly if they are counseled properly before it is implanted.[15, 47] Continuation rates as high as 91% have been reported; mean duration of use among adolescents is 26.5 months.[48] When, however, irregular menses, acne, hirsutism, or other signs of ovulatory dysfunction or androgen excess distress a Norplant user, another method, such as a combined OCP, may be a better choice. Removal of a Norplant device is best accomplished by a healthcare professional well trained in this procedure.

BARRIER METHODS

Male Condom

One third of women aged 18 to 19 years (and half of all males this age) report having had multiple sex partners in a 1-year period.[49] This percentage decreases as women get older, and, fortunately, condom use has increased in the United States among all women.[50] Condoms and spermicides are the most common nonhormonal methods used by teens aged 15 to 19.[9] Used properly and correctly, they provide excellent (although not 100%) protection against pregnancy and STDs, including HIV. Drawbacks are the need to interrupt foreplay and the required cooperation of the male partner. It is largely the male partners' unwillingness to consent to this method that results in its underutilization (Table 19–5).

One other reason given for not using condoms is latex allergy. Fortunately, a polyurethane male condom is now available that is FDA approved for protection against pregnancy and venereal disease transmission. Also, the polyurethane female condom (see later) is another useful alternative.

All adolescents who use other forms of birth control should be reminded to use condoms in

Table 19–5. Reasons Given for Failure to Use Condoms

Need to interrupt foreplay
Decreased penile and vaginal sensation during coitus
Coitus when or where a condom is not at hand
Ignorance of the potential for pregnancy or STD transmission
Female partner's misplaced trust in promise of coitus interruptus
Female partner's fear that request to use condom may cause partner to reject her
Latex allergy

---

addition, to prevent STDs. It is worth reminding patients that a negative blood test for AIDS does not rule out other STDs, such as herpesvirus or human papillomavirus (HPV). Some have recommended that a condom-using woman who becomes a "new start" OCP user not divulge her use of OCPs to her boyfriend, less he try to persuade her to stop using condoms. All condom users should also be aware of the availability and safety of EC (see earlier), in case of a broken condom or one that leaks or slips off during withdrawal.

Female Condom

The female condom is the only woman-controlled device that protects against both pregnancy and STDs, including HIV infection. A polyurethane sheath that is inserted into the vagina, it has a flexible internal plastic ring that holds the top of the sheath near the apex of the vaginal vault. The sheath extends to partially cover the external genitalia. Effectiveness rates approach 97%.[51] Disadvantages include its somewhat unusual appearance and the slight crackling sounds during coitus when it is used without a lubricant (now included in packaging), both of which may be more disconcerting to adolescents than to older patients. For highly motivated female adolescents, however, particularly those with a latex allergy or a less than fully cooperative partner, it remains a viable alternative.

Diaphragm

As a relatively inexpensive form of birth control that affords some STD protection, the diaphragm can be a suitable option for a well-motivated teen in a stable relationship. The diaphragm may disrupt foreplay to a lesser extent than condoms, although patients should be reminded that it is necessary to insert additional spermicide before each coital episode for optimal effectiveness (81% to 98%) and that the device must remain in place for 6 hours after sexual contact. Still, the requirement for an initial fitting by a healthcare professional and the attendant cost may be a hindrance, and the bulky packaging makes it difficult to camouflage discreetly. Some youngsters may choose to ignore the recommendation for yearly replacement, another potential failure factor.

Cervical Cap

The cervical cap is similar to the diaphragm, except that it covers only the cervix. For this reason, it is slightly more difficult to insert; many young patients will not be dexterous enough or comfortable enough with their own anatomy to check high in the vagina for proper cervical coverage or cap dislodgement. Forgetting to fill the cap (one-third full) with spermicide or removing the cap less than 8 hours after coitus are other possible causes of failure. Effectiveness varies from 88% to 94%,[7] so a backup method of contraception is recommended for the first one or two cycles. There is also a theoretical risk of accelerated cervical dysplasia, and the cap is contraindicated in the presence of an abnormal Pap smear or lower genital tract infection. Although no cases have been reported, the cap carries the same potential risk of toxic shock syndrome as the diaphragm[52] and should not be used during menstruation. All of these variables make the cervical cap a less than optimal choice for most teenagers.

Intrauterine Device

Two intrauterine devices (IUDs) are currently available in the United States. The Progestasert device contains progesterone and is approved for 1 year of use. The annual removal-reinsertion requirement limits its popularity.

The Paragard contains copper and is approved for 10 years of use, a feature that greatly enhances its appeal. It is very effective at preventing pregnancy; success rates are 98% to 99%.[53] Earlier concerns about the IUDs being abortifacient (rather than contraceptive) have been put to rest. Today, it is known to work by interfering with transport of viable sperm to the fallopian tube, thus preventing fertilization.[54]

Limiting IUD use to women at low risk for STDs has minimized (or even eliminated) the increased risk of pelvic inflammatory disease (PID) that was earlier associated with IUDs.[55]

Likewise, IUD use has not been found to compromise fertility.[56]

Despite these encouraging realizations, the recommended patient profile for IUDs excludes most adolescents. Patients should be in a mutually monogamous relationship and have no recent history or current risk factor for PID. Although many teenagers have no history of PID and believe themselves to be in a mutually monogamous relationship, the impossibility of ensuring that the male partner (of any age) is monogamous may be an obstacle. The IUD may be appropriate for an adolescent mother who has been unsuccessful with other methods of contraception, but the decision to use it must be made mutually by the patient and her clinician and tailored to her individual circumstances.

Enhancing Compliance

All reversible methods of contraception must be used correctly and consistently if their contraceptive effect is to be maximized. Spending extra time for patient education on the first visit increases the likelihood that a return visit for continued services will follow. Patients should be encouraged to involve their male partner in the discussion of contraceptive options and benefits, to enhance the couple's sense of mutual responsibility and maturity (Table 19–6, Fig. 19–1).

Sterilization

For certain mentally or severely physically handicapped young people, sterilization may be the best contraceptive option.

Patients in this category include those with permanent and extreme disability without hope of significant improvement whose capacity for self-care, learning, future independent living, and economic self-sufficiency is limited.[57] These patients are often partially or wholly institutionalized and, consequently, are at higher risk for sexual victimization than the average teenager. They lack the emotional maturity and the cognitive ability to distinguish between appropriate and inappropriate physical contact and typically have been counselled poorly, if at all, about sexual intimacy. Associated physical disabilities compound their dependency on their caretakers, their psychosocial isolation, and the inaccessibility of preventive health care.

Many of these young girls also suffer from menometrorrhagia (secondary to the oligoovulation that accompanies some chronic diseases) and difficulties with menstrual hygiene. Menses

Table 19–6 Enhancing Adolescents' Contraceptive Compliance

Remind patients that all interactions and records are confidential

Educate in additional benefits of their method (e.g., less dysmenorrhea with OCPs)

Reassure patients about perceived side effects of their chosen method (e.g., weight gain on OCPs) even when they do not inquire

Encourage patients to call with questions or when they need prescription refills, rather than discontinuing their method

Provide samples of OCPs, condoms, spermicides, whenever possible

On each visit, encourage concomitant condom use (latex type with spermicide) for teens who use other methods

Make teens aware of the availability and safety of the "morning-after pill" and its applications: after sexual assault, date rape, or contraceptive failure (e.g., broken condom)

Encourage patients to bring along their male partner to office visits to increase their involvement and sense of mutual responsibility

---

may also bring on an increased sense of frustration, especially in patients mentally incapable of understanding their physical condition. At times, this is compounded by inappropriate behavior, combativeness, catamenial seizures, and other variations of premenstrual syndrome (PMS) in the face of hormone fluctuations.

If it can be unequivocally concluded that the patient suffers from a devastating mental or physical handicap that is irremediable and renders her forever incapable of properly raising a child, sterilization is appropriate. In most cases, tubal ligation is the procedure of choice. When menstrual hygiene is an associated concern, endometrial ablation or hysterectomy (by laparoscopic approach whenever feasible) should be considered. Should catamenial seizures or other PMS-type symptoms be unusually difficult to control, concomitant bilateral salpingo-oophorectomy has been recommended, with postoperative estrogen replacement.

The tragic consequences of an undesired pregnancy in this special class of patients cannot be overstated; namely, inadequate prenatal care, possible transmission of a genetic or physical defect, possible congenital anomalies due to medications, risks of maternal morbidity and mortality, and incapacity to rear a child. In certain special instances, sterilization does not trample the rights of the individual; rather, it protects her.

The available contraceptive options are set forth in Table 19–7. The clinician must make an effort to provide the most clinically feasible

---

Table 19–7. Contraceptive Options for Adolescent Women with Medical Conditions

Patient Population	Contraceptive Options	Comments
Physically Disabled	Combination OC, Progestin-only OC DMPA, Progestin Implant, IUD	• Small pill packages require dexterity • Partner or caregiver can assist • Combination OC is contraindicated in patients with immobility or impaired circulation
Mental Disabilities and Psychiatric Illnesses	Combination OC, Progestin-only OC, DMPA, Implants, IUD	• Long-acting progestins may be recommended to improve successful use • May be at increased risk for STDs
Epilepsy/Seizure Disorders	Combination OC, DMPA, IUD	• Anticonvulsant therapy may increase catabolism in liver prompting use of a higher-dose combination OC • DMPA may decrease seizure frequency
Systemic Lupus Erythematosus	Progestin-only OC, DMPA, Implants, IUD	• Progestin-only OCs are not associated with increase in SLE flares
Chronically Anticoagulated Women	Combination OCs, Progestin-only OCs, DMPA, Progestin Implant, IUD	• Use combination OCs only if underlying condition is not an absolute contraindication for estrogen use • Use caution when using DMPA, progestin implant, and ID due to risk of bleeding
Hypercoagulable States Associated with: Cardiovascular disease; history of venous or arterial thrombus; coagulopathies (activated protein C resistance, antithrombin III deficiency)		
• Anticoagulated	Combination OC, Progestin-only OC, DMPA, Implants, IUD	• Use estrogen-containing OCs only if therapeutically anticoagulated • Give iron supplementation with IUD
• Not anticoagulated	Progestin-only OC, DMPA, Implants, IUD	• Use of estrogen-containing method is contraindicated
Cardiovascular Disorders: thrombophlebitis, thromboembolic disorders, coronary artery disease, myocardial infarction	Progestin-only OC, DMPA, Implants, IUD	• Estrogen promotes clotting and should not be used when patient is at increased risk for a thrombotic event
Dyslipidemia	Combination OC, Progestin-only OC, DMPA, Implants, IUD	• In women with hypertriglyceridemia; (TG ≤250 mg/dL) use less estrogen-dominant (lower estrogen dose or more androgenic progestin) combination OCs or other methods
Diabetes	Combination OC, Progestin-only OC, DMPA, Implants, IUD	• Use low-dose combination OCs in normotensive, well-controlled diabetic women • Diabetic women using hormonal contraception should have periodic HbA1c glucose levels, annual fasting lipid profile
History of Gestational Diabetes	Combination OC, IUD Progestin-only OC if not breastfeeding	• Select low-estrogen-dose OC with low dose of progestin • In breastfeeding women, do not use progestin-only OCs (associated with 3-fold increased risk of diabetes mellitus) • DMPA and implants are second-choice methods; if combination OCs are contraindicated, and long-acting progestin required for compliance, implants preferred over DMPA (due to lack of carbohydrate metabolic effect) • Postpartum and annual diabetes testing • Achieve ideal body weight; encourage daily exercise
Human Immunodeficiency Virus (HIV)	Combination OC, Progestin-only OC, DMPA, Implants	• Consistent and correct male condom use needed to prevent transmission of HIV
Migraine Headaches	Combination OC, Progestin-only OC, DMPA, Implants, IUD	• Combination OCs should not be used if migraine is with focal neurologic symptoms and there are other risk factors for stroke

*Barrier methods can be used by all women, but, due to high failure rates, barrier methods are often not optimal for women with medical conditions. IUD use should only be by monogamous women with no risk of pelvic inflammatory disease.

Kjos SL: Contraceptive selection in women with medical conditions. Dialogues Contracept 1999;5:1.

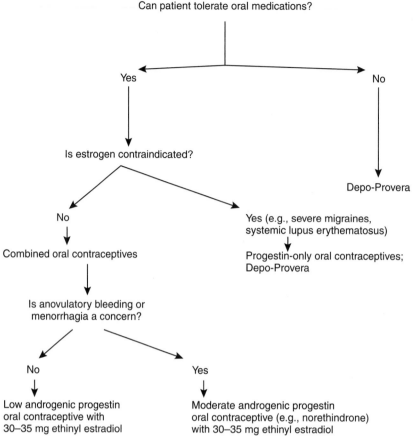

Figure 19–1. Contraception for women with medical conditions.

method of birth control and the type that is destined to promote maximum compliance.

REFERENCES

1. Kozlowski KJ, Ohlhausen WW, Warren AM, et al: Knowledge and attitudes of Norplant among adolescent females. J Adolesc Pediatr Gynecol 1994; 7:69.
2. Forrest JD: Timing of reproductive life stages. Obstet Gynecol 1993; 82:105.
3. Sex and America's Teenagers. New York: Alan Guttmacher Institute, 1994.
4. Moore KA, Nord CW, Peterson JL: Nonvoluntary sexual activity among adolescents. Family Plan Perspect 1989; 21:110.
5. Jaccard J: Adolescent contraceptive behavior: The impact of the provider and the structure of clinic-based programs. Obstet Gynecol 1996; 88:57.
6. Cheng TL, Savageau JA, Sattler AL, et al: Confidentiality in health care: A survey of knowledge, perceptions and attitudes among high school students. JAMA 1993; 269 (11):1404.
7. Emans SJ, Grace E, Woods ER, et al: Adolescents' compliance with the use of oral contraceptives. JAMA 1987; 257 (24):3377.
8. Repke JT: Adolescent pregnancy: Can we solve the problem? (Editorial). Mayo Clin Proc 1990; 65:1152.
9. Davis A: Contraceptive choices: The adolescent years. Dialogues Contracept 1995; 4(6):1.
10. Moore PJ, Adler NE, Kegeles SM: Adolescents and the contraceptive pill: The impact of beliefs on intentions and use. Obstet Gynecol 1996; 88(3):48S.
11. Peipert JF, Gutman J: Oral contraceptive risk assessment: A survey of 247 educated women. Obstet Gynecol 1993; 82:112.
12. Redmond GP, Olson WH, Lippman JS, et al: Norgestimate and ethinyl estradiol in the treatment of acne vulgaris: A randomized placebo-controlled trial. Obstet Gynecol 1997; 89(4):615.
13. Sullivan JM, Lobo RA: Considerations for contraception in women with cardiovascular disorders. Am J Obstet Gynecol 1993; 168 (6):2006.
14. Mestman JH, Schmidt-Sarosi C: Diabetes mellitus and fertility control: Contraception management issues. Am J Obstet Gynecol 1993; 168 (6):2012.
15. Sulak PJ, Haney AF: Unwanted pregnancies: Understanding contraceptive use and benefits in adolescents and older women. Am J Obstet Gynecol 1993; 168 (6):2042.
16. Robinson JC, Plichta S, Weisman CS, et al: Dysmenorrhea and use of oral contraceptives in adolescent women attending a family planning clinic. Am J Obstet Gynecol 1992; 166:578.
17. Hatcher RA, Trussel J, Stewart F, et al: Contraceptive Technology, 16th ed. New York: Irvington Publishers, 1994.
18. Potter SL: How effective are contraceptives? The deter-

mination and measurement of pregnancy rates. Obstet Gynecol 1996; 88:135.

19. Davis AJ: Teenagers, sexuality and contraception. Dialogues Contracept 1990; 3(2):1.

20. Speroff L, Glass RH, Kase NG (eds): Clinical Gynecologic Endocrinology and Infertility, 5th ed. Baltimore: Williams & Wilkins, 1994.

21. Kaunitz AM, Mishell DR: Progestin-only contraceptives: Current perspectives and future directions. Dialogues Contracept 1994; 4(2):1.

21a. Lucky J: J Am Acad Dermatol 1997; 37:746.

21b. Bradford-Hill: Principles of Medical Statistics, 9th ed. New York: Oxford University Press, 1971, p. 309.

21c. Redmond G, Olson W, Lippman J, et al: Obstet Gynecol 1997; 89; 615.

21d. Lemay A, Archer D, Roberts J, Harrison D: Gynecol Endocrinol 2000; 14(Suppl2), Abstract RT61.

22. Mishell DR, Carr BR, Comp PC, et al: Estrogen doses of oral contraceptives: What are the choices? Dialogues Contracept 1996; 4(8):1.

23. Mattson RH, Rebar RW: Contraceptive methods for women with neurologic disorders. Am J Obstet Gynecol 1993; 168:2027.

24. Yuzpe AA, Lancee WJ: Ethinyl estradiol and d-norgestrel as a postcoital contraceptive. Fertil Steril 1977; 28:932–936.

25. Tully B: Postcoital contraception—a study. Br J Fam Plan 1983; 8:119–124.

26. Luerti M, Tonta A, Ferla P, et al: Postcoital contraception by estrogen/progestagen combination of IUD insertion. Contraception 1986; 33:61–68.

27. Friedman EHI, Rowley DEM: Postcoital contraception—a two-year evaluation of a service. Br J Fam Plan 1987; 13:139–144.

28. Percival-Smith RKL, Abercombie B: Postcoital contraception with d-norgestrel/ethinyl estradiol combination: Six years experience in a student medical clinic. Contraception 1987; 36:287–293.

29. Bagshaw SN, Edwards D, Tucker A K: Ethinyl estradiol and d-norgestrel is an effective emergency contraceptive: A report of its use in 1200 patients in a family clinic. Aust NZ J. Obstet Gynecol 1988; 28:137–140.

30. Grou F, Rodriguez I: The morning-after pill—how long after? Am J Obstet Gynecol 1994; 171: 1529–1534.

31. Burton R, Savage W: Knowledge and use of postcoital contraception: A survey among health professionals in Tower Hamlets. Br J Gen Pract 1990; 40: 326–330.

32. Sawyer RG, Fong D, Stankus LR, McKeller LA: Emergency contraceptive pills: A survey of use and experiences at College Health Centers in the mid-Atlantic United States. J Am Coll Health 1996; 44:139–144.

33. Gold MA, Schein A, Coupey SM: Emergency contraception: A national survey of adolescent health experts. Adolesc Pediatr Gynecol 1995; 6:148.

34. Weisberg E, Fraser IS, Carrick SE, Wilde FM: Emergency contraception. General practitioner knowledge, attitudes and practices in New South Wales. Med J Aust 1995:162:136.

35. Harper C, Ellertson C: Knowledge and perceptions of emergency contraceptive pills among a college-age population: A qualitative approach. Fam Plan Perspect 1995; 27:149–154.

36. Harper CD, Ellerton CE: The emergency contraceptive pill: A survey of knowledge and attitudes among students at Princeton University. Am J Obstet Gynecol 1995; 173: 1438–1445.

37. Young L, McCowan LM., Roberts HE, Farquhar CM: Emergency contraception—Why women don't use it. NZ Med J 1995; 108:145–148.

38. Wessel J, Buscher U: Recent results regarding indications for the "morning after pill." Zentralbl Gynakol 1993; 115: 105–108.

39. George J, Turner J, Cooke E, et al: Women's knowledge of emergency contraception. Br J Gen Pract 1994; 44: 451–454.

40. Savonius H, Pakarinen P, Sjoberg L, Kajanoja PTI: Reasons for pregnancy termination: Negligence or failure of contraception? Acta Obstet Gynecol Scand 1995; 74:818–821.

41. Sawyer RG, Fong D, Stankus LR, et al: Feasibility of a telephone followup on use of emergency contraceptive pills in a college health center. J Am Coll Health 1996; 44:145–149.

42. Shirley B, Bundren JC, McKinnney S: Levonorgestrel as a postcoital contraceptive. Contraception 1995; 52:277–281.

43. Premakumara GA., Ratnasooriya WD, Tillekeratne LM: Studies on the postcoital contraceptive mechanisms of crude extract of Sri Lankan marine red algae, Gelidiella acerosa. Contraception 1995: 52:203–207.

44. Keshri G, Singh, MM, Lakshmi V, Kamboj VP: Postcoital contraceptive efficacy of the seeds of Nigella sativa in rats. Indian J Physiol Pharmacol 1995; 39:59–62.

44a. Management of anovulatory bleeding. American College of Obstetricians and Gynecologists Practice Bulletin #14, March 2000.

44b. Davis A, Godwin A, Lippman J, et al: Triphasic norgestimate-ethinyl estradiol for treating dysfunctional uterine bleeding. Obstet Gynecol 2000; 96:913–920.

45. Highlights from the Annual Clinical Meeting of the North American Society for Pediatric and Adolescent Gynecology, Atlanta, 2000.

46. Smith RD, Cromer BA, Hayes JR, et al: Medroxyprogesterone acetate (Depo-Provera) use in adolescents: Uterine bleeding and blood pressure patterns, patient satisfaction, and continuation rates. J Adolesc Pediatr Gynecol 1995; 8:24.

47. Hatcher RA, Trussel J: Contraceptive implants and teenage pregnancy. N Engl J Med 1994; 331(18): 1224.

48. Levine AS, Holmes MM, Haseldon C, et al: Subdermal contraceptive implant (Norplant) continuation rates among adolescents and adults in a family planning clinic. J Pediatr Adolesc Gynecol 1996; 9(2):67.

49. Forrest JD, Singh S: The sexual and reproductive behavior of American women, 1982–1988. Fam Plan Perspect 1990; 22(5):206.

50. Forrest JD, Fordyce RR: Women's contraceptive attitudes and use in 1992. Family Plan Perspect 1993; 25(4):175.

51. Trussel J, Sturgen K, Strickler J, et al: Comparative contraceptive efficacy of the female condom and other barrier methods. Family Plan Perspect 1994; 26:66.

52. Slupik RI: Toxic shock syndrome and contraceptive methods. In Sciarra JJ (ed): Gynecology and Obstetrics, Vol. 6. Philadelphia: JB Lippincott, 1990.

53. World Health Organization: The TCu 380A, TCu 220 C, Multiload 250, and Nova T IUDs at 3, 5 and 7 years of use—results from three randomized multicentre trials. Contraception 1990; 42:141.

54. Alvarez F, Brache V, Fernandez E, et al: New insights on the mode of action of intrauterine contraceptive devices in women. Fertil Steril 1988; 49:768.

55. Farley TMM, Rosenberg MJ, Rowe PJ, et al: Intrauterine devices and pelvic inflammatory disease: An international perspective. Lancet 1992; 339:785.

56. Vessey MP, Lawless M, McPherson K, et al: Fertility after stopping use of intrauterine contraceptive device. Br Med J 1983; 286:106.

57. Schor DP: Sex and sexual abuse in disabled adolescents. Semin Adolesc Med 1987; 3(1):1.

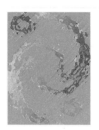

Chapter 20

Pregnancy in Adolescence

NATALIE PIERRE JOSEPH

Despite a recent decline in teen birth rates, unintended pregnancy continues to be a public health and social welfare problem among adolescents in the United States.[1, 2] The teen pregnancy rate in the United States is one of the highest among developed nations, and an estimated 78% of recent U.S. teen pregnancies are unplanned.[3, 4] More than one million teenagers become pregnant each year, resulting in 500,000 live births, of which about 200,000 are to girls aged 17 and younger.[5, 6] Most teen pregnancies are among older teenagers, those 18 or 19 years old.[7, 8] Three fourths of teen births are to first-time mothers, and 72% of these births are to single mothers. Approximately 51% of teenage pregnancies end in live birth, 35% end in induced abortion, and 14% in a miscarriage or stillbirth.[1, 2, 7–10] Other investigators reported similar findings (Table 20–1).

The children of teen mothers face heightened health and developmental risks, and have disproportionately high infant mortality rates and low birth weight (Table 20–2).[5, 9] In addition, adolescent fathers usually are not prepared to contribute financially to the support of their young children. Teen motherhood is associated with quitting school or delaying education, fewer employment opportunities, low wages, unstable marriages, and prolonged welfare dependency (Table 20–3).[11] The daughters of adolescent mothers are 83% more likely themselves to become mothers before age 18, and their sons are

Table 20–1. U.S. Statistics

56% of women and 73% of men have had intercourse by age 18.

Approximately 1 million teenage women become pregnant each year.

85% of teen pregnancies are unplanned.

Half the pregnancies occur within 6 months from first intercourse.

13% of all births are to teen mothers.

Table 20–2. Increased Risks to Infants of Teenage Mothers

Prematurity
Low birth weight
Death in first month of life
Death in first year of life
Exposure to sexually transmitted disease

2.7 times more likely to land in prison than the children of mothers who delay childbearing until their early 20s.[5] Owing to shifts in social norms, out-of-wedlock pregnancies have become more acceptable, and more common, even for older women (Fig. 20–1).

EPIDEMIOLOGY OF TEEN PREGNANCY (INCIDENCE/ STATISTICS)

Every 26 seconds, a teenager becomes pregnant in the United States.[7] Once a teenager has had one baby, she is at increased risk of having another. Historically, in the United States teenage birth rates were highest during the 1950s and 1960s, before the legalization of abortion and the development of many forms of contraception (see Fig. 20–1).[8, 12, 13] Until recently, data

Table 20–3. Consequence of Teen Pregnancy

Interrupted adolescent development
Interrupted education
Limited parenting skills
Limited career and earning potential
Premature marriage
Larger families for younger mothers
Poverty
Stigma of illegitimacy
Depression
Recurrent generation of early childbearing

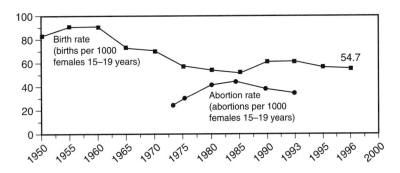

Figure 20–1. Trends in birth rates and abortion rates among adolescent females age 15 to 19 years. (From American Academy of Pediatrics. Adapted from Moore KA: Teen fertility in the United States: 1993 data. Facts at a glance. Child Trends, 1995.)

from the Alan Guttmacher Institute (AGI), The Centers for Disease Control and Prevention (CDC), and the news media showed encouraging trends in the teen pregnancy and birth rates. (Pregnancy rates include births, abortions, and miscarriages.) After a 7% increase between 1985 and 1990, the pregnancy rate for women aged 15 to 19 declined by 14% between 1990 and 1995, according to AGI data.[7] In 1994, for girls younger than 15, 81.7% of pregnancies that were carried to term were unintended. Fifty-nine percent of unintended pregnancies for these young women were aborted. Among women aged 15 to 19 years, 78% had an unintended pregnancy and 45% had an abortion. The proportion of all pregnancies that were unintended varied much by age, teenagers younger than 18 having the largest percentage (82% to 83%). The proportion decreased with age, dropping to 75% among women aged 18 and 19 years.[4] The U.S. teenage pregnancy rate in 1995 stood at 101.1 per 1000, the lowest level since the mid-1970s and down from a peak of 177 per 1000 in 1990.[6] Even more impressive, recent data from the 1997 CDC Youth Risk Behavior Surveillance system (YRBS) indicate that fewer high school students reported having had sexual intercourse—51% in 1991, 48% in 1997. Among adolescent males, the proportion who had ever had sex dropped from 57% in 1991 to 49% in 1997. Among those teenagers who were sexually active, condom use had increased from 46.2% in 1991 to 56.8% in 1997.[6, 14] Researchers attribute the declines in pregnancy to a combination of fewer teenagers' having sex and more effective contraception by those who do, greater condom use, and easier availability of injectable contraception (Table 20–4). Despite an encouraging decline in teen birth rates to 54.7 per 1000 in 1996, the rates in the United States are more than twice those of other industrialized nations, still higher than the rate for 1980.

INTERPRETATION OF THE TRENDS IN TEEN PREGNANCY RATES

There is no clear explanation for why pregnancy and birth rates have dropped.[4] Research-

ers say that recent trends in sexual activity and contraceptive use are the result of a confluence of factors, including greater emphasis on abstinence, more conservative attitudes about sex, fear of AIDS, the popularity of long-lasting methods such as implantable (Norplant) and injectable (Depo-Provera) contraceptives, and even the economy. Many experts believe that the strong economy and the associated availability of jobs at the lower end of the pay scale have contributed to reducing pregnancies among teenagers.[6]

CAUSES OF TEEN PREGNANCY

The causes of teen pregnancy in the United States are several and are related to economic, social, and cultural forces. The age of sexual debut has become progressively younger over the past century, while maturation—cognitive and in social relations—has been prolonged. A mismatch has developed between cognitive maturity (including an ability to anticipate future consequences of behaviors) and sexual maturity.[15] During the last 20 years, the age of initiation of sexual activity has declined. According to the 1997 U.S. YRBS, nationwide, 7.2% of students are younger than 13 at first sexual intercourse.[14] The percentage of American adolescents who are sexually active has increased significantly in recent years.[16–19] The average age of first intercourse dropped to 17 years for girls and 16 years for boys.[20] Approximately a quarter of youths report first intercourse by age 15 years.[17, 19] From 1995 to 1997 the percentage of high school stu-

Table 20–4. Trends in Teen Pregnancy

The teen pregnancy rate in the US decreased from 115/1000 in 1990 to 97.3/1000 in 1996.

35% of all pregnancies to 15–19-year-olds ended in abortion in 1996.

The rate of abortions to 15–19-year-olds decreased from 43.5/1000 in 1985 to 29.2/1000 in 1996.

dents who reported ever having had sexual intercourse decreased. In 1995, 54% of boys and 52% of girls reported ever having sexual intercourse, as compared with 49% of boys and 48% of girls in 1997.[16] Sixteen percent of students nationwide have had sexual intercourse with at least four sex partners. Younger teenagers are especially vulnerable to coercive and nonconsensual sex. Involuntary sexual activity has been reported in 74% of sexually active girls younger than 14 years and 60% of those younger than 15 years.[14]

Despite increasing use of contraceptives by adolescents at the time of intercourse,[18, 19, 21] 50% of adolescent pregnancies occur within 6 months after first sexual intercourse.[18] Adolescent women, like adult women, have changed their preferences for contraceptive methods in recent years: fewer use pills and more use injectable contraceptives.[22] Factors associated with more consistent contraceptive use among sexually active youths include academic success in school, anticipation of a satisfying future, and a stable relationship with a sexual partner.[7]

The CDC reported in the 1997 YRBS that 6.5% of high school students nationwide said they had been pregnant or had made someone else pregnant.[6] Overall, female students were significantly more likely to have been pregnant (8.5%) than male students were to have impregnated someone (4.7%).[6]

The CDC estimates that pregnancy rates declined for 18- to 19-year-olds in all 42 states that reported data for 1992 and 1995 and for 15- to 17-year-olds in all but two of these states. In most states, rates were considerably higher for black teens than for whites; however, between 1992 and 1995, in 24 of the 26 states that calculated rates by race, blacks reported greater declines than whites.[6] The teen birth rate declined not only for the nation as a whole but also in every state. In 1996, New Hampshire, Vermont, Maine, Minnesota, Massachusetts, and North Dakota had the lowest teen birth rates—about 29 to 32 per 1000, and Mississippi, Arkansas, Arizona, and Texas had the highest rates—about 74 to 76 per 1000.[6]

The decline in the birth rate, which varied considerably by race and age, is particularly noteworthy for black teenagers. The rate for blacks fell 21%, to a record low 91.4 per 1000 in 1996. In contrast, the rate for Hispanic teenagers barely changed between 1991 and 1995, although it fell 5% between 1995 and 1996, to 101.8 per 1000. Today, Hispanics have the highest teen birth rate. During the period between 1995 and 1996, for non-Hispanic whites, the birth rate declined 9%, to 48.1 per 1000.[6, 7] The decline in

birth rates varied less by age. The birth rate for teens aged 15 to 17 years fell 13% during the period 1995 to 1996 and 9% for 18- to 19-year-olds.[6] In 1996, the birth rate for girls aged 10 to 14 was 1.2 per 1000. Although that was down from 1.4 per 1000 in 1991, since 1970, the rate for this age group has been stable, between 1.1 and 1.4 per 1000.[6]

The percentage of teen pregnancies that ended in induced abortions has decreased every year, from 38% in 1990 (40% for girls aged 15 to 17 years and 36% for those aged 18 or 19 years) to 32% in 1995 (34% for women aged 15 to 17 years and 31% for those aged 18 to 19 years).[6] In each of the abortion rate years from 1990 through 1995, the abortion rate declined for both age groups. Thus, from 1991 to 1995, the abortion rate declined by 21% for the entire 15- to 19-year age group and by 16% for the sexually experienced ones.[3] This finding is consistent with longer-term trends in teen abortions. The percentage of teen pregnancies that end in abortion has been declining since 1987, as an increasing proportion of pregnant teenagers have chosen to give birth rather than terminate the pregnancy.[23–25] In addition, the decreased number of abortion providers and the increased number of state laws restricting teens' access to abortions may have affected teen abortion rates.[26, 27]

Patterns of abortion rates were distinctly different. The highest rates per 1000 women 15 to 19 years old were in Hawaii,[27a] California,[27b] and New York.[27c] The 10 highest rates were in California, Connecticut, Delaware, Florida, Hawaii, Maryland, Nevada, New Jersey, New York, and Washington. Abortion rates were lowest in relatively rural states (Kentucky, Louisiana, Oklahoma, West Virginia, Idaho, and Utah).[28]

Between 1988 and 1992, the national abortion rate among women aged 15 to 19 decreased by 18%. Only Mississippi and the District of Columbia registered increases, whereas nine states had declines of more than 30%—Iowa, Louisiana, Maine, Minnesota, New Hampshire, Ohio, Oklahoma, Utah, and Vermont.[4] The incompleteness of the abortion data limits the research that can be done and the conclusions that can be drawn.

RISK FACTORS FOR ADOLESCENT PREGNANCY

Several factors are associated with the high rates of pregnancy and childbearing among adolescents. Intrafamilial, sociocultural, intrapersonal, and biologic factors affect an adolescent's behavior and the risk of pregnancy.[29] Intrafamilial factors include parenting influences, a multigenerational history of teenage parenting, and parenting skill. Having a sibling who is a teenage parent increases the risk of pregnancy.[29] Sociocultural factors include the community and the social environment. Where prevalent, poverty and unemployment foster hopelessness, and adolescents develop the perception that few employment opportunities are available, that there is often little value in educational attainment, and that the benefits of either contraception or avoiding sexual activity are minimal.[29] Intrapersonal factors such as concrete cognitive level, poor self-esteem, depression, substance use, history of sexual abuse, and school failure all have been associated with adolescent pregnancy.[29, 30] Biologic and physical development are additional factors. Accompanying the trend toward earlier age of menarche, there has been a steady decline in age of sexual debut, which then occurs at a time that the adolescent's cognitive skills for decision making are still unsophisticated. There are several predictors of sexual intercourse during the early adolescent years, including early pubertal development, a history of sexual abuse, poverty, lack of attention and nurturing from parents, cultural and family patterns of early sexual experience, having no academic or career goals, and poor school performance or dropping out.[5, 15, 16, 18, 19, 31, 32] Factors associated with delayed initiation of sexual intercourse include living with both parents in a stable family environment, regular attendance at a place of worship, and increased family income.[16, 18, 19]

The greatest risk factors for pregnancy among teens are sexual inexperience, young age at first intercourse and delay in marriage,[33] large age discrepancy with the male partner, and unwanted intercourse.

SEXUALITY DECISIONS

Adolescents tend to use contraception sporadically and ineffectively; however, this does not imply that they are trying to become pregnant. Using contraception ineffectively despite not wanting to become pregnant has multiple roots, including ignorance of the "mechanics" of reproduction and contraception, limited access to family-planning and health services, and impulsivity.[15] Adolescents feel invulnerable and tend to be egocentric: they believe that they could not possibly become pregnant. Thus, preventive practices not considering the developmental

phases of the adolescent may also play a role, especially for teenagers at high risk.[15]

SEXUALITY ISSUES AMONG MALE ADOLESCENTS

Many of the factors that contribute to increasing births among adolescent girls have also affected adolescent boys. The age at first intercourse has declined for male adolescents in recent decades, and their use of contraceptives has increased. Nevertheless, many aspects of boys' role in teenage births are ill-understood. Males beyond their teens are also at risk of becoming involved in sexual relationships with teenage girls that lead to unwanted pregnancies. Vital statistics suggest that many or most of the fathers of children born to teen mothers are in their early 20s. In fact, the youngest girls seem to have the oldest partners.[34–36] This age discrepancy may create problems for the pregnant adolescent and her unborn child because of the differences in cognitive maturity, socioemotional development, and experience.[34, 37] Because, in some cultures, fathering a child is evidence of masculinity, these young men may be more likely to be involved in other activities, such as fighting and carrying weapons, that also symbolize masculinity.[38–40] Resnick and coworkers recently reported that male adolescents' involvement in pregnancy is associated with tobacco smoking, alcohol and drug use, fighting and gang involvement, and the belief that "getting a girl pregnant proves that you are a man."[39]

CONSEQUENCES OF TEEN PREGNANCY AND PARENTING

The consequences of unintended pregnancy are serious, imposing appreciable burdens on children and families.

Failure in school and welfare dependency are the most frequently reported and serious long-term sequelae among high school–aged girls.[41] Until recently, most studies on adolescent mothers concluded that early parenthood had a strong negative effect on their educational attainment, such that young mothers were unlikely to continue their education after childbirth and thus attained lower total levels of education than their peers who delayed childbirth. However, recent studies have found that this gap is narrowing, in part, because of availability of general equivalency degree programs, schooling requirements for welfare receipt, and more progressive school policies on accepting pregnant students.[15, 41] In addition, new methodologies have revealed that much of the difference in educational attainment between adolescent mothers and older mothers may be due, not to age, but rather to other differences between the groups.[15] The effects of teenage childbearing on educational attainment are also moderated by other variables, such as birth spacing and the decision to drop out of school.[7, 15] Finally, the increased availability of alternative schools with daycare programs and flexible hours has helped adolescent parents to complete their high school education, enter the job market at a young age, and become productive members of their communities.[42–44]

In addition to effects on educational attainment, teenage childbearing is also linked to different marital patterns. Young mothers are more likely to divorce and, thus, to spend more of their parenting years as single mothers than do women who delay childbearing.[15] Levels of educational attainment and the lack thereof, knowledge of parenting skills, and availability of parenting programs for teen fathers are other variables that can influence the fathers' level of involvement in the lives of their children.

In terms of parenting, adolescent mothers have been described as more concrete, punitive, and physically aggressive, and less interactive with their children.[45–47] Their parenting also reflects low confidence, high stress, and inappropriate values.[48] In addition, they have little understanding of child growth, development, and behavior. Young mothers also tend to provide a less stimulating home environment.[15] They are often idealistic, impulsive, and imitative, and seek immediate gratification of their own needs. They tend to focus on themselves, rather than their child. These normal but egocentric, inconsistent personality traits may compromise their ability to parent.

IMPACT OF TEEN PREGNANCIES ON FATHERS

Because of their own impoverished backgrounds, teen fathers are rarely a strong source of financial support for teen mothers and their children. Although most start out with a desire to provide for their children, their child support contributions are extremely small.[15] The amount of contact young fathers have with their children is quite variable. Somewhat surprisingly, given the low rate of marriage and high incidence of divorce among teenage mothers and their partners, 50% of teenage fathers live with their children for some time after birth, though often not for long.[7]

Consequences of Adolescent Pregnancy to the Offspring

Disproportionately high rates of maternal and neonatal mortality are associated with adolescent childbearing, especially for nonwhite adolescents younger than 15 years.[49] Given adequate prenatal care, however, adolescents aged 15 years and older have good outcomes.[50] During the first 2 years of life, infants born to young adolescents have a higher mortality rate than infants born to older adolescents or adults.[49] Infants are at greater risk for low birth weight, mental retardation, congenital malformations, neglect, physical abuse, and emotional and behavioral difficulties, and are twice as likely to die in the first year of life.[51] They are more likely to be placed in foster care than are children of older mothers, a risk that is greater for later born than for firstborn children of young mothers (see Table 20–2).[51]

Delays in cognitive development begin to emerge in the preschool years and persist into the school years.[15, 52] As adolescents, children of teenagers exhibit higher rates of repeating a grade, delinquency, incarceration (for boys), early sexual activity, and pregnancy than age-matched peers born to older mothers.[15]

Because of limited educational attainment, marital instability, and the poverty endemic to young parenthood, as adults, teenage mothers are likely to earn less and more likely than their peers who delay childbirth to be on welfare.[15, 53] The recent national welfare debate has highlighted the fact that adolescent pregnancies place a high financial burden on the United States. In 1990, the U.S. government spent more than $25 billion on behalf of all families whose first child was born when the mother was a teenager, and this figure does not include job training, housing subsidies, special education, foster care or daycare, or the Special Supplement Food Program for Women, Infants, and Children.[54] Preventing teen pregnancy was a critical part of the Clinton Administration's approach to welfare reform and the efforts to strengthen U.S. families.

DIAGNOSIS OF PREGNANCY

A newly pregnant teen must navigate a complex maze of medical, social, financial, and legal services. Teen pregnancy may be detected in a variety of clinical situations, including primary care sites, specialty clinics, and emergency departments. At the time of the medical visit, the chief complaint (or presenting problems) may vary from vague and nonspecific symptoms such as sore throat, abdominal pain, or urinary tract symptoms to more specific signs and symptoms characteristic of pregnancy.[55] Many postmenarchal young women have irregular ovulation and menstrual cycles and may thus be unaware of the possibility of pregnancy, or in denial. Urine ICON II hCG is an immunoenzymetric pregnancy assay for the semiquantitative determination of human chorionic gonadotropin (hCG). It is sufficiently sensitive to show a positive result as early as 1 week after implantation or 4 or 5 days before a first missed menses.[55, 56] A positive test result means that a urine specimen contains at least 10 to 25 mIU/ml of hCG. A serum beta-subunit hCG (β-hCG) assay may show a positive result as early as 1 week after conception. When there is clinical suspicion of pregnancy, a negative test result should be repeated in 1 to 2 weeks. A negative pregnancy test result affords the medical provider an opportunity for further counseling and prevention. While the pregnancy test is being processed, it is helpful to discuss with the teen what she hopes the outcome will be and what her plans are, should the result be positive (Table 20–5).

MEDICAL AND PSYCHOSOCIAL EVALUATION

Issues to be considered in counseling are personal history (social situation, educational and life goals, self-esteem, psychiatric history, financial status, insurance); medical, reproductive, and sexual history; and family, partner, or personal beliefs and attitudes about parenting, abortion, and adoption.[56] A calm, nonjudgmental approach is essential. The girl should know that her care provider has experience with others who have been in the same situation as hers and be reassured that he or she will support whatever decision she makes about the pregnancy. When working with teens it is important to remember that, developmentally, they are predominantly concrete thinkers, especially in stressful situations.

PERSONAL HISTORY. The initial assessment should investigate her social situation and support, which can be assessed with questions such as "who came with you to the clinic today? Who knows you are coming in for a pregnancy test today?" and "With whom have you discussed the possibility of being pregnant?" (parents? partner? a friend?).[56] Additional history should include educational and life goals, self-esteem and self-sufficiency, psychiatric history, and finances and insurance. Questions should be directed to finding out who provides emotional support for her, how she is feeling just then, and her risks for depression or suicide.

MEDICAL, REPRODUCTIVE, AND SEXUAL HISTORY. Her gynecologic history should include the number of previous pregnancy tests, previous pregnancies and their outcomes, and the number of children and their ages. A menstrual history, is helpful—date of last menstrual period, typical cycle length between menses, whether the last period was "on time," and its volume (normal or light). Similarly, the history of sexual experience, contraceptive use, and sexually transmitted diseases (STDs) needs to be collected. It is important to ask whether the girl wants to be pregnant and whether the intercourse that resulted in the pregnancy was consensual. Pregnancy may be the first clue to a rape or an abusive relationship in the family. Thus the provider needs to be sensitive when inquiring about the source of the pregnancy.[56] The medical history must include major illnesses; current medications, including prescription and over-the-counter drugs; and substance use during the last 30 days, including direct questions about tobacco, alcohol, and drugs (including marijuana).

COUNSELING

Adolescents often delay decision making or seek prenatal care late. The provider's awareness of the crucial elements of initial counseling and current legal constraints of confidentiality will be of great help to an adolescent girl through this time of decision. Whatever pregnancy option she chooses, she will benefit from early diagnosis. A pregnant patient's options should be outlined in a clear, straightforward manner. The client must be made aware that there is no perfect solution to an unintended pregnancy. Counseling must be unbiased, unhurried, and developmentally appro-

Table 20–5. Reasons for Delayed Diagnosis of Pregnancy

Unfamiliar with symptoms of pregnancy
Denial
Limited access to care
Fear of adult response
Conflict about options with parents
Ambivalence about options
Incest

priate. The clinician should be aware of the developmental differences between young, middle, and older adolescents. There are striking differences between 11- to 14-year-old and 17- or 18-year-old girls. Adolescents younger than 15 years may deny the pregnancy and not present until the second, or even the third, trimester. They sometimes have difficulty connecting with the idea of pregnancy and making decisions. Older adolescents are more likely to have better decision-making strategies. Several visits may be needed before the girl can make a decision.

The initial counseling focuses on a review of options. Pregnant teens have three: (1) continuing the pregnancy to parent the baby; (2) carrying the pregnancy to delivery and placing the baby up for adoption; (3) terminating the pregnancy.[7, 57] Often, such counseling can only be started at the initial visit and must be continued with close follow-up, preferably weekly appointments, until decisions are finalized and prenatal or termination services arranged. Financial need should not deprive a girl of her options for management of the pregnancy. The clinician should be knowledgeable about local funding resources for continuing or terminating a pregnancy. Many teenagers are unable to talk to their parents about the pregnancy, sometimes because of justified fear of physical or other abuse and sometimes out of fear that a pregnancy will announce to parents that they are sexually active. While the issue is still controversial, within institutions and among clinicians, legally, even though they are minors, adolescents, have rights to confidential reproductive health care. Teenagers who are unable to involve their parents should be informed by the clinician and counselors of legal alternatives to parental consent provisions in their state and neighboring states, including "judicial bypass," to ensure the constitutional rights of minors.[58] It is essential to encourage adolescents to talk to their parents and to offer assistance. The clinician should stay in contact with the teen—via clinic visits or telephone—until a final decision is made and the patient referred and connected with either a prenatal clinic or an abortion service.

If the adolescent decides to continue the pregnancy, the clinician should refer her for timely and appropriate prenatal care (Table 20–6). Adolescents who receive prenatal care in comprehensive adolescent pregnancy programs generally have had better outcomes than adolescents who were not in such a program, and clinicians may choose to refer preferentially to such programs, when they are available.[58] Adoption is an important option for the clinician or counselor to discuss with the adolescent. To make appropriate referrals, the physician should be familiar with the available medical, legal, counseling, and social service resources that facilitate arrangement of adoptions. If the adolescent decides to terminate her pregnancy, the clinician should be knowledgeable about community resources, considering the stage of pregnancy and any coexisting medical conditions. Abortion techniques that are suitable for adolescents include menstrual extraction, suction curettage, and medical techniques, which are becoming more widely available (first-trimester methotrexate/misoprostol). Because late second-trimester procedures (intraamniotic, intramuscular, or intravaginal) are generally physically and psychologically traumatic, every effort should be made to make a timely referral. The counseling practitioner should be familiar with referral sites and techniques and should consider the adolescent's financial resources and be aware of local or federal laws affecting the availability of services, prenatal notification, and consent.[58] Given the anticipated U.S. Food and Drug Administration's approval of drugs such as mifepristone, and the availability of prostaglandin analogues and methotrexate to induce early nonsurgical abortion, clinicians need to be aware of the nature and availability of these methods and have a clear understanding of their role in the counseling, provision of care, and referral.[58]

The likelihood of another pregnancy should be emphasized to those who choose abortion and those who choose to carry to term. Hence, introducing the topic of birth control during and after the pregnancy is essential, because many teenagers imagine that it won't happen again. The girl's anticipation of her feelings after the pregnancy is terminated or the birth of a newborn must be explored. For most, the overwhelming postabortion feeling is relief, although depression may be apparent, especially in adolescents with low self-esteem.

A full physical (including pelvic) examination is essential to the medical assessment of a pregnant teen. Determining the size of the uterus, to confirm an intrauterine pregnancy, is important, as dates adolescents provide may be inaccurate. A diagnosis can be made as early as the 6th week, during a pelvic examination. A 6-week uterus is about the size of a pear; an 8-week uterus about the size of an orange; and a 12-week uterus the size of a grapefruit and lying just at the brim of the symphysis pubis. A 16-week uterus generally can be palpated midway between the umbilicus and symphysis pubis; and a 20-week uterus at the umbilicus.[56] A Pap smear

Table 20–6. Prenatal Care

Initial Visit
History
  Identify risk factors

Physical examination
  General
  Blood pressure
  Height
  Weight (calculate body mass)
  Breast examination
  Abdominal examination
    Pelvic examination
    Identify risk factors
    Estimate gestational age

Laboratory evaluation
  Hemoglobin/Hematocrit
  Blood type, Rh factor
  Antibody screen
  Routine urinalysis
    Dipstick
    Sugar
    Protein
    Ketone bodies
  Pap smear
  Infections
    Cervical cultures
    Venereal Disease Research Laboratory test
    Antirubella antibodies
    Hepatitis screen
    HIV
  Genetic screen
  Drug screen

Week 6–8
History
  Update

Physical examination
  Blood pressure
  Weight
  Pelvic examination
  Fundal height (estimate gestational age)
  Fetal heart (e.g., fetoscopy, ultrasonography)

Laboratory evaluation
  Routine urinalysis
    Dipstick
    Sugar
    Protein
    Ketone bodies
    Culture and sensitivity
  Infections
    HIV (if appropriate)

Week 16–18
History
  Update

Physical examination
  Blood pressure
  Weight
  Fundal height (estimate growth)
  Fetal heart

Laboratory evaluation
  Screen for gestational diabetes
  Routine urinalysis
    Dipstick
    Sugar
    Protein
    Ketone bodies

Genetic screen
  Maternal serum α-fetoprotein screen
  Triple screen

Week 26–28
History
  Update

Physical examination
  Blood pressure
  Weight
  Fundal height (estimate growth)
  Assess fetal position
  Fetal heart

Laboratory evaluation
  Hemoglobin/Hematocrit
  Antibody screen
  Screen for gestational diabetes (if not done at 16–18
    weeks)
  Routine urinalysis
    Dipstick
    Sugar
    Protein
    Ketone bodies

Week 32
History
  Update

Physical examination
  Blood pressure
  Weight
  Fundal height (estimate growth)
  Fetal heart

Laboratory evaluation
  Screen for gestational diabetes (if appropriate)
  Routine urinalysis
    Dipstick
    Sugar
    Protein
    Ketone bodies

Week 36
History
  Update

Physical examination
  Blood pressure
  Weight
  Fundal height (estimate growth)
  Assess fetal position
  Fetal heart
Laboratory evaluation
  Routine urinalysis
    Dipstick
    Sugar
    Protein
    Ketone bodies

Week 38
History
  Update

Physical examination
  Blood pressure
  Weight
  Fundal height (estimate growth)
  Assess fetal position
  Fetal heart

Table continued on following page

Table 20–6. Prenatal Care *Continued*

Laboratory evaluation	***Week 40***
Routine urinalysis	**History**
Dipstick	Update
Sugar	**Physical examination**
Protein	Blood pressure
Ketone bodies	Weight
Week 39	Fundal height (estimate growth)
History	Assess fetal position
Update	Fetal heart
Physical examination	**Laboratory evaluation**
Blood pressure	Routine urinalysis
Weight	Dipstick
Fundal height (estimate growth)	Sugar
Assess fetal position	Protein
Fetal heart	Ketone bodies
Laboratory evaluation	
Routine urinalysis	
Dipstick	
Sugar	
Protein	
Ketone bodies	

and tests for gonorrhea and *Chlamydia* are appropriate. Transabdominal or transvaginal ultrasonography is useful when the uterus is larger or smaller than the date of the last menstrual period would suggest. Accurate dating will facilitate and direct treatment decisions later in pregnancy, e.g., management of prolonged pregnancy. Ultrasonography can confirm an intrauterine pregnancy, with cardiac motion demonstrable approximately 6 weeks after the last menstrual period.[56, 57] Additional tests include syphilis serology, purified protein derivative, rubella titer, complete blood count, blood typing with antibody screen, and HIV counseling and testing.

MEDICAL RISKS OF ADOLESCENT PREGNANCY (DISORDERS OF PREGNANCY)

Adolescent mothers experience more pregnancy and delivery problems and have less healthy babies overall than do older mothers, but these differences were less dramatic in recent research. First, the absolute degree of these differences seems to be decreasing, perhaps because of more or better health services for young mothers. Second, newer studies indicate that poor health outcomes are related more to the poverty and lack of prenatal care common to pregnant teenagers than to their age (except, perhaps, for adolescents younger than 15 years).[7] Pregnant adolescents younger than 17 years have a higher incidence of medical complications—for both mother and child—than do adult women,

although emerging data indicate that risks may be greatest for the youngest teenagers, those younger than 15. (Table 20–7).[7, 59] The incidence of low birth weight (less than 2500 gm) is more than double the rate for adult mothers, and the neonatal death rate (within 28 days after birth) is almost three times higher.[7, 59] The mortality rate for teenage mothers, although low, is twice that for pregnant women.[59] Adolescent pregnancy has been associated with other medical problems, including poor maternal weight gain, prematurity (birth before 37 weeks' gestation), pregnancy-induced hypertension, anemia, and STDs. Approximately 14% of births to adolescents aged 17 years or younger are premature, as compared with 6% for women 25 to 29 years old.[7] Adolescent mothers aged 14 years and younger are more likely than other age groups to give birth to low birth weight infants, and this complication is more prevalent among African Americans.[59]

Recent reports have addressed whether biologic or social factors account for most medical complications.[7, 59] The only biologic factors that have been associated consistently with negative

Table 20–7. Obstetric Risks for Teenage Mothers

Death (for girls <15 yr)
Low birth weight infant
Pregnancy-induced hypertension
Anemia
STD
Preterm labor
Poor nutritional status

pregnancy results are low maternal weight and height, parity, and poor pregnancy weight gain.[59] Many social factors have been associated with poor birth outcomes, including poverty, unmarried status, low education level, drug use, and inadequate prenatal care.[59] A combination of biologic and social factors may contribute to poor outcomes in adolescents.

During early pregnancy, adolescents can experience the same difficulties as adults, including ectopic pregnancy, molar pregnancy, and threatened, missed, or incomplete abortion. The difference is that adolescents may not have known they were pregnant before they come to the emergency department. Given the rising rates of STDs and pelvic inflammatory disease in adolescents, the clinician always needs to consider an ectopic pregnancy when evaluating adolescents with irregular bleeding and/or abdominal pain. Rarely, a girl has more than one diagnosis (e.g., ectopic pregnancy and pelvic inflammatory disease) at the time of presentation to the clinic.

The causes of tubal pregnancy include anatomic and functional ones: salpingitis, previous pelvic surgery, tubal surgery, previous ectopic pregnancy, history of intrauterine device use, and hormonal influences, among others.[60] Altered levels of estrogen or progesterone at the time of fertilization may be associated with increased risk of ectopic pregnancy, perhaps because of the effects of these levels on tubal motility. Embryonic causes include malformed embryo and chromosomal anomalies. The most common symptoms of ectopic pregnancy include irregular vaginal bleeding, abdominal or pelvic pain, and amenorrhea. Other symptoms are dizziness, fainting, pregnancy symptoms, and passage of tissue (decidual cast).[60] Supportive classic signs of ectopic pregnancy are abdominal tenderness, adnexal tenderness, and an adnexal mass. Orthostatic changes and fever are less common signs.

Diagnostic aids to identifying ectopic pregnancy include an hCG measurement, ultrasonography, and laparoscopy.[56] A sensitive urine pregnancy test can detect levels of hCG as low as 10 to 25 mIU/ml. Very early in its course, ectopic (or intrauterine) pregnancy can produce levels of hCG below 50 mIU/ml, but the likelihood of symptoms is low.[56] When the initial urine pregnancy test is negative but pregnancy is strongly suspected, a more sensitive test should be performed. The most sensitive and accurate test available, the serum immunoassay for the quantitative beta subunit of hCG, should be positive by 7 to 10 days after conception. Unusually low levels of hCG for gestational age frequently indi-

cate impending spontaneous abortion or ectopic pregnancy. Without definitive sonographic findings, a single hCG measurement is rarely diagnostic. A second test is usually appropriate within 48 hours. An increase in the beta-hCG subunit of 69% every 48 hours is normally expected, and of 100% every 72 hours.[56] Molar pregnancies, gestational trophoblastic neoplasia (GTN), and certain ovarian tumors and central nervous system dysgerminomas also produce hCG. Other adjunctive methods for identifying ectopic pregnancies include measuring the level of progesterone[27c, 56] and ultrasonography, particularly when it is used in conjunction with a discriminatory beta-hCG measurement. A serum progesterone value of 25 ng/ml (80 nmol/l) is associated with normal pregnancy 98% of the time, whereas a value of less than 5 ng/ml almost certainly signals an abnormal intrauterine pregnancy.[27c, 56] A discriminatory zone is the minimum level of hCG above which an intrauterine pregnancy can reliably be detected by ultrasonagraphy.[27c] A discriminatory zone is dependent on the operator and technique used in the lab, hence, clinicians are responsible for knowing the discriminatory zone at their institution.

Ultrasonography is very helpful in distinguishing between an intrauterine and an ectopic pregnancy. A gestational sac can be optimally visualized by abdominal ultrasonography using the latest scanning equipment at approximately 4000 to 6000 mIU/ml hCG (International Reference Preparation) (or 5 to 6 weeks after the last menstrual period) and at approximately 1000 to 1500 mIU/ml hCG by transvaginal sonography.[56] More than 98% of ectopic pregnancies implant in the fallopian tube, most in the ampullar portion (93%), followed by the isthmus (4%) and the cornual (interstitial) region (2.5%). Ovarian (0.5%), cervical (0.1%), and abdominal ectopics (0.03%) are rare.

When the situation is unclear and the physician continues to suspect an ectopic pregnancy, the matter can often be resolved by laparoscopy. It is possible to make a definitive diagnosis with laparoscopy in the vast majority of cases, but not always. Clinical management depends on the status of the patient, the hCG levels, the desire to continue an intrauterine pregnancy, and the ultrasound findings.[56]

Signs and symptoms of hydatidiform mole are bleeding in the first half of pregnancy, lower abdominal pain, toxemia before 24 weeks' gestation, hyperemesis gravidarum, uterus large for dates (a finding in 50% of cases), absence of fetal heart tones and fetal parts, and expulsion of vesicles.[60] Diagnostic studies include chest radiography, urinary hCG greater than 500,000 IU in 24 hours, ultrasonography, and amniocentesis and amniography if a fetus is present (rarely required). Systemic symptoms of molar pregnancy are most often seen in patients with metastatic disease.[60] Vaginal bleeding is a common symptom of molar pregnancy. Other systemic symptoms include amenorrhea due to hCG secretion. Hemoptysis, cough, or dyspnea may be associated with lung metastasis. A patient with central nervous system metastasis may complain of headaches, dizzy spells, "blacking out," or other symptoms referable to a space-occupying lesion in the brain. Rectal bleeding or dark stools could represent disease that has metastasized to the gastrointestinal tract.[60] Diagnostic tests for suspected metastases should include computed tomography (CT) of the abdomen, pelvis, and head. Lumbar puncture should be performed when brain CT findings are negative, because simultaneous evaluation of the beta-hCG titer in the cerebrospinal fluid and serum may allow very early detection of cerebral metastases.[61] Signs like those of GTN are common to many pathologic entities.

Threatened and missed abortion are two common types of spontaneous abortion. A threatened abortion is diagnosed when any bloody discharge appears to come from the pregnant uterus with a closed cervix and a viable pregnancy. Approximately 25% of pregnant women have vaginal spotting or heavier bleeding during the early months of gestation.[60] Other causes of early-pregnancy bleeding, including ectopic pregnancy and cervical lesions, should be excluded. There is no specific treatment for threatened abortion. Bed rest and progesterone have been suggested, but neither has been proven beneficial. Abstention from coitus during bleeding, and perhaps for 2 or more weeks thereafter, is usually recommended.[60]

The term *missed abortion* is used when an embryo is not viable but is retained in utero for at least 6 weeks. Subjective symptoms of pregnancy, such as nausea, breast tenderness, and urinary frequency, disappear. There is usually an intermittent brown vaginal discharge; uterine growth stops, and eventually the uterus shrinks. The pregnancy test result gradually becomes negative. Rarely, after prolonged retention of a dead second-trimester fetus, disseminated intravascular coagulation develops, and the patient may note bleeding from the nose, gums, or, especially, sites of trauma. Ultrasonography is diagnostic. In most cases of missed abortion, no treatment is required, as, ultimately, the abortus will be expelled.[60]

PREVENTING UNINTENDED TEEN PREGNANCY

In January 1996, President Clinton created the National Campaign to Prevent Teen Pregnancy to lead a national effort in the United States. This campaign has sought to highlight successful methods of pregnancy prevention. Findings to date emphasize the need for multidimensional programs using interventions that are developmentally appropriate for the targeted adolescent groups.[7, 9] Many models of adolescent pregnancy prevention programs have been devised.[27b, 53, 62] Most successful programs include multiple and varied approaches to the problem, such as promoting abstinence, making contraception accessible and available, sex education, school completion strategies, and job training. Both primary prevention (i.e., of a first pregnancy) and secondary prevention (repeat pregnancy) programs are needed that target the adolescents at highest risk of becoming pregnant, as are innovative programs that involve teenage boys.[27a, 63–65]

Effective approaches to teen pregnancy prevention based on social learning theory have been documented.[53, 66] They include (1) strong individual support from an adult; (2) emphasis on basic education achievement and cognitive skills; (3) attention to the world of work; (4) skills-building strategies aimed at preventing pregnancy; (5) involvement of community residents; (6) focus on peer pressures; and (7) starting interventions in the preteen years (since both girls and boys often initiate sexual activity very early).[53, 66] Program evaluations have identified futile interventions: (1) Imparting knowledge, alone, does not work; (2) no single intervention is effective; (3) no single intervention lasts throughout adolescence so several interventions must be implemented; (4) school-based clinics, alone, do not prevent teen pregnancy; (5) contraceptive availability is not enough; and (6) programs directed only toward abstinence are ineffective.[53, 66]

When designing an effective teen pregnancy prevention program, several additional facts must be recognized and incorporated into it. First, teen pregnancy is often multigenerational.[53] Second, risk behaviors for pregnancy often coexist with other risk behaviors, such as alcohol and drug abuse, violence, and school failure.[39, 40] Third, teens receive continuous messages about sexuality and pregnancy in the media. Fourth, because of generally worsening economic conditions in the last decade, some 25% of U.S. children are living in poverty. Fifth, shifts in social norms have made out-of-wedlock pregnancies more common and acceptable. Perceived fear of infertility is also prevalent in inner-city teens and may influence their sexual decision making.[66] Sixth, a history of sexual abuse is common among girls who become pregnant.[53] Finally, the role of males, especially young adult males, must be taken into consideration when planning teen pregnancy–prevention programs.[37, 38]

Programs aimed at delaying or reducing sexual activity have used a number of tactics: providing knowledge of sexual reproduction and access to contraceptives; reinforcing values and teaching abstinence; building decision-making and social skills; and increasing other life options.[5] Programs most successful in delaying sexual activity and increasing contraceptive use among adolescents generally take a two-pronged approach: (1) teaching that abstinence is best for preteens and young adolescents and (2) for older teens, providing information and access to contraceptives.[7, 53]

POLICY IMPLICATION: A FOCUS ON WELFARE REFORM

The most relevant and compelling current policy issue related to teenage pregnancy is welfare reform. The passage of the Personal Responsibility and Work Opportunity Reconciliation Act of 1996 is an extraordinary event in U.S. social policy toward impoverished children and their families, especially adolescent mothers and their offspring.[7]

The new welfare legislation was designed specifically to address adolescent and out-of-wedlock pregnancies and births. Several main provisions of the bill are likely to have a profound impact on young mothers: (1) entitlement to cash welfare benefits is abolished; (2) families can receive benefits for no longer than 5 years over their lifetime (shorter at the state's discretion; longer if states use their own funds); (3) after 2 years on welfare, recipients are required to work 20 to 30 hours per week; (4) minor mothers are required to live with a parent or a legal guardian and to stay in school; and (5) mothers are required to identify the fathers of their children and to cooperate with child support enforcement. States also may impose a family cap; that is, give no additional money for children born while mothers are receiving welfare.[8, 15]

The intense focus on teenage mothers and out-of-wedlock births in the new legislation is evidenced in several other provisions. As many as five states per year will each receive a $20-million "bonus" if they can show a decline in "illegitimacy" and abortion rates.[8, 19] In addition, substantial funds for states have been set aside for new abstinence education programs for adolescents.[15]

CONCLUSION

Recognizing that many adolescents trust physicians as authoritative sources of information, the American Medical Association has called on clinicians to include counseling on responsible sexual behavior, including abstinence and proper use of contraception, as part of annual preventive health visits.[67]

The Committee on Unintended Pregnancy (from the Division of Health Promotion and Disease Prevention, of the National Institute of Medicine) has concluded that reducing unintended pregnancies will require a new national understanding of the problem and consensus that pregnancy should be undertaken only with clear intent.[11] Accordingly, the committee urges, first and foremost, that the nation adopt a new social norm: All pregnancies should be intended—that is, they should be consciously and unquestionably desired at the time of conception.[11]

The U.S. Department of Health and Human Services, through its National Health Promotion and Disease Prevention Objectives, has urged that the proportion of all pregnancies that are unintended be reduced to 30% by the year 2000.[11, 53, 68] The committee endorses this goal and stresses that it is a realistic one that already has been reached by several other industrialized nations. Achieving this goal would mean, in absolute numbers, more than 200,000 *fewer* births each year that were unwanted at the time of conception, and about 800,000 fewer abortions each year.[11] To begin the long process of building national consensus around this norm, the committee recommends a multifaceted, long-term campaign with these objectives: (1) to educate the public about the major social and public health burdens of unintended pregnancy and (2) to stimulate a comprehensive set of activities at the national, state, and local levels to reduce such pregnancies.[11]

RECOMMENDATIONS BY AN AAP COMMITTEE ON ADOLESCENCE[7]

1. Pediatricians should encourage adolescents to postpone early sexual debut. Abstinence counseling is an important role for all pediatricians.

2. Pediatricians should be sensitive to issues relating to adolescent sexuality and be prepared to obtain developmentally appropriate sexual history on all adolescent patients.
3. Pediatricians should help ensure that all adolescents who are sexually active have knowledge of and access to contraception.
4. Pediatricians should encourage and participate in community efforts to prevent first and subsequent adolescent pregnancies. These efforts may vary widely from one community to another but should be directed to the specific needs of youth in that community.
5. Pediatricians should advocate for comprehensive medical and psychosocial support for all pregnant adolescents. Pregnant care should be tailored to the medical, social, nutritional, and educational needs of the adolescents and should include child care training.
6. Pediatricians should recommend that adolescent mothers not receive early postpartum discharge so that clinicians can ensure that the mother is capable of caring for her child and has resources available for assistance.
7. Pediatricians should advocate for the inclusion of the adolescent mother's partner and father of their child in teenage pregnancy and parenting programs with access to education and vocational training, parenting skills classes, and contraceptive education.
8. Pediatricians should serve as resources for pregnant teenagers and their infants, the teenager's family, and the father of the baby to ensure that optimal health care is obtained and appropriate support provided.

It is clear, now, that there is no single solution to the problem. No single curriculum has been found to reduce the high rate of pregnancies and births to teenagers nor has any single clinic-based or community-based approach. Healthy People 2000 objectives included reducing pregnancy by one third in the next 10 years, increasing the number of teens who delay sexual activity, and increasing contraceptive use (including safer sex practices that reduce STDs and HIV infections) by all adolescents.[68] Hence, to reach adolescent populations at risk for premature sexual activity and pregnancy, we must develop comprehensive efforts specially tailored to the unique needs of adolescents. We must build partnerships among national, state, and local organizations; schools; health and social services; businesses; religious institutions; federal, state, and local governments; and community and parents. Emphasizing personal responsibility for young people and providing them with opportunities for success are critical issues.

I am grateful to Dr. Marianne E. Felice, Dr. Jessica Daniel, and Dr. Sara Crane for editing this manuscript.

REFERENCES

1. Ventura SJ, Clarke SC, Matthews TJ: Recent declines in teenage birth rates in the United States: Variations by state, 1990–94. Mon Vital Stat Rep 1996; 45:1–6.
2. Spitz AM, Velebil P, Koonin LM, et al: Pregnancy, abortion, and birth rates among US adolescents: 1980, 1985, and 1990. JAMA 1996; 275:989–994.
3. Kaufmann RB, Spitz AM, Strauss LT, et al: The decline in US teen pregnancy rates, 1990–1995. Pediatrics 1998; 102(5):1141–1147.
4. Henshaw S: Unintended pregnancy in the United States. Fam Plann Perspect 1998; 30(1):24–29, 46.
5. Maynard R: Kids having kids: A Robin Hood Foundation Special report on the cost of adolescent childbearing. New York: Robin Hood Foundation, 1996.
6. Alan Guttmacher Institute: Falling Teen Pregnancy, Birthrates: What's Behind the Declines? New York: Alan Guttmacher Institute, 1998.
7. American Academy of Pediatrics, Committee on Adolescence: Adolescent Pregnancy—Current Trends and Issues: 1998. Pediatrics 1999; 103(2):516–519.
8. Moore KA: Teen Fertility the United States: 1993 data. Facts at a glance. Child Trends January 1996.
9. US Department of Health and Human Services: Secretary Shalala launches national strategy to prevent teen pregnancy: New state-by-state data show decline in teen birth rate. Human and Health Services News 1997; 1–3.
10. Smith SS: Teenage sex-cognitive immaturity increases the risk. BMJ 1996; 312:390–391.
11. Brown SS, Eisenberg L (eds): Consequences of unintended pregnancy. In The Best Intentions: Unintended Pregnancy and the Wellbeing of Children and Families. Washington, DC: Institute of Medicine, National Academy Press, 1995, pp 50–80.
12. Moore KA: Teen Fertility the United States: 1992 data. Facts at a glance. Child Trends February 1995.
13. Ventura SJ, Peters KD, Martin JA, et al: Births and Deaths: United States, 1996. Mon Vital Stat Rep 1997; 46:1–9.
14. Centers for Disease Control and Prevention: CDC Surveillance Summaries: Youth Risk Behavior Surveillance—United States, 1997. MMWR 1998; 47(SS-3):1–31.
15. Coley RL, Chase-Lansdale PL: Adolescent pregnancy and parenthood. Am Psychologist 1998; 53(2):152–166.
16. Brooks-Gunn J, Furstenberg FF Jr: Adolescent sexual behavior. Am Psychologist 1989; 44:249–257.
17. Forrest JD, Singh S: The sexual and reproductive behavior of American women, 1982–1988. Fam Plann Perspect 1990; 22:206–214.
18. Alan Guttmacher Institute: Sex and America's Teenagers. New York: Alan Guttmacher Institute, 1994.
19. Haffer DW (ed): Facing Facts: Sexual Health for America's Adolescents: The Report of the National Commission on Adolescent Sexual Health. New York: Sexuality Information and Education Council of the United States, 1995.
20. Centers for Disease Control and Prevention: Pregnancy,

Sexually Transmitted Diseases, and Related Risk Behaviors Among US Adolescents. Atlanta: Centers for Disease Control and Prevention, 1994.

21. Forrest JD: Timing of reproductive life stages. Obstet Gynecol 1993; 82:105–111.

22. Piccino LJ, Mosher WD: Trends in contraceptive use in the US:1982–1995. Fam Plann Perspect 1998; 46:4–10.

23. Hotz VJ, McElroy SW, Sanders SG: The impacts of teenage childbearing on the mothers and the consequences of those impacts for government. *In* Maynard R (ed): Kids Having Kids. Washington, DC: The Urban Institute Press, 1997.

24. Koonin LM, Atrash HK, Smith JC, et al: Abortion surveillance, 1986–1987. *In* CDC Surveillance Summaries, June 1990. MMWR 1990; 39(SS-2):23–56.

25. Koonin LM, Smith JC, Green CA: Abortion surveillance—United States, 1992. *In* CDC Surveillance Summaries, May 1996. MMWR. 1996; 45(SS-3):1–36.

26. Henshaw SK, Van Vort J: Abortion services in the United States, 1991 and 1992. Fam Plann Perspect 1994; 26:100–112.

27. Gober P: The role access in explaining state abortion rates. Soc Sci Med 1997; 44:1003–1016.

27a. Zabin LS, Emerson MR, Ringers PA, et al: Adolescents with negative pregnancy test results: An accessible at-risk group. JAMA 1996; 275:113–117.

27b. Peterson JL, Card JJ, Eisen MB, et al: Evaluating teenage pregnancy prevention and social programs: Ten stages of program assessment. Fam Plann Perspect 1994; 26:116–120.

27c. Spandorfer SD, Davis OK, Rosenwaks Z: Diagnosis of ectopic pregnancy. Hosp Physician 1998; 34:17–29.

28. AWHONN Lifelines: Teen birth rates declining. Aug 1998: 15.

29. Litt FI: Pregnancy in adolescence. JAMA 1996; 275:1030.

30. Cates W Jr: Contraception, unintended pregnancies, and sexual transmitted diseases:Why isn't a solution possible? Am J Epidemiol 1996; 143:311–318.

31. Carter DM, Felice ME, Rosoff J, et al: When children have children: The teen pregnancy predicament. Am J Prevent Med 1994; 10:108–113.

32. Jaskiewicz JA, McAnarney ER: Pregnancy during adolescence. Pediatr Rev 1994; 15:32–38.

33. Cherlin AC: Marriage, Divorce and Remarriage. Cambridge: Harvard University Press, 1992.

34. Laundry DJ, Forest JD: How old are US fathers? Fam Plann Perspect 1995; 27:159–161.

35. Fernandez M, Ruch-Ross HS, Montague AP: Ethnicity and effects of age gap between unmarried adolescent mothers and partners. J Adolesc Res 1993; 8:439–466.

36. Males M, Chew KSY: The age of fathers in California adolescent births, 1993. Am J Public Health 1996; 86:565–568.

37. Rickert VI, Wiemann CM, Berenson AB: Health risk behaviors among pregnant adolescents with older partners. Arch Pediatr Adolesc Med 1997; 151:276–280.

38. The Study Group on the Male Role in Teenage Pregnancy and Parenting. The Male Role in Teenage Pregnancy and Parenting: New Directions for Public Policy. New York: Vera Institute of Justice, 1990.

39. Resnick MO, Chambliss SA, Blum RW: Health and risk behaviors of urban males involved in a pregnancy. Fam Soc J Contemp Hum Serv 1993; 74:366–374.

40. Pierre N, Shrier AL, Emans SJ, et al: Adolescent males involved in pregnancy. J Adolesc Health 1998; 23:364–369.

41. Stevens-Simon C, Lowy R: Teenage childbearing: An

adaptive strategy for the socioeconomically disadvantaged or a strategy for adapting to socioeconomic disadvantage? Arch Pediatr Adolesc Med 1995; 149:912–915.

42. Hayes CD (ed): Risking the Future. Washington, DC: National Academic Press, 1987, p 1.

43. Stevens-Simon C, White M: Adolescent pregnancy. Pediatr Ann 1991; 20:322–331.

44. Stevens-Simon C, Beach R: Care of pregnant teenagers in school. J Sch Health 1992; 62:304–309.

45. McAnarney ER, Lawrence RA, Aten MJ, et al: Adolescent mothers and their infant. Pediatrics 1984; 73:358–362.

46. Elster AB, McArnaney ER, Lamb ME: Parental behavior of adolescent mothers. Pediatrics 1983; 71:494–501.

47. Seymore C, Frothingham TE, MacMillan J, DuRant RH: Child development knowledge, child rearing attitudes, and social support among first- and second-time adolescent mothers. J Adolesc Health 1990; 11:343–350.

48. East PL, Matthews KL, Felice ME: Qualities of adolescent mothers' parenting. J Adolesc Health 1194; 15:163–168.

49. American Academy of Pediatrics: Committee on Adolescent Pregnancy. Adolescent pregnancy. Pediatrics 1989; 83:132–134.

50. Buckerman B, Alpert JJ, Dooling E, et al: Neonatal outcome: Is adolescent pregnancy a risk factor? Pediatrics 1983; 71:489–493.

51. Witte K: Preventing teen pregnancy through persuasive communications: Realities, myths, and the hard-fact truths. J Community Health 1997; 22(2):137–153.

52. Brown SS, Eisenberg L (eds): Consequences of unintended pregnancy. *In* The Best Intentions: Unintended Pregnancy and the Wellbeing of Children and Families. Washington, DC: Institute of Medicine, National Academy Press; 1995, pp 21–49.

53. Pierre N, Cox J: Teenage pregnancy prevention programs. Curr Opin Pediatr 1997; 9:310–316.

54. Card BJ, Niego S, Mallari A, Farrell WS: The program archive on sexuality, health and adolescence: Promising "prevention programs in a box." Fam Plann Perspect 1996; 28:210–220.

55. Pierre N, Moy LK, Redd S, et al: Results of pregnancy testing protocol in adolescents undergoing surgery. J Pediatr Adolesc Gynecol 1998; 3:139–141.

56. Emans SJ, Laufer MR, Goldstein DP: Teenage pregnancy. *In* Callaghan P (ed): Pediatric and Adolescent Gynecology, 4th ed. Philadelphia: Lippincott-Raven, 1998, p 675.

57. American Academy of Pediatrics Committee on Adolescence: Counseling the adolescent about pregnancy options. Pediatrics 1998; 10:938–940.

58. American Academy of Pediatrics Committee on Adolescence: The adolescent's right to confidential care when considering abortion. Pediatrics 1996; 97:746–751.

59. Davinson NW, Felice ME: Adolescent pregnancy. *In* Friedman SB, Fisher M, Schonberg SK (eds): Comprehensive Adolescent Health Care. St. Louis: Quality Medical Publishing; 1992, pp 1026–1040.

60. Hacker NF, Moore JG: Ectopic pregnancy. Hacker NF, Moore JG (eds): Essentials of Obstetrics and Gynecology. Philadelphia: WB Saunders, 1986, p 336.

61. Hacker NF, Moore JG: Gestational trophoblastic neoplasia. Hacker NF, Moore JG (eds): Essentials of Obstetrics and Gynecology. Philadelphia, WB Saunders, 1986, p 509.

62. Greydanus DE, Pratt HD, Dannison LL: Sexuality education programs for youth: Current state of affairs and strategies for the future. J Sex Educ Ther 1995; 21:238–254.

63. Hardy JB, Zabin LS: Adolescent Pregnancy in an Urban Environment: Issues, Programs, Evaluation. Washington, DC: Urban Institute Press, 1991.

64. Fielding JE, Williams CA: Adolescent pregnancy in the United States: A review and recommendations for clinicians and research needs. Am J Prevent Med 1991; 7:47–52.

65. East PL, Felice ME: Pregnancy risk among the younger sisters of pregnant and childbearing adolescents. J Develop Behav Pediatr 1992; 13:128–136.

66. Philliber S, Namerow P: Trying to maximize the odds: Using what we know to prevent teen pregnancy. Document prepared for technical assistance workshop to support the Teen Pregnancy Program, Division of Reproductive Health, National Center for Chronic Disease Prevention and Health Promotion, Centers for Disease Control and Prevention, Atlanta, December 13–15, 1995.

67. American Medical Association: AMA Guidelines for Adolescent Preventive Services (GAPS): Recommendations and Rationale. Baltimore: Williams & Wilkins, 1994.

68. US Department of Health and Human Services, Public Health Service: National Health Promotion and Disease Prevention Objectives. Healthy People 2000. Boston: Jones & Barlett, Publishers 1996.

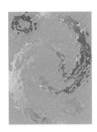

Chapter 21

Sexually Transmissible Diseases in Childhood

Kristi Morgan Mulchahey

The diagnosis of a sexually transmissible disease (STD) is, fortunately, a rare occurrence in childhood. However, STDs may be diagnosed in both symptomatic children with genitourinary complaints[1-3] and asymptomatic children who have been sexually abused.[4-6] In sexually abused children, survey studies have estimated the incidence of STDs to range from 1% to 26%, but most studies indicate rates of 1% to 5%. These findings appear to be consistent with those of international studies.[7, 8] All STDs that have been reported in adults have also been reported in the pediatric population.[9]

A clinician faced with the task of screening a symptomatic child or one child with a history of sexual abuse needs to consider many factors. The bulk of published data on STDs has been collected from adult populations; however, a number of factors are unique to childhood and are diagnostically and therapeutically important. From the perspectives of histology and physiology, the genital tract of children is markedly different from that of adults, and affects the presentation of STDs in childhood. The choice of an appropriate diagnostic test should take into account the unique characteristics of the pediatric age group. Mode of transmission is also an extremely important issue. Both perinatal (i.e., vertical) transmission and sexual transmission have been reported for pediatric STDs. The possibility of fomite or casual transmission must also be considered, although such cases appear to be quite uncommon.

GENITAL TRACT PHYSIOLOGY AND HISTOLOGY

The genital tract of the prepubertal girl is dramatically influenced by the presence or absence of estrogen. In the neonatal period, transplacental passage of maternal hormones results in a thickened vaginal epithelium in which intracellular glycogen accumulates. An acidic pH results from the metabolism of this glycogen by the abundant *Lactobacillus* organisms. The infant's normal vaginal flora is often similar to maternal vaginal flora. As the estrogens are metabolized, however, the vaginal epithelium takes on the characteristic thin appearance typical during childhood. On cytologic examination, the epithelial cells are smaller than the estrogenized epithelial cells of adults and have a higher nuclear-cytoplasmic ratio. On histologic examination, sections show a thinner epithelium with an alkaline pH and the basal and parabasal cells typical of the unestrogenized vaginal epithelium of postmenopausal women. With the onset of puberty and the production of estrogen, the vaginal epithelium again thickens and accumulates *Lactobacillus* organisms and glycogen, and the pH falls.[2]

There are also anatomic differences in the genital tracts of prepubertal and of postpubertal females.[10] In childhood, the cervix comprises a relatively larger portion of the uterus; with puberty, differential growth results in a relatively larger uterine fundus. In the estrogenized genital tract, the portio of the cervix contains endocervical glands, which are susceptible to infection by organisms such as *Neisseria gonorrhoeae* and *Chlamydia trachomatis*. In contrast, the prepubertal girl usually has no endocervical glands on the ectocervix, a condition that protects the upper genital tract from infection with these organisms.[1] The thin, unestrogenized vaginal epithelium is much more susceptible to infection that results in a true vaginitis with these organisms.[2]

TESTING

Most clinicians who frequently evaluate alleged pediatric sexual abuse selectively screen children for STDs, depending on symptoms and other perceived risks of infection.[11] Each clinician must balance cost effectiveness, risks of un-detected infection, and possible psychological trauma to the child when choosing "selected" versus universal STD screen for forensic evaluations.[12] The Centers for Disease Control and Prevention (CDC) recommends that decisions to screen pediatric patients for STDs be individualized and be mindful of minimizing psychological and physical pain. Screening is encouraged in certain high-risk situations: high-risk suspected offender, offender known to be infected with an STD, symptomatic child, high community prevalence of STDs, and a child whose sibling is an infected child or who demonstrates evidence of penetration of or ejaculation into the oral or genital orifice.

The diagnostic testing for STDs in the pediatric age group is another instance when clinical data collected from the adult population must be interpreted with caution. Children are anatomically and physiologically different from adults. For children, culture material must be collected from the sites where infection with sexually transmitted organisms is most likely. In prepubertal girls, culture material for gonococcal and chlamydial infection may be obtained from the vagina rather than the cervix. In prepubertal boys, the rectum is more likely than the urethra to be the site of infection.

Each clinical setting should have carefully developed protocols for each step of the microbiologic investigations; the procedures should begin with collection of the specimen and continue through generation of a report.[13] Culture or transport media should be chosen that minimize false-negative results. Care should be taken to avoid using swabs or bacteriostatic saline, which could affect results. Vaginal wash techniques appear to be at least as effective as a direct swab technique for the collection of specimens (Table 21-1).[14]

Antigen-detection testing methods have become increasingly popular in adult populations but are not recommended for forensic evaluation of children. These diagnostic tools are widely available, simple to perform, and cost-effective. They also offer more rapid results than the direct culture-testing methods. However, it is important to critically compare these indirect testing methods with the culture techniques that have long been the gold standard. Most of the sensitivity and specificity data that have been generated with the nonculture methods are from high-prevalence populations. Adults attending an STD clinic, for example, obviously have much higher rates of infection than children being screened for STDs because of genitourinary complaints or sexual abuse.[15] In addition, the use of nonculture

Table 21-1. CDC-Recommended Laboratory Procedures at Initial and Follow-up Evaluation of Sexually Abused Prepubertal Children

Gram stain of any genital or anal discharge°
Culture for *Neisseria gonorrhoeae*†
Culture for *Chlamydia trachomatis*†
Wet preparation of vaginal secretion for trichomonads
Culture of lesions for herpes simplex virus
Serologic test for syphilis
Serologic test for HIV‡
Frozen serum sample

°Care should be taken in the interpretation of results of any Gram stain of any anal discharge.
†Culture of pharynx, rectum, and vagina/urethra should be done.
‡Testing for HIV should be based on the prevalence of infection and on suspected risk.
Note. Syphilis and HIV serologic tests should be repeated in 12 weeks. All other tests should be repeated 10 to 14 days after the initial examination.
From Centers for Disease Control: 1989 sexually transmitted diseases treatment guidelines. MMWR 1989;38(S8):11-38.

methods in adults has been tested with material from anatomic sites such as cervix or urethra, sites different from those where infection is found in the pediatric age group. For these reasons, the nonculture testing methods are not recommended for use in children.[16] Nevertheless, Stewart's survey in 1993 still indicated frequent use of indirect testing methods in pediatric clinical settings.[11] More recent studies suggest that polymerase chain reaction (PCR) techniques may increase the yield for culture techniques in pediatric populations, although definitive studies have not been completed.[14]

SOURCES OF TRANSMISSION

In recent years, the role of nonsexual transmission of STDs in children has gained more attention. In 1982, the CDC's *Sexually Transmitted Disease Guidelines* stated, "Diagnosis of any sexually transmitted infection in a child who is prepubertal but not neonatal raises the strong possibility of sexual abuse unless proven otherwise. The presence of an STD may be the major or only physical evidence of sexual abuse and may be asymptomatic."[17] This might usefully be contrasted to the 1989 Sexually Transmitted Disease Guidelines: "The identification of a sexually transmissible agent from a child beyond the neonatal period suggests sexual abuse. However, exceptions do exist. . . . When the only evidence of sexual abuse is the isolation of an organism or the detection of antibodies, findings should be carefully confirmed."[18]

Whenever there is suspicion or a firm diagnosis of an STD in any child, it is essential to consider all possible sources of infection. Acquisition through sexual contact, vertical transmis-

Table 21–2. Transmission of STDs to Children

	Sexual	Perinatal	Casual/Fomite
N. gonorrhoeae	High	Possible	Rare
C. trachomatis	High	Common	Very rare
T. pallidum	High	Possible	Rare
Herpes simplex	Possible	Possible	?
Bacterial vaginosis	High	?	Rare
HPV	High	Possible	Uncommon
T. vaginalis	High	Possible	?

HPV, human papillomavirus.
Adapted from Ingram DL: Controversies about the sexual and nonsexual transmissions of adult STDs to children. *In* Krugman RD, Leventhal JM (eds): Child Sexual Abuse. Report of the 22nd Ross Roundtable on Critical Approaches to Common Pediatric Problems. Columbus, OH: Ross Laboratories, 1991, p 21.

sion at birth, nonsexual casual or fomite transmission should be considered (Table 21–2). It may be more realistic, especially in the pediatric age group, to use the phrase *sexually transmissible* rather than *sexually transmitted disease.*

GONORRHEA

Biology

N. gonorrhoeae is a gram-negative diplococcus responsible for some of the most commonly reported STDs of adults.[19] It is also one of the most extensively studied agents of sexually transmissible infection in childhood. This organism enters the body through mucous membrane surfaces like those in the mouth, urethra, vagina, endocervix, and anorectal canal.[20] For children, the most commonly infected sites are the vagina, rectum, pharynx, and conjunctiva. The vaginal epithelium of prepubertal girls is composed of relatively few layers of unestrogenized cells. Unlike the adult vaginal epithelium, which is resistent to infection with *N. gonorrhoeae*, the vaginal epithelium of the prepubertal child can be infected if exposed to this organism. However, the absence of endocervical glands on the ectocervix of the prepubertal child makes the cervix more resistant to infection. For this reason, ascending genital tract infection with *N. gonorrhoeae* is rare in children. Most of the reports of gonococcal peritonitis in children are from the era before widespread availability of antibiotics.[21] Infection of Bartholin's gland is also quite rare in prepubertal girls.

Demographics

The overall incidence of gonorrheal infection in children is relatively low, though it depends on the population of children being evaluated. The overall incidence of gonococcal infection in the 9 years and younger group was reported at 6.5 per 100,000 in both 1980 and 1985.[22] Among this group are neonates with gonococcal infection, most often ophthalmia neonatorum. As many as 7.5% of pregnant women attending public health obstetrics clinics have been found to have positive cervical cultures for *N. gonorrhoeae*, and their risk of neonatal transmission is 30%.[23, 24]

Occasionally, gonococcal infections are detected in both asymptomatic children and those with genitourinary complaints. In prepubertal girls with symptomatic vaginitis, culture of *N. gonorrhoeae* has been reported in 5% to 7%.[1, 25] In healthy children being screened during routine pediatric visits, the incidental finding of *N. gonorrhoeae* was very low—1% or less.[3, 26]

The possibility of gonococcal infection is greatest among children who are likely victims of sexual abuse. Among children being screened for STDs because of a report of suspected sexual abuse, the figures for positive gonococcal cultures have ranged from 2.6% to 11%. Older studies found incidences ranging from 4.7% to 11%, the greater ones in children who had other STDs,[27] a delay in reporting, multiple episodes of abuse, or whose siblings had positive cultures.[4–6, 28, 29] Ingram's recent prospective study of 1500 children evaluated by culture for possible sexual abuse reports gonorrhea rates of 2.6% for urethral or vaginal specimens and 1.8% and 0.14%, respectively, for anal and pharyngeal cultures.[30]

Some have suggested that the incidence of gonorrheal infections in children may be increasing; however, the increase in reported cases most likely represents more aggressive efforts at detection and better reporting of confirmed cases.[31]

Presentation

The incubation period for *N. gonorrhoeae* is roughly 1 week, and symptoms generally appear in 2 to 7 days. Neonates most commonly present within the first 3 to 4 days of life with ophthalmia neonatorum, although gonococcal arthritis, meningitis, and sepsis have also been reported.[23]

Children with symptomatic gonococcal infection usually present with vulvovaginitis accompanied by erythema, purulent vaginal discharge, and pruritus. Dysuria may result from the vulvitis or from urethritis. An 18-institution cooperative study of children with symptomatic gonococcal infection found erythema in 40%, pruritus in 22%, and dysuria in 8%.[32] If untreated, this purulent vaginal discharge may be replaced by a serous discharge, which can persist several months. Older studies of the natural history of untreated gonococcal vaginitis in girls have shown cases where the discharge resolved without treatment, leaving the children colonized (and, therefore, infectious) for as long as 6 to 7 months. After this time, some children became culture negative without treatment. Populations of children studied in the preantibiotic era also indicated a 9% incidence of peritonitis.[21]

Children colonized with *N. gonorrhoeae* sometimes have no symptoms. Several studies have reported a relatively high incidence of gonococcal infection in asymptomatic sexually abused children. In DeJong's 1986 review, 44% of positive gonococcal cultures were from asymptomatic children.[5] Along with other studies,[4] this points out the importance of "culturing" even asymptomatic children when the possibility of sexual abuse is being evaluated.

In prepubertal boys, urethritis may be the only symptom.[33] Pharyngitis and proctitis have also been reported in children of both sexes; although colonization of the pharynx or anorectum is more common than symptomatic infection.[34, 35] Gonococcal conjunctivitis beyond the neonatal period has also been reported and generally presents with a febrile illness accompanied by hyperpurulent conjunctivitis and periorbital cellulitis. This potentially severe infection may result in visual impairment if it is not diagnosed promptly and treated appropriately.[36]

Infection at more than one anatomic site is also quite common. In a series of 108 children, Nelson found that 50% of girls with positive vaginal cultures also had positive rectal cultures, and 15% had intercurrent positive vaginal and pharyngeal cultures. In only 3% were positive rectal cultures the sole finding.[32] Ingram found that 41% of girls with positive vaginal cultures were also colonized with *N. gonorrhoeae* in the anorectal canal and 19% had pharyngeal colonization.[33] In Silber's report of six children with asymptomatic pharyngeal gonorrhea, four of the children also had vaginal colonization with *N. gonorrhoeae*.[34] DeJong also reported, in his study of 532 sexually victimized children, that 32% of the positive cultures for *N. gonorrhoeae* were from samples from anatomic sites not disclosed in interviews.[5] This clearly demonstrates the importance of culturing material from all three sites (pharynx, vagina, rectum) when screening for *N. gonorrhoeae* and from other sites when, unexpectedly, a culture is positive.[27]

Transmission

Beyond the neonatal period, sexual contact is nearly always the cause of gonococcal infections in children. Because of the incubation period of *N. gonorrhoeae*, perinatally acquired infection usually presents in the first week(s) of life. In several carefully evaluated series, the strong likelihood of sexual transmission of pediatric gonococcal disease had been demonstrated. Among children aged 14 or younger, Branch and Paxton found a history of sexual abuse in 160 of 161 cases.[38] In a later study, Ingram found a history of sexual contact in all children between ages 5 and 12 years who had gonococcal infection. Among children younger than 4 years, he could document sexual abuse in only 35%. However, he stressed the difficulty of detecting sexual abuse in young children, especially during the preverbal years. For well-documented reasons, older children also may have difficulty disclosing sexual abuse. Only 17% of the older children in this study recounted a history of sexual abuse during the first interview after the gonococcal infection was diagnosed.[33] In fact, two of the children did not report sexual abuse until 8 years after completion of the study.[39] Farrell also stresses the need for a multidisciplinary approach to the evaluation of a child for gonococcal infection, because the majority of the sexually abused children in his study did not disclose that during the initial interview.[40]

When a child who is beyond the neonatal period but younger than 4 years presents with a gonococcal infection, sexual contact remains the most likely cause, although one difficult to prove. Especially in this age group, questions about transmission by fomites and close, nonsexual contact are often raised. *Gonococcus* organisms can remain viable in water for 2 hours and on towels for 24 hours.[39] There is only one documented case of an identified fomite transmitting *N. gonorrhoeae* to a child; the child of a laboratory worker developed pharyngeal gonococcal infection after eating a Thayer-Martin plate containing

N. gonorrhoeae colonies.[41] A question of fomite transmission was raised, but never identified, in an outbreak of gonococcal infection in infants contained on the same hospital ward in 1927.[42] Rice and colleagues failed to demonstrate either positive cultures from material collected from toilet seats or transmission to uninfected children in a hospital ward where children with untreated gonococcal vaginal discharge shared bathroom facilities with healthy children.[43]

The transmission of gonococcal infection from one child to another through genital exploratory behavior has been reported. Potterat described the case of a 5-year-old girl who infected her 4- and 7-year-old playmates.[44] This is probably an uncommon occurrence; an earlier study of 160 cases of pediatric gonococcal infection by Branch could identify no instances of children younger than 10 having been infected by peers.[38]

Although gonococcal conjunctivitis is the least common infection in children, it is possibly one exception to the strong relationship between infection with *N. gonorrhoeae* and sexual contact. Accidental gonococcal conjunctivitis has been reported in adult laboratory workers[45, 46]; however, most cases in adolescents and adults are attributed to direct contact with infected urine or genital secretions.[47, 48] Studies of childhood gonococcal conjunctivitis have been confounded by the unsuspected nature of the infection. Children were usually treated empirically with antibiotics before the pathogen was identified, a measure that rendered culturing of other sites useless. However, in a study of four children with gonococcal conjunctivitis, two parents were found to carry identical isolates. In each case, the child slept with the parent and no sexual contact could be documented.[36] Again, the inherent difficulties of obtaining an accurate history from small children warrant caution.

Diagnosis

Choosing the correct diagnostic test(s) is crucial to avoiding the possibility of either a false-negative or a false-positive result, as either error can have serious consequences. The use of indirect testing methods for *N. gonorrhoeae* is not recommended in children; both false-positive and false-negative results have been reported with monoclonal antibody and direct fluorescence antibody testing methods used in prepubertal children.[16, 49] Although the finding of gram-negative intracellular diplococci on Gram stain has been used by some as a diagnostic tool for *N. gonorrhoeae*, false-positive results have also

been reported with this method. Farrell found that 14% of his prepubertal patients with a positive Gram stain result had a negative culture.[40] For that reason, many suggest that Gram staining of secretions be reserved for situations when, in a symptomatic child, therapy must be instituted before culture results are received.[16]

Even with the culture techniques used to isolate *N. gonorrhoeae*, errors still sometimes occur. In a low-prevalence population, the use of presumptive criteria for identification of organisms from positive cultures also has little predictive value. Nongonococcal *Neisseria* organisms may be part of the normal flora in children, especially in the pharynx. The use of nonselective media is quite common, especially when gonococcal infection is not suspected. For this reason, confirmation of organisms presumptively identified as *N. gonorrhoeae* is necessary, using methods such as carbohydrate degradation, enzyme substrate, or immunologic testing. Of 40 pediatric gonococcal isolates submitted to the CDC for confirmatory testing, 14 were found to be nongonococcal *Neisseria* organisms. It is also recommended that isolates obtained from children be stored at $-70°C$, should additional confirmatory testing be necessary later.[16]

Treatment

The CDC currently recommends ceftriaxone for gonococcal infections in children. Children weighing more than 45 kg are treated as adults, and children weighing less than 45 kg with uncomplicated infection (vulvovaginitis, urethritis, pharyngitis, or proctitis) may be treated with a single 125-mg intramuscular dose of ceftriaxone. Intramuscular spectinomycin, 40 mg/kg, may be used in children who cannot tolerate ceftriaxone. It is recommended that children older than 8 years also receive a 7-day course of doxycycline. Children with a complicated gonococcal infection (conjunctivitis, peritonitis, arthritis, meningitis) should undergo a more prolonged course of parenteral ceftriaxone.[18]

Successful single-dose oral antibiotic therapy with amoxicillin and probenecid for culture-confirmed, uncomplicated childhood gonococcal infection has also been reported. In a multicenter study, this regimen was as efficacious as intramuscular penicillin G, procaine, and probenecid.[32] Although the endemic rise of penicillinase-producing *N. gonorrhoeae* may limit the usefulness of this therapy, the low cost and patient acceptance of an oral regimen are attractive in cases when culture and sensitivity results are available. Although some data from adults suggest that the oral regimen is less effective for pharyngeal and rectal gonococcal infections,[50] Nelson reported no treatment failures with his oral amoxicillin-probenecid regimen in children with positive pharyngeal or rectal cultures.[32]

For asymptomatic children being evaluated for possible sexual abuse, prophylactic treatment for gonococcal infection is not recommended.[5] Kramer and Jason have calculated that 96% of children receiving prophylactic treatment receive it unnecessarily.[51] Also, the rarity of upper tract genital disease in children supports this stance.

One final aspect of treatment of gonococcal infection in children that should be stressed is follow-up. Follow-up cultures after treatment are important to document complete eradication of the organism. Some authors have suggested a second set of follow-up cultures 6 to 8 weeks after documented cure to seek evidence of reinfection. This would seem especially important when the source of infection has not been identified or casual contact or fomite transmission is believed to be the source. In some cases, the assistance of Child Protective Services may be necessary. Farrell noted that 92% of children treated as outpatients were lost to follow-up.[40] Clearly, a multidisciplinary approach is helpful to ensure proper compliance and follow-up.

Chlamydia trachomatis

Biology

C. trachomatis is an obligate intracellular parasite, 15 serotypes of which have so far been identified. The less common serotypes, L1, L2, and L3, are responsible for lymphogranuloma venereum; serotypes D to K are responsible for inclusion conjunctivitis, pneumonia, vaginitis, nongonococcal urethritis, cervicitis, and salpingitis. This obligate intracellular organism can be cultured only in a living cell host, not in artificial culture media.

Inclusion conjunctivitis is principally a disease of the neonatal period, with *Chlamydia* pneumonitis occurring during infancy. In adults, genital tract infection is the usual clinical presentation. Beyond infancy, chlamydial infection in children is uncommon and generally affects the genital tract. *C. trachomatis* directly infects the squamo-columnar-columnar epithelial cells, causing extensive cell damage in its life cycle. In adults, the urethra of the man and the endocervix of the woman are the most common sites of primary infection. As with gonococcal infection of the

prepubertal genital tract, the "atrophic," unestrogenized vaginal epithelium can be directly infected with this organism, causing a true vaginitis. *C. trachomatis* is never considered part of the normal flora, but it often produces colonization without symptoms.[52]

Demographics

Infection with *C. trachomatis* is one of the most common STDs in adults, with an estimated 4 million new cases annually.[53] The significant cost and lack of availability of *Chlamydia* cell cultures have resulted in underdiagnosis of this infection in the adult population. The more recently developed antigen-detection methods have made diagnosis easier in adults, although these testing methods are not recommended for use in pediatric populations. It should also be remembered that in some areas infections with *C. trachomatis* are not "reportable" infections, and, so, underreporting seems very likely.

No overall figures are available for the incidence of chlamydial infection in children (as they are for gonococcal infection in children). A number of studies, however, have suggested that vertical transmission during the perinatal period is quite common. Many studies have found that some 6% to 10% of all pregnant women are infected with *C. trachomatis*, and, in high-risk populations, some 22% to 26%. Populations of pregnant adolescents have shown infection rates as high as 37%. Vertical transmission is very common in infants delivered through an infected genital tract. The risk of inclusion conjunctivitis ranges from 18% to 50%; chlamydial pneumonitis affects 22% to 10% of exposed infants; and 60% to 70% of exposed infants demonstrate serologic evidence of infection by 12 months of age.[23, 24, 54-56]

Infection of the genital tract is the most common presentation in children after infancy. As with gonococcal infection, the incidence varies greatly, according to the population being studied. Margaret Hammerschlag found a 1% incidence of positive vaginal *Chlamydia* cultures in her population of nonselected girls being screened in an ambulatory pediatric clinic as part of a study of normal vaginal flora.[3] Paradise found no positive *Chlamydia* cultures in her population of girls with vaginitis, although 2.8% of her control population of asymptomatic girls had positive cultures.[1] In a study by Bump, 20% of girls with symptoms of vaginitis were found to have chlamydial infection; there was a 44% positive culture rate in children whose presenting complaint was vaginal bleeding.[57]

When a population of suspected sexually abused children is examined, the overall incidence of chlamydial infection is generally reported to be between 2% and 6%.[5, 6, 58, 59] This relatively low incidence has led genital chlamydial infection in childhood to be described as "statistically nonsignificant but clinically important."[60] The incidence varies greatly in different areas, however, a finding that many authors have attributed to high rates of chlamydial infection in their adult population. The highest reported incidence was found by Keskey and colleagues, who reported 43% positive cultures in their preadolescent, sexually abused population.[61] Case-control studies have often been confounded by the appearance of chlamydial infection in the control population, whose unsuspected abuse was often detected after investigation.[58, 59]

As with gonococcal infection, multisite infection with *C. trachomatis* has been reported. In one population of suspected sexual abuse victims, 8% of children had positive vaginal cultures,[62] 2.4% positive rectal findings, and 0.8% positive pharyngeal cultures. In addition, 1.4% of pharyngeal cultures were positive in the investigators' population of children "at risk" for abuse.[62] An earlier study by the same author noted a 3% incidence of positive pharyngeal and concomitant vaginal and rectal cultures in a population of abused children.[58] Among children with a very high incidence of genital *Chlamydia* infections, 53% had positive culture results from several sites.[61] As with gonococcal infection, many of these positive cultures were obtained from anatomic sites not mentioned by children in their disclosures of abuse.

Presentation

In the neonatal period, infection with *C. trachomatis* most often presents as inclusion conjunctivitis at 5 to 7 days of age. Initially, a mucoid discharge is present, which may become purulent within a few days. Without treatment, colonization of the conjunctivae may persist as long as 2 years. Contrary to what was once thought, untreated conjunctival infection may produce chronic sequelae. Perinatal exposure to *C. trachomatis* can also result in pneumonitis at 3 to 11 weeks of age associated with a history of prolonged cough and congestion. Some but not all infants may have a history of conjunctivitis.[54]

Perinatal exposure may also result in colonization of the vagina and rectum.[63] Longitudinal studies of infants exposed to *C. trachomatis* at birth have shown carriage of the organism up to 55 weeks in the rectum and 53 weeks in the vagina.[64] A more recent study demonstrated rectal colonization as long as 2 years after perinatal exposure.[65] In these studies, the majority of the infants were asymptomatic.

C. trachomatis is also known to cause symptomatic vaginitis in infected children. Even before the organism was identified, case reports were published of vaginitis in prepubertal girls caused by the very organism responsible for inclusion conjunctivitis.[66] In adult women, this organism infects the squamocolumnar epithelium of the cervix, whereas prepubertal girls are infected in the atrophic, unestrogenized squamous epithelium of the vagina. When symptomatic, children usually present with vaginitis, urethritis, and/or pyuria.[57] *C. trachomatis* has also been reported as a cause of symptomatic urethritis in prepubertal boys.[67] From their series of children with genital chlamydial infection, Fuster and Neinstein found that 44% of children presented with vulvar erythema, 24% with vaginal discharge, 25% with rectal pain, and 12% with vaginal bleeding.[68] Bump found a 44% incidence of positive chlamydial cultures in children who presented with vaginal bleeding.[57] Many studies have confirmed that asymptomatic colonization is a common occurrence in children. In Ingram's study, 60% of children with positive vaginal cultures were asymptomatic. All of the girls in that study who had a positive oral or rectal culture were asymptomatic.[62]

Although nongonococcal urethritis in men usually develops within 2 weeks of exposure,[52] many reports of chlamydial infection in children have suggested the possibility of a long latent period. In the case-control study of Hammerschlag's group of prepubertal girls with chlamydial infection, the positive cultures in the control group were attributed to sexual abuse 3 years before the study.[59]

Children infected with *Chlamydia* organisms by sexual contact do not always exhibit evidence of vaginal penetration on physical examination. As with gonococcal infection in children, this suggests that the organism may be spread by vulvar contact with infected secretions or an infected body part. Ingram and colleagues found that 60% of the sexually abused children in one study who had positive vaginal *Chlamydia* cultures showed no evidence of vaginal penetration.[62] Fuster and Neinstein also found evidence of hymenal tears in only 26% of their population of prepubertal girls with positive vaginal chlamydial cultures.[68]

Intercurrent infection with *C. trachomatis* and *N. gonorrhoeae* has also been a fairly common finding. Many of the early reports of pediatric chlamydial vaginitis were in children whose symptoms persisted after they were treated for documented gonococcal vaginitis and who subsequently were found to have positive *Chlamydia* cultures. In a study of prepubertal children with gonococcal infection, Rettig and Nelson found 27% to be positive also for *C. trachomatis*.[67]

Transmission

The primary modes of transmission of *C. trachomatis* all involve direct contact, rather than a fomite. Given the obligate intracellular nature of this parasite, transmission via fomites is in theory extremely unlikely and has never been documented.

At birth, the neonate is inoculated by contact with infected secretions. Perinatal exposure has been well-documented to result in spread of the organism to the eyes, nasopharynx, vagina, and rectum. Vertical transmission at the time of cesarean section performed after the rupture of membranes has also been reported.[23, 24, 54–56] It appears that each site may be separately inoculated at birth; this mechanism is in addition to autoinoculation from one site to another. Bell and colleagues found that the majority of infants infected at birth with *Chlamydia* organisms demonstrated positive nasopharyngeal cultures several months before positive vaginal and/or rectal cultures were documented.[65]

The potential for prolonged colonization with perinatally acquired *C. trachomatis* may complicate determination of the source of infection in toddlers, because obtaining a history from the child is limited. Perinatal colonization up to 2 years of age has been reported, as it was in the case of a 16-month-old girl with symptomatic chlamydial vaginitis after untreated, perinatally acquired inclusion conjunctivitis.[60]

After 24 to 36 months of age, genital infection with *C. trachomatis* has been strongly associated with sexual abuse.[58] In the case-control study of Hammerschlag's group, the diagnosis of chlamydial vaginitis strongly correlated with a history of sexual abuse. Even in unsuspected cases of chlamydial vaginitis in her control group, careful investigation revealed histories of sexual abuse. It is important to remember that, like girls with gonococcal infection, sexual abuse victims may not report it at the first (or even second) interview. Bump found an initial history of sexual abuse in only 25% of the girls with chlamydial vaginitis; later interviewing discovered a history of abuse in all but one child.[57] Again, a multidisciplinary approach and high index of suspicion are in order.

Diagnosis

The choice of the correct diagnostic test is essential. Cell culture is regarded as the gold standard, and the optimal method of identifying this obligate intracellular organism. The most commonly employed technique involves a monolayer of susceptible cells (e.g., McCoy cells). Because this organism is intracellular, it is important to obtain epithelial cells for the culture, rather than simply to culture any discharge material.[19] In adults, this would involve a careful endocervical or urethral culture. In prepubertal children, a careful vaginal or urethral culture is necessary. Prepubertal girls can be infected with *C. trachomatis* without having any evidence of vaginal penetration or symptoms of vaginitis. Therefore, cultures should not be omitted simply because the child is asymptomatic or has normal hymenal anatomy. Culturing the pharynx does not often yield positive results, and it currently is not recommended.[18, 19]

The correct growth or transport media must be used to obtain accurate results. The choice of swab type is also important to avoid toxic effects on the cell culture.[71] Urethral swabs of calcium alginate (Calgi swabs) are often useful for collecting culture material from children because of their small diameter; these swabs may be batch tested to ensure they carry nothing toxic to the growth of *C. trachomatis* in cell culture. When positive culture results are obtained, freezing the organism at −70°C may be indicated. This is especially important if forensic confirmation may be necessary later.[71]

Antigen-detection testing has become increasingly popular in response to the expense and limited availability of cell cultures for *C. trachomatis*. These testing methods employ either a direct fluorescence monoclonal antibody (e.g., Microtrak) or an enzyme-linked immunoassay (ELISA, e.g., Chlamydiazyme). The antigen-detection methods were developed and sensitivity and specificity data generated in high-prevalence populations (such as adult STD clinic patients) and are used in the cervix and urethra.[19] The CDC recommends against the use of these testing methods in prepubertal children.[18] The low prevalence of *C. trachomatis* infection in sexually abused children and the need to test anatomic sites other than the cervix and urethra contribute to unacceptable sensitivity and specificity rates. False-positive and false-negative rates up to 50% have been reported with the use of antigen-detection methods in children. Specificity and sensitivity rates reported for adults are not applicable in children, because their prevalence rate for *C. trachomatis* infection is much lower, and cross-reacting organisms (e.g., *Escherichia coli*, group B streptococci, and *Acinetobacter*) are present in oral and fecal flora.[37, 68, 72, 73] Laboratories must also be able to distinguish between *C. trachomatis* and *C. pneumoniae*. Antigen-detection tests may fail to distinguish between these species when genus-specific antibodies are used.[74] Newer DNA amplification testing methods have not been sufficiently evaluated in children, but some experts consider them an alternative when cell culture is not available and confirmative testing is used.[69]

Serologic testing for the presence of antibodies to *C. trachomatis* has not been clinically useful in children. Seroconversion is common during the childhood years. In a study of well children, 15% of those between 9 months and 15 years demonstrated antibodies against *C. trachomatis*. Seropositivity increased with age: 2.7% of those younger than 6 years were positive, as compared with 23% of those between 6 and 15 years. This seroconversion is greater than would be expected from perinatal exposure.[75]

Treatment

The treatment of choice for pediatric genital *Chlamydia* infection is erythromycin for children 8 years and younger, and tetracycline is recommended for older children. *C. trachomatis* is also susceptible to sulfonamides and trimethoprim; however, trimethoprim had not been widely used for *C. trachomatis* because it lacks activity against other organisms known to cause genital disease, in particular, other STDs.

Prophylactic treatment of children for *C. trachomatis* is not indicated. As with gonococcal infection, the low prevalence and the minimal risk for the development of upper genital tract disease allows the practitioner to await culture results before instituting treatment. Given the high false-positive rates of antigen-detection methods, it would also seem reasonable to await a culture result before treating a child with a positive antigen-detection result. Because of the relatively frequent association of infection with *N. gonorrhoeae* and *C. trachomatis* in children,

coverage for *C. trachomatis* should be included in treatment for children with gonococcal infection if *Chlamydia* cultures are not available.[57]

After treatment, reevaluation should include a test of cure. Again, this should be performed by a cell culture method. Dead antigen could produce a false-positive test by the antigen-detection method. As with gonococcal infection, testing for reinfection in 2 to 3 months may be reasonable in prepubertal children with *C. trachomatis*. This would be especially helpful when abuse is suspected but not proven or when a perpetrator cannot be identified.

GENITAL MYCOPLASMAS

Genital mycoplasmas have not been studied in detail in prepubertal children; however, in adults, the presence of these organisms correlates well with sexual activity. Colonization of neonates with these organisms by vertical transmission has been documented and usually resolves spontaneously by the end of the first year of life. Genital mycoplasmas have also been reported as a cause of exudative vaginitis and recurrent urethritis in prepubertal children.[76, 77]

Genital mycoplasmas have been noted to colonize some 5% to 25% of well, asymptomatic children. In a case-control study by Hammerschlag and coworkers, *Mycoplasma hominis* and *Ureaplasma urealyticum* organisms were isolated significantly more often from the rectum and vagina of children with a history of sexual abuse than from control children with no known history of abuse. No association was found between colonization and symptoms in either group of children. Although genital mycoplasmas were isolated more frequently from abused children, the finding of these organisms in well children limits the usefulness of a positive culture in the forensic evaluation for sexual abuse.[78] These findings were further supported by Ingram and colleagues in a review of 452 prepubertal girls screened for genital mycoplasma during forensic evaluation. Colonization with these organisms did not correlate with history of abuse, type of sexual contacts, or evidence of hymenal injury. Along with other investigators, they concluded that genital mycoplasma colonization was not a useful marker for potential sexual abuse.[79]

TRICHOMONIASIS

Infection with the single-celled protozoan, *Trichomonas vaginalis*, is an uncommon finding in prepubertal children beyond the neonatal period. It appears that the unestrogenized vagina, with an alkaline pH, is relatively resistant to infection and colonization with this organism.[80, 81] A review of the literature since 1956 locates only scattered case reports of trichomoniasis in groups of symptomatic and asymptomatic girls.[9] Studies of pediatric vulvovaginitis by Paradise's and Gerstner's groups did not identify *T. vaginalis* among the symptomatic girls studied.[1, 26] The protozoan was found in only 1% of sexually abused girls studied by White.[4]

In contrast, the organism is a relatively common cause of vaginitis in the neonatal period, being isolated from 4% to 17% of babies examined because of vaginal discharge during the first few days of life.[82] This is probably attributable to the effect of maternal estrogen on the vagina of the neonate and the resulting acidic pH.

In Jones and coworkers' review of 18 girls with *T. vaginalis* isolated from the vagina, 65% were symptomatic. In two girls evaluated after being sexually abused, symptoms developed within 7 to 10 days of the abuse.[83] When symptomatic, girls usually present with a copious froth, discharge that is often described as yellow-gray. There are often accompanying complaints of vulvar itching and dysuria.[2] Since the prepubertal vagina is less likely to support the growth of this organism, the urinary tract may be the primary source of infection.[84] In these situations, the protozoan sometimes is not seen in vaginal specimens but is noted on urinalysis.[81] In neonates, isolation of *T. vaginalis* from both the vagina and the nasopharynx has been reported.[85]

Most of the older reports of trichomoniasis in children did not address the source of transmission; however, sexual transmission is the most common source of infection in both adults and children.[9, 81, 83, 86] Furthermore, perinatal acquisition is the most common form of nonvenereal transmission.[84] Approximately 5% of newborns of mothers with vaginal trichomoniasis become infected.[83, 87, 89] Many of these infections resolve spontaneously as maternal estrogen effect diminishes and vaginal pH rises. It is not known whether *T. vaginalis* infection in childhood could be related to neonatal exposure.[81]

The possible roles of fomite transmission and acquisition by nonsexual contact are unclear but appear unlikely. The organism is very sensitive to desiccation but may survive several hours on moist surfaces and in body fluids.[90] Although spread by way of wet, contaminated clothes in crowded, unhygienic conditions[86]; infected water from toilets[91]; and sleeping with an infected mother[42] has been suggested, well-documented cases of trichomoniasis in childhood as a result of fomite transmission have not been reported.[9, 84]

Diagnosis of trichomoniasis is usually made by the appearance of the motile organism on a wet preparation of secretions. At higher levels of magnification, the flagellum of the organism may be visualized. Significant numbers of leukocytes often accompany the organism, so careful inspection of the wet preparation is important.[19] Culture of the organism is both more sensitive and specific in making the diagnosis but not widely available or used.[93]

Metronidazole has been well-described as an effective method of treatment in adults, and initial concerns of carcinogenicity of this antibiotic do not appear clinically warranted.[94] Neonatal infection may often be managed expectantly, and the infection usually spontaneously subsides with loss of maternal estrogen. However, newborns may require treatment of more severe infections, such as those exacerbated by the presence of severe candidiasis.[95] In these infants as well as older children who require treatment, metronidazole may be given as three divided doses of 15 mg/kg per day (maximum dose 250 mg) for 7 days. The safety of metronidazole treatment for amebiasis in children has been evaluated. Single-dose treatment, frequently used in adults, has not been evaluated in children.[2, 96]

CONDYLOMATA ACUMINATA

Biology

In both adults and children, condylomata acuminata are caused by infection with the human papillomavirus (HPV). More than 50 subtypes of this double-stranded DNA virus have been identified to date. Each viral subtype is somewhat site specific for either skin or mucosal surfaces (Table 21–3). The virus infects the germinal layer of the epithelium, and it has been suggested that it enters through a traumatic break in the epithelium. Viral subtypes also differ in their association with the development of neoplasia.[97, 98]

Demographics

The prevalence of HPV infection in the population is difficult to determine. One conservative estimate suggests that 2% of the reproductive-aged women in the population are infected.[97] A dramatic increase in the number of clinical cases of HPV has been reported in adults. The number

Table 21-3. Human Papillomavirus: Types and Associated Lesions

Type	Lesion
1a–c	Plantar warts
2a–c	Common warts
3a,b	Flat warts
4	Plantar warts
10a, b	Flat warts
11a, b	Condylomata acuminata
	Cervical dysplasia
	Laryngeal papillomatosis
16, 18, 31, 33, 35	Condylomata acuminata
	Cervical dysplasia
	Squamous cell carcinoma

From Shah KV: Biology of human genital tract papillomaviruses. *In* Holmes KK (ed): Sexually Transmitted Diseases, 2nd ed. New York: McGraw-Hill, 1990, pp 425–431.

of private physician office visits for condylomata increased 459% in adults between 1966 and 1981. In women, this increase was 684%.[99] Although exact statistics are not known for the pediatric population, the recent proliferation of case reports of pediatric HPV infection suggests an increase paralleling that in adults.[100–106]

Presentation

Anogenital condylomas in children generally present as flesh-colored verrucous growths. Lesions have also been reported in the moist mucosal membranes of the urethra, bladder, mouth, and eyes.[107] The lesion may be friable and easily traumatized, especially in moist areas. The typical keratinized or "warty" appearance of the condyloma may not be present in diaper-aged children when the warts are continuously exposed to moisture. Condylomas generally present as asymptomatic lesions noted by the caretaker during diapering and bathing; however, the friable and vascular nature of pediatric condylomas may result in vaginal or rectal bleeding, dysuria, vaginal discharge, or painful defecation.[108]

The anatomic distribution of genital condylomas may vary between adults and children. In adults, labial lesions are most common in women and penile lesions in men. In contrast, prepubertal children are much more likely than adults to present with periurethral and perianal condylomas. In one study of prepubertal boys, 77% were found to have perianal condylomas; 16% had involvement of the urethral meatus, and only 3% had involvement of the penile shaft.[109] Similar findings have been noted in prepubertal girls: several authors have reported a 30% to 70%

incidence of perianal warts and a 19% to 33% incidence of periurethral warts.[110, 111]

The majority of women with external condylomas have upper genital tract disease; one study noted a 68% incidence of vaginal and cervical lesions in women with external condylomas.[109] This is a particular concern, given the association of certain HPV subtypes (16, 18, 31, and 33) with high-grade neoplasms of the vagina and cervix.[112–115] Studies of the upper genital tract of prepubertal girls for the presence of HPV, however, have shown this to be unusual.[111, 116] In contrast, the clinical finding of perianal condylomas has been strongly associated with the presence of additional HPV lesions in the anal canal.[111] This may represent a focus of untreated disease and a source for recurrence. Parallels drawn between cervical intraepithelial neoplasia and anal intraepithelial neoplasia in the adult population are an additional cause for concern in these children.[117] From these data, clinicians should consider the urethra and the anal canal as potential sites of infection.[119]

Sexually abused children with genital condylomas are also at significant risk for other STDs. Herman-Giddens and coworkers found a 50% incidence of other STDs in their population of sexually abused girls. The risk was greatest in the subset of girls who had had multiple abusers.[119] Genital condylomas that are refractory of standard treatment have also been reported in children with HIV infection.[120, 121]

Perioral condylomas have also been reported in children with documented sexual abuse. This is an unusual finding, representing only 3% of cases in a review of several series of case reports.[109] More common is juvenile laryngeal papillomatosis. It generally presents in children younger than 5 years with hoarseness and, rarely, respiratory obstruction. These HPV lesions are often asymptomatic, making a true estimate of their prevalence difficult. However, it has been suggested that this well-studied form of pediatric HPV infection may serve as a model for the study of genital HPV in children.[122]

Transmission

Vertical transmission at birth, casual transmission, and sexual transmission have all been implicated as possible means of HPV infection in children. Vertical transmission of juvenile respiratory papillomatosis has been the most thoroughly studied; the occasional case is also reported of HPV presented as vertically transmitted infantile conjunctival papillomas.[123] Nearly all pediatric laryngeal HPV lesions that have been typed were types 6 and 11, ones commonly responsible for genital disease. Epidemiologic studies of these children have shown that fewer than 1% were delivered abdominally and that as many as 60% of these mothers were known to have HPV lesions at the time of delivery.[124]

Genital HPV is a very common finding in women of child-bearing age. Cervical specimens are positive for HPV DNA in more than 10% of some obstetric populations. In a study of healthy mothers and infants without known HPV infections, HPV DNA was found in 4.3% of foreskin specimens obtained at circumcision from healthy newborns.[125] In these cases, exposure to the virus is believed to occur directly during passage through an infected genital tract. The possibility of hematogenous spread has been suggested by a case report of a premature newborn delivered by caesarean section, prior to known rupture of membranes, with genital condyloma noted at birth.[126–128] The risk of hematogenous spread must be exceedingly low, given the rarity of congenital condylomata acuminata and the widespread presence of genital HPV in obstetrical populations. In this case report, the possibility of occult rupture of fetal membranes as the cause of premature labor was not ruled out, making ascending infection a possible explanation.

Vertical transmission of HPV resulting in laryngeal lesions has been well-documented,[8, 127, 129] and probably occurs through aspiration of infected secretions into the upper airway of the newborn at birth. The overall risk of transmission appears to be quite low.[129] Presumed vertical transmission of genital HPV in infants and toddlers has also been reported. Although it is not clear why these anatomic sites are the most commonly reported sites of perinatally acquired HPV, it is possible that the mucosal surfaces are subjected to trauma at birth that results in epithelial cell damage and affords entry for the virus. Boyd found that 19% of cases of pediatric genital HPV infection had been attributed to perinatally acquired disease.[109] The majority of presumed perinatally transmitted HPV cases have been reported in children younger than 2 years,[104, 105] a finding in keeping with data suggesting an incubation period of up to 20 months in children.[110] It is important to remember the inherent difficulties of evaluating children of this age group for possible sexual abuse (i.e., preverbal children unable to give a history and the infrequent finding of genital trauma and other STDs in this age group). Weinberg and coworkers noted a 19% incidence of abuse discovered upon Child Protective Services' evaluation of children

with genital HPV when no abuse was suspected at the time of the referral.[130]

Sexual transmission of HPV has been well-documented in adults, and usual incubation periods are 4 weeks to 3 months.[131–133] In several reviews, transmission by sexual abuse was documented in 50% to 80% of children evaluated.[105, 109, 134] In series of children at least 2 years of age, abuse was documented in as many as 90% of those evaluated.[119] Demographic studies comparing route of delivery, maternal history of HPV, history of sexual abuse, evidence of genital trauma, and other STDs have shown significant differences between children with condylomas who are younger than 3 years and older ones.[135] Studies that "rule out" sexual abuse in older children with condylomas based on the presence of genital HPV lesions in parents should be interpreted with caution; it is well known that the mother's sex partner is frequently the perpetrator of sexual abuse, and partners of women with HPV are very frequently infected with the virus. The possibility of genital-oral contact resulting in pediatric laryngeal papillomatosis has also been raised.[136] It is essential to stress that regardless of age, each child who presents with condylomata acuminata deserves a thorough and careful evaluation for possible sexual abuse.[137, 138]

Reviews of cases of pediatric genital HPV have also included a significant number of children for whom the source of infection was not known (i.e., 10% to 37% of reported cases)[105, 109, 119, 139] and have raised questions about the possibility of casual spread of HPV or spread of warts by autoinoculation. In the adult population, the spread of genital condylomas via casual contact or autoinoculation is considered highly unlikely. Studies have failed to show an increased incidence of genital condylomas in adults with other cutaneous HPV lesions.[140] Whether these data are applicable to the pediatric population has recently been questioned. Some authors have lately suggested that casual contact may be responsible for some genital HPV lesions in childhood,[141] citing that normal contact involved in the care of small children is much less "casual" than contact between adults. Fleming reported one case of genital HPV in a 5-year-old boy that was attributed to autoinoculation from cutaneous warts.[142] Hansen also noted HPV-2 in genital warts of two children; sexual transmission was later documented in one of those cases. Another child in the series was also found to have both HPV-2 and HPV-18 in a single specimen.[105] Obalek and colleagues reported HPV-22 in 21% of their children evaluated for genital condylomas.[104] Since HPV-2 is generally associated with cutaneous warts, the investigators concluded that casual contact or autoinoculation was responsible for disease in these children. Again, caution is warranted when the possibility of abuse is ruled out on the basis of HPV DNA type alone. Factors such as cross-reactivity of HPV types on DNA probes, the knowledge that condylomas may express different viral types at different times, and the finding of HPV 1 and 2 in genital specimens of adults' condylomas are extremely important to consider.[143] Each child with genital condylomas deserves careful evaluation for possible sexual abuse.

Diagnosis

The diagnosis of genital condylomata acuminata in children generally can be made by careful clinical inspection. The application of 3% to 5% acetic acid on a compress for 10 to 15 minutes may elicit the classic acetowhite appearance of condylomas familiar to clinicians experienced in the care of adult HPV. A 3% acetic acid solution may be sufficient for mucosal lesions and causes less discomfort than the 5% solution frequently required to produce an acetowhite appearance in keratinized lesions.[109] On mucosal surfaces, the typical warty appearance is less common than a pink or red fleshy growth, often markedly vascular. Careful inspection of the perianal and periurethral area often reveals lesions initially missed.

The differential diagnosis of such genital lesions in children should include condylomata lata of secondary syphilis, generally having a less raised and a more "velvety" appearance; perineal tumors; urethral prolapse, easily confused with infected and traumatized periurethral condyloma; rhabdomyosarcoma (sarcoma botryoides); and molluscum contagiosum. Biopsy (facilitated by topical anesthetic agents, such as EMLA) may be indicated when the diagnosis is in question.[108] Children with rapidly progressive or quickly recurrent HPV should be evaluated for concurrent vertically or sexually acquired HIV infection.[144] When a general anesthetic is required for diagnosis or treatment, a thorough evaluation of the vagina, cervix, periurethral area, and anal canal should also be performed.

Microscopic examination of condylomas generally reveals classic findings of a hyperplastic squamous epithelium with acanthosis, hyperkeratosis, and parakeratosis. Koilocytosis is often present. Specimens should also be evaluated for findings of atypia. Immunoperoxidase staining has been used in an attempt to improve the specificity of the diagnosis by biopsy; however, as compared with testing for the HPV DNA, immunoperoxidase is relatively nonspecific. In pediatric populations, a positive immunoperoxidase stain has been reported in only 30% to 40% of lesions known to contain HPV DNA.[102, 135] Molecular biology techniques such as PCR are expected to improve the accuracy of histologic diagnosis.

Recent series have examined the role of DNA typing in the assessment of pediatric genital condylomas. In these cases, HPV-6/11 is reported most often, HPV-2 occasionally, and HPV-16/18 infrequently. The presence of an "as yet uncharacterized" HPV type has also been mentioned in several reports.[102–106, 109, 135] The clinical usefulness of HPV typing of pediatric lesions is not clearly defined. In adults, HPV typing is more specific than histologic examination alone for determining the diagnosis, although lesions with a classic appearance of condylomas occasionally fail to "type" with any available DNA probes. This may be due to the HPV types "as yet uncharacterized." Several investigators have used typing in an attempt to determine the source of transmission of the virus. Until more data are available, this should be done with great caution.[145] In adults, it is well-known that some cross-reactivity exists between different types and that a single wart may express different types of HPV DNA at different times. Although the viral subtypes are considered relatively site specific, HPV 1 and 2 have been reported in anogenital condylomas of adults.[143] HPV type 16 has also been reported in a series of periungual squamous cell carcinomas in adults.[146] Clearly, a great disservice may be done to a pediatric patient by relying on only one piece of information when drawing conclusions about this complex problem.

Although most of the HPV typing data collected to date from children have been positive for the "low-risk" viral types (HPV-6 and HPV-11), HPV-16 and HPV-18 have been reported in prepubertal children.[102, 103, 105] In adults, these viral types have been associated with increased risk of high-grade intraepithelial lesions and squamous cell carcinomas.[113, 114, 140, 147] There has been some concern that children infected with these viral types may be at a similarly increased risk for neoplasia. Two reports in the literature describe squamous cell carcinoma of the vulva in young, sexually inactive females. One report by Lister describes the development of vulvar carcinoma in a 14-year-old girl with a history of genital condylomas dating to infancy.[148] The previously discussed high incidence of anal canal disease in children with perianal condylomas,[135] and the similarities between cervical intraepithelial neoplasia and anal intraepithelial neoplasia in adults[117] are of great concern to clinicians who follow these infected children over the long term. Currently, no standard recommendations are available for follow-up of children exposed to HPV, although most concern centers around those exposed to the subtypes with oncogenic potential.[109] It is clear that these children deserve careful follow-up so that the long-term risks of neoplasia can be more clearly defined.[100]

Treatment

Any clinician experienced in the long-term care of adults infected with HPV is familiar with the frustrations associated with treatment. The special needs of children often compound these treatment difficulties. An ideal treatment for children would be inexpensive, effective, atraumatic, and widely available, but, unfortunately, all treatment regimens available to children are associated with relatively high recurrence risks, the need for close supervision by the clinician, and the possibility of physical discomfort or emotional trauma because of frequent genital examinations. Although spontaneous regression of condylomas has been well-described in adults, this is not generally chosen as a treatment of choice for children.[109]

Podophyllin is widely available as a 20% to 25% solution with tincture of benzoin, and its use has been described in the pediatric age group. When podophyllin is used in children, it is essential that the clinician be assured of careful compliance. The caretaker of the child must remove the solution by washing with soap and water approximately 4 hours after application. Systemic absorption of podophyllin with neurotoxicity has been described in adults and adolescents.[149–151] In pregnant adult women, deaths have been reported when large areas of abraded condylomas were painted with podophyllin and covered with an occlusive dressing.[152] These data should encourage clinicians to utilize podophyllin cautiously in children. Clinicians accustomed to treating adults should remember that painting a given surface area with podophyllin will expose a much greater percentage of the total body surface area of a child than of an adult. A 1-cm² patch of skin on an average-sized 3-year-old represents the same percentage of body surface area as a 3-cm² area on an adult. Systemic absorption may also be increased by the use of an occlusive dressing or disposable diapers. For this reason, it has been suggested that more dilute solutions

of podophyllin (e.g., 5% to 15%) may be more appropriate for use in children.[110] Newer products containing a gel suspension of podophyllin are also available; although not yet studied in children, these products may prove to be beneficial treatment modalities. As with adults, a relatively high recurrence rate has been reported; treatment failures or recurrences were noted in 43% of the pediatric population treated by Stringel and colleagues.[118, 153]

The use of cryotherapy with a probe or direct application of liquid nitrogen has also been described for the treatment of condylomas in adults and children. There is some theoretical concern about the effectiveness of cryotherapy in the treatment of condylomas, as data suggest that viable virus persists in tissue after treatment.[115] Like the topical application of caustic solutions, such as trichloroacetic or bichloroacetic acid, the therapeutic value of these agents is limited by the discomfort or actual pain involved in their use. An older child with a few condylomas may tolerate these treatment modalities well, although in children with more extensive disease, their usefulness will be limited by the need for frequent treatments. Again, newer topical anesthetic agents such as EMLA may expand the usefulness of these agents.

The topical use of 5-fluorouracil cream has been reported in adults as a cost-effective treatment for condylomas.[154] This relatively inexpensive drug may be applied externally by a parent or caretaker. Although careful follow-up by a clinician is necessary, less frequent follow-up may be required once treatment is under way and the parent has been educated in proper use. The most common side effect is inflammation of the skin surrounding the condylomas; however, this may be controlled by adjusting the amount of cream and frequency of use to a dose appropriate for a given child.

In the past, electrosurgical fulguration was commonly employed in the treatment of more severe condylomas. The anesthesia required increases both the medical risk and the cost of the procedure. Fulguration is not associated with a significantly lower recurrence rate than less invasive treatment methods, with up to a 50% recurrence rate noted.[105] Electrosurgical fulguration has also been associated with significant tissue damage and may cause scarring and stricture formation.[118, 153] Particularly in treatment planning for children with perianal and periurethral condylomas, the potential for damage from fulguration should be carefully weighed.

The carbon dioxide (CO_2) laser has become increasingly popular for the treatment of genital condylomas. Like electrosurgical fulguration, it requires general anesthesia; however, careful use of the laser allows control over depth of tissue destruction and avoids much of the scarring associated with electrosurgery.[109] The CO_2 laser may also be used to treat lesions in the periurethral and perianal areas and the anal canal, where other modalities are more difficult to use. Gale and Muram also noted fewer subjective complaints of postoperative discomfort in their series of children treated with the CO_2 laser. A 29% recurrence rate again supported laser over electrosurgical fulguration.[155]

The success of interferon in adults with genital condylomas has led several investigators to use it in children. The most extensive reports of interferon in children have addressed the treatment of laryngeal papillomatosis. In these children, the safety of interferon was demonstrated, although its use was associated with (reversible) elevation of liver enzymes and neutropenia. Clinical side effects—fever, anorexia, nausea, and vomiting—were noted. Linear growth was carefully followed and remained unaffected; however, 6-month follow-up of the groups, comparing surgical treatment and interferon, did not demonstrate any improvement in recurrence rate.[156] Persistence of viral infection during clinical remission after interferon treatment has been demonstrated in biopsy studies of laryngeal papillomatosis.[157]

Interferon treatment of genital condylomas in children has not yet been extensively studied, although case reports of its use are appearing in the literature. These case reports suggest that much of the data on interferon in laryngeal papillomatosis are applicable to children with condylomas. Similar laboratory and clinical side effects have been reported.[116, 120] There are no long-term studies of the effectiveness of interferon in children with genital condylomas; however, studies of adults suggest that significant numbers of patients will experience recurrence after the termination of treatment. Intralesional interferon has also been reported to be more effective than systemic dosing,[158] and the majority of studies that demonstrated efficacy in adults have used intralesional interferon. The difficulties associated with multiple intralesional injections in the pediatric age group and the lower effectiveness of systemic interferon may ultimately limit its usefulness in children.

Clinical experience and literature review clearly indicate that no single treatment is "correct" for children with condylomas. Instead, the clinician should be familiar with a number of treatment modalities so that therapy for each child may be individualized. Educating parents in the biology of the virus and the chronic nature of the infection may help them to deal with the natural frustrations associated with the high recurrence rate of lesions.

The oncogenic potential of the HPV is also a cause for concern in the long-term management of these children. Although no long-term studies have been conducted in children, findings in adults have raised concern about the risk of later development of neoplastic lesions in children exposed to HPV.[112, 113, 140] Many authors have emphasized the importance of long-term follow-up of these children, especially those exposed to the "high-risk" viral subtypes. However, until long-term studies have been performed, the exact nature of proper follow-up remains to be defined.[109]

GENITAL HERPES VIRUS INFECTION

Biology

Genital herpes is caused by infection with the double-stranded DNA herpes simplex virus (HSV), which occurs in two subtypes, HSV-1 and HSV-2.[159] Although it was once thought that HSV-1 produced only oral lesions and HSV-2 genital lesions, it has been thoroughly documented that infection with a particular HSV type is not site specific. Each HSV type generates a specific antibody response, and antibodies against one type do not confer immunity to the other type.[16]

Presentation

During childhood, HSV infection presents most often as gingivostomatitis. Taieb's series of 50 children with primary HSV infection reported oral lesions in 96%,[160] which can be mild gingivitis or a more severe infection with painful vesicular lesions of the lips and oral cavity that later will ulcerate. Pharyngitis also in a mild or a more severe, ulcerative form, sometimes develops. Both HSV-1 and -2 have been isolated from samples of childhood gingivostomatitis. Pharyngitis was reported in 10% of adults who had primary genital herpes.[161]

Multifocal disease appears to be surprisingly common in children with primary HSV infection. Taieb and coworkers found multifocal lesions in 36% of the children in their series. Herpetic whitlow presented as a painful vesicular lesion, usually along the edge of the nail. Lesions were also reported at other cutaneous sites.[160]

Genital herpes lesions, both HSV-1 and HSV-2, have been reported in children,[162–165] although in Taieb's series genital lesions accounted for only 6%.[160] The clinical presentation of primary genital herpes is very similar to that described in adults. After an incubation period of 2 to 20 days,[163] painful vesicular lesions develop, which subsequently ulcerate and are often accompanied by systemic symptoms. Inguinal adenopathy, fever, malaise, nausea, headache, and urinary retention may occur. The lesions of HSV-1 and HSV-2 infection can be clinically indistinguishable, but HSV-2 genital herpes is four times more likely to recur. Secondary lesions are generally associated with less viral shedding and no systemic symptoms.[19]

Transmission

HSV is transmitted by close contact with a person who is shedding the virus, which enters mucosal surfaces through an epithelial break.[161] The virus has been shown to survive in water and on plastic surfaces for several hours,[166] but fomite transmission has never been documented. Nonsexual transmission through close contact has been proposed as an explanation for the high incidence of antibodies to HSV-2 among children in certain geographic areas.[167] Casual transmission of genital herpes to a child through nonsexual contact has not been proven.

Perinatal transmission of HSV has been thoroughly studied. Congenital HSV infection from transplacental passage may occur but is uncommon. Vertical transmission of the virus during vaginal delivery has been well-described as the cause of the potentially devastating neonatal herpes infection.[19] Perinatal transmission is an uncommon cause of childhood genital herpes, but when the genitals are the site of neonatal cutaneous infection, the possibility for recurrent genital lesions exists.[30]

Autoinoculation from extragenital lesions has been documented as a source of genital herpes during childhood, but transmission by sexual contact is the most common source.[165, 168] Only small series of children with genital herpes have been reported in the literature; however, in Kaplan's study of six children, sexual contact was responsible for transmission in four.[164] In Nahmias's series of five children, three had a history of, or physical findings consistent with, sexual abuse.[162]

When a child presents with genital herpes, other sites should be carefully inspected for lesions, which are sometimes asymptomatic. The oropharynx and hands in particular should be carefully inspected. When both oral and genital lesions are present, the likelihood of autotransmission increases, although cases of sexual transmission have been documented in children with intercurrent simultaneous oral and genital herpes lesions.[162, 169]

Diagnosis

The diagnosis of genital herpes in a child is best made by viral culture of suspicious lesions. The differential diagnosis of ulcerative and vesicular lesions includes varicella and recurrent herpes zoster, ammonia dermatitis, trauma, syphilis, Stevens Johnson syndrome, condylomas, impetigo, erythema multiforme, and candidiasis, among others.[162]

Cell culture is the most accurate method of diagnosing genital herpes, but false-positive results may occur in children with herpes zoster owing to the similar cytopathic effects of herpes simplex and herpes zoster in cell culture. For that reason, it is recommended that positive herpes cultures in children be subjected to confirmatory testing.[16] False-negative findings may occur if specimens are obtained from lesions with less profuse viral shedding, such as recurrent lesions or ones that are ulcerated or crusted.[19]

Antigen-detection testing has not been evaluated in children and is not recommended. The concerns for specificity and sensitivity in testing are the same as for C. trachomatis.[16]

Treatment

No treatment guidelines are available for genital herpes infection in children. Data on antiviral agents, such as acyclovir, in adults applies to children with varicella. Acyclovir, a competitive inhibitor of viral DNA polymerase, inhibits viral DNA synthesis. The use of acyclovir has been demonstrated in adults to be effective in the symptomatic treatment of primary outbreaks and suppressive treatment of secondary lesions.[19] Since the therapeutic safety of acyclovir during childhood has been demonstrated with neonatal herpes simplex and childhood herpes zoster, some clinicians use it to treat children with genital herpes. Others prefer symptomatic treatment of the genital lesions with local care, sitz baths, and drying agents. Bacterial superinfection may require antibiotics, although it is uncommon except in immunocompromised persons[161] and those with epithelial skin breaks due to other dermatologic conditions such as atopic dermatitis or diaper dermatitis.[160]

BACTERIAL VAGINOSIS

Bacterial vaginosis (BV) generally presents as a thin, white vaginal discharge with a fishy odor. Culture of the discharge grows a mixed collection of organisms; these include *Gardnerella vaginalis*, anaerobes such as *Bacteroides* species and *Mobiluncus*, and sometimes genital mycoplasmas.[170]

In the mid-1980s, case reports began to appear describing a similar clinical presentation in children, especially sexually abused children.[171] In 1984, Muram and Buxton reported three cases of vaginitis due to *G. vaginalis* in prepubertal girls who had been sexually abused and suggested that "the isolation of *Gardnerella vaginalis* should alert the physician to the probability of sexual abuse."[172]

In both adults and children, BV is best diagnosed by the finding of clue cells on wet preparation accompanied by the release of an amine odor on application of an alkaline solution (potassium hydroxide). In adults, microscopic examination of a wet preparation was found to be the single most specific (94%) and sensitive (98%) method for diagnosis of BV. The specificity increased to 99% when the alkalinization of vaginal secretions was used. Gram stain was found to be less specific and less sensitive.[173] Diagnosis based solely on the isolation of *G. vaginalis* from culture of vaginal secretions has not been found to be accurate: *G. vaginalis* was isolated from 50% of adult women who did not otherwise meet diagnostic criteria for BV.[174] This appears also to be true of children. Hammerschlag and coworkers found a 13.5% incidence of vaginal colonization with *G. vaginalis* (then called *Corynebacterium vaginale*) in healthy asymptomatic children. The frequency of colonization was age dependent; 18% of children younger than 2 years were colonized, the incidence was 2.5% between age 3 and 10 years and 63% between 11 and 15 years.[175] Bartley also found clinical evidence of BV in only three of 25 prepubertal girls with cultures positive for *G. vaginalis*. He also found that the presence of *G. vaginalis* did not correlate with clinical symptoms such as pain or pruritus or clinical findings such as bleeding, discharge, or vulvar erythema.[176]

It is not clear exactly how often bacterial vaginosis is responsible for vaginitis in the pediatric age group. In Paradise and coworkers' study of symptomatic girls with vaginitis, no cases of BV or positive cultures for *G. vaginalis* were identified, although media selective for *G. vaginalis* were not used.[1] Other studies have identified cases of BV that met the clinical criteria described above in prepubertal children.[176, 177]

Controversy surrounds the mode of transmission of BV in postpubertal females. While the incidence of BV is higher in sexually experienced women, it may also be present in virginal women.[170] Bump and Bueschling found a 12% incidence of BV in their virginal adolescents[178]; however, when BV is studied in a prepubertal population, the data suggest that it is usually sexually transmitted. Hammerschlag's group studied sexually abused girls and a matched control population; they considered a diagnosis of BV "definite" when both clue cells and an amine odor were present and the diagnosis "possible" when either clue cells or an amine odor was present. They found a statistically significant difference in the incidence of BV in the two groups of girls—4% "possible" cases in the nonabused controls but no definite cases. Among the abused girls, they found a 25% incidence of "possible" or "definite" BV, and 12.9% met the criteria for "definite." They concluded that in prepubertal children BV, especially cases that met the "definite" criteria, is usually sexually transmitted in a prepubertal child.[177] It is not known whether BV can be transmitted perinatally.

Hammerschlag's study also suggests another interesting finding in the natural history of BV after sexual assault. None of the children who later exhibited the clinical criteria for BV had those findings on initial evaluation shortly after the episode(s) of abuse. On later evaluation, vaginal wash specimens demonstrated clue cells and an amine odor, and 60% of them had clinical symptoms.[177] This is very similar to Jenny's group's findings in adult women after sexual assault—a statistically significant increase in BV prevalence when initial and follow-up examinations were compared.[179]

No formal guidelines have been published for the treatment of bacterial vaginosis in the pediatric age group. Hammerschlag's group reported using metronidazole in their symptomatic children.[177] Use of ampicillin and amoxicillin has also been described in adults and may be of some benefit to children.[170]

SYPHILIS

Infection with *Treponema pallidum* has increased dramatically in the pediatric population, reflecting the increase in syphilis among women of child-bearing age. Perinatal transmission of syphilis occurs most often by hematogenous transplacental passage of the organism rather than direct exposure at birth.[180] Congenital and acquired syphilis can usually be distinguished by examining results of maternal serologic tests and cord blood or neonatal tests obtained at birth. There is a latent period between infection and conversion to positive serologic status, however. An infant delivered during this interval, may develop congenital syphilis despite negative perinatal serologic findings. This possibility should be considered when a child younger than 1 year presents with signs of acquired syphilis.[181, 182]

Primary syphilis has very similar presentations in children and adults, generally appearing as a painless genital chancre, on average 21 days after exposure. Condyloma latum, the most frequently described presentation, was noted in 85% to 90% of children in series by Lowry.[183] Primary lesions may also present in the oral cavity and perianal area. Perianal chancres have been confused with simple perianal fissures.[184] The differential diagnosis of these lesions includes condylomata acuminata, trauma, and ulcerative lesions such as those due to HSV.[185] At this stage, serologic results are frequently negative. It generally takes 4 to 8 weeks for nontreponemal tests, such as RPR and VDRL, to show positive results. These tests may be positive during the first week after the chancre appears. Treponemal serologies of MHA-TP and fluorescent treponemal antibody absorption tests may also be negative during the incubation period and early primary syphilis. For that reason, the clinician faced with a possible syphilitic chancre in a child should perform a dark-field examination.[182]

Secondary syphilis has also been reported in children. It often presents as a skin rash within several months of exposure. The differential diagnosis of such a rash includes pityriasis rosacea, psoriasis, tinea versicolor, viral illnesses, and drug reactions. Again, a relatively high index of suspicion is necessary to accurately diagnose the very infrequent condition of secondary syphilis in a child.[184]

In the absence of perinatal transmission, syphilis is nearly always sexually transmitted. Accidental transmission in laboratory accidents or during surgery on infection persons has been described.[86] Transmission during transfusion of blood, by contact with syphilitic lesions on the breast of a nursing mother, or by "nonsexual" kissing have all been described; however, these cases are very rare.

Syphilis in a child beyond the neonatal period is usually acquired through sexual abuse. Fortunately, this is one of the least common STDs among sexually abused children. White and coworkers' series reported six cases of positive serologic findings among 108 children screened, one of the highest syphilis rates reported in the literature.[4] Much lower prevalence rates have been reported in sexually abused children. One positive result was reported out of 532 children evaluated by DeJong.[5] Cupoli and Sewell found only one in 1059 positive serologic results.[6] The Center for Child Protection in San Diego found only two positive results in more than 6000 children screened.[186] This clearly indicates that syphilis is one of the most uncommon STDs transmitted to children during sexual abuse.[187]

The CDC currently recommends that cerebrospinal fluid samples be obtained from children to rule out congenital syphilis. They recommend that any child with congenital syphilis or evidence of neurologic involvement be treated with aqueous crystalline penicillin G (200,000 to 300,000 U/kg per day) for 10 to 14 days. If congenital and neurosyphilis can be ruled out, children may be treated with 50,000 U/kg of intramuscular benzathine penicillin, not to exceed 2.4 million U.

HUMAN IMMUNODEFICIENCY VIRUS

Acquired immunodeficiency syndrome (AIDS), caused by infection with the RNA retrovirus HIV, has been extensively described in the pediatric population.[188–192] Among the 1995 cases reported to the CDC as of February 1990 that met diagnostic criteria for AIDS, vertical transmission was responsible for 81% of infections. Transmission via transfusion of blood or its components was responsible for 11% of cases, and coagulation disorders for 5%, and 3% of children had idiopathic infections. In a 1985 editorial in the *Journal of the American Medical Association*, Osterholm raised the "unanswered question" of the possibility of HIV transmission to children from childhood sexual abuse.[193] Since that time, scattered case reports have described HIV-infected children thought to have been infected through sexual abuse.[186, 194–196]

It is difficult to determine the prevalence of HIV infection among childhood victims of sexual abuse. Dattel and coworkers reported only one HIV-positive child in their series of 161 children screened in San Francisco County; this was an adolescent male who had been sexually abused and subsequently worked as a prostitute and engaged in high-risk sexual behavior.[197] Gutman and associates recently reported a history of sexual abuse in 14.6% of 96 HIV-positive prepubertal children evaluated at Duke University. Of these 96 children, four were determined to have acquired their HIV infection from sexual abuse; for another six, abuse was a "possible" source; two had received infected blood components; and in the remaining three, vertical transmission was documented.[188] From a phone survey of child abuse programs, Gellert and colleagues identified six HIV-positive children in the 300 screens performed (from a total of 26,000 children evaluated by these centers).[199]

The few children described who acquired HIV infection from sexual abuse share many of the risk factors thoroughly described in the adult population.[200] Fischl and colleagues noted that 10% of the children in her series lived with caretakers who engaged in high-risk behaviors.[197] Gutman frequently identified the risk factors of substance abuse, alcoholism, prostitution, and poverty among the caretakers of the HIV-positive children in her series.[201] She also reported a higher incidence of HIV infection among children who were victims of anal-receptive or oral-receptive sexual activity, known risk factors among adults.[202, 203] Her HIV-positive patients also had a higher incidence of genital injury, as manifested by bleeding, discharge, and genital lesions.[198] Gellert's group reported that 37% of HIV-positive children presented with another STD and that only 50% of those infected children reported vaginal or rectal penetration.[204]

Observations such as these, along with recent recommendations from the CDC for the consideration of HIV screening in child abuse victims, have led to discussions about the development of protocols for HIV screening.[205] Gellert and Durfee conducted an extensive survey of child protection programs in 1990, and found that none had defined protocols in place at that time. It appeared, however, that screening was performed in selected cases at the discretion of the clinician. Testing appears to occur most frequently in situations of an alleged perpetrator known to be HIV positive or of high-risk sexual assault, such as anal intercourse. Based on their survey, they recommended a protocol for assessing the need for HIV screening among victims of child abuse (Table 21–4).[199]

Many authors have stressed the importance of a thoroughly evaluated testing program, informed consent of the parent and/or guardian, and the need for follow-up testing of abused children whose initial serologic test results are negative. As with much testing for STDs in chil-

Table 21–4. HIV Antibody Indicants in Sexually Abused Children

Victim
  Clinical profile consistent with AIDS/AIDS-related complex
  Behavioral profile of high-risk adolescent (e.g., prostitute, gay, drugs)
  Parent/adolescent insistent on test
Assailant
  HIV seropositive
  Clinical profile consistent with AIDS/AIDS-related complex
  High-risk behavioral profile (e.g., gay, drugs)

Adapted with permission from Child Abuse and Neglect. Vol. 14, Gellert GA, Durfee MJ, Berkowitz CD. Developing guidelines for HIV testing among victims of pediatric sexual abuse.© 1990. Pergamon Press.

dren, compliance with follow-up is poor. Dattel reported that only 5% of the children in need of follow-up HIV testing actually returned for care.[206] Another author has suggested that testing alleged perpetrators may be more appropriate, especially HIV-positive ones who admit to abusing multiple victims.[207] Since many programs selectively screen children based, at least in part, on the history, Hammerschlag has suggested obtaining a frozen serum sample from all children. This sample could be screened at a later date if the child disclosed additional risk history. Not all investigators agree that screening sexually abused children for HIV infection is advisable or cost-effective. Fost estimates that $25,000 would be spent in screening costs for each HIV-positive child identified.[208] He also points out that HIV screening of sexually abused children does not fulfill the standard criteria usually applied to screening programs.

CONCLUSIONS

The correct diagnosis of a pediatric STD involves a thorough understanding of the complexities of possible sources of transmission, unique aspects of the clinical presentation, correct diagnostic procedures, and special treatment issues. A multidisciplinary approach is also essential in the often difficult process of evaluating the possibility of sexual abuse. These children deserve a humane approach to their care and treatment, as many children have already faced sexual abuse. It is important to avoid retraumatizing them in the course of evaluating them.

REFERENCES

1. Paradise JE, Campos JM, Friedman HM, Frishmuth G: Vulvovaginitis in premenarcheal girls: Clinical features and diagnostic evaluation. Pediatrics 1982; 70:193–198.

2. Arsenault PS, Gerbie AB: Vulvovaginitis in the preadolescent girl. Pediatr Ann 1986; 15:577–585.
3. Hammerschlag MR, Alpert S, Rosner I, et al: Microbiology of the vagina in children: Normal and potentially pathogenic organisms. Pediatrics 1978; 62:57–62.
4. White ST, Loda FA, Ingram DL, Pearson A: Sexually transmitted diseases in sexually abused children. Pediatrics 1983; 72:16–21.
5. DeJong AR: Sexually transmitted diseases in sexually abused children. Sex Transm Dis 1986; 13:123–126.
6. Cupoli JM, Sewell PM: One thousand fifty-nine children with a chief complaint of sexual abuse. Child Abuse Neglect 1988; 12:151–162.
7. Hanson RM: Sexually transmitted diseases and the sexually abused child. Curr Opin Pediatrics 1993; 5:41–49.
8. Puranen M, Yliskoski M, Saarikoski S, et al: Vertical transmission of human papillomavirus from infected mothers to their newborn babies and persistence of the virus in childhood. Am J Obstet Gynecol 1996; 174:694–699.
9. Jenny C: Child sexual abuse and STD. In Holmes KK (ed): Sexually Transmitted Diseases, 2nd ed. New York: McGraw-Hill, 1990, pp 895–900.
10. Huffman JW: Anatomy and physiology. In Huffman JW, Dewhurst J, Capraro VJ (eds): The Gynecology of Childhood and Adolescence, 2nd ed. Philadelphia: WB Saunders, 1981, pp 24–69.
11. Stewart D, et al: STDs in child sexual abuse: who is being tested? Abstract. Presented at the Annual Meeting of North American Society for Pediatric Adolescent Gynecology. 1993.
12. Dattel BJ, et al: Isolation of Chlamydia trachomatis and Neisseria gonorrhoeae from the genital tract of sexually abused prepubertal females. Adolesc Pediatr Gynecol 1989; 2:217–220.
13. Dyson C, Hosein IK: The role of the microbiology laboratory in the investigation of child sexual abuse. J Med Microbiol 1996; 45:313–318.
14. Embree JE, Lindsay D, Williams T, et al: Acceptability and usefulness of vaginal washes in premenarcheal girls as a diagnostic procedure for sexually transmitted diseases. Pediatr Infect Dis J 1996; 15:662–667.
15. Schachter J: Rapid diagnosis of sexually transmitted diseases—speed has a price. Diagn Microbiol Infect Dis 1986; 4:195–199.
16. Whittington WL, Rice RJ, Biddle JW, Knapp JS: Incorrect identification of Neisseria gonorrhoeae from infants and children. Pediatr Infect Dis J 1988; 7:3–10.
17. Centers for Disease Control: Sexually transmitted diseases treatment guidelines. MMWR 1982; 31:595–605.
18. Centers for Disease Control: 1989 sexually transmitted diseases treatment guidelines. MMWR 1989; 38(S8):11–38.
19. Sweet RL, Gibbs RS: Sexually transmitted diseases. In Sweet RL, Gibbs RS (eds): Infectious Diseases of the Female Genital Tract, 2nd ed. Baltimore: Williams & Wilkins, 1990, pp 109–143.
20. Singleton AF: An approach to the management of gonorrhea in the pediatric age group. J Natl Med Assoc 1981; 73:207–218.
21. Benson RA, Steer A: Vaginitis of children. Am J Dis Child 1937; 53:806.
22. Gutman LT, Wilfert CM: Gonococcal diseases in infants and children. In Holmes KK (ed): Sexually Transmitted Diseases, 2nd ed. New York: McGraw-Hill, 1990, pp 803–810.
23. Frau LM, Alexander ER: Public health implications of sexually transmitted diseases in pediatric practice. Pediatr Infect Dis 1985; 4:453–467.
24. Alexander ER: Maternal and infant sexually transmitted diseases. Urol Clin North Am 1984; 11:131–139.
25. Lang WR: Pediatric vaginitis. N Engl J Med 1955; 253:1153.
26. Gerstner GJ, Grunberger W, Boschitsch E, Rotter M: Vaginal organisms in prepubertal children with and without vaginitis. Arch Gynecol 1982; 231:247–252.
27. Argent AC, Lachman PI, Hanslo D, Bass D: Sexually transmitted diseases in children and evidence of sexual abuse. Child Abuse Neglect 1995; 19:1303–1310.
28. Groothuis JR, Bischoff MC, Jauregui LE: Pharyngeal gonorrhea in young children. Pediatr Infect Dis 1983; 2:99–101.
29. Weiss JC, DeJong AR: Gonococcal infection and sexual abuse. Pediatr Infect Dis 1983; 2:415.
30. Ingram D, et al: Epidemiology of adult sexually transmitted disease agents in children being evaluated for sexual abuse. Pediatr Infect Dis J 1992; 11:945–950.
31. McClure EM, Stack MR, Tanner R, et al: Pharyngeal culturing and reporting of pediatric gonorrhea in Connecticut. Pediatrics 1986; 78:509–510.
32. Nelson JD, Mohs E, Dajani AS, Plotkin SA: Gonorrhea in preschool and school-aged children: Report of the prepubertal gonorrhea cooperative study group. JAMA 1976; 236:1359–1364.
33. Ingram DL, White ST, Durfee MF, Pearson AW: Sexual contact in children with gonorrhea. Am J Dis Child 1982; 136:994–996.
34. Silber TJ, Controni G: Clinical spectrum of pharyngeal gonorrhea in children and adolescents. J Adolesc Health Care 1983; 4:51–54.
35. Ingram D, White S, Durfee M: The association of gonorrhea (GC) in children and sexual contact. Ambulatory Pediatr Assoc Program Abstr 1982 number 33.
36. Lewis LS, Glauser TA, Joffe MD: Gonococcal conjunctivitis in prepubertal children. Am J Dis Child 1990; 144:546–548.
37. Grendeinglagen DH, et al: Gonorrhea in children: Epidemiologic unit analysis (Letter). Pediatr Infect Dis J 1992; 11:973–974.
38. Branch G, Paxton R: A study of gonococcal infections among infants and children. Publ Health Rep 1965; 80:347–352.
39. Ingram DL: The gonococcus and the toilet seat revisited. Pediatr Infect Dis 1989; 8:191.
40. Farrell MK, Billmire E, Shamroy JA, Hammond JG: Prepubertal gonorrhea: A multidisciplinary approach. Pediatrics 1981; 67:151–153.
41. Lipsitt HJ, Parmet AJ: Nonsexual transmission of gonorrhea to a child. N Engl J Med 1984; 311:470.
42. Cooperman MB: Gonococcal arthritis in infancy. Am J Dis Child 1927; 33:932–948.
43. Rice JL, Cohn A, Steer A, Adler EL: Recent investigation of gonococcic vaginitis. JAMA 1941; 117:1766–1769.
44. Potterat JJ, Markewich GS, King RD: Child-to-child transmission of gonorrhea: Report of asymptomatic genital infection in a boy. Pediatrics 1986; 78:712.
45. Diena BB, Wallace R, Ashton FE, et al: Gonococcal conjunctivitis: Accidental infection. CMA 1976; 115:609–610.
46. Bruins SC, Tight RR: Laboratory-acquired gonococcal conjunctivitis. JAMA 1979; 241:274.
47. Wan WL, Farkas GC, May WN, Robin JB: The clinical characteristic and course of adult gonococcal conjunctivitis. Am J Ophthalmol 1986; 102:575–583.
48. Legido A, Joffe M: Gonococcal conjunctivitis mimicking orbital cellulitis in a young adolescent. Am J Dis Child 1989; 143:443–444.

49. Hammerschlag M: Pitfalls in the diagnosis of sexually transmitted diseases in children. ASPAC News 1989; 4–5.
50. Hammerschlag MR, Rawstron SA, Bromberg K: A commentary on the 1989 sexually transmitted diseases treatment guidelines. Pediatr Infect Dis 1990; 9:382–384.
51. Kramer DG, Jason J: Sexually abused children and sexually transmitted diseases. Rev Infect Dis 1982; 4(suppl):S883–S890.
52. Schachter J: Biology of *Chlamydia trachomatis. In* Holmes KK (ed): Sexually Transmitted Diseases, 2nd ed. New York: McGraw-Hill, 1990, pp 167–180.
53. Sweet RL, Gibbs RS: Chlamydial infections. *In* Sweet RL, Gibbs RS (eds): Infectious Diseases of the Female Genital Tract, 2nd ed. Baltimore: Williams & Wilkins, 1990, pp 45–74.
54. Harrison HR, Alexander ER: Chlamydial infections in infants and children. *In* Holmes KK (ed): Sexually Transmitted Diseases, 2nd ed. New York: McGraw-Hill, 1990, pp 811–820.
55. Hammerschlag MR, Chandler JW, Alexander ER, et al: Longitudinal studies on chlamydial infections in the first year of life. Pediatr Infect Dis 1982; 1:395–401.
56. Schachter J, Grossman M, Sweet RL: Prospective study of perinatal transmission of *C. trachomatis.* JAMA 1986; 255:3374–3377.
57. Bump RC: *Chlamydia trachomatis* as a cause of prepubertal vaginitis. Obstet Gynecol 1985; 6:384–388.
58. Ingram DL, Runyan DK, Collins AD, et al: Vaginal *Chlamydia trachomatis* infection in children with sexual contact. Pediatr Infect Dis 1984; 3:97–99.
59. Hammerschlag MR, Doraiswamy B, Alexander ER, et al: Are rectogenital chlamydial infections a marker of sexual abuse in children? Pediatr Infect Dis 1984; 3:100–104.
60. Rettig PJ: Pediatric genital infection with *Chlamydia trachomatis:* Statistically nonsignificant, but clinically important. Pediatr Infect Dis 1984; 3:95–96.
61. Keskey TS, Suarez M, Gleicher N, et al: *Chlamydia trachomatis* infection in sexually abused children. Mt Sinai J Med 1987; 54:129–134.
62. Ingram DL, White ST, Occhiuti AR, Lyna PR: Childhood vaginal infections: Association of *Chlamydia trachomatis* with sexual contact. Pediatr Infect Dis 1986; 5:226–229.
63. Schachter J, Grossman M, Holt J: Infection with *Chlamydia trachomatis:* Involvement of multiple anatomic sites in neonates. J Infect Dis 1979; 139:232.
64. Bell TA, Stamm WE, Kuo CC: Chlamydial Infections. Cambridge, England: Cambridge University Press, 1986; pp 305–308.
65. Bell TA, Stamm WE, Kuo C-C, et al: Delayed appearance of *Chlamydia trachomatis* infections acquired at birth. Pediatr Infect Dis 1987; 6:928–931.
66. Thygeson P, Stone W: Epidemiology of inclusion conjunctivitis. Arch Ophthalmol 1942; 27:91.
67. Rettig PJ, Nelson JD: Genital tract infection with *Chlamydia trachomatis* in prepubertal children. J Pediatr 1981; 99:206–210.
68. Fuster CD, Neinstein LS: Vaginal *Chlamydia trachomatis* prevalence in sexually abused prepubertal girls. Pediatrics 1987; 79:235–238.
69. Centers for Disease Control and Prevention: 1998 guidelines for treatment of sexually transmitted diseases. MMWR 1998; 47:1–118.
70. Bell T, Stamm W, Wang S, et al: Chronic *Chlamydia trachomatis* infections in infants. JAMA 1992; 267:400.
71. Mahony JB, Chernesky MA: Effect of swab type and storage temperature on the isolation of *Chlamydia tra-*

chomatis from clinical specimens. J Clin Microbiol 1985; 22:865–867.
72. Alexander ER: Misidentification of sexually transmitted organisms in children: Medicolegal implications. Pediatr Infect Dis 1988; 7:1–2.
73. Hammerschlag MR, Rettig PJ, Shields ME: False positive results with the use of chlamydial antigen detection tests in the evaluation of suspected sexual abuse in children. Pediatr Infect Dis 1988; 7:11–14.
74. Bauwens JE, et al: *Chlamydia pneumoniae* (strain TWAR) isolated from two symptom-free children during evaluation for possible sexual abuse. J Pediatrics 1991; 19:591–593.
75. Black SB, Grossman M, Cles L, Schachter J: Serological evidence of chlamydial infection in children. J Pediatr 1981; 98:65–67.
76. Waites KB, et al: Association of genital mycoplasmas with exudative vaginitis in a 10 year old: A case of misdiagnosis. Pediatrics 1983; 71:250–252.
77. Shawn DH, Quinn PA, Prober C, Jadavji T: Recurrent urethritis associated with ureaplasm urealyticum in a prepubertal boy (Letter). Pediatr Infect Dis J 1987; 6:687–688.
78. Hammerschlag M, et al: Colonization of sexually abused children with genital mycoplasmas. Sex Transm Dis 1987; 14:23–25.
79. Ingram DL, White ST, Lyna P, et al: *Ureaplasma urealyticum* and large colony mycoplasma colonization in female children and its relationship to sexual contact, age, and race. Child Abuse Neglect 1992; 16:265–272.
80. Sweet RL, Gibbs RS: Infectious vulvovaginitis. *In* Sweet RL, Gibbs RS (eds): Infectious Diseases of the Female Genital Tract, 2nd ed. Baltimore: Williams & Wilkins, 1990, pp 216–228.
81. Ingram DL: Controversies about the sexual and nonsexual transmission of adult STDs to children. *In* Krugman RD, Leventhal JM: Child Sexual Abuse. 22nd Ross Roundtable on Critical Approaches to Common Pediatric Problems. Columbus, OH: Ross Laboratories, 1991, pp 14–27.
82. Lang WR: Premenarchal vaginitis. Obstet Gynecol 1959; 13:723.
83. Jones JG, Yamauchi T, Lambert B: *Trichomonas vaginalis* infection in sexually abused girls. Am J Dis Child 1985; 139:846.
84. Rein MF, Muller M: *Trichomonas vaginalis* and trichomoniasis. *In* Holmes KK (ed): Sexually Transmitted Diseases, 2nd ed. New York: McGraw-Hill, 1990, pp 481–492.
85. Blattner RJ: *Trichomonas vaginalis* infection in a newborn infant. J Pediatr 1967; 71:608.
86. Neinstein LS, Goldenring J, Carpenter S: Nonsexual transmission of sexually transmitted diseases: An infrequent occurrence. Pediatrics 1984; 74:67–76.
87. Al-Salihi FL: Neonatal *Trichomonas vaginalis*: Report of three cases and review of the literature. Pediatrics 1974; 53:196.
88. Bramley M: Study of female babies of women entering confinement with vaginal trichomoniasis. Br J Vener Dis 1976; 52:58.
89. Robinson SC, Halifax NS: Observations on vaginal trichomoniasis. I. In pregnancy. Can Med Assoc J 1961; 84:948.
90. Lossick JS: Trichomonads Parasitic in Humans. New York: Springer, 1989, p 237.
91. Burgess JA: *Trichomonas vaginalis* infection from splashing in water closets. Br J Vener Dis 1963; 39:248.
92. Orley J, Florian E, Juranji R: Vaginal discharge in puberty. Gynaecologia 1969; 168:191–202.

93. Fouts AC, Kraus SJ: Trichomonas vaginitis: Reevaluation of its clinical presentation and laboratory diagnosis. J Infect Dis 1980; 141:137–143.

94. Beard CM, Noller KL, O'Fallon WM: Lack of evidence for cancer due to use of metronidazole. N Engl J Med 1979; 301:519.

95. Williams TS, Callen JP, Owen LG: Vulvar disorders in the prepubertal female. Pediatr Ann 1986; 15:588–605.

96. Alchek A: Pediatric vulvovaginitis. J Reprod Med 1984; 29:359–375.

97. Sweet RL, Gibbs RS: Perinatal infections. In Sweet RL, Gibbs RS (eds): Infectious Diseases of the Female Genital Tract, 2nd ed. Baltimore: Williams & Wilkins, 1990, pp 290–319.

98. Shah KV: Biology of human genital tract papillomaviruses. In Holmes KK (ed): Sexually Transmitted Diseases, 2nd ed. New York: McGraw-Hill, 1990, pp 425–431.

99. Centers for Disease Control: Condyloma acuminatum—United States, 1966–1981. MMWR 1983; 32:306–308.

100. Bender ME: New concepts of condyloma acuminata in children. Arch Dermatol 1986; 122:1121–1123.

101. Seidel J, Zonana J, Totten E: Condylomata acuminata as a sign of sexual abuse in children. J Pediatr 1979; 22:553–554.

102. Vallejos H, Mistro AD, Kleinhaus S, et al: Characterization of human papilloma virus types in condylomata acuminata in children by in situ hybridization. Lab Invest 1987; 56:611–615.

103. Rock B, Naghashfar Z, Barnett N, et al: Genital tract papillomavirus infection in children. Arch Dermatol 1986; 122:1129–1132.

104. Obalek S, Jablonska S, Favre M, et al: Condylomata acuminata in children: Frequent association with human papillomaviruses responsible for cutaneous warts. J Am Acad Dermatol 1990; 23:205–213.

105. Hanson RM, Glasson M, McCrossin I, et al: Anogenital warts in childhood. Child Abuse Neglect 1989; 13:225–233.

106. Goerzen JL, Robertson DI, Inoue M, Trevenen CL: Detection of HPV DNA in genital condylomata acuminata in female prepubertal children. Adolesc Pediatr Gynecol 1989; 2:224–229.

107. Clark DP: Condyloma acuminata in children. Curr Concepts Skin Disord 1985; 6:10–17.

108. Cohen PR, Young AW: Genital warts in children: Diagnosis, treatment, and legal implications. Med Aspects Hum Sex 1989; Oct: 22–28.

109. Boyd AS: Condylomata acuminata in the pediatric population. Am J Dis Child 1990; 144:817–824.

110. DeJong AR, Weiss JC, Brent RL: Condyloma acuminata in children. Am J Dis Child 1982; 136:704–706.

111. Mulchahey KM: Genital findings in prepubertal girls with human papilloma virus infection (Abstract). Presented at the Fourth Annual Meeting of North American Society for Pediatric Adolescent Gynecology, 1990, Costa Mesa, CA.

112. McCance DJ: Human papillomaviruses and cancer. Biochem Biophys Acta 1986; 823:195.

113. Macnab B: Human papillomavirus in clinically and histologically normal tissue of patients with genital cancer. N Engl J Med 1986; 315:1052.

114. McCance DJ: Human papillomavirus types 16 and 18 in carcinomas of the penis in Brazil. Int J Cancer 1986; 37:55.

115. Nuovo GJ, Pedemonte BM: Human papillomavirus types and recurrent cervical warts. JAMA 1990; 263:1223–1226.

116. Trofatter KF, English PC, Hughes CE, Gall SA: Human lymphoblastoid interferon (Wellferon) in primary therapy of two children with condylomata acuminata. Obstet Gynecol 1986; 67:137–140.

117. Scholefield JH, Sonnex C, Talbot IC, et al: Anal and cervical intraepithelial neoplasia: Possible parallel. Lancet 1989; ii:765–769.

118. Stringel G, Mercer S, Corsini L: Condylomata acuminata in children. J Pediatr Surg 1985; 20:499–501.

119. Herman-Giddens ME, Gutman LT, Berson NL: Association of coexisting vaginal infections and multiple abusers in female children with genital warts. Sex Transm Dis 1988; 6:63–67.

120. Laraque D: Severe anogenital warts in a child with HIV infection. Letter. N Engl J Med 1989; 320:1220–1221.

121. Forman AB, Prendiville JS: Association of human immunodeficiency virus seropositivity and extensive perineal condylomata acuminata in a child. Arch Dermatol 1988; 124:1010–1011.

122. Kashima HK, Shah K, Goodstein M: Recurrent respiratory papillomatosis. In Holmes KK (ed): Sexually Transmitted Diseases, 2nd ed. New York: McGraw-Hill, 1990, pp 889–893.

123. Egbert JE, Kersten RC: Female genital tract papillomavirus in conjunctival papillomas of infancy. Am J Ophthalmol 1997; 123:551–552.

124. Shah K, Kashima H, Polk BF: Rarity of cesarean delivery in cases of juvenile-onset respiratory papillomatosis. Obstet Gynecol 1986; 68:795.

125. Fife KH, Rogers RE, Zwickl BW: Symptomatic and asymptomatic cervical infections with human papillomavirus during pregnancy. J Infect Dis 1987; 156:904.

126. Tang C-K, Shermeta DW, Wood C: Congenital condylomata acuminata. Am J Obstet Gynecol 1978; 131:912–913.

127. Puranen M, Yliskoski M, Saarikoski S, et al: Exposure of an infant to cervical human papillomavirus infection of the mother is common. Am J Obstet Gynecol 1997; 176:1039–1045.

128. Tseng C, Liang C, Soong Y, Pao C: Perinatal transmission of human papillomavirus in infants: Relationship between infection rate and mode of delivery. Obstet Gynecol 1998; 91:92–96.

129. Watts DH, Koutsky LA, Holmes KK, et al: Low risk of perinatal transmission of human papillomavirus: Results from a prospective cohort study. Am J Obstet Gynecol 1998; 178:365–373.

130. Weinberg R, et al: Outcome of CPS referral for sexual abuse in children with condylomata acuminata. Adolesc Pediatr Gynecol 1994; 7:19–24.

131. Oriel JD, Almeida JD: Demonstration of virus particles in human genital warts. Br J Vener Dis 1970; 46:37.

132. Oriel JD: Natural history of genital warts. Br J Vener Dis 1971; 47:1–13.

133. Teokharov BA: Non-gonococcal infections of the female genitalia. Br J Vener Dis 1969; 45:334–340.

134. Goldenring JM: Condylomata acuminata: Still usually a sexually transmitted disease in children (Letter). Am J Dis Child 1991; 145:600–601.

135. Mulchahey KM: Characteristics of children with genital human papilloma virus infection. North American Society for Pediatric Adolescent Gynecology, 1990, Costa Mesa, CA.

136. Yoshpe NS: Oral and laryngeal papilloma: A pediatric manifestation of sexually transmitted disease? Int J Pediatr Otorhinolaryngol 1995; 31:77–83.

137. Gutman L, Herman-Giddens M, Prose NS: Diagnosis of child sexual abuse in children with genital warts (Letter). Am J Dis Child 1991; 145:126.

138. Schachner L, Hankin D: Assessing child abuse in child-

hood condyloma acuminatum. J Am Acad Dermatol 1985; 12:157–160.

139. Handley J, Dinsmore W, Maw R, et al: Anogenital warts in prepubertal children: Sexual abuse or not? Int J STD AIDS 1993; 4:271–279.

140. Gissman L, Schwartz E: Papillomaviruses. New York: John Wiley, 1986, p 190.

141. Pacheco BP, et al: Vulvar infection caused by human papillomavirus in children and adolescents without sexual contact. Adolesc Pediatr Gynecol 1991; 4:136–142.

142. Fleming KA: DNA typing of genital warts and a diagnosis of sexual abuse in children. Lancet 1987; ii:454.

143. Krzyzek RA, Watts SL, Anderson DL, et al: Anogenital warts contain several distinct species of human papillomavirus. J Virol 1980; 36:236–244.

144. Brown J, Hauger SB, Clare FS, Rogers AR: Human immunodeficiency virus (HIV), human papillomavirus (HPV), and sexual abuse. Adolesc Pediatr Gynecol 1995; 8:208–212.

145. Norins AL, Caputo RV, Lucky AW, Krafchik BR: Genital warts and sexual abuse in children: American Academy of Dermatology Task Force on Pediatric Dermatology. J Am Acad Dermatol 1984; 11:529–530.

146. Moy RL, Eliezri YD, Nuovo GJ, et al: Human papillomavirus type 16 DNA in periungual squamous cell carcinomas. JAMA 1989; 261:2669–2673.

147. Marx JL: How DNA viruses may cause cancer. Science 1989; 243:1012–1013.

148. Lister UM, Akinla O: Carcinoma of the vulva in childhood. J Obstet Gynecol Br Comm 1972; 79:470–473.

149. Stoehr GP: Systemic complications of local podophyllin therapy. Ann Intern Med 1978; 89:362.

150. Slater GE: Podophyllin poisoning: Systemic toxicity following cutaneous application. Obstet Gynecol 1978; 52:94.

151. Moher LM, Maurer SA: Podophyllin toxicity: Case report and literature review. J Fam Pract 1979; 9:237.

152. Ward JW, Clifford WS, Monaco AR, Bickerstaff HJ: Fatal systemic poisoning following podophyllin treatment of condyloma acuminatum. S Med J 1954; 47:1204–1206.

153. Stringel G, Spence J, Corsini L: Genital warts in children. Can Med Assoc J 1985; 132:1397–1398.

154. Pride GL: Treatment of large lower genital tract condylomata acuminata with topical 5-fluorouracil. J Reprod Med 1990; 35:384–387.

155. Gale C, Muram D: The surgical treatment of condyloma acuminata in children. Adolesc Pediatr Gynecol 1990; 3:189–192.

156. Healy GB, Gelber RD, Trowbridge AL, et al: Treatment of recurrent respiratory papillomatosis with human leukocyte interferon. N Engl J Med 1988; 319:401–407.

157. Steinberg BM, Topp WC, Schneider PS, Abramson AL: Laryngeal papillomavirus infection during clinical remission. N Engl J Med 1983; 308:1261–1264.

158. Friedman-Kien AE, Eron LJ, Conant M, et al: Natural inferferon alfa for treatment of condylomata acuminata. JAMA 1988; 259:533–538.

159. Sweet RL, Gibbs RS: Herpes virus infection. In Sweet RL, Gibbs RS (eds): Infectious Diseases of the Female Genital Tract, 2nd ed. Baltimore: Williams & Wilkins, 1990, pp 144–157.

160. Taieb A, Body S, Astar I, et al: Clinical epidemiology of symptomatic primary herpetic infection in children. Acta Paediatr Scand 1987; 76:128–132.

161. Corey L: Genital herpes. In Holmes KK (ed): Sexually Transmitted Diseases, 2nd ed. New York: McGraw-Hill, 1990, pp 391–413.

162. Nahmias AJ, Dowdle WR, Naib ZM, et al: Genital infection with herpesvirus hominis types 1 and 2 in children. Pediatrics 1968; 42:659–666.

163. Gardner M, Jones J: Genital herpes acquired by sexual abuse of children. J Pediatr 1984; 104:243–244.

164. Kaplan KM, Fleisher GR, Paradise JE, Freidman HN: Social relevance of genital herpes simplex in children. Am J Dis Child 1984; 138:872–874.

165. Gushurst CA: The problem of genital herpes in prepubertal children. Am J Dis Child 1985; 139:542–545.

166. Nerurkar LS, West F, May M, et al: Survival of herpes simplex virus in water specimens collected from hot tubs in spa facilities and on plastic surfaces. JAMA 1983; 250:3081–3083.

167. Douglas JM, Corey L: Fomites and herpes simplex viruses: A case of nonvenereal transmission? JAMA 1983; 250:3093.

168. Hibbard RA: Herpetic vulvovaginitis and child abuse. Am J Dis Child 1985; 139:542.

169. Miller RG, Whittington WL, Coleman RM, Nigida SM: Acquisition of concomitant oral and genital infection with herpes simplex virus type 2. Sex Transm Dis 1987; 14:41–43.

170. Hillier S, Holmes KK: Bacterial vaginosis. In Holmes KK (ed): Sexually Transmitted Diseases, 2nd ed. New York: McGraw-Hill, 1990, pp 547–559.

171. DeJong AR: Vaginitis due to Gardnerella vaginalis and to Candida albicans in sexual abuse. Child Abuse Neglect 1985; 9:27–29.

172. Muram D, Buxton BH: Gardnerella vaginalis in children: An indicator of sexual abuse. Pediatr Adolesc Gynecol 1984; 2:197–200.

173. Thomason JL, Gelbert SM, Anderson RJ, et al: Statistical evaluation of diagnostic criteria for bacterial vaginosis. Am J Obstet Gynecol 1990; 162:155–160.

174. Eschenbach D: Diagnosis and clinical manifestation of bacterial vaginosis. Am J Obstet Gynecol 1988; 158:819.

175. Hammerschlag MR, Alpert S, Rosner I, et al: Microbiology of the vagina in children: Normal and potentially pathogenic organisms. Pediatrics 1978; 62:57–62.

176. Bartley DL, Morgan L, Rimsza ME: Gardnerella vaginalis in prepubertal girls. Am J Dis Child 1987; 141:1014–1017.

177. Hammerschlag MR, Cummings M, Doraiswamy B, et al: Nonspecific vaginitis following sexual abuse in children. Pediatrics 1985; 75:1028–1031.

178. Bump RC, Bueschling WJ: Bacterial vaginosis in virginal and sexually active adolescent females: Evidence against exclusive sexual transmission. Am J Obstet Gynecol 1988; 159:935.

179. Jenny C, Hooton TM, Bowers A, et al: Sexually transmitted diseases in victims of rape. N Engl J Med 1990; 322:713–716.

180. Zenker PN, Berman SM: Congenital syphilis: Trends and recommendations for evaluation and management. Pediatr Infect Dis 1991; 10:516–522.

181. Dorfman DH, Glaser JH: Congenital syphilis presenting in infants after the newborn period. N Engl J Med 1990; 323:1299–1302.

182. Sanchez P, Wendal G, Norgard MV: Congenital syphilis associated with negative results of maternal serologic tests at delivery. Am J Dis Child 1991; 145:967–969.

183. Lowy G: Sexually transmitted diseases in children. Pediatr Dermatol 1991; 4:329–334.

184. Ginsburg CM: Acquired syphilis in prepubertal children. Pediatr Infect Dis 1983; 2:232–234.

185. Horowitz S, Chadwick DL: Syphilis as a sole indicator of sexual abuse: Two cases with no intervention. Child Abuse Neglect 1990; 14:129–132.

186. Gellert GA, Durfee MJ: HIV infection and child abuse. N Engl J Med 1989; 321:685.

187. Bays J, Chadwick D: The serologic test for syphilis in sexually abused children and adolescents. Adolesc Pediatr Gynecol 1991; 4:148–151.

188. Ammann AJ: The acquired immunodeficiency syndrome in infants and children. Ann Intern Med 1985; 103:734–737.

189. Shannon KM, Ammann AJ: Acquired immune deficiency syndrome in childhood. J Pediatr 1985; 106:332–342.

190. Rogers MF: AIDS in children: A review of the clinical, epidemiologic and public health aspects. Pediatr Infect Dis 1985; 4:230–236.

191. Okeske J, Minnefor A, Cooper R, Thomas K: Immune deficiency syndrome in children. JAMA 1983; 249:2345–2349.

192. Gutman LT, et al: Pediatric acquired immunodeficiency syndrome: Barriers to recognizing the role of child sexual abuse. Am J Dis Child 1993; 147:775–780.

193. Osterholm MT, MacDonald KL: Facing the complex issues of pediatric AIDS: A public health perspective. JAMA 1987; 258:2736–2737.

194. Leiderman IZ, Grimm KT: A child with HIV infection. JAMA 1986; 256:3094.

195. Rubinstein A: Pediatric AIDS. Curr Probl Pediatr 1986; 16:362–409.

196. Thomas PA, Lubin K, Miblerg J, et al: Cohort comparison study of children whose mothers have acquired immunodeficiency syndrome and children of well inner city mothers. Pediatr Infect Dis 1987; 6:247–251.

197. Dattel BJ, Coulter K, Grossman M, Hauer LB: Presence of HIV antibody (Ab) in sexually abused children (SAC). IV International Conference on Aids, 1988.

198. Gutman LT, St Claire KK, Weedy C, et al: Human immunodeficiency virus transmission by child sexual abuse. Am J Dis Child 1991; 145:137–141.

199. Gellert GA, Durfee MJ, Berkowitz CD: Developing guidelines for HIV testing among victims of pediatric sexual abuse. Child Abuse Neglect 1990; 14:9–17.

200. Siegal R, et al: Incest and *Pneumocystis carinii* pneumonia in a twelve-year-old girl: A case for early human immunodeficiency virus testing in sexually abused children. Pediatr Infect Dis 1992; 11:681–682.

201. Gutman L, et al: Sexual abuse of human immunodeficiency virus-positive children: Outcomes for perpetrators and evaluation of other household children. Am J Dis Child 1992; 146:1185–1189.

202. Fischl MA, Dickinson GM, Scott GB, et al: Evaluation of heterosexual partners, children, and household contacts of adults with AIDS. JAMA 1987; 257:640–644.

203. Padian N, Marquis L, Francis DP: Male-to-female transmission of human immunodeficiency virus. JAMA 1987; 258:788–790.

204. Gellert GA, et al: Situational and sociodemographic characteristics of children infected with human immunodeficiency virus from pediatric sexual abuse. Pediatrics 1993; 91:39–44.

205. Rimza ME: Words too terrible to hear: Sexual transmission of human immunodeficiency virus to children. Am J Dis Child 1993; 147:711–712.

206. B. J. Dattel, MD, personal communication.

207. Fuller AK, Bartucci RJ: HIV transmission and childhood sexual abuse. JAMA 1988; 259:2235–2236.

208. Fost N: Ethical considerations in testing victims of sexual abuse for HIV infection. Child Abuse Neglect 1990; 14:5–7.

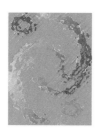

Chapter 22
Sexually Transmitted Diseases in Adolescents

David Muram

The increasing incidence of sexually transmitted diseases (STDs) among persons 13 to 19 years of age raises significant concerns about the reproductive health of adolescents overall in the United States. Epidemiologic surveys of teenagers indicate that the initiation into sexual activity is occurring earlier than before and often is not accompanied by measures to prevent pregnancy and STDs (Fig. 22–1).[1] Adolescents who initiate sexual intercourse at younger ages are more likely to have multiple partners, thus increasing their chances of becoming infected with an STD. In one study, the incidence of gonorrhea among very young adolescents was 34.0 cases per 1000 person-months, and the median time from initiation of intercourse to first positive culture was 4.6 months.[2]

Every year, 2.5 million teenagers are infected with an STD; this number represents approximately one of every six sexually active adolescents. Risk-taking behavior, such as denial of the possibility of harm, increases sexual risk-taking behavior as well.

While the reported incidence of gonorrhea decreased by 71.3% between 1981 and 1996, women aged 15 to 19 years had the highest rates, almost twice that of the general population.[3] Furthermore, many teenagers are ignorant of the symptoms and signs of acute infections and, so, are less likely to seek treatment for an STD. The sequelae of undiagnosed and untreated STDs (i.e., pelvic inflammatory disease (PID), infertility, ectopic pregnancy, cervical cancer, and inadvertent transmission of HIV) exact considerable cost. Even so, the health consequences and costs associated with the high prevalence of STDs in adolescents remain largely hidden.[4] Risky behavior and threats to health are amplified by alcohol, drugs, and tobacco, which often compromise adolescents' ability to make sound judgments about sex and contraception and place them at increased risk of pregnancy or infection. In this chapter the current status of the major STDs of adolescents is addressed.

EPIDEMIOLOGY

Because of reporting ability and numerical significance, the best estimates of STD morbidity patterns among adolescents are extrapolated from data for gonorrhea. In 1991, approximately 609,459 cases of gonorrhea (233 per 100,000 population) were reported to the Centers for Disease Control (CDC), reflecting a continuing decline since 1980.[5] Rates for adolescents have declined more slowly than those in any other age group, however, and actually increased (from 881 to 954 per 100,000) in black adolescent males.[5] A more recent study showed that, while the incidence of reported gonorrhea decreased from 431.5 to 124.0 cases per 100,000 between 1981 and 1996, 15- to 19-year-old women had the highest rate 716.6 cases per 100,000 in 1996.[3] A racial trend is apparent; incidences for black male and female teenagers are nearly 44 and 16 times greater, respectively, than those for white teenagers. Some speculate that prevention messages have been less successful and that diverted partner notification efforts and overburdened public clinics have disproportionately affected minority populations.[6] Furthermore, the use of illicit drugs, particularly crack cocaine, is associated with frequent sexual activity and risk taking. In one study, a third of black adolescent male crack users reported having had at least 10 sex partners in the preceding year.[3, 7]

Chlamydia trachomatis infection, one of the most prevalent STDs in the United States, affects an estimated 4 million people each year.[5] Among adolescents, *Chlamydia* infections are diagnosed more often than gonorrhea.[8] In one study, *Chlamydia* organisms were detected in 8% to 40% of teenage females during the routine gynecologic examination, a rate twice that for gonorrhea.[9]

357

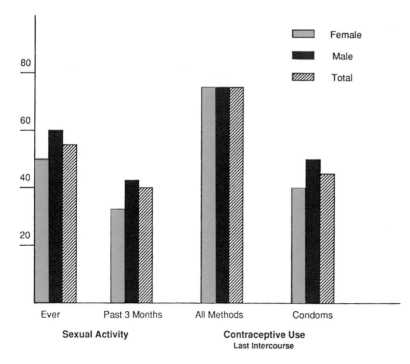

Figure 22–1 Prevalence of sexual intercourse and use of contraceptives in U.S. high school students. (From Centers for Disease Control: Sexual behavior among high school students, United States, 1990. MMWR 1992; 40:885–888).

Because infections caused by chlamydiae are not reportable diseases throughout the United States, the true incidence is unknown, a fact that further complicates efforts at control and increases the risk for associated complications such as PID, ectopic pregnancy, and infertility.

Infections caused by viral STDs—human papillomavirus (HPV), and herpes simplex virus (HSV)—are probably the most common ones in the United States. Using sensitive detection techniques, studies of the prevalence of HPV report infection rates as high as 38% to 46% in adolescents and sexually active young women.[10, 11] Additionally, asymptomatic cervical infection is nearly three times more common than reported external genital warts.[12] Serologic studies of HSV antibody have revealed widespread asymptomatic infections among a representative cohort of patients in the United States.[13] Approximately 4% of white teenagers and 17% of black teens have been infected (as determined by HSV-2 antibody) by the age of 19.

Clearly, adolescents participate in significant risk-taking behavior. To reduce the incidence of human immunodeficiency virus (HIV) infections and STDs, programs and policies must address adolescents' decision making about sexual activity and the psychosocial dynamics that affect these decisions. Chapter 23 contains a discussion of risk determinants of STDs and HIV infections in adolescents.

GONORRHEA

Gonorrhea is an infection of the mucous membrane of the urethra and genital tract caused by *Neisseria gonorrhoeae*, a gram-negative diplococcus. Clinical illness caused by *N. gonorrhoeae* was described in ancient literature as early as 2637 BC. The organism itself was described by Albert Neisser from stained smears of exudates from urethras, cervices, and neonatal ophthalmic tissue and was first cultured by Leistkow in 1882.[14] Because the gonococcal organisms infect columnar and transitional epithelia, the adult vaginal mucosa is resistant to infection with *N. gonorrhoeae*.

The incubation period for *N. gonorrhoeae* is roughly 1 week; symptoms generally appear 2 to 7 days after exposure. Asymptomatic infections are not uncommon, particularly in women; only 10% to 20% of those affected have a mucopurulent cervical discharge.[15] Other related symptoms in women include urethritis, increased vaginal discharge, dysuria, intermenstrual bleeding, and menorrhagia.[16, 17] Urogenital involvement in females may extend to the vestibular glands, Skene's glands, and Bartholin's ducts and glands, in which case purulent secretions may be expressed from the infected site (Fig. 22–2). In males, local complications include epididymitis, posterior urethritis, lymphangitis, and prostatitis. The majority of infections of the anal canal pro-

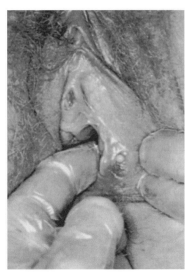

Figure 22–2 Gonococcal bartholinitis.

duce nonspecific symptoms such as irritation and tenesmus, if any. The natural history of these infections is ill-understood, but isolated rectal infections in women are uncommon (prevalence less than 5% of patients with gonorrhea).[18] Rectal infection is relatively common in patients with urogenital infections, however. Prevalences are 35% to 50% for female patients with cervicitis[19, 20] and 40% for sexually active homosexual men.[21, 22] Most rectal infections in females are assumed to occur by local spread of infected cervical secretions, whereas in male homosexuals, rectal gonorrhea is due to direct inoculation through receptive anal intercourse.

DNA-specific probes for *N. gonorrhoeae* and polymerase chain reaction (PCR) tests are also quite useful in adolescents: reported sensitivity and specificity rates are 97% and 99%, respectively. In addition, DNA probes can be reliable tests for cure.[23] Ligase chain reaction tests were also found to be quite sensitive for *N. gonorrhoeae*.[24–26] The presence of morphologically typical, gram-negative, intracellular diplococci is sufficiently sensitive (90% to 95%) and specific (95% to 100%) to establish the diagnosis of gonorrhea in symptomatic males.[27] Gram-stained smears are relatively insensitive in women (30% to 60%), and interpretation may be confounded by vaginal bacterial contamination.[18, 20] For this reason, the use of Gram-stained smears to determine treatment should be confined to patients at high risk whose therapy *must* be instituted before culture results are received[15]—those suspected to have PID, or who have a history of exposure to gonorrhea and a mucopurulent cervical discharge. Likewise, findings from stained smears

of urethral and anal specimens, with the exception of mucopurulent anal discharge, are too nonspecific for routine use. Because of the expense of confirmation, the absence of symptoms, and the often self-limited nature of the infection, an argument has been made for foregoing routine culture from the pharynx.[15]

DISSEMINATED GONOCOCCAL INFECTION

Disseminated gonococcal infections (DGIs) occur in 0.5% to 3% of patients with untreated urogenital gonorrhea.[27, 29] It is the most common systemic complication of acute gonorrhea. Clinical manifestations, in addition to malaise and fever, include skin lesions, arthralgia, and tenosynovitis. Typically, the arthritis is migrating polyarthritis involving the wrists, metacarpals, ankles, and knees. The typical skin lesion of DGI consists of a necrotic pustule on an erythematous base (Fig. 22–3). The number of lesions may vary, but most patients have fewer than 30, and these may evolve from or present as macules, pustules, ecchymoses, petechiae, or bullae.[30, 31] DGI is more common in females, and the onset of symptoms follows the menstrual period in approximately 50% of patients.[28–32] Pregnancy and pharyngeal gonorrhea have also been cited as risk factors. Gonococcal strains that become bloodborne tend to be nutritionally deficient auxotypes, AHU/1A-1 and AHU/1A-2.[17] These strains are more likely to cause asymptomatic infections and to be susceptible to penicillin, are more difficult to culture, and are more resistant to the complement-mediated bactericidal activity of human sera.[28, 30, 33]

Definitive diagnosis of DGI depends on isolating the gonococcus from the blood, skin lesions,

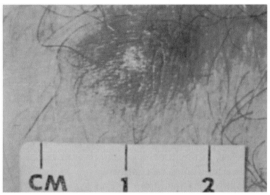

Figure 22–3 Hemorrhagic pustule of disseminated gonococcal infection.

synovial fluid, or cerebrospinal fluid; this can be done early in the disease course in 10% to 30% of patients.[28-31] In some patients, the diagnosis is established from observing the typical clinical manifestations and concurrently isolating *N. gonorrhoeae* from the lower genital tract, the rectum, or, at times, from a sexual partner.

TREATMENT

Although the incidence of gonorrhea has been declining since 1975, the emergence of antimicrobial drug–resistant gonorrhea has created a complex problem for clinicians and monitors of resistant patterns. By 1990, antimicrobial-resistant strains accounted for 8.4% of all reported cases of gonorrhea.[5] Gonococcal resistance to antimicrobial agents has been evolving since the sulfonamides and penicillin became available in the 1940s. In 1976, penicillinase-producing *N. gonorrhoeae* (PPNG) was discovered, marking an accelerated trend toward antibiotic resistance because of the mechanism by which resistance is acquired: a new plasmid that carried genes for production of a β-lactamase capable of disrupting the β-lactam ring of the penicillin molecule. Plasmid-mediated resistance is responsible for the increasing numbers of tetracycline-resistant gonorrhea (TRNG) strains and combined PPNG-TRNG resistance. Resistant gonorrhea resulting from random selection of mutants from the huge gonoccocus population has been termed *chromosome-mediated resistant gonorrhea* (CRNG). Recognizing the importance of these changing microbial trends, the Centers for Disease Control (CDC) created a sentinel surveillance system to monitor antimicrobial-resistant *N. gonorrhoeae*. The Gonoccocal Isolate Surveillance Project (GISP) consists of 24 sentinel STD clinics that monthly submit isolates to five regional laboratories for susceptibility testing.

Because of widespread and steadily increasing resistance to penicillin, the CDC's *1998 STD Treatment Guidelines* recommended using a penicillinase-resistant regimen (e.g., ceftriaxone combined with doxycycline).[34] As a result, treatment regimens consisting of second- and third-generation cephalosporins (cefuroxime axetil, ceftizoxime, cefotaxime) and fluorinated quinolones (ciprofloxacin, norfloxacin) have become standard throughout the United States. For patients who cannot take ceftriaxone, the preferred alternative is spectinomycin, 2 gm intramuscularly in a single dose.[33] Amoxicillin combined with probenecid is still useful when the pathogen

is *known* not to be penicillin resistant. The recommended treatment for patients with systemic infections (DGI, meningitis, endocarditis) is high-dose, intravenous ceftriaxone or an equivalent β-lactam–resistant antibiotic.

ADDITIONAL CONSIDERATIONS

Patients infected with gonorrhea are at risk for other STDs. Thus, the detection of one infection should prompt a search for concurrent infections. Patients should submit to serologic testing for syphilis and should be offered counseling and testing for HIV infection. Patients with incubating syphilis may be cured by β-lactam antibiotics combined with tetracycline. Patients treated with regimens utilizing spectinomycin or fluoroquinolone's, however, require further testing and as appropriate therapy for syphilis.

PREVENTION

Treatment of asymptomatic carriers and of sexual partners may reduce the pool of infected persons, who in turn might infect others. Routine screening for cervical gonococcal infection was found to be cost-effective in communities where the prevalence of asymptomatic infections was high.[34] The study supported widespread gonococcal screening as an essential part of a prevention program. In addition, patients who received treatment that is not effective against PPNG must be tested for cure. Concurrent treatment with doxycycline or tetracycline for intercurrent *Chlamydia* infection is recommended.[28] Because STDs are indicators of unsafe sex practices and risk-taking behavior, educational programs must be developed to alter such behavior.

CHLAMYDIAL INFECTIONS

In the United States, *C. trachomatis* infection is the most common of the bacterial STDs. Conservative estimates indicate that at least 4 million new cases occur each year.[36] As many as 75% of women and 25% of men with uncomplicated chlamydial infection have no symptoms or signs of it. Recognition of the association between *C. trachomatis* infection and tubal infertility and subfertility (in the form of ectopic pregnancy) has been one of the most important advances in reproductive health. In addition, perinatal *Chlamydia* infections are a common cause of infant pneumonia and the most common cause of neonatal conjunctivitis. Because of these complications, wide availability of screening programs is crucial for preventing chlamydial infection. Control measures, however, are severely hampered by the expense of laboratory tests for the organism, a constraint that limits the ability to screen effectively in facilities where funding is limited. Also, because *C. trachomatis* infections are not a reportable disease in all states, the impact of traditional disease intervention efforts and partner notification for treatment are seriously limited. Thus, spread of asymptomatic infections, with profound long-term consequences, particularly in females and infants, is common.

C. trachomatis is an obligate intracellular parasite with 17 different currently identified immunotypes.[37, 38] Types A, B, Ba, and C are most often associated with ocular trachoma, and types L1, L2, and L3 are the agents of lymphogranuloma venereum. Immunotypes D through K are responsible for the majority of sexually transmitted infections; types D, E, and F are the most common.[39] A detailed discussion of the biology, host response, and pathogenesis of chlamydial infections is beyond the scope of this chapter. Interested readers are encouraged to consult Schachter's work.[40]

CLINICAL MANIFESTATIONS

In females, the endocervix is the organ most often infected with *C. trachomatis*. Most of these infections are asymptomatic and can be detected only by screening pelvic examinations. (The majority of *Chlamydia* infections of the endocervix fail to demonstrate inflammation sufficient to produce clinical signs.[41]) When clinical signs are present, the most common ones are a yellow or green mucopurulent endocervical discharge[42] and hypertrophic ectropion (Fig. 22–4).[43] (*Hypertrophic ectopy* describes an area of cervical ectopy that is edematous, congested, and bleeds easily on manipulation.) These clinical signs have been correlated with the number of polymorphonuclear (PMN) leukocytes (10 to 30 per 1000 fields) obtained from a carefully collected endocervical Gram-stained smear.[41–44]

Results of screening studies in STD clinics have shown that the urethra is a common site of *C. trachomatis* infection.[45, 46] Among women with symptoms of dysuria and frequency of urination, urine cultures for other common urinary tract pathogens are often negative, whereas chlamydial organisms can be isolated in as many as 65% of patients.[47] Studies have shown that simultaneously culturing both the urethra and the cervix

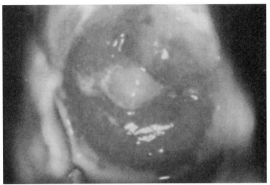

Figure 22–4 Mucopurulent cervicitis due to *C. trachomatis*.

increases the yield of culture-positive females by as much as 20%.[48]

UPPER GENITAL TRACT INFECTION

C. trachomatis may ascend from the endocervix into the upper genital tract to produce asymptomatic or symptomatic PID. Early studies of patients with symptomatic PID showed that cervical cultures of many grew *C. trachomatis*.[49] In later studies utilizing laparoscopy to obtain specimens directly from the fallopian tubes, *C. trachomatis* was recovered from about 30% of patients.[50] Clinically, the presentation of *C. trachomatis* PID is similar to that of *N. gonorrhoeae* PID, although the symptoms may be less severe,[51] consisting only of menorrhagia and metrorrhagia.[52] Serologic studies have suggested that *C. trachomatis* is also a common cause of perihepatitis.[53]

Diagnosis

In most circumstances, the diagnosis is based solely on clinical findings and any reported risk factors—young age, nonwhite race, single marital status, and use of oral contraceptive pills (OCPs).[45, 54–56] The incidence of *Chlamydia* infections is also high in pregnant women, women with acute PID or mucopurulent cervicitis, and sex partners of men who have urethritis. Screening should be extended to include sexually active young women who have had a new sex partner or more than two partners in the previous 2 months.[57]

Antigen detection testing has become increasingly popular in response to the expense and limited availability of cell cultures for *C. tracho-*

matis. These methods employ one of these: a direct flourescence monoclonal antibody (e.g., Microtrak), an enzyme-linked immunosorbent assay (ELISA; e.g., Chlamydiazyme), DNA probes (e.g., Pace 2, Gen-Probe), PCR (e.g., Amplicor), ligase chain reaction (LCR), and transcription-mediated amplification (Gen Probe Amplified). These tests are most useful in adolescents and other high-risk populations and have high sensitivity and specificity rates.[58, 59, 65]

Although *Chlamydia* culture is expensive and technically difficult, it remains the gold standard for clinical purposes and the procedure against which new diagnostic methods are measured. Some 70% to 80% of untreated patients have positive results when cultured repeatedly, and culture-negative patients usually remain so on repeated cultures.[60–62] The low sensitivity of *Chlamydia* culture is affected by several factors, including specimen collection techniques, sites of sampling, the number of sites sampled, and specimen transport and storage conditions.[63] Newer techniques using vortexing and sonication of specimens improved recovery of organisms from as many as 96% of specimens.[64] Serologic testing has little or no role in the diagnosis of acute chlamydial infections.

Several published studies sought to identify the most cost-effective method for detecting urogenital *Chlamydia* infections. In one decision analysis model that compared culture, ELISA, nonamplified DNA probe, and ligase and polymerase chain reaction techniques, the most cost-effective strategy was DNA amplification techniques—using cervical specimens from those women who received pelvic examinations and collected urine specimens from those who did not have an indication for pelvic examination (i.e., asymptomatic women).[66] Shafer reported that urine-based LCR screening was the most cost-effective strategy in asymptomatic, sexually active adolescent girls, because of better acceptance of urine testing than of routine pelvic examinations.[67]

Treatment

Drugs with the greatest activity against *C. trachomatis* in tissue culture are rifampin and the tetracyclines, followed by macrolides and azalides, sulfonamides, some fluoroquinolones, and clindamycin.[68] Azithromycin, 1 gm orally in a single dose, or doxycycline, 100 mg twice daily for 7 days, is recommended for children aged 8 years and older.[35, 69]

In contrast to *N. gonorrhoeae,* no clinically

significant evidence of *C. trachomatis* resistance has been noted. Alternatively, an erythromycin base or an equivalent (sulfisoxazole or amoxicillin) is recommended. Considerable interest has been generated by published studies of single-dose oral azithromycin for uncomplicated genital chlamydial infections.[70, 71]

The recommended drugs for *Chlamydia* infection during pregnancy is an erythromycin base or equivalent, 500 mg orally four times daily for 7 days. In the 1998 CDC sexually transmitted diseases treatment guidelines, azithromycin was listed as an alternative regimen for pregnant women. A recent study suggested that azithromycin may be the treatment of choice. As compared with regimens that contain erythromycin or tetracycline, azithromycin therapy was associated with a lower failure rate (21% and 4.5%, respectively), and fewer side effects.[72] Oral clindamycin has also demonstrated effectiveness in eradicating cervical chlamydial infection in pregnant patients.[74]

LYMPHOGRANULOMA VENEREUM

Lymphogranuloma venereum (LGV) is an uncommon infection caused by *C. trachomatis* immunotypes L1 through L3. Fewer than 100 cases are reported each year.[75] Although LGV is included in the differential diagnosis of genital ulcer disease, ulcers are a minor feature of LGV. The incidence of acute LGV in males is greater than that in females by as much as 5:1,[76] principally because, in females, infections much less often produce symptoms. The ulcer can take several different forms but typically is small, shallow, and painless; in females, the endocervix appears to be the most common initial site of infection.[77] Lymphadenopathy is the principal feature of LGV and appears 7 to 30 days after the ulcer. Inguinal adenopathy occurs as a result of multiple enlarged, matted, and tender nodes, which may coalesce with suppuration and bubo formation (Fig. 22–5). Left untreated, these swollen glands can rupture and form draining sinuses. Systemic signs—fever, malaise, myalgia—are common at this stage. In addition, women infected with LGV often develop acute proctocolitis, with fever, tenesmus, and rectal pain. Even without treatment, most LGV infections resolve spontaneously after this stage. In some patients, however, healing is associated with scarring and fibrosis that may lead to rectal strictures and to chronic genital edema (elephantiasis). Genital ulcers and sinuses may persist. Such deformities may require extensive reconstructive surgery.

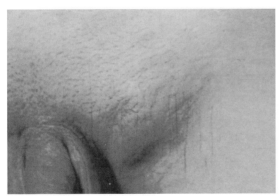

Figure 22–5 Inguinal bubo caused by lympho-granuloma venereum.

The diagnosis can often be established from the typical clinical features, when present, but usually a complement fixation serologic titer of at least 1:64 is diagnostic.[64] The specific diagnosis requires isolation of *C. trachomatis* from infected tissue and subsequent immunotyping or microimmunofluorescence to identify type-specific immune responses. Despite their limitations, other techniques (e.g., monoclonal antibodies or histologic identification of *C. trachomatis* in infected material) may also be used. A recent study tested sera for type-specific anti-*Chlamydia* antibodies using purified chlamydial antigens (*C. trachomatis* A–C (CTA-C), *C. trachomatis* D–K (CTD-K), LGV (LGVI-3), and *C. pneumoniae* (CPn), in a microimmunofluorescence (micro-IF) test. The investigators reported that the micro-IF test is a useful epidemiologic tool for identifying antibodies to *Chlamydia* and distinguishing between genital and extragenital infections.[78]

Effective treatment of LGV consists of oral tetracyline and erythromycin therapy. It is recommended that the treatment period be extended to 3 weeks, regardless of what regimen is used.[79] Alternative medications include sulfisoxazole, chloramphenicol, and rifampin. Reconstructive surgery may be required to correct anogenital deformities.

PELVIC INFLAMMATORY DISEASE

Acute PID, a major public health problem, affects 1 of 10 American women during their reproductive years.[80] It has been estimated that 1 million females are treated annually for PID, at a cost of $4.2 billion dollars when the costs of the sequelae are included.[81] Currently, a 1%

increase in the incidence of PID increases this cost twofold. As a complication of sexual transmission of pathogens, PID exacts a more significant toll on adolescent females, in the form of the sequelae of tubal infertility, ectopic pregnancy, and chronic pelvic pain that develop at an earlier stage of reproductive life.[82]

PID is an acute syndrome attributed to the ascending spread of microorganisms from the vagina and endocervix to the endometrium, fallopian tubes, and contiguous structures. The particular pathogen demonstrates geographic variations and also depends on what sites are cultured. Various studies have shown that *N. gonorrhoeae* may be recovered from 5% to 81% of patients with acute PID and that *C. trachomatis* has been recovered from 6% to 68% of such patients.[83] Studies utilizing laparoscopy for recovery of organisms from the fallopian tube, however, have demonstrated that mixed bacteria are often present.[84–87] The most common aerobic organisms include *Escherichia coli*, *Haemophilus influenzae*, group B streptoccoci, and *Gardnerella vaginalis*. Anaerobic bacteria recovered most frequently include the *Bacteroides* spp. and *Peptostreptococcus* and *Peptococcus* organisms. Genital mycoplasmas have been recovered infrequently from patients with acute PID, and their exact role in the causation of PID has not been determined.

Several other factors may influence the ability of microorganisms to ascend from the endocervix into the uterus and fallopian tubes. Cervicovaginal bacteria are introduced into the uterus and tubes during menses. Specific mucosal immune mechanisms (e.g., secretory immunoglobulin A) may be inactivated by *N. gonorrhoeae* proteases, thus immobilizing an important host defense.[88] The relationship between use of an IUD and the development of PID remains controversial, inspite of the fact that more than 25 studies have addressed the question.[77] The presence of an IUD tail and its ability to "wick" bacteria into the uterine cavity, the formation of microulcers, the conversion of the vaginal (bacterial) flora to predominantly anaerobic organisms, and the foreign body inflammatory reaction produced by the device have all been postulated as mechanisms for increased risk of upper genital tract infection.[83] Recognized risk factors for the development of PID are summarized in Table 22–1.

CLINICAL MANIFESTATIONS

Patients who present with PID may be asymptomatic or have severe peritonitis. Abdominal

Table 22–1. Risk Indicators Associated with the Development of Pelvic Inflammatory Disease

Demographic and social indicators
　Age
　Socioeconomic status
　Single marital status
Contraceptive practice
　Intrauterine contraceptive device
Healthcare behavior
　Evaluation of symptoms
　Compliance with treatment instructions
　Partner notification
Others
　Douching
　Smoking
　Temporal relationship to menstrual cycle

From Centers for Disease Control: Sexually transmitted diseases: Treatment guidelines. MMWR 1998; 47(RR-1):1–116.

Table 22–2. Diagnostic Criteria for Pelvic Inflammatory Disease

Routine
　Oral temperature >38.3°C
　Abnormal cervical or vaginal discharge
　Elevated erythrocyte sedimentation rate and/or C-reactive protein
　Culture or nonculture* evidence of cervical infection with N. gonorrhoeae or C. trachomatis
Elaborate
　Histopathologic evidence on endometrial biopsy
　Tuboovarian abscess on sonography
　Laparoscopic evidence

*Gram stain antigen detection assay.
From Centers for Disease Control: Sexually transmitted diseases: Treatment guidelines. MMWR 1998; 47(RR-1):1–116.

pain, usually of less than 10 days' duration, is the most common symptom. Others of varying significance include recent onset of menses, increased dysmenorrhea with the most recent period, irregular menses (menorrhagia), recent pelvic dyspareunia, and symptoms of proctitis. Gastrointestinal tract symptoms such as nausea and vomiting, diarrhea, and anorexia are related to bowel inflammation caused by free pus in the abdomen.

Clinical signs that have the strongest correlation with laparoscopically proven PID include abnormal vaginal discharge, temperature above 38°C, and a palpable adnexal mass.[90, 91] Additionally, as many as 15% of patients with PID present with perihepatitis (Fitz-Hugh-Curtis syndrome) as part of the clinical picture.

CLINICAL DIAGNOSIS

The clinical diagnosis of acute PID is based primarily on a history of abdominal pain and tenderness to motion of the cervix and adnexae on bimanual examination. When signs of a lower genital tract infection (more leukocytes than any other cell type on a wet-mount specimen) are present, along with abdominal pain and motion tenderness, the diagnosis of PID is correct in only 60% of patients.[92] For all patients, cervical cultures should be grown for N. gonorrhoeae and cultures or nonculture tests for C. trachomatis. Additional criteria useful for the diagnosis of PID are listed in Table 22–2. The lack of substantial clinical signs dictates that clinicians maintain a high index of suspicion when they evaluate young women at risk for PID. Atypical features such as menorrhagia, mucopurulent cervicitis, or both in

women who do not use OCPs should be considered signs of upper genital tract infection,[52] and an indication for a more thorough workup and therapy.

MANAGEMENT

An appropriate management plan requires thorough assessment of the severity of infection. Hospitalization should be utilized liberally, although there is no objective evidence that parenteral antimicrobial therapy produces better long-term outcomes. Indications for hospitalization are listed in Table 22–3. Because bacteriologic data suggest a mixed infection in many patients, administration of broad-spectrum antibiotics is necessary, along with adequate support with intravenous fluids and analgesia. Patients managed as outpatients require close follow-up (within 72 hours) to check response to therapy and compliance with medication instructions.[93] This visit affords an opportunity to emphasize the need to avoid sexual intercourse and to refer sexual partners for evaluation and treatment.

Table 22–3. Indications for Hospitalization for Pelvic Inflammatory Disease

Uncertain diagnosis
Suspected pelvic abscess
Pregnancy
Adolescent patient
Severe illness precluding outpatient treatment
Inability to tolerate or comply with outpatient regimen
Failure to respond to outpatient treatment
Clinical follow-up within 72 hours if starting antibiotics cannot be arranged

From Centers for Disease Control: Sexually transmitted diseases: Treatment guidelines. MMWR 1998; 47(RR-1):1–116.

Treatment and Prevention

Many different treatment regimens have been evaluated and proven to be very effective in achieving clinical cure. No single regimen has been shown to be clearly superior, but two basic regimens have been recommended by the CDC to provide broad-spectrum coverage for the pathogens most likely to be encountered (Table 22–4). A discussion of treatment considerations is provided in Peterson's paper.[94]

Effective stategies are crucial for preventing PID—thereby protecting women from the adverse reproductive consequences and avoiding substantial economic losses. The best strategies for preventing PID are prevention of lower genital tract infection with *C. trachomatis* and *N. gonorrhoeae*, in men and women alike.[93] If prevention fails, early detection, followed by prompt

Table 22–4. Recommended Treatment of Hospitalized Patients with Pelvic Inflammatory Disease

Oral and IM treatment guidelines for acute PID
  Regimen A
    Ofloxacin, 400 mg orally, twice daily for 14 days,
          plus
    Metronidazole, 500 mg orally, twice daily for 14 days
  Regimen B
    Ceftriaxone, 250 mg IM as a single dose,
          or
    Cefoxitin, 2 gm IM, plus probenecid, 1 gm orally in a single dose, given concurrently
          or
    Other parenteral third-generation cephalosporins (e.g., ceftizoxime)
          plus
    Doxycycline, 100 mg orally, twice daily for 14 days
Inpatient treatment guidelines for patients with acute PID
  Recommended Regimen A
    Cefoxitin, 2 gm IV every 6 hours, or cefotetan, 2 gm IV every 12 hours
          plus
    Doxycycline, 100 mg PO or IV every 12 hours
  Recommended Regimen B
    Clindamycin (900 mg IV every 8 hours)
          plus
    Gentamicin (2.0 mg/kg loading dose followed by a 1.5-mg/kg maintenance dose every 8 hours)
  Intravenous regimens are given for at least 48 hours after the clinical signs and symptoms have improved.
    Following discharge, patients should be given:
    Doxycycline, 100 mg PO every 12 hours
          or
    Clindamycin, 450 mg PO every 6 hours
IV therapy may be discontinued 24 hours after clinical improvement. Oral doxycycline, 100 mg twice daily, should be continued for a total of 14 days of therapy.

From Centers for Disease Control. Sexually transmitted diseases: Treatment guidelines. MMWR 1998; 47(RR-1):1–116.

and effective treatment of lower genital tract infections, is mandatory.

SYPHILIS

Historically, syphilis has been a major cause of morbidity and mortality worldwide. The implementation of public health initiatives and the availability of penicillin initially led to a significant decline in syphilis-related complications; however, since 1986, the incidences of primary and secondary syphilis have increased every year, to a rate of 20 per 100,000, the highest since 1949.[95, 95a] These most recent increases have been most prevalent in nonwhite heterosexuals and have been closely linked to use of illicit drugs, particularly crack cocaine.[95a] Although rates of early syphilis are highest in adults aged 20 to 24 years, in women the rate of increase has been greater for adolescent females during the 1990s.[6] A grave concern is the risk of congenital syphilis in a population in which pregnancy rates continue largely unabated. The association between increased risk of HIV transmission and genital ulcer disease in heterosexuals[8] amplifies the current risk environment for both teenagers and adults.[95b, 96, 98]

Syphilis is caused by *Treponema pallidum*, a spirochete that measures 6 to 20 μm by 0.1 to 0.18 μm, and, so, is too narrow to be seen by light microscopy.[97] It has a characteristic corkscrew motility that allows identification by darkfield examination. Because the spirochete cannot survive outside the body, the disease is rarely contracted except through intimate contact. The organism usually enters the body through invisible breaks in the skin or through intact mucous membranes lining the mouth, rectum, or genital tract. Approximately one third of those exposed to a sexual partner with syphilis contract the disease.[99] Other potential routes of transmission include perinatal transmission and transmission through transfusion of infected blood. Because serologic tests for syphilis are performed routinely in blood banks, transfused blood and blood products are rare modes of transmission. Hematogenous spread through infected needles shared by intravenous drug users is, theoretically, a concern. Syphilis in children is discussed in detail in Chapter 20.

CLINICAL MANIFESTATIONS

The clinical features of untreated syphilis are divided into a series of clinical stages that are used as indicators of the length of infection and as a guide for therapy. Overlap among the various stages is frequent, however, and, at times, the features of a given stage are mild—and sometimes even absent.

Primary Syphilis

Approximately 3 weeks after inoculation, the patient develops a macule or papule at the site of entry.[100] The lesion is usually around the genitalia but is sometimes on the lips or mouth, on the breasts, or around the rectum. The ulcer is a painless, usually solitary lesion, with raised, well-defined borders and a clean, indurated base. The chancre contains large numbers of spirochetes and is highly infectious. It is usually associated with nontender regional adenopathy, which may be unilateral or bilateral. Although the external genitalia is the most common site for ulcers in females, the cervix and vagina are frequently involved (Fig. 22–6).[101] Even without treatment, the chancre heals slowly over several weeks; the spirochetes, however, spread throughout the body.

Secondary Syphilis

Between 4 and 10 weeks after the appearance of the chancre, secondary syphilis develops. This stage is characterized by an array of clinical manifestations. Systemic complaints such as low-grade fever, myalgia, and arthralgia are common, as is generalized adenopathy. The most prominent feature is a painless, nonpruritic maculopapular rash that typically affects the limbs, including the palms and soles, and the trunk (Fig. 22–7). Alternatively, lesions described as pustular, eczematous, nodular, and plaquelike may

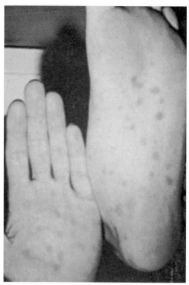

Figure 22–7 Palmar-plantar rash of secondary syphilis.

present in secondary syphilis. Mucous patches form in the mouth and around the vagina and anus. Other anogenital lesions, called *condylomata lata*, are broad-based, flat, beefy lesions that are pearly gray in color and highly infectious (Fig. 22–8). The reader is urged to consult a dermatology reference or a comprehensive review of syphilis for further discussion, including ocular and neurologic manifestations. These symptoms and the lesions eventually resolve, and the disease enters its latent phase.

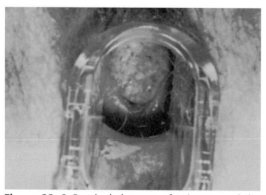

Figure 22–6 Cervical chancre of primary syphilis.

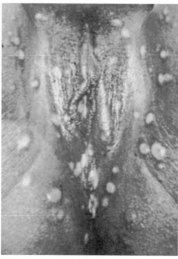

Figure 22–8 Condylomata lata of secondary syphilis involving the perineum.

Latent Syphilis

During latency, serologic tests for syphilis are reactive but there are no clinical signs of the disease. Latent syphilis of less than 1 year's duration is considered *early latent*, whereas *late latent syphilis* is marked by a latent phase longer than 1 year. The World Health Organization (WHO) designates a 2-year period for differentiation of early and late syphilis. Differentiation of these two phases is designed to reflect differences in infectivity and to serve as a guide for therapy. Recurrent early manifestations are seen primarily in the first year after secondary syphilis, and the infectious potential for sexual partners during that year is assumed to be greater; infectious potential is less for partners of patients with disease of long standing.[92] The rationale for more prolonged therapy for patients with late latent syphilis is that treponemes are assumed to be dividing at a slower rate and thus require higher levels of antibiotic.

Tertiary Syphilis

Tertiary syphilis is almost never seen in adolescents. The following is included for completeness. Approximately two thirds of syphilitic patients who enter late latency have no further clinical illness and are no longer infectious, although the disease may cause serious complications several months to years later. The more common cardiovascular manifestations of tertiary syphilis include aortic aneurysm, aortic insufficiency, and coronary ostial occlusion. Gummas, the chronic inflammatory lesions of tertiary syphilis, affect principally the skin, subcutaneous tissues, and bone. Initially, they are nodules, and slowly they progress to form granulomatous lesions, which sometimes ulcerate. These lesions destroy normal surrounding tissues, and the clinical features vary with the organs affected. Central nervous system (CNS) involvement occurs at all stages of syphilis. Asymptomatic CNS disease, confirmed by cerebrospinal fluid cell and serologic abnormalities, may also be present in some persons. Involvement of the brain and spinal cord (neurosyphilis) occurs in some persons and impairs mentation and creates difficulties with sensation and movement. The reader is encouraged to seek a more comprehensive review of cardiovascular and CNS manifestations of late syphilis for a detailed discussion of these subjects.

DIAGNOSIS

The diagnosis of syphilis is based on characteristic clinical features in conjunction with positive results on appropriate serologic tests. During the primary and secondary stages, *T. pallidum* can be observed on dark-field examination of chancres, condylomata lata, and mucous patches. Reactive nonspecific serologic tests (the rapid plasma reagin [RPR] or the Venereal Disease Research Laboratory [VDRL] test) must be confirmed with specific antibody tests for *T. pallidum*. Commonly employed specific tests include the fluorescent treponemal antibody absorption test (FTA-ABS), the microhemagglutination–*T. pallidum* test (MHA-TP), or the hemagglutination treponemal test for syphilis (HATTS). Suspected CNS involvement may require evaluation of the cerebrospinal fluid.

TREATMENT

Penicillin remains the cornerstone of therapy for syphilis. It has remained effective because of the persistent sensitivity of *T. pallidum* to penicillin. The benzathine formulation readily achieves the sustained, moderately low serum levels required to eradicate the spirochete, which has a long division time. Treatment regimens are based on the stage of the disease at diagnosis. Benzathine penicillin, 2.4 million U intramuscularly in two separate injections, is the recommended treatment for primary, secondary, and early latent disease.[79] For patients who are allergic to penicillin, doxycycline, 100 mg orally twice daily for 14 days, or tetracycline, 500 mg orally four times daily for 14 days, may be used. Patients with late latent syphilis, syphilis of unknown duration, or tertiary syphilis other than neurosyphilis should receive a longer course of therapy, for the reasons mentioned earlier. Benzathine penicillin, 7.2 million U administered in 2.4 million-U doses at weekly intervals for 3 weeks, is currently recommended.[67] Patients who are allergic to penicillin are treated with doxycycline or tetracycline, although 4 weeks of such therapy is recommended.[67] Patients with neurosyphilis should be given aqueous crystalline penicillin G, 12 to 24 million U intravenously daily (2 to 4 million U intravenously every 4 hours) for 10 to 14 days, or procaine penicillin G, 2.4 million U intramuscularly daily, given together with probenecid, 500 mg orally four times daily, for the same length of time.

Recent reports of neurosyphilis and invasion of cerebrospinal fluid by *T. pallidum* in patients with HIV infection have called into doubt the adequacy of the recommended penicillin G benzathine therapy for early syphilis. A recent study, however, showed that clinically defined failure was uncommon after treatment for primary or secondary syphilis.[102]

ADDITIONAL CONSIDERATIONS

Pregnant adolescents with syphilis should be given penicillin in doses appropriate for the stage of disease.[79] Because tetracyclines are contraindicated in pregnancy and because of unacceptably high rates of failure to prevent congenital syphilis when using alternative drugs (erythromycin), pregnant women who are allergic to penicillin should undergo skin testing and desensitization to receive penicillin.[92]

Patients should be cautioned about Jarisch-Herxheimer reactions after treatment for early syphilis. The self-limited manifestations include myalgias, chills, headache, and postural hypotension. Management consists of hydration and aspirin. Pregnant patients may experience preterm labor or fetal distress and should be observed for such.

To assess response to treatment, follow-up serologic testing should be performed 3, 6, and 12 months after treatment. At least a fourfold (two-dilution) decline in titer is generally regarded as an appropriate response.[103, 104] Sex partners of persons with early syphilis should be assumed to have incubating syphilis and, so, should be treated as if they had early disease. All infected persons and their sexual contacts should be encouraged to seek HIV counseling and testing.

GENITAL HERPES SIMPLEX INFECTION

Genital HSV infection is a common viral STD in all populations of sexually active persons.[13, 105] Although symptomatic disease in adults is self-limiting, the first episode of genital HSV may be associated with considerable medical morbidity, including hospitalization for aseptic meningitis and urinary retention. Recurrent episodes exact a significant toll, psychological and economically.[106] A large portion of seropositive persons in both high- and low-prevalence populations have unrecognized HSV-2 infection.[107] In addition, current strategies for diagnosing genital HSV infections, including colposcopy, Pap smears, and viral cultures of lesions, fail to identify many cases.[108] Without greater emphasis on prevention

and risk reduction, the spread of this incurable disease may remain unchecked and could have significant implications for the transmission of HIV.

HSV is a member of the herpesvirus family, which includes the Epstein-Barr, and varicella zoster viruses and cytomegalovirus. Two major serotypes of HSV cause genital infections in humans: HSV-1, responsible primarily for oral (and some genital) infections, and HSV-2. The subtypes are similar in their DNA content but exhibit different infective properties and clinical manifestations.[109] Although the majority of genital infections are caused by HSV-2, HSV-1 can be isolated from 10% to 25% of genital lesions in persons with primary, first-episode HSV and in 1% of patients with nonprimary, first-episode HSV.[106] HSV has a predilection for cutaneous and mucous membrane sensory ganglia and persists in this neural tissue in a dormant state. The risk of recurrence after primary, first-episode genital herpes is more than 80% for HSV-2 infection and approximately 50% for HSV-1.[106, 110]

HSV is transmitted by close contact with a person who is shedding the virus, which enters mucosal surfaces through an epithelial break.[58] Infectivity may be as high as 50%.[111] Primary infection occurs in patients not previously exposed to HSV, who, thus, have no circulating HSV antibodies. The initial episode is associated with significant vulvar pain, dysuria, and, at times, urinary retention. Tender inguinal lymphadenopathy typically is present. Systemic symptoms are common; patients complain of fever, headaches, malaise, and myalgia. Severe complications such as meningitis are rare. Early in the course of the disease, the infected area shows vesicular lesions with associated inflammation and edema. With time, these vesicles break, forming ulcerative lesions with an erythematous base, that often are covered with a purulent exudate (Fig. 22–9). The ulcers may coalesce and form a larger ulcer with a covering crust. Complete healing of the lesions usually occurs within 2 weeks, although it may take as long as 4 to 6 weeks. Typically, recurrent episodes of the disease are less painful and have minimal systemic signs, a smaller mean number of lesions, and a shorter mean duration of viral shedding.

HSV types 1 and 2 may cause perianal infections. These infections are often associated with pain of acute onset bloody or mucoid discharge, tenesmus, constipation, fever, malaise, myalgia, and urinary retention. External lesions may be visible on only 50% of those infected. Anoscopy or sigmoidoscopy may reveal friability of the lower 10 cm of the rectum and occasionally dem-

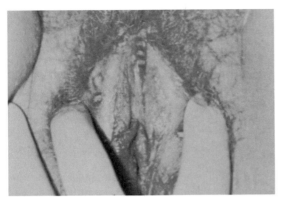

Figure 22–9 First episode of genital herpes of the vulva.

onstrates discrete ulcerations. The differential diagnosis includes herpes zoster, syphilis, chancroid, trauma, Behçet's disease, and other less common disorders.

DIAGNOSIS

Viral culture of the lesions is the most sensitive and specific method of diagnosis of mucocutaneous HSV.[93] Vesicles and pustular lesions have the highest viral isolation rates; as many as 90% contain material that produces positive cultures.[95] Ulcer material grows positive cultures in 70% of cases; crusted lesions in only 30% of cases.[95] Cytologic examination of lesional exudate using Tzanck preparations or Papanicolaou smears is much less sensitive and provides less definitive information on the viral type. Serologic testing is not useful for the diagnosis of HSV in adults, because commercially available tests do not reliably differentiate between type-specific and type-common antigens.[112]

Serologic diagnosis is most useful for detecting previous infection or to show that the current infection is primary. It may be a helpful adjunct to culture or immunologic diagnosis. It may be particularly useful when lesions are cultured in the ulcerative stages. Paired sera must be obtained if there are indications of active or recent infection. The absence of antibodies in two samples collected 2 to 3 weeks apart excludes the diagnosis. A rise in immunoglobulin M (IgM) antibodies followed by a rise in IgG antibodies indicates recent infection. The antibody testing performed by many commercial laboratories has cross-reactivity between HSV-1 and HSV-2. Thus, a fourfold increase in the titer is difficult to interpret, as it could represent a significant new infection or a new infection with another virus type.

A recent study illustrates the advantage of rapid PCR diagnosis of HSV and varicella zoster virus in vesicle fluids. The investigators tested vesicular fluid from 132 patients using PCR technique. PCR did not differentiate between HSV-1 and -2, but its sensitivity and specificity were 100%. The sensitivities of virus isolation and electron microscopy for detection of HSV were 56% and 80%, respectively.[113]

TREATMENT

Antiviral therapy with oral or parenteral acyclovir is currently recommended for primary genital herpes infections. Acyclovir has been shown to accelerate healing of genital lesions and reduce the duration of viral shedding, and parenteral therapy has been shown to limit local and systemic symptoms.[114] Treatment should be instituted as soon as the diagnosis is suspected, as the benefits of treatment usually outweigh the risks of waiting for culture results, and the toxicity of acyclovir is quite low, especially with oral therapy. Acyclovir, 400 mg orally three times a day for 7 to 10 days or 200 mg five times a day for 7 to 10 days; famciclovir, 250 mg orally three times a day for 7 to 10 days; and valacyclovir, 1 gm orally twice daily for 7 to 10 days, have been demonstrated in adults to be effective for the treatment of primary herpes. Regimens for suppressive treatment of secondary lesions contain lower doses of these drugs: acyclovir, 400 mg orally twice daily; famciclovir, 250 mg orally twice daily; valacyclovir, 500 mg or 1 gm daily. The results of a randomized controlled trial of famciclovir documented its clinical utility in suppressing recurrences of genital herpes.[115] An accompanying editorial notes that famciclovir appears to be more effective than acyclovir or valacyclovir, as judged from the recurrence rate at 1-year follow-up, although famciclovir is more costly than similar regimens of acyclovir and valacyclovir.[116]

A recent study evaluated the efficacy and safety of parenteral interferon alfa-2-alpha (IFN-$\alpha_2\alpha$) for the treatment of recurrent HSV infection. A total of 97 patients, each having had at least five recurrences of genital herpes during the previous 12 months, were treated with IFN-$\alpha_2\alpha$ (3×10^6 IU) by subcutaneous injection, three times weekly for 4 weeks; the same schedule was repeated at 3 and 6 months. The investigators reported that prophylactic administration of IFN-$\alpha2\alpha$ prevented recurrences of genital

HSV infection in 51 of the 97 patients, and hastened healing—from 8.5 days (before treatment) to 2.5 days (after treatment). The authors concluded that this regimen may have value for routine treatment of recurrent herpes.[117]

Local adjunctive treatment of the vulvovaginal lesions is important. Sitz baths using tepid water and Burow solution soothe the inflamed perineum. Wet areas are patted dry or dried with a hair dryer on a low setting, and topical lidocaine gel or ointment is applied. Patients can be advised to void in the bathtub to limit urine contamination of the lesions. Catheterization is needed when urinary retention is present or appears likely.

With recurrent genital HSV infection, initiation of oral therapy at the first sign of prodrome or lesions is only moderately effective in reducing the number of symptomatic days.[118] Episodic therapy should be reserved for patients who have infrequent recurrences that are moderate or very protracted. Patients who have frequent recurrences generally benefit from prolonged suppressive therapy, regardless of the severity of recurrences.[119, 120]

HUMAN PAPILLOMAVIRUS INFECTION

The incidence of HPV infections has increased dramatically since the 1970s. Using more sensitive detection techniques like PCR, it has been estimated that at least 24 million persons are currently infected.[5] First visits to private physicians for a genital wart, a likely indicator of new cases, nearly tripled between 1966–1970 and 1986–1990.[5] It has been estimated that genital warts account for approximately 5% of all STD clinic visits, and in some clinics cases of genital warts outnumber cases of gonorrhea.[5] More than 60 subtypes of HPV have been identified to date, and approximately 20 of them have been associated with genital infection.[121] Research into the biology of HPV has revealed that certain serotypes of the virus are powerful carcinogens and are likely to induce premalignant and malignant lesions in previously infected areas. The long-term potential for genital or anal neoplasia is of particular concern for affected persons.

Papillomaviruses are members of the papovavirus family, which also includes simian virus 40 and the polyomaviruses. Structurally, they are unencapsulated, have an icosahedral virion capsid, and contain a double-stranded DNA genome. The early transcription regions, E6 and E7, are important for transformation, and the late (L) region is responsible for viral capsid formation.[122] Although it is known that the virus is transmitted sexually, the exact mechanism of infection at the molecular level is unknown. It is assumed that the virus gains entry to the basal cell layer of the surface epithelium through microscopic abrasions, leading to transformation of one or more basal cells.[123] Genital lesions usually appear after an incubation period of approximately 3 months (range, 3 weeks to 8 months). The natural history of HPV infection is remarkably variable, ranging from spontaneous regression to persistent infection and, in some cases, neoplastic progression.[123] Evidence of a role for host cell–mediated immunity in controlling HPV infections has been gained from examining immunodeficient patients. Several studies have documented an increased incidence of genital neoplasms in renal transplant patients and in patients with lymphoma, Hodgkin's disease, chronic lymphocytic leukemia, and HIV infection.[124] It is well-known that HPV infections get worse during pregnancy, but it is not clear whether this is due to alterations in cell-mediated immunity, hormonal changes, or other factors.[125]

CLINICAL MANIFESTATIONS

HPV produces overt infection in 30% of cases and subclinical infection in 70%. The virus can also persist in a latent state, during which it can be identified only by recombinant DNA techniques. The *lesions* are usually multifocal and frequently involve large areas of the genital tract. The most common sites in females are the posterior fourchette, adjacent labia and perineum, vaginal introitus, vagina, and cervix. Approximately 5% of men and women with genital warts also have perianal and anal warts, which may or may not be associated with anal intercourse.[126] Three types of lesions are common: exophytic warts, papules, and macules (flat condylomas). Condyloma acuminatum is the most widely recognized manifestation of anogenital HPV infection. A disorder characterized by a subset of pigmented condylomatous papules is referred to as *bowenoid papulosis*; these lesions are associated with low-grade intraepithelial neoplasia.[127] The giant condyloma (Buschke-Löwenstein tumor) is an uncommon, locally invasive, nonmetastasizing tumor originating from genital warts.

DIAGNOSIS

HPV has not yet been grown in tissue culture; thus, diagnostic methods are limited to more indirect methods such as light microscopy and DNA, and radioactive probes. Traditionally, the diagnosis in sexually active adolescents and adults has been visual inspection, often aided by colposcopy; biopsy is reserved for perplexing cases and those that do not respond to therapy. Inspection with the unaided eye readily discerns the typical cauliflower-like projections—and, occasionally, flat, papular lesions. Application with 5% acetic acid for 5 minutes may enhance flat lesions that are not readily apparent.[128, 129] Tissue infected with HPV often undergoes epithelial hyperplasia and has a shiny white appearance (acetowhitening) after soaking with acetic acid (Fig. 22–10). Distal urethroscopy is important for the diagnosis of meatal and distal urethral warts in men. Anoscopy and proctoscopy are often necessary for the diagnosis of anal warts, which can extend beyond the dentate line. Biopsy specimens of exophytic or papular lesions or scrapings of flat lesions can be sent for light microscopy and DNA subtyping. Vaginal washing may be used to identify viral particles from infected children.[130] Amplification of small quantities of viral DNA can be achieved by PCR techniques.[131, 132] In adolescents, cytology has been the method most commonly used for HPV detection in cervical scrapings (Pap smear); however, a significant number of false negatives confound this technique. Histopathologic methods include hematoxylin and eosin staining of biopsy specimens looking for the characteristic koilocytosis. Histopathologic detection of HPV through koilocytosis is a fairly sensitive and specific technique for HPV in expert hands, but in forensically sensitive cases, this method should be combined with a DNA identification method that can identify subtypes (e.g., Southern blot, in situ hybridization, Vira-Pap, Vira-Type, and PCR). The Southern blot is an extremely time-consuming and costly method that requires biopsy material. It is the gold standard against which all other methods are compared.

In situ hybridization is useful for examining paraffin-embedded biopsy specimens, though exfoliated cell scrapings have been used. It lacks some sensitivity as compared with the Southern blot. The Vira-Pap identifies the presence of HPV DNA using a radiolabeled nucleic acid probe. It is a commercial kit designed to be used as the Pap smear is. The Vira-Type identifies the specific genital subtype of HPV DNA. The PCR amplification method is useful when only small quantities of DNA are available. False-positive results are possible, if contamination occurs. It should be noted that all DNA hybridization tests can have false-negative results for many reasons. If a false-negative result is suspected, analysis should be repeated with a new clinical sample.

TREATMENT

Studies have shown that HPV lesions resolve spontaneously in many patients. Of 608 college women followed at 6-month intervals for 3 years, 43% had HPV infections. The median duration of new infections was 8 months; persistence longer than 6 months was associated with oncogenic HPV types and multiple other HPV types, but not with smoking. Squamous intraepithelial lesions were uncommon (31 of 608 subjects), but only two were of high grade.[133] In another study, the investigators followed 618 young women who were positive for HPV DNA from urogenital sites. They reported that 70% of lesions had regressed by 24 months and that those with low-risk HPV type were more likely to regress. The majority (88%) of women with persistent HPV had not developed high-grade squamous intraepithelial neoplasia on cytologic examination.[134]

The goal of therapy should be symptomatic—to eradicate lesions and associated symptoms. There are no data to suggest that any therapy alters the long-term consequences of HPV infections. HPV has been demonstrated in normal tissue adjacent to laser-excised lesions and frequently recurs even when the original lesions are treated. Patient preference, physician experience, and available resources guide the selection of a treatment modality.

In general, treatment modalities are divided into two major groups: patient-applied and provider-applied (Table 22–5).

Patient Applied Treatment

Patient-applied therapy consists of the application of podofilox, 0.5% solution or gel, to the

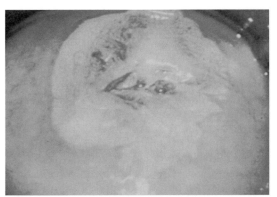

Figure 22–10 Acetowhitening of the transformation zone with application of acetic acid, caused by HPV infection.

Table 22–5. Treatment for Genital Warts

Topical keratolytic agents
  Podophyllin, 10% to 25% solution
  Podophyllotoxin, 0.5% solution
  Trichloroacetic acid, 80% to 90% solution
Topical cytotoxic agents
5-Fluorouracil (5-FU), 5% cream
Surgical therapy
  Cryotherapy
  Electrocautery
  Loop electrocautery excision procedure (LEEP)
  Laser
Immunomodulators
  Injectable interferon
  Imiquimod cream
  Dinitrochlorobenzene (DNCB)

Modified from Gall SA: Human papillomavirus infection. Contemporary Ob/Gyn 1999; 8:15–35.

visible lesions. The patient applies the medication twice daily for 3 days then uses no therapy for 4 days. This 7-day cycle should be repeated for no more than four cycles. Another treatment is imiquimod, 5% cream. The patient applies the medication at bedtime, three times a week for as long as 16 weeks.

Provider-Applied Therapy

1. Topical tricholoroacetic acid (TCA) or bicholoroacetic acid (BCA), 80% to 90%, is applied by the physician. These agents may be used for external genital/perianal, vaginal, and anal warts. Lesions may be treated as frequently as 3 times per week. Treatment-associated discomfort can be managed with wet towels, a topical gel, and a hand-held fan. Although effective, TCA treatment can be painful and may not be optimal for very young patients or those who have extensive lesions.
2. Cryotherapy with liquid nitrogen has been used for anogenital warts in children and adolescents. The cryoprobe may be used for external exophytic or cervical warts. Freezing should be continued until the iceball is 1 to 2 mm larger than the diameter of the wart. Topical/local anesthetic should be used, because cryotherapy is painful. Cryotherapy should probably not be used in infants or children with extensive lesions.
3. Podophyllin in tincture of benzoin has been used to treat external genital or perianal warts. A 10% to 25% solution is usually applied. Because podophyllin is potentially neurotoxic, the CDC recommends that, at one treatment session, no more than 0.5 ml should be ap-

plied and an area no larger than 10 cm² of keratinized skin or 2 cm² of vaginal mucosa should be treated. It should be washed off in 1 to 4 hours and reapplied once a week. Some experts caution against vaginal application of podophyllin because of concern for systemic absorption. Podophyllin is contraindicated during pregnancy and is not recommended for lesions in densely vascular tissue, such as cervical, anal, and oral warts. Use in small children should be judicious; many centers do not use podophyllin for children. Podophyllin is a resin with a high degree of variability of concentration. If results are poor, a new bottle should be opened. It may also be used in conjunction with other therapies, for example, immediately after cryotherapy or TCA.
4. Surgical removal—by electrosurgery, sharp excision, or laser ablation—may be necessary for extensive lesions, for patients whom topical therapy failed, or for young patients who require general anesthesia for removal of warts. Some centers prefer to use the carbon dioxide laser in the superpulse mode for all prepubertal children, noting that this technique minimizes the amount of eschar and adjacent tissue damage and hastens healing.[135]

Some centers employ interferon, either when other therapies fail or in combination with other modalities. Systemic interferon is not effective. It must be injected subcutaneously into muscle or directly into the lesions. Because of the inconvenient routes of administration, interferon is not recommended for routine use.

Vaginoscopy or anoscopy may be indicated for refractory disease. All adults and adolescent women with anogenital warts should have a Pap smear at least in the entry year. Some clinicians recommend follow-up every 6 months.

MEDICAL IMPLICATIONS

STDs in adolescents are important because of the high rates of infections in this group, many of which will have their greatest health impact sometime in the future. Many teenagers infected with STDs are asymptomatic, do not recognize symptoms when they are present, or fail to associate symptoms with a disease that has potentially severe complications. Lower genital tract infections and their sequelae affect females and their reproductive potential disproportionately. In females, several biologic characteristics function to increase susceptibility to STDs and their sequelae.

Female teenagers comprise approximately 20% of the 1 million women diagnosed annually with PID in the United States.[138] Sexually active adolescents have a particularly high rate of PID when rates are statistically adjusted for sexual activity. Conversely, women age 15 to 24 with PID appear to have less PID-associated tubal damage and infertility than do older women with PID[90, 139]; however, the infertility rate increases approximately threefold with each recurrent infection. Along with age-related sexual behaviors, physiologic characteristics that increase the risk for PID in adolescents are a lower prevalence of anti-*Chlamydia* antibodies and greater penetrability of cervical mucus.[82]

During adolescence, the squamocolumnar junction is extruded onto the portio of the cervix. This zone of ectopy (or ectropion) consists primarily of columnar epithelial cells, which are particularly susceptible to both chlamydial and gonococcal infections. Cervical mucus acts as a mechanical barrier to the ascent of pathogens into the upper genital tract. This function is enhanced by the progestin component of oral contraceptives, which promote formation of thick, tenacious mucus. Secretory immunoglobulin A (SigA) in cervical mucus impedes the attachment of bacteria to epithelial cells and neutralizes bacterial activity. Conversely, oral contraceptive use promotes ectopy and thus increases the risk of cervical infection with *C. trachomatis*.[41] Because cervicitis is often asymptomatic or is not recognized by patients and practitioners, the infection sometimes serves as a reservoir for pathogens that may ascend to cause upper genital tract infection (e.g., PID, chorioamnionitis, post-partum endometritis).[140] The alteration of humoral defenses by STD pathogens may be the first phase of lower genital tract infection—and of subsequent extension to the upper genital tract.

The relationship between oral contraceptive use and risk of genital tract infection is complex. A two- to threefold increase in the recovery of *C. trachomatis* from the cervix of oral contraceptive users has been documented repeatedly[41, 139, 140]; however, rates of PID are reduced by as much as 50% in oral contraceptive users as compared with other women.[142] This apparent paradox is explained by the effect of oral contraceptives on the development of cervical ectopy, which entrances the attachment and subsequent recovery of *Chlamydia* organisms. Conversely, the thick cervical mucus and relative atrophy of the endometrial cavity produced by oral contraceptives act to reduce upper genital tract invasion and proliferation of pathogens. Local immune

responses and mucosal cell susceptibility may be altered by oral contraceptive use.[143]

The prevalence of cervical ectopy in adolescent females and the association between cervical infections and ectopy have important implications for the transmission of HIV. Prospective studies of sexually active women in Africa have shown that HIV seroconversion is nearly six times more likely in women who have cervical infections caused by STD pathogens (including *C. trachomatis* and *N. gonorrhoeae*) than in women without these infections.[144, 145] The use of oral contraceptives and adolescent age have been independently associated with HIV infection.[145, 146] In addition, a cross-sectional study of couples in Kenya demonstrated that, after controlling for confounding variables, cervical ectopy remained the only independent predictor of HIV seropositivity.[147] The authors hypothesized that vascularity of ectopy and the ease of bleeding with trauma may facilitate entry of the virus into the bloodstream or the target cells of the mucosa or surrounding tissue. The prevalence of cervical ectopy during pregnancy and the increased risk of HIV transmission during pregnancy, and of subsequent perinatal transmission, thus are significant issues.

Evidence linking genital ulcer disease (GUD; e.g., syphilis, chancroid, HSV) with HIV infection is more compelling than its association with nonulcerative STDs. Although a detailed discussion of this subject has been published,[148] it is important to emphasize that both prospective and cross-sectional studies of GUD have shown a strong association between HIV seroconversion and GUD.[144, 149, 150] In addition, evidence of an increased number of clinical recurrences or persistent lesions, atypical lesions, and treatment failures with recommended antimicrobial therapy has emerged from studies of heterosexual and homosexual cohorts.[121] The relatively recent resurgence of genital ulcer–producing diseases in heterosexuals in the United States and the increases in new cases of genital HSV raise the specter of HIV-related illnesses that may overwhelm all efforts for control.[151]

The relationship between HPV infection and the development of genital neoplasia raises particular concerns for adolescents. The alarming prevalence (nearly 50%) in a cohort of sexually active teenagers indicates that subclinical infections account for the majority of HPV infections.[152] Current theory identifies HPV as an essential prerequisite for neoplasia.[152] Other factors, including cigarette smoking, HPV DNA type (e.g., 16, 18, 31, 33, 35), oral contraceptive use, and host immune-mediated alterations are associated with genital neoplasia.[152, 153] Prospective studies of the risk of cervical cancer after cytologic detection of HPV demonstrate increased risk of progression to cervical cancer for women younger than 25 years.[154, 155]

The limitation of Pap smears in detecting HPV disease was demonstrated in a study of 9000 women who had normal Pap smears, 10% of whom tested positive for HPV-16.[156] In 70% of patients, in situ hybridization failed to detect persistent HPV-16 on follow-up Pap smears, and, subsequently, some patients with negative smears tested positive for HPV.[157] These findings amplify concerns about latent viral infections acquired relatively early in life and the potential for neoplastic transformation at an earlier age.

Infection with HIV can affect the natural history of HPV infection in two principal ways. First, infection with multiple HPV types and the development of multicentric lesions has been described in women.[158-160] Second, HIV-related immunosuppression may promote development of anogenital neoplasia. Despite the confounding influence that stage of infection may have on HPV detection, several studies have shown a significant association between abnormal results on cervical cytologic tests and infection with HIV.[161-163] Although well-designed prospective studies are needed to establish the nature of these interactions, implications for the health of sexually active persons are a grave concern.

REFERENCES

1. Committee on Adolescence: Sexually transmitted diseases. Pediatrics 1994; 94:568.
2. Burnstein GR, Waterfield G, Joffe A, et al: Screening for gonorrhea and *Chlamydia* by DNA amplification in adolescents attending middle school health centers. Opportunity for early intervention. Sex Transm Dis 1998; 25:395–402.
3. Fox KK, Whittington WL, Levine WC, et al: Gonorrhea in the United States, 1981–1996. Demographic and geographic trends. Sex Transm Dis 1998; 386–393.
4. Eng TR, Butler WT (eds): The Hidden Epidemic: Confronting Sexually Transmitted Diseases. Washington, DC: Institute of Medicine, 1996.
5. Centers for Disease Control: Division of STD/HIV Prevention Annual Report, 1991. Atlanta: US Department of Health and Human Services, Public Health Service, 1992.
6. Cates W: Teenagers and sexual risk taking: The best of times and the worst of times. J Adolesc Health 1991; 12:84–94.
7. Fullilove RE, Fullilove MT, Bowser BP, et al: Risk of sexually transmitted disease among black adolescent crack users in Oakland and San Francisco, California. JAMA 1990; 263:851–855.
8. Batteiger BE, Jones RB: *Chlamydia* infections. Infect Dis Clin North Am 1987; 1:55–81.
9. Shafer MA, Moscicki AB: Sexually transmitted diseases. *In* Hendee WR, Wilford B (eds): Health of Adolescents: Adolescent Health Issues. San Francisco: Jossey-Bass, 1991.
10. Rosenfeld WD, Vermund SH, Wentz SJ, et al: High prevalence rate of human papillomavirus infection and associated abnormal Papanicolaou smears among sexually active adolescents. Am J Dis Child 1989; 143:1443–1447.
11. Bauer HM, Ting Y, Greer CE, et al: Genital human papillomavirus infection in female university students as determined by a PCR-based method. JAMA 1989; 265:472–477.
12. Stone KM: Epidemiologic aspects of genital HPV infection. Clin Obstet Gynecol 1989; 32:112–116.
13. Johnson RE, Nahmias A, Madger LS, et al: A seroepidemiologic survey of the prevalence of herpes simplex virus type 2 infection in the United States. N Engl J Med 1989; 321:7–12.
14. Kampareier RH: Identification of the gonococcus by Albert Neisser. Sex Transm Dis 1978; 5:71–73.
15. Judson FN: Gonorrhea. Med Clin North Am 1990; 74:1353–1366.
16. McCormack M, Stumacher RJ, Johnson K, Donner A: Clinical spectrum of gonococcal infection in women. Lancet 1977; 1:1182–1185.
17. Hook EW, Hansfield HH: Gonococcal infections in the adult. *In* Holmes KK, Mardh PA, Sparling PF (eds): Sexually Transmitted Diseases, 2nd ed. New York: McGraw-Hill, 1990, pp 149–165.
18. Barlow D, Phillips I: Gonorrhea in women: Diagnostic, clinical, and laboratory aspects. Lancet 1978; 1:761–764.
19. Schmake JD, et al: Observation on the culture diagnosis of gonorrhea in women. JAMA 1969; 210:312–315.
20. Thin RN, Shaw EJ: Diagnosis of gonorrhea in women. Br J Vener Dis 1979; 55:434–438.
21. Lebedoff DA, Hochman EB: Rectal gonorrhea in men: Diagnosis and treatment. Ann Intern Med 1980; 92:463–467.
22. Quinn TC, Stamm WE, Goodell SE, et al: The polymicrobial origin of intestinal infections in homosexual men. N Engl J Med 1983; 309:576–582.
23. Hanks JW, Scott CT, Butler CE, Wells DW: Evaluation of a DNA probe essay (Gen-Probe PACE 2) as the test of cure for *Neisseria gonorrhoeae* genital infections. J Pediatrics 1994; 125(1):161–162.
24. Liebling MR, Arkfeld DG, Michelini GA, et al: Identification of *Neisseria gonorrhoeae* in synovial fluid using the polymerase chain reaction. Arthritis Rheum 1994; 37(5):702–709.
25. Ching S, Lee H, Hook EW 3rd, et al: Ligase chain reaction for detection of *Neisseria gonorrhoeae* in urogenital swabs. J Clin Microbiol 1995; 33(12):3111–3114.
26. Smith KR, Ching S, Lee H, et al: Evaluation of ligase chain reaction for use with urine for identification of *Neisseria gonorrhoeae* in females attending a sexually transmitted disease clinic. J Clin Microbiol 1995; 33(2):455–457.
27. Jacobs NF, Krans SJ: Gonococcal and nongonococcal urethritis in men: Clinical and laboratory differentiation. Ann Intern Med 1975; 82:7–11.
28. O'Brien JA, Goldenberg DL, Rice PA: Disseminated gonococcal infection. A prospective analysis of 49 patients and a review of the pathophysiology and immune mechanisms. Medicine 1983; 62:395–406.
29. Hook EW 3rd, Holmes KK: Gonococcal infections. Ann Intern Med 1985; 102:229–243.
30. Handsfield HH, Wiesner PJ, Holmes KK: Treatment of the gonococcal arthritis-dermatitis syndrome. Ann Intern Med 1976; 84:661–667.

31. van Overbeek JJ: Gonorrheal infections in the oropharynx. Arch Otolaryngol 1976; 102:94–96.
32. Weisner PJ, et al: The clinical spectrum of pharyngeal gonococcal infections. N Engl J Med 1973; 288:181–185.
33. Dice PA, Goldenberg DL: Clinical manifestations of disseminated gonococcal infection caused by *Neisseria gonorrhoeae* are linked to differences in bacterial reactivity of infecting strains. Ann Intern Med 1985; 95:175–180.
34. Pederson AHB, Bonin P: Screening females for asymptomatic *Gonorrhea* infection. Northwest Med 1971; 70:255–259.
35. Centers for Disease Control: Sexually transmitted diseases: Treatment guidelines. MMWR 1998; 47(RR-1):1–116.
36. Centers for Disease Control: Division of STD/HIV Prevention Annual Report, 1990. Atlanta: US Department of Health and Human Services, Public Health Service, 1991.
37. Wang SP, Grayston JT: Immunological relationship between genital TRIC, lymphogranuloma venereum, and related organisms in the new microtiter indirect immunofluorescence test. Am J Ophthalmol 1970; 70:367–371.
38. Wang SP, Kno CC, Barnes RC, et al: Immunotyping of *Chlamydia trachomatis* with monoclonal antibodies. J Infect Dis 1985; 152:791–794.
39. Kuo CC, Wang SP, Holmes KK, et al: Immunotypes of *Chlamydia trachomatis* isolates in Seattle, Washington. Infect Immun 1983; 41:865–868.
40. Schachter J: Biology of *Chlamydia trachomatis*. In Holmes KK (ed): Sexually Transmitted Diseases, 2nd ed. New York: McGraw-Hill, 1990, pp 167–180.
41. Harrison JR, Costia M, Meder JB, et al: Cervical *Chlamydia trachomatis* infection in university women: Relationship to history, contraception, ectopy and cervicitis. Am J Obstet Gynecol 1985; 153:244–249.
42. Brunham RC, Paavonen J, Stevens CE, et al: Mucopurulent cervicitis: The ignored counterpart in women of urethritis in men. N Engl J Med 1984; 311:1–8.
43. Rees E, Tait IA, Hobson D, et al: *Chlamydia* in relation to cervical infection and pelvic inflammatory disease. In Hobson D, Holmes KK (eds): Nongonococcal Urethritis and Related Infections. Washington, DC: American Society for Microbiology, 1977, p 67.
44. Katz BP, Caine VA, Jones RB: Diagnosis of mucopurulent cervicitis among women at risk for *Chlamydia trachomatis* infection. Sex Transm Dis 1988; 16:103–106.
45. Brunham RC, et al: Epidemiologic and clinical correlates of *C. trachomatis* and *N. gonorrhoeae* infection among women attending an STD clinic. Clin Res 1981; 29:474–494.
46. Paavonen J: *Chlamydia trachomatis*–induced urethritis in female partners of men with nongonococcal urethritis. Sex Transm Dis 1979; 6:69–72.
47. Stamm WE, Wagner KF, Amsel R, et al: Causes of the acute urethral syndrome in women. N Engl J Med 1980; 303:409–414.
48. Jones RB, Katz BP, Vanderpol B, et al: Effect of blind passage and multiple sampling in recovery of *Chlamydia trachomatis* from urogenital specimens. J Clin Microbiol 1986; 24:1029.
49. Eschenbach DA, Buchanan TM, Pollock HM, et al: Polymicrobial etiology of acute pelvic inflammatory disease. N Engl J Med 1975; 293:166–171.
50. Mardh PA, Ripa KT, Svensson L, et al: *Chlamydia trachomatis* infection in patients with acute salpingitis. N Engl J Med 1977; 296:1377.
51. Svensson L, Westrom L, Ripa KT, et al: Differences in some clinical and laboratory parameters in acute salpingitis related to culture and serologic findings. Am J Obstet Gynecol 1980; 138:1017–1021.
52. Wolner-Hansen P, Kiviat N, Holmes KK: Atypical pelvic inflammatory disease: Subacute, chronic or subclinical upper genital tract infection in women. In Holmes KK (ed): Sexually Transmitted Diseases, 2nd ed. New York: McGraw-Hill, 1990, pp 615–620.
53. Wang SP, Eschenback DA, Holmes KK, et al: *Chlamydia trachomatis* infection in Fitz-Hugh-Curtis syndrome. Am J Obstet Gynecol 1980; 138:1034–1038.
54. Richmond J, Paul ID, Taylor PK: Value and feasibility of screening women attending STD clinics for cervical *Chlamydia* infections. Br J Vener Dis 1980; 56:92–96.
55. Sultz GR, et al: *Chlamydia trachomatis* infections in female adolescents. J Pediatric 1981; 98:981–989.
56. Bowie WR, et al: Prevalence of *C. trachomatis* and *N. gonorrhoeae* in two populations of women. Can Med Assoc J 1981; 124:1477–1481.
57. Handsfield HH, Jasman LL, Roberts PL, et al: Criteria for selective screening for *Chlamydia trachomatis* infection in women attending family planning clinics. JAMA 1986; 255:1730–1738.
58. Clarke LM, Sierra MR, Diadone BJ, et al: Comparison of the Syva Micro Trak enzyme immunoassay and Gen-Probe PACE 2 with cell culture for diagnosis of cervical *Chlamydia trachomatis* infection in a high-prevalence female population. J Clin Microbiol 1993; 31(4):968–971.
59. Schachter J, Stamm WE, Quinn TC, et al: Ligase chain reaction to detect *Chlamydia trachomatis* infection of the cervix. J Clin Microbiol 1994; 32(10):2540-0–3.
60. Schachter J: Chlamydial infections. N Engl J Med 1978; 298:428–434.
61. Paavonen J, Kousa M, Saikku P, et al: Treatment of nongonococcal urethritis with trimethoprim-sulphadiazine and with placebo. A double-blind partner-controlled study. Br J Vener Dis 1980; 56:101–104.
62. Stamm WE, Running K, McKevitt M, et al: Treatment of the acute urethral syndrome. N Engl J Med 1981; 304:956–958.
63. Martin DH: Chlamydial infections. Med Clin North Am 1990; 74:1367–1387.
64. Barnes RC: Laboratory diagnosis of human chlamydial infections. Clin Microbiol Rev 1989; 2:119–131.
65. Stamm WE: Diagnosis of *Chlamydia trachomatis* genitourinary infection. Ann Intern Med 1988; 108:710–720.
66. Howell M, Quinn T, Brathwaite W, Gaydos C: Screening women for *Chlamydia trachomatis* in family planning clinics. Sex Transm Dis 1998; 2:108–117.
67. Shafer MA, Pantell R, Schachter J: Is the routine pelvic examination needed with the advent of urine-based screening for sexually transmitted diseases? Arch Pediatr Adolesc Med 1999; 153:119–125.
68. Stamm WE, Holmes KK: *Chlamydia trachomatis* infections of the adult. In Holmes KK (ed): Sexually Transmitted Diseases, 2nd ed. New York: McGraw-Hill, 1990, pp 181–193.
69. Toomey KE, Barnes RC: Treatment of *Chlamydia trachomatis* genital infection. Rev Infect Dis 1990; 12(Suppl 6):5645–5653.
70. Stamm WE: Azithromycin in the treatment of uncomplicated genital chlamydial infection. Am J Med 1991; 91(Suppl A):195–205.
71. Martin DH, Mroczkowski TF, Dalu ZA, et al: A controlled trial of a single dose of azithromycin for the treatment of chlamydial urethritis and cervicitis. N Engl J Med 1992; 327:921–925.

72. Wehbeh HA, Mary RR, Shahem S, et al: Single-dose azithromycin for *Chlamydia* in pregnant women. J Reprod Med 1998; 43:509–514.

73. Cromblehome WR, Schachter J, Grossman M, et al: Amoxicillin therapy for *Chlamydia trachomatis* infection in pregnancy. Am J Obstet Gynecol 1990; 75:752–756.

74. Alger LS, Lovchik JC: Comparison of efficacy of clindamycin versus erythromycin in eradication of antenatal *Chlamydia trachomatis*. Am J Obstet Gynecol 1991; 165:23–27.

75. Schmid G. Approach to the patient with genital ulcer disease. Med Clin North Am 1990; 74:1556–1572.

76. Schachter J: Lymphogranuloma venereum and other nonocular *Chlamydia trachomatis* infections. *In* Hobson D, Holmes KK (eds): Nongonococcal Urethritis and Related Infections. Washington, DC: American Society for Microbiology, 1977, pp 91–97.

77. Perina P, Osoba AD: Lymphogranuloma venereum. *In* Holmes KK (ed): Sexually Transmitted Diseases, 2nd ed. New York: McGraw-Hill, 1990, pp 195–204.

78. Duncan ME, Jamil Y, Tibaux G, et al: Chlamydial infection in a population of Ethiopian women attending obstetric, gynaecological and mother and child health clinics. Central Afr J Med 1996; 42(1):1–14.

79. Centers for Disease Control: 1989 Sexually transmitted diseases treatment guidelines. MMWR 1989; 38:27–39.

80. Aral SO, Mosher WD, Cates W Jr: Self-reported pelvic inflammatory diseases in the United States. JAMA 1991; 266:2570–2573.

81. Washington AE, Katz D: Cost and payment services for pelvic inflammatory disease: Trends and projections, 1983 through 2000. JAMA 1981; 266:2581–2586.

82. Cates W, Rolfs RT, Aral SO: Sexually transmitted diseases, pelvic inflammatory disease and infertility: An epidemiologic update. Epidemiol Rev 1990; 12:199–220.

83. Eschenbach DA: Acute pelvic inflammatory disease. *In* Sciarra J (ed): Gynecology and Obstetrics, Vol. I. Hagerstown: Harper & Row, 1988.

84. Eschenbach DA, Buchanon TM, Pollock HM, et al: Polymicrobial etiology of acute pelvic inflammatory disease. N Engl J Med 1975; 293:166.

85. Paavonen J, Teisala K, Heinoven PK, et al: Microbiological and histopathological findings in acute pelvic inflammatory disease. Br J Obstet Gynaecol 1987; 94:454–460.

86. Wasserheit JN, Bele TA, Kivrat NB, et al: Microbiological causes of proven pelvic inflammatory disease and efficacy of clindamycin and tobramycin. Ann Intern Med 1986; 104:187–193.

87. Sweet RL, Mille J, Hadley K, et al: Use of laparoscopy to determine the microbiologic etiology of acute salpingitis. Am J Obstet Gynecol 1979; 134:781.

88. Rice DA, Schachter J: Pathogenesis of pelvic inflammatory disease: What are the questions? JAMA 1991; 266:2587–2593.

89. Washington AE, Aral SO, Wolner-Hanssen P, et al: Assessing risk for pelvic inflammatory disease and its sequelae. JAMA 1991; 266:2581–2586.

90. Jacobson L, Wertrom L: Objectivized diagnosis of acute pelvic inflammatory disease: Diagnostic and prognostic value of laparoscopy. Am J Obstet Gynecol 1969; 105:1088–1098.

91. Kahn JG, Walker CK, Washington AE, et al: Diagnosing pelvic inflammatory disease: A comprehensive analysis and considerations for developing a new model. JAMA 1991; 266:2594–2604.

92. Westrom L, Mardh PA: Acute pelvic inflammatory disease (PID). *In* Holmes KK (ed): Sexually Transmitted Diseases, 2nd ed. New York: McGraw-Hill, 1990, pp 593–613.

93. Centers for Disease Control: Pelvic inflammatory disease: Guidelines for prevention and management. MMWR 1991; 40(RR-5):1–25.

94. Peterson HB, Walker CK, Kahn JG, et al: Pelvic inflammatory disease: Key treatment options. JAMA 1991; 266:2605–2611.

95. Centers for Disease Control: Primary and secondary syphilis—United States, 1981–1990. MMWR 1991; 40:314–315.

95a. Rolff RT, Nakashima AK: Epidemiology of primary and secondary syphilis in the United States, 1981–1989. JAMA 1990; 264:1432–1437.

95b. Centers for Disease Control and Prevention: Primary and secondary syphilis—United States, 1997. JAMA 1998; 280:1218–1219.

96. St. Louis ME, Wasserheit JN: Elimination of syphilis in the United States. Science 1998; 281:353–354.

97. Hutchins CM, Hook EW: Syphilis in adults. Med Clin North Am 1990; 74:1389–1416.

98. Primary and secondary syphilis, United States, 1997. MMWR 1998; 47:493–497.

99. Schroeter AL, Turner RH, Lucas JB, et al: Therapy for incubating syphilis: Effectiveness of gonorrhea treatment. JAMA 1971; 218:711–713.

100. Chapel TA: The variability of syphilitic chancres. Sex Transm Dis 1978; 5:68–70.

101. Mindel A, Tovey SJ, Timmins DJ, et al: Primary and secondary syphilis, 20 years' experience. 2. Clinical features. Genitourin Med 1989; 65:1–3.

102. Rolfs RT, Joesoef MR, Hendershot EF, et al: A randomized trial of enhanced therapy for early syphilis in patients with and without human immunodeficiency virus infection. The Syphilis and HIV Study Group. N Engl J Med 1997; 337(5):307–314.

103. Fiumara NJ: Treatment of secondary syphilis: An evaluation of 204 patients. Sex Transm Dis 1977; 4:92–95.

104. Fiumara NJ: Treatment of seropositive primary syphilis: An evaluation of 196 patients. Sex Transm Dis 1977; 4:96–99.

105. Siegal D, Golden E, Washington AE, et al: Prevalence and correlates of herpes simplex infections: The Population-based AIDS in Multiethnic Neighborhoods Study. JAMA 1992; 268:1702–1708.

106. Corey L, Adams HG, Brown ZA, et al: Genital herpes simplex virus infections: Clinical manifestations, course, and complications. Ann Intern Med 1983; 98:958–972.

107. Koutsky LA, Ashley RL, Holmes KK, et al: The frequency of unrecognized type 2 herpes simplex infection among women. Sex Transm Dis 1990; 17:90–94.

108. Koutsky LA, Stevens CE, Holmes KK, et al. Underdiagnosis of genital herpes by current clinical and viral-isolation procedures. N Engl J Med 1992; 326:1533–1539.

109. Mertz GJ: Genital herpes simplex virus infections. Med Clin North Am 1990; 74:1433–1454.

110. Reeves WC, Corey L, Adams HG, et al: Risk of recurrence after first episodes of genital herpes: Relationship to HSV type and antibody response. N Engl J Med 1981; 305:315–319.

111. Corey L: Genital herpes. *In* Holmes KK, Mardh PA, Sparling PF (eds): Sexually Transmitted Diseases, 2nd ed. New York: McGraw-Hill, 1990, pp 391–413.

112. Fife KH, Corey L: Herpes simplex virus. *In* Holmes KK (ed): Sexually Transmitted Diseases, 2nd ed. New York: McGraw-Hill, 1990, pp 941–952.

113. Beards G, Graham C, Pillay D: Investigation of vesicu-

lar rashes for HSV and VZV by PCR. J Med Virol 1998; 54(3):155–157.

114. Corey L, Benedetti JK, Critchlow C, et al: Treatment of primary first-episode genital herpes simplex virus with acyclovir: Results of topical, intravenous and oral therapy. J Antimicrob Chemother 1983; 12(Suppl B):79.

115. Diaz-Mitoma F, Sibbald G, Shafran SD, et al: Oral famciclovir for the suppression of recurrent genital herpes: A randomized controlled trial. JAMA 1998; 280:887–892.

116. Engel J: Long-term suppression of genital herpes. JAMA 1998; 280:928–929.

117. Cardamakis E, Relakis K, Kotoulas IG, et al: Treatment of recurrent genital herpes with interferon alpha-2-alpha. Gynecol Obstet Invest 1998; 46(1):54–57.

118. Reichman RC, Badger GJ, Mertz GJ, et al: Treatment of recurrent genital herpes simplex infections with oral acyclovir: A controlled trial. JAMA 1984; 251:2103–2108.

119. Mertz GJ, Eron L, Kaufman R, et al: Prolonged continuous versus intermittent acyclovir treatment in normal adults with frequently recurring genital herpes simplex virus infection. Am J Med 1988; 85(Suppl 2A):14–19.

120. Mertz GJ, Jones CC, Mills J, et al: Long-term acyclovir suppression of frequently recurring genital herpes simplex virus infection. A multicenter double-blind trial. JAMA 1988; 260:201–206.

121. de Villers E-M: Heterogeneity of the human papillomavirus group. J Virol 1989; 63:4898–4903.

122. Neary K, Horwitz BH, DiMaio D: Mutational analysis of open reading frame E4 of bovine papillomavirus type 1. J Virol 1987; 61:1248–1252.

123. Oriel JD: Natural history of genital warts. Br J Vener Dis 1971; 47:1–13.

124. Brown DR, Fife KH: Human papillomavirus infections of the genital tract. Med Clin North Am 1990; 74:1455–1485.

125. Schwartz DB, Greenberg MD, Daoud Y, et al: The management of genital condylomas in pregnancy. Obstet Gynecol Clin North Am 1987; 14:589–599.

126. Oriel D: Genital human papillomavirus infection. In Holmes KK (ed): Sexually Transmitted Diseases, 2nd ed. New York: McGraw-Hill, 1990, pp 433–441.

127. Stoltz E, Memke HE, Vuzeviski VD: Other genital dermatoses. In Holmes KK (ed): Sexually Transmitted Diseases, 2nd ed. New York: McGraw-Hill, 1990, pp 717–735.

128. Aho M, Vesterinen E, Myer B, et al: Natural history of vaginal intraepithelial neoplasia. Cancer 1991; 68:195–202.

129. Cone R, Beckmann A, Aho M, et al: Subclinical manifestations of vulvar human papillomavirus infections. Int J Gynecol Pathol 1991; 10:26–31.

130. Gutman LT, St. Claire K, Herman-Giddens ME, et al: Evaluation of sexually abused and non-abused young girls for intravaginal human papillomavirus infection. Am J Dis Child 1992; 146(6):694–699.

131. Gutman LT, St. Claire KK, Everett VD, et al: Cervical-vaginal and intraanal human papillomavirus infection of young girls with external genital warts. J Infect Dis 1994; 170(2):339–344.

132. Pakarian F, Kaye J, Cason J, et al: Cancer associated human papillomaviruses: Perinatal transmission and persistence. Br J Obstet Gynaecol 1994; 101(6):514–517.

133. Ho GY, Bierman R, Beardsley L, et al: Natural history of cervicovaginal papillomavirus infection in young women. N Engl J Med 1998; 338:423–428.

134. Moscicki A-B, Shiboski S, Broering J, et al: The natural history of human papillomavirus infection as measured by repeated DNA testing in adolescent and young women. J Pediatrics 1998; 132:277–284.

135. Davis AJ, Emans SJ: Human papillomavirus infection: The pediatric and adolescent patient. J Pediatrics 1989; 115:1–9.

136. Koss LG, Durfee GR: Unusual patterns in squamous epithelium of the uterine cervix and pathologic study of koilocytotic atypia. Ann NY Acad Sci 1956; 63:1245–1251.

137. Shibata DK, Arnheim N, Martin WJ: Detection of human papillomavirus in paraffin embedded tissue using the polymerase chain reaction. J Exp Med 1988; 167:225–230.

138. Washington AE, Sweet RL, Shafer M-A: Pelvic inflammatory disease and its sequelae in adolescents. J Adolesc Health Care 1985; 6:298–310.

139. Westrom L: Influence of sexually transmitted diseases on sterility and ectopic pregnancy. Acta Eur Fertil 1985; 16:21–32.

140. Holmes KK: Lower genital tract infections in women: Cystitis, urethritis, vulvovaginitis, and cervicitis. In Holmes KK, Mardh PA, Sparling PF (eds): Sexually Transmitted Diseases, 2nd ed. New York: McGraw-Hill, 1990, pp 527–545.

141. Cromer BA, Heald FP: Pelvic inflammatory disease associated with Neisseria gonorrhoeae and Chlamydia trachomatis: Clinical correlates. Sex Transm Dis 1987; 14:125–129.

142. Washington AE, Gove S, Schachter J, Sweet RL: Oral contraceptives, Chlamydia trachomatis infection, and pelvic inflammatory disease: A word of caution about protection. JAMA 1985; 253:2246–2250.

143. Wolner-Hanssen P, Eschenbach DA, Paavonen J, et al: Decreased risk of symptomatic pelvic inflammatory disease associated with oral contraceptive use. JAMA 1990; 263:54–59.

144. Laga M, Nzila N, Manoka AT, et al: Nonulcerative sexually transmitted diseases (STD) as risk factors for HIV infection. Abstract Th.C.97. In Program and Abstracts: Sixth International Conference on AIDS, San Francisco, June, 1990.

145. Plummer FA, Simonsen NJ, Cameron DW, et al: Cofactors in male-to-female transmission of human immunodeficiency virus type I. J Infect Dis 1991; 163:233–239.

146. N'Galy B, Ryder RW: Epidemiology of HIV infection in Africa. J Acquir Immune Defic Syn 1988; 1:551–558.

147. Moss GB, Clemetson D, D'Costa L, et al: Association of cervical ectopy with heterosexual transmission of human immunodeficiency virus: Results of a study of couples in Nairobi, Kenya. J Infect Dis 1991; 164:588–591.

148. Wasserheit JN: Epidemiological synergy: Interrelationships between human immunodeficiency virus infection and other sexually transmitted diseases. Sex Transm Dis 1992; 19:61–77.

149. Cameron DW, Lourdes JD, Gregory MM, et al: Female-to-male transmission of human immunodeficiency virus type 1: Risk factors for seroconversion in men. Lancet 1989; 2:403–407.

150. Holmberg SD, Stewart JA, Gerber AR, et al: Prior herpes simplex virus type 2 infection as a risk factor for HIV infection. JAMA 1988; 59:1048–1050.

151. Aral SO, Holmes KK: Sexually transmitted diseases in the AIDS era. Sci Am 1991; 264:62–69.

152. Wright TC, Richart RM: Review: Role of human papillomavirus in the pathogenesis of genital tract warts and cancer. Gynecol Oncol 1990; 37:151–164.

153. Ritter DB, Kadish AS, Vermund SH, et al: Detection

of human papillomavirus deoxyribonucleic acid in exfoliated cervicovaginal cells as a predictor of cervical neoplasia in a high-risk population. Am J Obstet Gynecol 1988; 159:1517–1525.

154. Mitchell H, Drake M, Medley G: Prospective evaluation of the risk of cervical cancer after cytological evidence of human papillomavirus infection. Lancet 1986; 1:573–575.

155. Kurman RJ, Schiffman MH, Lancaster WD, et al: Analysis of individual papillomavirus types in cervical neoplasia: A possible role for type 18 in rapid progression. Am J Obstet Gynecol 1987; 156:212–216.

156. De Villers EM, Wagner D, Schneider A, et al: Human papillomavirus infections in women with and without abnormal cervical cytology. Lancet 1987; 1:703–705.

157. Moscicki A-B, Winkler B, Irwin CE Jr, Schachter J: Differences in biological maturation, sexual behavior, and sexually transmitted disease between adolescents with and without cervical neoplasia. J Pediatrics 1989; 115:487–493.

158. Byrne MA, Taylor-Robinson D, Munday PE, et al: The common occurrence of human papillomavirus infection and intraepithelial neoplasia in women infected with HIV. AIDS 1989; 3:379–382.

159. Caube P, Poulques H, Katlama C: Multifocal human papillomavirus infection of the genital tract in HIV seropositive women. NY State J Med 1990; 90:162–163.

160. Feingold AR, Vermund SH, Burk RD, et al: Cervical cytologic abnormalities and papillomavirus infection in women infected with human immunodeficiency virus. J Acquir Immune Defic Syn 1990; 3:2911–2916.

161. Schrager LK, Friedland GH, Maude D, et al: Cervical and vaginal squamous abnormalities in women infected with human immunodeficiency virus. J Acquir Immune Defic Syn 1989; 2:570–575.

162. Vermund SH, Kelley DF, Burk RD, et al: Risk of human papillomavirus (HPV) and cervical intraepithelial lesions (SIL) highest among women with advanced HIV disease. Abstract No. S.B. 517. In Program and Abstracts: Sixth International Conference on AIDS. San Francisco, June, 1990.

163. Crocchiolo P, Lizioli A, Goisis F, et al: Cervical dysplasia and HIV infection. Lancet 1988; 2:238–239.

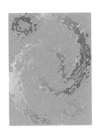

Chapter 23

Human Immunodeficiency Virus Infection in Adolescents

Angela M. Hagy and Sten H. Vermund

Risk for HIV infection typically begins in the years of adolescence. The magnitude of the risk varies with sexual activity, use of barriers (i.e., condoms), use of alcohol and drugs, and background seroprevalence in the community. Disease manifested in adolescence depends on its own set of factors: baseline immune status, exposure to specific opportunistic infections, timing of HIV testing (i.e., early vs. late recognition), access to and compliance with medical care, substance abuse, and host and viral factors inherent in infection. While not all relevant issues can be presented in a chapter, we seek to highlight those of greatest interest to providers of adolescent gynecologic care.

EPIDEMIOLOGY

HIV-related death in (U.S.) women has its greatest impact on young and middle-aged adults, especially racial and ethnic minorities. Even in the age of highly active antiretroviral therapy (HAART), HIV was the seventh leading cause of death in the United States for women aged 15 to 24 years in 1998. HIV was the fourth leading cause of death in women between 25 and 44 years, many of them having become infected as teenagers.[1] HIV-related illnesses were the second leading cause of death among African American women and the third leading cause among Hispanic women aged 25 to 44. The proportion of all AIDS cases reported in the United States among adolescent women ages 13 to 19 rose from 29% in 1993 to 40% in 1998, while the proportion of AIDS cases in women 20 to 24 years rose from 34% to 51% during the same period (Fig. 23–1).[2–7] It is estimated that at least half of all new HIV infections in the United States affect people younger than 25 and that

the majority of young people are being infected through sexual contact.[8]

A Centers for Disease Control and Prevention (CDC) study using data collected from 25 states with integrated HIV and AIDS reporting systems for the period between January 1994 and June 1997 found that young people (ages 13 to 24) accounted for a much greater proportion of HIV than of AIDS cases. While the overall incidence of AIDS was declining, there was no comparable decline in the number of newly diagnosed HIV cases among youth.[9] In 1998, among persons from the 30 states where confidential HIV reporting exists for adults and adolescents, females comprise 48% of HIV cases in Americans ages 13 to 24, and 62% among those ages 13 to 19. This reflects the risk of heterosexual acquisition of HIV among young women and the increasingly frequent testing of females, especially during pregnancy. Young African Americans are most heavily affected, accounting for 56% of all HIV cases reported among people ages 13 to 24 from 1981 to 1998 in the United States, nearly three times the proportion of the population they represent.[2]

Young disadvantaged women, particularly African American women, are being infected with HIV at younger ages and more frequently than their male counterparts, an observation from entrants to the U.S. Job Corps program from 1990 to 1996. The Job Corps is a federally funded job training program for economically and educationally disadvantaged out-of-school youths from all 50 states and the U.S. territories. The study tested more than 350,000 16- to 21-year-olds and found HIV incidence rates of 2.8 per 1000 for women and 2.0 per 1000 for men. Infection rates were dramatically higher among women ages 16 to 18 years than among their male age peers, whereas, for 19- to 21-year-olds, rates were simi-

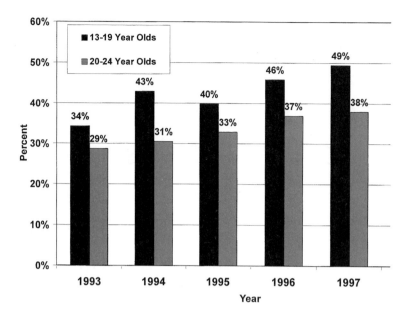

Figure 23–1 Percentage of AIDS cases among adolescent females, 1993–1998, CDC year-end data.[2–7]

lar in both genders. Young African American women had the highest HIV infection rate of any group, 4.9 per thousand, more than seven times higher than that for young white women (0.7 per 1000) and young Hispanic women (0.6 per 1000). At age 20, the HIV infection rate for African American women in the study was 7 per 1000. These data suggest that HIV prevalence among disadvantaged young women is highest in the District of Columbia (10.3 per 1000), Florida (9.8 per 1000), Maryland (9.1 per 1000), South Carolina (8.2 per 1000), and Louisiana (5.1 per 1000) among all the states and territories.[10] The high rates in the Baltimore-Washington area and in the southeastern United States may be associated with high overall STD rates.[11]

The estimated number of all young persons ages 13 to 19 who are living with AIDS is highest in New York, Florida, California, Texas, and New Jersey (Fig. 23–2).[12] The next highest estimated numbers of persons living with AIDS are clustered in the southeastern United States and scattered through the Middle Atlantic states and the Midwest. Together, the high seroprevalence rates among Job Corps recruits and the highest estimated number of young people living with AIDS are evidence of the emerging epidemic in the southeastern United States.

TRANSMISSION

Since 1997, heterosexual contact has been the most common mode of transmission of HIV in females ages 13 to 24 years.[2, 7] In 1998, 1798 persons ages 13 to 24 were reported to have AIDS, for a cumulative total of 27,860 cases through 1998.[2] In 1998, 51% of affected young males were men who have sex with men (MSM); 10% were injection drug users (IDUs); and 9% were infected through heterosexual contact; for the remaining 22%, risk factors were not known. For women ages 13 to 24 years, 47% were infected through heterosexual activity, 14% were IDUs, and 39% knew of no risk factor at the time of reporting in 1998.[2] Most unknown "risk" cases in young women are eventually determined to be of heterosexual origin.

A variety of behavioral and biologic factors can put sexually active teenage girls at greater risk for STDs and for HIV infection, including lifetime number of sex partners, high prevalence of HIV and other STDs among sex partners, and high rates of substance use or abuse and unprotected sex.[13] Risk behaviors associated with HIV infection occur within the context of adolescents' social and sexual relationships.[14] Often, adolescents are serially monogamous: they engage in a series of exclusive relationships of relatively short duration. A significant number of female adolescents are sexually involved with older men. For girls, large age discrepancies between partners are associated with younger age at first intercourse and less frequent condom use (and consequently higher risk of HIV infection).[15] Teenage girls are often unable or unwilling to negotiate abstinence or safer sex practices with their male partners to reduce their STD and HIV risk.[16]

The 1997 Youth Risk Behavior Survey found

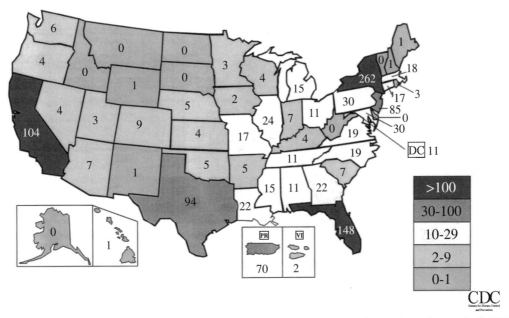

Figure 23–2 Estimated number of persons ages 13–19 years living with AIDS at the end of 1997 as modeled by CDC with data as of September 1998.[12]

that, by the 12th grade, 62% of female students surveyed in the United States had had sexual intercourse, 4.5% of them before age 13. Some 14.1% reported having had four or more partners during their lifetimes. Of note, 43.2% of sexually active students, male and female, had not used a condom for their last sexual intercourse encounter. Among female high school seniors, 82% reported having tried alcohol and 33.5% reported periodic heavy drinking. Injection drug use was higher among 12th-grade males; 2.0% reported ever having injected an illegal drug, as compared with 0.8% of 12th-grade females.[17] The study used self-reports and is therefore likely to underreport the actual rates of sexual behaviors and substance use among female adolescents in the United States. The study did not include out-of-school teens such as runaways and homeless youths and the data underrepresents inner-city youths, whose rates of unsafe sexual behavior and substance use are higher.[18]

In a separate study conducted by the Youth Risk Board looking at 12th-grade students in eight large city school districts from 1991 to 1997, the proportion of sexually experienced students and the prevalence of multiple sex partners declined over time and condom use increased. In all but one of the districts, the proportion of students who reported currently being sexually active declined.[19] The decrease in the percentage of urban students who reported sexual activity and multiple sex partners parallels recent na-

tional trends in these health risk behaviors, which represent a reversal of the increasing national trend during the "sexual revolution" of the 1970s and 1980s.[19–21]

In 1998, injection drug use was the second most often reported source of infection among young women in the United States. In addition to the direct risks associated with drug injection (sharing needles, syringes, and drug paraphernalia), behavior associated with use of other substances is also fueling heterosexual spread of the epidemic. Many American women infected heterosexually, including some who initially reported having no risk factors, are infected through sex with an IDU.[2] This suggests that women may be unaware of their partners' risk factors or that healthcare providers are not documenting such risks. Poor judgment associated with drinking alcohol and trading sex for money or drugs associated with crack cocaine and IDU contribute to heterosexual risk. In the adolescent age group, drinking alcohol is especially common.[17] From 1994 to 1996, 2414 minority women ages 12 to 24 years who attended a community-based health center in South Central Los Angeles were asked about alcohol use and sex practices. The study found that young women who used alcohol were twice as likely as those who have not used alcohol to have had unprotected vaginal intercourse in the past year (odds ratio 2.34).[22]

Persons who have an STD are at greater risk than others for HIV infection.[13, 23] Compared with their male partners, adolescent females are physiologically more susceptible to many STDs, including HIV.[13] Young women may be at comparably higher risk of HIV infection for a given number of exposures.[24] Immature adolescent vaginal mucosa with relatively large cervical ectopy zones may be more susceptible to trauma (i.e., bleeding) during sex and may be prone to infection with STDs because of the exposed transformation zone.[25–28] The presence of an STD in an HIV-negative partner disrupts the normal mucosal barriers and allows more efficient transmission of the virus.[27, 29, 30] It is not widely appreciated that, when sexually active persons are in the denominator of the rate, adolescents have the highest STD rates of any population.[24] Genital ulcers and a friable cervix in the HIV-negative partner confer special risk for HIV; syphilis, genital herpes, and chancroid are associated with a 2.3- to 11.3-fold increase in the risk of transmission. Inflammatory STDs such as gonorrhea, *Chlamydia* infection, bacterial vaginosis, and trichomoniasis also increase risk, by a factor of 1.9 to 9.8.[27] Recruitment of CD4+ target cells can be substantial.[31] Given that inflammatory STDs are more common than ulcerogenic ones, the population attributable risk for HIV is substantial. Up-regulation of CCR5 co-receptors in the cervical mucosa of women with active STDs may facilitate HIV transmission and is yet another reason for synergy between other STDs and HIV.[32] STD control can be expected to help reduce the risk.[33–35]

HIV transmission may be promoted by sexual activity that involves exposure to blood, as during menses,[36,37] rape,[38–42] or a first coitus.[25] Women who engage in receptive anal intercourse are at higher risk of transmission, most likely due to trauma to the rectal mucosa, the absorptive capacity of the descending colon, and the presence of infectible target cells in the gastrointestinal mucosa.[43–45] The increased concentration of HIV in cervicovaginal fluid during pregnancy may be a mechanism for female-to-male and female-to-infant transmission.[46] It is likely that female genital mutilation is a traumatic risk factor for HIV among adolescents in parts of Africa and Asia.

The role of oral contraceptives in the transmission of HIV is still unclear. Oral contraceptives can cause cervical ectopy and thus may increase the risk of transmission.[47] Progesterone is associated with an increase in CCR5 co-receptor activity for CD4+ target cells, providing another possible mechanism for increased transmission.[48] Since oral contraceptives are oftentimes used as an alternative to condoms, it is difficult to determine whether the documented increase in seroprevalence in oral contraceptive users[49] is attributable to the oral contraceptive or to failure to use condoms.

Not surprisingly, higher viral load in the infected partner has been demonstrated to increase the risk of transmission.[50–52] Greater viral loads in HIV-infected mothers increase the rate of perinatal transmission.[53–56] In addition, the clade, or subtype, of HIV may also play a role in the sexual transmission of HIV. In a study of the relative tropisms of various clades of HIV for Langerhans cells that line the uterine cervix and the male foreskin, clade E, the predominant subtype of HIV in Thailand, was more infectious than clade B, the subtype most common in the United States.[57] Confirmation of this observation has been elusive, and it remains an open question.[58]

DISEASE RECOGNITION

The symptoms and signs of initial HIV infection are quite nonspecific, as described in studies consisting almost exclusively of men.[59] In a study of female commercial sex workers in Mombasa, Kenya, fever, arthralgia, myalgia, diarrhea, vomiting, and swollen glands were associated with primary HIV infection. The only physical finding that distinguished acute HIV infection from other common infections in these women was lymphadenopathy, particularly in extrainguinal sites. Another feature that distinguished the women with acute HIV infection was the relative severity of these nonspecific symptoms that caused approximately 40% of these impoverished women to stay away from work.[60]

The most common reason that HIV-infected women first seek medical attention is recurrent vaginitis due to *Candida albicans*. In a study of U.S. women in the pre-HAART era, recurrent vaginal yeast infections were the initial complaint that prompted 37% to seek medical care.[61] Lymphadenopathy was the next most common initial manifestation. For 13%, it was bacterial pneumonia, and for 7%, acute retroviral syndrome. Some 7% initially had systemic symptoms, including fever, drenching night sweats, or weight loss. Other "first manifestations" included oral thrush (5%), thrombocytopenic purpura (5%), oral hairy leukoplakia (3%), and multidermatomal herpes zoster (1%).[61]

Since the early symptoms of HIV infection are so nonspecific, health care workers have turned to using risk factor assessments to decide whom to test for HIV. The problem with using risk factors as the sole determinant of whether to test for HIV is that, in women, risk factors are often overlooked or are not known, especially in young women. In 1989, a study was conducted to determine the rate of recognition of HIV infection and associated features in women and men by emergency department personnel. The records of 2102 consecutive patients at least 13 years of age were reviewed and only those patients undergoing venipuncture (excluding patients who had AIDS) were included in the study (N = 856). Discarded blood samples were tested for HIV in a linked, anonymous fashion. HIV infection was recognized by emergency room staff in 13.2% of women and 27.0% of men. Among infected women, doctors recognized HIV infection only in the 25- to 44-year old group, missing both younger and older infected women. HIV infection was recognized in men of all age groups. Risk assessments were recorded less frequently for women (11.2%) than for men (15.9%).[62] The problem of underrecognition of HIV has been overcome somewhat by expanded pregnancy-related testing[63] as per the 1998 recommendation of an Institute of Medicine panel that all willing pregnant women be tested for HIV.[64]

DISEASE PROGRESSION AND MORTALITY

Conflicting evidence has been produced as to whether gender is an isolated factor for disease progression or death. One recent study reports faster disease progression among women than among men,[65] but other studies have not reported gender differences.[66-72] Poorer outcomes for women could be attributable to limited access to health care, lower socioeconomic status, and less social support, all variables demonstrated to affect disease progression and mortality.[73-76] In addition, in socioeconomically disadvantaged women the infection tends to be diagnosed later.[77] Pregnancy probably does not accelerate the course of HIV disease.[78, 79]

Women and adolescent girls with HIV infection are statistically less likely to receive medical services than infected men, including medications, hospital admissions, and outpatient visits.[80-84] Women with asymptomatic HIV infection, even after adjustment for income, race, insurance, and geographic differences between the sexes, are 20% less likely than men to receive zidovudine and 20% less likely than male AIDS patients to be hospitalized for AIDS-related conditions.[83] The Women's Interagency HIV Study (WIHS) evaluated the use of antiretroviral agents

in 2015 HIV-infected women. At the baseline visit (1994 to 1995), 64% reported that they were not taking antiretroviral therapy, including 52% of those with CD4+ cell counts below 200 cells/mm^3.[85]

GYNECOLOGIC MANIFESTATIONS

Gynecologic abnormalities are extremely common among HIV-infected women; at a routine visit performed as part of the HERS study, as many as 63% had at least one such problem.[84] At the time of hospitalization, 83% of HIV-infected women had at least one gynecologic condition, although only 5% were actually admitted for that reason. Several other studies observed gynecologic diseases in HIV-seropositive women to be as high as 42%.[76, 86] Although the infections reported are also common in HIV-negative women, HIV-positive women frequently have recurrent infections that tend to be more severe and are more refractory to treatment than a comparable infection in an immunocompetent woman. Adolescents with HIV will have been infected recently, and their immunosuppression relatively less profound. In addition, immunosuppressed long-term survivors of HIV acquired from perinatal transmission occasionally present in adolescence.[87]

Vaginal Candidiasis

Recurrent vaginal candidiasis, the most common gynecologic infection in HIV-infected women, affects some 7% to 89% of them.[61, 88, 89] Vaginal candidiasis is also the most common initial manifestation of HIV infection in women, its prevalence varying from 24% to 71%.[61, 88-92] In a recent study of 66 HIV-infected women, healthcare providers had failed to recognize recurrent vaginal candidiasis as a potential indicator of HIV, and, for approximately 26% of subjects, diagnosis was delayed, even though these women were at high risk for HIV.[86] Furthermore, because half of these women would have met all criteria for initiation of antiretroviral therapy, the delay in HIV diagnosis may have had a detrimental effect on subsequent prognosis and survival. Factors that predispose to recurrent vaginal candidiasis in immunocompetent women include broad-spectrum antibiotics, corticosteroids, or oral contraceptives; women with underlying HIV infection are at high risk for candidiasis due to their HIV infection alone.[93]

Women with recurrent *Candida* vaginitis often have nearly normal CD4+ lymphocyte counts. As the HIV infection progresses, *Candida* infections of the oropharynx and esophagus become more prevalent, especially when the CD4+ lymphocyte count drops below 50 cells/mm[3].[86] Women with a history of recurrent candidiasis should have a thorough HIV risk assessment and be encouraged to be tested for HIV. Several other factors, including hormonal changes, tight-fitting synthetic clothes, antibiotic use, and diabetes mellitus, can also contribute to recurrent vaginal *Candida* infections.[94]

Candida vaginitis can be treated with either topical antifungal agents (e.g., miconazole, clotrimazole, or terconazole) or with oral fluconazole. Although single-dose fluconazole (150 mg) is approved for the treatment of vaginal candidiasis, immunocompromised women often require a longer course (5 to 7 days) to control the infection.[95] Studies have found that treatment of male sex partners or aggressive attempts to clear the fungus from the gastrointestinal tract do not significantly reduce the incidence of reinfection.[96,97] Fungal prophylaxis to reduce frequent or severe episodes of vaginitis is controversial. The development of resistant *Candida* species with prolonged use of fluconazole is well documented; therefore, prophylaxis of vaginitis with fluconazole should probably be avoided.[98] Since candidiasis occurs even with higher CD4+ cell lymphocyte counts, it is common in HIV-infected adolescents (Reach project, unpublished data).

PELVIC INFLAMMATORY DISEASE

When pelvic inflammatory disease (PID) occurs in HIV-seropositive women, it tends to be more clinically severe.[99] HIV seropositivity rates up to 13.6% have been reported in women admitted to a New York hospital for PID.[99] Both PID and HIV risk are associated with failure to use barrier contraception, early sexual activity, and multiple sex partners. Unlike *Candida* vaginitis, PID may have different clinical signs in women who have intercurrent HIV infection. In immunocompetent women, PID typically presents with marked leukocytosis, pelvic pain, fever, cervical motion tenderness, and an adnexal mass. In immunosuppressed HIV-infected women with PID, abdominal pain and leukocytosis may be far less prominent.[99-102] No obvious differences have been identified in the pathogenes of PID in HIV-positive and HIV-negative women. Lower rates of recovery of *Neisseria gonorrhoeae* and *Chlamydia trachomatis* have

been reported in a small series of 23 HIV-infected patients admitted with PID.[102] The implication of this finding is that endogenous lower genital tract pathogens, such as anaerobes and *Mycoplasma hominis*, which are normally controlled by local immune mechanisms, may play a more prominent role in HIV-infected patients. Also, HIV-infected patients are often taking various antibiotics that may alter cervical culture results.

Studies have reported conflicting results as to whether or not PID in an HIV-infected woman is more likely to require surgery. A study of 349 women who were hospitalized with PID found that the HIV-infected women presented with more severe PID, with a prolonged clinical course and longer duration of fever and hospital stay, and were more likely to require a change in antibiotic therapy.[101] In contrast, a smaller study found that HIV-infected women were less likely to respond to medical therapy (e.g., antibiotic therapy) and were more likely to require surgical intervention (17% in HIV-seropositive women versus 4% for seronegative ones).[102]

CDC/STD Treatment Guidelines recommend that all HIV-infected women with PID be admitted to the hospital for intravenous antibiotic therapy.[103] Regimens used in immunocompetent women can be used in HIV-positive women as well: cefoxitin or cefotetan plus doxycycline or clindamycin plus gentamicin. Although inpatient management is recommended, outpatient treatment with cefoxitin/probenecid or ceftriaxone plus doxycycline or ofloxacin plus metronidazole or clindamycin can be used for certain patients with milder illness (low-grade fever, no nausea or vomiting, and low suspicion for pelvic abscess) for whom careful follow-up can be ensured. These patients must be reexamined within 72 hours to ensure clinical improvement.[103] Clinical care for lower tract gonorrhea and chlamydia is the same for HIV-infected and uninfected persons.

TRICHOMONIASIS AND BACTERIAL VAGINOSIS

Bacterial vaginosis and trichomoniasis are more common in HIV-infected women; *Trichomonas* is identified in 28% of HIV-infected patients, as compared with 16% of HIV-negative ones.[61,92] Use of *Trichomonas* culture (TVPouch) improves sensitivity, but saline wet prep is far more commonly used. Clinical diagnosis of bacterial vaginosis (Amsel criteria) is less specific than microscopic characterization (Nugent criteria).[104] Whether common risk factors are responsible for high rates of intercurrent infection or whether immunosuppression increases the risk of infection or its duration is not known. Initial treatments do not differ between HIV-infected and uninfected persons.

HERPES

Genital infection by Herpes simplex virus type 2 (HSV-2) is relatively common in HIV-infected women. Lesions can persist long and recur frequently or present with an atypical presentation.[105] Serologic studies have estimated that as many as 77% of HIV-positive patients harbor HSV infection[106, 107] though, overall, these prevalence figures are likely to be lower in the adolescent age group. Chronic or recurrent genital herpes may be associated with extensive ulcerative disease in HIV-infected women. As immune dysfunction progresses, patients often experience more prolonged and severe HSV disease. Chronic lesions may become quite large and atypical in appearance, causing significant local erosion. Immunosuppressed persons are also at higher risk for nongenital HSV disease, including pneumonitis, esophagitis, and disseminated skin involvement. In 1987, the CDC diagnostic criteria were revised to include chronic mucocutaneous HSV (ulcers persisting for more than 1 month) and pneumonitis, bronchitis, or esophagitis caused by HSV as AIDS-defining illnesses.[108] Chronic perianal herpes infection serves as the initial AIDS-defining condition in approximately 2% of women.[61, 92] The most common site of recurrent herpetic infection in women is the labia majora, followed by labia minora, sacrum, and anus and buttocks.[109]

Treatment of HSV with antiviral agents like acyclovir can reduce the duration or number of recurrences. The diagnosis is usually based on clinical suspicion, but viral cultures should be used where available and are quite sensitive when fresh lesions are sampled. The yield is lower on lesions that have been present for several days. The use of cultures in the outpatient setting is limited because specimens may become nonviable during transport and, typically, results are not available for several days. A Tzanck smear of an unroofed vesicle showing multinucleate giant cells suggests the diagnosis. HIV-infected persons may require higher than usual doses of antiviral medication to control HSV outbreaks. Acyclovir (400 mg) 3 to 5 times per day, has been found to be useful. Therapy should be continued until clinical resolution of the lesion

occurs. Intravenous acyclovir (5 mg/kg) every 8 hours, may be required in severe cases.[103] Famciclovir is an alternative to acyclovir and has good oral absorption. Although valacyclovir is commonly used to treat HSV infections in immunocompetent patients, its use is discouraged in immunocompromised patients because of a small apparent risk of thrombotic thrombocytopenic purpura and hemolytic uremic syndrome.[110]

Failure to respond to high-dose acyclovir suggests the possibility of acyclovir-resistant HSV. Such strains are also resistant to ganciclovir but may respond to foscarnet. When foscarnet is used to treat acyclovir-resistant HSV, intravenous administration is required. Some patients are unable to tolerate the drug because of a severe "flushed" feeling and paresthesias, and the drug has been associated with renal toxicity and electrolyte abnormalities. Topical use of (S)-1-(3-hydroxy-2-phosphonylmethoxypropyl) cytosine (HPHMPC) cured acyclovir-resistant perineal lesions in one HIV-infected patient.[111]

SYPHILIS

Syphilis is important to recognize in HIV-infected women, since primary or secondary infection may progress more rapidly to neurosyphilis, presumably owing to the immune deficits caused by HIV. Since syphilis and HIV are transmitted in the same manner, and since the presence of syphilis may predispose exposed persons to HIV infection, all women who have either disease should be tested for the other. Serologic profiles related to syphilis are the same in HIV-positive and HIV-negative women at risk, with similar rates of false-positive results (2%) on the rapid plasma reagin test (RPR).[112] Double intramuscular doses of benzathine penicillin (4.8 M units) have been used in immunosuppressed women.[103]

HUMAN PAPILLOMAVIRUS

Human papillomavirus (HPV) is the agent of anogenital warts (condylomata acuminata), most squamous intraepithelial lesions, and nearly all invasive squamous cancers of the anogenital region. Seropositive women have higher rates of HPV infection and are more likely to be symptomatic and to have persistent infection.[113-118] A study of 133 HIV-positive women and 55 HIV-negative ones aged 13 to 19 years participating in the REACH cohort were studied with cervical cytologic examination, cervicovaginal HPV testing by PCR, CD4+ count, and HIV viral load. Use of HAART, other sexually acquired infections, substance use, and smoking were assessed. Most of the HIV infections were acquired through heterosexual contact. When they entered the study, 62% of the women had not yet begun HAART. HPV infection was more prevalent in the HIV-positive women (77%) than in HIV-negative ones (54%) (RR, 1.4, CI 1.1–1.8).[119] These very high rates were detected with a sensitive cell sampling technique, cervicovaginal lavage,[120, 121] and with PCR, which is very sensitive and specific.

As CD4+ cell counts decrease and viral levels increase, women are at greater risk for HPV infection, persistent infection, cervical dysplasia, and neoplasm.[113, 114, 118, 122, 123] Women with CD4+ counts greater than 200/mm³ with an HIV viral load of less than 20,000 copies per milliliter have a lower risk for HPV infection. CD4+ counts less than 200 cells/mm³ with an HIV viral load greater than 20,000 copies per milliliter are associated with increased risk, whereas those whose CD4+ counts less than 200 cells/mm³ are at greatest risk for HPV infection.[123] HPV infection was five times more common in HIV-infected women whose CD4+ counts were below 200 cells/mm³ than it was in women whose CD4+ counts were higher.[114] This may reflect lack of local immunity after recent infection, behavioral risk, and possible direct HIV contributions to the pathogenic process.[124]

Given that HPV is more common with HIV, it follows that the incidence rates of HPV-associated cervical squamous intraepithelial lesions (SIL) and biopsy-confirmed cervical intraepithelial neoplasia (CIN) are higher among HIV-positive women than HIV-negative ones. In the REACH cohort of 13- to 19-year-olds, the young women with normal Pap smears had high HPV prevalence even if they were HIV-negative, demonstrating the very high background rates of infection among sexually active adolescents. Among girls with abnormal Pap smears, HIV-infected youth had higher HPV rates at every level of abnormality than HIV uninfected youth. HPV was more prevalent in high-grade squamous intraepithelial lesions (SIL) than low-grade SIL or atypical cells of undetermined significance (ASCUS) both in HIV-infected and uninfected youth (Fig. 23–3).[119]

The prevalence of CIN is five times greater in seropositive women than in matched seronegative ones. CIN progresses more rapidly in HIV-infected women than in HIV-negative women and recurs more often after primary therapy. During the pre-HAART era, HIV-positive women were significantly more likely than the HIV-negative women to have persistent SIL.[124, 125] As with HPV infection, increased viral load and decreased CD4+ cell counts have been associated with increases in SIL.[122]

Anal cytologic examination and anoscopy should be considered for HIV-positive women, because multisite involvement is common.[126, 127] Odds ratios of anogenital neoplasia range from

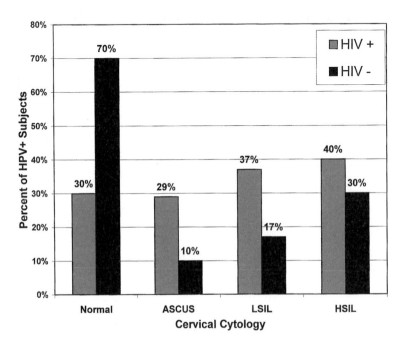

Figure 23–3 Cervical cytology and HIV status among HPV-positive adolescents in the REACH cohort. ASCUS = atypical cells of undetermined significance; LSIL = low-grade squamous intraepithelial lesions; HSIL = high-grade intraepithelial lesions. 1<.001 for difference between cytologic categories (Adapted from Moscicki A, Ellenger J, Vermund S, et al: Prevalence and risks for cervical human papillomavirus infection and squamous intraepithelial lesions in adolescent women: Impact of infection with human immunodeficiency virus. Arch Pediatr Adolesc Med 2000; 18:939–945.)

3.5 to 10 in HIV-positive persons.[127] Anogenital neoplasia rates 9 to 14 times those of matched controls have been reported in female renal transplant patients.[128, 129] Prevalence of HPV anal infection and anal intraepithelial neoplasia are higher in HIV-infected women.[130] A significant increase in reported cases of invasive cervical cancer in HIV-positive women has been noted in New York State[131]; however, it sometimes takes several years for SIL to progress to invasive cancer, and the advent of newer therapies for HIV that are prolonging survival may, paradoxically, increase the risk of progression of SILs to cancer by prolonging life unless the highly active antiretroviral therapies cause SIL to regress.

Cervical cytologic examination is an adequate screening tool for CIN in HIV-positive women, but the high recurrence rate and multifocal nature of the disease reinforce the need for regular screening (at least once a year).[132] Cervical cancer in this population can have an aggressive clinical course with a high recurrence rate and poor response to therapy. Failure rates of 40% after primary therapy have been reported.[133] Surgical therapy is an option that should be considered if the patient is a good candidate, regardless of her HIV status. Radiation and chemotherapy may be used when indicated, but a poor response to radiation therapy and suppressed number and function of T cells may lead to poor outcomes.[134] Since 1993, invasive cervical carcinoma has been an AIDS-defining illness.[135] The clinician should consider offering HIV testing to all younger patients newly diagnosed with cervical cancer. A 19% HIV seropositivity rate was noted in Brooklyn, New York, among women younger than 50 who had cervical cancer.[136]

The current recommendations for Pap smears for HIV-infected women are as follows: all women should have a baseline Pap smear and comprehensive gynecologic examination. If the initial Pap smear results are normal, another Pap smear should be taken after 6 months. If the second examination is normal, then Pap smears should be repeated annually.[103] For women who have a CD4+ cell count below 200 cells/mm³ or a history of HPV, continued semiannual exams should be seriously considered. If the initial Pap smear shows inflammation with reactive squamous cellular changes, any identified cause (e.g., *Trichomonas*) should be treated and the Pap smear repeated after 3 months. If the initial Pap smear shows dysplastic changes or ASCUS, the patient should be referred for colposcopy.

MENSTRUATION

Although gynecologic abnormalities occur with HIV infection, HIV-infected women do not seem very different from uninfected women of similar age and social backgrounds. One study evaluated the potential effect of HIV infection on the duration of the menstrual cycle.[137] In data on the menstrual cycles from more than 1000 women, 802 of them HIV-positive, HIV infection had little effect on the duration of cycles. Women with fewer than 200 CD4+ cells/mm³ had a tendency to have longer cycles (more than 40 days), but age, ethnicity, and body mass index play far more important roles in the determination of cycle length.

OTHER OPPORTUNISTIC INFECTIONS AND MALIGNANCIES

It is unusual to see opportunistic infections (OIs) or malignancies in adolescents. Since they have been infected recently, they tend to have higher CD4+ cell counts, though children with hemophilia (nearly all male) and long-term survivors of perinatally acquired infection (half female) may reach adolescence with substantial immunodeficiency. We may anticipate more such patients in the near future, given the fact that surviving infants infected in the 1980s and early 1990s are aging into adolescence in the early 21st century. Only three clinical case series of HIV-infected adolescents have been published. In New Orleans, Louisiana, 92 young women ages 13 to 21 were studied.[138] At least one STD was diagnosed in 75% of adolescent women, and SILs were seen in 55% on at least one Pap smear. As among adults, opportunistic infections (OIs) were seen when CD4+ cells dropped below 200/mm³. HIV disease progression was associated with oral and dermatologic manifestations, oral hairy leukoplakia, thrush, and herpes zoster. In New York City, 17 young women ages 13 to 21 were reported.[139] STDs were also very common: 88% had or had had salpingitis and 76% reported multiple STDs. In a relatively short follow-up, 41% of females had a newly acquired STD after HIV diagnosis. OIs among females were not reported separately from males; thrush, fevers, sepsis, pneumonia, and generalized lymphadenopathy were seen in the 13 patients—male and female—whose CD4+ counts were under 200/mm³. The final case series is by far the largest; 258 HIV-infected females are currently being studied at 16 clinical sites in 13 U.S. cities (Table 23–1).[119, 140] Details of the Reaching for Excellence in Adolescent Care and Health (REACH) Project in the Adolescent Medicine HIV/AIDS Research Network as well

Table 23–1. Characteristics of the REACH Cohort

	HIV Positive n = 138	HIV Negative n = 59
Mean age (SD)	16.8 (1.2)°	16.3 (1.3)°
	N (%)	*N (%)*
Race: African American	104 (75.9)	40 (67.8)
Age of 1st consenting vaginal sex ≤12 years	28 (25.9)	9 (20)
No. of lifetime sexual partners		
0–4	42 (31.6)	23 (41.8)
5–10	47 (35.3)	20 (36.4)
>10	44 (33.1)	12 (21.8)
Last intercourse unprotected	48 (36.9)†	30 (54.6)†
Smokes ≥20 cigarettes per day	12 (9.2)	4 (7.8)
Currently on hormonal therapy	53 (38.7)	24 (40.7)
Currently pregnant	8 (5.8)	1 (1.8)
C. trachomatis and/or *N. gonorrhoeae* infection	27 (19.7)	8 (14.0)
Bacterial vaginosis	19 (15.8)	8 (14.8)
Dropped out of school	35 (35.6)	8 (13.6)
Viral load (NASBA)		
<400	25 (18.4)	
400–9999	67 (49.3)	
10,000–50,000	28 (20.6)	
>50,000	16 (11.7)	
CD4+ cell counts		
>500	68 (50.0)	
200–499	59 (43.4)	
<200	9 (6.6)	
Current antiretroviral therapy use:		
No therapy	86 (62.3)	
Therapy without PI	36 (26.1)	
Therapy with PI	16 (11.6)	

°$p < 0.005$.
†$p < .05$.
In calculating percentages, denominators vary due to missing values.
Adapted from Douglas SD, Rudy B, Muenz L, et al: Peripheral blood mononuclear cell markers in antiretroviral therapy—naive HIV infected and high-risk seronegative adolescents. Adolescent Medicine HIV/AIDS Research Network. AIDS 1999; 13:1629–1635.

as clinic care (Project Treat) and adolescent outreach programs (Project Access) are available from us (SHV). It is anticipated that data on reproductive system and opportunistic infections and neoplasms in HIV-infected adolescents will be forthcoming from this relatively large cohort.

Pneumocystis carinii pneumonia remains the most common AIDS-defining opportunistic infection among both men and women (prevalence 35.7% and 33.7% respectively in 1998). Men are more likely to present with Kaposi's sarcoma (KS), extrapulmonary cryptococcosis, and cytomegalovirus (CMV) disease, whereas women are more likely to present with esophageal candidiasis, recurrent pneumonia, pulmonary tuberculosis, and chronic herpes simplex. Overall, the incidences of KS, CMV disease, and extrapulmonary cryptococcosis are higher in males than in females, but, among IDUs and persons exposed to HIV through heterosexual contact, women actually have higher OI risks.[141] Overall, the incidences of pulmonary tuberculosis, chronic her-

pes simplex disease, and extrapulmonary tuberculosis were higher in females than in males; however, among IDUs, extrapulmonary tuberculosis was more prevalent in males than in females.[141] The HHV-8, the agent of KS, seems to circulate in higher concentrations among men than among women.[142, 143]

PSYCHOSOCIAL ISSUES

Adolescent women are especially vulnerable to contracting HIV.[76, 144, 145] Complex economic and social factors, along with the persistence of the gender power imbalance, all contribute to this vulnerability.[146] The same factors impede their access to care. Adolescents' economic dependence often interferes with their obtaining appropriate housing, nutrition, physical protection, and medical care.[76, 145, 147] Young women are also often isolated and stigmatized in their own communities as a result of their HIV status. Con-

Table 23–2. Approved Antiretroviral HIV Drugs[149]

Drug Name	Trade Name
Zidovudine (AZT, ZDU)	Retrovir
Didanosine (ddI)	Videx
Zalcitabine (ddC)°	Hivid
Stavudine (d4T)	Zerit
Lamivudine (3TC)	Epivir
Saquinavir (hard gelatin capsule)°	Invirase
Ritonavir	Norvir
Indinavir°	Crixivan
Nevirapine	Viramune
Nelfinavir	Viracept
Delavirdine°	Rescriptor
Zidovudine and Lamivudine°	Combivir
Saquinavir (soft gelatin capsule)°	Fortovase
Sustiva	Efavirenz
Ziagen	Bacavir
Agenerase	Amprenavir

°No pediatric labeling was available as of October 1, 1999.
From Food and Drug Administration. Antiretroviral HIV Drug Approvals and Pediatric Labeling Information. www.foa.gov/htm.

fidentiality is a major concern for many women, especially in smaller rural communities, because the social consequences of the disclosure of status can have a profound impact. An important report from the U.S. Surgeon General on services for adolescents with HIV disease is available as a resource guide.[148]

Psychosocial issues significantly complicate the provision of care to many HIV-infected girls. Much effort must be spent addressing the basic needs of housing, nutrition, personal safety, and child care, particularly for homeless or runaway youth.[148]

TREATMENT OF HIV

As of April 16, 1999, 16 drug products (14 drug substances) were approved by the U.S. Food and Drug Administration (FDA) for the treatment of HIV infection.[149] Eight drug products have pediatric information in the approved product labeling (Table 23–2). The 16 products are of three drug families:

- Nucleoside reverse transcriptase inhibitors (NRTIs)
- Nonnucleoside reverse transcriptase inhibitors (NNRTIs)
- Protease inhibitors (PIs)

Adult guidelines for antiretroviral therapy are appropriate for postpubertal adolescents, because the clinical course of HIV infection in

adolescents infected sexually or (rarely) through IDU is more like that of adults than that of children.[150] Medications for HIV infection and opportunistic infections should be prescribed according to Tanner staging of puberty, not on the basis of age.[151] Dosing for adolescents in early puberty (i.e., Tanner stage I or II) should follow pediatric schedules, whereas for those in late puberty (i.e., Tanner stage V), it should follow adult schedules. Youths in the growth spurt for girls Tanner stage III and for boys stage IV should be closely monitored for medication efficacy and toxicity when using adult or pediatric dosing guidelines.[152, 153] Assessment of blood drug levels is now feasible at many centers.

Puberty is a time of somatic growth and sex differentiation, when females develop more body fat and males more muscle mass. While, theoretically, these physiologic changes could affect pharmacokinetics (especially for drugs with a narrow therapeutic index that are used in combination with protein-bound medicines or hepatic enzyme inducers or inhibitors), no clinically consequential difference between adolescents and adults has been observed.[154] Clinical experience with protease inhibitors and nonnucleoside reverse transcriptase inhibitor antiretroviral drugs is more limited.

The current standard of care for HIV is HAART, a combination of drugs from at least two of the three drug families, including at least one PI. The US Department of Health and Human Resources recommendations for treatment of established HIV infection can be seen in Table 23–3. Ideally, antiretroviral therapy should maxi-

Table 23–3. Suggested Antiretroviral Regimen for HIV-Infected Adolescents: 1999*[150]

Column A	Column B
Indinavir	ZDV + ddl
Nelfinavir	d4T + ddl
Ritonavir	ZDV + ddC
Saquinavir-SGC°	ZDV + 3TC
Ritonavir + Saquinavir-SGC or Saquinavir-HGC+	d4T + 3TC

SGC = soft gel capsule; HGC = hard gel capsule.
°One choice each from column A and column B. Drugs are listed in random order. Combinations of drugs less likely to provide sustained virus suppression:
    1 NNRTI (Nevirapine) + 2 NRTIs (column B)
    Saquinavir-HGC + 2 NRTIs (column B)
Not recommended:
    Monotherapies
    Dual therapies (e.g., 2 NRTIs).
From Guidelines for the use of antiretroviral agents in HIV-infected adults and adolescents. Department of Health and Human Services and Henry J. Kaiser Family Foundation. MMWR 1998; 47:43–82.

Table 23–4. Risks and Benefits of Early Institution of Antiretroviral Therapy in Asymptomatic HIV-Infected Patients[150]

Potential benefits
  Control of viral replication and mutation; reduction of viral burden
  Prevention of progressive immunodeficiency; potential maintenance or reconstitution of a normal immune system
  Delayed progression to AIDS and prolongation of life; decreased risk of selecting resistant virus
  Decreased risk of drug toxicity
Potential risks
  Reduction in quality of life from adverse drug effects and inconvenience of current maximally suppressive regimens
  Earlier development of drug resistance
  Limitation in future choices of antiretroviral agents secondary to development of resistance
  Unknown long-term toxicity of antiretroviral drugs
  Unknown duration of effectiveness of current antiretroviral therapies

From Guidelines for the use of antiretroviral agents in HIV-infected adults and adolescents. Department of Health and Human Services and Henry J. Kaiser Family Foundation. MMWR 1998; 47:43–82.

mally suppress viral replication below levels capable of being detected with HIV RNA assays.

Opinions differ on the correct time to initiate therapy for asymptomatic adolescents. Adolescents are likely to be more recently infected, so the efficacy of HAART is reinforced by a less compromised immune system.[155] In addition, preliminary evidence in a cohort being studied by clinicians in REACH suggests that adolescents may have a greater capacity than adults for immune reconstruction because of persistent thymic tissue.[155] Finally, because teens may be early in the infection process, they may harbor fewer resistant viruses, and thus respond better to treatment. Early institution of therapy is not without potential risks, especially selection for drug-resistant HIV in adolescents who do not comply strictly with the medication schedule (Table 23–4). The U.S. Department of Health and Human Services, in its Guidelines for the use of antiretroviral agents in HIV-infected adults and adolescents, published information based on CD4+ count and HIV RNA levels to help clinicians determine when best to institute treatment.[156] Table 23–5 reflects the current lack of consensus among leading clinicians on this matter.

Symptomatic adolescents should receive maximally suppressive regimens of HAART. Overlapping drug toxicities and drug interactions are compounded by the greater number of drugs required for advanced HIV disease. Initiation of therapy for advanced-stage disease may be postponed because of clinical considerations related to treatment of an acute illness. Once patients are being maintained on an antiretroviral regimen, however, they should not discontinue therapy during an acute opportunistic infection or malignancy, except in cases of drug toxicity, intolerance, or interactions.

Young women with HIV who present during pregnancy should have their immune status assessed in the same way as other adolescents.[156] The treatment goals are to maintain the health of the mother-to-be and to prevent perinatal transmission. In a 1998 report, a panel of the Institute of Medicine recommended testing all pregnant woman.[64] In addition, a course of HAART (or at least zidovudine [AZT] if HAART is not tolerated) should be administered to prevent perinatal transmission. Until 1998, AZT was the only antiretroviral shown to be effective in preventing perinatal HIV. Recent study has demonstrated that nevirapine, combination therapies,

Table 23–5. Indications for the Institution of Antiretroviral Therapy in the HIV-Infected Patient

Clinical Category	CD4+ T Cell Count and HIV RNA	Recommendation
Symptomatic	Any value	Treat
Asymptomatic	CD4+ T cells <500/mm³ or Strength of HIV RNA >10,000 (bDNA) or >20,000 (RT-PCR)	Treatment should be offered. Recommendation is based on prognosis for disease-free survival and patient willingness to accept therapy.°
Asymptomatic	CD4+ T cells >500/mm³; HIV RNA <10,000 (bDNA) or <20,000 (RT-PCR)	Many experts would delay therapy and observe; some would treat.

°Some experts would observe patients whose CD4+ T cell counts are between 350 and 500/mm³ and HIV RNA levels <10,000 (bDNA) or <20,000 (RT-PCR).
Adapted from Guidelines for the use of antiretroviral agents in HIV-infected adults and adolescents. MMWR 1998; 47:1–31.

and a short course of AZT also have the potential to prevent perinatal transmission.[157–161] Efavirenz and indinavir are not recommended during pregnancy.

Consensus recommendations have been developed using plasma HIV RNA measurements to guide changes in antiretroviral therapy for HIV-infected adults and adolescents. For adults, they recommend that health care providers consider changing therapy:

1. If the HIV RNA level drops less than three-fold (0.5 log 10) after 4 weeks of therapy and less than 10-fold (1.0 log 10) after 8 weeks of therapy

                    or

2. If HIV RNA has not decreased to undetectable levels after 4 to 6 months of therapy.

ADHERENCE

After any discussion of therapeutic regimens, one point is critical. Antiretrovirals work only when taken properly. Adherence to complex, multiple-antiretroviral therapy is particularly problematic, so a simple regimen should be used—one that has few pills, small pills, few (and flexible) dosing times per day, and no dietary or intake requirements or restrictions. An invaluable guide for helping HIV-infected adolescents to adhere to antiretroviral therapy was published in 1999.[162]

HIV-infected adolescents have particular compliance problems. Comprehensive systems of care are required to serve both their medical and psychosocial needs, because they are frequently inexperienced with health care systems. Many HIV-infected adolescents face challenges in adhering to medical regimens for psychosocial reasons that have little to do with the biomedical side effects of the drugs. These include denial and fear of their HIV infection; misinformation; mistrust of the medical establishment; fear and skepticism about the effectiveness of medications; low self-esteem; unstructured and chaotic lifestyles; and frequently a lack of familial and social support. Treatment regimens for adolescents must balance the goal of prescribing a maximally potent antiretroviral regimen with realistic assessment of existing and potential support systems to promote compliance. It is especially common for adolescents to avoid colposcopy, and many centers have made it possible for gynecologists to go to adolescent HIV clinics to offer one-stop care.

Developmental issues make caring for adolescents unique. Their approach to illness is often different from adults. The thought processes of adolescents make it difficult for them to take medications when they are asymptomatic, particularly medications that have side effects. Adherence with complex regimens is particularly challenging at a time when adolescents do not want to be different from their peers. Greater challenges face adolescents who live with parents to whom they have not yet disclosed their HIV status, or who are homeless or whose transience results in the lack of a stable place to store medicine.

Failure to comply with prescribed regimens and subtherapeutic levels of antiretroviral medications may promote the development of drug resistance. Data indicate that the development of resistance to one of the available PIs reduces susceptibility to all of the other available PI drugs and, thus, substantially reduces the treatment options. This also applies to NNRTIs and, to a lesser extent, NRTIs. Therefore, infected adolescents and their caregivers must be educated when therapy is instituted in the importance of compliance with the prescribed regimen and the lessons should be reinforced at subsequent visits. Many strategies can be used to promote compliance, including intensive patient education over several visits before therapy is instituted, cues and reminders for administering drugs, a patient-focused treatment plan that accommodates the patient's particular needs, and mobilization of social and community support services.

PREVENTION, INTERVENTION, AND RISK REDUCTION

Knowing about preventive behaviors and the importance of practicing them is critical for each and every generation of young women. Prevention programs should be comprehensive, and parents and the educational system should participate. Community-based programs must reach out-of-school youths in such settings as detention centers and shelters for runaways. Programs should address the intersection of drug use and sexual HIV transmission; develop and widely disseminate effective female-controlled preventive methods[163]; and improve adolescents' access to medical services, including STD services. Adequate time must be spent in the clinical setting to fully develop a trusting clinician–patient relationship.

Research has shown that early, clear communication between parents and young people about sex is important in helping adolescents to adopt and maintain protective sexual behaviors. Parents need to discuss condom use before their adolescent's first intercourse. Condom use increased only among teens whose mother talked to them before first intercourse: they were three times more likely to use a condom than those whose parent had never discussed condoms or discussed them after the first act of intercourse. Teens who use condoms at first intercourse are 20 times more likely to use them in subsequent acts.[164]

School-based programs are important for reaching youths before dangerous behaviors have been established. Research has clearly shown that the most effective programs are comprehensive ones that promote delaying sexual behavior and provide information on how sexually active young people can protect themselves. Making condoms available in high schools has been very controversial and has produced mixed results. Several studies have been published on this topic, and they all agreed that making condoms available in schools did not increase sexual activity among teens.[165–168] The studies are evenly divided on whether making condoms available increased their *use*. The largest of the studies, the only one to collect baseline data and adequate comparison groups, found no difference in condom use.[165]

Young adults are also at risk for HIV from IDU. Currently, there is a ban on federal support for needle-exchange programs in the United States, even though six separate government-sponsored reports have concluded that such programs help to reduce HIV infection and do not increase drug use.[169] IDU is not common in the adolescent group; however, alcohol, marijuana, and occasionally crack cocaine are risks because they disinhibit sexual activity.

Whether the prevention is centered in the home, school, or community, the message should be a balance of abstinence and condom use. Condoms need to be made more accessible and their use and purchase more socially acceptable. Prevention education needs to be provided in the context of broader services, including housing, social services, general education, employment, and other holistic approaches. Finally, societal misconceptions about the impact of making condoms available to teens and implementing needle-exchange programs must be addressed if these programs are ever to see widespread use.

IMPLICATIONS FOR PREVENTION

Looking at changes in HIV prevalence over time can provide an indication of the impact of prevention efforts. Referring again to U.S. Job Corps study of economically and educationally disadvantaged youth discussed in the introduction to this chapter, researchers found that, from the beginning of the study period to the end, HIV prevalence among young people in the Job Corps was cut in half. HIV prevalence among women dropped from 4 per 1000 in 1990 to 2 per 1000 in 1996, and among men dropped from 3 per 1000 in 1990 to 1.5 per 1000 in 1996. These and other data suggest that HIV prevention has contributed to significant slowing of the spread of the HIV epidemic in the United States. International successes include Uganda and Thailand. Both nations have reported declining HIV incidence and prevalence among adolescents and young adults as a consequence of prevention activities.

Comprehensive HIV prevention efforts for young people must be sustained and must include programs targeted to those who are neither in school nor at work. Several community-based programs for disadvantaged inner-city young people have been found effective in reducing risk behaviors. It is critical that effective approaches be replicated more widely, particularly in areas of high HIV prevalence among young people. Despite signs of success, much remains to be done to reduce the toll of the epidemic among our nation's youngest and most vulnerable populations. Clinicians can optimize medical HIV-prevention efforts with adolescent girls by forming caring and appropriate relationships based on an understanding of adolescent development relative to needs for HIV education. HIV prevention should be a part of regular clinical care for adolescent females and should be integrated into history taking and ongoing health counseling. Skilled clinicians can support teenage girls in the process of making informed choices about their personal behaviors.

REFERENCES

1. Centers for Disease Control and Prevention: National Vital Statistics Report. 1999; 47(16).
2. Centers for Disease Control and Prevention: HIV/AIDS Surveillance Report. 1998; 10(2).
3. Centers for Disease Control and Prevention: HIV/AIDS Surveillance Report. 1993; 5(4).
4. Centers for Disease Control and Prevention: HIV/AIDS Surveillance Report. 1994; 6(2).
5. Centers for Disease Control and Prevention: HIV/AIDS Surveillance Report. 1995; 7(2).
6. Centers for Disease Control and Prevention: HIV/AIDS Surveillance Report. 1996; 8(2).
7. Centers for Disease Control and Prevention: HIV/AIDS Surveillance Report. 1997; 9(2).
8. Rosenberg PS, Biggar RJ: Trends in HIV incidence

among young adults in the United States. JAMA 1998; 279:1894–1899.

9. Centers for Disease Control and Prevention: Diagnosis and reporting of HIV and AIDS with integrated HIV and AIDS surveillance—United States. MMWR 1998; 47(15):309–314.

10. Valleroy LA, MacKellar DA, Karon JM, et al: HIV infection in disadvantaged out-of-school youth: Prevalence for U.S. Job Corps entrants, 1990 through 1996. J Acquir Immune Defic Syndr Hum Retrovirol 1998; 19:67–73.

11. Centers for Disease Control and Prevention: Division of STD Prevention. Sexually Transmitted Disease. Surveillance Report. 1998;

12. Department of Health and Human Services, Centers for Disease Control and Prevention: HIV/AIDS Surveillance Supplemental Report. 1999; 5(1).

13. Institute of Medicine (U.S.): Committee on Prevention and Control of Sexually Transmitted Diseases. The hidden epidemic: Confronting sexually transmitted diseases. In Eng TR, Butler WT (eds): Washington: National Academy Press, 1997, pp xii, 432.

14. AMA Guidelines for Adolescent Preventive Services (GAPS) Recommendations and Rationale. In Retford D (ed): Baltimore: Williams & Wilkins; 1994.

15. Miller KS, Clark LF, Moore JS: Sexual initiation with older male partners and subsequent HIV risk behavior among female adolescents. Fam Plann Perspect 1997; 29:212–214.

16. Rotheram-Borus M, Jemmott L, Jemmott J: Preventing AIDS in female adolescents. In O'Leary A, Jemmott L (eds): Women at Risk: Issues in the Primary Prevention of AIDS. New York: Plenum, 1995; pp 103–109.

17. Kann L, Kinchen SA, Williams BI, et al: Youth risk behavior surveillance—United States, 1997. MMWR 1998; 47:1–89.

18. Centers for Disease Control and Prevention: Health risk behaviors among adolescents who do and do not attend school—United States, 1992. MMWR 1997; 43(08); 192–132.

19. Centers for Disease Control and Prevention: Trends in HIV-related sexual risk behaviors among high school students-selected US cities, 1991–1997. MMWR 1999; 48:440–443.

20. Centers for Disease Control and Prevention: Trends in HIV-related sexual risk behaviors among high school students-selected US cities, 1991–1997. MMWR 1998; 47:749–752.

21. Abma JC, Chandra A, Mosher WD, et al: Fertility, family planning, and women's health: New data from the 1995 National Survey of Family Growth. Vital Health Stat 1997; 23:1–114.

22. Stoyanoff SR, Weber MD, Gatson B, et al: Factors associated with unprotected vaginal intercourse among minority, heterosexual females 12–24 years of age attending a community-based health center in Los Angeles. Natl Conf Women HIV 1997; 142:4.

23. Centers for Disease Control and Prevention: HIV prevention through early detection and treatment of other sexually transmitted diseases—United States. 1998; 47:1–24.

24. Aval SO, Schaffer JE, Mosher WD, et al: Gonorrhea rates: what denominator is most appropriate? Am J Public Health 1988; 78:702–703.

25. Bouvet E, De Vincenzi I, Ancelle R, Vachon F: Defloration as risk factor for heterosexual HIV transmission (Letter). Lancet 1989; 1:615.

26. Lehner T, Hussain L, Wilson J, Chapman M: Mucosal transmission of HIV (Letter; Comment) Nature 1991; 353:709.

27. Fleming DT, Wasserheit JN: From epidemiological synergy to public health policy and practice: The contribution of other sexually transmitted diseases to sexual transmission of HIV infection. Sex Transm Infect 1999; 75:3–17.

28. Schwarz SK, Bolan GA, Fullilove M, et al: Crack cocaine and the exchange of sex for money or drugs. Risk factors for gonorrhea among black adolescents in San Francisco. Sex Transm Dis 1992; 19:7–13.

29. Wasserheit JN: Epidemiological synergy: Interrelationships between human immunodeficiency virus infection and other sexually transmitted diseases. Sex Transm Dis 1992; 19:61–77.

30. Grosskurth H, Mosha F, Todd J, et al: Impact of improved treatment of sexually transmitted diseases on HIV infection in rural Tanzania: Randomised controlled trial (see Comments). Lancet 1995; 346:530–536.

31. Levine WC, Pope V, Bhoomkar A, et al: Increase in endocervical CD4 lymphocytes among women with nonulcerative sexually transmitted diseases. J Infect Dis 1998; 177:167–174.

32. Spear GT, Sha BE, Saarloos MN, et al: Chemokines are present in the genital tract of HIV-seropositive and HIV-seronegative women: Correlation with other immune mediators. J Acquir Immune Defic Syndr Hum Retrovirol 1998; 18:454–459.

33. Cohen MS, Miller WC: Sexually transmitted diseases and human immunodeficiency virus infection: Cause, effect, or both? (Editorial; Comment). Int J Infect Dis 1998, 3:1–4.

34. Cohen M: Natural history of HIV infection in women. Obstet Gynecol Clin North Am 1997; 24:743–758.

35. Cohen MS, Hoffman IF, Royce RA, et al: Reduction of concentration of HIV-1 in semen after treatment of urethritis: Implications for prevention of sexual transmission of HIV-1. AIDSCAP Malawi Research Group. Lancet 1997; 349:1868–1873.

36. Lazzarin A, Saracco A, Musicco M, Nicolosi A: Man-to-woman sexual transmission of the human immunodeficiency virus. Risk factors related to sexual behavior, man's infectiousness, and woman's susceptibility. Italian Study Group on HIV Heterosexual Transmission (Published erratum appears in Arch Intern Med 1992 Apr; 152[4]:876). Arch Intern Med 1991; 151:2411–2416.

37. Vogt MW, Witt DJ, Craven DE, et al: Isolation patterns of the human immunodeficiency virus from cervical secretions during the menstrual cycle of women at risk for the acquired immunodeficiency syndrome. Ann Intern Med 1987; 106:380–382.

38. Murphy SM: Rape, sexually transmitted diseases and human immunodeficiency virus infection ([Editorial]; [see Comments]). Int J STD AIDS 1990; 1:79–82.

39. Irwin KL, Edlin BR, Wong L, et al: Urban rape survivors: Characteristics and prevalence of human immunodeficiency virus and other sexually transmitted infections. Multicenter Crack Cocaine and HIV Infection Study Team. Obstet Gynecol 1995; 85:330–336.

40. Glaser JB, Hammerschlag MR, McCormack WM: Epidemiology of sexually transmitted diseases in rape victims. Rev Infect Dis 1989; 11:246–254.

41. Vermund SH, Alexander-Rodriguez T, Macleod S, et al: History of sexual abuse in incarcerated adolescents with gonorrhea or syphilis (Published erratum appears in J Adolesc Health Care 1991 Mar; 12[2]:214). J Adolesc Health Care 1990; 11:449–452.

42. Zierler S, Feingold L, Laufer D, et al: Adult survivors of childhood sexual abuse and subsequent risk of HIV infection. Am J Public Health 1991; 81:572–575.

43. Padian N, Marquis L, Francis DP, et al: Male-to-female

transmission of human immunodeficiency virus. JAMA 1987; 258:788–790.

44. Royce RA, Sena A, Cates W Jr, Cohen MS: Sexual transmission of HIV (Published Erratum appears in N Engl J Med 1997; 11:337[11]:799). N Engl J Med 1997; 336:1072–1078.

45. Risk factors for male to female transmission of HIV. European Study Group. Br Med J 1989; 298:411–415.

46. Henin Y, Mandelbrot L, Henrion R, et al: Virus excretion in the cervicovaginal secretions of pregnant and nonpregnant HIV-infected women (see Comments). J Acquir Immune Defic Syndr 1993; 6:72–75.

47. Baulieu EE, Benagiano G, Brosens I, et al: Sexual behavior, contraception and the risk of contracting HIV. Int J Gynaecol Obstet 1993; 40:101–103.

48. Patterson BK, Landay A, Andersson J, et al: Repertoire of chemokine receptor expression in the female genital tract: Implications for human immunodeficiency virus transmission. Am J Pathol 1998; 153:481–490.

49. Wang CC, Kreiss JK, Reilly M: Risk of HIV infection in oral contraceptive pill users: A meta-analysis. J Acquir Immune Defic Syndr 1999; 21:51–58.

50. Operskalski EA, Stram DO, Busch MP, et al: Role of viral load in heterosexual transmission of human immunodeficiency virus type 1 by blood transfusion recipients. Transfusion Safety Study Group. Am J Epidemiol 1997; 146:655–661.

51. Pedraza MA, del Romero J, Roldan F, et al: Heterosexual transmission of HIV-1 is associated with high plasma viral load levels and a positive viral isolation in the infected partner. J Acquir Immune Defic Syndr 1999; 21:120–125.

52. Ragni MV, Faruki H, Kingsley LA: Heterosexual HIV-1 transmission and viral load in hemophilic patients. J Acquir Immune Defic Syndr Hum Retrovirol 1998; 17:42–45.

53. Garcia PM, Kalish LA, Pitt J, et al: Maternal levels of plasma human immunodeficiency virus type 1 RNA and the risk of perinatal transmission. Women and Infants Transmission Study Group (Comments). N Engl J Med 1999; 341:394–402.

54. Mofenson LM, Lambert JS, Stiehm ER, et al: Risk factors for perinatal transmission of human immunodeficiency virus type 1 in women treated with zidovudine. Pediatric AIDS Clinical Trials Group Study 185 Team (Comments) N Engl J Med 1999; 341:385–393.

55. Mazza C, Ravaggi A, Rodella A, et al: Influence of maternal CD4 levels on the predictive value of virus load over mother-to-child transmission of human immunodeficiency, virus type 1 (HIV-1). Study Group for Vertical Transmission. J Med Virol 1999; 58:59–62.

56. Shaffer N, Roongpisuthipong A, Siriwasin W, et al: Maternal virus load and perinatal human immunodeficiency virus type 1 subtype E transmission, Thailand. Bangkok Collaborative Perinatal HIV Transmission Study Group. J Infect Dis 1999; 179:590–599.

57. Soto-Ramirez LE, Renjifo B, McLane MF, et al: HIV-1 Langerhans' cell tropism associated with heterosexual transmission of HIV (see Comments). Science 1996; 271:1291–1293.

58. Hu DJ, Buve A, Baggs J, et al: What role does HIV-1 subtype play in transmission and pathogenesis? An epidemiological perspective (editorial). AIDS 1999; 13:873–881.

59. Daar ES, Bai J, Hausner MA, et al: Acute HIV syndrome after discontinuation of antiretroviral therapy in a patient treated before seroconversion. Ann Intern Med 1998; 128:827–829.

60. Lavreys L, Martin H, Manoaliya K, et al: Primary HIV-1 infection: Clinical manifestations among women in Mombasa, Kenya. Int Conf AIDS (Abstract no. 333/12186) 1998; 12:48.

61. Carpenter CC, Mayer KH, Stein MD, et al: Human immunodeficiency virus infection in North American women: Experience with 200 cases and a review of the literature. Medicine (Baltimore) 1991; 70:307–325.

62. Schoenbaum EE, Webber MP: The underrecognition of HIV infection in women in an inner-city emergency room. Am J Public Health 1993; 83:363–368.

63. Fiscus SA, Adimora AA, Schoenbach VJ, et al: Trends in human immunodeficiency virus (HIV) counseling, testing, and antiretroviral treatment of HIV-infected women and perinatal transmission in North Carolina. J Infect Dis 1999; 180:99–105.

64. Reducing the Odds: Preventing Perinatal Transmission of HIV in the United States. In Soto M, Alamario D, McCormick M (eds): Committee on Perinatal Transmission of HIV, Institute of Medicine. National Academy Press, 1999, p 416.

65. Farzadegan H, Hoover DR, Astemborski J, et al: Sex differences in HIV-1 viral load and progression to AIDS (see Comments). Lancet 1998; 352:1510–1504.

66. Ellerbrock TV, Bush TJ, Chamberland ME, Oxtoby MJ: Epidemiology of women with AIDS in the United States, 1981 through 1990. A comparison with heterosexual men with AIDS. JAMA 1991; 265:2971–2975.

67. Moroni M: Sex differences in HIV-1 viral load and progression to AIDS. ICONA Study Group. Italian cohort of HIV-1 positive individuals (Letter; Comment). Lancet 1999; 353:589–590.

68. Selwyn PA, Alcabes P, Hartel D, et al: Clinical manifestations and predictors of disease progression in drug users with human immunodeficiency virus infection N Engl J Med (Published erratum appears in N Engl J Med 1993; 328[9]:671). 1992; 327:1697–1703.

69. Ronald PJ, Robertson JR, Elton RA: Continued drug use and other cofactors for progression to AIDS among injecting drug users. AIDS 1994; 8:339–343.

70. Hanson DL, Horsburgh CR Jr, Fann SA, et al: Survival prognosis of HIV-infected patients. J Acquir Immune Defic Syndr 1993; 6:624–629.

71. Junghans C, Ledergerber B, Chan P, et al: Sex differences in HIV-1 viral load and progression to AIDS. Lancet 1999; 353:589.

72. Chaisson RE, Keruly JC, Moore RD: Race, sex, drug use, and progression of human immunodeficiency virus disease (see Comments). N Engl J Med 1995; 333:751–756.

73. Bastian L, Bennett CL, Adams J, et al: Differences between men and women with HIV-related *Pneumocystis carinii* pneumonia: Experience from 3,070 cases in New York City in 1987. J Acquir Immune Defic Syndr 1993; 6:617–623.

74. Phillips AN, Antunes F, Stergious G, et al: A sex comparison of rates of new AIDS-defining disease and death in 2554 AIDS cases. AIDS in Europe Study Group. AIDS 1994; 8:831–835.

75. Moore RD, Hidalgo J, Sugland BW, Chaisson RE: Zidovudine and the natural history of the acquired immunodeficiency syndrome (see Comments). N Engl J Med 1991; 324:1412–1416.

76. Hankins CA, Handley MA: HIV disease and AIDS in women: Current knowledge and a research agenda. J Acquir Immune Defic Syndr 1992; 5:957–971.

77. Anastos K, Greenblatt R: Clinical update: HIV in women: Epidemiology and natural history. HIV: Advances in Research and Therapy, 1994; pp 11–20.

78. Tuomala RE, Kalish LA, Zorilla C, et al: Changes in

total, CD4+, and CD8+ lymphocytes during pregnancy and 1 year postpartum in human immunodeficiency virus–infected women. The Women and Infants Transmission Study. Obstet Gynecol 1997; 89:967–974.

79. Vermund SH, Galbraith MA, Ebner SC, et al: Human immunodeficiency virus/acquired immunodeficiency syndrome in pregnant women. Ann Epidemiol 1992; 2:773–803. (Published erratum appears in Ann Epidemiol 1993 3[6]:653.)

80. Turner BJ, Markson LE, McKee LJ, et al: Health care delivery, zidovudine use, and survival of women and men with AIDS. J Acquir Immune Defic Syndr 1994; 7:1250–1262.

81. Stein MD, Piette J, Mor V, et al: Differences in access to zidovudine (AZT) among symptomatic HIV-infected persons. J Gen Intern Med 1991; 6:35–40.

82. Turner JC, Korpita E, Mohn LA, Hill WB: Reduction in sexual risk behaviors among college students following a comprehensive health education intervention. J Am Coll Health 1993; 41:187–193.

83. Hellinger FJ: The use of health services by women with HIV infection. Health Services Res 1993; 28:543–561.

84. Solomon L, Stein M, Flynn C, et al: Health services use by urban women with or at risk for HIV-1 infection: The HIV Epidemiology Research Study (HERS). J Acquir Immune Defic Syndr Hum Retrovirol 1998; 17:253–261.

85. Currier J, Richardson J, Masari L, Levine AM: Prevalence and determinants of non-use of antiretroviral therapy among women: Women's Interagency HIV Study (WIHS) (Abstract no. 42288). Int Conf AIDS 1998; 12:831.

86. Imam N, Carpenter CC, Mayer KH, et al: Hierarchical pattern of mucosal *Candida* Infections in HIV-seropositive women (see Comments). Am J Med 1990; 89:142–146.

87. Schrager L, Young J, Fowler M, (ed): Long-term survivors of HIV-1 infection: Definitions and research challenges. AIDS 1994; 8:S95–S108.

88. Rhoads JL, Wright DC, Redfield RR, Burke DS: Chronic vaginal candidiasis in women with human immunodeficiency virus infection. JAMA 1987; 257:3105–3107.

89. White MH: Is vulvovaginal candidiasis an AIDS-related illness? Clin Infect Dis 1996; 22(Suppl 2):S124–127.

90. Morlat P, Parneix P, Dourad D, et al: Women and HIV infection: A cohort study of 483 HIV-infected women in Bordeaux, France, 1985–1991. The Groupe d'Epidemiologie Clinique du SIDA en Aquitaine. AIDS 1992; 6:1187–1193.

91. Baker DA: Management of the female HIV-infected patient. AIDS Res Hum Retroviruses 1994; 10:935–938.

92. Carpenter CC, Mayer KH, Fisher A, et al: Natural history of acquired immunodeficiency syndrome in women in Rhode Island. Am J Med 1989; 86:771–775.

93. Duerr A: Gynaecological conditions in HIV-positive women (Abstract 385). 12th World AIDS Conference. Geneva, Switzerland; 1998.

94. Sobel JD: Pathogenesis and treatment of recurrent vulvovaginal candidiasis. Clin Infect Dis 1992; 14(Suppl): S148–153.

95. Minkoff HL, DeHovitz JA: Care of women infected with the human immunodeficiency virus (Comments). JAMA 1991; 266:2253–2258.

96. Sobel JD: Management of recurrent vulvovaginal candidiasis with intermittent ketoconazole prophylaxis. Obstet Gynecol 1985; 65:435–440.

97. Milne JD, Warnock DW: Effect of simultaneous oral and vaginal treatment on the rate of cure and relapse in vaginal candidosis. Br J Vener Dis 1979; 55:362–362.

98. Maenza JR, Keruly JC, Moore RD, et al: Risk factors for fluconazole-resistant candidiasis in human immunodeficiency virus–infected patients. J Infect Dis 1996; 173:219–225.

99. Hoegsberg B, Abulafia O, Sedlis A, et al: Sexually transmitted diseases and human immunodeficiency virus infection among women with pelvic inflammatory disease. Am J Obstet Gynecol 1990; 163:1135–1139.

100. Safrin S, Dattel BJ, Hauer L, Sweet RL: Seroprevalence and epidemiologic correlates of human immunodeficiency virus infection in women with acute pelvic inflammatory disease. Obstet Gynecol 1990; 75:666–670.

101. Barbosa C, Macasaet M, Brockmann S, et al: Pelvic inflammatory disease and human immunodeficiency virus infection. Obstet Gynecol 1997; 89:65–70.

102. Korn AP, Landers DV, Green JR, Sweet RL: Pelvic inflammatory disease in human immunodeficiency virus–infected women. Obstet Gynecol 1993; 82:765–786.

103. Centers for Disease Control and Prevention: 1998 Guidelines for the treatment of sexually transmitted disease. MMWR 1998; 47:1–118.

104. Schwebke JR, Hillier SL, Sobel JD, et al: Validity of the vaginal Gram stain for the diagnosis of bacterial vaginosis. Obstet Gynecol 1996; 88:573–576.

105. Maier JA, Bergman A, Ross MG: Acquired immunodeficiency syndrome manifested by chronic primary genital herpes. Am J Obstet Gynecol 1986; 155:756–758.

106. Safrin S, Arvin A, Mills J, Ashley R: Comparison of the Western immunoblot assay and a glycoprotein G enzyme immunoassay for detection of serum antibodies to herpes simplex virus type 2 in patients with AIDS. J Clin Microbiol 1992; 30:1312–1314.

107. Siegel D, Golden E, Washington AE, et al: Prevalence and correlates of herpes simplex infections. The population-based AIDS in Multiethnic Neighborhoods Study. JAMA 1992; 268:1702–1708.

108. Centers for Disease Control and Prevention: Revision of the CDC surveillance case definition for acquired immunodeficiency syndrome. MMWR 1987; 36(suppl): 1S–15S.

109. Wickett WH Jr, Miller RD. Sites of multiple lesions in recurrent genital herpes. Am Fam Physician 1985; 32:145–152.

110. Valacyclovir. Med Lett Drugs Ther 1996; 38:3–4.

111. Snoeck R, Andrei G, Gerard M, et al: Successful treatment of progressive mucocutaneous infection due to acyclovir- and foscarnet-resistant herpes simplex virus with (S)-1-(3-hydroxy-2-phosphonylmethoxypropyl) cytosine (HPMPC). Clin Infect Dis 1994; 18:570–578.

112. Rompalo A, Astenborsky J, Klein R, et al: Syphilis: Serologic patterns among women with or at risk for HIV. 6th Conference on Retroviruses and Opportunistic Infections. Chicago, IL; 1999.

113. Vermund SH, Kelley KF, Klein RS, et al: High risk of human papillomavirus infection and cervical squamous intraepithelial lesions among women with symptomatic human immunodeficiency virus infection. Am J Obstet Gynecol 1991; 165:392–400.

114. Johnson JC, Burnett AF, Willet GD, et al: High frequency of latent and clinical human papillomavirus cervical infections in immunocompromised human immunodeficiency virus–infected women. Obstet Gynecol 1992; 79:321–317.

115. Six C, Heard I, Bergeron C, et al: Comparative prevalence, incidence and short-term prognosis of cervical squamous intraepithelial lesions amongst HIV-positive and HIV-negative women. AIDS 1998; 12:1047–1056.

116. Sedlacek TV: Advances in the diagnosis and treatment of human papillomavirus infections. Clin Obstet Gynecol 1999; 42:206–220.

117. Andieh L, Munoz A, Vlahov D, et al: Cervical neoplasia and the persistence of HPV infection in HIV + women (Abstract 463). 6th Conference on Retroviruses and Opportunistic Infections. Chicago, IL; 1999.

118. Hankins C, Coutlee F, Lapointe N, et al: Persistence of human papilloma virus (HPV) infection in HIV-positive and HIV-negative women. Canadian Women's HIV Study Group (Abstract no. 22303). Int Conf AIDS 1998; 12:323.

119. Moscicki A, Ellenger J, Vermund S, et al: Prevalence and risks for cervical human papillomavirus infection and squamous intraepithelial lesions in adolescent women: Impact of infection with human immundeficiency viruc. Arch Pediatr Adolesc Med 2000; 18(3):939–945.

120. Goldberg GL, Vermund SH, Schiffman MH, et al: Comparison of Cytobrush and cervicovaginal lavage sampling methods for the detection of genital human papillomavirus. Am J Obstet Gynecol 1989; 161:1669–1672.

121. Vermund SH, Schiffman MH, Goldberg GL, et al: Molecular diagnosis of genital human papillomavirus infection: Comparison of two methods used to collect exfoliated cervical cells. Am J Obstet Gynecol 1989; 160:304–308.

122. Shah K, Farzadegan H, Daniel R, et al: Relationship of HIV-1 RNA copies in plasma and CD4 counts to human papillomavirus (HPV) prevalence and cervical dysplasia (Abstract no. 22317). Int Conf AIDS 1998; 12:326.

123. Palefsky JM, Minkoff H, Kalish LA, et al: Cervicovaginal human papillomavirus infection in human immunodeficiency virus-1 (HIV)-positive and high-risk HIV-negative women [see comments]. J Natl Cancer Inst 1999; 91:226–236.

124. Vermund SH, Kelley KF, Burk RD, et al: Risk of human papillomavirus (HPV) and cervical squamous intraepithelial lesions (SIL) highest among women with advanced HIV disease (Abstract no. S.B.517). Int Conf AIDS 1990; 6:215.

125. La Ruche G, Leroy V, Mensah-Ado I, et al: Short-term follow up of cervical squamous intraepithelial lesions associated with HIV and human papillomavirus infections in Africa. Int J STD AIDS 1999; 10:363–368.

126. Williams AB, Darragh TM, Vranizan K, et al: Anal and cervical human papillomavirus infection and risk of anal and cervical epithelial abnormalities in human immunodeficiency virus–infected women. Obstet Gynecol 1994; 83:205–211.

127. Palefsky J: Human papillomavirus (HPV) infection and HPV-associated neoplasias in the immunocompromised host. 2nd National AIDS Malignancy Conference. Bethesda, Md: 1998.

128. Penn I: Cancers of the anogenital region in renal transplant recipients. Analysis of 65 cases. Cancer 1986; 58:611–616.

129. Porreco R, Penn I, Droegemueller W, et al: Gynecologic malignancies in immunosuppressed organ homograft recipients. Obstet Gynecol 1975; 45:359–364.

130. Palefsky JM: Human papillomavirus infection and anogenital neoplasia in human immunodeficiency virus–positive men and women. J Natl Cancer Inst Monogr 1998; 23:15–20.

131. Chiasson M, Kelley K, Vazquez F, et al: Increased incidence of invasive cervical cancer (ICC) in HIV + women in New York City (Abstract 4). 2nd National AIDS Malignancy Conference. Bethesda, Md; 1998.

132. Shah KV, Solomon L, Daniel R, et al: Comparison of PCR and hybrid capture methods for detection of human papillomavirus in injection drug–using women at high risk of human immunodeficiency virus infection. J Clin Microbiol 1997; 35:517–519.

133. Maiman M: Cervical neoplasia in women with HIV infection. Oncol (Huntingt) 1994; 8:83–89.

134. Agarossi A, Muggiasca ML, Ravasi L, et al: HIV infection and CIN (Abstract no. PoB 3045). Int Conf AIDS 1992; 8:B94.

135. Centers for Disease Control and Prevention: 1993 Revised classification system for HIV infection and expanded surveillance case definition for AIDS among adolescents and adults. JAMA 1993; 269:460.

136. Maiman M, Fruchter RG, Serur E, et al: Human immunodeficiency virus infection and cervical neoplasia. Gynecol Oncol 1990; 38:377–382.

137. Harlow S, Schuman P, Cohen M, et al: Menstrual function and HIV serostatus (Abstract 461). 6th Conference on Retroviruses and Opportunistic Infections. Chicago, IL, 1999.

138. Fuller C, Clark RA, Kissinger P, Abdalian SE: Clinical manifestations of infection with human immunodeficiency virus among adolescents in Louisiana. J Adolesc Health 1996; 18:422–428.

139. Futterman D, Hein K, Reuben N, et al: Human immunodeficiency virus–infected adolescents: The first 50 patients in a New York City program (Comments). Pediatrics 1993; 91:730–735.

140. Rogers AS, Futterman DK, Moscicki AB, et al: The REACH Project of the Adolescent Medicine HIV/AIDS Research Network: Design, methods, and selected characteristics of participants. Adolesc Health 1998; 22:300–311.

141. Centers for Disease Control and Prevention: Surveillance for AIDS-defining opportunistic illnesses, 1992–1997. 1999; 48:1–22.

142. Chang Y, Cesarman E, Pessin MS, et al: Identification of herpesvirus-like DNA sequences in AIDS-associated Kaposi's sarcoma (Comments). Science 1994; 266:1865–1869.

143. Lennette ET, Blackbourn DJ, Levy JA: Antibodies to human herpesvirus type 8 in the general population and in Kaposi's sarcoma patients (Comments). Lancet 1996; 348:858–861.

144. Ancelle-Park R, De Vincenzi I: Epidemiology and natural history of HIV/AIDS in women. In Johnson M, Johnstone F (eds): HIV Infection in Women. Edinburgh: Churchill Livingstone, 1993, px, 290.

145. Hankins CA: Issues involving women, children, and AIDS primarily in the developed world. J Acquir Immune Defic Syndr 1990; 3:443–438.

146. Lawson M, Katzenstein D, Vermund S: Emerging biomedical interventions. In Gibney L, DiClemente R, Vermund S (eds): Preventing HIV Infection in Developing Countries. New York: Kluwer Academic 1999, p 43–69.

147. Legg JJ: Women and HIV. J Am Board Fam Pract 1993; 6:367–377.

148. Ensign J, Gittelsohn J: Health and access to care: Perspectives of homeless youth in Baltimore City, U.S.A. Soc Sci Med 1998; 47:2087–2099.

149. Food and Drug Administration. Antiretroviral HIV Drug Approvals and Pediatric Labeling Information 1999. www.foa.gov/eashi/aids/pedlbl.htm.

150. Guidelines for the use of antiretroviral agents in HIV-infected adults and adolescents. Department of Health and Human Services and Henry J. Kaiser Family Foundation (published erratum appears in MMWR Rep 1998; Jul 31; 47:619). MMWR 1998; 47:43–82.

151. Department of Health and Human Services: Guidelines for the Use of Antiretroviral Agents in Pediatric HIV Infection. MMWR 1998; 47:1–31.

152. Hein K, Futterman D: Guidelines for the care of children and adolescents with HIV infection. Medical management in HIV-infected adolescents. J Pediatrics 1991; 119:S18–20.
153. Hein K: Introduction to the special issue on pharmacokinetics and pharmacodynamics in adolescents. J Adolesc Health 1994; 15:609–611.
154. Palumbo PE, Kwok S, Waters S, et al: Viral measurement by polymerase chain reaction-based assays in human immunodeficiency virus-infected infants. J Pediatr 1995; 126:592–595.
155. Douglas SD, Rudy B, Muenz L, et al: Peripheral blood mononuclear cell markers in antiretroviral therapy–naive HIV infected and high risk seronegative adolescents. Adolescent Medicine HIV/AIDS Research Network. AIDS. 1999; 13:1629–1635.
156. Department of Health and Human Services: Guidelines for the use of antiretroviral agents in HIV-infected adults and adolescents. MMWR 1998; 47:43–82.
157. Wiktor SZ, Ekpini E, Karon JM, et al: Short-course oral zidovudine for prevention of mother-to-child transmission of HIV-1 in Abidjan, Cote d'Ivoire: a randomised trial. Lancet 1999; 353:781–785.
158. Science, ethics, and the future of research into maternal infant transmission of HIV-1. Perinatal HIV Intervention Research in Developing Countries Workshop participants [see comments]. Lancet 1999; 353:832–835.
159. Gray RH, Wawer MJ, Serwadda D, et al: Population-based study of fertility in women with HIV-1 infection in Uganda. Lancet 1998; 351:98–103.
160. Musoke P, Guay LA, Bagenda D, et al: A phase I/II study of the safety and pharmacokinetics of nevirapine in HIV-1-infected pregnant Ugandan women and their neonates (HIVNET 006). AIDS 1999; 13:479–486.
161. Money D, Burdge D, Forbes J: An analysis of a cohort of 75 HIV infected pregnant women: Antiretroviral effects, obstetrical and neonatal outcomes. International Conference on AIDS, 1998; p. 566.
162. Health and Human Resources Administration: Helping adolescents with HIV adhere to HAART. Rockville, MD, HIV/AIDS Bureau, 1999.
163. Rosenberg MJ, Gollub EL: Commentary: Methods women can use that may prevent sexually transmitted disease, including HIV. Am J Public Health 1992; 82:1473–1478.
164. Miller KS, Levin ML, Whitaker DJ, Xu X: Patterns of condom use among adolescents: The impact of mother-adolescent communication. Am J Public Health 1998; 88:1542–1544.
165. Kirby D, Brener ND, Brown NL, et al: The impact of condom availability [correction of distribution] in Seattle schools on sexual behavior and condom use [published erratum appears in Am J Public Health 1999; 89(3):422]. Am J Public Health 1999; 89:182–187.
166. Furstenberg FF Jr, Geitz LM, Teitler JO, Weiss CC: Does condom availability make a difference? An evaluation of Philadelphia's health resource centers. Fam Plann Perspect 1997; 29:123–127.
167. Kirby DB, Brown NL: Condom availability programs in U.S. schools. Fam Plan Perspect 1996; 28:196–202.
168. Guttmacher S, Lieberman L, Ward D, et al: Condom availability in New York City public high schools: Relationships to condom use and sexual behavior. Am J Public Health 1997; 87:1427–1433.
169. Lurie P, Drucker E: An opportunity lost: Estimating the number of HIV infections due to the US failure to adopt a national needle exchange policy. *International Conference on AIDS,* Vancouver, 1996.

Chapter 24
Child Sexual Abuse

DAVID MURAM

Child sexual abuse is recognized as a common and serious problem that affects children of every age, sex, socioeconomic class, and geographic location.[1] Children from infancy to young adulthood have been victims of abuse; the average reported age at first incident ranged between 8 and 11 years.[1, 2] Other investigators have suggested that younger children (4 to 9 years) may be at a higher risk because of a naive and trusting attitude toward adults and vulnerability to being misled about the meaning of various sexual activities.[3] In the National Incidence Study conducted from 1993, 300,200 children were classified as sexually abused (incidence 45 cases per 100,000 children).[4] It is well accepted, however, that the number of reported incidents of child sexual abuse represents only a portion of the actual number of victims. Retrospective studies showed that as many as 38% of all females younger than 18 have reported having been abused.[2, 5–8]

Some states have introduced child protection laws. One example is Tennessee, which introduced such a law in 1985. Among its provisions, the law requires that "Any person, physicians included, who knows or has reasonable cause to suspect, that a child has been sexually abused shall report such knowledge or suspicion." During the first 2 years of the registry, the number of validated incidents of abuse involving minors rose from an average of 15 reports per month in 1984 to 60 validated incidents per month in 1986.[9] Such an increase in the number of reported cases was also seen at the national level.[4] During the next 3 years, from October 1986 through September 1989, however, the number of validated incidents of abuse remained relatively stable at about 30 to 35 per month.[9] Reported abuse rates were higher for girls than for boys; of 1985 separate incidents involving minors, 1600 involved females and 385 involved males. Other investigators also found that the incidence of sexual abuse remained stable over time.[10]

In a number of areas throughout the country,

special multidisciplinary facilities have been developed to care for these young victims of abuse.[11, 12] Many agencies prefer to refer children to such facilities,[13] which provide consistent and standardized medical evaluation, and make evaluators available and willing to participate in legal proceedings later. Still, many of these children are brought to emergency department facilities or to their private physician's office for evaluation. Many physicians have difficulty identifying and managing victims of child sexual abuse.[14–18] It is also possible that the physician may be reluctant to broach the subject of sexual abuse with the family. The American Medical Association suggested in its Diagnostic and Treatment Guidelines on Child Sexual Abuse that evaluating for sexual abuse may conflict with the traditional role of the primary care provider and his or her relationship with the family.[19]

DEFINITIONS

The literature contains many variations and inconsistencies in the descriptions and definitions of child sexual abuse and incest. Terms such as *molestation*, *sexual abuse*, *child rape*, *sexual victimization*, and *incest* have often been used interchangeably and loosely. Furthermore, sexual interaction between two minors is considered by many to represent sexual experimentation, not abuse. Some authors have suggested that a 5-year age difference between two minors is sufficient for the activity to be considered abusive,[20] but an exact age discrepancy for determination of abuse has not been established.

In an effort to reduce the inconsistency and confusion, the NCCAN adopted the following definition of child sexual abuse[21]:

Contact or interaction between a child and an adult, when the child is being used for the sexual stimulation of that adult or another person. Sexual abuse may also be committed by another minor, when that person is either significantly older than the victim or when the abuser is in a position of power or control over that child.

Illustrations in this chapter are courtesy of Dr. David Muram.

This definition was written with the intention that it would encompass all forms of sexual abuse and exploitation perpetrated on children by adults.

Incest, a major subcategory of sexual abuse, consists of inappropriate sexual behavior within the context of a preexisting family relationship. It includes relatives of various types and degrees and of the same or the opposite sex. Because the stepparent and stepchild relationships are frequently indistinguishable from those with natural parents, sexual activity between established steprelatives is often defined as incest. Abuse by sexual partners of a parent, such as a common law spouse or a paramour living in the home, is called *incest* only when there is a long-standing relationship and that person is functioning as a surrogate parent. Such inclusion has practical implications, because, in incestuous relationships, the home becomes an unsafe environment for the victim.

Although the legal definitions for crimes of sexual assault vary from state to state, most authorities agree that, for rape to have taken place, the following four criteria must be met:

1. A victim
2. Unwillingness to consent or inability to consent (e.g., young age, mental disability)
3. Threats of force or use of force
4. Penetration

Not all sexual assaults are defined as rape.[1] Physicians who treat victims of sexual assault should be familiar with the various definitions recognized by their state. (A list of definitions is included in Appendix 1.)

THE ABUSIVE RELATIONSHIP

Child sexual abuse is a sexual relationship imposed on a child by a powerful and dominant perpetrator. Authority and power enable the perpetrator to coerce the child into compliance. Though in some instances, the perpetrator selects the victim by chance (e.g., abduction), in most cases the perpetrator has known the child for some time, has easy access to him or her, and has opportunities to be alone with the victim. By using inducements (e.g., small gifts or special attention) the perpetrator engages the child in a relationship that gradually evolves into sexual behavior. Physical force is rarely used by a family member but is sometimes used by a perpetrator who is not known to the child.

Initially, the sex acts are limited to exposure, light touching, and the like. These rapidly progress to overt sexual acts, the most common of which is oral penetration. If another area of the child's body is to be penetrated, the next most likely opening is the anus. Vaginal penetration in very young children is limited, but perpetrators often rub the penis against the genital area of the child, an act known as *dry intercourse*. The hymen and the fossa navicularis may be injured during dry intercourse, but the extent of these injuries is rather limited. Direct penetration of the vagina of a young girl by an erect penis will, however, cause significant injury.

As the incestuous relationship develops, the perpetrator persuades or presses the child to keep the activity secret. The child is made to feel guilty, ashamed, and responsible for this illicit relationship. At times, threats, demonstration of force, or even the use of force is used to secure the child's silence. Usually, children do not reveal details of the abusive relationship.

Disclosure of the abuse is often accidental, and the secret is usually revealed as a result of external circumstances. Someone may observe an abnormal pattern of behavior, or physical injury may bring the child to a physician's attention. Less frequently, the child conscientiously tells an outsider about the abuse, either to share the experience or because the youngster wishes to discontinue the abusive relationship. After disclosure, the child may be under pressure to suppress publicity, information, and intervention, particularly if he or she has been a victim of *incest*. The perpetrator and other family members induce feelings of guilt and isolation in the child with the intention of forcing him or her to withdraw the complaint and stop cooperating with outsiders.

MEDICAL EVALUATION

HISTORY

When the victim is a young child, additional information is required. Because victims of physical or sexual abuse must be removed from an unsafe environment, it is extremely important to know who the perpetrator is and how the child sustained the injury. The questions must be open-ended, not leading. For example, it is preferable to ask, "Why are you here?" instead of "Who hurt you?" The American Professional Society on the Abuse of Children (APSAC) issued detailed guidelines on the proper way to interview children.[22] An abbreviated version is included in Appendix 2. The information should be recorded carefully, using the victim's own

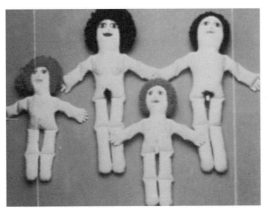

Figure 24–1. Anatomically detailed dolls.

Table 24–2. Nonspecific Signs of Sexual Abuse in Children

Behavioral

Anxiety, fearfulness
Sleep disturbances
Withdrawal
Somatic complaints
Increased sexual play
Inappropriate sexual behavior
School problems
Acting out behaviors
Self-destructive behaviors
Depression, low self-esteem

Physical

Unexplained vaginal injuries
Unexplained vaginal bleeding
Bruises, bites, scratches
Pregnancy
Sexually transmitted disease
Recurrent vaginal infections
Pain in the anal or genital area
Recurrent atypical abdominal pain

words, not adult language. Audio or video recording may be used to document the interview. Although a detailed history is desirable, the patient should not be made to repeat the story of the incident over and over again. To overcome deficiencies that arise from the limited verbal skills of young victims, other interviewing techniques, such as drawings, play interviews, and anatomically detailed dolls have been developed (Fig. 24–1).[23–25] When these techniques are used, the interviewer must be experienced, ask open-ended questions, and avoid leading the child to predetermined answers (Table 24–1).[26]

Even with these techniques, it is sometimes impossible to obtain a detailed history from a very young victim. The physician is then compelled to accept an account of the incident from a relative, police officer, neighbor, or other chil-

dren. Throughout the encounter with the child, the physician should be aware of signs and symptoms commonly associated with child abuse (e.g., night terrors, change in sleeping habits, clinging behavior). The examiner should note the child's composure, behavior, and mental state, as well as the child's interaction with parents and other persons (Table 24–2).

PHYSICAL EXAMINATION

Most children can be fully evaluated in an office that is properly equipped to examine young children. Most children tolerate the evaluation well.[27] In rare instances, often after penile penetration of the vagina, a significant degree of trauma is present (Fig. 24–2) and a properly equipped operating room and general anesthesia are necessary for a thorough evaluation and repair.[28, 29] In most children the physical findings are less dramatic or are absent altogether. Some forms of abuse do not cause injury, and in these circumstances an examination is not expected to detect any physical evidence of abuse.[30–32]

Even when injured, many abused children may not be seen for weeks, months, or even years after the incident. This delay allows semen and debris to be washed away and most, if not all, injuries to heal. Physical findings, when present, vary with the extent of trauma. Minimal trauma produces injuries that heal in a short time and leave no permanent scars. Deep lacerations take longer to heal and often leave scars that can be seen, even relatively long afterward.

Table 24–1. Obtaining a History from a Child Victim of Sexual Abuse

General Measures

Provide a comfortable environment.
Use developmentally appropriate language and technique.
Allow sufficient time to avoid any coercive quality to the interview.
Establish rapport with the child.

Questioning

The initial questions should be nondirective, to elicit spontaneous responses.
Leading questions should be avoided. If such questions are used, responses should be carefully evaluated.
Nonverbal tools (e.g., anatomically detailed dolls or drawings) may be used to help the child to communicate.
Anatomically detailed dolls should be used primarily for the identification of body parts and clarification of previous statements.
Psychological testing is not required to prove sexual assault.
At some point, the child should be questioned directly about the abusive relationship.

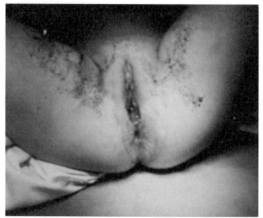

Figure 24–2. A significant vaginal injury from sexual assault in a 20-month-old girl.

The use of magnifying devices to enhance anogenital inspection is well accepted. Investigators have reported using a simple magnifying glass, otoscope, or colposcope (Fig. 24–3). The colposcope currently appears to be the instrument of choice for the examination of child victims of sexual abuse.[33–37] Colposcopy affords detailed magnified inspection of the vulva for physical signs of abuse that may have escaped detection by the naked eye (Fig. 24–4). In this technique, the external genitalia are inspected through a colposcope under magnification. The labia are gently retracted downward and laterally to expose the hymenal ring and the posterior vaginal wall.[38] The Valsalva maneuver and the knee-chest position can be used in some patients to better visualize the lower vaginal walls. The genitalia are inspected both under regular illumination and through a green filter, which better

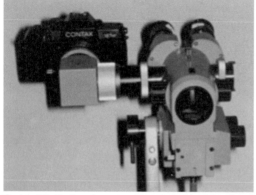

Figure 24–3. A colposcope equipped with photographic equipment. The attachment allows the physician to use any type of camera, including a video camera.

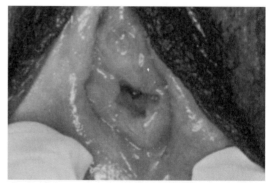

Figure 24–4. A colposcopic photograph of the external genitalia. An intact hymen is noted.

demonstrates vascular patterns. No solutions or dyes need to be applied to the genitalia during the examination.

The evaluation of child sexual abuse victims and the use of a colposcope require experience and training; otherwise, misdiagnosis is likely to occur.[16] Small areas of skin irritation and superficial abrasions that cannot be detected with the naked eye may be identified under magnification. Some of these lesions may not be the result of sexual abuse. Vulvar irritation is fairly common in small children as a result of poor local hygiene, maceration of the skin secondary to wetness from diapers, or the child's scratching a local infection (Fig. 24–5). Such nonspecific findings, enhanced by the colposcope, should not be regarded as definitively diagnostic of sexual abuse. Despite its limitations, colposcopy improves the examiner's diagnostic skills by providing an opportunity to review the physical findings under magnification. In addition, when equipped with a camera attachment, the colposcope enables the physician to gather photographs that can then be added to the medical record or used for education or peer review. Finally, should legal action be taken, these pictures can be reviewed to refresh the examiner's memory and to be introduced as evidence. It is strongly recommended that, whenever sexual abuse is a possibility, photographic documentation be obtained during each assessment. This can be done either through the colposcope or with an adequate camera equipped with a macro lens attachment.[39]

Some investigators have found the colposcope to be extremely useful.[36, 37] In one series, only colposcopic examination was able to identify signs of genital trauma in 59 of 500 (11.8%) patients. That particular series was composed primarily of adult patients, however, and it is difficult to extrapolate from this series the usefulness of colposcopy in children.[36] In a prospec-

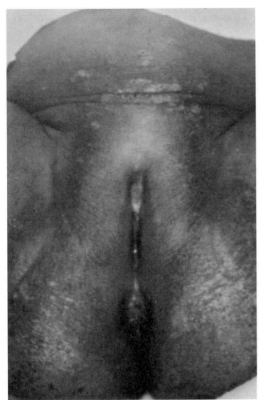

Figure 24–5. In a 14-month-old infant referred for evaluation of possible sexual abuse, severe diaper rash was mistaken for genital injuries.

tive study limited to prepubertal children, other investigators have concluded that colposcopy does not substantially enhance the rate of detection of signs of sexual abuse in prepubertal children, as compared with a careful unaided physical examination.[33] Most important, regardless of whether a colposcope is used, the physician must conduct a thorough examination and objectively record the findings. Unfortunately, consensus has not been reached on the meaning of the various specific findings observed in child victims of abuse.[40]

Abnormal Physical Findings

There are no accepted criteria by which to classify physical findings that are diagnostic of sexual abuse. A simplified classification of the physical findings observed in prepubertal girls has been developed (Table 24–3). This classification distinguishes nonspecific findings from those that are highly suggestive or definitively related to abuse and has proven useful in subsequent

legal proceedings. All physical findings are classified into one of four categories[41, 42]:

1. Normal-looking genitalia.
2. Nonspecific findings—abnormalities of the genitalia that could have been caused by sexual abuse but are also often seen in girls who are not victims of sexual abuse (e.g., inflammation and scratching). These findings may be the sequelae of poor perineal hygiene or nonspecific infection. Included in this category are redness of the external genitalia (Fig. 24–6), increased vascular pattern of the vestibular and labial mucosa, purulent discharge from the vagina, small skin fissures or lacerations in the area of the posterior fourchette (Fig. 24–7), and agglutination of the labia minora (Fig. 24–8).
3. Specific findings—one or more abnormalities strongly suggestive of sexual abuse. Such findings include recent or healed lacerations of the hymen and vaginal mucosa (Figs. 24–9, 24–10), proctoepisiotomy (a laceration of the vaginal mucosa extending to the rectal mucosa as in Figure 24–2), and indentations in the skin (bite marks). This category also includes laboratory evidence of a sexually transmitted disease. However, when the only evidence of sexual abuse is isolation of a sexually transmissible organism or detection of antibodies to one, the findings should be confirmed and the implications considered carefully.
4. Definitive findings—sperm or confirmed pregnancy in a young adolescent.

Modifications of this initial classification have evolved in other centers.[43]

Table 24–3. Medical Evaluation: Classification of Abnormal Findings

Category	Abnormalities
Normal examination	No abnormalities detected
	Variations of normal
Nonspecific abnormalities	Redness, irritation, abrasions
	Friability of the posterior fourchette
	Labial adhesions, hymenal tags, hymenal bumps and clefts
	Nonspecific infections
	Bruising of the external genitalia
Specific findings	Hymenal-vaginal tear
	Hymenal-perineal tear
	Sexually transmitted disease
	Bite marks on the genitalia
Definitive abnormalities	Presence of sperm
	Pregnancy in an adolescent

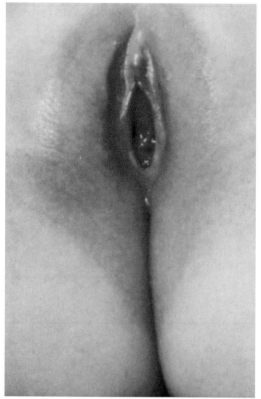

Figure 24–6. Vulvar redness and irritation caused by nonspecific vulvovaginitis.

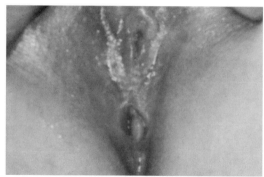

Figure 24–8. Agglutination of the labia minora.

who were determined by child protective services to be victims of sexual abuse were evaluated. Sixty five (32%) had normal-looking genitalia and failed to show any sign of previous injury. Nonspecific abnormalities were present in 45 (22%), and 95 (46%) had abnormalities considered specific for sexual abuse. Hymenal vaginal lacerations were detected in 68 of these young girls (Table 24–4). In three, the examination revealed extensive lacerations through the posterior vaginal wall, with extension into the rectum. Two patients were found to have motile sperm in the vaginal fluid or on the vulvar skin. Venereal disease was noted in 31 girls; 25 of them had no other sign of genital injury (see Table 24–4).[42]

In general, the external genitalia and the anal area can be manipulated by oral, digital, and genital contact. Unless vaginal penetration occurs, injury is limited to the vulvar region. When the perpetrator rubs his penis on the child's vulva (dry intercourse), erythema, swelling, skin bruis-

Many injuries are superficial and often are limited to the vulvar skin. Within a few days healing is complete, and, when the child is examined later, the anatomic features of the anogenital area appear normal.[42] It has been shown that, even in girls in whom sexual abuse has been documented, the medical evaluation fails to reveal specific findings in 50% of victims.[42, 44] In a large prospective study, 205 prepubertal girls

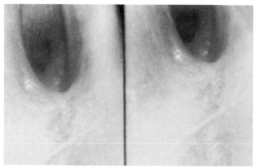

Figure 24–7. Friability of the posterior fourchette. Notice the fissures caused by separation of the labia.

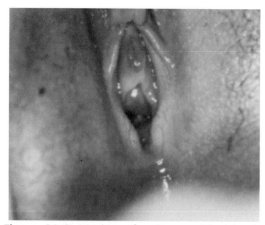

Figure 24–9. Vagina of a 9-year-old girl who was assaulted 2 weeks before the examination. Notice a healing tear of the hymen and vaginal wall.

Table 24–4. Genital Findings in 205 Prepubertal Girls Who Were Victims of Sexual Abuse

Category	Findings	Number of Patients
1	No abnormalities	65
2	Redness and irritation	16
	Redness, irritation, and skin lacerations	12
	Skin lacerations only	8
	Labial adhesions	8
	Redness, irritation, and labial adhesions	1
3	Laceration of hymen	28
	Veneral disease	24
	Lacerations of hymen and hymenal opening ≥ 1 cm	12
	Laceration of hymen, redness, and irritation	6
	Laceration of hymen, venereal disease	5
	Laceration of hymen, redness, irritation, and skin lacerations	5
	Proctoepisiotomy	3
	Laceration of hymen and skin lacerations	3
	Laceration of hymen, venereal disease, and labial adhesions	2
	Laceration of hymen, redness, irritation, and labial adhesions	2
	Laceration of hymen, enlarged hymenal opening, and irritation	2
	Bite marks	1
4	Motile sperm in vaginal fluid and laceration of hymen	1
	Semen on vulva; redness, and irritation	1

From Muram D: Child sexual abuse—genital tract findings in prepubertal girls. I. The unaided medical examination. Am J Obstet Gynecol 1989; 160(2):328–333.

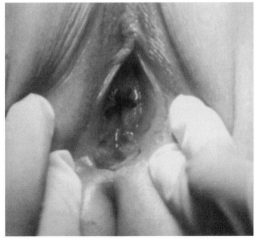

Figure 24–10. Fresh laceration of the hymen and vagina after an assault.

ally abused girls.[46] In another study, Adams and colleagues reported average hymen orifice diameters exceeding 6 mm in 23 abused girls who denied penetrating sexual contact (Table 24–5).[47] The investigators observed that hymenal orifice diameters increased as a function of both advancing age and degree of sexual contact. Emans and associated noted that a group of sexually abused girls had larger hymen orifice diameters than a group who had not been abused.[48] The average difference in diameter between the two groups was 1.6 mm, which is, perhaps, within the range of measurement error. Furthermore, only 7% of the abused girls had measurements exceeding the range observed in the nonabused girls.[48] In another study the investigators noted that 53% of sexually abused girls, including 26% of those who specifically described digital or penile pene-

ing, and excoriations are found on the labia and vestibule. Similar findings can be expected when the perpetrator digitally manipulates the vulva or introitus without vaginal penetration. These injuries are superficial and often limited to the vulvar skin. Within a few days, healing is complete, and, when the child is examined later, the anatomic features of the anogenital area appear normal.[42, 44]

The relationship between the size of the hymenal aperture and sexual abuse allegations remains controversial, and normative data on nonabused children are few or inadequate. Observations by Cantwell documented that 74% of female pediatric victims whose hymenal orifice diameters were more than 4 mm had a history of sexual abuse.[45] The same author later described a decrease in hymenal orifice diameter, attributed to healing, after reexamination of 20 sexu-

Table 24–5. Mean Hymenal Diameter Related to Age and Type of Abuse Alleged

Type of Abuse	Age (yr)		
	1–5	6–9	10–12
Total group	N = 42	N = 29	N = 15
	0.54 ± 0.35 cm	0.97 ± 0.41 cm	1.17 ± 0.39 cm
Fondling only	n = 10	n = 12	n = 3
	0.62 cm	0.85 cm*	0.90 cm
Digital penetration	n = 3	n = 5	n = 3
	0.75 cm	0.91 cm	1.17 cm
Penile penetration	n = 2	n = 12	n = 5
	1.10 cm	1.29 cm*	1.45 cm

*Significant difference $p < .0002$.
From Adams J, Ahmad M, Phillips P: Anogenital findings and hymenal diameter in children referred for sexual abuse examination. Adolesc Pediatr Gynecol 1988; 1:123–127.

tration, had hymenal orifice diameters smaller than 4 mm. The study concluded that introital diameter is a specific (better than 90%) but not very sensitive (6% to 48%) test.[49]

The absence of physical findings should not be construed to mean that the history obtained from the child is incorrect. One study correlated the physical findings and histories from the victims with confessions obtained from the perpetrators.[44] The study documented the reliability of the histories obtained from the children. In only six instances did the assailant not confirm the child's story, but even in these instances, the assailant admitted to sexually assaulting the child and confirmed penile contact, although penetration was denied. All the patients in that study were confirmed victims of sexual abuse by the perpetrators' admission, but the medical examination failed to detect abnormalities in 29% of them. Of all abnormal findings, hymen vaginal tear (HVT) was the most common finding in girls who described penile or digital penetration. Of the 18 girls who described vaginal penetration, only 11 were found to have HVT (Table 24–6).[44]

Anal abuse is a common form of sexual assault against children, especially boys.[50, 51] Although genital injuries are often recognized as possible signs of abuse, anal and perianal injuries are sometimes dismissed by physicians as being associated with common bowel disorders (e.g., constipation or diarrhea).[52, 53] A number of studies have examined the issue of perianal abnormalities caused by sexual assault. In one study,[54] the authors attempted to collect normative data regarding anogenital anatomy from a sample of 267 nonabused prepubertal children ranging in age from 2 months to 11 years. In a significant number of these children, the investigators observed

Table 24–6. Relationship Between Genital Findings and Confession of Vaginal Penetration by the Perpetrator

| | Vaginal Penetration | | |
Findings	Yes	No	Total
Normal-looking genitalia	2	7	9
Nonspecific abnormalities (e.g., inflammation, labial adhesions)	5	3	8
Abnormalities suggestive of abuse (e.g., vaginal tears, venereal disease)	11	3	14
Total	18	13	31

Reprinted from Muram D: Child sexual abuse: Relationship between sexual acts and genital findings. Child Abuse Negl 1989; 13(2):211–216. Copyright 1989, with kind permission from Pergamon Press Ltd, Headington Hill Hall, Oxford OX3 OBW, UK.

perianal erythema, increased pigmentation, smooth areas on or near the anal verge in the midline, and skin tags or folds. They failed to notice fissures, abrasions, lacerations, or hematomas in any of the subjects. Interestingly, the investigators observed anal dilatation, which became more pronounced the longer the child remained in the knee-chest position. With this dilatation, the investigators observed the loss of the slightly puckered anal verge and the flattening or smoothing out of the folds, which was attributed to the relaxation of anal sphincter muscles (Table 24–7).

Other investigators have associated anal dilatation and soft tissue changes with sexual abuse. In one study (Table 24–8), 143 children were evaluated and the following abnormalities observed: fissures or tears (53), redness and other minor skin changes (53), reflex anal dilatation (42), laxity of the sphincter (38), venous congestion (24), scars or skin tags (8), and human papillomavirus (HPV) lesions (4).[51] Further observations allowed the authors to conclude that virtually complete healing may be expected even in very young children. This may take weeks to years, and sometimes the appearance of the anus remains permanently abnormal and scarred. Swelling of the anal margin largely disappears within 7 to 10 days. Anal dilatation commonly disappears in 1 to 6 weeks, deep fissures may take months to heal, and distended veins are one of the last signs to disappear. In some children anal dilatation persists many months after abuse has ceased.[51]

Similar abnormalities were observed in another group of 310 sexually abused children[55]: 104 had abnormal findings (34%); 61 anal dilatation (19.7%); 44 skin tags (14.2%); 33 rectal tears (10.6%); 15 sphincter tears (4.8%); four HPV lesions (1.3%); two perineal scarring (0.6%); and one bite marks (0.3%). Anal and perianal abnormalities were observed in 59 of 70 children (84%) with obvious evidence of anal assault, but in only 25 of 175 (14%) who denied such abuse. Failure to document perianal abnormalities in almost two thirds of the patients may be the result of healing.

Other disorders can cause perianal abnormalities.[56] For example, they are often seen in children suffering from Crohn's disease or Hirschsprung's disease. In children with significant constipation, the anal canal gapes when the buttocks are gently drawn apart. This is a normal anorectal reflex initiated by the distended rectum. Usually, stool can be seen in the anal canal. After defecation, minor small fissures may be seen for 2 to 3 weeks (Fig. 24–11). Reddening

Table 24–7. Frequency of Perianal Findings in Nonabused Children

Findings	Number of Subjects Observed°	Subjects with Positive Findings	Percentage with Positive Findings
Erythema	168	68	41
Pigmentation	251	74	30
Venous congestion			
Beginning	113	8	7
Midpoint	113	59	52
End	113	83	73
Anal dilatation	267	130‡	49
Intermittent anal dilatation	130†	81‡	62
Configuration during dilatation			
Oval	94	84	89
Round	94	8	9
Irregular	94	2	2
Smooth area	81	21	26
Dimple/depression	81	15	18
Skin tags	164	18	11
Scars	240	4‡	2

°The number of observed subjects varied because of missing data as a result of changes over time in the number of variables assessed.
†Includes only those subjects whose anus dilated.
‡May include "smooth area" on anal verge, no photographs available to recheck findings.
Note: No abrasions, hematomas, fissures, or hemorrhoids were discovered in the 267 subjects.
Reprinted from McCann J, Simon M, Voris J, Wells R: Perianal findings in prepubertal children selected for nonabuse: A descriptive study. Child Abuse Negl 1989;13:179–193. Copyright 1989, with kind permission from Pergamon Press Ltd, Headington Hill Hall, Oxford OX3 OBW, UK.

of the perianal area may be noted in children with fecal soiling.[54] Unfortunately, children who have been abused often suffer from functional constipation, and a damaged anal sphincter often causes fecal soiling.

The absence of abnormal perianal findings is easily explained. Many victims of anal assault do not sustain significant physical injuries, because the anal sphincter and anal canal are capable of dilatation. Penetration, even by an adult male penis, can occur without significant injury. The pain that follows anal assault sometimes causes spasm of the anal sphincter and, consequently, functional constipation. This explains the child's complaints of pain and rectal bleeding. Most child victims do not disclose incidents of sexual abuse immediately, and many are not brought for an examination—for weeks, months, or even years—after the abuse occurs. By that time, the injuries often have healed completely, and the physical examination reveals few, if any, abnormalities. Although the literature documents large series of children who were evaluated after anal assault, it is difficult to say which ones' findings were the result of abuse. More controlled studies are required to identify the findings specific to anal assault.

It is estimated that the likelihood that a sibling of an abused child has also been abused at some

Table 24–8. Percentage Frequency of Anal Signs in Sexually Abused Children

Physical Sign	All Ages (N = 143)	0–5 (N = 69)
Fissures or tears	53	59
Reflex and dilatation	42	53
Reddening, skin changes	53	43
Laxity	38	37
Venous congestion	24	21
Tear	8	19
Scars/tags	8	3
Warts	4	6

Reprinted from Hobbs CJ, Wynne JM: Sexual abuse of English boys and girls: The importance of anal examination. Child Abuse Negl 1989; 13:195–210. Copyright 1991, with kind permission from Pergamon Press Ltd, Headington Hill Hall, Oxford OX3 OBW, UK.

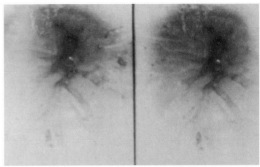

Figure 24–11. Fine perianal fissures indicative of mucocutaneous injury. In this particular instance, the origin of the injury was unknown.

Table 24–9. Genital Findings in Siblings and Friends of Child Victims of Sexual Assault

Findings	Entire Group (N = 247)	Primary Victims (N = 188)	Associates (N = 59)
Specific	119 (48%)	79 (42%)	40 (68%)
Nonspecific	55 (22%)	50 (27%)	5 (8%)
Normal	73 (30%)	59 (31%)	14 (24%)

Reprinted from Muram D, Speck P, Gold S: Genital abnormalities in female siblings and friends of child victims of sexual abuse. Child Abuse Negl 1991; 15:105–110. Copyright 1989, with kind permission from Pergamon Press Ltd, Headington Hill Hall, Oxford OX3 OBW, UK.

time is 20%.[56] Within families, incestuous fathers may abuse more than one child, and cases have been cited in which the father begins with the oldest child and abuses other children as they reach a certain age. In one study of 59 young females who were closely associated with known victims of sexual abuse, 76% had abnormal genital findings (Table 24–9).[57] Reports of sexual molestation in ritualistic settings documented that multiple children may have been victimized.[58, 59] These findings suggest that the examiner should consider evaluating an entire family, rather than only the "index case."

Collection of Evidence

Although the primary objective of the physical examination is to attend to the medical needs of the victim, the examination has a secondary purpose: to collect samples that can later be used as evidence. For proper medical management, specimens may be collected from the child and sent to the hospital laboratory. If the assault occurred within 72 hours of the examination, a second set of samples should be collected for the forensic laboratory and handled according to the following protocol. They must be identified in the record: the anatomic site where they were collected and any associated findings (e.g., saliva collected from the patient's neck near a bite mark). All items collected must be individually packaged and clearly labeled, and the containers and envelopes sealed and signed by the examiner. The evaluator may wish to use a commercially marked collection kit (Fig. 24–12). Each label must include these data:

Patient identification
Specimen
Site from which the specimen was collected
Date and time collected
Examiner's initials

These specimens must be placed in containers and sealed with special-evidence tape, properly labeled, and affixed with a routing slip. The physician may wish to use commercially available kits designed esspecially for this purpose. The kit is then given to the police investigator, who signs for it in the record and on the routing slip. All persons who handle the materials must sign the routing slip. Such a system is necessary to maintain the chain of evidence; otherwise, results obtained from these specimens may not be admissible in court. If the kit *must* be stored in the physician's office, it should be inaccessible (preferably locked up) until it can be given to the

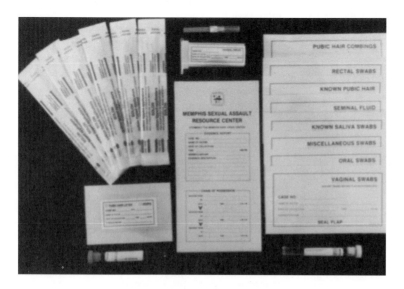

Figure 24–12. Commercially available kit for the collection of evidence of sexual assault. The kit includes swabs, glass slides, envelopes, containers, labels, and sealing tape.

police investigator or the forensics laboratory. The specimens required are listed in Table 24–10.

The clothing worn by the patient during the assault is collected and placed in a properly labeled bag. A description of the clothes and of their condition should be attached. During the general inspection, all foreign material (e.g., sand, grass) should be removed and placed in clearly labeled envelopes. Scrapings are collected from underneath the fingernails and loose hairs on the skin. A Wood lamp can be used to detect seminal fluid on the patient's body, as the ultraviolet light causes semen to "fluoresce." The stain

Table 24–10. Specimens to Be Collected for Forensic Evaluation

General

Outer and underclothing worn during or immediately after the assault
Fingernail scrapings
Dried and moist secretions and foreign material on the patient's body; use Wood lamp to detect semen

Oral Cavity

Swabs (two) for semen within 6 hours of the assault
Culture for gonorrhea and other sexually transmitted diseases
Saliva (for reference)

Genital Area

Dried and moist secretions and foreign material
Comb pubic hair; collect all loose hair and foreign material
Vaginal swabs (three)
Wet mount
Dry-mount slides (two)
Culture for gonorrhea and other sexually transmitted diseases

Anus

Dried and moist secretions and foreign material
Rectal swabs (two)
Dry-mount slides (two)
Culture for gonorrhea and other sexually transmitted diseases

Blood

Blood typing
Rapid plasma reagin test
Pregnancy test (blood or urine)
Alcohol/toxicology evaluation (blood or urine)

Urine

Urinalysis

Blood or Urine

Pregnancy test
Alcohol/toxicology evaluation

Other

Saliva: Use clean gauze or filter paper
Head hair: Cut and remove sample
Pubic hair: Cut and remove sample

Table 24–11. Indications for Screening Children for STDs

1. Signs or symptoms of an STD.
2. Signs or symptoms of a genital infection that could have been transmitted through sexual contact.
3. A known offender is known to harbor an STD.
4. A known offender is very likely (at high risk) to harbor an STD.
5. High prevalence of STDs in the community.
6. History of penetration or ejaculation.
7. A known STD or signs or symptoms of an STD in a sibling or other member of the child's household.

Modified from Centers for Disease Control: Sexually transmitted diseases treatment guidelines. MMWR 1998; 47(RR-1):1–116.

may be lifted off the skin with moistened cotton swabs for further analysis.

If vaginal penetration is suspected, vaginal fluid is collected and sent for culture, wet preparation, cytologic examination, and acid phosphatase determination. An immediate wet-mount preparation performed by the examining physician may help to detect motile sperm. Culture swabs are collected from the rectum, vagina, urethra, and pharynx, even when the patient denies orogenital contact. When the cost is prohibitive, selective cultures may be obtained from asymptomatic children with a remote history of abuse.

The decision to evaluate any child for STDs must be individualized to that child's circumstances. It may be unnecessary to evaluate asymptomatic children whose history suggests low risk for an STD.[60] STD screening is indicated when the probability that the child might have contracted an STD is increased (Table 24–11). Serologic testing for HIV should likewise be considered case by individual case, and every patient requires repeat evaluations. Data on the safety and efficacy of postexposure prophylaxis for HIV in children are insufficient.

For children or adolescents who are evaluated very soon after a single assault, the CDC recommends that the tests listed in Table 24–12 be done initially and be repeated within 2 weeks. The serologic tests for syphilis and HIV should be repeated in 3 months and, for HIV again in 6 months. A single examination may be sufficient if the last episode of abuse occurred long before the medical evaluation. Some states now allow testing of the alleged perpetrator for communicable diseases such as syphilis and HIV infection. If the abuse has been ongoing and if circumstances permit, the alleged offender may be evaluated in the manner just described, and follow-up care

Table 24–12. Recommended Laboratory Procedures for Initial Evaluation of Sexually Abused Children

Test	Collection Site	
	Girls	*Boys*
Inspection	Body	Body
	Oral cavity	Oral cavity
	Genitalia	Genitalia
	Anal and perianal areas	Anal and perianal areas
Cultures for	Vaginal	Urethral°
N. gonorrhoeae	Anal	Anal
	Oral	Oral
Cultures for	Vaginal	Urethral°
C. trachomatis	Anal	Anal
Culture	Vaginal fluid	
Wet mount for *T. vaginalis*, amine test, clue cells, other indicators of bacterial vaginosis (BV)		
Serum for serologic testing—syphilis, hepatitis, HIV		

°Meatal specimen is sufficient when discharge is present.

for the child or adolescent can be modified accordingly.

TREATMENT

Certain objectives must be addressed when treating a child victim of sexual abuse:

1. Repair injuries and treat sexually transmitted disease.
2. Protect against further abuse.
3. Provide psychiatric support for the victim and the family.

REPAIR OF INJURIES

Many sexual assault victims do not sustain serious physical injury, particularly those who were sexually active before the assault. Superficial injuries (bruises, edema, local irritation) resolve within a few days and require no special treatment. Meticulous perineal hygiene is important to prevent secondary infections. Sitz baths should be utilized to remove secretions and contaminants to some patients with extensive skin abrasions, broad-spectrum antibiotics should be given as prophylaxis. In most patients, vulvar hematomas do not require special treatment. Usually, small hematomas can be controlled by pressure with an ice pack, and even massive swelling of the vulva usually subsides promptly when cold packs and external pressure are applied (Fig. 24–13). Occasionally, large hemato-

mas continue to increase in size; such lesions should be incised, the clots removed, and bleeding points identified and ligated. Large vulvar tears require suturing, which is best accomplished under general anesthesia, using fine, absorbable suture material.

Bite wounds should be irrigated copiously and necrotic tissue cautiously débrided. Often, an uninfected fresh wound can be closed primarily, but most bite wounds should be left open. Closure is completed when granulation tissue has formed. After 3 to 5 days, secondary débridement may be required to remove necrotic tissue. Antitetanus immunization should be provided if the child has not already been immunized. Broad-spectrum antibiotics should be prescribed for therapy rather than prophylaxis.

Although vulvar injuries are easily accessible for repair, injuries of the vagina or rectum may present surgical difficulties because of the small caliber of the organs involved. Special instruments, as well as proper exposure and assistance, are required. Many vaginal lacerations are superficial and limited to the mucosal and submucosal tissues. Such tears are repaired with fine suture material after complete hemostasis is secured. Vaginal wall hematomas form when bleeding persists underneath the repaired vaginal mucosa. The internal pressure created by the blood clot often controls the bleeding. If the bleeding continues, the overlying mucosa is incised, the blood clot evacuated, and the bleeding points identified and ligated.

TREATMENT OF SEXUALLY TRANSMITTED DISEASE

If the child has no symptoms, prophylactic antibiotic therapy is not necessary. Instead, treatment should be deferred until the results of cultures and serologic tests for syphilis become available so that optimal therapy can be instituted. If vulvovaginitis is clinically suspected on the initial visit, appropriate antibiotic therapy is administered. When the infection is severe, a short course of topical estrogen cream promotes healing of vulvar and vaginal tissues. When irritation is intense, hydrocortisone cream (1%) may be necessary to alleviate the pruritus. A repeat Venereal Disease Research Laboratory (VDRL) test is required 6 weeks later to check for seroconversion.

PROTECTION AGAINST FURTHER ABUSE

It is imperative that the child's safety be ensured. Is the perpetrator known? Can the child

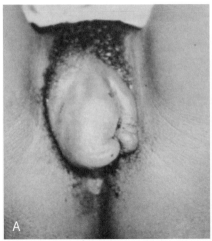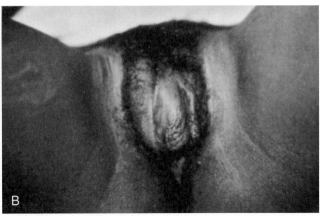

Figure 24–13. *A,* A large vulvar hematoma. *B,* The same hematoma resolved spontaneously within 36 hours.

be safely discharged home? Sometimes it is advisable to admit the child to the hospital or provide temporary placement until these questions can be confidently answered. All suspected victims of child sexual abuse should be referred to child protective services for further evaluation.

PSYCHOLOGICAL SUPPORT FOR THE VICTIM AND FAMILY

In the period immediately following sexual assault or disclosure, the victim and family often require intensive day to day support, counseling, and guidance. The therapist must be prepared to assist them to cope with the examination, the medical treatment, the investigative interviews, child protective services, and law enforcement agencies.

After sexual abuse, child victims often complain of depression, feelings of guilt, fear, and low self-esteem. The major thrust of emotional therapy involves strengthening the child's ego, improving self-image, and enabling him or her to learn to trust others and feel secure again. Appropriate referral for counseling is imperative. To begin the strengthening process, children need to realize that they are victims. They must ventilate their feelings of anger and hurt so that these feelings may later be expressed without experiencing additional guilt. Children often have both positive and negative feelings toward the perpetrator and often require help in sorting out these feelings. Sometimes children blame their parents for not protecting them. The parent-child relationship and intrafamilial structure are critical areas that require restructuring. After

this crisis intervention phase, a treatment program of individual and peer group therapy is instituted. The patient and family should be offered treatment as required.[31, 61, 62]

REFERENCES

1. Kemp C: Sexual abuse, another hidden pediatric problem. Pediatrics 1978; 62:382.
2. Kemp C: Incest and other forms of sexual abuse. *In* Kemp CE, Helfer RE (eds): The Battered Child. Chicago: University of Chicago Press, 1980.
3. Gelinas D: The persisting negative effects of incest. Psychiatry 1983; 46:312.
4. Sedlak AJ, Brooadhurst DB: Third National Study of Child Abuse and Neglect. Washington, DC: US Government Printing Office, 1996.
5. Russell D: The incidence and prevalence of intrafamilial and extrafamilial sexual abuse of female children. Child Abuse Negl 1983; 7:133.
6. Sarafino E: An estimate of nationwide incidence of sexual offenses against children. Child Welfare 1979; 58:127.
7. Weinberg S: Incest Behavior. New York: Citadel, 1955.
8. Muram D, Weatherford T: Child sexual abuse in Shelby county. Two years of experience. Adolesc Pediatr Gynecol 1988; 1:114–118.
9. Muram D, Dorko B, Brown J, Tolley E: Child sexual abuse in Shelby county, Tennessee: A new epidemic? Child Abuse Negl 1991; 15:523–529.
10. Wyatt GE, Loeb TB, Solis B, et al: The prevalence and circumstances of child sexual abuse: Changes across a decade. Child Abuse Negl 1999; 23(1):45–60.
11. Muram D, Rivara F, Buxton B: Comment on current practice: Management of sexual abuse in prepubertal children. Pediatr Adolesc Gynecol 1984; 2:191.
12. Stovall T, Muram D, Wilder M: Sexual abuse and assault: A comprehensive program utilizing a centralized system. Adolesc Pediatr Gynecol 1988; 1:248–251.
13. Hibbard RA: Triage and referrals for child sexual abuse medical examinations from the sociolegal system. Child Abuse Negl 1998; 22:503–513.
14. Ladson S, Johnson C, Doty R: Do physicians recognize sexual abuse? Am J Dis Child 1987; 141:411–415.

15. Orr D: Limitations of emergency room evaluations of sexually abused children. Am J Dis Child 1978; 132:873.

16. Brayden R, Altemeier W, Yeager T, Muram D: Interpretation of colposcopic photographs: Evidence for competence in assessing sexual abuse? Child Abuse Negl 1991; 15:69–76.

17. DeJong AR, Finkel MA: Sexual abuse of children. Curr Probl Pediatr. St. Louis: Mosby–Year Book, 1990.

18. Finkel MA: Child sexual abuse continues to present many dilemmas for the practicing pediatrician. Child Abuse and Neglect 1996; 20:93–94.

19. American Medical Association: Diagnostic and Treatment Guidelines on Child Sexual Abuse. Chicago, American Medical Association, 1992.

20. Finkelhor D: Sexually Victimized Children. New York: Free Press, 1979.

21. National Center on Child Abuse and Neglect (NCCAN): Child sexual abuse: Incest, assault and exploitation. Special report. Washington, DC: HEW, Children's Bureau, 1978.

22. Guidelines for the psychosocial evaluation of suspected sexual abuse in children. Chicago: The American Professional Society on the Abuse of Children, 1990.

23. Eaddy VB, Gentry GC: Play with purpose. Public Welfare 1981; 39:43.

24. Goodwin J: The use of drawings in incest cases. *In* Goodwin J (ed): Sexual Abuse Incest Victims and Their Families. Boston: John Wright PSG, 1982.

25. Cohn DS: Anatomical doll play of preschoolers referred for sexual abuse and those not referred. Child Abuse Negl 1991; 15:455–466.

26. Use of Anatomical Dolls in Child Sexual Assessment. Chicago: The American Professional Society on the Abuse of Children, 1995.

27. Dubowitz H: Children's response to the medical evaluation for child sexual abuse. Child Abuse Negl 1998; 22:581–584.

28. Muram D: Pediatric and adolescent gynecology. *In* De Cherney AH, Pernol ML (eds): Current Gynecologic and Obstetric Diagnosis and Treatment, 8th ed. Norwalk: Appleton & Lange, 1994, pp 633–661.

29. Muram D: Genital tract injuries in the prepubertal child. Pediatr Ann 1986; 15(8):616–620.

30. Adams JA, Knudson S: Genital findings in adolescent girls referred for suspected sexual abuse. Arch Pediatr Adolesc Med 1996; 15:850–857.

31. Adams JA, Harper K, Knudson S, Revilla J: Examination findings in legally confirmed child sexual abuse: It's normal to be normal. Pediatrics 1994; 94(3):310–317.

32. Bays J, Chadwick D: Medical diagnosis of the sexually abused child. Child Abuse and Neglect 1993; 17:91–110.

33. Muram D, Elias S: Child sexual abuse—genital tract findings in prepubertal girls. II. Comparison of colposcopic and unaided examinations. Am J Obstet Gynecol 1989; 160(2):333–335.

34. McCann J: Use of the colposcope in childhood sexual abuse examinations. Pediatr Clin North Am 1990; 37(4):863–880.

35. Slaughter L, Brown C: Colposcopy to establish physical findings in rape victims. Am J Obstet Gynecol 1992; 166:83–86.

36. Teixeira W: Hymenal colposcopic examination in sexual offenses. Am J Forens Med Pathol 1981; 2:209–215.

37. Heger A: Child Sexual Abuse: A Medical View. Los Angeles: United Way Children's Institute International, 1985.

38. McCann J, Voris J, Simon M, Wells R: Comparison of genital examination techniques in prepubertal girls. Pediatrics 1990; 85(2):182–187.

39. The American Professional Society on the Abuse of Children: Chicago: Photographic Documentation of Child Abuse, 1995.

40. Adams J, Phillips P, Ahmad M: The usefulness of colposcopic photographs in the evaluation of suspected child sexual abuse. Adolesc Pediatr Gynecol 1990; 3:75–82.

41. Muram D: Classification of genital findings in prepubertal girls who are victims of sexual abuse. Adolesc Pediatr Gynecol 1988; 2:149.

42. Muram D: Child sexual abuse—genital tract findings in prepubertal girls. I. The unaided medical examination. Am J Obstet Gynecol 1989; 160(2):328–333.

43. Adams JA, Harper K, Knudson S: A proposed system for the classification of anogenital findings in children with suspected sexual abuse. Adolesc Pediatr Gynecol 1999; 5(1):73–75.

44. Muram D: Child sexual abuse: Relationship between sexual acts and genital findings. Child Abuse Negl 1989; 13(2):211–216.

45. Cantwell H: Vaginal inspection as it relates to child sexual abuse in girls under thirteen. Child Abuse Negl 1983; 7:171–176.

46. Cantwell H: Update on vaginal inspection as it relates to child sexual abuse in girls under thirteen. Child Abuse Negl 1987; 11:545–546.

47. Adams J, Ahmad M, Phillips P: Anogenital findings and hymenal diameter in children referred for sexual abuse examination. Adolesc Pediatr Gynecol 1988; 1:123–127.

48. Emans SJ, Woods E, Flagg N: Genital findings in sexually abused, symptomatic, and asymptomatic girls. Pediatrics 1987; 79:778–786.

49. White S, Ingram D, Lyna PR. Vaginal introital diameter in the evaluation of sexual abuse. Child Abuse Negl 1989; 13:217–224.

50. Hobbs CJ, Wynne JM: Buggery in childhood—a common syndrome of child abuse. Lancet 1986; II:792–796.

51. Hobbs CJ, Wynne JM: Sexual abuse of English boys and girls: The importance of anal examination. Child Abuse Negl 1989; 13:195–210.

52. Clayden G: Anal appearances and child sexual abuse. Lancet 1987; I:620–621.

53. Roberts R: Examination of the anus in suspected child sexual abuse. Lancet 1986; II:1100.

54. McCann J, Simon M, Voris J, Wells R: Perianal findings in prepubertal children selected for nonabuse: A descriptive study. Child Abuse Negl 1989; 13:179–193.

55. Muram D: Anal and perianal abnormalities seen in prepubertal victims of abuse. Am J Obstet Gynecol 1989; 161:278–281.

56. Bays J, Jenny C: Genital and anal conditions confused with child sexual abuse trauma. Am J Dis Child 1990; 144:1319–1322.

57. Muram D, Speck P, Gold S: Genital abnormalities in female siblings and friends of child victims of sexual abuse. Child Abuse Negl 1991; 15:105–110.

58. Haugaard J, Reppucci N: The Sexual Abuse of Children. San Francisco: Jossey Bass, 1988, pp 155–156.

59. Green A: Special issues in child abuse. *In* Schetcky D, Green A (eds): Child Sexual Abuse: A Handbook for Health Care and Legal Professionals. New York: Brunner/Mazel, 1988, pp 133–134.

60. Centers for Disease Control: Sexually transmitted diseases treatment guidelines. MMWR 1998; 47(RR-1):1–116.

61. Sgroi S: Handbook of Clinical Intervention in Child Sexual Abuse. Lexington, Mass: Lexington Books, 1982.

62. Berkowitz CD: Medical consequences of child sexual abuse. Child Abuse Neglect 1998; 22:541–550.

Definitions

Intimate parts include the primary genital area, groin, inner thigh, buttock, or breast of a human being.

Sexual contact includes the intentional touching of the victim's, the defendant's, or any other person's intimate parts or the intentional touching of the clothing covering the immediate area of the victim's, the defendant's, or any other person's intimate parts, if that intentional touching can be reasonably construed as being for the purpose of sexual arousal or gratification.

Sexual penetration means sexual intercourse, cunnilingus, fellatio, anal intercourse, or any intrusion, however slight, of any part of a person's body or of any object into the genital or anal openings of the victim's, the defendant's, or any other person's body; emission of semen is not required. In some states, **sodomy** is no longer separated from the above definition. It remains a legal term pertaining to a variety of sexual acts involving orifices other than the vagina.

Rape is the unlawful sexual penetration of the victim by the defendant, or of the defendant by the victim.

Sexual battery is unlawful sexual contact of the victim by the defendant, or vice versa.

Statutory rape is the sexual penetration of the victim by the defendant, or of the defendant by the victim, when the victim is at least 13 but less than 18 years of age and the defendant is at least 4 years older than the victim.

Medical Interview of Sexually Abused Children

1. Obtain information from the parent, social worker, or significant other, without the child present. Ask about the child's terminology for genitalia.
2. Interview the child alone, in a nonthreatening room, preferably not an examination room. Establish rapport: let the child color, play with toys, etc. Be unhurried, calm, nonjudgmental.
3. Begin the actual interview:

   "Do you know why you are here?"

   or

   "Some children who come to see me tell me that someone has touched them in a way that made them uncomfortable. Has anything like that happened to you?"

   or

   "I am a doctor who looks at little girl/boy parts. We're concerned that someone has touched (hurt) your girl/boy parts that you didn't want to. Would anything like that have happened to you?"
4. *"What happened?"* Use dolls. *"Can you show me what happened?"* *"Did he/she touch you here or here?"* *"And then what happened?"* *"What were you wearing?"* *"Did he (she) take your clothes off?"* *"Were you on your side? your back? your tummy?"*
5. *"Who did this?"* Even 2-year-olds can identify people. Repeat the question later in the interview for clarification.
6. *"Where did this happen?"* Four- to 5-year-olds are the youngest children who are able to answer *where?* *"Where was your mother when this happened?"* *"Where were your family members when this happened?"*
7. *"When did this happen?"* Seven- to 8-year-olds are the youngest children who are able to answer *when?* Ask younger patients, *"Was it light or dark outside?"* Use holidays—Christmas or summer, for instance—for reference points.
8. Reassure the patient after the interview: *"Thank you for telling me."* *"I believe what you said."* Acknowledge that the patient is not at fault but will need to tell more people so that it doesn't happen again.
9. Explain the examination: *"We need to check your girl/boy parts to make sure they are okay. Can you help with that?"*

Note

1. Do *not* ask leading questions (i.e., ones that start with *Is, Are, Were, Do, Did*).
2. Dictate the history verbatim. Quote the child's answers in his or her own words.

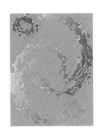

Chapter 25
Eating Disorders

PAULINE S. POWERS

Eating disorders affect at least seven million people in the United States. Women are more likely to develop eating disorders, and many have medical complications that require treatment by a primary care physician. The most common eating disorder, bulimia nervosa, has a prevalence of 1% to 2% among the general population.[1, 2] The prevalence among college-aged women is about 5% and among males about 0.4%.[3] Among the general population, the incidence of anorexia nervosa ranges from 0.45 to 1.6 per 100,000[4]; however, among adolescent girls the prevalence has been estimated to be 0.7%.[5] Although anorexia nervosa is uncommon overall, it is the most common cause of weight loss among adolescent girls in the United States.

At least 80% of bulimia nervosa patients and 95% of anorexia nervosa patients are female. Conventional wisdom has held that eating disorders principally affect upper socioeconomic groups, although there is currently evidence that, for bulimia nervosa, the opposite may be the case and little evidence that anorexia nervosa occurs primarily among upper socioeconomic classes.[6]

Anorexia nervosa has the highest premature mortality rate of any psychiatric disorder; follow-up studies after 15 to 20 years document that 12% to 16% have died.[7, 8] A metaanalysis found the crude rate of mortality from all causes for anorexia nervosa was 5.6% per decade.[9] The long-term consequences of unresolved anorexia nervosa include osteoporosis, infertility, and cardiac and renal disease. The long-term outcome of bulimia nervosa is unclear, but the premature mortality rate is lower (less than 0.5%), but, in about 50% of patients, it appears to be a chronic relapsing and remitting condition, with or without treatment.[10]

DIAGNOSIS

KEY SCREENING QUESTIONS

Although it is usually easy to diagnose anorexia nervosa, some patients with bulimia may be of normal weight and may not volunteer sufficient information to reveal the diagnosis. The key factors to be evaluated to establish an eating disorder diagnosis include weight and diet history, possible binge eating or purging behavior, body image, exercise patterns, and, in females, menstrual history. Table 25–1 lists the key screening questions that usually determine whether a patient is likely to have an eating disorder.

ANOREXIA NERVOSA

The current DSM-IV criteria[11] for anorexia nervosa include weight 15% or more below ideal body weight (IBW), morbid fear of obesity, body image disturbance (e.g., misperception of size as larger than in reality, or negative attitudes toward one's appearance), and, in females, amenorrhea of at least 3 months' duration (Table 25–2). A woman is considered to have amenorrhea if her menses occur only after hormone administration. In patients whose weight loss (or failure to gain weight) starts before or during the adolescent growth spurt, linear growth may be impaired. There are two types of anorexia nervosa: restricting and binge eating–purging.

Although the usual age of onset is between 10 and 25 years, patients as young as 4 years[12] and as old as 94[13] have been described. The rate of

---

Table 25–1. Key Screening Questions

Has there been any change in your weight?
What did you eat yesterday?
Do you ever binge?
Have you ever used self-induced vomiting, laxatives, diuretics, or enemas to lose weight or compensate for overeating?
How much do you exercise in a typical week?
How do you feel about how you look?
Are your menstrual periods regular?

From Powers PS: Initial assessment and early treatment options for anorexia nervosa and bulimia nervosa. Psychiatric Clin North Am 1996; 19:640.

Table 25–2. Diagnostic Criteria for Anorexia Nervosa (DSM-IV)

Weight loss of 15% below minimum normal weight
Intense fear of becoming fat
Body image disturbance
In postmenarchal females, three consecutive missed menstrual periods

Types

Restricting: No binge eating or purging
Binge eating–purging: Regular binge eating and/or purging

recovery is similar for prepubertal patients and those with anorexia of later onset, but even among patients who improve, menarche and growth in stature are typically delayed, and as adults they may be shorter than their normal peers.[14]

BULIMIA NERVOSA

Bulimia is characterized by episodes of binge eating, and the use of various methods to compensate for its effects, that occur at least twice weekly for 3 months. Self-evaluation is influenced unduly by body shape and weight. There are purging and nonpurging types. Patients with the purging type utilize self-induced vomiting or other forms of purging (e.g. laxative, diuretic, or enema abuse), and those with the nonpurging type either fast or exercise to excess (Table 25–3). Patients are normal or overweight. Those whose weight is more than 15% below IBW who have symptoms of bulimia are classified as having anorexia nervosa, binge eating–purging type.

The diagnostic criteria specify that binge eating is characterized by eating a larger than normal amount of food in a discrete period of time *and* a sense of lack of control over eating during the episode. Some patients consider a

Table 25–3. Diagnostic Criteria for Bulimia Nervosa (DSM-IV)

Recurrent episodes of binge eating
   Large quantities consumed in discrete time period
   Sense of lack of control over eating during the episode
Recurrent inappropriate compensatory behavior to prevent weight gain (self-induced vomiting, laxative, or diuretic abuse)
Binge eating and compensatory behavior twice weekly for 3 months
Self-evaluation influenced by size and shape

Types

Purging type
Nonpurging type

normal small snack to be a binge, whereas, to others, binge eating is defined as very large amounts. Although the diagnostic criteria require a large amount of food to qualify as a binge, the patient's self-perception often determines whether or not purging will follow.

The usual age of onset for bulimia is typically several years later than for anorexia nervosa.[15] Bulimia usually begins in the late teens or 20s, but prepubescent patients with symptoms typical of bulimia nervosa have been described.

EATING DISORDER NOT OTHERWISE SPECIFIED

A final category is eating disorders not otherwise specified (EDNOS), which includes subsyndromal and atypical eating disorders. The binge eating disorder and the female athlete triad are included in this category.

The changes in the psychiatric nomenclature that have occurred during the last decade have helped to promote better understanding of full syndromal anorexia nervosa and bulimia nervosa that have led to improvements in treatment, but the changes have also had negative effects. For example, at least one fourth of patients who present to eating disorder clinics have EDNOS.[16] The physiologic complications associated with atypical eating disorders are just as serious as those of the full-blown syndromes.[17] Furthermore, some chronically ill patients may at some point during their illness meet the criteria for all the eating disorder diagnoses. As Marya Hornbacher wryly states in her autobiography, *Wasted*,[18] "I became bulimic at the age of 9, anorexic at the age of 15. I couldn't decide between the two and veered back and forth from one to the other until I was 20. And now, at 23, I am an interesting creature, an Eating Disorder Not Otherwise Specified" (p 2).

BINGE EATING DISORDER

The DSM-IV includes proposed criteria for the binge eating disorder (Table 25–4). It has been estimated that 25% of women in weight control programs have binge eating disorder.[19] Little is known about the age of onset or course of binge eating disorder, but it appears to be a chronic condition frequently associated with obesity. Since, by definition, patients do not use inappropriate behaviors to compensate for weight gain following binge eating, many of the

Table 25–4. Binge Eating Disorder (Proposed Criteria)

Recurrent episodes of binge eating
Binge eating associated with three or more of following:
  Rapid eating
  Eating until uncomfortably full
  Eating large amounts when not hungry
  Eating alone because embarrassed about amount eaten
  Negative feelings after overeating
Marked distress over binge eating
Occurs at least twice weekly for 6 months
Not associated with inappropriate compensatory behavior

physiologic complications are the chronic ones associated with obesity.

FEMALE ATHLETE TRIAD

The female athlete triad is characterized by disordered eating, osteoporosis, and amenorrhea.[20] This condition is probably best conceptualized as subsyndromal anorexia nervosa. Certain groups of female athletes, including gymnasts, figure skaters, and distance runners, have a higher prevalence of eating disorders, including the female athlete triad, than the general young female population.[21] Williamson and colleagues[22] have developed a model for identifying athletes at risk (Fig. 25–1). They postulate that special antecedent factors impinge on the athlete, including anxiety about athletic performance and the athlete's own self-appraisal. When the athlete

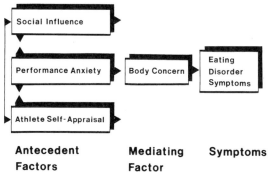

Antecedent Factors   Mediating Factor   Symptoms

Figure 25–1. The antecedent factors include social influence, anxiety about athletic performance, and negative self-appraisal. These antecedent factors may lead to body concern, which mediates the development of eating disorder symptoms. (From Williamson DA, Netmayer RG, Jackman LP, et al: Structural equation modeling for risk factors for the development of eating disorders: Symptoms in female athletes. Int J Eat Disord 1995; 17:287.)

becomes concerned about her performance and negative in her own self-appraisal, then body concern may occur. This mediating factor (body concern) may then result in an overt eating disorder.

The gynecologist is likely to be consulted when an athlete develops amenorrhea. Multiple interactive factors may contribute to the development of amenorrhea, including weight loss, stress, exercise, dietary changes, and alterations in hormones and neurotransmitters (Fig. 25–2). Although amenorrhea in female athletes was once considered benign and related solely to extreme exercise, it is now known that weight loss and amenorrhea, for even relatively brief periods (less than a year), can be associated with osteopenia.[23]

PHYSIOLOGIC ABNORMALITIES: CLINICAL FINDINGS

Multiple physiologic abnormalities have been identified in both anorexia and bulimia nervosa patients. Because many patients with anorexia nervosa have the binge eating–purging type,[24] signs and symptoms of semistarvation, binge eating, and purging are often observed in the same individual.

The severity of the physiologic complications depends on the innate vulnerability of the patient and on the duration and intensity of the abnormal behavior. For example, a 16-year-old who was 5 ft 3 in (1.6 m) tall, lost weight (from 115 to 88 lb or 52.3 to 40 kg) in 6 months by severely restricting her food intake and exercising intensively. She presented with amenorrhea, cachexia, dehydration, low serum potassium, superventricular tachycardia, the "euthyroid sick syndrome," low serum protein, mitral valve prolapse, and both pneumothorax and pneumomediastinum. Another patient, aged 32, who had a 16-year history of bulimia nervosa and subsyndromal anorexia nervosa, was 5 ft 2 in (1.57 m) tall and weighed 98 lb (44.5 kg) with infertility, menstrual irregularities, enlarged parotid glands, mild cachexia, but no dehydration, normal serum electrolytes and protein, elevated parotid amylase isoenzyme, and osteopenia.

The difference in these two patients' presentation is related partly to the different methods used to achieve or maintain low body weight and the duration of the disorder. Patients with rapid weight loss or very severe binge eating or purging are more likely to develop acute problems such as cardiac arrhythmias and electrolyte disturbances. Patients with slow weight loss or pro-

POTENTIAL INTERACTIVE FACTORS
MEDIATING AMENORRHEA

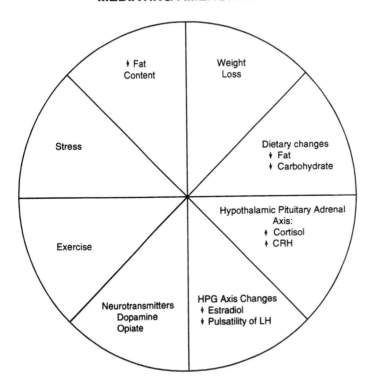

Figure 25–2. Multiple factors contribute to the development of amenorrhea, including exercise, weight loss, stress, decrease in body fat, dietary changes, hormonal changes, and neurotransmitters. CRH = corticotropin-releasing hormone; HPG = hypothalamic pituitary gonadal; LH = luteinizing hormone.

longed but less intensive binge eating or purging are more likely to develop chronic problems such as parotid gland enlargement, hyperamylasemia, or osteoporosis. The nature of the purge behavior is also very significant. For example, extensive use of laxatives or diuretics is likely to be associated with electrolyte or cardiac problems.

The physiologic complications of anorexia nervosa and bulimia nervosa are reviewed in terms of semistarvation, abnormal food or fluid intake, purging behavior, and excessive exercise. For each of these abnormal behaviors aimed at weight loss, the common complications and the relationship to presenting signs, symptoms, or laboratory data will be discussed.

SEMISTARVATION

Cardiac abnormalities are common in patients who are underweight.[25, 26] Prolonged QT intervals and ventricular arrhythmias are the most dangerous of these and are usually associated with electrolyte disturbances, especially low potassium. Purging, particularly by laxative or diuretic abuse, can also result in electrolyte disturbances, which are often reflected in low serum potassium

levels. Total body potassium may fall significantly before the serum level does.[27] Electrocardiographic changes include ST-T wave abnormalities and U waves when serum potassium is low. Decreased cardiac performance and decreased exercise tolerance also occur.

Classic endocrine abnormalities that are related, at least in part, to semistarvation include the euthyroid sick syndrome; amenorrhea associated with decreased serum levels of luteinizing hormone (LH), follicle-stimulating hormone (FSH), and estradiol; and elevated cortisol levels. Skeletal complications, including early osteopenia and osteoporosis with pathologic fractures, are also common. The most frequent gastrointestinal consequence of semistarvation is delayed gastric emptying[28]; the associated postprandial discomfort often promotes further weight loss.

Imaging studies of the brain have documented mild to moderate cerebral atrophy and enlarged ventricles in as many as a third of patients[29]; these abnormalities normalize in some, but not all, patients after they achieve normal weight.[30] One positron emission tomographic study of five anorexic patients who did not binge or purge found glucose hypermetabolism in the head of the caudate that normalized with weight gain.[31]

Although neuropsychological abnormalities[32] have been found in anorexics, it is not known whether these abnormalities correlate with the changes noted in various radiographic studies of the brain.

Hematologic abnormalities[33] include leukopenia, anemia, mild thrombocytopenia, and bone marrow hypoplasia. Immunologic studies have found a wide variety of abnormalities, including low complement factor 3, often not associated with decreased albumin.[34] Some semistarved anorexia nervosa patients are resistant to viral infections until weight falls below 60% of IBW.[35] Decreased fat and muscle content are hallmarks of the disorder and are causally related to a number of the physiologic and cognitive complications, including skeletal, cardiac, and (probably) central nervous system changes.

ABNORMAL FOOD AND FLUID INTAKE

Binge eating large quantities of food can result in gastric dilatation or perforation.[36] Binge-eating carbohydrates contributes to the dental caries associated with bulimia.[37] Benign parotid hypertrophy[38, 39] may also develop; this condition produces swollen cheeks and is usually, but not always, painless. Binge eating usually results in an increase in fat content, even when associated with purge behavior, since purging depletes primarily the components of lean body mass.

Unusual eating habits aimed at attenuating hunger can also produce significant complications. For example, some patients drink large quantities of water and decrease the concentrating capacity of the kidneys.[40] Eating large quantities of low-calorie foods containing carotene (e.g., green vegetables) may result in a yellowish skin tone, particularly on the soles and palms, and an elevated serum carotene level.[41]

PURGE BEHAVIOR

The wide range of purge behaviors have a variety of clinical presentations. Electrolyte abnormalities may include hypokalemia, hyponatremia, and hypomagnesemia. Dental complications include loss of enamel and dentin on teeth that touch the lingual surfaces of the tongue.[37] Buccal erosions may develop from regurgitated hydrochloric acid. Dry mouth, associated with decreases in pH, buffering capacity, and quantity and quality of the saliva, can also occur,[42] and benign parotid hypertrophy sometimes develops

secondary to repeated vomiting.[38] Pneumothorax, pneumomediastinum, or subcutaneous emphysema may result from increased intrathoracic pressure caused by induced vomiting.[43]

MENSTRUAL FUNCTION: ENDOCRINE AND NEUROCHEMICAL PARAMETERS

Part of the fascination with the endocrine changes that occur in anorexia nervosa is the fact that patients who were semistarved and regain weight often progress from prepubertal through pubertal to adult stages of hormonal development and thus provide a clinical model for understanding puberty. Boyer and colleagues[44] demonstrated a regression in the circadian secretory pattern of LH to prepubertal levels at the nadir of weight loss. As the subjects gained weight, the change in the LH secretory pattern progressed from the prepubertal pattern, to early premenarchal patterns, to late pubertal patterns, and finally to the normal adult pattern.

HYPOTHALAMIC-PITUITARY-OVARIAN AXIS IN ANOREXIA NERVOSA

Abnormalities of the hypothalamic-pituitary-ovarian (HPO) axis include low estradiol and gonadotropin levels (LH and FSH).[45] The response of LH and FSH to gonadotropin-releasing hormone (GnRH) may be normal but delayed or manifested only after repeated injections of GnRH.[46]

Although weight loss may partly explain the endocrine changes, there is evidence that other factors are involved. Weiner[46] has estimated that weight loss alone accounts for only half of the variance in response to GnRH. Vigersky and colleagues[47] found that dieting women who lost an average of 19.5% of IBW and developed amenorrhea had normal LH levels. In another study of five healthy women who fasted for 21 days (average weight loss 8 kg), two continued to have adult LH patterns.[48] Other factors that may contribute to the endocrine abnormalities include leptin levels, changes in body fat content, carbohydrate restriction, vitamin deficiencies, binge eating, irregular eating, electrolyte imbalance, volume depletion, hyperactivity, sleep disturbance, and psychic distress. Substance abuse (including diet pills, thyroid medications, diuretics, and laxatives), using alcohol, and drinking too much caffeine, to suppress hunger, may also contribute to endocrine abnormalities. The duration, rate, and extent of weight loss, and purging by vomiting, may also affect hormone levels.

Several problems have beset studies of the resumption of menses. First, some patients have been declared "weight restored" even at 15% below IBW. Second, it is not clear whether the critical weight for normal endocrine function varies from person to person (i.e. that some may have a physiologic set point that is above normal on the standard height-weight tables); thus, their weight may not actually be restored just because it is in the so-called IBW range. Meyer and colleagues found that weight-restored anorexics whose menses resume have fewer preoccupations with food and weight than those who do not regain menses.[49]

LEPTIN AND ANOREXIA NERVOSA

Leptin, a product of the *Ob* gene synthesized by the white fat cells, has been implicated in key findings of anorexia nervosa. Low leptin levels increase food intake with associated weight gain, and high leptin levels depress consumption of food, and increase motor activity, energy metabolism, and body temperature, resulting in weight loss. In anorexia nervosa, leptin levels are low, but, as weight is gained, they peak higher than those of controls matched for BMI.[50] The finding that leptin levels peak before all weight is regained may account for the frequently premature cessation of weight gain.

Low leptin levels also predict amenorrhea in underweight women.[51] In animals, elevations of adrenocorticotropin (ACTH) and cortisol (well-known biologic markers of anorexia nervosa) can be lowered with exogenous leptin.[52] Furthermore, in humans, rapid fluctuations in plasma levels of leptin are inversely related to those of ACTH and cortisol.[53] In *ObOb* mice, repeated administration of leptin corrects sterility and results in ovulation.[54] Thus, leptin may act as a signal that triggers puberty, a theory that supports the hypothesis that fat accumulation enhances maturation of reproductive function. A critical level of leptin may also be necessary for maintenance of normal menstrual function.

HYPOTHALAMIC-PITUITARY-OVARIAN AXIS IN BULIMIA NERVOSA

Menstrual irregularities occur in 20% to 64% of bulimics. In one study,[55] 18 of 28 female bu-

limic patients had a history of an episode of amenorrhea lasting 3 months or longer. Pirke and colleagues[56] found inadequate follicular development, as evidenced by low estradiol levels, in mildly underweight bulimia patients. In normal and slightly overweight bulimic patients, they found luteal phase dysfunction, evidenced by low serum progesterone levels.

Reports on LH and FSH in bulimia nervosa patients have conflicting findings. For example, normal plasma LH and FSH levels have been reported in women who purge by vomiting, but elevated levels have been reported in women who purge with laxatives.[57] In another study,[58] no significant differences were found between bulimics and normal controls in nocturnal secretion of LH, but differences in the secretion of FSH were very significant. In addition, plasma LH and FSH levels were significantly reduced in bulimics with evidence of decreased calorie intake. Kiriike and coworkers[59] observed low basal LH levels in four of nine bulimics with oligomenorrhea or amenorrhea, but normal responses of LH to GnRH; there was a significant correlation between basal LH level and body weight.

Part of the difficulty in assessing these findings is that bulimia nervosa occurs across the weight spectrum with varying degrees of semistarvation determined only in part by weight.[58, 59] For example, in the study by Fichter and colleagues,[58] the weight range was 84% to 113% of IBW, which might include patients who would meet the criteria for anorexia nervosa. They found lower levels of LH and FSH in bulimics who had low triiodothyronine (T_3) levels and low calorie intake during the week preceding the testing. Another complicating factor is a history of anorexia nervosa. For example, Russell[60] reported that, when weight-recovered anorexia nervosa patients develop bulimic symptoms, age-inappropriate LH patterns persist. FSH secretion has also been studied in bulimia nervosa by Schweiger and coworkers.[61] In a series of 22 normal-weight bulimic patients, the rate of ovarian dysfunction was increased and pulsatile LH secretion decreased. Furthermore, it was hypothesized that the observed increase in serum cortisol levels reflected activation of the hypothalamic-pituitary-adrenal axis and was believed to be associated with the pathogenesis of gonadal dysfunction in bulimics.

Thus, there is some evidence that HPO axis abnormalities occur in bulimia nervosa patients, although generally the abnormalities are less pronounced and less consistent than those in anorexia nervosa patients. A history of anorexia nervosa or an existing state of semistarvation (not necessarily related to whether the patient is at or near IBW) confounds interpretation of these studies.

PREMENSTRUAL EXACERBATION OF BINGE EATING

Some bulimia patients' binge eating increases before menses. Animal studies have documented a relationship between food intake and the menstrual cycle.[62] In a pilot study of eight normal women, the average daily calorie increase during the 10 days after ovulation was 500 calories as compared with the 10 days before.[63] Gladis and Walsh[64] documented a modest but statistically significant premenstrual exacerbation of binge eating.

OTHER ENDOCRINE ABNORMALITIES

HYPOTHALAMIC-PITUITARY-THYROID AXIS ABNORMALITIES

The hypothalamic-pituitary-thyroid (HPT) axis has been studied particularly thoroughly in its relation to anorexia nervosa.[55] Most patients have the euthyroid sick syndrome—characterized by a T_3 value in the hypothyroid range, elevated reverse T_3 (rT_3, the metabolic inactive isomer of T_3), normal or slightly decreased serum thyroxine (T_4) level but normal free T_4, and a normal baseline thyroid-stimulating hormone (TSH) value. Low concentrations of T_3 are the most frequently encountered abnormality in nonthyroidal disease and have been correlated with degree of weight loss. About 80% to 90% of T_3, which is the more active thyroid hormone, is derived from the peripheral conversion of T_4. The low serum T_3 level represents a protective metabolic adaptation of the body to starvation or carbohydrate restriction. Most of these changes return to normal with nutritional rehabilitation.

The thyrotropin-releasing hormone (TRH) stimulation test is abnormal in some anorexia nervosa patients. The normal response to TRH is a surge of TSH, which peaks in 15 to 20 minutes. In about 50% of anorexics the response is delayed, and in about 15%, blunted.[55] Findings have been variable in bulimia nervosa patients, with some studies showing normal baseline T_3, T_4, rT_3, and TSH levels and other studies finding significantly lower levels. One important difference between anorexia nervosa and bulimia nervosa is that rT_3 levels are not elevated in bulimia nervosa.[65] Another difference is that the TSH

response to TRH is not usually delayed but is blunted more often than in anorexia nervosa patients.[66, 67] Blunting of the TSH response to TRH has been associated with other psychiatric disorders, particularly depression.[68]

ABNORMALITIES OF THE HYPOTHALAMIC-PITUITARY-ADRENAL AXIS

Clear-cut abnormalities of the hypothalamic-pituitary-adrenal (HPA) axis have been demonstrated for anorexia nervosa patients, but abnormalities among bulimia norvosa patients are less common. Elevated free urinary cortisol levels[69] and elevated mean 24-hour total cortisol levels[70] have been documented in anorexia nervosa patients. The 24-hour secretory pattern of cortisol is also disturbed: levels are elevated during the evening and the first half of the night, when normally, values are low or undetectable. The plasma half-life of cortisol is prolonged[71] as a result of decreased hepatic metabolism of cortisol. It may be that the cortisol production rate does not increase absolutely but rather in relation to body weight and surface area, although this phenomenon would not account for the changes in the secretory pattern.[72] The precise location of the abnormality in the HPA axis is not known, but the normal adrenal response to exogenous ACTH, coupled with normal pituitary responses to glucocorticoids,[73] suggests that it is at the level of the hypothalamus or above.

The overnight dexamethasone suppression test (DST) for HPA overactivity is easily performed. By the DST, more than 90% of patients with anorexia nervosa demonstrate failure to suppress; usually suppression is restored to normal with only a 10% weight gain.[71, 74] These studies, taken together, provide convincing evidence for HPA hyperactivity in anorexia nervosa patients.

In bulimia nervosa patients, nonsuppression of the DST is demonstrated in 20 to 50%.[55, 75] This rate of nonsuppression is very similar to that associated with major depression.[76] In a study comparing 24 women with bulimia to normal controls, Fichter and colleagues[58] did not find nocturnal elevation in plasma cortisol levels.

FAT CONTENT

CRITICAL FAT CONTENT THEORY

Frisch[77] has argued that adequate body fat content, rather than adequate body weight *per se*, is the crucial regulator of menstrual function. Frisch and Revelle[78] found that the average weight at onset of menses (47 kg, or 103 lb) was the same for both early and late maturers. After studying body fat content among these girls and using calculations based on height and weight measures, the investigators found that, at menarche the average body fat content was 24%.

Frisch and McArthur[79] found that, if menarche was to occur, young girls whose height growth was nearly complete (which is usually the case before menarche) had to gain enough weight in relation to their height to reduce the water content of their body to 59.8%, which would correlate with at least 17% of their weight being fat. These investigators also found that women with secondary amenorrhea after simple weight loss needed to weigh about 10% more than the menarchal threshold if normal ovulation was to be restored and sustained. For these patients, fat accounted for about 22% of total body weight. The investigators concluded that a minimum of 17% body fat is required to support menarche, and 22% body fat for normal ovulation at the end of growth in height (about age 18). Normal adolescents gain fat between menarche and age 18, when, typically, they have completed the phase of adolescent subfertility during which the ovary, uterus, and fallopian tubes are still growing and anovulatory cycles are not uncommon. Frisch[77] proposed a nomogram to predict the minimum weight a girl of a given height must attain to have menarche and the probability of regaining menses after secondary amenorrhea at certain weights (Fig. 25–3). Frisch also hypothesized[80] that both the relative and absolute fat content are important, because the woman must be large enough to reproduce.

The main drawback is that Frisch's theory[81] uses formulas that depend solely on measures of height and weight, and that such measures do not necessarily reflect fat content. For example, using standard height and weight tables, Welham and Behnke[82] studied football players who were clearly overweight and found that these athletes had a lower than average body fat content. Similarly, Abraham and colleagues[83] studied a group of ballet dancers with higher than normal muscle content who were of normal weight but had little body fat.

FAT CONTENT IN EATING DISORDER PATIENTS

Several observations regarding fat content in anorexics and bulimics are relevant to integrating the concept of Frisch's critical fat content into the determination of target weights for these patients. Normal-weight bulimics often weigh more than they did before the onset of their disorder, have a higher fat content than age- and weight-matched peers, and require significantly fewer calories to maintain their weight (about 200 fewer per day[84]) than do controls. These data have been interpreted in a variety of ways, but one likely contributing factor is that the result of repeated weight gain–weight loss cycles (associated with binge-purge episodes) is continuously increasing body fat content, which requires fewer calories to maintain.

Many methods are available to assess fat content, including underwater weighing, electrical impedance, and skinfold measures. Of these techniques, skinfold measures are both easiest and least expensive to use, at least in normal and underweight subjects. Skinfolds are measured at four sites—triceps, biceps, subscapular, and suprailiac—and total fat content for females aged 16 to 50 can be determined using the nomogram devised by Durnin and Womersely (Table 25–5).[86] Proposed reference values using the four-site caliper method in younger girls have been published by Westrate and Deurenberg (Table 25–6).[86] Estimation of fat content in this study utilized formulas dependent on certain unproven assumptions about the relationship between body density and skinfold measures; however, as a first estimate, Table 25–6 is a useful guide for determining the fat content of younger girls by skinfold measures. The issue of what constitutes "normal" fat content in younger girls is even less well understood. The data that Fomon and colleagues[87] reported for girls aged 10 and younger (Table 25–7) are also useful.

Although a number of technical errors can occur with the caliper method (including misplacement of the calipers) in experienced hands, the measures are replicable. A more serious problem is that the nomograms make certain assumptions about the relationship between peripheral fat content (as estimated by skinfold measures) and visceral fat content. These assumptions may not be applicable to eating disorder patients, particularly during quick weight changes.

In summary, body fat content is probably an important factor in the regulation of menses and ovulation. Frisch's theory that 17% total body fat is necessary for menarche and 22% total body fat for normal ovulation is an elegant hypothesis that deserves further study. Height and weight measures (including the currently popular BMI)

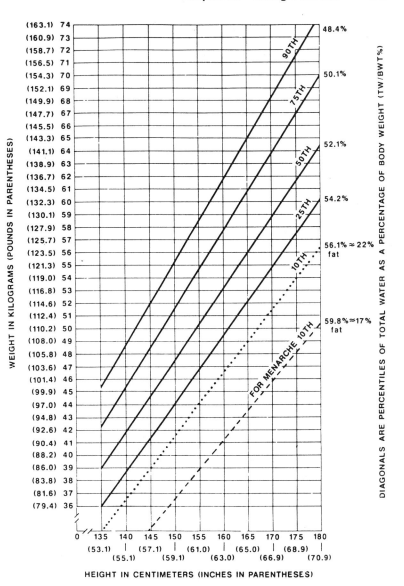

Figure 25–3. Nomogram proposed by Frisch and McArthur indicating the threshold, or minimum weight, that a female of agiven completed height must attain to have normal menstrual cycles. The dashed line shows the minimum weight necessary for menarche. The dotted line shows minimum weight for correcting secondary amenorrhea. The top five diagonal lines indicate percentiles of total water as a percentage of weight—which is an index of fatness—for fully grown, mature women in a normal sample; the dotted line is the 10th percentile. The dashed line represents the 10th percentile for the same sample at menarche. The 50th percentile line indicates the normal weight for height of mature women aged 18 to 25 years. (Adapted from Frisch RE: Fatness and fertility. Sci Am 1988; 258:88.)

will not be adequate to prove or disprove the theory.

OVARIAN AND UTERINE CHANGES

Treasure and colleagues[88, 89] have studied ovarian and uterine changes during weight gain in girls with anorexia nervosa. The changes in ovarian structure and size were found to replicate normal pubertal development, albeit more rapidly. Three stages of ovarian development were identified during weight restoration: amorphous, multifollicular (previously termed *multicystic* or *polycystic*), and finally a single dominant follicle.

Characteristic endocrine findings were noted in each stage. In the amorphous stage, LH, FSH, and estradiol levels were low; in the multifollicular stage, FSH rose significantly, but LH levels increased only moderately, and estradiol levels remained low. In the single–dominant follicle stage, LH increased, FSH increases were small or absent, and estradiol levels rose (until follicular size was greater than 22 mm) and then fell. In this study, 41% of the patients who were discharged with multifollicular ovaries (and at lower weights than patients with a single dominant follicle) were readmitted with a severe relapse, whereas only 16% who were discharged with a dominant follicle (and at higher weights) were readmitted. It was proposed that a critical

Table 25–5. Percentage of Body Weight as Fat in Females Aged 13 and Older*

Skinfolds (mm)	Age (yr)			
	16–29	*30–39*	*40–49*	*50 +*
15	10.5			
20	14.1	17.0	19.8	21.4
25	16.8	19.4	22.2	24.0
30	19.5	21.8	24.5	26.6
35	21.5	23.7	26.4	28.5
40	23.4	25.5	28.2	30.3
45	25.0	26.9	29.6	31.9
50	26.5	28.2	31.0	33.4
55	27.8	29.4	32.1	34.6
60	29.1	30.6	33.2	35.7
65	30.2	31.6	34.1	36.7
70	31.2	32.5	35.0	37.7
75	32.2	33.4	35.9	38.7
80	33.1	34.3	36.7	39.6
85	34.0	35.1	37.5	40.4
90	34.8	35.8	38.3	41.2
95	35.6	36.5	39.0	41.9
100	36.4	37.2	39.7	42.6
105	37.1	37.9	40.4	43.3
110	37.8	38.6	41.0	43.9
115	38.4	39.1	41.5	44.5
120	39.0	39.6	42.0	45.1
125	39.6	40.1	42.5	45.7
130	40.2	40.6	43.0	46.2
135	40.8	41.1	43.5	46.7
140	41.3	41.6	44.0	47.2
145	41.8	42.1	44.5	47.7
150	42.3	42.6	45.0	48.2
155	42.8	43.1	45.4	48.7
160	43.3	43.6	45.8	49.2
165	43.7	44.0	46.2	49.6
170	44.1	44.4	46.6	50.0
175	—	44.8	47.0	50.4
180	—	45.2	47.4	50.8
185	—	45.6	47.8	51.2
190	—	45.9	48.2	51.6
195	—	46.2	48.5	52.0
200	—	46.5	48.8	52.4
205	—	—	49.1	52.7
210	—	—	49.4	53.0

*The equivalent fat content, as a percentage of body weight, for a range of values for the sum of four skinfolds (biceps, triceps, subscapular, and suprailiac) of females of different ages.

Modified from Durnin J, Womersely J: Body fat assessed from total body density, and its estimation from skinfold thickness: Measurements on 481 men and women aged from 16 to 72 years. Br J Nutr 1974;32:77.

nutritional threshold must be achieved before a dominant follicle can develop.

Treasure[89] also studied 20 normal-weight bulimics (weight ranging from 85% to 105% IBW) with amenorrhea and observed decreased ovarian volume, multifollicular ovaries, and a marked decrease in uterine volume. Five normal-weight bulimics with oligomenorrhea had normal-sized ovaries with one dominant, developed follicle

Table 25–6. Percentage of Body Fat in Females*

Age (yr)	Skinfolds (mm)				
	15%	*20%*	*25%*	*30%*	*35%*
0	17	22	30	40	52
1	18	24	32	43	58
2	18	25	34	45	60
4	18	25	34	46	62
6	19	25	35	47	63
8	19	26	35	48	65
10	19	27	37	51	69
12	21	30	42	58	80
14	23	33	47	66	92
16	25	37	53	75	106
18	27	40	58	85	122

*Data from 2285 Dutch children aged 0 to 18 years. Skinfolds (in millimeters) are the sum of biceps, triceps, suprailiac, and subscapular skinfold thicknesses.

From Westrate JA, Deurenberg P: Body composition in children: Proposal for a method for calculating body fat percentage from total body density or skinfold thickness measurements. Am J Clin Nutr 1989; 50:1104. © American Society for Clinical Nutrition.

but failed to ovulate and had inadequate corpus luteum function.

INFERTILITY AND EATING DISORDERS

Bates and colleagues[90] studied 47 females aged 16 to 36 years who presented to a reproductive endocrinology clinic for assessment for infertility or menstrual dysfunction. Weights of

Table 27–7. Percentage of Body Weight as Fat in Females from Birth to Age 10 Years

Age	Length/Height		Weight		Fat
	(cm)	**(in)**	**(kg)**	**(lbs)**	**(%)**
Birth	50.5	19.98	3.325	7.315	14.9
1 mo	53.4	21.02	4.131	9.098	16.2
3 mo	59.6	23.46	5.743	12.63	23.8
6 mo	65.8	25.91	7.250	15.95	26.4
9 mo	70.4	27.72	8.270	18.19	25.0
12 mo	74.3	29.25	9.180	20.20	23.7
18 mo	80.2	31.57	10.78	23.72	21.8
24 mo	85.5	33.66	11.91	26.20	20.4
3 yr	94.1	37.05	14.10	31.02	18.5
4 yr	101.6	40.0	15.96	35.11	17.3
5 yr	108.4	42.68	17.66	38.85	16.7
6 yr	114.6	45.12	19.52	42.94	16.4
7 yr	120.6	47.48	21.84	48.05	16.8
8 yr	126.4	49.76	24.84	54.65	17.4
9 yr	132.2	52.05	28.46	62.61	18.3
10 yr	138.3	54.45	32.55	71.61	19.4

From Fomon SJ, Ziegler EE, Nelson SE: Body composition of reference children from birth to age 10 years. Am J Clin Nutr 1982; 35:1169. © American Society for Clinical Nutrition.

those in the infertile group were, on average, 9% below IBW and of those with menstrual irregularities, on average 11% below IBW. Four patients were diagnosed as having anorexia nervosa. Among the women who agreed to gain weight to predicted IBW, 19 of 26 infertile women conceived spontaneously, and 9 of 10 with secondary amenorrhea resumed menstruation. Eleven women refused to accept underweight as a cause of reproductive failure and refused to participate in the study.

In a study by Stewart and colleagues,[91] 11 of 66 women aged 21 to 39 years evaluated in a university hospital fertility clinic had eating disorders (one had anorexia nervosa, four had bulimia nervosa, and six had atypical eating disorders). The 12 amenorrheic women in the sample had a higher prevalence of eating disorders (58%) than did women with normal cycles (7%). These eating disorder prevalences are significantly higher than the 4% reported in a careful survey of women aged 16 to 35 attending a family practice clinic.[92] Thus, infertile women with menstrual abnormalities may be particularly likely to have an eating disorder.

PREGNANCY

ONSET DURING PREGNANCY

Although, typically, eating disorders begin in adolescence, they may begin at any age. Often, onset of an eating disorder is triggered by a crucial developmental step, such as pregnancy. In one study of 100 women from an unselected community sample who were pregnant for the first time, five developed an eating disorder.[93] Two had a history of bulimia nervosa that had resolved before the pregnancy. Another study[94] found that pregnant women had lower scores on the drive for thinness and body dissatisfaction subscales of the Eating Attitudes Inventory, but there was no evidence of any relaxation of body image ideal during pregnancy. In a study of 97 primagravidas, followed 6 months post partum, a marked increase in behaviors and attitudes characteristic of eating disorders were noted.[95] Since pregnancy and the postpartum period may be associated with increased risk, the obstetrician may be in a unique position to recognize an emerging eating disorder.

EFFECT OF PREGNANCY ON A PATIENT WITH A PREEXISTING EATING DISORDER

Although most women with anorexia nervosa do not become pregnant and invariably have amenorrhea, when pregnancy does occur the effect can be devastating for both the patient and her fetus. For patients with chronic anorexia nervosa, body fat content may increase even if weight remains low, and fertility may be reestablished. Thus, a chronic anorexia nervosa patient may unexpectedly become pregnant. Since patients with anorexia nervosa may not gain weight, detection of pregnancy may be belated. Two extreme cases in which recognition of pregnancy occurred at weeks 25 and 26 have been described.[96]

Among anorexia nervosa patients who do become pregnant, weight gain is typically inadequate and complications of pregnancy and birth are very common. Maternal complications include inadequate weight gain, hyperemesis, and vaginal bleeding[97, 98] Fetal and birth complications include low birth weight and prenatal death. With treatment and supervised adequate weight gain, delivery can be normal and birth weight of the infant may be normal.[98]

Patients with bulimia nervosa are more likely to be fertile, and they often become pregnant. The frequency of binge eating and purging often decreases during pregnancy, perhaps because the woman has the ego strength to avoid behaviors that might injure the child. It may also be that the enlarging uterus makes binge eating more difficult and uncomfortable. Unfortunately, after delivery at least two thirds of patients resume binge eating and purging.[99, 100]

EFFECTS ON THE FETUS

Disordered eating behavior can have teratogenic effects. In one study, the risk of fetal loss was nearly twice as high for bulimic mothers as for normal controls.[101] Failure to gain weight during pregnancy may result in fetal death or low birth weight. Nonprescription drugs abused by patients to promote weight loss may be teratogenic. For example, diet pills containing phenylpropanolamine have been associated with clubfoot and inguinal hernia. Table 25–8 shows possible fetal effects of over-the-counter diet pills, diuretics, laxatives, and the purgative, ipecac. In addition, patients with eating disorders sometimes abuse certain prescription medica-

Table 25–8. Possible Teratogenic Effects of Nonprescription Drugs Abused by Eating Disorder Patients

Drug Type	Brand Name	Active Ingredient(s)	Possible Fetal Effects
Diet pills	Acutrim	Phenylpropanolamine	? Clubfoot, inguinal hernia[1]
	Dexatrim	Phenylpropanolamine	
Diuretics	Aqua Ban	Caffeine	Withdrawal symptoms after birth,[2] low birth weight[3]
		Ammonium chloride	? Inguinal hernia, cataract, benign tumor[4]
Laxatives	Correctol	Bisacodyl	None[5]
		Docusate	? Neonatal hypomagnesemia[6]
	Ex-Lax	Anthraquinone glucosides	None[4]
	Senokot	Anthraquinone glucosides	None[4]
Purgative	Ipecac (brand and generic name)	Mixture of alkaloids	Probably none[1]

Note: The information in this table was obtained from the University of South Florida Teratogen Information Service.
1. Data from Heinonen OP, Sloan D, Shapiro SC: Birth Defects and Drugs in Pregnancy. Littleton, Mass: Publishing Sciences Group, 1977.
2. Data from Devoe LD, Yousif A, Murray C, Arnaud M: Maternal caffeine consumption and fetal behavior in normal third-trimester pregnancy. Am J Ob Gyn 1993; 168:1105.
3. Data from Godel JC, Johnson KE, Pabst HF, et al: Smoking and caffeine and alcohol intake during pregnancy in a Northern population, effect on fetal growth. Can Med Assoc J 1992; 147:181.
4. Data from Reproductive Toxicology Center (producer). Reprotox database (machine-readable data file). Washington, DC: Producer, 1988.
5. Data from Berkowitz RL: Handbook for Prescribing Medications During Pregnancy. 2nd ed. Boston: Little, Brown, 1986.
6. Data from Briggs GG (ed): Drugs in Pregnancy and Lactation, 4th ed. Baltimore: Williams & Wilkins, 1994.

This table adapted and used with permission from Powers PS: Management of patients with co-morbid conditions. *In* Garner DM, Garfinkel PE (eds): Handbook of Treatment for Eating Disorders, 2nd ed. New York: Guilford Press, 1997, p 432.

tions. For example, some patients misuse furosemide or chlorthiazide in the mistaken belief that they will lose fat. Both drugs are in the U.S. Food and Drug Administration (FDA) category C (i.e., fetal risk cannot be ruled out). Many patients with eating disorders develop physiologic complications that require treatment with drugs that may confer fetal risk (for example, cisapride used to treat delayed gastric emptying is in category C). Since comorbid psychiatric disorders are very common among eating disorder patients, various psychotropic medications may also be necessary. Table 25–9 shows the common prescription drugs used or abused by

eating disorder patients and their estimated fetal risks.

EFFECTS ON THE CHILD

Several studies have shown long-term physiologic and psychological problems in the children of eating disorder patients. One group[102] found that mothers with eating disorders were more intrusive with their infants during mealtimes. Another group found that some women with anorexia nervosa underfeed their children.[103] An occasional infant with failure to thrive may have

Table 25–9. Possible Teratogenic Risks of Prescription Medications Used or Abused by Eating Disorder Patients

Generic Name	Brand Name	Use or Abuse	Category*
Metoclopramide	Reglan	Facilitator of gastric emptying	B
Cisapride	Propulsid	Facilitator of gastric emptying	C
Fluoxetine	Prozac	Antidepressant	B
Paroxetine	Paxil	Antidepressant	B
Sertraline	Zoloft	Antidepressant	B
Lithium	Eskalith, others	Antimanic	D
Amphetamine	Dexedrine, others	Appetite suppressant	C
Furosemide	Lasix	Purge method	C
Chlorothiazide	Diuril	Purge method	C

*FDA categories: A, controlled studies show no risk; B, no evidence of risk in humans; C, risk cannot be ruled out; D, positive evidence of risk.
Reprinted with permission from Powers PS: Management of patients with co-morbid conditions. *In* Garner DM, Garfinkel PE (eds): Handbook of Treatment for Eating Disorders, 2nd ed. New York: Guilford Press, 1997, p 432.

a mother with an eating disorder whose ambivalence about eating compromises her feeding the child. In a report of 12 patients who had anorexia nervosa or bulimia nervosa, significant disturbances in parenting were noted, and two of the patients abandoned their children.[104]

TREATMENT OF THE PREGNANT PATIENT WITH AN EATING DISORDER

Since patients with eating disorders usually resume disturbed eating after delivery, it is best to counsel the patient to postpone pregnancy until she has fully recovered. Patients who do become pregnant while they are still ill require intensive multidisciplinary treatment. A first step is to educate the mother and her partner about the possible teratogenic effects of inadequate weight gain and various purge methods.

Comprehensive management usually requires an obstetrician who specializes in high-risk pregnancies, a psychiatrist, and a nutritionist. Psychoeducation during pregnancy can be particularly helpful in arresting dangerous behavior. For example, the patient may be able to gain weight if the composition of weight gain (Fig. 25–4) is explained and she realizes that only a small portion of the weight is fat. Individual therapy can help the patient to recognize and adapt to changes that will be required when she is a mother. This circumstance often triggers memories of inadequate parenting the patient received as a child; coming to terms with her own early development may be helpful. The father of the baby can be a powerful influence to help the patient to abandon dangerous behavior during pregnancy and after delivery.

BONE MINERAL DEFICIENCY

Bone mineral deficiency is common in anorexia nervosa patients and in bulimia nervosa patients who have a history of anorexia nervosa. Males with anorexia nervosa also develop osteoporosis. Patients with bone mineral deficiency have reduced total bone mass and bone density. Recent studies have shown that, during early adolescence, an episode of anorexia nervosa as brief as 1 year may result in long-lasting bone mineral deficiency.[23] *Osteopenia* is defined as mineral deficiency that is 1 to 2.5 standard deviations below the value for age-matched controls. *Osteoporosis* is bone mineral deficiency greater than 2.5 standard deviations below age-matched controls and is often associated with pathologic fractures.

PHYSIOLOGY OF BONE

Most bone mineral mass is deposited by age 15, but smaller increases occur until age 30 when peak bone mass is achieved. Then, bone mass begins to decline. The balance between bone formation and bone resorption is a dynamic one that is influenced by both nutritional and hormonal factors. Bone formation requires adequate nutritional intake, including calcium and vitamin D (required for osteoblast activity). For estrogen to be effective, an adequate body fat store is required. Patients with anorexia nervosa are malnourished, often have an inadequate fat store, and have calcium deficiency. Bone resorption is increased by elevated glucocorticoid levels (for example, cortisol) and deficient estrogen.

The effect of exercise on bone is complex. Moderate exercise may be useful in preventing

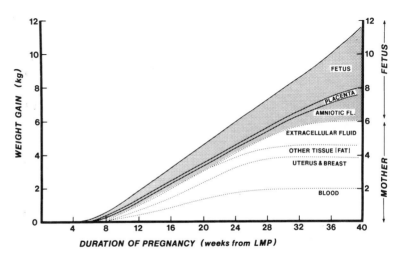

Figure 25–4. Components of weight gain during pregnancy. Pattern and components of average weight gain during pregnancy. Shaded areas represent the fetal components. LMP = last menstrual period. Note that only a small percentage of weight gain is fat tissue. (From Pitkin RM: Nutritional support in obstetrics and gynecology. Clin Obstet Gynecol 1976; 19:489. Reprinted with permission.)

bone loss, whereas strenuous exercise may promote it. High-impact sports can increase the risk of fractures.[105]

OSTEOPOROSIS AND ANOREXIA NERVOSA

The bone mineral deficiency that occurs in anorexia nervosa is different from postmenopausal osteoporosis, which is due primarily to estrogen deficiency and, to some extent, calcium deficiency. The osteoporosis that occurs in anorexia nervosa is due to a combination of deficient bone formation and increased bone resorption.[106] Among anorexia nervosa patients, type 1 collagen carboxyl terminal propeptide (ICTP), a marker of bone resorption, is high and type 1 procollagen carboxyl terminal propeptide (PCTP), a marker of bone formation, is low. With weight gain, ICTP decreases and PICP increases.

Multiple interacting factors contribute to the development of osteoporosis in anorexia nervosa patients. Although estrogen deficiency is involved in reducing bone mineral mass, the mechanism is unclear. All of the following conditions can contribute to bone mass deficiency: inadequate dietary calcium, vitamin D deficiency, decreased body fat and body weight, deficient estrogen, elevated cortisol, and excessive strenuous high-impact exercise (Table 25–10). Bone mineral density is reduced primarily in the hip joints and in the lumbar spine.[23]

ASSESSMENT

Patients with anorexia nervosa or a history of it should be assessed for osteoporosis. Many patients with an EDNOS are also at risk, since they may have had intermittent episodes of amenorrhea or underweight even though they have not met strict criteria for anorexia nervosa. The history should include an assessment of the duration of low weight and amenorrhea as well as a history of pathologic fractures (i.e., fractures

Table 25–10. Factors Contributing to Decreased Bone Density In Anorexia Nervosa

- Underweight
- Decreased fat stores
- Inadequate calcium
- Inadequate vitamin D
- Elevated cortisol
- Estrogen deficiency
- Excessive strenuous exercise

occurring without apparent stress). Nutritional assessment includes calories, calcium, and vitamin D. Details of exercise history are also needed. A dual-energy x-ray absorptiometry (DEXA) image should be obtained; estradiol levels should be obtained at the same time. In the future, monitoring bone formation and bone resorption markers may be feasible.

TREATMENT OF OSTEOPENIA OR OSTEOPOROSIS

Educating the patient and her family is the key to successful treatment. Patients often deny that their behavior has consequences. Gentle confrontation with an abnormal DEXA may permit the patient to accept her diagnosis and comply with treatment.

The goal of treatment is adequate nutritional intake with weight restoration and increase in total body fat stores. The proportion of body fat should be about 17% for adolescent girls and 22% to 25% for young adult women. The normal calcium requirement is 1200 mg/day but should be 1500 mg/day in recovering anorexia nervosa patients. Nutritional assessment can be used to estimate calcium intake in food and supplements prescribed as necessary. Vitamin D supplementation may be necessary if the patient is rarely out of doors.

Estrogen supplementation *does not* prevent further loss of bone mineral stores in anorexia nervosa patients who do not gain weight.[107] Nonetheless, after a period of 6 months of anorexia nervosa in a patient who is in treatment, estrogen supplementation may be wise.

Other treatments have been proposed but have not yet been shown to be effective. Alendronate (Fosamax) is a form of biphosphonate that has been helpful in treating patients with postmenopausal osteoporosis, but it has gastrointestinal side effects that may make it difficult to use in anorexia nervosa patients. A recent report[108] has found that recombinant insulin-like growth factor (rhIGF-1) increases bone formation in anorexia nervosa patients, however, this osteotrophic hormone requires daily injections and its long-term effects are not known.

A recent report[109] found that anorexia nervosa patients who were weight-restored for a mean of 21 years had decreased femur bone mineral density, but lumbar spine bone mineral density was similar to that of controls.

SEXUAL ABUSE: EFFECTS ON PATIENT CARE

Because about 30% of patients who have an eating disorder also have a history of sexual abuse,[110] the primary care physician who assesses a patient with anorexia nervosa or bulimia should keep this possibility in mind. Patients may volunteer the information, but much more often they do not. Asking the patient if she has been sexually or physically abused often prompts her to acknowledge this history. The physician's initial response should be to validate the reality of the abuse and to acknowledge that these experiences may have had an effect on the patient's life, including her sexual functioning. The physician can then inquire about any anxiety about the pelvic examination that might relate to this history and suggest various strategies for relieving the anxiety, including the presence of a relative, a detailed description of the examination, among others.

Some patients who have been abused do not acknowledge it, even when questioned in an empathic and understanding manner. Usually, this means that the patient is not emotionally prepared to cope with her feelings about the experience, and the physician should not query the patient further.

GENERAL PRINCIPLES OF TREATMENT

Both anorexia nervosa and bulimia nervosa require prompt psychiatric intervention. It is well-known that, with anorexia nervosa, the prognosis dims progressively with the duration of the illness and the extent of weight loss.[111, 112] The development of binge eating or purging in a patient with anorexia nervosa makes the prognosis still bleaker. In some semistarved patients, binge eating starts when the drive to eat overwhelms the patient. In other anorexia patients, the onset of binge eating or purging is related to iatrogenic factors. Patients who are urged to gain weight without resolving the psychological issues may comply at first but then begin purging when they are no longer under medical observation.

Most patients with anorexia nervosa require inpatient treatment at some point during recovery. Weight restoration is a crucial aspect of treatment. Several methods have been used, but the effectiveness of behavior modification programs based on operant conditioning is well-established.[113] Long-term individual psychotherapy, starting in the hospital and usually continuing for

several years after hospitalization, is an essential part of treatment. Family therapy is another important aspect of a comprehensive treatment plan.[114, 115] Patients with the binge eating–purging type of disorder whose weight is 25% or more below IBW, who have been ill for more than 6 months, or who have any of the well-known physiologic complications of semistarvation need hospitalization to achieve and maintain IBW and to establish a positive relationship with an individual therapist. With appropriate treatment for adolescent anorexia nervosa patients, full recovery occurs in nearly 76% within 5 to 6 years after the index hospitalization.[116]

Patients whose weight has been restored and who then start taking fluoxetine have a lower risk of relapse.[117]

Patients with bulimia nervosa can usually be treated as outpatients with a combination of individual or group psychotherapy and antidepressant medication. There is a strong link between bulimia nervosa and major depression,[118] but not all patients with bulimia are depressed. Antidepressants are a mainstay of treatment; fluoxetine is the one best studied. In a multicenter trial of more than 200 patients, a significant reduction in the frequency of binge eating was achieved with 60-mg doses of fluoxetine daily, regardless of whether the patient met criteria for major depression.[119] Fluoxetine is currently the only medication approved by the FDA for bulimia nervosa. The outcome of bulimia nervosa is poorly understood.

ROLE OF THE PHYSICIAN

The physician rendering care to young, underweight, amenorrheic females should have a high index of suspicion for anorexia nervosa and, in such cases, should facilitate prompt assessment and treatment by mental health professionals. One of the most effective strategies available is to stress to the patient (and her family) the long-term physiologic complications of eating disorders. Although the long-term psychological consequences are equally devastating, early in the course of these conditions (at the very time when intervention is likely to be most effective), the patient may feel better because the underlying psychodynamic conflicts have been temporarily alleviated by the symptoms.

REFERENCES

1. Pyle RL, Mitchell JE: The epidemiology of bulimia. *In* Blinder BF, Chaitin BF, Goldstein RS (eds): The Eating

Disorders: Medical and Psychological Bases of Diagnosis and Treatment. New York: PMA Publishing, 1988, p 259.

2. Gotestam KG, Agras WS: General population-based epidemiological study of eating disorders in Norway. Int J Eat Disord 1995; 18:119.

3. Heatherton TF, Nichols P, Mahamedi F, Keel P: Body weight, dieting, and eating disorder symptoms among college students, 1982–1992. Am J Psychiatry 1995; 152:1623.

4. Willie J, Grossman S: Epidemiology of anorexia nervosa in a defined region of Switzerland. Am J Psychiatry 1982; 140:564.

5. Steinhausen HC, Winkler C, Meier M: Eating disorders in adolescence in a Swiss epidemiological study. Int J Eat Disord 1997; 22:147.

6. Gard MC, Freeman CP: The dismantling of a myth: A review of eating disorders and socioeconomic status. Int J Eat Disord 1996; 20:1.

7. Halmi K, Brodland G, Luney J: Prognosis in anorexia nervosa. Ann Intern Med 1973; 78:907–909.

8. Ratnasuriya RH, Eisler I, Szmukler GT, Russell GF: Anorexia nervosa: outcome and prognostic factors after 20 years. Br J Psychiatry 1991; 158:495–502.

9. Sullivan PF: Mortality in anorexia nervosa. Am J Psychiatry 1995; 152:1073.

10. Keel PK, Mitchell JE: Outcome in bulimia nervosa. Am J Psychiatry 1997; 154:313.

11. Diagnostic and Statistical Manual of Mental Disorders, 4 ed (DSM-IV). Washington, DC: American Psychiatric Association, 1994 pp 539–550; 729–731.

12. Gislason I: Eating disorders in childhood. In Blinder BJ, Chaitin BF, Goldstein RD (eds): The Eating Disorders: Medical and Psychological Bases of Diagnosis and Treatment. New York: PMA Publishing, 1988, p 285.

13. Bernstein IC: Anorexia nervosa: 94-year-old woman treated with electroshock. Minn Med 1972; 55:552.

14. Goodman S, Blinder BJ, Chaitin BF, Hagman J: Atypical eating disorders. In Blinder BJ, Chaitin BF, Goldstein RS (eds): The Eating Disorders: Medical and Psychological Bases of Diagnosis and Treatment. New York: PMA Publishing, 1988, p 393.

15. Soundy TJ, Lucas AR, Suman VJ, Melton LJ 3rd: Bulimia nervosa in Rochester, Minnesota from 1980 to 1990. Psychol Med 1995; 25:1065.

16. Garfinkel PE, Kennedy SH, Kaplan AS: Views on classification and diagnosis of eating disorders. Can J Psychiatry 1995; 40:445.

17. Garfinkel PE, Lin E, Goering P, et al: Should amenorrhea be necessary for the diagnosis of anorexia nervosa. Evidence from a Canadian community sample. Br J Psychiatry 1996; 168:500.

18. Hornbacher M: Wasted. A Memoir of Anorexia and Bulimia. New York: Harper Collins, 1998.

19. deZwaan M, Mitchell JE, Raymond NC, Spitzer RL: Binge eating disorder: Clinical features and treatment of a new diagnosis. Harvard Rev Psychiatry 1994; 1:310–325.

20. American College of Sports Medicine position stand: The Female Athlete Triad. Med Sci Sports Exerc 1997; 29:i–ix.

21. Thompson RA, Sherman RT: Helping Athletes with Eating Disorders. Champaign, Ill: Human Kinetics, 1993.

22. Williamson DA, Netemeyer RG, Jackman LP, et al: Structural equation modeling for risk factors for the development of eating disorder symptoms in female athletes. Int J Eat Disord 1995; 17:287.

23. Bachrach LK, Guido D, Katzman D, et al:. Decreased bone density in girls with anorexia nervosa. Pediatrics 1990; 86:440.

24. Pryor T, Wiederman MW, McGilley B: Clinical correlates of anorexia nervosa subtypes. Int J Eat Disord 1996; 19:371.

25. Schocken DD, Holloway JD, Powers PS: Weight loss and the heart. Arch Intern Med 1989; 149:877.

26. Powers PS, Schocken DD, Feld J, et al: Cardiac function during weight restoration in anorexia nervosa. Int J Eat Disord 1991; 10:521.

27. Powers PS, Tyson IB, Stevens BA, Heal AV: Total body potassium and serum potassium among eating disorder patients. Int J Eat Disord 1995; 18:269.

28. Dubois A, Gross HA, Ebert MH, Castell DO: Altered gastric emptying and secretion in primary anorexia nervosa. Gastroenterology 1979; 77:319.

29. Kohlmeyer K, Lehmkuhl F, Poustka F: Computed tomography in patients with anorexia nervosa. Am J Neuroradiol 1983; 4:437.

30. Heinz ER, Martinez J, Haenggeli A: Reversibility of cerebral atrophy in anorexia nervosa and Cushing's syndrome. J Comput Assist Tomogr 1977; 1:415.

31. Herholz K, Krieg JC, Emrich HM, et al: Regional cerebral glucose metabolism in anorexia nervosa measured by positron emission tomography. Biol Psychiatry 1987; 22:43.

32. Fox C: Neuropsychological correlates of anorexia nervosa. Int J Psychiatry Med 1981; 11:285.

33. Kay J, Stricker R: Hematologic and immunologic abnormalities in anorexia nervosa. South Med J 1983; 76:1008.

34. Palmblad JA, Fohlin L, Nurberg R: Plasma levels of complement factors 3 and 4. Acta Paediatr Scand 1979; 6G8:617.

35. Pertschuk M, Crosby L, Barot L, Mullen J: Immunocompetency in anorexia nervosa. Am J Clin Nutr 1982; 35:968.

36. Mitchell JE, Pyle RL, Miner RA: Gastric dilatation as a complication of bulimia. Psychosomatics 1982; 23:96.

37. Wolcott RB, Yager J, Gordon G: Dental sequelae to the binge-purge syndrome (bulimia): Report of cases. J Am Dent Assoc 1984; 109:723.

38. Levin P, Falko J, Dixon K, et al: Benign parotid enlargement in bulimia. Ann Intern Med 1980; 93:827.

39. Blinder BJ, Hagman J: Serum salivary isoamylase levels in patients with anorexia nervosa, bulimia or bulimia nervosa. Hillside J Clin Psychiatry 1986; 8:152.

40. Mecklenburg R, Loriaux D, Thompson R, et al: Hypothalamic dysfunction in patients with anorexia nervosa. Medicine 1974; 523:147.

41. Casper R, Kirschner B, Sanstead H, et al: An evaluation of trace metals, vitamins and taste function in anorexia nervosa. Am J Clin Nutr 1980; 33:1801.

42. Levinson NA: Oral manifestations of eating disorders: Indications for a collaborative treatment approach. In Blinder BJ, Chaitin BF, Goldstein RS (eds): The Eating Disorders: Medical and Psychological Bases of Diagnosis and Treatment. New York: PMA Publishing, 1988, p 405.

43. Al-Muffy N, Bevan D: A case of subcutaneous emphysema, pneumomediastinum and pneumothorax associated with functional anorexia. Br J Clin Pract 1977; 31:160.

44. Boyar RM, Katz JL, Finkelstein JW, et al: Anorexia nervosa: Immaturity of the 24-hour luteinizing hormone secretory pattern. N Engl J Med 1974; 291:861.

45. Wakeling A, DeSouza VFA: Differential endocrine and menstrual responses to weight changes in anorexia nervosa. In Darby PL, Garfinkel PE, Garner DM, Coscina

DV (eds): Anorexia Nervosa: Recent Developments in Research. New York: Alan R. Liss, 1983, p 271.

46. Weiner H: Psychoendocrinology of anorexia nervosa. Psychiatr Clin North Am 1989; 12:187.

47. Vigersky RA, Anderson AE, Thompson RH, Loriaux DL: Hypothalamic dysfunction in secondary amenorrhea associated with simple weight loss. N Engl J Med 1977; 297:1141.

48. Pirke KM, Fichter MM, Warnhoff M, et al: Hypothalamic regulation of gonadotropin secretion in anorexia nervosa and starvation. Int J Eating Dis 1983; 2:151.

49. Meyer A, von Holtzapfel B, Deffner G, et al: Psychoendocrinology of amenorrhea in the late outcome of anorexia nervosa. Psychother Psychosom 1986; 45:174.

50. Hebebrand J, Blum WF, Barth N, et al: Leptin synthesis in patients with anorexia nervosa is reduced in the acute stage and elevated upon short-term weight restoration. Molec Psychiatry 1997; 2:330–334.

51. Köpp W, Blum W, vonPrittwitz S, et al: Low leptin levels predict amenorrhea in underweight and eating disordered females. Molec Psychiatry 1997; 2:335–340.

52. Ahima RS, Prabakaran D, Mantzoros C, et al: Role of leptin in the neuroendocrine response to fasting. Nature 1996; 382:250–252.

53. Lucinio J, Mantzoros C, Megrão AB, et al: Human leptin levels are pulsatile and inversely related to pituitary-adrenal function. Nature Med 1997; 3:575–579.

54. Chehab FF, Lim ME, Lu R: Correction of the sterility defect in homozygous obese female mice by treatment with the human recombinant leptin. Nature Genet 1996; 12:318–320.

55. Hudson JI, Hudson MS: Endocrine dysfunction in anorexia nervosa and bulimia: Comparison with abnormalities in other psychiatric disorders and disturbances due to metabolic factors. Psychiatr Dev 1984; 4:237.

56. Pirke KM, Fichter MM, Chlond C, et al: Disturbances of the menstrual cycle in bulimia nervosa. Clin Endocrinol 1987; 27:245.

57. Friedman EJ, Stolar M, Kramer M, Gerner RH: Psychological and endocrine evaluation of bulimia. Presented at the Annual Meeting of the American Psychiatric Association, Los Angeles, 1984.

58. Fichter MM, Pirke KM, Pöllinger J, et al: Disturbances in the hypothalamo-pituitary-adrenal and other neuroendocrine axes in bulimia. Biol Psychiatry 1990; 27:1021.

59. Kiriike N, Nishiwaki S, Nagata T, et al: Gonadotropin response to LH-RH in anorexia nervosa and bulimia. Acta Psychiatr Scand 1988; 77:420.

60. Russell G: Bulimia nervosa: An ominous variant of anorexia nervosa. Psychol Med 1979; 9:429.

61. Schweiger U, Pirke KM, Laessle RC, Ficther MM: Gonadotropin secretion in bulimia nervosa. J Clin Endocrinol Metab 1992; 74:1122.

62. Czaja JA: Food rejection by female rhesus monkeys during the menstrual cycle and early pregnancy. Physiol Behav 1975; 14:579.

63. Dalvit SP: The effect of the menstrual cycle on patterns of food intake. Am J Clin Nutr 1981; 34:1811.

64. Gladis MM, Walsh BT: Premenstrual exacerbation of binge-eating in bulimia. Am J Psychiatry 1987; 144:1592.

65. Kiyohara K, Tamai H, Kobayaski N, Nakagawa T: Hypothalamic-pituitary axis alterations in bulimic patients. Am J Clin Nutr 1988; 47:805.

66. Vigersky RA, Loriaux DL, Anderson AE, Lipsett MB: Anorexia nervosa: Behavioral and hypothalamic aspects. Clin Endocrinol Metab 1976; 5:517.

67. Mitchell JE, Bantle JP: Metabolic and endocrine investigations in women at normal weight with the bulimic syndrome. Biol Psychiatry 1983; 18:355.

68. Targum SD, Sullivan AC, Byrnes SM: Neuroendocrine interrelationships in major depressive disorder. Am J Psychiatry 1982; 139:282.

69. Walsh BT, Katz JK, Levin J, et al: Adrenal activity in anorexia nervosa. Psychosomat Med 1978; 40:499.

70. Boyar RM, Hellman LD, Roffwarg H: Cortisol secretion and metabolism in anorexia nervosa. N Engl J Med 1977; 296:190.

71. Doerr P, Fichter M, Pirke KM, Lund R: Relationship between weight gain and hypothalamic pituitary adrenal function in patients with anorexia nervosa. J Steroid Biochem 1980; 13:529.

72. Weiner J, Katz JL: The hypothalamic-pituitary-adrenal axis in anorexia nervosa: A reassessment. In Darby PL, Garfinkel PE, Garner DM, Coscina DV (eds): Anorexia Nervosa: Recent Developments in Research. New York: Alan R Liss, 1983, p 249.

73. Gold PW, Gwirtsman H, Augerinos PC: Abnormal hypothalamic-pituitary-adrenal function in anorexia nervosa. N Engl J Med 1986; 314:1335.

74. Gerner RH, Gwirtsman HE: Abnormalities of dexamethasone suppression test and urinary MHPG in anorexia nervosa. Am J Psychiatry 1981; 138:650.

75. Gwirtsman HE, Roy-Byrne P, Yager S, Gerner RH: Neuroendocrine abnormalities in bulimia. Am J Psychiatry 1983; 140:559.

76. Gwirtsman HE, Gerner RH, Sternback H: The overnight dexamethasone suppression test: Clinical and theoretical review. J Clin Psychiatry 1982; 43:321.

77. Frisch RE: Fatness and fertility. Sci Am 1988; 258:88.

78. Frisch RE, Revele R: The height and weight of adolescent boys and girls at the time of peak velocity of growth in height and weight: Longitudinal data. Hum Biol 1969; 41:536.

79. Frisch RE, McArthur JW: Menstrual cycles: Fatness as a determinant of minimum weight for height necessary for their maintenance or onset. Science 1974; 185:949.

80. Frisch RE: The right weight: Body fat, menarche and ovulation. Clin Obstet Gynecol 1990; 4:419.

81. Mellits ED, Cheek DB: The assessment of body water and fatness from infancy to childhood. Monogr Soc Res Child Dev 1970; 35:12.

82. Welham WC, Behnke AR: The specific gravity of healthy men; body weight divided by volume and other physical characteristics of exceptional athletes and of naval personnel. JAMA 1942; 118:498.

83. Abraham SF, Beaumont PJV, Fraser TS, Llewellyn-Jones D: Body weight, exercise and menstrual status among ballet dancers in training. Br J Obstet Gynaecol 1982; 89:507.

84. Kaye W, Hansen D: Introduction to the psychobiology of eating disorders: Part II. Presented at the annual meeting of the ANAS, Columbus, OH, 1989.

85. Drunin J, Womersley J: Body fat assessed from total body density and its estimation from skinfold thickness: Measurements on 481 men and women aged from 16 to 72 years. Br J Nutr 1974; 32:77.

86. Westrate JA, Deurenberg P: Body composition in children: Proposal for a method for calculating body fat percentage from total body density or skinfold-thickness measurements. Am J Clin Nutr 1989; 50:1104.

87. Fomon SJ, Haschke F, Ziegler EE, Nelson SE: Body composition of reference children from birth to age 10 years. Am J Clin Nutr 1982; 35:1169.

88. Treasure JL, Gordon PA, King EA, et al: Cystic ovaries: A phase of anorexia nervosa. Lancet 1985; 2:1379.

89. Treasure JL: The ultrasonographic features in anorexia

nervosa and bulimia nervosa: A simplified method of monitoring hormonal states during weight gain. J Psychosom Res 1988; 32:623.

90. Bates GW, Bates SR, Whiteworth NS: Reproductive failure in women who practice weight control. Fertil Steril 1982; 37:373.

91. Stewart DE, Robinson GE, Goldbloom DS, Wright C: Infertility and eating disorders. Am J Obstet Gynecol 1990; 163:1196.

92. King MB: Eating disorders in general practice. Br Med J 1986; 293:1412.

93. Fairburn CG, Stein A, Jones R: Eating habits and eating disorders during pregnancy. Psychosom Med 1992; 54:665.

94. Davies K, Wardle J: Body image and dieting in pregnancy. J Psychosom Res 1994; 38:787.

95. Stein A, Fairburn CG: Children of mothers with bulimia nervosa. Br Med J 1989; 299:777.

96. Bonne OB, Rubinoff B, Berry EM: Delayed detection of pregnancy in patients with anorexia nervosa: Two case reports. Int J Eat Disord 1996; 20:423.

97. Namiri S, Melman KN, Yager J: Pregnancy in restricter-type anorexia nervosa: A study of pregnancy in six women. Int J Eat Disord 1986; 51:837.

98. Rand CSW, Willis DC, Kuldau JM: Pregnancy after anorexia nervosa. Int J Eat Disord 1987; 6:671.

99. Lacey H, Smith G: Bulimia nervosa: The impact of pregnancy on mother and baby. Br J Psychiatry 1987; 150:777.

100. Lemberg R, Phillips J: The impact of pregnancy on anorexia nervosa and bulimia. Int J Eating Disord 1989; 8:285.

101. Mitchell JE, Seim JC, Glotter D, et al: A retrospective study of pregnancy in bulimia nervosa. Int J Eating Disord 1991; 10:209.

102. Stein A, Woolley H, Cooper SD, Fairburn CG: An observational study of mothers with eating disorders and their infants. J Child Psychol Psychiatry 1994; 35:733.

103. Smith SM, Hanson R: Failure to thrive and anorexia nervosa. Postgrad Med J 1972; 48:382.

104. Woodside DB, Skekter-Wolfson LF: Parenting by patients with anorexia nervosa and bulimia nervosa. Int J Eating Disord 1990; 9:303.

105. LaBan MM, Wilkins JC, Sackeyfio AH, Taylor RS: Osteoporotic stress fractures in anorexia nervosa: Etiology, diagnosis, and review of four cases. Arch Phys Med Rehab 1995; 76:884.

106. Serpell L, Stefanis N, Treasure J: The osteopenia of anorexia. Presented at the Eating Disorders Research Society meeting. Pittsburgh, Pa., 1996.

107. Hergenroeder AC: Bone mineralization, hypothalamic amenorrhea, and sex steroid therapy in female adolescents and young adults. J Pediatrics 1995; 126:683.

108. Grinspoon S, Baum H, Lee K, et al: Effects of short-term recombinant human insulin-like growth factor I administration on bone turnover in osteopenic women with anorexia nervosa. J Clin Endocrin Metab 1996; 81:3864.

109. Hartman D, Crisp A, Rooney B, et al: Bone density of women who have recovered from anorexia nervosa. Int J Eat Disord 2000; 28:107.

110. McClelland L, Mynors-Wallis L, Fahy T, Treasure J: Sexual abuse, disturbed personality and eating disorders. Br J Psychiatry 1992; 10 (Suppl):63.

111. Hsu LKG, Crisp AH, Harding B: Outcome of anorexia nervosa. Lancet 1979; 1:61.

112. Morgan HG, Purgold J, Welbourne J: Management and outcome in anorexia nervosa: A standardized prognostic study. Br J Psychiatry 1983; 143:282.

113. Powers PS: Anorexia nervosa: Evaluation and treatment. Compr Ther 1990; 16:24.

114. Minuchin S, Rosman BL, Baker L: Psychosomatic Families: Anorexia Nervosa in Context. Cambridge: Harvard University Press, 1978.

115. Selvini-Palazzoli M, Viaro M: The anorectic process in the family: A six-stage model as a guide for individual therapy. Fam Process 1988; 17:129.

116. Strober M, Freeman R, Morrell W: The long-term course of severe anorexia nervosa in adolescents: Survival analysis of recovery, relapse, and outcome predictors over 10 to 15 years in a prospective study. Int J Eat Disord 1997; 22:339.

117. Kaye W: Anorexia nervosa: Different stages of treatment require different strategies of intervention. Presented at Eighth International Conference on Eating Disorders, April 25, 1998, New York, NY.

118. Strober M, Katz JL: Do eating disorders and affective disorders share a common etiology? Int J Eating Disord 1987; 6:171.

119. The Fluoxetine Bulimia Nervosa Collaborative Study Group. Fluoxetine in the treatment of bulimia nervosa: A multicenter placebo-controlled, double-blind trial. Arch Gen Psychiatry 1992; 49:139.

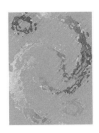

Chapter 26

Depression, Suicide, and Substance Abuse

CYNTHIA HOLLAND AND PAMELA J. MURRAY

Adolescence is a developmental period characterized by physical maturation and the achievement of certain cognitive, emotional, and psychosocial milestones. The ability for abstract thinking and decision making is refined, egocentrism gradually gives way to the appreciation of others' points of view, and separation from parents occurs. As teens oscillate between childlike and adult thought processes and behaviors, others may view them as being "irrational" or "moody," but the belief that normal adolescence is characterized by severe mood swings and emotional turmoil is erroneous. In fact, most teens report being happy most of the time. When this is not the case, caregivers must consider the possibility of a mood or substance use disorder.

DEPRESSION

Depression is a frequent diagnosis in adolescents, which very often goes unrecognized, untreated, or undertreated. It may occur as a primary condition or as a response to personal or environmental stressors. Depression carries substantial morbidity and often goes unrecognized until the adolescent's functioning becomes significantly impaired. Like adults, teens with mood disorders sometimes present with somatic symptoms. Clinicians who treat teens must therefore be trained to recognize and address these issues.

Epidemiologic studies suggest that disorders of mood, including major depression, have become more common with each successive generation.[1, 2] Over the past decades, the age at which children are diagnosed with these disorders has also fallen.[3] Depression is now clearly described in school-aged children and has even been recognized in infants. The prevalence of mood disorders in adolescents is difficult to assess. A 1992 review of the epidemiologic literature by McCracken found reported rates of depressive disorders in community samples of nonreferred adolescents to vary from 1.2% to 8.8%, depending on the definitions and methods used.[4] It is estimated that fewer than half of all affected teens receive treatment. Although the prevalence varies with socioeconomic factors and race, depression remains a significant problem across demographic subgroups. The average age of onset in adolescents is 15 years[5]; however, development of symptoms seems to be more closely related to puberty and physical maturation than to chronologic age. Females are affected approximately twice as often as males.

DIAGNOSIS

Specific mood disorders have strict diagnostic criteria, which are published in the American Psychiatric Association's *Diagnostic and Statistical Manual of Mental Disorders (DSM-IV)*. Table 26–1, while it does not provide complete diagnostic criteria, summarizes the characteristic features of a variety of common syndromes. Depression is characterized by a dysphoric mood and a loss of interest and pleasure in activities that formerly were enjoyable. A general sense of unhappiness, pessimism, and decreased energy or motivation is common. Depressed adolescents may present with irritability and anger rather than sadness, and they may report hypersomnia rather than insomnia. Decreased appetite may lead to weight loss or failure to gain weight appropriately in a young teen. Patients may report decreased sexual or romantic interest. Female patients are more likely to report "atypical" symptoms such as weight gain and hypersomnia.

In general, manifestations of depression are more behavioral and less neurovegetative in teens than in adults.[3] Substance abuse, high-risk sexual practices, and suicidal gestures are all more common among depressed youth. Adolescence is normally a time of separation from the parents during which healthy teens often engage

Table 26–1. Characteristic Features of Mood Disorders

Major Depressive Disorder
Depressed or irritable mood most every day for at least 2 weeks
Diminished interest or pleasure in activities
Significant appetite or weight changes
Insomnia or hypersomnia
Fatigue or loss of energy
Feelings of guilt or worthlessness
Bipolar Disorder
Cyclic episodes of major depression and manic or hypomanic episodes
Manic episode: abnormally and persistently elevated, expansive, or irritable mood lasting a week or more, including one or
   more of the following:
     Racing thoughts
     Decreased need for sleep
     Pressured speech
     Excessive involvement in pleasurable activities that have potentially negative consequences
Dysthymic Disorder
Depressed or irritable mood most days for at least 1 year
Sleep or appetite disturbances
Fatigue or loss of energy
Poor concentration
Hopelessness
Adjustment Disorder with Depressed Mood
Depressive symptoms within 3 months of the onset of an identifiable stressor
Symptoms in excess of what is expected or associated with functional impairment
Resolution of symptoms no longer than 6 months after termination of the stressor (or its consequences)
Depression with Seasonal Pattern (Seasonal Affective Disorder)
Symptoms of a major depressive episode during the fall and/or winter months for at least 2 years
Full remission of symptoms in summer
Symptoms not due to season-related psychosocial stressors (e.g., school)
Premenstrual Dysphoric Disorder
Symptoms present during most cycles for at least 1 year
Depressed mood, anxiety, or tension
Marked affective lability, irritability
Decreased interest in usual activities
Sleep or appetite changes
Absence of symptoms the week post menses
Postpartum Mood Disorder
Meets criteria for depression or bipolar disorder
Occurs within the first 4 weeks post partum

Adapted from American Psychiatric Association. Diagnostic and Statistical Manual of Mental Disorders, 4th ed. Washington, DC: American Psychiatric Association, 1994.

in some risk-taking behaviors. When good judgment is used in choosing these activities, they play an important role in the development of autonomy and independence. What distinguishes these normal behaviors from the pathologic disorders is the *persistent impairment of functioning* associated with mood disorders (see Table 26–1). This may include impaired functioning in the family, poor academic performance, or problematic social functioning among peers or in other settings outside the family. Similarly, the egocentrism that characterizes the normal adolescent may lead to severe distress after a humiliation or loss, such as a breakup with a boyfriend. Excessive or persistent *distress beyond what is considered normative* in this population, such as suicidality, suggests the presence of an underlying mood disorder that previously may have been unrecognized.

Major depressive disorder (MDD) may be diagnosed when symptoms listed in Table 26–1 are present for 2 weeks or more. One of the symptoms must be either a depressed or irritable mood or loss of interest or pleasure in activities that were formerly enjoyable. Several other symptoms must also be present. The estimated prevalence of MDD in adolescents is 4% to 8% and the cumulative incidence by 18 years of age is approximately 20%.[6] *Bipolar disorder* includes both major depressive and manic episodes, which may occur simultaneously or in cycles. Mania may be the initial manifestation, or it may not develop until years after the first major depressive episode. It is estimated that 20% to 30% of persons with MDD develop bipolar disorder within 5 years of the onset of depressive symptoms.[7] *Dysthymic disorder* is a chronic depressed mood that lasts a year or more, in which symptoms are not sufficient for diagnosis of MDD. As many as 8% of teens are affected,[3] and morbidity is significant. Dysthymic disorder persists for an average of 3 to 4 years. So-called double depression occurs when a major depressive episode is superimposed on dysthymic disorder; this often occurs 2 to 3 years after the onset of dysthymia.

Several variations of depressive disorders are common in young people. *Adjustment disorder with depressed mood* occurs in response to an identifiable psychosocial stressor and resolves within 6 months of the termination of that stressor or of its consequences. The depressive symptoms do not fulfill the criteria for MDD, which can also be precipitated by stressful events. Adjustment disorders are generally self-limited (mean duration 7 months, recovery rate 97%). The occurrence of an adjustment disorder is not predictive of future mood disorders or dysfunction.[8] *Depression with seasonal pattern*, commonly known as *seasonal affective disorder* (SAD), is more prevalent in northern climates. Depressive symptoms and increased sleeping occur in the fall, worsen during the winter, and begin to resolve as the days lengthen in the spring. Patients feel completely well during the summer. Four times more females are affected than males. Bright-light therapy is often a successful treatment for this disorder.[9] It is important to distinguish seasonal affective disorder from depressive symptoms that constitute a response to a temporally associated psychosocial stressor such as school. *Uncomplicated bereavement* generally occurs in response to the death of a loved one. There may be temporary impairment of functioning, and symptoms may be sufficient for a diagnosis of MDD. Gradual improvement occurs over time. MDD generally is not diagnosed unless symptoms persist longer than 2 months, are accompanied by excessive and inappropriate feelings of guilt and preoccupation with one's own death, or lead to severe and prolonged functional impairment.

Premenstrual dysphoric disorder (PDD) occurs in 3% to 5% of menstruating adult women.[10, 11] Prevalence in adolescents is not known. PDD differs from premenstrual syndrome (PMS) in that the affective symptoms in the former are comparable to those of MDD and are marked by significant functional impairment. Symptoms occur principally during the last week of the luteal phase, remit a few days after the onset of the follicular phase, and resolve completely by the week after menses. While hormonal factors in general may influence the onset of a depressive disorder, there is no clear pathway to demonstrate their effect on neuro-

transmitters in depressive disorders; nor have consistent abnormalities in sex steroids or gonadotropins been demonstrated in depressed women. Oral contraceptives and injectable and implantable progestins have been associated with depression and mood lability in some studies, though this is not a consistent finding.[12, 13] A baseline history of depressive symptoms should therefore be assessed before instituting hormone therapy, to more accurately assess the effect of estrogens and progestins on mood.

RISK FACTORS

Risk factors for mood disorders are summarized in Table 26–2. Strong genetic components for MDD and for bipolar disorder have been clearly demonstrated by adoption and twin studies. Children of parents with affective disorders have as much as a threefold greater risk of developing a mood, anxiety, or conduct disorder; these disorders tend to develop at a young age and have prolonged symptoms.[14] Stressful life events often precipitate initial episodes of depression. Medical illness and disability are also associated with increased risk of developing a mood disorder. In particular, persons with chronic illnesses characterized by frequent, unpredictable or uncontrollable exacerbations and those with associated loss of function are at risk. Other personal factors that predispose to mood disorders include poor social skills, low self-esteem, and low self-efficacy. Learning disabilities, developmental delays, attention deficit disorder, and other conditions that negatively affect learning and school performance may therefore be associated with depressive symptoms. Environmental factors can have a significant impact, intrafamilial problems

Table 26–2. Risk Factors for Mood Disorders

Genetic
Mood disorder in first-degree relative
Personal
Medical illness or disability
Developmental delay
Learning disability
Poor self-esteem
Poor socialization skills
Gender identity issues or homosexuality
Environmental
Stressful life events
Family dysfunction
Parent-child conflict
Physical or sexual abuse
Serious illness in family member
Maternal separation
Divorce or other alteration of family structure

being the most important. Parent-adolescent conflict and poor attachment are particularly strong risk factors. Although adolescents with mood disorders have high rates of substance abuse, a causal relationship cannot be established. Some teens may become depressed secondary to substance addiction; others may initially feel depressed and turn to illicit drugs in an attempt to self-medicate. Other risky behaviors, such as sexual promiscuity, delinquency, and running away from home are also associated with depression. Factors that protect against mood disorders include high self-esteem, a good mother-child relationship, and strong intra- and extrafamilial supports.

ASSESSMENT

Several clinical features may lead a provider to inquire about a mood disorder, and providers should not hesitate to do so. Although many depressed teens readily admit to feelings of sadness that they perceive as "depression," others deny depressed feelings. Alternatively, they may admit to feeling anger, irritability, or boredom. Other manifestations of depression include cognitive distortions, such as pessimism and negativity, that persist despite objective evidence that the situation is not so hopeless. Vague somatic complaints, such as fatigue, sleep disturbance, chronic headache, and abdominal pain, are often the presenting symptoms of the depressed teen. Pelvic pain also has a strong association with depression. In one series, 60% of women who were evaluated for pelvic pain were found to have depression.[15] It must be kept in mind, however, that chronic pain can also be a *cause* of depression, so it is important to determine the timing of both the physical symptoms and mood alterations.

Several screening tools help to identify adolescents with mood disorders. The Beck Depression Inventory is a 21-item self-report scale that has been widely used with adults and is appropriate for adolescents as well.[16] The Depression Self-Rating Scale is a similar screening tool that can be rapidly administered and has been shown to be sensitive and specific for moderate to severe depression in children and adolescents.[17] Although these easily administered instruments are useful for *screening* for depression and monitoring changes over time, they are not useful for the *diagnosis* of specific mood disorders, which requires a more extensive interview and evaluation process.[3] PRIME-MD, a rapid screening and diagnostic tool for mental disorders designed for administration by primary care physicians, has been validated in large studies that included adolescent patients[18] but has not been evaluated exclusively in this age group.

Teen and parent should be interviewed, both together and separately, since mothers and their daughters have been shown to have poor agreement on symptoms and diagnoses and each may be more comfortable discussing certain issues in private.[19, 20] Parents may also offer different perspectives on family functioning and relationships. Many depressed teens are grateful to be asked how they are feeling and speak willingly about it. In this case, the clinician should assess the specific symptoms, their duration, and the degree of functional impairment. A history of recent losses or other adverse life events should be elicited and the patient questioned about physical or sexual abuse. Inquiry about risk-taking behaviors such as substance abuse and unsafe sexual practices is crucial, since these behaviors are more common in depressed teens and may place them in immediate danger. Every depressed teen must be asked directly whether he or she has had suicidal thoughts or plans.

Teens who deny that there is a problem may become angry and defiant and refuse to answer questions. In such a case, the examiner must remain nonjudgmental and express the desire simply to understand the teen's point of view. The patient must be informed that the clinician is obligated to act on disclosures of abuse or suicidality but assured that any other feelings and behaviors that she chooses to reveal will remain confidential. When a teen persists in her refusal to discuss these issues, the clinician should respect her right to privacy yet continue to present himself or herself as a supportive figure who is available for such discussions or to make appropriate referrals in the future, should the teen change her mind.

Comorbid conditions often confound the diagnosis of a mood disorder. Depression may accompany serious medical problems such as cancer, anemia, systemic lupus erythematosus, hypothyroidism, epilepsy, and diabetes mellitus. Various studies of depressed youths have demonstrated comorbitity rates of 40% to 90% with other mental health disorders, most notably anxiety, conduct, and oppositional-defiant disorders. Dysthymia, attention deficit disorder, and substance abuse also have strong associations with mood disorders.[3] It is not clear whether these disorders generally antedate the onset of depression, are consequences of depression, or develop concurrently.

Laboratory studies are not routinely indicated in the evaluation of mood disorders. A complete blood count, sedimentation rate, and urinalysis are generally sufficient to rule out serious disease in patients who present with fatigue or vague, diffuse somatic complaints. Thyroid function studies may be included if the history supports a possible thyroid disorder. Although patients with depression demonstrate abnormalities on dexamethasone suppression tests, thyroid and growth hormone stimulation tests, and electroencephalography (EEG), currently none of these studies is clinically useful.

MANAGEMENT

Recommendations for treating mood disorders in adolescents are based on a limited number of rigorous studies. Caution must be exercised when extrapolating from findings of adult studies to children and adolescents, whose developmental stage may figure importantly in their responses to various treatment modalities. Both psychotherapeutic and pharmacologic treatments have been shown to be beneficial in adolescents; which should be used first, or whether the two should be initiated in combination, is fraught with controversy.[3] It is generally recommended that some form of counseling or psychotherapy be included in the management of all adolescents with depression. Outpatient management is usually adequate. Inpatient admission may be indicated in the presence of suicidality, severe mania with out-of-control behaviors, or severe functional impairment. Treatment must begin with educating patient and family in the likely course of the illness. Caregivers must learn how to respond appropriately to the child's behaviors and how to recognize and react to suicidality.

For mild to moderate depression, psychotherapy alone may be effective. Although there are many psychotherapeutic approaches to treatment, cognitive-behavioral therapy is the best-studied in adolescents and has demonstrated efficacy.[21] Cognitive therapy focuses on changing maladaptive thought patterns such as persistent negativity and low self-esteem. Behavioral therapy focuses on developing specific coping skills, adaptive strategies, and behavioral changes. This is within the capability of many primary care providers who choose to seek specific training in this area. Family, group, and other modes of therapy, which also are employed, merit further investigation in this age group.

Pharmacotherapy is often indicated in conjunction with counseling for patients with more severe symptoms. Psychologists and counselors who cannot prescribe medications may seek a primary care physician's assistance and input in starting antidepressant therapy. It is therefore desirable for the physician to develop some comfort with the use of these medications. Before one is prescribed, the likelihood of compliance to a medication regimen must be assessed through inquiries about the patient's attitudes toward medications in general and, specifically, psychoactive medications. Certain medications may have adverse effects when taken erratically or stopped abruptly; this should be made clear to the patient. Since specific complaints such as insomnia and decreased libido and sexual satisfaction can be either primary symptoms of depression or side effects of an antidepressant medication, it is important to document the presence or absence of these symptoms before initiating medication. Caregivers should be involved and should take responsibility for holding medications secure and for dispensing them to patients at risk of suicide.

Selective serotonin-reuptake inhibitors (SSRIs) are now the first-line pharmacologic choice for adolescents with MDD. They have clearly been shown to be efficacious in this population, although the majority of patients do not demonstrate complete remission.[22] Efficacy has also been demonstrated for SSRIs in the treatment of premenstrual dysphoric disorder in adult women,[23–25] but they have not been studied in teens. Antidepressants of this class have gained popularity because of low side-effect profiles and relatively low lethality in overdose. SSRIs are neither sedating nor addictive. Reported side effects include gastrointestinal symptoms, restlessness, headache, anxiety, sleep disturbances, and sexual dysfunction in both genders.[26] There are also reports of SSRIs' inducing manic episodes or other forms of "behavioral activation," including suicidality. Fluoxetine (Prozac) has a half-life of 2 to 3 days and its pharmacologically active metabolite, norfluoxetine, a half-life of 7 to 9 days. Sertraline (Zoloft) is preferred by many for its shorter half-life of 24 hours and its less active metabolites. It is often tolerated by patients who are unable to tolerate fluoxetine. Paroxetine (Paxil) is also short-acting and has no active metabolites; withdrawal symptoms, including dizziness, nausea, and anxiety, have been reported on abrupt discontinuation. Fluoxetine and paroxetine inhibit the cytochrome P_{450} isoenzyme system and thus impair the metabolism of certain other drugs; sertraline does not interfere with this system. No baseline or monitoring laboratory studies are necessary when administering an SSRI.

Tricyclic antidepressants (TCAs) act by blocking the reuptake of both norepinephrine and serotonin, but their primary action is on norepinephrine. Although TCAs are useful for treating adults with depression, they have not been shown to be any more effective than placebo in adolescents.[27] They are still used in some cases as second-line treatment. Side effects can be significant, including anticholinergic symptoms, weight gain, and sedation. Cardiac toxicity is responsible for the high lethality of overdose. Concomitant administration of combination oral contraceptives increases plasma concentrations of unbound TCAs. Before TCA treatment is instituted, a baseline electrocardiogram should be obtained and heart rate and blood pressure documented. These studies should be repeated, along with serum TCA levels (1) when steady-state dosing is achieved, (2) after any dose increase, and (3) after the addition of an agent that could have a pharmacokinetic interaction with a TCA.[28]

Other commonly prescribed psychopharmacologic agents include bupropion hydrochloride (Wellbutrin), a monocyclic antidepressant whose mechanism of action is not known. Its efficacy, in general, is comparable to that of TCAs. Bupropion has a low incidence of anticholinergic side effects, orthostatic hypotension, seizure, and cardiac arrhythmia. The incidence of seizure is increased in patients with anorexia nervosa or bulimia who take bupropion and it is therefore contraindicated in the treatment of these disorders. Heterocyclic antidepressants such as trazodone also have efficacy and side effect profiles comparable to TCAs', although the side effects are less severe. Trazodone causes significant sedation and is often used to treat the insomnia associated with depression or antidepressant use. Since antidepressants can induce mania in a patient with bipolar disorder or depression with psychotic features, such patients are often started on mood-stabilizing drugs such as lithium carbonate, carbamazepine, or valproic acid. These have only modest antidepressant effects but reduce the risk of cycling. Carbamazepine decreases the efficacy of combination oral contraceptives by enhancing the metabolism of estrogen. The treating physician should, therefore, consider prescribing a progestin-only contraceptive or a combination oral contraceptive containing 50 μg of estrogen, closely monitoring cycle control as an indicator of ovarian suppression. The use of barrier methods should also be encouraged in girls on this medication. Valproic acid is associated with ovarian hyperandrogenism and polycystic ovarian syndrome; this effect is particularly marked in adolescent patients.[29]

Hypericum perforatum, commonly known as *St. John's wort*, is often prescribed in Europe for the treatment of depression and has recently gained popularity in the United States. The pharmacologically active component and the mechanism of action are unclear. Meta-analysis of 23 studies performed in Europe concluded that hypericum extracts were significantly superior to placebo in the treatment of mild or moderate depression, and apparently had few short-term side effects.[30] Individual studies varied much in their methods, diagnostic criteria for depression, and specific preparations. Long-term side effects have not been studied. A large randomized trial comparing *H. perforatum* to placebo and to an SSRI is currently under way in the United States, where St. John's wort is sold as a nutritional supplement and is not regulated by the U.S. Food and Drug Administration.

The decision to primarily manage patients with mood disorders or to refer them to specialists depends on the severity of symptoms and the comfort and experience of the clinician. Adjustment disorder can often be handled by a skilled and willing primary care provider. When psychiatric referral resources are limited, it may be appropriate for patients with MDD and dysthymic disorder to be managed by an experienced primary care provider, either alone or in collaboration with a mental health specialist. Potentially suicidal patients, however, must be able to reach their provider or another trained professional 24 hours a day. Patients who do not show improvement within 6 to 8 weeks, who are suicidal, or who have bipolar disorder or psychotic features to their mood disorder should be referred to a mental health professional. Clinicians should gain familiarity with the mental health resources in their communities for both urgent care (i.e., acute crisis intervention) and routine mental health services. When possible, working relationships should be established with persons skilled at counseling children and adolescents. Subspecialists should feel comfortable enlisting the assistance of the patient's primary care provider in arranging mental health follow-up, but care should be taken to make sure patients at risk are not lost to follow-up.

OUTCOMES

Depressive disorders are often chronic and recurrent. Major depressive episodes last, on average, 32 weeks in children and adolescents who are referred for care, and 4 to 8 weeks in community samples. Ninety-two percent recover from the acute episode within 18 months. Recurrence rates up to 70% have been reported within 5 years of the first major depressive episode.[31] Probability of relapse is increased with onset at an early age, a family history of MDD in a first-degree relative, cormorbid substance abuse or an anxiety disorder, low socioeconomic status or other psychosocial challenges, or a history of suicidality.[5] All patients with mood disorders (other than acute adjustment disorders) should receive 6 to 12 months of continuous therapy. Patients who have had two or more episodes of major depression should continue treatment for 1 to 3 years. Since many patients are not adherent to prolonged courses of treatment, it is important for medical providers to stress the importance of follow-up, even after the resolution of the acute disturbance. They must also watch for signs of recurrence and inquire routinely about mood at subsequent visits. Unfortunately, some of the psychosocial consequences of depression, such as impaired family and social relationships, poor school performance, and substance abuse, may persist after the acute depressive episode has resolved.[32]

SUICIDE

Suicide is the third leading cause of death, after motor vehicle accidents and homicide, for teenagers and young adults of both genders in the United States.[33] In the 1997 *Youth Risk Behavior Survey*, 27% of female high school students reported that they had seriously considered attempting suicide in the past 12 months. Twenty percent had made a specific plan, and nearly 12% had attempted suicide during the past year.[34] A review of the adolescent suicide literature by Bell and Clark found, on average, 15 to 20 nonfatal suicide attempts for each completion.[35] Although males are more likely than females to be suicide completers, females are far more likely to make nonfatal attempts. This is due in part to the more lethal means males use, such as hanging and firearms. A female attempter is more likely to slash her wrists or overdose on medication, methods that afford more time for discovery and rescue. An alarming trend over the past decades, however, shows an increase in the use of firearms in suicide attempts for both genders. Alcohol is often involved in these episodes.[36] Most suicides occur in the child's home.

Cluster suicide describes the phenomenon of one adolescent's suicide being followed within weeks by the suicide of one or more others who live in the same area. Although this is a clearly recognized and disturbing phenomenon, we must not be misled by the excessive media coverage afforded such events. Far more suicides occur in isolation than in relation to other suicides.

Despite the high prevalence of suicidal thoughts among adolescents, clinicians often neglect to explore this subject while taking a medical and psychosocial history. In a survey of teens attending a general medical clinic, 14.5% reported a previous suicide attempt; however, only 17% of those subjects' medical records documented any indication that the physician had addressed this issue.[37] The same study found that suicide attempters were more likely to be female, to keep the appointment without a parent or guardian, and to have a chief complaint related to a sexually transmitted disease or other gynecologic problem. Clinicians who provide reproductive health services must therefore be comfortable inquiring about, assessing, and initiating interventions with suicidal teens.

RISK FACTORS FOR SUICIDE ATTEMPTS

Factors associated with suicidality, many of which overlap with the risk factors for depression and other psychiatric disorders, are listed in Table 26–3. Reviews by Bell and others conclude that, in the absence of a psychiatric disorder, suicide is rare among adolescents.[35] Depression, bipolar disorder, substance abuse, and conduct disorder are consistently found to be prevalent among teens who ultimately commit suicide. Unfortunately, many of these diagnoses go unrecognized or mislabeled, and fewer than half seek treatment from a mental health professional.[38] Previous attempts are another strong predictor

Table 26–3. Risk Factors for Suicide

Prior suicide threat or attempt
Psychiatric disorder
Substance abuse disorder
Chronic illness
History of aggressive or impulsive behavior
History of physical or sexual abuse
Feeling of hopelessness
Low self-esteem
Desire to die
Family disruption
Family history of suicide
Family history of mood disorder
Firearm in the home
Residence in a correctional facility

for future suicide. It is estimated that more than 40% of adolescent suicide victims have made previous attempts.[39] The majority of teens who make nonfatal suicide attempts state that their objective was to die, to seek relief from a terrible state of mind, and to escape, rather than to manipulate or elicit responses from other people.[40] The desire to die is, itself, a strong risk factor for suicide. Even low-risk suicidal gestures should be taken seriously, because the adolescent's *perception* of the lethality of a suicidal act may be more important than the actual danger it poses. More serious attempts may follow. Alternatively, a teen may underestimate the lethality of a suicidal gesture (e.g., acetaminophen ingestion) and should be counseled about the potentially serious consequences of such actions.

Several characteristic behaviors have been observed in suicide completers during the days and weeks before the event. The teen may become fixated on thoughts and discussions of death and suicide, though not necessarily her own death. A depressed teen may experience a sudden calmness or mood elevation, for no clear reason. She may contact friends or relatives who are important to her, give away prized possessions, and generally "put her affairs in order." Recent family or other interpersonal conflicts commonly precede suicidal acts. The absence of these behaviors or risk factors, however, does not preclude suicidality.

ASSESSING RISK

As always, a successful interview with an adolescent patient begins with establishing rapport and helping the adolescent to feel safe and comfortable discussing sensitive issues. Confidentiality should be addressed. It must be made clear that the primary responsibility of a health care provider is to keep any patient safe and alive. The patient needs to understand that a disclosure may compel the provider to share information or concerns with her parent or guardian or take other action to ensure her safety. Open-ended (not leading) questions are helpful in allowing suicidal patients to disclose such thoughts without embarrassment or fear of being seen as "crazy"; however, direct, unambiguous questions about suicidal thoughts are also critical. The belief that such direct inquiry may increase the likelihood of future suicidal acts has not been substantiated. In fact, most teens who are considering suicide express relief at the opportunity to disclose these feelings. Table 26–4 provides examples of directed questions that may be use-

Table 26–4. Questions for Assessing Suicidality

Are things ever so bad that you just feel like giving up?
Do you ever get so down that you think about hurting or killing yourself?
Have you ever tried to do something to end your own life?
Are you having any thoughts or plans of killing yourself now?

ful in this setting. When a teen discloses that she is having suicidal thoughts, a skilled clinician does not express shock or anxiety. It is more productive to approach this as an acute problem to be addressed and solved together with the patient.

Clinicians who wish to enhance their skills in caring for suicidal patients may do so by participating in continuing medical education courses designed for this purpose. It is also appropriate to contact the patient's primary care provider, school counselor, or a mental health provider to seek assistance in managing acute suicidality or depression. For uninsured adolescents, mental health resources are available in many schools and communities, and it is worthwhile for clinicians to become familiar with the resources available in their community.

When a teen does admit to suicidal thoughts, the clinician who assumes responsibility for her care must assess the immediate risk and determine the likelihood that she will act on those thoughts. A patient who demonstrates some lightening of her mood and who is willing to form a "No Suicide" contract with the provider (described later) may be considered at lower risk of imminent suicide. In contrast, a patient who demonstrates no mood elevation or who at the end of the interview persists in her desire to die is at high and immediate risk. A suicide plan that is specific, feasible, and lethal is further cause for concern. A patient who has a history of manic depression, schizophrenia, or psychosis, or who experiences auditory hallucinations commanding her to harm herself is at great risk and should be referred immediately to a mental health specialist.

INTERVENTION

An experienced clinician may play a part in the care of a suicidal patient who is at low risk of an imminent suicide attempt. The patient's parents or caregivers must be contacted and made aware of the situation before the teen leaves the office. Confidentiality issues rarely present a problem in this setting, since most teens are relieved to have their parents involved. When at all possible, a parent or responsible adult should come to meet the child in the office. Immediate, close supervision must be available on a continuous basis. Stressful environmental factors should be altered or removed when possible. The provider and caregivers should enter into a *written* "No Suicide" contract with the patient (elements are listed in Table 26–5). For the benefit of both the patient and the provider, a list of community resources available to suicidal teens, such as local mental health agencies, child welfare services, 24-hour crisis hotlines, and crisis intervention centers should be readily available. Close follow-up is mandatory, and referral to a mental health specialist is indicated when suicidality or a mood disorder persists or recurs.

Immediate psychiatric referral is indicated for all teens who attempt suicide, for anyone at high risk for imminent suicide, and for those teens whose caregivers are unable to provide appropriate support and supervision. Developing working relationships with psychiatrists, clinical psychologists, and other therapists experienced at dealing with children and adolescents is crucial. Inpatient management may be required to treat the medical sequelae of a suicide attempt. Many recommend at least a brief inpatient stay for observation and assessment of all suicide attempters. One-on-one supervision is generally indicated in these situations. Patients who have not committed a suicidal act but who display the high-risk profile described above may also be candidates for inpatient management by a psychiatrist. Voluntary or involuntary admission to a psychiatric facility is sometimes indicated in these situations, and providers should become familiar with the state regulations regarding this type of admission process. Last, it is important to recall that treatment of any underlying psychiatric diagnosis may be the most important measure in managing a suicidal patient.

SUBSTANCE ABUSE

Persons who abuse drugs and alcohol generally initiate these behaviors during adolescence. Clinicians may be in a position to intercede during the evolution of these behaviors, identifying and interrupting a pattern of escalating substance abuse. Drug or alcohol use contributes to poor decision making, particularly with regard to sexual activity, aggressive behavior, and other risky or self-destructive behavior. The teen substance abuser places herself, and others, at increased risk of both physical and emotional harm. She is more likely to experience interpersonal violence and to have difficulty with interpersonal relationships. Drug and alcohol abuse contribute significantly to adolescent accidents, homicide, and suicide, the top three causes of death in persons 15 to 24 years of age.

GENERAL TRENDS

The prevalence of adolescent substance abuse has been determined largely from data from several large national surveys of high school students.[34, 41] Given that severe substance abuse is associated with school absenteeism and dropping out, it is reasonable to assume that the adolescents at highest risk are underrepresented in these surveys. Abuse of illegal drugs became widespread among teenagers in the early 1970s and peaked in the early 1980s. There were slow declines in use throughout the remainder of that decade, and reported drug use reached a low point in 1992. Since then, however, the number of adolescent users of drugs and alcohol has steadily increased and shows no appreciable leveling off. Adolescents' perceived risks associated with regular use of certain substances such as marijuana have correspondingly diminished during this period (Fig. 26–1).

In 1997, more than 90% of high school seniors had tried alcohol at some point in their lives,[34] and almost 50% had used marijuana. Nearly a third had used an illicit drug other than alcohol or marijuana.[41] Although the overall numbers are smaller, the proportions of teens who report monthly or daily substance use are similarly increasing. Substance use is becoming more widespread among younger adolescents as well: more than a third of eighth graders report use of some illicit substance other than alcohol. This trend of

Table 26–5. Elements of a "No Suicide" Contract

Time and date of contract
Patient has no immediate plans to commit suicide
Patient agrees to call health care provider if suicidal thoughts return
Patient agrees to inform designated person (e.g., parent) if suicidal thoughts return
Firearms and other means of potential self-harm will be removed from the home
Provider ensures 24-hour availability of self or another provider by telephone
Patient agrees to follow-up with provider and/or behavioral health specialist as arranged (specify date and time)
Contract signed by all involved parties

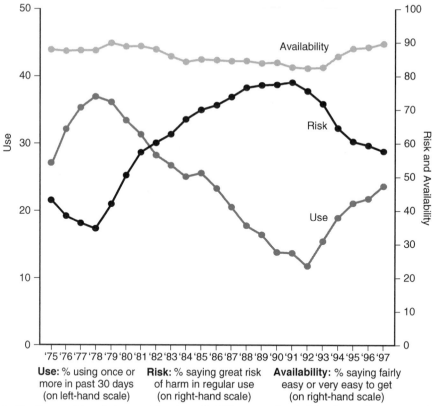

Use: % using once or more in past 30 days (on left-hand scale)   **Risk:** % saying great risk of harm in regular use (on right-hand scale)   **Availability:** % saying fairly easy or very easy to get (on right-hand scale)

Figure 26–1. Marijuana: Trends in perceived availability, perceived risk of regular use, and prevalence of use in past thirty days for twelfth graders. (Johnston LD, Bachman JG, O'Malley PM: National Survey Results on Drug Use from the "Monitoring the Future" Study, 1975–1997; Vol 1, Secondary School Students. Rockville, MD: National Institute on Drug Abuse, 1998, p 236.)

earlier experimentation with drugs showed signs of slowing in the late 1990s. Substance abuse spans all races and socioeconomic strata and is somewhat more prevalent in males than in females. Exceptions to this gender discrepancy include sedatives, amphetamines, and barbiturates, which are more often used by females.[42]

ROLE OF THE HEALTH CARE PROVIDER

The physician can play an important role in the identification and assessment of a substance-abusing teen. In a survey of adolescents in drug rehabilitation facilities, only half recalled having been asked by their physician about drug use, despite having been seen during the time that they were using.[43] Since gynecologic care is the most frequent type of health care routinely sought by many adolescent girls, physicians who provide this care must inquire about these issues and become comfortable addressing them.

Numerous risk factors have been described

that may predispose a teen to substance abuse (Table 26–6). Family characteristics, including parental substance abuse and dysfunctional parenting styles, often contribute.[44] Exposure to drugs at an early age and disorders of mood or behavior, such as depression, attention deficit–hyperactivity disorder, conduct disorder, or oppositional-defiant disorder, are also risk factors.[45] When considering an adolescent girl seeking gy-

Table 26–6. Risk Factors for Substance Abuse

Parental alcoholism
Family history of alcohol or other drug use
Permissive or authoritarian parenting style
Family conflict
Use of drugs or alcohol by peers
History of physical or sexual abuse
Low self-esteem
Mood disorder or other psychopathology
School failure or truancy
Early antisocial behavior
Early experimentation with alcohol or other drugs
Early initiation of sexual activity

necologic care, one must recall that sexual activity in teenagers can be associated with other risky behaviors, including substance abuse.

For some, drug use and sexual behaviors are interdependent.[46] A teen with a history of sexual abuse or other unresolved issues about sexuality may use drugs to modify her sexual experiences; their numbing or dissociative effects may allow her a psychological escape from the situation. Some drugs intensify sexual feelings and sensations, and most reduce anxiety and inhibition. This may lead to increased self-confidence, sexual aggressiveness, and sexual experimentation. An adolescent under the influence of alcohol or drugs may be more likely to make poor decisions with regard to condom use, choice of sexual partners, and contraception.[47] Drug addiction may lead to the exchange of sex for drugs or money; the result may be unintended pregnancy or sexually transmitted infections, including HIV. Chronic use of most illicit substances ultimately leads to decreased libido and sexual performance.

ASSESSMENT

Discussion of substance use should occur in a confidential, "safe" setting; parents should not be present. Before the discussion, the clinician should explain to the teen his or her policies on confidentiality as well as those circumstances in which confidentiality would be breached. A provider who conveys understanding and remains nonjudgmental builds better rapport and obtains a more accurate history than one who demonstrates shock or disapproval. One may begin by inquiring about risk factors and about general attitudes toward drug use. Inquiring about peer behavior may be less threatening to a teen than immediately asking about her own experiences with substance use. Examples of questions that may be used to initiate a conversation about substance use are given in Table 26–7. The history must include what drugs the adolescent

Table 26–7. Questions to Initiate a Discussion of Substance Abuse

Do any of the kids in your school/neighborhood use drugs?
What drugs have your friends tried in the past?
Do any of your friends use drugs regularly?
Have you ever tried drugs yourself? Which ones?
Have you ever tried cigarettes or drinking alcohol?
Have you ever inhaled anything to get high?
Have you ever taken anything to help you gain or lose weight?

Table 26–8. CAGE Questions for Alcohol Abuse

- Have you ever tried to *Cut down* on your alcohol use because it was getting out of hand?
- Have you ever become *Angry* with people who criticize your alcohol use?
- Have you every felt *Guilty* about your patterns of use?
- Have you every had a drink in the morning (*Eye opener*) to overcome a hangover?

uses, how much and how often, and the settings in which they are used. The extent to which the patient's home life, social life, employment, and education are disrupted by substance use must be determined. Her perceptions of the impact of substance use on her decision making, with regard to sexual activity, condom use, and other risky behaviors, should be determined, and she should be screened for symptoms of depression or other psychiatric comorbidity, since dual diagnoses are common. If parents are present, they should be interviewed separately. In addition to questioning them about the child's substance use, they should be asked, in a nonaccusatory fashion, about family dynamics and their own patterns of substance use or abuse. A family mental health history should be gathered.

Several brief screening questionnaires are available for administration in the office. These include instruments that focus specifically on substance abuse, such as Schwartz's Drug and Alcohol Problem Quick Screen,[48] and those that cover a variety of risky behaviors, such as the Problem-Oriented Screening Instrument for Teenagers (POSIT).[49] Simple mnemonics have also been devised to assist in assessing the extent of substance use and addiction, such as the CAGE questions (Table 26–8). There are generally no abnormal findings on physical examination, even in teens who chronically abuse drugs or alcohol.

DRUG TESTING

Urine screening tests are widely available for the illicit substances most commonly used. Blood tests are generally used to quantitate alcohol intoxication. The utility of drug testing is limited. At best, this technique gives information only about recent use at the time of screening. It gives no information about the adolescent's pattern of use, drug addiction or dependency, or the degree of psychosocial impairment caused by substance use. A negative drug screen is not conclusive evidence that a teen is not using drugs.

It is imperative that a physician ordering a

drug test understand the specific technique being used for testing and its associated limitations. Generally, *screening tests* with high sensitivity are performed first, testing for a panel of metabolites of illicit substances. Immunoassays such as the enzyme-multiplied immunoassay test (EMIT), which is based on antigen recognition by antibodies, are most commonly used for this purpose and can detect nanogram quantities of drug metabolites. Predetermined cutoff values, which vary from one laboratory to another, determine a positive or negative result. Positive screen results for cannabinoids, cocaine, and alcohol are generally reliable indicators of use. Positive findings for opiates, amphetamines, and phencyclidine are inconclusive owing to cross-reactivity with other medications and foodstuffs (Table 26–9). In either case, *confirming tests* are indicated. Gas chromatography/mass spectrometry (GC/MS) is the reference standard for confirmatory testing. In the United States, this method of testing, which maximizes specificity, is the only one acceptable for forensic analysis.

Table 26–9. Potential Cross-Reactive Medications in Immunoassay Tests

Test Substance	Possible Cross-Reactors
Amphetamines	Diethylpropion
	Dopamine
	Ephedrine
	Fenfluramine
	p-Hydroxyamphetamine
	Isoxsuprine
	Methamphetamine
	Methylphenidate
	Nylidrin
	Phentermine
	Phenylephrine
	Phenylpropanolamine
	Pseudoephedrine
Barbiturates	Glutethimide
	Phenytoin
Opiates	Chlorpromazine
	Codeine
	Dextromethorphan
	Diphenoxylate
	Hydromorphone
	Meperidine
	Oxycodone
	d-Propoxyphene
Phencyclidines	Chlorpromazine
	Dextromethorphan
	Diphenhydramine
	Doxylamine
	Meperidine
	Thioridazine

Used with permission of the American Academy of Pediatrics and Center for Advanced Health Studies: Use of the laboratory. *In* Schoenberg SK (ed): Substance Abuse: A Guide for Health Professionals. Elk Grove Village, Ill: American Academy of Pediatrics, 1988, p 59.

Table 26–10. Approximate Duration of Detectability of Selected Drugs in Urine

Drug	Approximate Duration of Detectability* in Urine
Amphetamine	48 h
Methamphetamine	48 h
Barbiturates	
Short-acting	24 h
Long-acting	≥7 d
Benzodiazepines	3 d†
Cocaine metabolites	2–3 d
Methadone	≈3 d
Codeine	48 h
Cannabinoids	
Single use	3 d
Chronic, heavy use	21–27 d
Phencyclidine	
Chronic use	≈8 d

Adapted with permission of the American Academy of Pediatrics and Center for Advanced Health Studies: Use of the laboratory. In Schoenberg SK (ed): Substance Abuse: A Guide for Health Professionals, p 55. Elk Grove Village, IL, American Academy of Pediatrics, 1988.

*Interpretation of the duration of detectability must take into account many variables, such as drug metabolism and half-life, subject's physical condition, fluid balance and state of hydration, and route and frequency of ingestion. These are general guidelines only.

How long after substance use a urine test remains positive varies with the particular substance and the pattern of use (Table 26–10). Generally speaking, metabolites remain detectable longer in persons with a history of prolonged, heavy use. This is particularly notable for marijuana, which is detectable in the urine for only 2 to 3 days after a single use. Persons with a history of long-term, daily marijuana use, however, may have positive urine tests for a month or more following their last use. Passive inhalation of marijuana, under normal circumstances, does not produce a positive urine result; however, some studies conducted in very small, unventilated rooms or sealed automobiles have demonstrated positive urine screens after passive inhalation.[50]

The ethical considerations surrounding drug testing in adolescents are substantial. The concept of "voluntary screening" is problematic, given that adolescents are not generally considered competent to provide consent. Some teens may feel coerced and fear that refusing to be tested will be interpreted as an admission of drug use. Conversely, substance users will likely decline testing if it is truly voluntary. Involuntary testing is also considered inappropriate for adolescents with decisional capacity, according to the American Academy of Pediatrics, even with parental consent.[51] Involuntary testing should only be undertaken in the presence of strong medical indications or legal requirements. Like any diagnostic test, drug testing should be used judiciously, in situations where the patient's history and physical findings are consistent with drug abuse, her behaviors are placing her at serious risk of harm, and her treatment might be altered by the outcome of the test. To maintain an optimal therapeutic relationship with the patient, a physician should avoid testing for purposes of incrimination in the legal system, except when required by a court order.

Once the decision to perform drug testing is made, numerous practical considerations arise. An early morning urine specimen is preferred, since the concentrations of drug metabolites will be highest at this time. Opportunities for the patient to contaminate the specimen must be minimized. This can be accomplished by having a same-sex monitor (other than the physician) present during urine collection. Coloring the toilet water or measuring the temperature or specific gravity of the specimen are other means of detecting dilution. Once collected, the specimen should be stored in the refrigerator or freezer. Wrapping the container in foil is recommended, since certain substances, such as D-lysergic acid diethylamide (LSD), degrade on prolonged exposure to light.

INTERVENTION

A variety of treatment options are available for substance use problems. These range from office management by the primary care provider to intensive inpatient services and detoxification. It is thus crucial for all physicians who may encounter substance-abusing teens to identify a consultant with expertise in this area and to feel comfortable making referrals as they would to any other subspecialist.

A patient's primary care physician may manage milder forms of substance abuse that do not cause major psychosocial disruption. Counseling should focus on the immediate risks and sequelae of substance abuse, such as personal injuries and poor decision making about risky sexual behavior. Patients and providers may develop written contracts that address specific behaviors, such as using condoms or not driving while using alcohol or drugs, or total abstinence. Drug testing may be used on a voluntary basis to monitor abstinence. In some cases, this can provide a teen who wishes to abstain with an "excuse" to resist peer pressure to continue using. Voluntary testing can also play a part in reestablishing trust between a teen and her parents. Frequency and extent of substance use and its impact on psychosocial functioning are the major determinants

of treatment needs. Patients known or suspected to have a dual diagnosis of mood, conduct, or anxiety disorders should be evaluated by a behavioral health specialist.

Treatment in an inpatient or residential facility is indicated in the following situations:

1. The patient is unable to discontinue use despite a trial of appropriate outpatient management.
2. The patient is no longer in control and demonstrates abusive or dangerous behavior toward herself or others.
3. She demonstrates runaway behavior or suicidality.
4. Her physical and emotional condition has deteriorated to a level that threatens her life.[52]

Residential treatment may be hospital based and run by medical personnel or may occur in a nonmedical therapeutic community setting (typically one staffed by former substance abusers). Care in a medical setting is indicated for management of withdrawal symptoms or active psychiatric disorders. Components of different treatment options vary greatly, largely owing to the paucity of long-term outcome studies demonstrating the benefits of one approach over others. Many are traditional Twelve-Step programs with little variability or consideration for the developmental needs of the adolescent. The Provisional Committee on Substance Abuse of the American Academy of Pediatrics compiled a list of desirable characteristics for adolescent substance abuse treatment programs.[52] These include a demand for total abstinence, in which any use is considered abuse; a medical staff knowledgeable in adolescent development and in chemical dependency; recognition of the importance of treating the whole family and provision of individual, family, and group therapy; and the integration of support groups into treatment. Follow-up and continuing outpatient therapy are crucial for success.

Treatment efficacy is difficult to study methodologically; research findings are even less conclusive for adolescents than for adults. An extensive review of the treatment literature by Catalano and colleagues led to the following conclusions:

1. Some treatment is better than no treatment.
2. The superiority of one treatment modality over another has not been clearly determined.
3. Marijuana and alcohol were the drugs most strongly associated with poorer outcomes.
4. More controlled outcome studies are needed.[53]

Another review described several pretreatment characteristics that are predictive of poor treatment outcomes, such as extent and frequency of use, psychiatric symptoms, peer influence, family pathology, and work, school, or legal problems prior to treatment.[54] Studies of the Twelve-Step Alcoholics Anonymous (AA) and Narcotics Anonymous (NA) treatment model have shown that completion of a treatment program is associated with higher rates of recovery in the short term, but not always over the long term.[55]

Relapse rates are likewise difficult to assess; estimates vary from 15% to 65%.[53] Specific factors associated with relapse have not been rigorously studied, but some literature suggests that components of treatment and the patient's posttreatment environment have a greater impact on outcome than pretreatment factors.[53] Since adolescents are even more sensitive than adults to environmental influences such as peer pressure and other psychosocial stressors, it may be that posttreatment factors, such as time spent with nonusing friends, are, in this age group, even more critical for success. Other social resources have similarly been associated with lower relapse rates.[56] Continuing outpatient therapy after discharge from a treatment program is strongly associated with ongoing success.[57, 58] Recovering substance abusers who more frequently attend AA or NA meetings show higher rates of abstinence,[55] although a causal relationship has not been demonstrated. Personal characteristics, such as poor coping skills, low self-efficacy, and behavioral problems, also compromise the long-term prognosis.[59]

DRUGS OF ABUSE

Tobacco

Tobacco is the substance most commonly abused by adolescents: 25% of high school seniors report daily use.[41] Smoking rates are higher for whites than for nonwhites, with no clinically significant differences between males and females. Although tobacco is less likely to lead to severe psychosocial impairment than other illicit substances, its long-term medical sequelae are a major public health concern and expense. In addition to the well-publicized strong associations with lung cancer, cardiovascular disease, and stroke, cigarette smoking was shown to be associated with high-grade cervical intraepithelial neoplasia in women with abnormal cervical smears.[28, 60] Infants born to mothers who smoke are more likely to be premature or have low birth weight. Smoking is also associated with the abuse of other substances and tobacco is generally the first substance used by adults who go

on to develop chemical dependencies. Although smoking cessation is challenging, patients do respond to the advice of their health care provider. Effective treatment modalities exist, including behavior modification, nicotine replacement therapies, and bupropion hydrochloride to reduce cravings. These are often used in combination with one another in adults. Although it is reasonable to consider using all of these approaches in older adolescents, the pharmacologic treatments have not yet been extensively studied or approved for patients younger than 18 years.

Alcohol

Alcohol use is widespread among adolescents: more than 90% of high school seniors have tried it at some point. Perhaps more concerning is that 30% of seniors report binge drinking, stating that they had five or more drinks on a single occasion during the 2 weeks prior to the survey.[41] Binge drinking is prevalent in early adolescents of both genders as well.[34] A family history of alcohol abuse is a strong predictor of use and abuse by an adolescent. Adoption and twin studies demonstrate a genetic predisposition to alcoholism in addition to strong environmental influences.

Alcohol is rapidly absorbed from the gastrointestinal tract, with onset of action approximately 10 minutes after ingestion. CNS depression and disinhibition occur. While a blood alcohol level of 0.10% or higher generally defines legal intoxication, levels of 0.05% are sufficient to cause intoxication, especially in new users. Even lower levels of alcohol can impair judgment and reaction time. Tolerance develops with frequent use. Acute alcohol effects in adolescents are similar to those in adults, including erosive gastritis and pancreatitis. Adolescents rarely have enough cumulative alcohol consumption to cause long-term effects such as cirrhosis and nutritional deficiencies. Alcohol withdrawal in the adolescent may be associated with minor symptoms of restlessness, tremors, and mild diaphoresis, but the major withdrawal syndrome of delirium tremens seen in adults is rare in adolescents. Fetal alcohol effects in infants of mothers who drink include mild to moderate mental retardation, microcephaly, attention problems, and a characteristic facies. These effects appear to be dose related, but no amount of alcohol ingestion during pregnancy has been demonstrated to be safe, and adolescents should be counseled to abstain completely when pregnant or planning to become pregnant.

The adverse behavioral outcomes associated with teen alcohol abuse far outweigh its physiologic impact. In 1997, more than a third of high school students stated that within the past month they had ridden in a car when the driver had been drinking alcohol, and 17% had driven after drinking alcohol themselves.[34] Alcohol is frequently involved in motor vehicle accidents involving teens and in teen homicides and suicides. For this reason, alcohol is considered by some to be the leading cause of death in this age group, as well as being associated with numerous nonfatal injuries. Alcohol addiction in adolescents is characterized by daily or nearly daily use, the occurrence of blackouts, accidents, school failure, and other psychosocial impairment secondary to alcohol use. Far more common is the adolescent "problem drinker" who engages in episodic binge drinking associated with accidents or other negative consequences, including legal consequences. In these situations, inpatient treatment is rarely indicated, and the goal is to interrupt the pattern of drinking and the associated adverse behaviors, and to initiate long-term maintenance therapy.

Marijuana

Marijuana is the most abused illegal substance. More than 20% of high school seniors report regular use, and almost 6% report daily use.[41] The perceived risks of marijuana use decreased as its use became more prevalent during the 1990s.[41] Marijuana is derived from the leaves and seeds of the hemp plant *Cannabis sativa*. The psychoactive metabolites, such as delta-9-tetrahydrocannabinol (THC) and other cannabinoids, are present in variable concentrations in the different forms of the drug. The dried tops and leaves of the plant are most commonly sold as "weed." This is the least potent form of marijuana and is smoked in "joints" or "blunts," pipes, or water-cooled smoking chambers ("bongs"). Hashish is the dried resin secreted by the flowers of the female plant and is several times more potent. It may be smoked or ingested. Hash oil is derived from hashish and is the most potent form of the drug. Adulterants, including hallucinogens, are commonly added to marijuana. Onset of action occurs within minutes of inhaling. Physiologic effects include tachycardia, conjunctival vasodilatation, and slowed reaction time. Psychoactive effects vary and range from euphoria and intensification of auditory and visual stimuli to frank hallucinations and dysphoric reactions. Perceptions of time, speed, and distance are distorted. Occasional use of unadulterated marijuana rarely causes serious physiologic consequences, but frequent and long-term use can be associated with pulmonary irritation, impairment of attention and short-term memory, menstrual irregularity in females, and possibly, in both genders, impaired fertility mediated by a decrease in pituitary gonadotropins.[61] This last appears to be reversed with discontinuation of the drug. THC crosses the placenta and has been associated with fetal growth retardation and congenital anomalies in some studies, but no teratogenic effect has consistently been demonstrated in humans.[62] Although marijuana does not cause physiologic addiction or a withdrawal syndrome, psychological addiction is common. The "amotivational syndrome" of apathy, loss of energy, and decreased goal-directed activity may be seen in frequent users.

Stimulants

COCAINE

Cocaine use peaked in the 1980s, before its dangerous and addictive nature was widely recognized, and has decreased significantly since that time. Nonetheless, use is not uncommon among adolescents and has been slowly increasing again since the early 1990s. Nearly 9% of high school seniors have tried cocaine, and, since heavy use is strongly associated with school absence, the actual prevalence of use is probably greater. Cocaine hydrochloride, derived from the leaves of the South American *Erythoxolon coca* plant, most often is inhaled through the nose ("snorting") but can also be administered subcutaneously or intravenously. Crack cocaine, the smokable freebase formulation of the drug, is rapidly absorbed and delivered to the brain in high concentrations. Its availability, highly addictive nature, and rapid emergence of tolerance have led to serious problems with escalating use and addiction in some communities.

Cocaine intoxication rapidly produces euphoria, decreased fatigability, and increased motor activity. Other acute physiologic effects include tachycardia, vasoconstriction, and hypertension. Rare but serious medical complications include cardiac arrhythmias, stroke, and respiratory arrest. The nasal mucosa may become ulcerated or infected due to local vasoconstriction. Sexual interest and performance may initially be enhanced but are adversely affected with long-term use. Neuroendocrine effects have been described in animal studies, but reproductive effects in humans are unclear.[63] Pregnant women using cocaine are at increased risk of preterm labor, abruptio placentae, and spontaneous abortion. Infants born to addicted mothers often display irritability and decreased interactive behavior in the neonatal period. Although several teratogenic effects have been described, no consistent clinical syndrome secondary to prenatal cocaine exposure has been described.[64] No clear cocaine abstinence syndrome has been described, but intoxication may be followed by depression, agitation, and intense cravings for more drug. This can lead to poor academic performance, decreased goal-directed behavior, and prostitution or other criminal behavior to support a habit.

METHAMPHETAMINE

Like cocaine, other stimulants are less widely used than in the early 1980s, but lifetime prevalence of use remains more than 15% for high school seniors.[41] Some individuals utilize methamphetamine to increase alertness or promote weight loss; others take the drug for its euphoric and hypomanic effects. Methamphetamine may be inhaled, injected, or taken orally. The crystallized form of the potent D-methamphetamine known as *ice* or *crystal meth* may be smoked. Serious medical complications are similar to those of cocaine, but less common. Overdose and chronic use can cause insomnia, agitation, and repetitive or stereotyped behaviors. Hypersexuality may be seen. Grandiosity and increased motor activity may lead to injury. Withdrawal is associated with depression, somnolence ("crash"), and suicidal or homicidal behaviors.

OTHER STIMULANTS

Numerous other legal and illegal stimulants are available and widely used. In large doses, some have effects similar to those of methamphetamine. Sales of 3,4-methylenedioxymethamphetamine (MDMA, or Ecstasy), an amphetamine with hallucinogenic properties, were banned in 1995, but it remains widely available. It is commonly used for its aphrodisiac effect, and has been implicated in some date rapes. So-called herbal ecstasy, sold in health food stores and by mail order, now generally contains benign ingredients with little psychoactive effect. Ephedra, another herbal product available in many health food stores, contains ephedrine alkaloids with marked alpha-adrenergic effects. It is used for its euphoric effects and is believed to have caused a number of deaths, many in young people. Numerous amphetamine "look-alikes" are

widely available through the illicit drug market and are often the first stimulants young adolescents use. They often contain caffeine, ephedrine, or phenylpropanolamine but may contain a variety of (often legal) substances. Overdose can cause stroke or cardiotoxicity.

Hallucinogens

A variety of different compounds are used for their hallucinogenic effect, and their pharmacologic properties differ greatly. Use of hallucinogens increased during the 1990s and now approaches the level of use in the early 1970s, 4% of high school seniors reporting regular use.[41] LSD is most often abused, and produces alterations in sensory perceptions, distortions of reality, and depersonalization. Doses used by teens today are generally significantly smaller than those used in the 1960s, and fewer adverse reactions are therefore seen. LSD is taken orally, and effects persist several hours. The greatest acute risk associated with use is engaging in dangerous behaviors, prompted by either delusions of omnipotence and invulnerability or by an acute panic reaction or "bad trip." Chronic use may result in depression or drug-induced psychosis, including persistent perceptual disorders. Flashbacks to prior LSD experiences may occur in some persons. Phencyclidine piperidine (PCP) is used less often but is slowly regaining popularity among adolescents. It is a dissociative anesthetic that is rapidly but erratically absorbed when inhaled or ingested, resulting in delusions and hallucinations, sensations of prominent body distortions, and loss of contact with reality. Bizarre and aggressive behaviors may lead to traumatic injury. Acute and chronic medical complications of PCP abuse are more prominent than those associated with LSD and include prolonged depression or psychosis, hypertension, and cardiac arrest. Other hallucinogens include mescaline, psilocybin mushrooms, morning glory seeds, and other ("designer") compounds. These compounds often contain LSD or PCP as the psychoactive substance and may be adulterated with other drugs.

Opioids

In addition to its increasing reported use by high school and college students, heroin is used disproportionately by those adolescents who do not attend school and whose use is therefore not reflected in school-based surveys. Inhalation is the most common route of delivery in this age group, but the drug can also be injected or taken orally. Methadone, meperidine, and other commonly prescribed oral narcotics (Dilaudid, MS Contin, Percocet, Vicodin) are even more commonly abused. All are capable of producing analgesia and euphoria. Immediate medical effects are most common with heroin use, and include miosis, respiratory depression, and decreased gastrointestinal motility. Anovulation and amenorrhea may occur in females. Pregnancy may be complicated by spontaneous abortion and fetal growth retardation. A well-described fetal abstinence syndrome includes irritability, feeding problems, diarrhea, and seizure; it may occur hours to weeks after delivery.

Other serious health consequences are related to the route of delivery, such as skin abscesses or cellulitis from subcutaneous use. Intravenous use poses the risk of systemic infection, including hepatitis B or C, infectious endocarditis, and HIV infection. Subcutaneous carbon deposits or "tracks" on the skin are remnants of attempts to sterilize needles with a flame. A characteristic withdrawal syndrome occurs after prolonged regular use of opioids, and includes flulike symptoms, anxiety, dilated pupils, yawning, diarrhea, and lacrimation. Withdrawal from chronic use should be managed by an experienced professional and may include the use of methadone or other medications. Continued support after detoxification is critical, and relapse is common. Adolescents with chronic pain syndromes requiring prolonged opiate use generally do not experience the complete withdrawal syndrome, and anxiety may be their worst symptom.

Sedatives

CNS depressants, including benzodiazepines and barbiturates, are used by adolescents less commonly today than in the past. Benzodiazepines are often obtained by prescription, written either for the patient herself or for a family member. Initial use may be therapeutic or semi-therapeutic. Tolerance develops gradually, though true physiologic dependency and withdrawal rarely occur in adolescents. Signs of acute toxicity include excessive sedation, respiratory depression, ataxia, and slurred speech. Flunitrazepam (Rohypnol) is a benzodiazepine that deserves special mention owing to its recent notoriety as the "date-rape drug." Though not approved for use in the United States, flunitrazepam is inexpensive and widely available. It produces sedation, amnesia, and muscle relaxation. These effects are accentuated by the use of alcohol in conjunction with the

drug, and the effects last several hours. Flunitrazepam is often undetectable on routine urine screens for benzodiazepines. If its presence is suspected, the laboratory should be notified and specific testing requested. Barbiturate use is somewhat uncommon but is increasing in adolescents. Withdrawal from chronic use is similar for benzodiazepines and barbiturates, and includes anxiety, insomnia, and seizure. A characteristic neonatal abstinence syndrome includes hyperactivity, hyperreflexia, sneezing, and hiccups.

Inhalants

Inhalants have the second highest lifetime prevalence of use, after marijuana. Current use is most common among early adolescents.[41] Substances inhaled include volatile solutions such as gasoline, lighter fluid, and numerous other glues, solvents, and cleaning fluids, many of which contain hydrocarbons. They may be inhaled directly from the container ("sniffing"), or placed on a cloth ("huffing") or in a plastic bag, which is then placed over the nose and mouth ("bagging"). Other substances, ranging from nitrous oxide (purchased in balloons or from compressed whipped cream containers) to typewriter correction fluid, are regularly abused as well. Most youth underestimate the medical risks associated with inhalant abuse. Inhalation rapidly produces a sense of euphoria and stimulation, which may be followed by CNS depression. This decreased level of consciousness may predispose to suffocation or aspiration pneumonia. Sudden death and acute organ toxicity have also been reported after hydrocarbon inhalation. Inhalant use is often discontinued at an early age and at that time may be replaced by alcohol or marijuana use. Abuse of inhalants by older adolescents and adults is often associated with a comorbid psychiatric condition.

Anabolic Steroids

Although steroid abuse is more common among males than females, 2% of female high school students state that they have used steroids illegally (i.e., without a doctor's prescription) at some time.[34] Steroids may be injected or taken orally, and are generally used to improve athletic performance. Girls who abuse steroids may present with menstrual irregularity or virilizing effects such as acne, hirsutism, change of body habitus, and clitoromegaly. Gonadotropin levels are often decreased. If physical maturation is not yet complete at the time of steroid abuse, an adolescent may undergo premature closure of the epiphyseal growth plates, leading to shorter adult stature. Steroids are not detected by routine urine screens for drugs of abuse in most laboratories.

CONCLUSION

Any provider who cares for adolescent patients may encounter teens with mood disorders, suicidality, or substance abuse problems. It is best to anticipate these situations and to gain familiarity with available mental health resources—at a medical center, in the larger medical community, or in the schools. Crisis intervention services for teens exist in many communities and often provide 24-hour access. National organizations that address these issues can often be of assistance in identifying appropriate local resources. Several of these resources are listed below. Once a useful referral system has been established, many providers become more comfortable at identifying and addressing these challenging issues.

RESOURCES

- Youth Crisis Hotline: 800–448–4663
- National Runaway Hotline: 800–621–4000
- National Mental Health Association: 800–969–6642
- American Association of Suicidology: 202–237–2280; URL: http://www.suicidology.org
- The American Academy of Child & Adolescent Psychiatry: 202–966–7300; URL: http://www.aacap.org
- The Center for Substance Abuse Treatment's National Drug and Treatment Routing Service: 800–662-HELP
- National Clearinghouse for Alcohol and Drug Information: 800–729–6686; URL: http://www.health.org

REFERENCES

1. Klerman GL, Weissman MM: Increasing rates of depression. JAMA 1989; 261:2229–2236.
2. Ryan ND, Williamson DE, Iyengar S, et al: A secular increase in child and adolescent onset affective disorder. J Am Acad Child Adolesc Psychiatry 1992; 31:600–605.
3. American Academy of Child and Adolescent Psychiatry: Practice parameters for the assessment and treatment of children and adolescents with depressive disorders. J Am Acad Child Adolesc Psychiatry 1998; 37:63S–83S.
4. McCracken JT: The epidemiology of child and adolescent mood disorders. Child Adolesc Psychiatr Clin N Am 1992; 1:53–72.
5. Lewinsohn PM, Clarke GN, Seeley JR, et al: Major depression in community adolescents: Age at onset, episode duration, and time to recurrence. J Am Acad Child Adolesc Psychiatry 1994; 33:809–818.
6. Lewinsohn PM, Hops H, Roberts RE, et al: Adolescent psychopathology, I: Prevalence and incidence of depression and other DSM-III-R disorders in high school students. J Abnorm Psychol 1993; 102:133–144.
7. Kovacs M: Presentation and course of major depressive disorder during childhood and later years of the life span. J Am Acad Child Adolesc Psychiatry 1996; 35:705–715.
8. Kovacs M, Gatsonis C, Pollock M, et al: A controlled prospective study of DSM-III adjustment disorder in childhood: Short-term prognosis and long-term predictive validity. Arch Gen Psychiatry 1994; 51:535–541.
9. Swedo SE, Allen AJ, Glod CA, et al: A controlled trial of light therapy for the treatment of pediatric seasonal affective disorder. J Am Acad Child Adolesc Psychiatry 1997; 36:816–821.
10. American Psychiatric Association: Diagnostic and Statistical Manual of Mental Disorders, Fourth Edition. Washington, DC: American Psychiatric Association, 1994.
11. Rivera-Tovar AD, Frank E: Late luteal phase dysphoric disorder in young women. Am J Psychiatry 1990; 147:1634–1636.
12. Westhoff C: Depot medroxyprogesterone acetate contraception: Metabolic parameters and mood changes. J Reprod Med 1996; 41:401–406.
13. Cromer BA, Smith RD, Blair JM, et al: A prospective study of adolescents who choose among levonorgestrel implant (Norplant), medroxyprogesterone acetate (Depo-Provera), or the combined oral contraceptive pill as contraception. Pediatrics 1994; 94:687–694.
14. Beardslee WR, Keller MB, Lavori PW, et al: The impact of parental affective disorder on depression in offspring: A longitudinal follow-up in a nonreferred sample. J Am Acad Child Adolesc Psychiatry 1993; 32:723–730.
15. Steege JF, Stout AL, Somkuti SG: Chronic pelvic pain in women: Toward an integrative model. J Psychosom Obstet Gynecol 1991; 12(Suppl):3–30.
16. Marton P, Churchard M, Kutcher S, et al: Diagnostic utility of the Beck Depression Inventory with adolescent psychiatric outpatients and inpatients. Can J Psychiatry 1991; 36:428–431.
17. Birleson P, Hudson I, Buchanan DG, et al: Clinical evaluation of a self-rating scale for depressive disorder in childhood (Depression Self-Rating Scale). J Child Psychol Psychiatry 1987; 28:43–60.
18. Spitzer RL, Williams JBW, Kroenke K, et al: Utility of a new procedure for diagnosing mental disorders in primary care: The PRIME-MD 1000 study. JAMA 1994; 272:1749–1756.
19. Andrews VC, Garrison CZ, Jackson KL, et al: Mother-adolescent agreement on the symptoms and diagnoses of adolescent depression and conduct disorders. J Am Acad Child Adolesc Psychiatry 1993; 32:731–738.
20. McGee R, Feehan M, Williams S, et al: DSM-III disorders in a large sample of adolescents. J Am Acad Child Adolesc Psychiatry 1990; 29:611–619.
21. Brent DA, Kolko DJ, Birmaher B, et al: Predictors of treatment efficacy in a clinical trial of three psychosocial treatments for adolescent depression. J Am Acad Child Adolesc Psychiatry 1998; 37:906–914.
22. Emslie GJ, Rush AJ, Weinberg WA, et al: A double-blind, randomized, placebo-controlled trial of fluoxetine in children and adolescents with depression. Arch Gen Psychiatry 1997; 54:1031–1037.

23. Steiner M, Steinberg S, Stewart D, et al: Fluoxetine in the treatment of premenstrual dysphoria. N Engl J Med 1995; 332:1529–1534.

24. Eriksson E, Hedberg MA, Andersch B, et al: The serotonin reuptake inhibitor paroxetine is superior to the noradrenaline reuptake inhibitor maprotiline in the treatment of premenstrual syndrome. Neuropsychopharmacology 1995; 12:167–176.

25. Yonkers KA, Halbreich U, Freeman E, et al: Symptomatic improvement of premenstrual dysphoric disorder with sertraline treatment. JAMA 1997; 278:983–988.

26. Labellarte MJ, Walkup JT, Riddle MA: The new antidepressants: Selective serotonin reuptake inhibitors. Pediatr Clin North Am 1998; 45:1137–1155.

27. Hazell P, O'Connell D, Heathcote D, et al: Efficacy of tricyclic drugs in treating child and adolescent depression: A meta-analysis. BMJ 1995; 310:897–901.

28. Daly JM, Wilens T: The use of tricyclic antidepressants in children and adolescents. Pediatr Clin North Am 1998; 45:1123–1135.

29. Isojarvi JIT, Laatikainen TJ, Pakarinen AJ, et al: Polycystic ovaries and hyperandrogenism in women taking valproate for epilepsy. N Engl J Med 1993; 329:1383–1388.

30. Linde K, Ramirez G, Mulrow CD, et al: St. John's wort for depression—an overview and meta-analysis of randomised clinical trials. BMJ 1996; 313:253–258.

31. Kovacs M, Feinberg TL, Crouse-Novak M, et al: Depressive disorders in childhood: II. A longitudinal study of the risk for a subsequent major depression. Arch Gen Psychiatry 1984; 41:643–649.

32. Rao U, Ryan ND, Birmaher B, et al: Unipolar depression in adolescents: Clinical outcome in adulthood. J Am Acad Child Adolesc Psychiatry 1995; 34:566–578.

33. Anderson RN, Kochanek KD, Murphy SL: Report of final mortality statistics, 1995. Monthly vital statistics report; Vol 45, No 11, Supp 2, Table 7. Hyattsville, Md: National Center for Health Statistics, 1997.

34. Centers for Disease Control and Prevention: CDC Surveillance Summaries, August 14, 1998. MMWR 1998; 47:1–89.

35. Bell CC, Clark DC: Adolescent suicide. Pediatr Clin North Am 1998; 45:365–380.

36. Clark DC: Suicidal behavior in childhood and adolescence: Recent studies and clinical implications. Psychiatr Ann 1993; 23:271–283.

37. Slap GB, Vorters DF, Khalid N, et al: Adolescent suicide attempters: Do physicians recognize them? J Adolesc Health 1992; 13:286–292.

38. Shaffer D, Gould MS, Fisher P, et al: Psychiatric diagnosis in child and adolescent suicide. Arch Gen Psychiatry 1996; 53:339–348.

39. Shafii M, Carrigan S, Whittinghill JR, et al: Psychological autopsy of completed suicide in children and adolescents. Am J Psychiatry 1985; 142:1061–1064.

40. Boergers J, Spirito A, Donaldson D: Reasons for adolescent suicide attempts: Associations with psychological functioning. J Am Acad Child Adolesc Psychiatry 1998; 37:1287–1293.

41. Johnston LD, Bachman JG, O'Malley PM: National Survey Results on Drug Use from the Monitoring the Future Study, 1975–1997, Vol. 1, Secondary School Students. Rockville, Md: National Institute on Drug Abuse, 1998.

42. O'Malley PM, Johnston LD, Bachman JG: Adolescent substance use and addictions: Epidemiology, current trends, and public policy. Adolescent Med 1993; 4:227–248.

43. Friedman LS, Johnson B, Brett AS: Evaluation of substance-abusing adolescents by primary care physicians. J Adolesc Health Care 1990; 11:227–230.

44. Simcha-Fagan O, Gersten JC, Langner TS: Early precursors and concurrent correlates of patterns of illicit drug use in adolescence. J Drug Issues 1986; 16:7–28.

45. Hawkins JD, Fitzgibbon JJ: Risk factors and risk behaviors in prevention of adolescent substance abuse. Adolesc Med: State of the Art Reviews 1993; 4:249–262.

46. MacKenzie RG: Influence of drug use on adolescent sexual activity. Adolesc Med: State of the Art Reviews 1993; 4:417–422.

47. Hingson R, Alpert J, Day N, et al: Effects of maternal drinking and marijuana use on fetal growth and development. Pediatrics 1982; 70:539–546.

48. Schwartz RH, Wirtz PW: Potential substance abuse: Detection among adolescent patients. Clin Pediatrics 1990; 29:38–43.

49. Fuller PG, Cavanaugh RM: Basic assessment and screening for substance abuse in the pediatrician's office. Pediatr Clin North Am 1995; 42:295–315.

50. Schwartz RH: Urine testing in the detection of drugs of abuse. Arch Intern Med 1988; 148:2407–2412.

51. Committee on Substance Abuse, American Academy of Pediatrics: Testing for drugs of abuse in children and adolescents (RE9628). Pediatrics 1996; 98:305–307.

52. Provisional Committee on Substance Abuse, American Academy of Pediatrics: Selection of substance abuse treatment programs. Pediatrics 1990; 86:139–140.

53. Catalano RF, Hawkins JD, Wells EA, et al: Evaluation of the effectiveness of adolescent drug abuse treatment, assessment of risks for relapse, and promising approaches for relapse prevention. Int J Addict 1991; 25:1085–1140.

54. Shoemaker RH, Sherry P: Post-treatment factors influencing outcome of adolescent chemical dependency treatment. J Adolesc Chemical Dependency 1991; 2:89–106.

55. Alford GS, Koehler RA, Leonard J: Alcoholics Anonymous–Narcotics Anonymous model inpatient treatment of chemically dependent adolescents: A two-year outcome study. J Stud Alcohol 1991; 52:118–126.

56. Richter SS, Brown SA, Mott MA: The impact of social support and self-esteem on adolescent substance abuse treatment outcome. J Subst Abuse 1991; 3:371–385.

57. Harrison PA, Hoffman NG: CATOR 1987 Report: Adolescent Residential Treatment Intake and Follow-up Findings. St. Paul, Minn: Ramsey Clinic, 1987.

58. Hoffman NG, Kaplan RA: CATOR Report: One-year Outcomes Results for Adolescents: Key Correlates and Benefits of Recovery. St. Paul, Minn: New Standards, 1991.

59. Myers MG, Brown SA: Coping responses and relapse among adolescent substance abusers. J Subst Abuse 1990; 2:177–189.

60. Kanetsky PA, Gammon MD, Mandelblatt J, et al: Cigarette smoking and cervical dysplasia among non-Hispanic black women. Cancer Detect Prev 1998; 22:109–119.

61. Smith CG, Asch RH: Acute, short-term, and chronic effects of marijuana on the female primate reproductive function. NIDA Res Monogr 1984; 44:82–96.

62. Lee MJ: Marijuana and tobacco use in pregnancy. Obstet Gynecol Clin North Am 1998; 25:65–83.

63. Mello NK, Mendelson JH: Cocaine's effects on neuroendocrine systems: Clinical and preclinical studies. Pharmacol Biochem Behav 1997; 57:571–599.

64. Plessinger MA, Woods JR: Cocaine in pregnancy: Recent data on maternal and fetal risks. Obstet Gynecol Clin North Am 1998; 25:99–118.

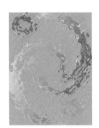

Chapter 27
Diagnostic Imaging

LUIGI FEDELE, MILENA DORTA,
AND ANTONELLA PORTUESE

The use of invasive instrumental diagnostic investigations such as hysterosalpingography, hysteroscopy, and pelvic pneumography in children and adolescents is limited, but occasionally a serious organic disease or a congenital malformation demands a precise diagnosis so that definitive therapy can be planned and inappropriate interventions avoided. In such situations, ultrasonography (US) should be part of the pelvic exploration. US has limitations, however, especially in the precise characterization of tissues. The vaginal probe is of limited benefit in young patients because it is invasive. This explains the use in pediatric gynecology, of abdominal US and more sophisticated imaging methods such as magnetic resonance imaging (MRI), and the frequent recourse to diagnostic endoscopy despite its invasiveness and cost.

IMAGING OF THE NORMAL FEMALE PELVIS IN CHILDREN AND ADOLESCENTS

US provides immediate real-time images of the pelvic structures in multiple planes. Real-time, preferably convex, probes of 3.5, 5, 7.5, or 10 MHz are used, depending on the patient's habitus. Generally, sagittal or transverse images are obtained, but angling the transducer on the sagittal, coronal, and transverse planes may generate additional images. Children usually have minimal perivisceral fat and thus are excellent subjects for US. The absence of ionizing radiation means that the examination can be repeated without using biologic effects.

An inconvenience of abdominal US is the need for a full bladder to act as a sonic window. It elevates the small bowel, which, when filled with air, reflects the echoes and obscures the posterior structures. If necessary, sterile water can be instilled as contrast medium to outline the bladder, vagina (water vaginography), or rectum (water enema technique). It can also be used to

fill other structures, such as a cloaca or utricle. Patients should be well-hydrated before the examination to facilitate the procedure, and bladder filling by catheterization can be avoided. Neonates should be placed comfortably on an examination table and the room well heated to prevent rapid loss of body heat.

Another difficulty of pediatric US is patient movement. A parent should be allowed to remain close to the child during the examination. Sedation is occasionally required; chloral hydrate, 50 mg/kg by mouth 30 minutes before the study begins, may be used. Often, however, the best sedation for a neonate or small child is a full stomach.

Transvaginal US does not require a full bladder. It uses a 6.5-MHz transducer placed in the vagina, and, thus, cannot be used in children or in adolescents with an intact hymen. These high-frequency probes provide excellent resolution 2 to 7 cm from the transducer. This pelvic US modality is an important advance and often fundamental to the evaluation of cul-de-sac masses and the adnexa. It is not affected by the patient's habitus or abdominal surgical scars, and the probe can be placed very close to the structures to be investigated. With a transvaginal probe, it is easy to differentiate solid masses from cystic ones and to delineate septa, excrescences, and calcifications in cystic masses.

US has limitations in the evaluation of large tumors in which the organ of origin cannot be determined, and a complete evaluation of tumor spread may be difficult. The lack of good identifiable reference landmarks makes US less helpful to the surgeon than CT or MRI scans. Image quality, delineation of anatomic structures, and lesion detection are operator and machine dependent.

Color-flow and duplex Doppler US are useful for demonstrating vascular structures in the pelvis and providing information about flow characteristics. They can help to differentiate between benign and malignant lesions and sometimes to identify ectopic pregnancy or adnexal torsion.

Computed tomography (CT) generally provides poor density resolution of the reproductive organs. It does offer some advantages: great spatial resolution, short imaging time, and low cost. It uses ionizing radiation and requires patient preparation, such as opacification of the gastrointestinal tract and intravenous iodinated contrast material. Complete opacification of the small bowel and colon is essential, as the intestine occupies a large portion of the pelvis and the most common error in interpreting CT images is mistaking nonopacified intestinal loops for a pelvic mass. Patients of average habitus should imbibe 500 to 700 ml of a diluted barium solution before the examination. If the patient is reluctant to drink such a large amount of liquid, she may be given 40 to 50 ml diatrizoate meglumine (Gastrografin). Rectal contrast medium is sometimes administered via enema. A slender tampon, which provides air density, may be inserted in the vagina to enhance the distinction between vagina and cervix and between paracervical and parametrial regions. Intravenous contrast medium may also be used. When pelvic disease is suspected, transaxial images are obtained at 10-mm slice thickness. Thin or repeated sections are occasionally required to better delineate suspected abnormalities.

Spiral (helical) CT is the latest technologic advance in CT. Spiral CT involves continuous, simultaneous patient translation and x-ray rotation during data acquisition. This is made possible by a slip-ring gantry system, improved detector efficiency, and greater tube-cooling capability. This new technique has markedly increased imaging speed and made possible volume-acquisition CT. When spiral CT is used, the necessity for sedating children has been shown to decrease by as much as 45% to 49%. The short scan time also makes it possible to perform contrast-enhanced studies during peak contrast enhancement. This is particularly important in the evaluation of tumor viability and for optimal vascular enhancement.

MRI has been a viable imaging technique since the early 1980s. It is noninvasive, provides excellent tissue contrast, and uses no ionizing radiation. The examination takes some time, however, and children may be afraid of being placed in the machine. In addition, it may be difficult for a child to lie still for a long time, and young patients should not be made to suffer claustrophobia. For any of these reasons, sedatives may be used. Girls younger than 5 years should be sedated as a matter of routine; chloral hydrate, 50 to 70 mg/kg, may be used.

Unfortunately, the physical principles on which MRI is based are considerably different from those of radiographic and US imaging. MRI is based on the interaction of tissue immersed in a static magnetic field with radiofrequency (RF) pulses that create perturbations of short duration on nuclei oriented by the static magnetic field. At cessation of the RF pulse, the nuclei restore the energy they absorbed in the form of signals that are received by the same RF coil in reception phase. The MR signal is then amplified and converted from analog to digital, to be processed by the computer, which reconstructs the image by localizing and interpreting the signal from each unit of volume. Some physical characteristics of the tissues and other variables controlled by the operator affect the signals emitted by the tissues. Specifically, the density of protons of hydrogen nuclei; the relaxation times (time it takes protons to return to equilibrium after excitation); the velocity of blood flow; and the presence of paramagnetic substances (e.g., iron) that shorten relaxation times all influence the formation of the image. The dependence of the signals on the relaxation times is particularly important. Relaxation time reflects the water content and the dynamics of water in the tissues. There are two types of relaxation processes. T1 expresses the interaction of the hydrogen nucleus with the surrounding molecular environment; T2 expresses the magnetic interaction among the protons. The operator can make the images "T1-" or "T2-weighted" by varying the pulse sequences, a maneuver that accentuates contrasts among the various tissues with different T1 and T2.

By reducing the T1 relaxation time, static gadolinium-enhanced studies are useful for the evaluation of neoplasms, because they can define areas of increased vascularity (which suggests viable tumor) and of decreased intensity (which may suggest a necrotic tumor).

In MRI, the bladder serves as a reference for signal characterization in the pelvis. Cysts that demonstrate a signal like that of urine are classified as simple (serous). Urine is isointense in T1 and hyperintense in T2 images, because the short T2 of smooth muscle contrasts with the long T2 of the adjacent urine and perivesical fat. In the images, white signifies high signal intensity and black low signal intensity. Solid formations show low signal intensity in both T1- and T2-weighted images. Fluid tissues with abundant free water (urine, stagnant blood) have low and high signal intensities in T1- and T2-weighted images, respectively. Proteinaceous fluids are distinguished by intermediate signal intensity in T1-weighted images and by high signal in T2-weighted ones. Flowing blood is characterized by the absence of signals (i.e., black images). In T1-weighted images, tissues with a short relaxation time show elevated signal (i.e., fat), whereas in T2-weighted images the tissue components with a long relaxation time show high signal intensity (i.e., urine).

VAGINA

On US the vaginal canal is evident as a central linear echo created by the reflective interface of the opposing walls of the structure and of fluid in the canal. MRI clearly defines the vagina in T2-weighted images. The mucus in the lumen has high signal intensity, which contrasts with the low signal intensity of the muscular walls.

UTERUS

The neonatal uterus is relatively large as a result of residual stimulation from maternal hormones. Nussbaum and Orsini and coworkers reported a mean craniocaudal length of 3.4 cm (range, 2.5 to 4.6 cm) based on US findings in 35 neonates in the first 7 days of life.[1, 2] In most cases, the uterus is tubular or spade-shaped. The anteroposterior diameter of the cervix is as long as or longer than that of the fundus. Up to age 7 years, the size of the uterus is not related to age, and the cervix is larger than the corpus, so that the organ has an inverted pear shape (Fig. 27–1). The ratio between the anteroposterior diameters of the corpus and cervix is 1:1 (Fig. 27–2). Beginning at age 7 years, the diameter and the volume of the uterus increase in relation to age. Because the increase in total length and in the anteroposterior diameter of the corpus is more pronounced than the increase in the anteroposterior diameter of the cervix, the organ gradually acquires the typical pear shape of the adult uterus by age 12 to 13 years (Fig. 27–3).

MYOMETRIUM

As compared with the full bladder, the myometrium on US is very echogenic because of the abundance of muscular, fibrous, and vascular components. On CT, the best definition of the myometrium is obtained when intravenous contrast, which clearly differentiates this tissue from all other reproductive structures, is used. On MRI the myometrium, like other smooth muscles, has a long T1 and short T2. In an adolescent with normal menses its thickness varies from 1.5 to 2 cm. Its appearance varies during the

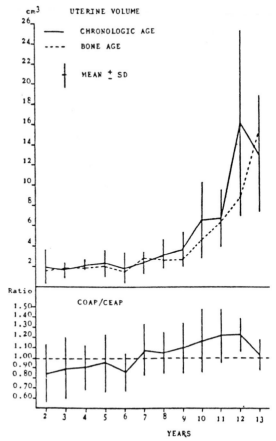

Figure 27–1. Uterine volume (*top*) and the relationship between the anteroposterior diameters of the corpus (COAP) and the cervix (CEAP, *bottom*), as determined by ultrasonography, from ages 2 to 13. (From Orsini L, Salardi S, Pilu G, et al: Pelvic organs in premenarchal girls: Real-time ultrasonography. Radiology 1984; 153:113–116.)

menstrual cycle, although this variation is less pronounced than that of the endometrium. It increases in thickness by 2.2% daily during the follicular phase of the menstrual cycle and by 1.8% daily during the secretory phase.

ENDOMETRIUM

On US, the endometrium appears as an elliptical shadow with distinct borders (believed to represent the basalis-myometrial junction). A longitudinal central line is evident that represents the interface of the anterior and posterior superficial endometrial layers (Figs. 27–3, 27–4, 27–5). The endometrium is seen as a high-signal layer in T2-weighted MR images because of its tortuous vessels and abundant mucus. In the neonate the

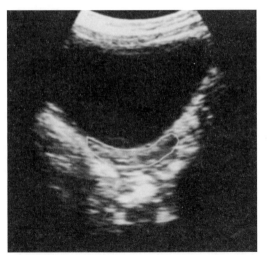

Figure 27–2. Sagittal ultrasound scan of the uterus in a 5-year-old girl. The ratio between the anteroposterior diameters of the corpus and cervix is 1:1.

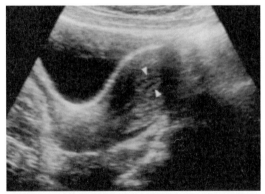

Figure 27–4. Sagittal ultrasound scan of the uterus showing the endometrium in the proliferative phase. A three-striped elliptical shadow is seen (*arrowheads*).

endometrial cavity is easily demonstrated by US because of the stimulated endometrium and the mucus and secretions frequently present in the cavity (Fig. 27–6). Anatomic studies of neonatal uteri have shown that the cavity is often filled with blood, epithelial residue and denuded stroma[3] that are attributable to residual maternal hormone stimulation. In normally menstruating adolescents, physiologic changes in the stratum ba-

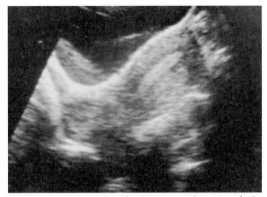

Figure 27–5. Sagittal ultrasound scan of the uterus showing the secretory phase in the same case shown in Figure 27–4. The endometrium appears as a thickened echogenic area.

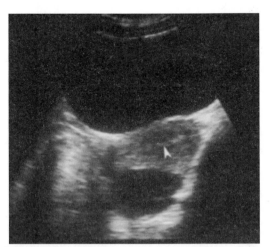

Figure 27–3. Sagittal ultrasound scan of the uterus of a 13-year-old girl. The anteroposterior diameter of the corpus is more pronounced than that of the cervix. The endometrium appears as a linear cavity echo of high amplitude in the initial proliferative phase (*arrowhead*). As a related finding, an ovarian cyst is seen in the pouch of Douglas.

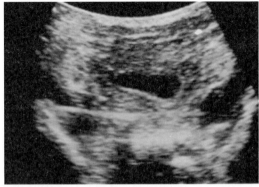

Figure 27–6. Sagittal ultrasound scan showing the endometrial cavity in a neonate. The cavity is dilated and surrounded by stimulated endometrium, which appears as a thin, hyperechogenic line.

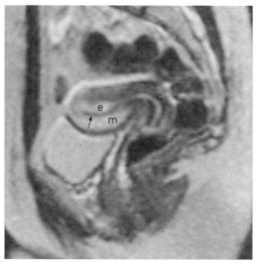

Figure 27–7. Sagittal T2-weighted image (TR = 2000 ms; TE = 60 ms) demonstrating the uterine anatomy: c, cervix; e, endometrium; m, myometrium. The arrow indicates the junctional zone.

salis and stratum functionalis are reflected in the width and degree of definition of the stripe on both US and MRI.[4]

On both US and MRI, a thin stripe is identified in the interface between the endometrium and myometrium. This stripe has low signal intensity (short T2) on MRI (Fig. 27–7) and is echogenic on US. The nature of this so-called junctional zone is still a mystery. It was visible on 29% of neonatal US scans performed by Nussbaum and coworkers, who also reported that it was 2 to 3 mm thick in postpubertal uteri.[1] In adolescents with normal menses who are taking oral contraceptives, the junctional zone is very difficult to identify.

CERVIX

The cervix has an echogenicity similar to that of the myometrium. Inside the cervix, a mixed hypo- and hyperechoic stripe representing endocervical secretions is often seen. MRI of the cervix demonstrates a stripe of high intensity, corresponding to the endocervical glands and mucus, and an external zone with low signal intensity that represents the fibrous stroma and is continuous with the junctional zone of the corpus. A third layer, of undefined origin and with moderate signal intensity, has been described in continuation with the myometrium.

OVARIES

The ovaries are readily demonstrated by US and MRI. It is sometimes difficult to recognize them because of their small size and the neonate's inability to maintain a full bladder for very long. Anatomic studies have demonstrated that neonatal ovaries vary from 0.5 to 1.5 cm in length and from 0.3 to 0.4 cm in thickness.[3] In prepubertal girls, the ovaries generally are solid and homogeneous and stable in size up to age 6 years (Fig. 27–8). After that point, growth is age-related, and microcystic aspects become increasingly frequent, although on US homogeneous ovaries remain prevalent until age 11.

Small cysts (mean <7.5 mm in diameter) can be seen in slightly more than 80% of ovaries of girls aged 1 to 24 months. Cysts have also been noted in 68% of ovaries in premenarcheal girls between 2 and 12 years of age. Some 90% to 95% of these follicles are smaller than 9 mm in diameter (average follicle or cyst size being 6 mm). The remaining girls have ovarian cysts with diameters greater than 9 mm, termed *macro-*

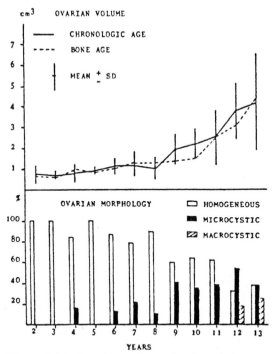

Figure 27–8. Ovarian volume (*top*) and changes in ovarian morphology (*bottom*), as determined by ultrasonography, from ages 2 to 13. (From Orsini L, Salardi S, Pilu G, et al: Pelvic organs in premenarchal girls: Real-time ultrasonography. Radiology 1984; 153:113–116. Reprinted with permission of the Radiological Society of North America.)

cysts. The reasons for the presence of cystic follicles in premenarcheal children has not been definitely established, but it is postulated that pulsatile secretions of low levels of gonadotropin-releasing hormone stimulate ovarian maturation before clinical signs of puberty develop.

Multiple ovarian cysts can also be found in children with primary hypothyroidism or cystic fibrosis. Bilateral ovarian enlargement with discrete cysts has also been seen in children with McCune-Albright syndrome.

At puberty, the ovaries attain their adult size and features. Ovarian volume may be calculated using the formula for ellipsoids. Before puberty ovarian volume is about 1 ml. The size increases with age. Ovarian volume is about 6 ml in normally menstruating adolescents.

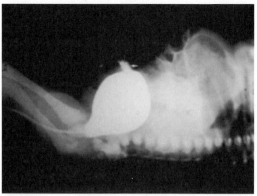

Figure 27–9. Vaginogram in a neonate. The contrast medium opacifies the dilatation of the vagina and endocervix (*arrow*).

IMAGING OF CONGENITAL ABNORMALITIES

HYDROCOLPOS

Hydrocolpos is a collection of fluid in the vagina and, possibly also the uterus (hydrometrocolpos) (Table 27–1). It is observed in neonates but also occurs later in childhood.[6] It is usually caused by a vaginal obstruction such as an imperforate hymen or a septum of varying thickness occluding the vaginal introitus.

Correct early diagnosis of hydrocolpos by US makes laparotomy unnecessary. US is not only safe but also reliable and specific for investigating both abdominal masses and the urinary tract, and

it is therefore strongly recommended before any radiologic examinations are performed. Plain radiographs of the abdomen are rarely indicated when US reveals a "cystic" hypogastric mass. However, if the fluid in the vagina contains debris, the mass may appear "complex" or even "solid" and, thus, the findings are equivocal. The uterus may be slightly dilated by the vaginal fluid (Fig. 27–9). Cystography should be performed to exclude (1) reflux from a megaureter and (2) ureterocele. Because obstruction of the lower urinary outlet is very rare in females,[7] it is crucial to distinguish ovarian tumors from hydrocolpos immediately after birth. With US it is usually possible to identify the vagina as the origin of the "cystic" mass with reasonable accuracy (Fig. 27–10). The association of such a mass with hy-

Table 27–1. Hydrocolpos and Hemato(metro)colpos: Clinical Features

	Hydro(metro)colpos	Hemato(metro)colpos
Age	Neonate mainly	Adolescent
	Child	
Cause	Transverse vaginal septum	Same
	Imperforate hymen	
Uterine involvement	Possible	Possible
Symptoms	Range from no pain to acute pelvic pain	Cyclic acute pelvic pain
	Retention of urine	Dysuria
	Intestinal occlusion	Retention of urine
Signs	Distended hymen	Same
Diagnostic studies		
Ultrasonography	Hypogastric anechoic fluid collection	Hypogastric corpuscular or complex fluid collection, or solid mass
		Possibly associated with dilated uterine cavity (hematometra)
Abdominal radiography	—	Useful if solid mass at ultrasonography
Vaginography/cystography	To exclude megaureter and ureterocele	Same
Barium enema	To exclude intestinal occlusion	Same
Differential diagnosis	Ovarian tumor	Same
	Lower urinary tract obstruction	

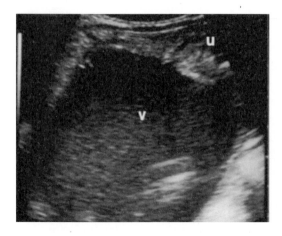

Figure 27–10. Sagittal ultrasound scan demonstrating hydromucometrocolpos in the neonate shown in Figure 27–9. The vagina (v) is very dilated and contains fine debris, and the endometrial cavity is slightly dilated. u, Uterus.

dronephrosis and obstructive megaureter should be easy to recognize and is pathognomonic for hydrocolpos. On the other hand, it is unlikely that a complex or a solid mass is a hydrocolpos, rather than a tumor. Barium enemas may be required to evaluate suspected intestinal involvement, such as duplication or obstruction.

IMPERFORATE HYMEN

With an imperforate hymen, vaginal distention may be so great that a mass is clearly evident in the lower abdomen (Fig. 27–11).

TRANSVERSE VAGINAL SEPTUM

A low complete or suprahymenal septum may first manifest itself early in infancy (hydromuco-

colpos); or after the start of cyclic endometrial activity (similar to symptoms and signs of an imperforate hymen; Fig. 27–12A). High complete septa are less common and generally are located at the junction of the middle and upper thirds of the vagina. US is useful to demonstrate a normal cervix and for precise localization of the obstructing septum (see Fig. 27–12B).

CERVICAL AGENESIS

The pure form of cervical agenesis (Buttram and Gibbons class IB; Table 27–2) is rare, and the clinical picture is always confused with that of a high complete vaginal septum.[8] Differential diagnosis is fundamental and can be readily performed by US (Fig. 27–13). The various surgical attempts to create a stable uterovaginal commu-

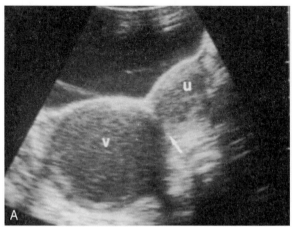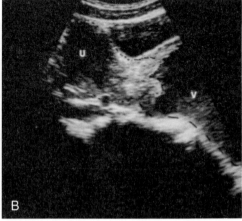

Figure 27–11. Hematometrocolpos resulting from an imperforate hymen in a young adolescent. *A,* This sagittal pelvic sonogram shows a dilated uterine cavity (u) filled with echogenic debris (blood) and communicating via a wide endocervix (*arrow*) with the obstructed vagina (v), which is also filled with debris. *B,* Ultrasound image of the imperforate hymen. The cervix, with conserved morphology, projects into the large hematocolpos on the right. The uterus and the endometrial cavity are conserved (*black broken lines*). u, Uterus; v, vagina.

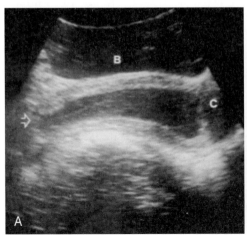
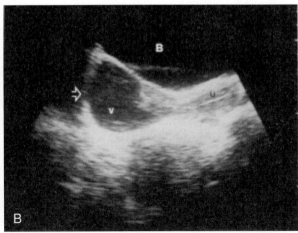

Figure 27–12. Transverse vaginal septa. *A,* A small hematocolpos resulting from a suprahymenal transverse vaginal septum. This sagittal sonogram of the pelvis demonstrates a collection of fine debris (blood) under the bladder (B), delineated at the bottom by the suprahymenal septum (*arrow*) and at the top by the uterine cervix (C). *B,* Pelvic cyst in a 13-year-old girl. This sagittal ultrasound scan shows a normal cervix projecting into the dilated vagina (v) and containing fine debris (blood) that has accumulated as a result of a high complete transverse vaginal septum (*arrow*). B, Bladder; u, uterus.

Table 27–2. Cervical Agenesis: Clinical Features

Prevalence	Sympotms	US Findings	Differential Diagnosis
Rare	Primary amenorrhea Cyclic pelvic pain	Dilated uterine cavity but no cervix Regular vaginal echoes	Complete transverse vaginal septum

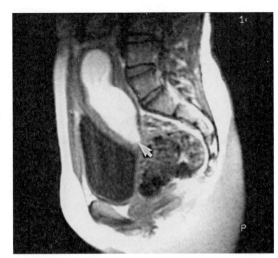

Figure 27–13. Total vaginal agenesis and cervical hypoplasia shown by T1-weighted sagittal MRI scan. The uterine cavity is dilated and funnel-shaped owing to a large hematometra.

Table 27–3. Diagnostic Studies for Suspected Uterovaginal Agenesis

Study	Capability
Ultrasonography	Demonstrates uterovaginal agenesis
	Recognizes cavitation of the müllerian remnants
Laparoscopy	Offers a panoramic view of the internal genital system
Magnetic resonance	Recognizes site and cavitation of the müllerian remnants and ovaries (sometimes extrapelvic)
	Evaluates the subperitoneal structures (complete or partial vaginal agenesis?)
	Demonstrates presence/absence of the cervix?
	Demonstrates fibrous cord?

nication often entail or are complicated by the onset of an ascending infection.

AGENESIS OF THE VAGINA AND UTERUS

The most frequent type of congenital absence of the vagina is known as *Rokitansky syndrome* (Buttram and Gibbons class IE) (Fig. 27–14; Table 27–3). The typical physical features, in conjunction with imaging findings, are often sufficient to establish the diagnosis. Laparoscopy

is rarely necessary for diagnostic purposes. The finding are quite typical (Fig. 27–15). Furthermore, US or MRI studies help to determine the characteristics of the müllerian rudiments and whether they are cavitary (Fig. 27–16). MRI provides equally good images of superficial and deep planes, is not affected by the patient's body habitus, and does not require a full bladder. In addition, MRI is more precise than US in tissue discrimination.

In a study of six girls suspected to have Rokitansky syndrome,[9] it was noted that more precise information was obtained with MRI than with US or laparoscopy (Fig. 27–17A). The greater diagnostic reliability of MRI as compared with laparoscopy, was due to the finding that laparoscopy provided no information on subperitoneal structures. In fact, in Rokitansky syndrome, vaginal agenesis may be only partial; the cervix may be present, or there may be a fibrous, partially cavitary cord (Fig. 27–17B). The importance of such findings is not just theoretical; the surgeon may use this information to plan reconstruction of a functional vagina.[10] MRI easily demonstrates an endometrial cavity within the müllerian remnants as a high-intensity signal on T2-weighted images (Fig. 27–17C). The clinical importance of these endometrial islands in the myometrium of müllerian rudiments is not clear, but surgical removal is indicated when they are large and cause cyclic pelvic pain.

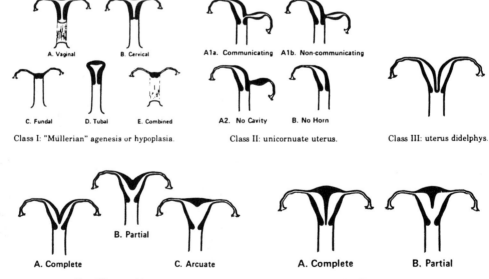

Figure 27–14. Müllerian anomalies, classes I through V. (From Buttram VC Jr, Gibbons WE: Müllerian anomalies: A proposed classification [an analysis of 144 cases]. Fertil Steril 1979; 32:40–45. Reprinted with permission of the American Society for Reproductive Medicine, formerly the American Fertility Society.)

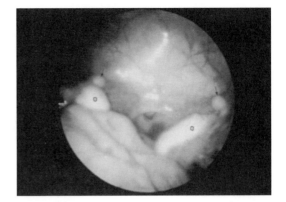

Figure 27–15. Mayer-Rokitansky-Küster-Hauser syndrome. This laparoscopic image shows the absence of the uterus. Two small müllerian rudiments (*arrows*) are seen at the upper poles of the ovaries (O).

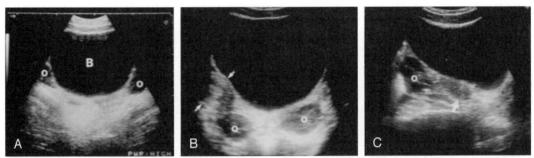

Figure 27–16. Transverse ultrasound scans of the pelvis demonstrating Mayer-Rokitansky-Küster-Hauser syndrome. *A,* Two normal ovaries (O) can be visualized behind the full bladder (B); the uterus is absent. *B,* A cavitary müllerian rudiment (*arrows*) can be visualized at the center, above the left ovary (O), with the endometrium appearing as a hyperechoic area. *C,* Longitudinal scan of the pelvis. A noncavitary müllerian rudiment (*arrow*) is visible below a micropolycystic ovary (O).

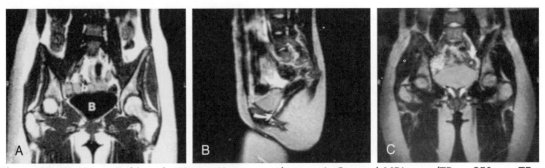

Figure 27–17. Mayer-Rokitansky-Küster-Hauser syndrome. *A,* Coronal MRI scan (TR = 350 ms; TE = 20 ms). No uterine structure can be detected. The bowel (b) can be seen over the bladder (B). *B,* Medial sagittal scan (TR = 1510 ms; TE = 100 ms). A fibrous structure (*arrow*) appears between the rectum and the bladder. *C,* Coronal scan (TR = 1380 ms; TE = 100 ms) demonstrating a markedly lateralized cavitary müllerian rudiment (*arrow*). (From Fedele L, Dorta M, Brioschi D, et al: Magnetic resonance imaging in Mayer-Rokitansky-Küster-Hauser syndrome. Obstet Gynecol 1990; 76(4):593–596. Reprinted with permission from the American College of Obstetricians and Gynecologists.)

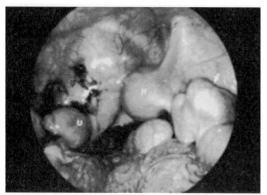

Figure 27–18. Unicornuate (*left*) uterus (U), Buttram and Gibbons subclass AIb. This laparoscopic view reveals a large, dilated rudimentary horn (H) in communication with a large hematosalpinx (*arrow*). Free blood is present in the pouch of Douglas, and endometriosis can be identified on the bladder peritoneum.

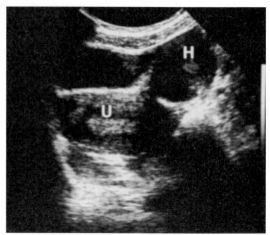

Figure 27–19. Plain transverse sonogram of the pelvis with a partially full bladder shows a unicornuate uterus (U) with a large, round, cavitary rudimentary horn (H). Endometrium is seen as a hyperechoic area located centrally in the unicornuate uterus and cavitary horn.

UNICORNUATE UTERUS WITH NONCOMMUNICATING CAVITARY RUDIMENTARY HORN

This anomaly (Buttram and Gibbons class IIA1b) may cause severe symptoms as a result of retained menstrual blood (Fig. 27–18; Table 27–4). Retention does not always occur, because, in most cases, the endometrium of rudimentary horns exhibits only partial and attenuated cyclic modifications that do not produce true menstrual bleeding.[11] The diagnosis may be delayed or confused with other diseases, particularly ovarian cysts and a "double" uterus with an imperforate hemivagina.

US demonstrates the unicornuate uterus and its banana-shaped cavity.[12] Scans of the hemipelvis contralateral to the hemiuterus reveals the presence of a large, rounded rudimentary horn that has the same echogenicity as the myometrium and contains a thickened and hyperechoic zone that resembles secretory endometrium (Fig. 27–19). MRI identifies the rudimentary horn lateral to the unicornuate uterus, and the high–signal intensity central zone on T2-weighted images denotes cavitation (Fig. 27–20).[13]

Independently of menstrual retention, US and

Table 27–4. Diagnostic Techniques for Suspected Uterine Malformations

Technique	Utility
Ultrasonography	
Pelvic	To detect the presence of a uterine
Transabdominal	structure and endometrium
Transvaginal	Better in premenstrual period
Transrectal	
Urinary tract	To detect associated kidney anomalies (absence or pelvic location)
Magnetic resonance	Better spatial resolution
imaging	To detect secretive endometrium
Hysterography	In girls with sexual experience
	To assess the morphology of uterine cavity
Laparoscopy	When imaging findings are equivocal
	Therapy

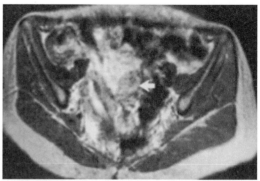

Figure 27–20. MRI scan of the same unicornuate uterus shown in Figure 27–19 (T2-weighted image; TR = 2000 ms; TE = 100 ms). In the rudimentary horn, the central high signal zone (*arrow*) denotes cavitation. (From Fedele L, Dorta M, Brioschi D, et al: Magnetic resonance imaging of unicornuate uterus. Acta Obstet Gynecol Scand 1990; 69:5911–513. Reprinted with permission of the Scandinavian Association of Obstetricians and Gynecologists.)

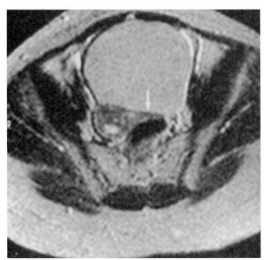

Figure 27–21. MRI scan of a unicornuate (*right*) uterus with a small left rudimentary horn (TR = 1447 ms; TE = 50 ms). In the small rudimentary horn (*arrow*), the high-signal central zone denoting cavitation is absent. (From Fedele L, Dorta M, Brioschi D, et al: Magnetic resonance imaging of unicornuate uterus. Acta Obstet Gynecol Scand 1990; 69:511–513. Reprinted with permission of the Scandinavian Association of Obstetricians and Gynecologists.)

MRI can both demonstrate unicornuate uterus of subclasses IIA1b, IIA2, and IIB in an adolescent (i.e., to detect the presence of a rudimentary horn [Fig. 27–21] and establish whether it is cavitary [Fig. 27–22]). Axial and paraxial scans

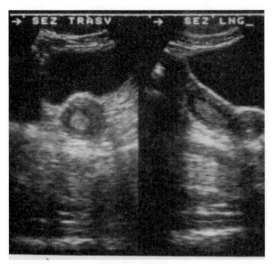

Figure 27–22. A simple unicornuate uterus, Buttram and Gibbon subclass B. *Left,* A transverse sonogram shows the uterus with a cylindric form. *Right,* On a longitudinal scan, the endometrium appears banana-shaped.

oriented to contain the plane passing through the tubal ostium and internal uterine os allow simultaneous visualization of the entire endometrial cavity and the external profile of the uterus, and thus clearly delineates the architecture of the organ. To visualize any endometrium inside the rudimentary horns, T2-weighted sequences optimize the contrast between different tissue layers. Unlike laparoscopy, US and MRI do not demonstrate endometriosis, nor do they afford assessment of the fallopian tubes.

"DOUBLE" UTERUS WITH AN OBSTRUCTED HEMIVAGINA

A double uterus—didelphic, bicornuate, or septate—is generally associated with a complete or partial vaginal septum, but occasionally a developmental abnormality of the urogenital sinus causes a complete vaginal diaphragm with an imperforate hemivagina to form. This müllerian anomaly is always associated with ipsilateral renal agenesis. Three anatomic varieties of the anomaly have been described, according to whether there is a communication between the two hemiuteri and whether the vaginal obstruction is complete or incomplete.[14]

In the noncommunicating type, the imperforate vagina and "its uterus" constitute a cavity completely separate from the contralateral vagina and uterus. The only communication is with the peritoneal cavity through the corresponding salpinx. In the communicating form, the communication is between the two hemiuteri, generally at the level of the isthmus. In these two varieties, the imperforate vagina swells progressively with successive menstrual flows after menarche, and hematometra and hematosalpinx develop. In the type with incomplete vaginal obstruction, the septum is perforated at one or more points, so formation of a true hematocolpos is prevented. The clinical picture is characterized by a triad of symptoms (dysmenorrhea, pelvic mass, and ipsilateral renal agenesis), which, considering the usual age of presentation of the patient, is sufficiently pathognomonic.

In patients in whom hysterosalpingography can be performed, this may provide sufficiently characteristic images. Contrast medium, placed through the only demonstrable cervix, provides visualization of the hemiuterus contralateral to the pelvic mass; if there is an isthmic communication between the two hemiuteri, it may opacify the imperforate hemivagina (Fig. 27–23). Opacification of the hemiuterus, corresponding to the imperforate hemivagina, may occur if the interisthmic communication is wide (Fig. 27–24).

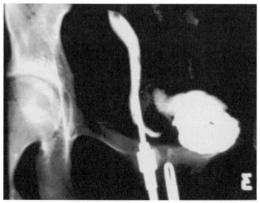

Figure 27–23. Hysterosalpingography of a "double" communicating uterus with an obstructed right hemivagina. The contrast medium delineates a uterine horn above the cannulated cervix and the contralateral obstructed hemivagina. Opacification of the hemiuterus corresponding to the imperforate hemivagina is not possible because of the narrowness of the interisthmic communication.

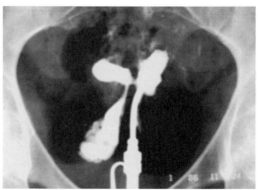

Figure 27–24. Hysterosalpingogram of a "double" communicating uterus with an obstructed right hemivagina. Three cavities are visualized (1) in a uterine horn directly above the cannulated cervix, (2) in a right horn communicating with the contralateral horn via a small isthmus, and (3) under the right uterine horn (obstructed hemivagina).

Hysterosalpingography is useful in documenting an interisthmic communication between the two hemiuteri but shows only the internal profile of the uterus, whereas it is obviously equally essential to visualize the external morphology of the organ to classify the malformation precisely.

When a "double" uterus with imperforate hemivagina is suspected, US is an excellent method of diagnosis (Fig. 27–25). The imperforate hemivagina caudad to the uterus appears as a sac delineated by a structure whose echogenicity is similar to that of the myometrium (vaginal wall) and containing hyperechoic fine debris or mixed hyper- and hypoechoic material. The nature of this material cannot be determined by US, but MRI has shown it to be blood alone or blood mixed with mucus and pus. Occasionally, US images of the two cervices and the normal vagina are poor. In contrast, MR images are more panoramic and detailed (Fig. 27–26) and afford

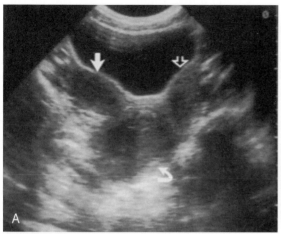
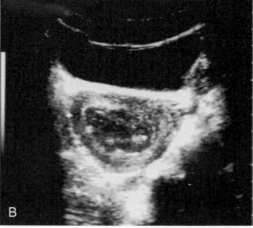

Figure 27–25. "Double" uterus with an imperforate left hemivagina. *A,* A transverse sonogram of the pelvis shows a "double" uterus with a deep fundal notch. The right hemiuterus is of normal size (*open arrow*); the left is dilated and contains debris (hematometra, *solid arrow*). A predominantly cystic mass (hematocolpos) is seen below the uterus (*curved arrow*). *B,* A sonogram with a partially full bladder visualizes the hematocolpos more clearly (*calipers*). The wall of the imperforate hemivagina circumscribes hyper- and hypoechoic material (blood and mucus, respectively).

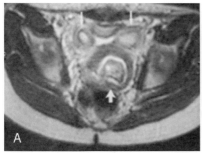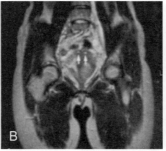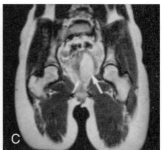

Figure 27–26. MRI scan of a didelphic uterus with an imperforate left hemivagina. *A,* Transverse section (TR = 2000 ms; TE = 100 ms). Two distinct uterine bodies are visible (*small arrows*), the left with a dilated endometrial cavity. Below the left hemiuterus is a vast saccular collection of high–signal intensity fluid (*large arrow*), consistent with a hematocolpos. *B,* Coronal section (TR = 2000 ms; TE = 100 ms). Two uterine cervices are seen with central high-intensity areas that delineate two cervical canals (*double arrows*). Beneath them, two vaginas can be detected, the left one dilated and containing a collection of blood. *C,* Coronal section (TR = 2000 ms; TE = 100 ms). The right hemivagina is normally patent (*small arrow*), and the left one ends blind (*large arrow*). (From Fedele L, Dorta M, Brioschi D, et al: Magnetic resonance evaluation of gynecologic masses in adolescents. Adolesc Pediatr Gynecol 1990; 3:83–88.)

visualization of the two vaginas, one normal and the other transformed into an abundant saccular collection of fluid with high signal intensity consistent with blood. The two endometrial cavities are clearly identifiable, as is blood in cases of hematometra of the uterine body communicating with the imperforate hemivagina.

US must be performed in the second half of the menstrual cycle. Fundal scanning parallel to the frontal planes of the uterus and with a half-full bladder is the only way to visualize the area surrounding the fundus and to determine myometrial thickness and conformation of the endometrial cavity.[15] Once the orientation of the uterus is established, the organ is examined with MRI, using slices paralleling, as much as possible, the anatomic plane containing the tubal ostia and internal uterine os. These images are usually T2 weighted for greater contrast between peritoneal fat and the external contour of the uterus, but, in some instances, T1-weighted slices are also obtained.[16]

Bicornuate- and didelphic uterus are differentiated from partial- and complete septate uterus on US and MRI by a fundal indentation deeper than 10 mm and associated with an angle between the medial margins of the hemicavities of at least 60 degrees (Fig. 27–27 through 27–29). These parameters are arbitrary but have been found to be reliable in several studies.[15] The level of the lower apex of the myometrial septum in the cervical canal or uterine cavity is used to differentiate a didelphic from a bicornuate uterus and complete from partially septate uterus (Fig. 27–30).

Ovarian cysts and neoplasms must be considered in the differential diagnosis of a pelvic mass in an adolescent who menstruates regularly. Pelvic examination may be misleading because of certain intrinsic difficulties at this age. The finding of renal agenesis is indicative of "double" uterus with an obstructed hemivagina, as are US findings, showing duplication of the uterine body. Another common diagnostic error arises from confusion of this condition with Gartner duct cysts because of the characteristics of Gartner duct cysts and their location on the lateral wall of the vagina. Even exploratory puncture of the cysts does not resolve doubts easily unless it yields a mucosanguineous fluid that is more characteristic of hematocolpos.

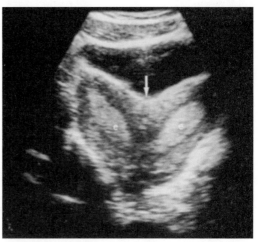

Figure 27–27. Bicornuate uterus. This ultrasound scan shows a sagittal fundal notch larger than 10 mm (*arrow*). The endometrial cavity (e) is bifid.

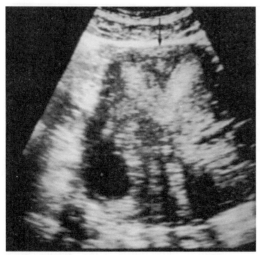

Figure 27–28. Subseptate uterus. In this sonogram the peritoneal fundal profile of the uterus is regular (*arrow*); the endometrial cavity is bifid.

IMAGING OF BENIGN DISEASE

HYMENAL CYSTS

Hymenal cysts are occasionally found in a newborn (Table 27–5). It is important for the diagnostician to establish with certainty whether the vaginal introitus is patent. If it is not, hydromucocolpos is likely. US may be helpful.

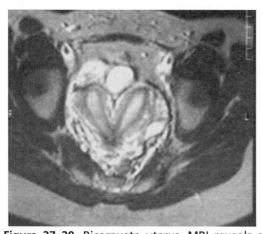

Figure 27–29. Bicornuate uterus. MRI reveals a deep peritoneal fundal notch. The two hemicavities are somewhat asymmetric, the left one slightly wider than the right. (From Fedele L, Dorta M, Brioschi D, et al: Magnetic resonance evaluation of double uteri. Obstet Gynecol 1989; 74:844–847. Reprinted with permission from The American College of Obstetricians and Gynecologists.)

VAGINAL CYSTS

US and MRI may be useful for identifying an obstructed hemivagina by studying the cyst content and excluding a concomitant uterine malformation and renal agenesis. Sonographically, vaginal cysts appear as fluid-filled structures in the vagina (Fig. 27–31; Table 27–5). Other vaginal cystic masses include paraurethral cysts, inclusion cysts, and paramesonephric (müllerian duct) cysts.

BENIGN UTERINE TUMORS

Benign uterine tumors are very rare in children and adolescents. Uterine leiomyomas are infrequent, but those in adolescents can be large (Fig. 27–32).

OVARIAN CYSTS

Ovarian cysts account for most pelvic masses in neonates. Neonatal ovarian cysts result from exaggerated normal follicular development caused by stimulation in utero by maternal hormones. The result is a pelvic or abdominal mass. A cyst can be discovered incidentally on prenatal sonography, or it can present as a palpable mass in a newborn. The sonographic appearance of an ovarian cyst varies, depending on whether it is complicated by hemorrhage or torsion. On US, an uncomplicated ovarian cyst is an anechoic, thin-walled mass with through-transmission. A complicated cyst contains a fluid-debris level or septations. If the cyst is large, it can extend into the upper abdomen and be mistaken for

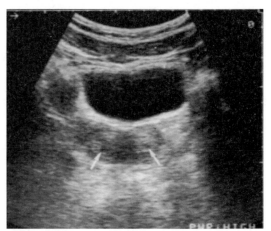

Figure 27–30. Transverse sonogram of the pelvis with a partially full bladder reveals two cervices. The two small anechoic areas surrounded by a hyperechogenic border are the two cervical canals (*arrows*) separated by a wide septum.

Table 27–5. Vaginal Cysts: Differential Diagnosis

Cyst Type	Ultrasonographic Finding (Location)	Differential Diagnosis
Paraurethral	Between the vagina and the lower tract of the urethra	Hydrocolpos Gartner cysts Müller cysts
Inclusion	Vulva	—
Gartner	Lateral vaginal wall	Cystocele Pelvic mass Paraurethral cysts Imperforate hymen
Paramesonephric (Müller)	Higher third of the vagina, near the cervix	Paraurethral cysts
Hymenal	—	Hydromucocolpos
Imperforate hemivagina	Associated with uterine malformation	Gartner cysts

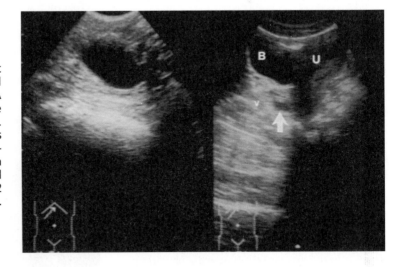

Figure 27–31. Gartner's duct cyst. *Right,* Transabdominal sonogram of the pelvis. A small anechoic mass is visible under the normal uterus (U). B, Bladder, v, vagina. *Left,* This transvaginal sonogram visualizes the anechoic formation better. Located in the vaginal wall, it has a diameter of 2 cm and thin, regular margins.

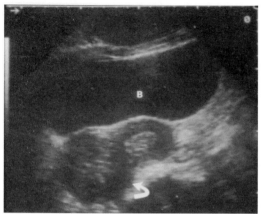

Figure 27–32. Uterine myoma. This is a transverse ultrasound section of the uterus with a subserous fibroma. Typically, this is seen as a large mass arising from the uterus with characteristically weak internal echoes and poor sound transmission (*arrow*). B, Bladder.

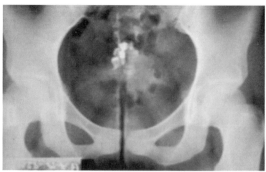

Figure 27–33. Benign cystic teratoma. In this plain film of the pelvis, structured radioopacities—calcified masses resembling teeth—can be seen in the mass.

a mesenteric or omental cyst. In asymptomatic infants, serial US studies are reasonable, because some cysts resolve spontaneously. In symptomatic patients, cystectomy or percutaneous aspiration may be necessary.

Nonneoplastic masses of the ovary, although benign, may cause serious general symptoms in children and adolescents because of the marked tendency toward torsion of the adnexa—and, occasionally, associated endocrine alterations.

BENIGN CYSTIC TERATOMA

Formerly termed *dermoid tumor*, benign cystic teratoma is the most common benign ovarian neoplasm in female children and adolescents (38.6% of all such lesions).[17] Approximately 50% are diagnosed incidentally during laparotomy or pelvic radiography (Fig. 27–33).

The US appearance of teratomas depends on their internal composition.[18] Most often, they are complex adnexal masses, often with echogenic internal components (fat and hair; Fig. 27–34). Some teratomas are completely solid and echogenic; others have cystic areas, with or without internal septa (Fig. 27–35). This explains why teratomas are sometimes confused with the rest of the adnexa or mistaken for intestinal loops containing gas.

On MRI (Fig. 27–36), these lesions typically produce bright signals on both T1- and T2-weighted images, as a result of the sebaceous contents.[19] Endometriomas and hemorrhagic cysts may also produce these findings. The hair,

teeth, and debris contained in benign cystic teratomas generate foci of very low signal intensity with both types of pulse sequences. Lesions that are predominantly cystic, however, may appear hypointense on T1-weighted images because their contents are principally fluid, rather than lipid. Thus, they are indistinguishable from other cystic ovarian masses.

FOLLICULAR AND LUTEIN CYSTS

Together with parovarian cysts, follicular and lutein cysts account for 35.9% of all ovarian lesions treated surgically in children and adolescents.[20] In children, functional cysts are not rare, since the follicular system of the developing ovary is hyperactive. Functional cysts have also

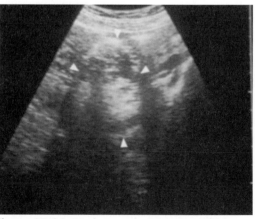

Figure 27–34. Benign cystic teratoma. This transabdominal sonogram reveals a mixed formation, predominantly solid, with a hyperechoic area and ill-defined margins as a result of a posterior cone of shade (*arrowheads*).

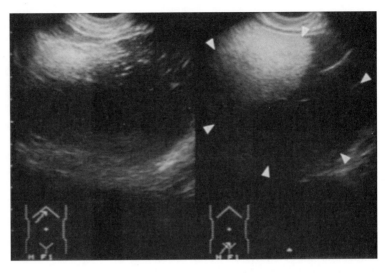

Figure 27–35. Benign cystic teratoma. Transabdominal longitudinal (*left*) and transverse (*right*) ultrasound scans show a mixed mass, predominantly cystic (*arrowheads*). Attached to the cyst wall is a bright, entangled echogenic area representing hair.

been described in neonates, as a consequence of dysequilibrium of maternal gonadotropins.

A functional cyst appears as a "roundish" transonic formation having thin margins with posterior intensification (Figs. 27–37, 27–38). MRI demonstrates follicular cysts as well-circumscribed and smoothly marginated lesions with a thin wall. Because of their principally fluid contents, they have low and high signal intensity on T1- and T2-weighted images, respectively (Fig. 27–39).

When a lutein cyst is hemorrhagic, the sonogram demonstrates an internal echogenic area (Fig. 27–40). The cyst's contents generally become less echogenic as fibrinolysis takes place in the coagulum. It must be remembered that, in newborns, ovarian cysts sometimes lie outside the pelvis, frequently in the upper abdomen. On MRI, if hemorrhage is present, the cysts may be bright on both T1- and T2-weighted sequences and may be indistinguishable from other hemorrhagic cysts, endometriomas, and teratomas (Fig. 27–41).

ENDOMETRIOSIS

Recent studies have demonstrated that endometriosis in adolescents is not rare. Its preva-

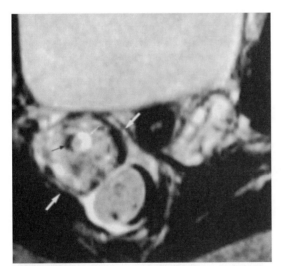

Figure 27–36. MRI scan of the benign cystic teratoma shown in Figure 27–34 (TR = 2000 ms; TE = 25 ms). This coronal view of the pelvis reveals a mixed septate formation that is well-encapsulated (*large arrows*), with a central area of low signal intensity owing to bone formation (*black arrow*) and an area of high signal intensity resulting from fat (*small white arrow*) lateral to the uterine cervix.

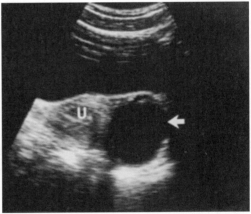

Figure 27–37. Functional ovarian cyst in an adolescent. In this transverse sonogram of the pelvis, a transonic mass with regular wall (*arrow*) and smooth inner lining is visible lateral to the uterus (U).

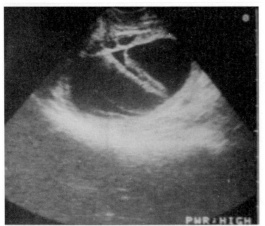

Figure 27–38. Multiseptate follicular cyst. This ultrasound image shows an ovary containing a transonic formation transversed by two thick, parallel septa. Three small follicles can be seen in the residual ovarian parenchyma.

lence is simply underestimated.[21] Early diagnosis allows prompt treatment and may forestall progression of the disease and consequent impaired fertility.

On US, small endometriotic implants on the uterosacral ligaments or on the serous surface of the peritoneum and bowel are difficult to detect. Depending on the conformation and content of an endometrioma, any of a variety of US images is produced.[22] When endometriomas become larger than 1 or 2 cm, they may be identified on US as multiple cystic masses (Fig. 27–42, 27–43). Low-level echoes observed in some endometriomas reflect the clotted blood they contain.

MRI usually demonstrates endometriosis as a high-intensity image suggestive of blood on both T1- and T2-weighted scans (Fig. 27–44). Often, low-intensity regions are noted at the margins of the endometrioma. The lesions may have a hypointense fibrous capsule and be multilocular or multifocal. They can be confused with benign teratomas, which are also bright on both T1- and T2-weighted sequences. MRI has been reported to be sufficiently specific for endometriotic ovarian cysts, but, overall, the best diagnostic tool for this disease is still endoscopy.[23] As Zawin and colleagues suggested, for monitoring treatment response, MRI is probably more useful than laparoscopy, once the diagnosis of endometriosis is conclusive.[24]

POLYCYSTIC OVARY

Polycystic ovaries are usually enlarged to a volume of more than 10 ml. Multiple immature or atretic follicles are observed along their periphery (Figs. 27–45, 27–46). As many as a third of adolescents with this disorder, however, have normal-sized ovaries.[18] On MRI, low–signal intensity cysts are revealed at the periphery of the gonads on T1-weighted images; typically, these are bright on T2-weighted images (Fig. 27–47). At the center of the ovaries, the signal intensity is low, probably because of fibrous luteinization.

Multiple ovarian cysts can also develop in children with primary hypothyroidism and children with cystic fibrosis. Bilateral ovarian enlargement with discrete cysts has been reported in girls with McCune-Albright syndrome.

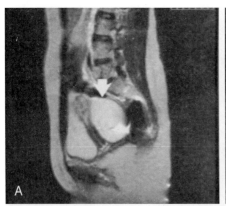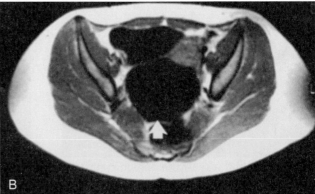

Figure 27–39. MRI scan of a mesosalpingeal cyst. *A,* Medial sagittal section (TR = 2000 ms; TE = 100 ms). Posterior to the uterus and vagina, a cyst (*arrow*) with high–signal intensity contents occupies the entire pelvis. *B,* This transverse T1-weighted image of the cyst (*arrow*) shows low signal intensity similar to that of the bladder, indicating serous contents (TR = 500 ms; TE = 20 ms). (From Fedele L, Dorta M, Brioschi D, et al: Magnetic resonance evaluation of gynecologic masses in adolescents. Adolesc Pediatr Gynecol 1990; 3:83–88.)

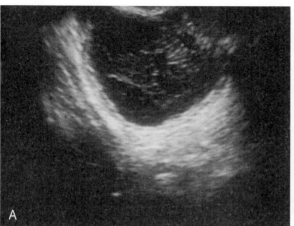

Figure 27–40. Hemorrhagic corpora lutea in an adolescent. These transvaginal ultrasound images show A, an irregularly shaped and echogenic trabecular structure surrounded by a sonolucent area of fluid and B, a similar structure that is more echogenic and dense at the upper pole.

Figure 27–41. A multilocular serohemorrhagic cyst (*arrow*) as shown by a medial sagittal MRI scan (TR = 550 ms; TE = 20 ms). (From Fedele L, Dorta M, Brioschi D, et al: Magnetic resonance imaging in Mayer-Rokitansky-Küster-Hauser Syndrome. Obstet Gynecol 1990; 76:593–596. Reprinted with permission from The American College of Obstetricians and Gynecologists.)

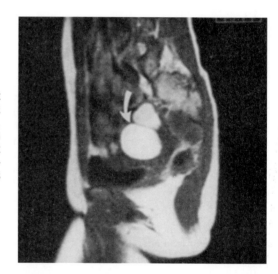

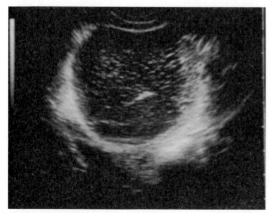

Figure 27–42. Endometrioma in an adolescent. This transvaginal ultrasound scan demonstrates a cyst with rare, thin, internal echoes; part of the ovarian parenchyma is conserved.

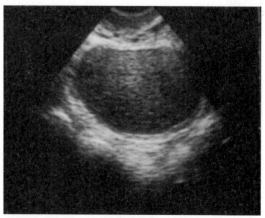

Figure 27–43. A large endometrioma scanned with 6.5-MHz transvaginal probe. The uniformly echogenic thick blood in the cyst is seen.

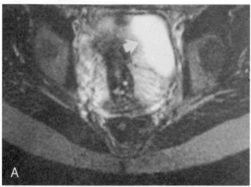
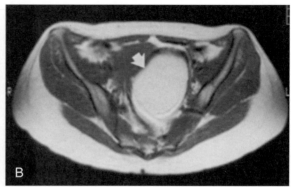

Figure 27–44. An ovarian cyst filled with blood. This MRI scan demonstrates the left adnexal region occupied by a round structure (*arrow*) with clear outlines, no septation, and uniformly elevated signal intensity on T2-weighted sequences. *A*, Transverse section (TR = 2120 ms; TE = 100 ms); *B*, transverse section (T1-weighted image, TR = 500 ms; TE = 20 ms). (From Fedele L, Dorta M, Brioschi D, et al: Magnetic resonance evaluation of gynecologic masses in adolescents. Adolesc Pediatr Gynecol 1990; 3:83–88.)

OVARIAN TORSION

Enlarged ovaries or ones that contain a neoformation may develop torsion involving the tube, the ovary, or both. In the initial stages, only venous and lymphatic drainage are impaired, but in a few days, the ovary increases markedly in volume and appears on US as a solid mass, the result of vascular engorgement and stromal edema (Fig. 27–48). If the torsion is intermittent, ovarian enlargement may regress rapidly. When torsion is associated with an ovarian mass, US generally demonstrates a pelvic-abdominal mass of complex echogenicity (Fig. 27–49). Intraperitoneal fluid is sometimes evident, the result of hemorrhagic or exudative processes.[18] The differential diagnosis of ovarian enlargement should consider "nongynecologic" abdominal diseases, including mesenteric cysts and gastrointestinal duplication cysts. Typically, mesenteric cysts develop at the base of the mesentery and contain several septa. The septa derive from the distal small intestine and may or may not communicate with the intestinal lumen.

DISORDERS OF PUBERTY

US may be useful in the evaluation of a girl known or suspected to have a disorder of puberty. It is performed as an adjunct to a detailed history, physical examination, complete endocrine profile, chromosome analysis, and determi-

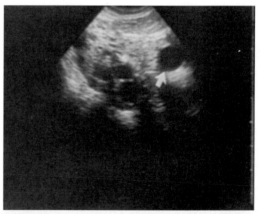

Figure 27–46. Micropolycystic ovary as shown by a transvaginal ultrasound scan with a 6.5-MHz probe. The ovary is normal in size with multiple discrete cysts smaller than 1 cm in diameter. There is a small hydatid cyst of Morgagni medial to the ovary but completely separate from it (*arrow*).

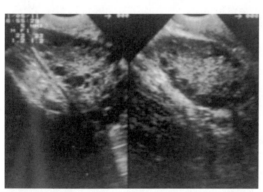

Figure 27–45. Micropolycystic ovaries scanned with a 5-MHz probe. The ovaries are enlarged and round, with small follicles along the periphery.

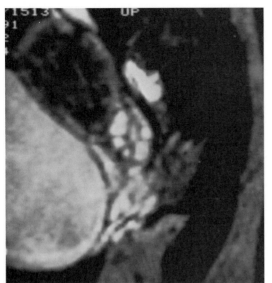

Figure 27–47. MRI scan of a micropolycystic ovary (T2-weighted image, TR = 2000; TE = 90). The follicles present as small cysts with high signal intensity at the ovarian periphery.

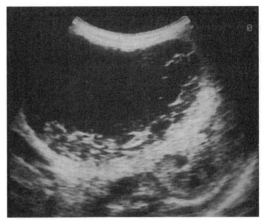

Figure 27–49. Ovarian torsion due to a neonatal cyst in a 1-month-old girl. This transverse ultrasound scan shows the abdomen occupied by a large cyst containing dyshomogeneous echoes in the lower part.

nation of bone age. Ovarian and uterine volume and US characteristics are important indicators of pubertal change.[25]

True precocious puberty is the result of premature maturation of the hypothalamic-pituitary-ovarian axis. In one study of 44 patients with this condition, large-for-age or adult-sized ovaries were detected on US.[25] The ovarian enlargement occurs early, whereas the size of the uterus varies from intermediate to adult, depending on the duration of precocious puberty. US has been used to monitor changes in ovarian and uterine size in patients treated with gonadotropin-releasing hormone (GnRH) analogues.

Precocious pseudopuberty includes a series of clinical conditions such as premature thelarche, premature adrenarche, congenital adrenal hyperplasia, and neurofibromatosis (see Chapter 5). It may also be caused by exogenous estrogens. Adrenal and ovarian tumors are rare causes of isosexual pseudopuberty but are detectable with US.

Delayed puberty is sometimes due to an extragonadal cause, such as juvenile hypothyroidism. One study of five women with hypothyroidism demonstrated ovarian cysts 1 to 4 cm in diameter in every case.[26] A transitory cyst larger than 3 cm was found in 43% of 13 patients with cystic fibrosis.[27] More often, delayed puberty is due to gonadal dysgenesis or a variant. In Turner syndrome, US ovarian findings describe a wide range, from absent to infantile to normal adult size (Fig. 27–50, 27–51). Normal ovaries can be predicted in Noonan syndrome. US has been used to monitor the effectiveness of hormone therapy for Turner syndrome by examining changes in uterine shape.[18]

MENOMETRORRHAGIA IN THE ADOLESCENT

Menometrorrhagia is due to continuous, although variable, estrogen stimulation of the endometrium, which on histologic examination gen-

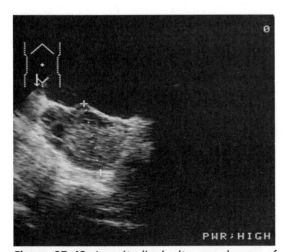

Figure 27–48. Longitudinal ultrasound scan of ovarian torsion in a 10-year-old girl. The ovary is enlarged, and the echostructure of the lower half is dyshomogeneous.

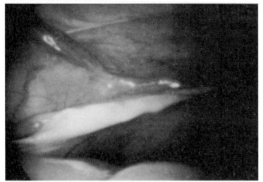

Figure 27–50. Turner syndrome. This laparoscopic image shows a small left ovarian streak.

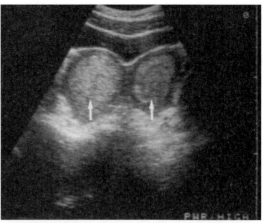

Figure 27–52. Endometrial hyperplasia in the bicornuate uterus of a 13-year-old girl. A transverse ultrasound scan of the pelvis reveals two asymmetric, widely separated, enlarged uterine horns; thin myometrium; and hyperechogenic, markedly thickened (about 4 cm) endometrium (*arrows*).

erally appears to be in the proliferative phase or is hyperplastic. Diagnosis is based on ruling out other causes that sometimes have the same clinical picture. US is useful for excluding concomitant pelvic disease and is indispensable as a noninvasive study of the endometrium. It assesses endometrial thickness to within 1 mm of the measurement obtained on histopathologic examination. A diagnosis of endometrial hyperplasia must be established when the endometrium is thicker than 10 mm (Fig. 27–52). US may also be useful in monitoring the endometrium after institution of hormone therapy (Fig. 27–53).

HYDROSALPINX AND TUBOOVARIAN ABSCESSES

Pelvic inflammatory disease is a serious complication of sexually transmitted diseases in adolescent girls. Generally, the presenting symptom is acute lower abdominal and pelvic pain. Appendicitis is the first condition to be considered in

the differential diagnosis. Initially, the inflammatory fluid distends the fallopian tube, and US identifies an anechoic adnexal mass and changes in the uterus consistent with endometritis. (Swayne and colleagues described patients with an entirely normal pelvic sonogram, however.[28]) In the presence of a true tuboovarian abscess, US reveals a pelvis completely filled with disorganized heterogeneous echoes mixed with solid and cystic areas (Fig. 27–54). In the series of Fedele and associates, the contribution of MRI to the imaging of pelvic inflammatory disease was modest, although investigators using T1-weighted images have reported that regions of low intensity may be seen along the uterine surface and within pelvic peritoneal recesses as a result of purulent

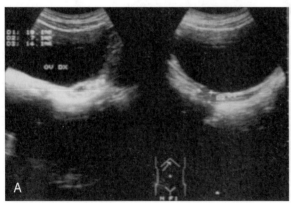
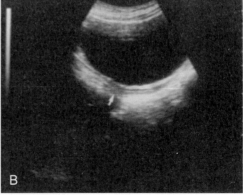

Figure 27–51. Ultrasound scans from the patient shown in Figure 27–50 demonstrating *A*, a small, elongated ovary without evident follicular formation behind the bladder (*calipers*) and *B*, a hypotrophic uterus (*arrow*).

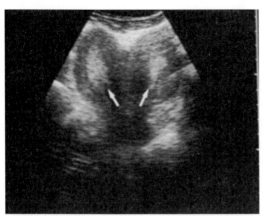

Figure 27–53. Fundal scan of the malformed uterus of the same patient shown in Figure 27–52 after hormone therapy. The notch of the external profile is evident. The myometrium is less thin, and the width of the endometrial cavity is normal (*arrows*).

fluid accumulation.[19, 23] Laparoscopy affords a precise picture of the extent of the disease; a sample of intraperitoneal exudate may be collected to plan therapy.

IMAGING OF MALIGNANT NEOPLASMS

Malignant tumors of the genital tract are unusual in children and adolescents. Although all types of neoplasms found in adults have been reported, in this age group neoplasms are usually embryonal tumors or teratomas.

VAGINAL NEOPLASMS

Vaginal neoplasms include two important lesions: mixed mesodermal tumor (rhabdomyosarcoma) and clear-cell adenocarcinoma. In infants, rhabdomyosarcoma typically is manifested as a botryoid sarcoma. In adolescents, it originates in the vagina.

Clear-cell adenocarcinoma almost always derives from malignant transformation of vaginal adenosis. More than 500 cases have been reported in the literature; the age range is 7 to 30 years (peak incidence at 19 years).[17] On US, these tumors appear as solid, homogeneous masses filling the vaginal cavity (Fig. 27–55). On MRI, T2-weighted images have high signal intensity and correct tumor staging is, theoretically, possible.[29] In stage I, the signal intensity of the vaginal wall and the high signal intensity of the paravaginal fat are preserved. In stage II, the low-intensity vaginal wall is no longer recognized, and the interface between vaginal wall and fat is indistinct. In stage III, the normal low intensity of the pelvic side wall muscles is distorted, and in stage IV, T1-weighted scans demonstrate obliteration of the normal fat signals and planes and extension into the bladder or rectum. Furthermore, MRI has clear advantages over other conventional imaging techniques in evaluating patients after radiotherapy or surgery, because it differentiates fibrotic tissue from recurrent tumor.

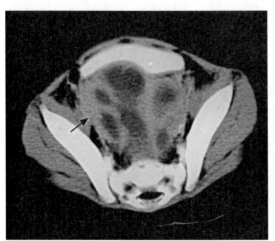

Figure 27–54. Pelvic abscess. CT scan with intravenous contrast medium. Transverse scan of the true pelvis reveals a large, multilocular retrovesicular formation containing fluid (*arrow*) referable to a collection in the pouch of Douglas. The bladder is deformed and displaced anteriorly.

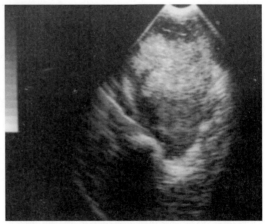

Figure 27–55. Pelvic rhabdomyosarcoma. This ultrasound image demonstrates a solid homogeneous mass with an irregular outline. (Courtesy of Professor C.A. Dell'Agnola, University of Milan.)

OVARIAN CANCERS

Ovarian malignancies are rare in children and adolescents (prevalence ~ 1% of all malignant tumors before age 17 years).[20] In children, most ovarian tumors arise from germ cells; in adult women, some 80% to 90% have an epithelial origin.

Dysgerminoma

Dysgerminomas account for 16% of germ cell tumors and 11% of all ovarian tumors of children and adolescents.[20] Usually, a dysgerminoma is a large, solid, encapsulated mass with central hypoechoic areas that represent hemorrhage, necrosis, and cystic degeneration (Fig. 27–56).

Malignant Teratoma

Malignant transformation of an ovarian teratoma occurs in 1% of all ovarian neoplasms, most commonly in the first two decades of life.[30] Teratomas in children and adolescents should always be very carefully examined. Clinically, they are characterized by rapid growth, weight loss, and abdominopelvic pain. US findings resemble those of benign teratoma.

Sertoli-Leydig-Stromal Cell Tumors

These neoplasms contain Sertoli cells, Leydig cells, fibroblasts, or all three in varying proportions. Androgenic activity may be exhibited (thus, the term *androblastoma*), but many lack endocrine manifestations although few produce estrogen or progesterone. They vary in size from microscopic to large masses but usually have a diameter of 5 to 15 cm. In general, they are cystic and contain large, edematous papillae like those of serous papillary tumors (Fig. 27–57).

Granulosa and Thecal Cell Tumors

Granulosa cell and thecal cell tumors are the most common ovarian tumors responsible for isosexual precocious puberty,[31] which in children is manifested as rapid development of secondary sex characteristics. In adolescents, the effects of hormonal stimulation are less important but can

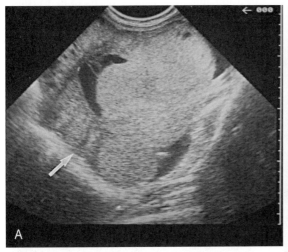
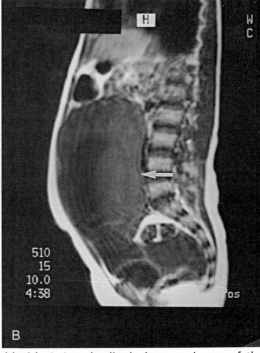

Figure 27–56. Ovarian dysgerminoma in a 10-year-old girl. *A,* Longitudinal ultrasound scan of the true pelvis reveals an enormous mass (*arrow*) that occupies the entire abdomen, has irregular margins and mixed structure, mainly solid, hyperechoic, with central liquid areas surrounded by a thin ascitic rim. *B,* In the T1-weighted sagittal MRI scan, the mass (*arrow*) extends from the epigastric region to the true pelvis, causing craniad dislocations of the intestinal loops.

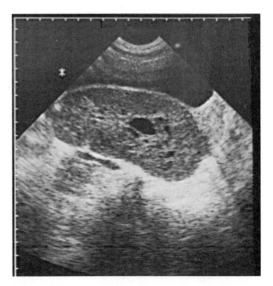

Figure 27–57. Granulosa cell tumor in an 8-year-old girl with signs of precocious puberty. A longitudinal ultrasound scan shows a large oval ovarian mass with regular margins behind the bladder. The mass is solid with small central liquid areas.

include hypermenorrhea (75%), amenorrhea (25%), or ascites (20%), which may delay diagnosis. The gross aspect is generally mixed (i.e., both solid and cystic), and the cyst sometimes contains hemorrhagic fluid. The appearance on US is nonspecific; such tumors have been variously reported as homogeneously solid or as solid with a central anechoic area.

Cystadenomas and Cystadenocarcinomas

Tumors of epithelial origin constitute 17% of all ovarian neoplasms diagnosed during the first two decades of life.[20] When papillary, they present as solid areas and vegetations inside the cystic cavity. Generally, the more solid and irregular its internal morphology, the more likely a cystadenoma is to be malignant. In the presence of ascites, the tumor has probably spread beyond the capsule. Ascites is rarely associated with benign tumors such as ovarian fibroma (Meig syndrome). Cystadenomas and cystadenocarcinomas cannot be distinguished by MRI.[19] Solid tumor nodules are, more often than not, associated with malignancy but are also observed in benign mucinous cystadenomas (Fig. 27–58). MRI provides accurate delineation of the neoplasm as well as details of the adjacent structures (Figs. 27–59 to

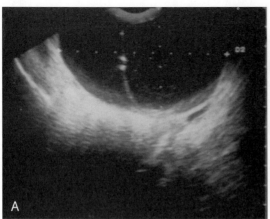
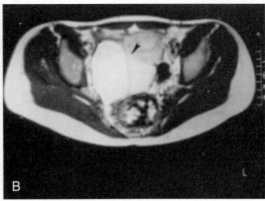

Figure 27–58. Mucinous cystadenoma. *A,* A transvaginal image shows a large, septate cystic structure with scanty internal echoes (*calipers*). The septum is thickened and hyperechogenic. *B,* A transverse MRI scan (TR = 1585 ms; TE = 70 ms) shows the right hemipelvis, which contains a cystic structure with a maximum diameter of 10 cm (*arrowhead*), thin walls, and a vertical septum that divides it into two cavities. The lateral cavity is larger and contains serous fluid; the medial one has a different signal, and its contents are probably mucoid.

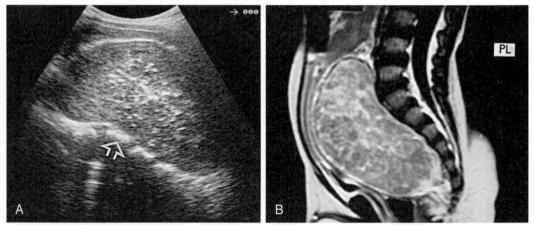

Figure 27–59. Pelvic neuroblastoma in a 10-year-old girl. *A,* Longitudinal ultrasound scan of the true pelvis. The bladder is displaced anteriorly by a solid oval mass with multiple microcalcifications and regular outline adhering to sacrum (*arrow*). *B,* In this T1-weighted sagittal MRI scan the pelvis is occupied by an enormous solid mass of dyshomogeneous structure adhering to the sacrum.

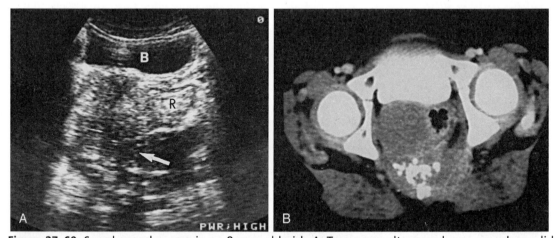

Figure 27–60. Sacral ependymoma in an 8-year-old girl. *A,* Transverse ultrasound scan reveals a solid neoformation with large irregular calcifications, which originates from the sacrum. The mass displaces the bladder (B) and the rectum (R) anteriorly. *B,* This axial CT scan confirms the sacral origin of the mass and the anterior displacement of the rectum toward the left.

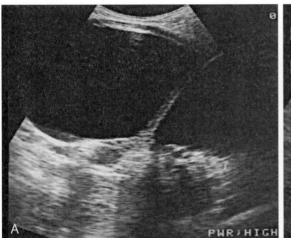

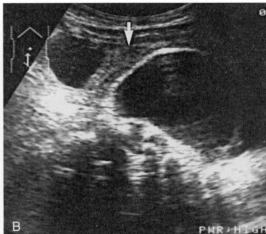

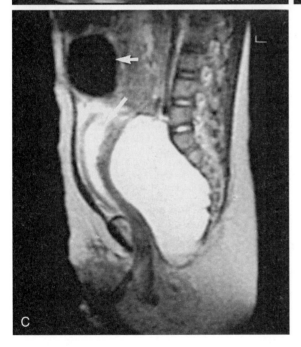

Figure 27–61. Anterior meningocele in a 5-month-old girl. *A,* Longitudinal ultrasound scan of the true pelvis showing two formations containing fluid separated by a thin septum. *B,* Another longitudinal scan reveals that, after urination, the more craniad of the two formations has emptied, whereas the caudad one has not. The thin septum separating the two cysts is seen to be the rectal ampulla (*arrow*). *C,* The anterior meningocele of sacral origin displaces the rectum (*long arrow*) and the bladder (*short arrow*) anteriorly in this T1-weighted MRI image.

27–61). Such detail is of paramount importance when planning surgical intervention.

REFERENCES

1. Nussbaum AR, Sanders RC, Jones MD: Neonatal uterine morphology as seen on real-time ultrasound. Radiology 1986; 160:641.
2. Orsini LF, Solardi S, Pilu G, et al: Pelvic organs in premenarchal girls: Real-time ultrasonography. Radiology 1984; 153:113.
3. Krantz KE, Atkinson JP. Gross anatomy. Ann NY Acad Sci 1967; 142:575.
4. McCarthy S, Tauber C, Gore J: Female pelvic anatomy: MR assessment of variations during the menstrual cycle and with use of contraceptives. Radiology 1986; 160:119.
5. Sample WF, Lippe BM, Gyepes MT: Gray-scale ultrasonography of the normal female pelvis. Radiology 1977; 125:477.
6. Dell'Agnola CA, Fedele L, Zamberletti D, et al: The management of hydrocolpos. Acta Eur Fertil 1984; 15:51.
7. Johnston JH: Female genital tract anomalies. In Williams DI, Johnston JH (eds): Pediatric Urology. London: Butterworths, 1982, p 500.
8. Buttram VC Jr, Gibbons WE: Müllerian anomalies: A proposed classification. Fertil Steril 1979; 32:40.
9. Fedele L, Dorta M, Brioschi D, et al: Magnetic resonance imaging in Mayer-Rokitansky-Kuster-Hauser syndrome. Obstet Gynecol 1990; 76:593.
10. McIndoe A: The treatment of congenital absence and obliterative conditions of the vagina. Br J Plast Surg 1950; 2:254.
11. Fedele L, Marchini M, Carinelli S, et al: Endometrium of cavitary rudimentary horns in unicornuate uteri. Obstet Gynecol 1990; 75:437.
12. Fedele L, Dorta M, Vercellini P, et al: Ultrasound in the diagnosis of subclasses of unicornuate uterus. Obstet Gynecol 1988; 71:274.
13. Fedele L, Dorta M, Brioschi D, et al: Magnetic resonance imaging of unicornuate uterus. Acta Obstet Gynecol Scand 1990; 69:511.
14. Rock JA, Jones HW: The double uterus associated with an obstructed hemivagina and ipsilateral renal agenesis. Am J Obstet Gynecol 1980; 138:339.
15. Fedele L, Ferrazzi E, Dorta M, et al: Ultrasonography in the differential diagnosis of "double" uteri. Fertil Steril 1988; 50:361.
16. Fedele L, Dorta M, Brioschi D, et al: Magnetic resonance evaluation of "double" uteri. Obstet Gynecol 1989; 74:844.
17. Kleinhaus S, Sheran M: Surgical gynecology. In Boley SJ, Cohen MI (eds): Surgery of the Adolescent. Orlando, FL: Grune & Stratton, 1986, p 89.
18. Fleischer AC, Shawker TH: The role of sonography in pediatric gynecology. Clin Obstet Gynecol 1987; 30:735.
19. Fishman-Javitt MC, Lovecchio JL, Syein HL: The ovary. In Fishman-Javitt MC, Stein HL, Lovecchio JL (eds): Imaging of the Pelvis: MRI with Correlations to CT and Ultrasound. Boston: Little, Brown, 1990, p 109.
20. Breen J, Maxon WS: Ovarian tumors in childhood and adolescence. Clin Obstet Gynecol 1977; 20:923.
21. Vercellini P, Fedele L, Arcaini L, et al: Laparoscopy in the diagnosis of chronic pelvic pain in adolescent women. J Reprod Med 1989; 34:829.
22. Fleischer AC: Pelvic sonography. In Fisher MR, Krieum ME (eds): Imaging of the Pelvis. Rockville, Md. Aspen, 1989, p 151.
23. Fedele L, Dorta M, Brioschi D, et al: Magnetic resonance evaluation of gynecologic masses in adolescents. Adolesc Pediatr Gynecol 1990; 3:83.
24. Zawin M, McCarthy S, Scoutt L, Comite F. Endometriosis: Appearance and detection at MR imaging. Radiology 1989; 171:693.
25. Lippe BM: Primary ovarian failure. In Kaplan SA (ed): Clinical Pediatric and Adolescent Endocrinology. Philadelphia: WB Saunders, 1982, p 286.
26. Riddlesberger MM, Kuhn JP, Munschauer RW: The association of juvenile hypothyroidism and cystic ovaries. Radiology 1981; 139:77.
27. Showker T, Hubbard V, Reicher C, et al: Cystic ovaries in cystic fibrosis: An ultrasound and autopsy study. J Ultrasound Med 1983; 2:439.
28. Swayne LC, Love MB, Karasik SR: Pelvic inflammatory disease: Sonographic pathologic correlation. Radiology 1984; 151:751.
29. Stein HL, Lovecchio JL, Fishmen-Javitt MC: The vulva and vagina. In Fishman-Javitt MC, Stein HL, Lovecchio JL (eds): Imaging of the Pelvis: MRI Correlations to CT and Ultrasound. Boston: Little, Brown, 1990, p 37.
30. Talerman J: Germ cell tumors of the ovary. In Kurman RJ (ed): Blaunstein's Pathology of the Female Genital Tract, 3rd ed. New York: Springer-Verlag, 1989, p 660.
31. Thompson J, Dockerty M, Symmonds R, Hayles A: Ovarian and paraovarian tumors in infants and children. Am J Obstet Gynecol 1967; 97:1059.

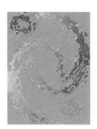

Chapter 28
Delayed Consequences of Childhood Malignancies

David Muram

Modern therapy for childhood malignancies has prolonged disease-free intervals and improved cure rates: five forms of childhood cancer had a 5-year relative survival rate of 85% or better.[1] Although outcomes for all types of neoplasms have improved, the increased survival rates for patients with non-Hodgkin's lymphoma, bone tumors, and rhabdomyosarcoma (sarcoma botryoides) are particularly striking.[2] It was estimated that, in 1990, one of every thousand 20-year-olds was a survivor of childhood cancer.[3–5] This estimate is based on the incidences of the various malignancies occurring between birth and age 15 years, and an estimated overall cure rate of 60% (Table 28–1).[2, 4] Incidence and survival data from the National Cancer Institute's Surveillance, Epidemiology, and End Results (SEER) Program reveal that childhood cancer incidence rates remained relatively stable during the 1980s, with an overall incidence of 127 per million children. For all forms of cancer combined, the 5-year relative survival rate was 57%. The 5-year relative survival rate exceeded 80% for fibrosarcomas, retinoblastomas, Hodgkin's disease, and gonadal and germ cell tumors (Figs. 28–1 through 28–3),[2] although these figures may be even higher, because the annual cancer rate in infants is still increasing.[6] For example, the reported incidence of primary malignant brain tumors among children in the United States increased by 35% during the period from 1973 through 1994.[7] Another study found similar increases.[8]

While the increasing number of pediatric cancer survivors is gratifying, the lifelong sequelae of childhood cancer must be considered. Most of them are relatively minor, but some patients have severe disabilities in function—physical, emotional, or intellectual. Some complications are therapy specific, but many are general and related to the nature of the illness, its treatment, and fears related to potential recurrences.

As these children are cured of their malignancy, they are no longer treated by the oncologist but instead are referred back into the community health care system. Thus, the primary care physician becomes responsible for their care and, therefore, should be familiar with the various complications that often develop among survivors of childhood cancers.

Many variables affect the long-term consequences of the cancer and its therapy: the primary malignancy, its location, the type of therapy, and the interval between therapy and the onset of possible complications. Often, the abnormality caused by the cancer therapy is obvious (e.g., when amputation is required to remove an osteosarcoma); in other cases, it may be subtle and appear so remote in time from therapy that the physician may not recognize the connection (e.g., hypothyroidism after irradiation for Hodgkin's disease). Special attention must be given to physical growth and development and the sexual maturation of children who have survived cancer.

The gynecologist may be asked to evaluate survivors of childhood cancer because of growth abnormalities, delayed sexual maturation, or aberrant reproductive tract development. Because the gonads are particularly vulnerable to radiation and chemotherapeutic agents, impaired gonadal function is a fairly common complication of cancer therapy.[9, 10] The long-term effects of childhood malignancy on growth, sexual maturation, and reproductive function must be understood by the clinician.

GROWTH AND DEVELOPMENT

Therapy for cancer during childhood frequently affects the growth of bones and soft

Table 28–1. Kaplan-Meier Estimates of Survival and Event-Free Survival Over Time*

	Survival			Event-Free Survival		
	2-Year	*3-Year*	*5-Year*	*2-Year*	*3-Year*	*5-Year*
Non-T, non-B, noninfant ALL						
1976–80 (848 patients, 204/yr)	77 (1.5)	69 (2.0)	56 (1.8)	69 (1.7)	57 (3.8)	43 (1.8)
1980–81 (177 patients, 236/yr)	81 (3.1)	75 (3.2)	68 (3.7)	69 (3.6)	64 (3.7)	54 (3.9)
1981–86 (1504 patients, 336/yr)	87 (0.9)	80 (1.0)	73 (1.5)	75 (1.1)	69 (1.2)	56 (1.6)
1986–89 (1511 patients, 394/yr)	92 (1.1)	88 (2.3)	—	85 (1.5)	80 (2.7)	—
T-cell ALL						
1976–78 (61 patients, 27/yr)	54 (6.5)	48 (6.5)	39 (6.6)	48 (6.5)	41 (6.4)	34 (6.5)
1978–81 (71 patients, 28/yr)	59 (6.0)	49 (6.1)	47 (6.1)	49 (6.0)	46 (6.0)	45 (6.0)
1981–86 (283 patients, 57/yr)	87 (2.8)	58 (3.0)	50 (3.6)	54 (3.0)	49 (3.0)	43 (3.1)
1986–89 (300 patients, 78/yr)	75 (4.0)	60 (7.8)	—	64 (4.3)	56 (7.4)	—
Infant ALL						
1976–81 (31 patients, 6/yr)	54 (9)	36 (9)	24 (9)	27 (9)	19 (8)	13 (9)
1981–84 (32 patients, 9/yr)	44 (9)	34 (8)	31 (11)	22 (7)	16 (6)	13 (7)
1984–89 (83 patients, 20/yr)	45 (7)	36 (8)	—	30 (6)	28 (7)	—
ANLL						
1977–81 (195 patients, 52/yr)	37 (3.6)	27 (3.3)	24 (3.3)	26 (3.3)	21 (3.1)	18 (2.9)
1981–84 (266 patients, 89/yr)	41 (3.1)	34 (3.0)	28 (3.7)	34 (2.9)	25 (2.7)	23 (3.4)
1984–88 (293 patients, 72/yr)	48 (3.4)	37 (4.9)	—	39 (3.3)	32 (4.8)	—
Advanced lymphoblastic NHL						
1976–79 (41 patients, 15/yr)	73 (7)	63 (8)	57 (8)	71 (7)	58 (8)	53 (8)
1979–83 (77 patients, 19/yr)	67 (6)	59 (6)	52 (6)	55 (6)	49 (6)	45 (6)
1983–86 (53 patients, 20/yr)	76 (6)	64 (7)	64 (11)	66 (7)	60 (7)	58 (11)
1986–89 (130 patients, 34/yr)	73 (6)	73 (10)	—	75 (6)	69 (10)	—
Advanced DUL						
1979–81 (24 patients, 10/yr)	41 (10)	36 (10)	36 (13)	33 (10)	33 (10)	33 (10)
1981–86 (124 patients, 25/yr)	69 (4)	69 (5)	68 (7)	65 (4)	65 (5)	64 (7)
1986–89 (66 patients, 21/yr)	79 (11)	—	—	75 (12)	—	—
Advanced large-cell NHL						
1976–79 (18 patients, 7/yr)	56 (12)	56 (12)	56 (12)	56 (12)	56 (12)	56 (12)
1979–81 (32 patients, 13/yr)	72 (8)	72 (8)	68 (9)	63 (9)	63 (9)	63 (9)
1981–86 (28 patients, 6/yr)	68 (9)	68 (9)	—	54 (9)	54 (10)	54 (14)
1986–89 (61 patients, 19/yr)	77 (13)	—	—	67 (15)	—	—
Limited-stage NHL						
1976–79 (27 patients, 10/yr)	93 (5)	89 (6)	85 (7)	82 (7)	78 (8)	74 (9)
1979–83 (75 patients, 19/yr)	91 (3)	85 (4)	79 (5)	89 (4)	78 (8)	75 (5)
1983–87 (145 patients, 35/yr)	94 (2)	94 (2)	94 (5)	92 (2)	91 (3)	90 (6)
1987–89 (94 patients, 38/yr)	93 (10)	—	—	89 (15)	—	—
Osteosarcoma						
1982–84 (117 patients, 59/yr)	77 (4)	70 (5)	58 (7)	54 (5)	50 (5)	44 (6)
1984–86 (96 patients, 41/yr)	84 (4)	79 (6)	—	74 (5)	72 (6)	—
1986–89 (64 patients, 20/yr)	82 (11)	—	—	60 (14)	—	—
Neuroblastoma						
1981–84 (145 patients, 46/yr)	20 (3)	18 (3)	13 (3)	10 (3)	8 (2)	6 (3)
1984–87 (147 patients, 61/yr)	45 (4)	27 (4)	—	35 (4)	21 (4)	—
1987–89 (157 patients, 59/yr)	36 (10)	—	—	35 (9)	—	—

*Values represent percentages, with SE in parentheses. Annual accrual is month specific.

ALL, Acute lymphocytic leukemia; ANLL, acute nonlymphocytic leukemia; DUL, diffuse undifferentiated NHL; NHL, non-Hodgkin's lymphoma.

From The Pediatric Oncology Group: Progress against childhood cancer: The Pediatric Oncology Group experience. Pediatrics 1992; 89:597–600.

tissues. The determinants of growth operate through both local and central mechanisms. Sequelae involving the latter include growth hormone (GH) deficiency with subsequent diminished somatomedin production, thyroid hormone deficiency, gonadal dysfunction, malnutrition secondary to chronic illness, and psychological factors. Sequelae involving the former are due predominantly to radiation therapy and its effects on bone and associated soft tissues and blood vessels.[11] These effects are dose related and are more pronounced in fast-growing tissue. In general, the younger the patient and the higher the radiation dose, the more pronounced are the long-term effects.[12–16]

Irradiation to bone may cause arrested chondrogenesis, deficient absorption in calcified bone and cartilage, and altered periosteal activity and

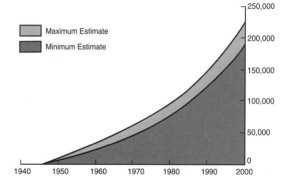

Figure 28–1. Cumulative number of childhood cancer survivors in the United States, 1945–2000. (From Bleyer WA: The impact of childhood cancer on the United States and the world. CA 1990; 40:355–367.)

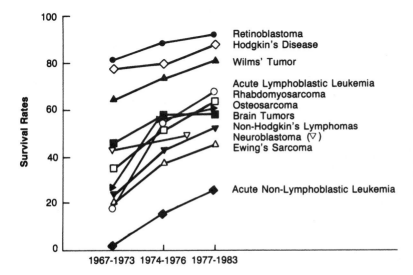

Figure 28–2. Increased survival rates for individual types of childhood cancer. (From Bleyer WA: The impact of childhood cancer on the United States and the world. CA 1990; 40:355–367.)

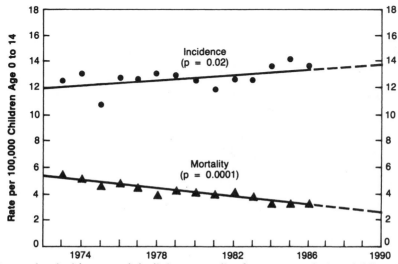

Figure 28–3. Increasing incidence and declining mortality from cancer during childhood. (From Bleyer WA: The impact of childhood cancer on the United States and the world. CA 1990; 40:355–367.)

bone modeling.[17] Radiographically, growth arrest lines and epiphyseal irregularities may be observed.[18] Decreased bone growth is also associated with decreased muscle and soft tissue mass.[19]

The spinal column is also affected by irradiation, and multiple abnormalities of the spine may affect final height. These include impairment or irregularity of growth at the vertebral end plates, decreased vertebral body height, and changes in contour (Fig. 28–4), among others.[18]

GH deficiency is a well-known complication causing growth abnormality in cancer survivors, particularly children who received cranial irradiation. After external irradiation, the damage to the hypothalamic-pituitary axis is at the level of the hypothalamus, whereas patients who undergo pituitary ablation with interstitial radiotherapy or heavy particle beams sustain direct damage to the pituitary gland.[20]

In one study of 27 prepubertal and postpubertal children with brain tumors who had normal GH levels before therapy, impaired GH response

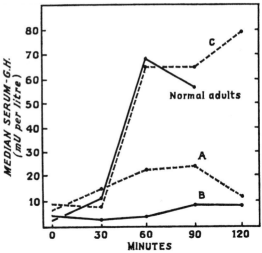

Figure 28–5. Growth hormone levels during insulin-induced hypoglycemia. Group A and group B represent children treated for malignancy. Group C are controls. (From Shalet SM, Morris-Jones PH, Beardwell CG, et al: Pituitary function after treatment of intracranial tumors in children. Lancet 1975; ii:104–107.)

to hypoglycemia was found in 10 of them after chemotherapy and cranial irradiation (Fig. 28–5).[21] More recent studies showed similar abnormalities.[22] Although radiation doses were not reported, it is estimated that these patients received at least 3500 rad to the pituitary gland. When the radiation dose is lower, pituitary function is less likely to be affected. One study of 14 children with acute lymphocytic leukemia (ALL) who were treated with chemotherapy and cranial radiation therapy (2000 to 2500 rad) found only minor dysfunction of the hypothalamic-pituitary axis.[23] The relationship among radiation dose, pituitary damage, and subsequent GH deficiency was further supported by Shalet and Beardwell, who suggested that the total dose of radiation appears to be a more significant determinant of future pituitary function than the number of fractions and the dose given per fraction.[24]

GH deficiency affects principally children who have received cranial irradiation. Studies of the effects of chemotherapy on children who did not receive cranial radiation show a normal GH response. Consequently, in children with ALL, growth in height was abnormally slow after cranial radiation, whereas in those who received chemotherapy alone, the growth pattern was normal.[25] A similar study of 12 patients noted no difference between irradiated and nonirradiated patients with respect to GH secretion and height. These patients, however, received total radiation doses of 2400 rad, doses lower than the 3500 rad

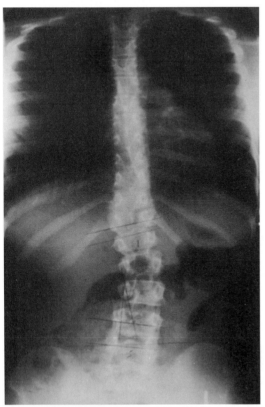

Figure 28–4. Spinal column abnormalities caused by irradiation during childhood. Notice the decreased vertebral body height and changes in contour causing severe scoliosis. (Courtesy of Dr. David Muram.)

reported to cause hypothalamic-pituitary dysfunction, which was noted to be associated with an abnormal GH response.[26] Low-dose total-body irradiation may also affect growth adversely. The majority of children who were treated with cyclophosphamide and single-fraction total-body irradiation (900 to 1000 rad) before a bone marrow transplant exhibited growth failure as a result of multiple endocrinopathies, including gonadal failure.[27]

The overall effects of therapy on growth pattern appear to be slight after chemotherapy, radiation therapy, or both, provided that the total radiation dose does not exceed 2500 rad. When radiation therapy is extended to include abdominal and gonadal radiation, however, children have shown abnormal growth.[28, 29] In one study, investigators concluded that any patient who receives a total irradiation dose of 2000 rad or more to the hypothalamic-pituitary axis is at risk for hypopituitarism, although the threshold dose may be lower. Furthermore, these patients are at increased risk of developing multiple deficiencies. A higher fraction size increases the risk of anterior pituitary failure.[13]

Some investigators have shown that treatment with GH increases growth velocity in children who were adversely affected by cranial irradiation.[30] Other investigators, however, found that such therapy failed to correct growth abnormalities after cranial irradiation but did benefit children when a surgical excision had resulted in GH deficiency.[31] In fact, a study comparing patients with GH deficiency after central nervous system (CNS) radiation therapy and normal subjects revealed no significant differences in growth rate, somatomedin activity, or bone age.[32] Thus, many physicians currently do not use GH therapy to treat these children.[32–35]

Hypothyroidism, which may occur after radiation therapy to the head and neck region, may also impair linear growth during childhood. Affected children have reduced thyroxine (T_4) and/or elevated thyroid-stimulating hormone (TSH) levels. In a long-term follow-up study of patients treated with neck irradiation in childhood, more than half demonstrated some abnormality of T_4 or TSH or thyroid gland nodularity. Lymphangiography and a radiation dose of 3000 rad or more increased patients' risk of developing palpable thyroid nodules and of thyroid hypofunction as demonstrated by elevated TSH levels. Thyroid hyperfunction may follow neck irradiation, with or without clinical signs of hyperthyroidism.[36, 37] Thyroid dysfunction can also interfere with the normal menstrual cycle.

Less is known about the effects, if any, of chemotherapy on thyroid function. In one study, 28 children were treated for Hodgkin's disease—four with chemotherapy alone, 15 with radiation alone (estimated thyroid dose 4570 rad), and nine with chemotherapy combined with radiation (estimated thyroid dose 4000 rad). None of the four children treated with chemotherapy alone developed hypothyroidism.[38] In comparison, 21 of the 24 children who received radiation therapy, with or without chemotherapy, developed thyroid dysfunction.

The physician who follows cancer survivors should measure and weigh them regularly. Plotting these measurements over time on growth charts and growth velocity charts is essential for detecting growth abnormalities. When patients appear to have growth failure, referral to an endocrinologist is warranted for possible treatment with recombinant GH. If it is clear that poor growth is related only to local damage caused by the irradiation, intervention may not be necessary.

In a recent study, the investigators found that approximately half the survivors of childhood leukemia become obese young adults. At final height, 23 of 51 male patients (45%) and 30 of 63 female patients (47%) were obese. That girls became obese between diagnosis and the end of chemotherapy ($p = .02$) and subsequently had no further increase, indicated that chemotherapy may have contributed to their obesity. Boys had a progressive and gradual increase in body mass index until they stopped growing. The obesity did not appear to be associated with GH deficiency, disproportionate growth, or abnormal timing of puberty.[39] The authors suggest that children who are treated for cancer be advised of this risk and be encouraged to adopt a more active lifestyle and a healthy diet in an attempt to reduce the risk of obesity.

GONADAL FUNCTION

Cancer therapy can adversely affect gonadal function, both hormone production and the viability of germ cells. Apparent predictors of long-term effects include the sex of the patient, the type of therapy (radiation or chemotherapy), the dosage and duration of therapy, and, to a lesser degree, the age and sexual maturity of the patient. Amenorrhea and gonadal failure often follow fractionated total-body irradiation. Amenorrhea developed within 3 months of irradiation in all females, and gonadotropin levels were elevated in all patients.[29] The endocrine sequelae of total-body irradiation are often limited to gonadal failure, which requires estrogen replacement therapy.[29, 40] It has been estimated that the median lethal dose (LD_{50}) for the human oocyte does not exceed 400 rad.[40] After irradiation, 20% of prepubertal girls with leukemia had no follicle growth and 80% had incomplete follicular development. Another study showed a marked decrease in antral, primordial, and primary follicles.[10, 41, 42]

It is currently a common practice in young females to suspend the ovaries out of the planned radiation field (oophoropexy) to decrease their exposure to the damaging effects of ionizing radiation and thus prevent the long-term sequela of ovarian failure. Future normal ovarian function is inversely related to the amount of radiation absorbed by the gonads, and how much is absorbed depends on distance from the radiation field. In one study, 71% of the patients undergoing ovarian transposition maintained ovarian function. Preservation of ovarian function was directly related to the estimated scatter dose to the ovaries. Of patients whose calculated ovarian dose was 300 rad or less, only 11% had gonadal failure, as compared with 60% of patients whose ovarian dose was more than 300 rad.[43] Lateral transposition of the ovaries reduces the radiation dose to the gonad, but if this measure is to be effective, the ovaries should be positioned above the iliac crest.[43] Patients who undergo ovarian transposition, however, are prone to develop symptomatic ovarian cysts, which may occur in as many as 25% of patients secondary to vascular compromise.[43] In one study, computed tomography (CT) was found to have value in the prognosis for ovarian function after transposition: When the ovaries were visualized on pelvic scans, ovarian function was likely to have been preserved (Figs. 28–6, 28–7).[44]

The gonads are very sensitive to irradiation damage, and radiation doses to the ovary of 400 to 700 rad often causes ovarian failure. In one study, however, investigators reported that only 17 of 25 girls developed ovarian failure when both ovaries were exposed to doses of 1200 to 5000 rad (mean 3200 rad). They concluded that younger women are less susceptible to the deleterious effects of irradiation.[45] Puberty is usually, but not always delayed by such treatment.[46]

Cancer chemotherapy, most notably alkylating agents, can cause menstrual irregularities or amenorrhea, loss of libido, menopausal symptoms, and, possibly, osteoporosis.[47, 48] The incidence of gonadal dysfunction after chemotherapy seems to be strikingly high and is 80% greater in women treated for Hodgkin's disease than in normal women.[23] Although lasting gonadal dysfunction may follow the use of a single chemotherapeutic agent, in general, chemotherapy-induced gonadal damage is related to the amount of cytotoxic agent administered.[49] Available data indicate that, gonadal dysfunction is due to gonadal—rather than hypothalamic-pituitary—damage. Basal gonadotropin levels were elevated in 98% of affected persons, and gonadotropin response to gonadotropin-releasing hormone (GnRH) stimulation tests was consistent with primary gonadal dysfunction in 99% of patients with abnormal gonadal function.[49]

Although these symptoms of gonadal dysfunction in postpubertal females are well-known, the effects of similar therapy during the prepubertal years are not as well documented. Many studies have been designed to assess the relationship

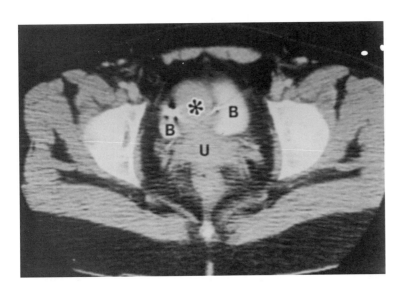

Figure 28–6. Ovarian tissue *(asterisk)* can be identified indenting the bladder. Marker clips are seen laterally. B = bladder; U = uterus. (From Winer-Muram HT, Muram D, Salazar J, Thompson E: Ovariopexy—clinical and radiologic correlation. Adolesc Pediatr Gynecol 1988; 1:239–243.)

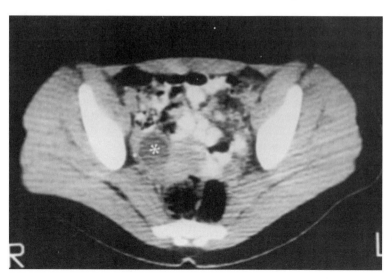

Figure 28–7. A CT scan shows a functional ovarian cyst *(asterisk)* in a transposed ovary. (From Winer-Muram HT, Muram D, Salazar J, Thompson E: Ovariopexy—clinical and radiologic correlation. Adolesc Pediatr Gynecol 1988; 1:239–243.)

of gonadal activity and chemotherapy-induced gonadal damage. Some have shown that prepubertal status affords some protection from such damage. Cyclophosphamide administered to prepubertal and pubertal females produced no gonadal dysfunction, as measured by plasma levels of gonadotropins.[50, 51] One literature review of 30 studies evaluated gonadal function after either cyclophosphamide therapy for renal disease or combination chemotherapy for Hodgkin's disease or acute lymphocytic leukemia.[49] The data were stratified according to sex, illness, chemotherapeutic regimen and dose, and pubertal stage at the time of treatment. The likelihood of developing chemotherapy-induced damage depended on the drugs and the dose and was directly related to the degree of gonadal activity at the time of treatment.[49]

If chemotherapy-induced damage varies according to pubertal status, it might be assumed that it is related to gonadal activity at the time of treatment. Specifically, it would be expected that prepubertal children with inactive gametogenesis would have a lower incidence of chemotherapy-induced damage than would similarly treated adults and that adolescents who experience a progressive increase in gonadal activity would have an incidence of gonadal dysfunction intermediate between that of children treated before and those treated after puberty.

In recent years, prevention of chemotherapy-induced gonadal damage has received significant attention. The basic premise is that artificial gonadal suppression may render the gonads more resistant to the deleterious effects of chemotherapy or irradiation therapy. The potential for preserving reproductive function through the

suppression of ovarian activity with oral contraceptives has shown some success.[52] In one study, preservation of ovarian function was documented in five of five females treated for Hodgkin's disease concurrently with oral contraceptives.[53] Other investigators reported that fertility rates were greater among women who had taken oral contraceptives during treatment of Hodgkin's disease than among those who did not take them[54]; however, in that particular study the patients who took oral contraceptives were younger than those who did not take them.[54]

Medroxyprogesterone acetate (Depo-Provera, or DMPA), a long-acting progestin, was also used to suppress gonadal function before treating males with chemotherapeutic agents.[55] A second group was not given MPA and was treated only with chemotherapy. In this particular study, there was no difference between the groups with respect to recovery of sperm cell production after chemotherapy. DMPA-induced medical castration during intensive chemotherapy in male patients appeared not to protect the testis against treatment-induced damage to spermatogenesis, at least when hormone treatment was provided simultaneously with chemotherapy.[55]

The hypothesis that a "down-regulated" gonad is less vulnerable to the effects of cytotoxic chemotherapy has been investigated, with conflicting results. In one study, the investigators were able to demonstrate that treatment of rats with long-acting GnRH analogues diminished histologically evident testicular damage secondary to chemotherapy.[56] A subsequent study evaluated the protective effect of the GnRH agonist leuprolide acetate (Lupron). Animals were treated with cyclophosphamide in combination with Lupron, progesterone, or placebo. Both Lupron and progesterone were shown to protect the gonad from the negative effects of cyclophosphamide.[57] Other investigators, however, using GnRH agonists with chemotherapy failed to preserve fertility in patients treated for Hodgkin's disease.[58]

Life-saving therapy may require agents that have toxic effects on the gonads. Because chemotherapy-induced gonadal damage is related to gonadal activity, further study is required to develop preventive strategies, and, despite the conflicting data, it may be advisable to achieve gonadal quiescence to increase the resistance of the gonads to the side effects of therapy.

The natural history of gonadal dysfunction after chemotherapy has not been extensively described. Current evidence suggests that complete recovery of normal gonadal function generally does not occur.[49] In one study of female patients treated for Hodgkin's disease, 49% were amenorrheic soon after therapy, 34% had irregular menstrual cycles, and 17% had normal ovarian function.[47] During 16 months of continued observation, however, progressive loss of ovarian function was observed in 30% of those who had had either normal or irregular menstrual cycles after treatment. None of the women with amenorrhea regained normal ovarian function.[47] Unfortunately, at the present time there are no medical means by which gonadal healing may be promoted or accelerated.[9, 10, 47]

The potential for chemotherapeutic agents to induce genetic abnormalities in offspring has not been determined. Radiation therapy is known to produce germ cell effects. In humans, a gonadal dose of 200 roentgen equivalents in man (rem) in childhood increases the risk of genetic damage about 1%. As the dose of radiation therapy increases up to 1000 rem, there is a linear increase in the genetic effects. Gonadal radiation therapy beyond 1000 rem usually produces sterility, and the risk of a genetic abnormality is approximately 1% to 5%, depending on the dose.[5] Pregnancy outcome, however, usually is not affected, and, when compared with a control group, there is no significant increase in the rates of spontaneous abortions or abnormal offspring among survivors whose childhood cancer was treated with either chemotherapy or irradiation.[50, 51] In Holmes and Holmes' series, however, the group treated with a combined modality did have significantly higher incidences of spontaneous abortions or abnormal offspring.[71] In the series of Blatt and colleagues, there was no increase in the rate of abortions. Follow-up studies of children born to previously treated mothers showed no increase in the prevalence of congenital abnormalities.[72, 73]

Infertility appears to be the principal concern. In one study of 103 women who were treated for Hodgkin's disease with radiation and chemotherapy, the pregnancy rate was considerably lower than the expected rate adjusted for age.[74] The likelihood of becoming infertile was directly related to the radiation absorbed dose (rad) to the gonads. Gonadal dysfunction after therapy commonly results in decreased fertility rates.[75] Recent advances currently permit some women with gonadal failure to conceive after receiving an egg or an embryo from a donor. The recipient's endometrium is synchronized with the donor's use of estrogen and progesterone. After fertilization of the donor's egg, a preembryo is transferred into the recipient's uterus.[76]

LATE CONSEQUENCES OF CURE

Survivors of childhood malignancies are at risk for developing a second malignancy, often 10 years or more after completion of therapy for the primary neoplasm. Although the exact risk has not been determined, it is estimated to be 3% to 12% for children diagnosed and treated before 1971. For children treated more recently, the prevalence is estimated to be about 8%.[59–61] These rates represent 10 to 20 times greater risk for these patients as compared with the general population.[62–70]

FERTILITY AND PREGNANCY OUTCOME

A potential mutagenic effect may be produced by chemotherapy or radiation therapy. It can harm germ cells and, subsequently, the offspring of cancer survivors. The ultimate genetic effect, however, is determined by the sex and age of the exposed patient, because germ cells exist at different developmental stages in the two sexes and at the various stages of pubertal development. Oogonial mitosis is completed in fetal life; the ova are therefore less vulnerable than spermatogonia to point mutations but more susceptible to nondisjunction. Offspring of treated females are at increased risk for chromosomal aneuploidy, whereas offspring of treated males are more likely to sustain single-gene mutations or structural rearrangements than aneuploidy.[5]

NEOPLASMS IN THE OFFSPRING

Offspring of cancer survivors are at greater risk than the general population for developing cancer.[77] Carcinomas in offspring of survivors occur in two ways: some offspring inherit the genes that caused the parent's cancer; others acquire new genetic abnormalities induced in parental germ cells by therapeutic agents.[77, 78] The first possibility, inheritance, is most likely in the offspring of parents who in childhood had a genetic form of embryonal tumor, such as retinoblastoma, Wilms tumor, and neuroblastoma.[73, 77–79]

PSYCHOSOCIAL ADJUSTMENT

In addition to the medical complications of therapy, many survivors suffer adverse psychological sequelae. Various studies have attempted to explore such issues, but the results have varied—and at times have been controversial.[80–87] Scholastic problems may arise as a result of absenteeism secondary to therapy, a decrease in intellectual performance after cranial irradiation, or social isolation of these children by their peers. A decrease in school performance may lead to dropping out and its sequelae. Occasionally, physical impairment after amputation demands adjustments, both psychosocial and physical.

Special efforts must be made to allow these children to lead as normal a life as possible. Tutorial services should be provided in the hospital so that they can maintain their class standing. Counseling with parents and families can help to resolve conflicts that often arise after the diagnosis; fears of dying and cancer recurrence must also be dealt with during therapy.[88] Counseling with peers who survived similar disease may also be beneficial. The combination of adolescence and cancer creates a high risk for emotional disturbances and psychosocial difficulties. Every effort must be made to permit survivors of childhood cancer to lead normal and fulfilling lives.

Finally, survivors of childhood cancer often worry about the impact of the treatment modalities on their future health, their reproductive ability, and their offspring. Intensive counseling is vital for cancer patients and must address these issues.

REFERENCES

1. Miller RW, Young JL Jr, Novakovic B: Childhood cancer. Cancer 1995; 75(1 Suppl):395–405.
2. Young JL, Ries LG, Silverberg E, et al: Cancer incidence, survival, and mortality for children younger than age 15 years. Cancer 1986; 58(Suppl):598–602.
3. Jenkin D, Berry M: Hodgkin's disease in children. Semin Oncol 1980; 7:202–211.
4. The Pediatric Oncology Group: Progress against childhood cancer: The Pediatric Oncology Group experience. Pediatrics 1992; 89:597–600.
5. Meadows AT, Silber J: Delayed consequences of therapy of childhood cancer. CA 1985; 35:271–286.
6. Kenney LB, Miller BA, Ries LA, et al: Increased incidence of cancer in infants in the U.S.: 1980–1990. Cancer 1998; 82(7):1396–1400.
7. Smith MA, Freidlin B, Ries LA, Simon R: Trends in reported incidence of primary malignant brain tumors in children in the United States. J Natl Cancer Inst 1998; 90(17):1269–1277.
8. Gurney JG, Davis S, Severson RK, et al: Trends in cancer incidence among children in the U.S. Cancer 1996; 78(3):532–541.
9. Chapman RM: Effect of cytotoxic therapy on sexuality and gonadal function. Semin Oncol 1989; 9:84–94.
10. Mackie EJ, Radford M, Shalet SM: Gonadal function following chemotherapy for childhood Hodgkin's disease. Med Pediatr Oncol 1996; 27(2):74–78.
11. Vaeth JM, Levitt SH, Jones MD, et al: Effects of radiation therapy in survivors of Wilms' tumor. Radiation 1962; 79:560–568.
12. Donaldson SS, Kaplan HS: Complications of treatment of Hodgkin's disease in children. Cancer Treat Rep 1982; 66:977–989.
13. Muller HL, Klinkhammer-Schalke M, Kuhl J: Final height and weight of long-term survivors of childhood malignancies. Exp Clin Endocrinol Diabetes 1998; 106(2):135–139.
14. Ogilvy-Stuart AL, Shalet SM: Effect of chemotherapy on growth. Acta Paediatr 1995; 411(Suppl):52–56.
15. Davies HA, Didcock E, Didi M, et al: Growth, puberty and obesity after treatment for leukaemia. Acta Paediatr 1995; 411(Suppl):45–50.
16. Didcock E, Davies HA, Didi M, et al: Pubertal growth in young adult survivors of childhood leukaemia. J Clin Oncol 1995; 13(10):2503–2507.
17. Parker RG, Berry HC: Late effects of therapeutic irradiation on the skeleton and bone marrow. Cancer 1976; 37:1162–1171.
18. Riseborough EJ, Grabias SL, Burton RI, et al: Skeletal alterations following irradiation for Wilms tumor: With particular reference to scoliosis and kyphosis. J Bone Joint Surg 1976; 58:526–536.
19. Rubin P, Duthie RB, Young LW: The significance of scoliosis in postirradiated Wilms' tumor and neuroblastoma. Radiology 1962; 79:539–559.
20. Littley MD, Shalet SM, Beardwell CG: Radiation and hypothalamic-pituitary function. Clin Endocrinol Metab 1990; 4:147–175.
21. Shalet SM, Morris-Jones PH, Beardwell CG, et al: Pituitary function after treatment of intracranial tumors in children. Lancet 1975; 2:104–107.
22. Brennan BM, Rahim A, Mackie EM, et al: Growth hormone status in adults treated for acute lymphoblastic leukaemia in childhood. Clin Endocrinol 1998; 48(6):777–783.
23. Swift PGF, Kearney PJ, Dalton RG, et al: Growth and hormonal status of children treated for acute lymphoblastic leukemia. Arch Dis Child 1978; 53:890–894.
24. Shalet SM, Beardwell CG: Endocrine consequences of treatment of malignant disease in childhood: A review. J R Soc Med 1979; 72:39–41.
25. Wells RJ, Foster MB, D'Ercole AJ, et al: The impact of cranial irradiation on the growth of children with acute lymphocytic leukemia. Am J Dis Child 1983; 137:37–39.
26. Hakami N, Mohammad A, Meyer JW: Growth and growth hormone of children with acute lymphocytic leu-

kemia following central nervous system prophylaxis with and without cranial irradiation. Am J Pediatr Hematol Oncol 1980; 2:311–316.

27. Leiper AD, Stanhope R, Lau T, et al: The effect of total body irradiation and bone marrow transplantation during childhood and adolescence on growth and endocrine function. Br J Haematol 1987; 67:419–426.

28. Robison LL, Nesbit ME Jr, Sather HN, et al: Height of children successfully treated for acute lymphoblastic leukemia: A report from the Late Effects Study Committee of Children's Cancer Study Group. Med Pediatr Oncol 1985; 13:14–21.

29. Littley MD, Shalet SM, Morgenstern GR, Deakin DP: Endocrine and reproductive dysfunction following fractionated total body irradiation in adults. Q J Med 1991; 78:265–274.

30. Romshe CA, Zipf WB, Miser A, et al: Evaluation of growth hormone release and human growth hormone treatment in children with cranial irradiation–associated short stature. J Pediatr 1984; 104:177–181.

31. Winter RJ, Green OC: Irradiation-induced growth hormone deficiency: Blunted growth response and accelerated skeletal maturation to growth hormone therapy. J Pediatr 1985; 106:609–612.

32. Shalet SM, Price DA, Breadwell CG, et al: Normal growth despite abnormalities of growth hormone secretion in children treated for acute leukemia. J Pediatr 1979; 94:719–722.

33. Fisher JN, Aur RJA: Endocrine assessment in childhood acute lymphocytic leukemia. Cancer 1982; 49:145–151.

34. Ogilvy-Stuart AL, Stirling HF, Kelnar CJ, et al: Treatment of radiation-induced growth hormone deficiency with growth hormone–releasing hormone. Clin Endocrinol 1997; 46(5):571–578.

35. Ogilvy-Stuart AL, Shalet SM: Growth and puberty after growth hormone treatment after irradiation for brain tumours. Arch Dis Child 1995; 73(2):141–146.

36. Kaplan MM, Garnick MB, Gelber R, et al: Risk factors for thyroid abnormalities after neck irradiation for childhood cancer. Am J Med 1983; 74:272–280.

37. Wasnich RD, Grumet CF, Payne RO, et al: Graves' ophthalmopathy following external neck irradiation for nonthyroidal neoplastic disease. J Clin Endocrinol Metab 1973; 37:703–713.

38. Devney RB, Sklar CA, Nesbit ME Jr, et al: Serial thyroid function measurements in children with Hodgkin's disease. J Pediatr 1984; 105:223–227.

39. Didi M, Didcock E, Davies HA, et al: High incidence of obesity in young adults after treatment of acute lymphoblastic leukemia in childhood. J Pediatrics 1995; 127(1):63–67.

40. Wallace WH, Shalet SM, Hendry JH, et al: Ovarian failure following abdominal irradiation in childhood: The radiosensitivity of the human oocyte. Br J Radiol 1989; 62:995–998.

41. Nicosia SV, Matus-Ridley M, Meadows AT: Gonadal effects of cancer therapy in girls. Cancer 1985; 55:2364–2372.

42. Shalet SM: Endocrine sequelae of cancer therapy. Eur J Endocrinol 1996; 135(2):135–143.

43. Chambers SK, Chambers JT, Kier R, Peschel RE: Sequelae of lateral ovarian transposition in irradiated cervical cancer patients. Int J Radiat Oncol Biol Phys 1991; 20:305–308.

44. Winer-Muram HT, Muram D, Salazar J, Thompson E: Ovariopexy—clinical and radiologic correlation. Adolesc Pediatr Gynecol 1988; 1:239–243.

45. Stillman RJ, Schinfeld JS, Schiff I: Ovarian failure in long-term survivors of childhood malignancy. Am J Obstet Gynecol 1981; 139:62–66.

46. Barrett A, Nichols J, Gibson B: Late effects of total body irradiation. Radiother Oncol 1987; 9:131–135.

47. Chapman RM, Sutcliffe SB, Malpas JS: Cytotoxic-induced ovarian failure in women with Hodgkin's disease. I. Hormone function. JAMA 1979; 242:1877–1881.

48. Chapman RM, Sutcliffe SB, Malpas JS: Cytotoxic-induced ovarian failure in women with Hodgkin's disease. II. Effects on sexual function. JAMA 1979; 242:1882–1884.

49. Rivkees SA, Crawford SD: The relationship of gonadal activity and chemotherapy-induced gonadal damage. JAMA 1988; 259:2123–2125.

50. Pennisi AJ, Grushkin CM, Lieberman E: Gonadal function in children with nephrosis treated with cyclophosphamide. Am J Dis Child 1975; 129:315–318.

51. Etteldorf JN, West CD, Pitcock JA, et al: Gonadal function, testicular histology, and meiosis following cyclophosphamide therapy in patients with nephrotic syndrome. J Pediatrics 1976; 88:206–212.

52. Chapman RM, Sutcliffe SB: Protection of ovarian function by oral contraceptive use in women receiving chemotherapy for Hodgkin's disease. Blood 1981; 58:849–851.

53. King DJ, Ratcliffe MD, Dawson DD, et al: Fertility in young men and women after treatment for lymphoma: A study of a population. J Clin Pathol 1985; 38:1247–1251.

54. Siris ES, Leventhal BG, Vaitukaitis JL: Effects of childhood leukemia and chemotherapy on puberty and reproductive function in girls. N Engl J Med 1976; 294:1143–1146.

55. Fossa SD, Klepp O, Norman N: Lack of gonadal protection by medroxyprogesterone acetate–induced transient medical castration during chemotherapy for testicular cancer. Br J Urol 1988; 62:449–453.

56. Glode LM, Robinson J, Gould SF: Protection from cyclophosphamide induced testicular damage with analogue of gonadotropin-releasing hormone. Lancet 1981; 1:1132–1134.

57. Montz FJ, Wolff AJ, Gambone JC: Gonadal protection and fecundity rates in cyclophosphamide-treated rats. Cancer Res 1991; 51:124–126.

58. Waxman JH, Ahmed R, Smith D, et al. Failure to preserve fertility in patients with Hodgkin's disease. Cancer Chemother Pharmacol 1987; 19:159–162.

59. Tucker MA, Meadows AT, Boice JD Jr, et al: Cancer risk following treatment of childhood cancer. In Boice JD, Fraumeni JF Jr (eds): Radiation Carcinogenesis: Epidemiology and Biological Significance. New York: Raven Press, 1984, pp 211–224.

60. Li F: Second malignant tumors after cancer in childhood. Cancer 1977; 40:1899–1902.

61. Miké V, Meadows AT, D'Angio GJ: Incidence of second malignant neoplasms in children: Results of an international study. Lancet 1982; 2:1326–1331.

62. Goss PE, Sierra S: Current perspectives on radiation-induced breast cancer. Journal of Clinical Oncology 1998; 16(1):338–347.

63. Miyahara H, Sato T, Yoshino K: Radiation-induced cancers of the head and neck region. Acta Oto-Laryngologica 1998; 533(Suppl):60–64.

64. Enrici RM, Anselmo AP, Iacari V, et al. The risk of non-Hodgkin's lymphoma after Hodgkin's disease, with special reference to splenic treatment. Haematologica 1998; 83(7):636–644.

65. Mohney BG, Robertson DM, Schomberg PJ, Hodge DO: Second nonocular tumors in survivors of heritable retinoblastoma and prior radiation therapy. Am J Ophthalmol 1998; 126(2):269–277.

66. Karlsson P, Holmberg E, Lundell M, et al: Intracranial

tumors after exposure to ionizing radiation during infancy: A pooled analysis of two Swedish cohorts of 28,008 infants with skin hemangioma. Radiation Res 1998; 150(3):357–364.

67. Kimball Dalton VM, Gelber RD, Li F: Second malignancies in patients treated for childhood acute lymphoblastic leukemia. J Clin Oncol 1998; 16(8):2848–2853.

68. Cutuli B, Dhermain F, Borel C, et al: Breast cancer in patients treated for Hodgkin's disease: Clinical and pathological analysis of 76 cases in 63 patients. Eur J Cancer 1997; 33(14):2315–2320.

69. Bhatia S, Robison LL, Oberlin O, et al: Breast cancer and other second neoplasms after childhood Hodgkin's disease. N Engl J Med 1996; 334(12):745–751.

70. Travis LB, Curtis RE, Boice JD Jr, et al: Second malignant neoplasms among long-term survivors of ovarian cancer. Cancer Res 1996; 56(7):1564–1570.

71. Holmes GE, Holmes FF: Pregnancy outcome of patients treated for Hodgkin's disease: A controlled study. Cancer 1978; 41:1317–1322.

72. Blatt J, Mulvihill JJ, Ziegler JL, et al: Pregnancy outcome following cancer chemotherapy. Am J Med 1980; 69:828–832.

73. Kenney LB, Nicholson HS, Brasseux C, et al. Birth defects in offspring of adult survivors of childhood acute lymphoblastic leukemia. A Childrens Cancer Group/National Institutes of Health Report. Cancer 1996; 78(1):169–176.

74. Horning SJ, Hoppe RT, Kaplan HS, et al: Female reproductive potential after treatment for Hodgkin's disease. N Engl J Med 1981; 304:1377–1382.

75. Chapman RM: Reproductive potential after treatment for Hodgkin's disease (Letter). N Engl J Med 1981; 305:891.

76. Navot D, Laufer N, Kopolovic R, et al: Artifically induced endometrial cycles and establishment of pregnancies in the absence of ovaries. N Engl J Med 1986; 314:806–811.

77. Knudson AG Jr: Genetics and the child cured of cancer. *In* van Eys J, Sullivan MP (eds): Status of the Curability of Childhood Cancers. New York: Raven Press, 1980, pp 295–305.

78. Knudson AG Jr: Genetics and the etiology of childhood cancer. Pediatr Res 1976; 10:513–517.

79. Lewis EB: Possible genetic consequences of irradiation of tumors in childhood. Radiology 1975; 114:147–153.

80. Mulvihill JJ, Connelly RR, Austin DF, et al: Cancer in offspring of long-term survivors of childhood and adolescent cancer. Lancet 1987; 2:813–817.

81. Greenberg HS, Kazak AE, Meadows AT: Psychologic function in 8- to 16-year-old cancer survivors and their parents. J Pediatrics 1989; 114:488.

82. Lannering B, Marky I, Lundberg A, Olsson E: Long-term sequelae after pediatric brain tumor: Their effect on disability and quality of life. Med Pediatr Oncol 1990; 18:304–310.

83. Mulhern RK, Wasserman AL, Friedman AG, et al: Social competence and behavioral adjustment of children who are long-term survivors of cancer. Pediatrics 1989; 83:18.

84. Tebbi CK, Bromberg C, Piedmonte M: Long-term vocational adjustment of cancer patients diagnosed during adolescence. Cancer 1989; 63:213.

85. Carr-Gregg M, Hampson R: A new approach to the psychological care of adolescents with cancer. Med J Austr 1986; 145:580, 582–583.

86. Spirito A, Stark LJ, Cobiella C, et al: Social adjustment of children successfully treated for cancer. J Pediatr Psychol 1990; 15:359–371.

87. Wasserman AL, Thompson EI, Wilimas JA, et al: The psychological status of survivors of childhood/adolescent Hodgkin's disease. Am J Dis Child 1987; 141:626.

88. Zeltzer LK, Chen E, Weiss R, et al: Comparison of psychologic outcome in adult survivors of childhood acute lymphoblastic leukemia versus sibling controls: A cooperative Children's Cancer Group and National Institutes of Health study. J Clin Oncol 1997; 15(2):547–556.

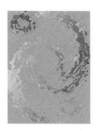

Chapter 29

Sports-Related Problems in Reproductive Function

ROBERT W. REBAR

The notion that participation in sports in the adolescent years can affect reproductive function is commonly accepted today. Extrapolating to typical teenagers from data obtained from the study of elite adolescent and adult athletes engaged in endurance training may, however, be more difficult. Nevertheless, data are accumulating that indicate that, for adolescent athletes at all skill levels, reproductive disorders are associated with their preoccupation with sports. In this chapter the initial focus is the impact of strenuous training on reproductive development and function. Then, I will attempt to integrate this information into the care of more typical adolescent girls.

REPRODUCTIVE DISORDERS ASSOCIATED WITH EXERCISE

DELAYED MENARCHE

Malina and coworkers[1, 2] were the first to report an association between menarcheal delay and competition in track and field sports. In general, the more skilled the athlete, the later was her age at menarche (Fig. 29–1). These investigators were extremely cautious in drawing any conclusions from their data (obtained from histories). They suggested that it was possible that the physical build associated with better performance in track and field events (i.e., tall stature and long limbs) might confer a selection bias that is quite independent of any effect of exercise on pubertal development. One other historical study suggested that delayed menarche is associated with success in competitive running because it promotes tallness and thinness, attributes that can be used to advantage in certain sports.[3] Furthermore, in a given age group, early sexual maturation may influence socialization that does not value physical activity.

That endurance training itself does affect the

pubertal process is supported by several subsequent studies. Frisch and her colleagues[4] documented that intensive training of runners in the premenarcheal years delays menarche. In addition, both Frisch's group[5] and Warren[6] noted that menarche is delayed for dedicated ballet dancers who begin strenuous training before adolescence. Warren further noted that menarche is not delayed in serious musicians, who might be expected to suffer a comparable degree of mental stress.

Thus, it is likely that strenuous exercise before menarche contributes to its delay, but the mechanism remains unclear. It has been suggested that, because endurance training promotes thinness athletic girls do not attain the "critical" percentage of body fat required for menarche.[7] Body composition cannot be the only contributor to menarcheal delay: ballet dancers whose weight and body fat content exceed the "critical" values do not attain menarche until they cut back physical training.[6] Thus, prospective studies of the effects of exertion on menarche still will be necessary to identify the mechanisms of delayed menarche.

LUTEAL PHASE DEFECTS

Suggestions that endurance training might lead to luteal phase abnormalities in elite athletes first appeared in the late 1970s. Perhaps the best of these early reports noted that four skilled teenage swimmers had shorter luteal phases than nonexercising girls.[8] Failure of progesterone levels in the swimmers to increase, despite a luteinizing hormone (LH) surge, suggested nonluteinization of the follicle. The follicle-stimulating hormone (FSH)–LH ratio was reduced in the swimmers, a finding that might account for the luteal phase inadequacy. The data may suggest that a central mechanism is responsible for the relative decrease in FSH which leads to inade-

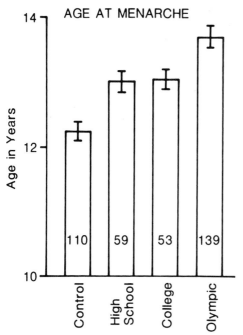

Figure 29–1. Recalled age of menarche (± standard error) in nonathletes and in track-and-field athletes of varying competitive abilities. The Olympic athletes participated in the 1976 Games. The numbers in each bar refer to the number of athletes in each group. (Data from Malina et al.[1, 2] Reprinted with permission from Cumming DC, Rebar RW: Exercise and reproductive function in women: a review. Am J Int Med 1983; 4:113. Copyright © 1983. Reprinted by permission of Wiley-Liss, a division of John Wiley and Sons.)

quate follicular maturation. In a single case study of a 30-year-old woman runner, shorter luteal phases and lower midluteal progesterone levels were recorded during menstrual cycles in which the individual trained more extensively.[9] On the basis of basal body temperature changes, Prior and associates[10] reported luteal phase defects in two women training for a marathon, which resolved after the race. Based on additional basal body temperature data, Prior[11] suggested that luteal dysfunction may occur in as many as 50% of long-distance runners.

More recent studies have examined progesterone secretion in the luteal phase in greater detail. Schweiger and colleagues[12] reported that 14 of 18 endurance-trained athletes with cyclic gonadal function had reduced levels of circulating estradiol and progesterone during the luteal phase. Ellison and Lager[13] documented lower salivary progesterone levels in ovulatory recreational women runners.

Hoffman and coworkers examined daily first morning urinary pregnanediol glucuronide (PDG) excretion during two successive menstrual cycles in a select group of elite eumenorrheic runners (running 35 or more miles per week) with no history of menstrual irregularities.[14] PDG excretion in the nine runners differed from that in the seven age- and weight-matched control subjects in 14 of the 18 cycles examined. Each of the runners had at least one aberrant cycle, whereas for five both cycles were altered. Compared to the cycles in the controls, those in the runners could be divided into three distinct groups: cycles whose luteal phase was shortened (n = 7), those whose PDG excretion was decreased despite normal length (n = 7), and those whose luteal phase length and PDG excretion were similar to the controls (n = 4). Three runners who voluntarily reduced their training to 30 miles or less per week had increased PDG excretion in the very next menstrual cycle. Thus, these data indicate that luteal phase alterations are common even in eumenorrheic women engaged in endurance training.

More recently, Beitins and her colleagues[15] enrolled a group of athletic college women with normal menstrual cycles who did not participate in aerobic training but wished to devote a summer to exercise training. During the first month the women ran 5 days a week, starting at 4.0 miles per day during the first week and advancing by 1½ miles during each successive week, reaching 10.0 miles per day by the fifth week. In addition to running, the subjects participated in 3½ hours of moderate intensity sports activities, including bicycling, tennis, and volleyball. During the second month, the running distance was held constant at 10.0 miles per day with the subjects' heart rates corresponding to 70% to 80% of their Vo_2 max. During the control month and the two exercise months, all subjects collected daily overnight urine samples for determination of hormone excretion. Of the 28 participants, 18 women were identified who had a total of 20 cycles with urinary hormone excretion patterns consistent with an inadequate or short luteal phase. Four women developed inadequate luteal phase cycles during the first exercise month, 10 developed short luteal phase cycles, two developed inadequate luteal phase cycles, and four, short luteal phase cycles during the second exercise month. Two women had luteal phase defects in both exercise months. This study, too, indicates that initiation of strenuous endurance training in previously ovulating untrained women frequently leads to corpus luteum dysfunction. Because the midcycle LH surge was delayed in spite of increased estrogen secretion, the authors further suggested that exercise induces alterations in the neuroendocrine system.

It is true that almost all of the studies of luteal function were conducted in women older than 18 years; however, it is highly likely that similar defects would develop in young adolescents engaged in endurance training.

AMENORRHEA

Feicht and her colleagues[16] first reported that long-distance runners are especially prone to become amenorrheic. From a questionnaire they determined that 6% to 43% of collegiate runners were amenorrheic and that the incidence increased directly with the training mileage (Fig. 29–2). Several other investigators subsequently confirmed the observation that the incidence of amenorrhea is higher in runners than in the typical adult female population.[17–19] The inci-

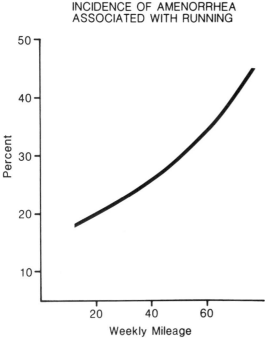

Figure 29–2. The relationship between the incidence of amenorrhea (defined as fewer than three cycles in the preceding 12 months) and weekly running mileage of 20 to 80 miles. (Adapted from Feicht et al.[16] Reprinted from Cumming DC, Rebar RW: Exercise and reproductive function in women: A review. Am J Int Med 1983; 4:113. Copyright © 1983. Reprinted by permission of Wiley-Liss, a division of John Wiley and Sons, Inc.)

dence of amenorrhea also appears to be increased in ballet dancers[5, 6] and in swimmers and cyclists.[20] In view of the fact that adolescents and older women may be involved in endurance training, it is reasonable to conclude that whatever mechanisms are involved in producing amenorrhea in athletes can operate in women of any age.

A CONTINUUM OF REPRODUCTIVE DEFECTS?

It is possible that endurance training can lead to luteal dysfunction first and later to amenorrhea in women who have already menstruated. In contrast, younger girls engaged in endurance training may have delayed puberty. In other words, there appears to be a continuum of reproductive defects in susceptible women who engage in endurance training. What makes certain ones susceptible and others relatively resistant is not clear, but a number of factors appear to play some role in causing these disorders.

THE FEMALE ATHLETIC TRIAD

In 1992 the American College of Sports Medicine coined the term *female athletic triad* to describe three disorders recognized as occurring together in athletic females: disordered eating, amenorrhea, and osteoporosis.[6a] These disorders, much more common than is generally recognized, represent serious health risks to women athletes.

FACTORS INVOLVED IN EXERCISE-ASSOCIATED REPRODUCTIVE DYSFUNCTION

To date, most studies of reproductive dysfunction associated with exercise have been retrospective. Despite limitations of such studies, it has been possible to identify a number of distinct factors that appear to be implicated in the etiology of exercise-associated reproductive dysfunction.

Specifically, several changes typically occur during the course of athletic training. In association with regular aerobic exercise, women may lose weight,[18, 19] have changes in body composition,[18, 21] alter their diets,[18, 22] experience changes in several hormone secretion patterns,[18, 23, 24] and may be subject to physical and emotional stresses associated with their training.[5, 18]

BODY COMPOSITION AND WEIGHT LOSS

In a cross-sectional survey of women runners, Schwartz and colleagues[18] noted that amenorrheic runners had less body fat than eumenorrheic runners, who were, in turn, leaner than sedentary women (Fig. 29–3). In addition, it has been reported that ballet dancers with secondary amenorrhea are significantly leaner than those who are eumenorrheic.[5] Furthermore, women who became amenorrheic after beginning to run regularly also stated that they had lost more weight since starting to exercise than those who remained eumenorrheic (Fig. 29–4).[18] Total body water as a proportion of total weight, as an estimate of thinness, decreases in women runners as the prevalence of amenorrhea increases.[20] Last, it is now recognized that young girls who volunta-

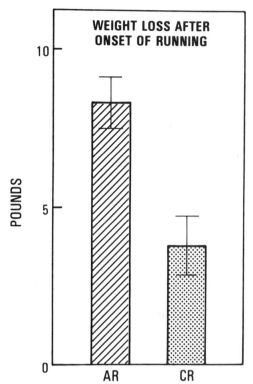

Figure 29–4. Mean (± standard error) weight loss after taking up running. The amenorrheic runners (AR) stated they had lost significantly more weight ($p < .05$) than did the eumenorrheic control runners (CR). (Modified from Schwartz B, Cumming DC, Riordan E, et al: Exercise-associated amenorrhea: A distinct entity? Am J Obstet Gynecol 1981; 141:662.)

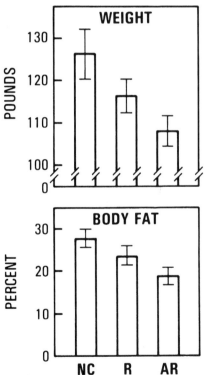

Figure 29–3. Mean (± standard error) weights and percentage body fat of women runners and nonrunners. NC = normal sedentary controls; R = eumenorrheic control runners; AR = amenorrheic runners. AR weighed significantly less ($p < .01$) and had less body fat ($p < .05$) than the other two groups. (Modified from Schwartz B, Cumming DC, Riordan E, et al: Exercise-associated amenorrhea: A distinct entity? Am J Obstet Gynecol 1981; 141:662.)

rily restrict their weight will delay pubertal progression and menarche.[25]

All of these observations are consistent with the hypothesis developed by Frisch and McArthur[7] that a minimum height for weight is required for the onset and maintenance of regular menstrual cycles. However, if weight and body fat are the most important causal factors in exercise-associated amenorrhea, then Warren's longitudinal observations[6] in amenorrheic ballet dancers defy explanation. She noted that young dancers failed to undergo menarche or had secondary amenorrhea despite weights and body fat percentages that far exceeded the minimum quantities suggested by Frisch and McArthur.[7] Only with injuries preventing exercise, and without any gain in weight or body fat, did menarche occur or cyclic menses resume. Thus, Warren's research indicates that other factors, perhaps commonly associated with weight loss and thinness, lead to exercise-associated amenorrhea.

Her observations suggesting the importance of factors other than body fat should not be surprising, in view of the fact that menarche is a late event in pubertal development. Moreover, her data are consistent with other reports that some athletes with as little as 4% body fat can still sustain menstrual function.[25]

DIET

Abundant evidence now indicates that persons engaged in endurance training typically alter their diet. If anything, one would suspect this change would be more prominent in teens. Long-distance runners are more apt than sedentary persons to eat less lean red meat and to be vegetarian. Prospective dietary histories confirm significant differences in diet between eumenorrheic and amenorrheic runners.[4, 18, 26] In fact, disordered eating apparently affects some 16% to 72% of female athletes.[26a–c] There is a wide spectrum of disordered eating patterns among athletes, including anorexia and bulimia nervosa. In most cases, the main goal appears to be weight loss, an independent risk factor for reproductive dysfunction. Putukian[26d] has reported that approximately a third of collegiate athletes practice some form of pathogenic weight control behavior, and many consider such behavior harmless. She also noted that athletic females may begin controlling their weight very early, between ages 9 and 14 years.

How and why dietary changes may lead to amenorrhea is not clear. An inadequate supply of nutrients may trigger protective mechanisms to prevent pregnancy. It is possible that changes in diet also lead to changes in thyroid and steroid hormone metabolism.

PREVIOUS MENSTRUAL PATTERNS AND OBSTETRIC HISTORY

Persons who develop amenorrhea with endurance training are more apt to have had irregular menses before beginning their training.[17, 18] More than half the women who developed amenorrhea after starting to run had a history of menstrual irregularity.[18] In contrast, fewer than 15% of eumenorrheic runners had such a history. Amenorrhea is also more common in younger runners[27] and those who are nulliparous.[17, 18]

The higher incidence of amenorrhea in younger runners suggests that menstrual dysfunction may be attributable in part to the relative immaturity of the hypothalamic-pituitary-ovarian axis or to greater susceptibility of younger athletes. In view of the observation that pretraining menstrual irregularity is associated with beginning to run at an earlier age and with running sooner after menarche,[19] it is possible that some factor promoting menstrual irregularity may inspire women to begin running.

"STRESS" ASSOCIATED WITH EXERCISE

Endurance training is commonly believed to be physically and mentally "stressful." The observation that menses may begin or resume in young ballet dancers during injury-imposed respites from training[6] supports this contention. So, too, does the observation that almost half of the first class of women recruits to the U.S. Military Academy were amenorrheic after just 6 months of classes and physical conditioning.[28]

In an effort to investigate the psychological stress of exercise, Schwartz and associates[18] utilized a number of psychometric instruments to measure depression, hypochondriasis, psychasthenia, obsessive-compulsive tendencies, and recent stressful life events in eumenorrheic and amenorrheic runners and sedentary control subjects. No differences were identified among the three groups; however, when the runners were asked to evaluate subjectively the stress associated with running on a scale of 0 to 10 (10 being maximal), the amenorrheic runners reported significantly more stress than did the eumenorrheic ones, despite the fact that they did not run more or faster and did not engage in more competitive events.

Warren's observation[6] that menarche is delayed approximately 3 years in ballet dancers than in musicians preparing for professional careers suggested to her that the menarcheal delay in the dancers was "not entirely related to stress." She pointed out that the goal-oriented lifestyles of both groups provided similar stress.

Hormonal changes associated with exercise are more difficult to interpret but may well be indicative of stress. Because it is known that endogenous opiates within the hypothalamus inhibit GnRH neurons and thus LH secretion and reproductive function,[29] it has been tempting to speculate a role for endorphins in exercise-associated amenorrhea. Carr and coworkers[30] reported that basal circulating levels of cortisol and opioid peptides increased with progressive aerobic training in women. The same investigators also reported that naloxone, an opioid antagonist given as an intravenous bolus, increased circulating LH pulses and levels in one of three amenorrheic runners tested.[31] However, Dixon and colleagues[32] failed to observe an increase in LH in any of seven amenorrheic runners, a finding confirmed by other investigators in male runners.[33] Together, then, these data suggest that endogenous opiates in the CNS do not play a major role in the causation of exercise-associated amenorrhea. The increases in opiates observed peripherally by Carr and coworkers[30] may not originate in the hypothalamus and may not directly affect hypothalamic-pituitary function.

It is well-documented that both circulating cortisol levels[34, 35] and 24-hour urinary free cortisol secretion[34] are increased in both eumenorrheic and amenorrheic runners, as compared with sedentary control subjects (Fig. 29–5). Because increases in serum cortisol in response to exogenous corticotropin, the disappearance of exogenous cortisol from the circulation and circulating corticoid-binding globulin concentrations are similar in runners and other women,[34] it is reasonable to conclude that corticotropin secretion is increased in women. Further, it would seem that increased corticotropin-releasing hormone (CRH) secretion increases corticotropin secretion. If this is true, then the data become more

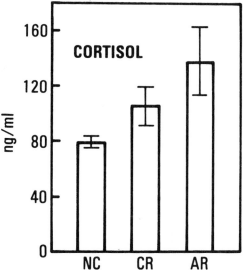

Figure 29–5. Basal morning serum cortisol levels (± standard error) in women runners and non-runners. Values in the normal sedentary controls (NC) were significantly lower than those in either the eumenorrheic control runners (CR) or the amenorrheic runners (AR). It is important to note that all values are in the normal range. (Data from Schwartz B, Cumming DC, Riordan E, et al: Exercise-induced amenorrhea: A distinct entity? Am J Obstet Gynecol 1981; 141:662.)

difficult to explain: both corticotropin and the opioid peptides are synthesized from a common precursor, and the release of corticotropin by exogenous CRH is associated with contemporaneous release of the opioid peptides.

How might CRH, corticotropin, and cortisol interact to affect reproductive function? Although any such relationship is poorly understood, it is possible to formulate a hypothesis to link the hypothalamic-pituitary-adrenal axis and reproductive function.

Administration of exogenous corticotropin or glucocorticoids can inhibit LH release or ovulation in experimental animals and humans.[36–40] Further, intracerebral administration of CRH to rats[41, 42] and peripheral administration to monkeys[43] inhibits LH secretion. In ovariectomized rats CRH can inhibit release of gonadotropin-releasing hormone (GnRH) into the portal circulation.[44] That inhibition of GnRH can be reversed by a CRH antagonist in rats both in vitro[45] and in vivo[46] suggests that CRH-induced GnRH suppression is receptor mediated. In addition, that inhibition of LH can be reversed by naloxone in rats[47, 48] and monkeys[49] indicates a relationship between CRH and endogenous opiates. That the effect of CRH on GnRH-LH secretion is direct is suggested by inhibition of LH secretion even in adrenalectomized animals.[41, 50]

Barbarino and colleagues have reported that exogenous CRH inhibits LH secretion during the midluteal phase of the menstrual cycle[51] and that inhibition is blocked by naloxone.[52] Thomas and associates,[53] however, failed to document any decrease in LH in response to exogenous CRH in agonadal women. Thus, the effect of CRH on LH secretion in humans remains to be defined. In considering all of these studies together, however, it is tempting to postulate that stress, defined strictly as hypercortisolism, is a major pathophysiologic mechanism of exercise-associated menstrual dysfunction. A reasonable hypothesis is that activation of the hypothalamic-pituitary-adrenal axis inhibits the hypothalamic-pituitary-ovarian axis. It is important to note, however, that cortisol levels in amenorrheic athletes are still well within the normal range; thus, cortisol measurements have no role in the evaluation of athletes who are amenorrheic.

HORMONAL CHANGES ASSOCIATED WITH BRIEF INTENSIVE AND LONG-TERM EXERCISE

A defined series of hormonal changes occur in both men and women exercising at maximal capacity for a short time (Fig. 29–6).[24, 54–56] Cortisol levels are increased in the 2 hours before the onset of known exercise. Both LH and testosterone levels increase dramatically in the 5 minutes before exercise begins. Because no other hormone increases likewise in anticipation of exercise, it would seem that the changes in LH and testosterone are specific. Moreover, in view of the abrupt and coincident secretion of both hormones, it is difficult to believe that testosterone secretion is stimulated by the increased LH secretion. It is possible that the increase in testosterone is due to adrenergic innervation of hilar cells in the ovary and Leydig cells in the testis. This possibility is supported by the observation that testosterone does not increase in anticipation of exercise in oophorectomized women.[56]

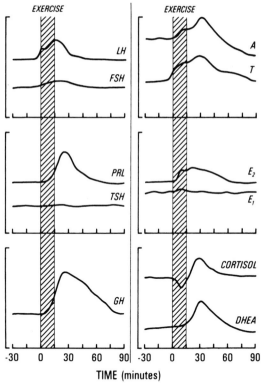

Figure 29–6. Diagram of hormonal changes observed before, during, and after symptom-limited incremental exercise on a bicycle ergometer in eumenorrheic untrained women. LH = luteinizing hormone; FSH = follicle-stimulating hormone; PRL = prolactin; TSH = thyroid-stimulating hormone; GH = growth hormone; A = androstenedione; T = testosterone; E₂ = estradiol; E₁ = estrone; DHEA = dehydroepiandrosterone. (From Rebar RW: Effects of exercise on reproductive function in females. *In* Givens JR [ed]: The Hypothalamus, Chicago: Year Book Medical, 1984, pp 245–262.)

Thus, the changes in testosterone associated with exercise appear to be due to increased gonadal hormone secretion.

Virtually every pituitary peptide and gonadal and adrenal steroid hormone examined increases with exercise.[24, 54, 55] The differences in the time courses of the increases of cortisol and dehydroepiandrosterone (of adrenal origin) from that of testosterone again suggest separate adrenal and gonadal secretion. It is tempting to speculate that the dramatic increases in these hormones with exercise allow humans to better respond to exercise. It is also possible that repeated episodes of acute exercise, with these associated hormonal changes, may precipitate menstrual dysfunction in susceptible individuals.

It has been suggested that the recurrent hyperprolactinemia associated with recurrent exercise may contribute to menstrual dysfunction.[57] No data support this hypothesis. In fact, it has been reported that amenorrheic runners who perform strenuous exercise exhibit no increase in serum prolactin levels, in contrast to eumenorrheic runners and sedentary (control) women.[58] Thus, no available data support any role for prolactin in exercise-associated amenorrhea.

HYPOTHALAMIC DYSFUNCTION

The pulsatile secretion of LH is decreased in both eumenorrheic and amenorrheic runners as compared with normal sedentary women.[22] These data suggest that diminished GnRH secretion in the hypothalamus is associated with endurance training. This observation also supports the notion that exercise-associated amenorrhea is "hypothalamic amenorrhea." That the hypothalamic dysfunction is minimal is suggested by the finding that temperature regulation is normal in amenorrheic women runners[32] and profoundly abnormal in women with anorexia nervosa and weight loss–associated amenorrhea.[59, 60]

MULTIFACTORIAL CAUSATION?

Together, the data suggest that the cause of exercise-associated reproductive dysfunction is complex and ultimately involves hypothalamic dysfunction (Fig. 29–7). Although the hypothalamic dysfunction may well result from metabolic alterations in the periphery, a central cause for the amenorrhea cannot be excluded. Exercise-associated changes in reproductive function in women appear to result from the complex interaction of physical, hormonal, nutritional, psycho-

Figure 29–7. Diagram of some of the factors involved in the pathophysiology of exercise-associated amenorrhea. (From Rebar RW: Effects of exercise on reproductive function in females. *In* Givens JR [ed]: The Hypothalamus. Chicago: Year Book Medical, 1984, pp 245–262.)

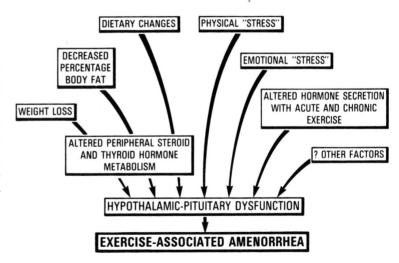

logical, and environmental factors. Weight loss, decreased body fat, and voluntary changes in diet may induce changes in peripheral steroid and thyroid hormone metabolism. Altered feedback signals transmitted to the hypothalamic-pituitary unit might then contribute to reproductive dysfunction. Other factors described in this chapter, may be important as well. At present, it seems overly simplistic to suggest that exercise-associated reproductive dysfunction has a single cause. In addition, it seems appropriate to regard exercise-associated amenorrhea as a form of hypothalamic amenorrhea, related and similar to yet distinct from, psychogenic amenorrhea, anorexia nervosa, and amenorrhea associated with malnutrition (Fig. 29–8). "Pure" forms of each of these can be identified, and some women suffer from "overlapping" forms.

OSTEOPOROSIS AS A CONSEQUENCE OF REPRODUCTIVE DYSFUNCTION

Bone-mass increases in response to exercise but decreases in hypoestrogenic women. Thus, several studies have shown that spinal bone mineral density is increased in athletes who have normal menses but is decreased in those with exercise-associated amenorrhea.[61–64]

Although it is not yet clear precisely why there is this association between exercise-associated amenorrhea and decreased bone mass, several factors might play a role. The decrease could be due to delayed skeletal maturation, accelerated bone loss, or both. Individuals more likely to become amenorrheic generally begin endurance training at an earlier age than do the others, so

Figure 29–8. Theoretical representation of the associations among various forms of functional hypothalamic amenorrhea. These disorders appear to be closely related. (From Rebar RW: The reproductive age: Chronic anovulation. *In* Serra G [ed]. Comprehensive Endocrinology. The Ovary. New York: Raven Press, 1983, pp 241–256.)

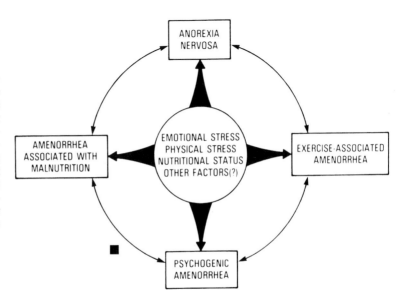

they may never acquire as much bone mass as eumenorrheic athletes. In addition, athletes' diets may not supply enough calcium relative to the needs of some.

From the study of Drinkwater and colleagues,[65] it appears that the osteopenia in amenorrheic athletes is reversible. In seven amenorrheic athletes whose menses returned (probably owing to a decrease in the severity of the exercise), the bone mineral density in the lumbar spine increased by an average of 6.3% over 15.5 months, as compared with a decrease of 0.3% in seven regularly menstruating athletes. It would seem that the return of ovarian function, when it occurs within several years of the onset of amenorrhea, results in an increase in bone mass. It is not yet known if the bone loss is irreversible in women whose amenorrhea persists for many years. What appears to be the case is that the hypoestrogenic hypogonadism in women with exercise-associated amenorrhea interferes with the normally beneficial effects of exercise on bone mass. There can be little doubt that the bone loss also is accelerated by the nutritional disturbances so common in amenorrheic athletes.

Warren and her colleagues have extended these observations in young ballet dancers.[66] In a survey of 75 professional dancers, the prevalence of scoliosis was 24%. Dancers with scoliosis were much more apt to have had delayed menarche (to age 14 years or later). The incidence of fractures (61%) also rose with age at menarche. The incidence of secondary amenorrhea was twice as high among the dancers with stress fractures as among those who did not give such a history. Thus, their data, too, suggest that delayed menarche and prolonged intervals of hypoestrogenic amenorrhea may predispose ballet dancers to scoliosis and stress fractures.

Together, these data indicate the importance in recognizing and treating young athletes with hypoestrogenism. It would seem prudent to discourage women who train for endurance from doing so to the extent that menstrual function is impaired.

EVALUATION AND TREATMENT OF ATHLETES WITH REPRODUCTIVE DYSFUNCTION

Women who appear to be at particularly high risk for exercise-associated amenorrhea include runners, gymnasts, ballet dancers, cyclists, and lightweight rowers.[67] Regardless of their sport, however, athletes with menstrual dysfunction should be evaluated in the same way as any woman who presents with similar complaints. Because most competitive athletes begin training in childhood, these reproductive disorders are common in adolescents. It is important to resist the temptation to ascribe an athlete's reproductive dysfunction to her exercise without first evaluating her. Exercise-associated reproductive dysfunction must be a diagnosis of exclusion.

DELAYED PUBERTY

Puberty is generally defined as *delayed* when no secondary sexual characteristics have developed by age 13, or menarche has not occurred by age 16, or 5 years after breast budding.

In any teenager with delayed puberty, any possible serious cause must be excluded. It is particularly important in young athletes to consider the age of onset and type and intensity of endurance training. Anorexia nervosa and bulimia also warrant consideration. It is important to ask about the dietary patterns of athletic teens with delayed puberty. Any evidence of a central neurologic disturbance, thyroid dysfunction, adrenal or pituitary disorders, or diabetes mellitus should be sought. An obstructed outflow tract should be apparent on pelvic examination and should be suspected if there is a history of intermittent abdominal pain and—especially primary amenorrhea—in a girl with normally developed secondary sexual characteristics.

In the absence of an obvious cause, minimal laboratory evaluation includes measurement of circulating FSH, TSH, and prolactin concentrations. Radiographic estimation of bone age is generally indicated. A karyotype is warranted when genetic abnormalities are possible and for girls with elevated levels of FSH.

Girls with delayed puberty as a result of endurance training have no significant abnormalities on evaluation. FSH concentrations are generally low to normal and are typical of those in normal prepubertal children, as are those for LH if it, too, is determined. The bone age may be delayed. It is important to ensure that the diet is adequate and, because of the risk of osteopenia, especially calcium intake. Reassurance, counseling, and adjustment of training patterns should prompt resumption of pubertal development. It is important to follow affected girls closely to be certain that a significant abnormality is not overlooked.

SECONDARY AMENORRHEA OR OLIGOMENORRHEA

In general, exercise-associated amenorrhea is characterized by low to normal levels of circulating FSH, LH, and prolactin. Radiographic assessment of the sella turcica is indicated whenever both FSH and LH levels are less than 10 mIU/ml, even in the absence of normal serum prolactin levels, to rule out pituitary adenoma.

The nutritional status of women engaged in endurance training must always be investigated. Those who begin such training without close professional supervision seem more apt to change their diets and suffer from unrecognized mineral (especially calcium and iron) deficiencies. As a consequence, a dietary history and complete blood count and basic blood chemistries are indicated whenever exercise-associated amenorrhea is the presumptive diagnosis. Dietary calcium, iron, and protein appear especially likely to be diminished.[18, 25a] Despite advice that adolescents and young adults consume 1200 mg of elemental calcium each day, very few young women get this much calcium from their diet alone. The National Health and Nutrition Examination Survey II found a mean calcium intake of 764 mg/day for girls between 15 and 17 years of age.[67a] For young women aged 18 to 24 years, the mean intake was 679 mg/day.

In view of the very real risk of osteopenia, calcium supplementation is warranted and exogenous estrogen should be encouraged in women with exercise-associated amenorrhea. Because vitamin D deficiency predisposes to osteoporosis, it is not unreasonable to recommend ingestion of 400 IU of vitamin D each day. Low-dose oral contraceptives maintain bone density in hypoestrogenic amenorrheic athletes and will provide contraception as well. For women who are not sexually active, cyclic estrogen and progestin may be provided as an alternative. There is no evidence that suppression of the hypothalamic-pituitary axis by exogenous steroids has any adverse effect on subsequent reproductive function, however, women must be informed that their amenorrhea may persist after exogenous steroids are withdrawn. Thus, ovulation induction may be necessary when pregnancy is desired. Despite the advantages of therapy, many amenorrheic athletes refuse exogenous estrogen, sometimes citing concerns about a decline in performance and sometimes complaining of the side effects of hormone therapy, including breast tenderness, bloating, nausea, and mood swings. It appears that, for most women, the effects on performance are inconsequential.[67b] Amenorrheic ones who refuse exogenous estrogen should have periodic estimates of spinal bone density to monitor for accelerated bone loss.

If exercise-associated menstrual dysfunction describes a continuum from luteal dysfunction, to oligomenorrhea, to euestrogenic amenorrhea, and finally to hypoestrogenic amenorrhea, athletes with oligomenorrhea and euestrogenic amenorrhea (though these stages appear to be brief) should be at increased risk for endometrial hyperplasia. Women seem either to progress to hypoestrogenic amenorrhea or to resume regular menses. No report has yet been published of any woman with exercise-associated amenorrhea developing endometrial hyperplasia.

Despite the relative hypoestrogenism of most amenorrheic athletes, complaints of signs and symptoms of estrogen deficiency are few. Thus, it is possible that the accelerated bone loss reported is due as much to dietary calcium inadequacy as to hypoestrogenism. It is difficult to believe that athletes so in tune with their bodies would fail to note the vaginal dryness, hot flushes, and emotional lability associated with hypoestrogenism.

Amenorrheic athletes who refuse to use oral contraceptives should be advised to utilize some other form of contraception if they are sexually active and do not want to become pregnant. For the majority of women with exercise-associated amenorrhea menses resume, and in many cases they ovulate before any menstruation. Often, minor changes in diet or training promote resumption of ovulation and cyclic menses.

CONCLUSIONS

An understanding of the reproductive abnormalities that can accompany endurance training in women is necessary to counsel and treat women athletes properly. Although the causes of these reproductive disorders are not understood, it is nevertheless possible to make rational recommendations to amenorrheic women. It is important to reassure the patient that the disorder is not serious if treated properly. Failure to treat an amenorrheic athlete, however, can have permanent sequelae. It is also important to remember that accumulating data indicate that male athletes who engage in endurance training can also have relative hypogonadism.

REFERENCES

1. Malina RM, Harper AB, Avent HH, Campbell DE: Age at menarche in athletes and non-athletes. Med Sci Sports 1973; 5:11.
2. Malina RM, Spirduso WW, Tate C, Baylor AM: Age at menarche and selected characteristics in athletes at different competitive levels and in different sports. Med Sci Sports 1978; 10:218.

3. Shangold MM, Kelly M, Berkeley AS, et al: The relationship between menarcheal age and adult height. South Med J 1989; 82:443.

4. Frisch RE, Gotz-Welbergen AV, McArthur JW, et al: Delayed menarche, irregular cycles and amenorrhea of college athletes in relation to the age of onset of training. JAMA 1981; 246:1559.

5. Frisch RE, Wyshak G, Vincent L: Delayed menarche and amenorrhea in ballet dancers. N Engl J Med 1980; 303:17.

6. Warren MP: The effects of exercise on pubertal progression and reproductive function in girls. J Clin Endocrinol Metab 1980; 51:1150.

6a. American College of Sports Medicine: The female athlete triad: Disordered eating, amenorrhea, and osteoporosis. Call to action. Sports Med Bull 1992; 27:4.

7. Frisch RE, McArthur J: Menstrual cycles: Fatness as a determinant of minimum weight for height necessary for their maintenance or onset. Science 1974; 185:949.

8. Bonen A, Belcastro AN, Ling WY, Simpson AA: Profiles of selected hormones during menstrual cycles of teenage athletes. J Appl Physiol 1981; 50:545.

9. Shangold M, Freeman R, Thysen B, Gatz M: The relationship between long distance running, plasma progesterone and luteal phase length. Fertil Steril 1979; 31:130.

10. Prior JC, Ho Yuen B, Bowie L, et al: Reversible luteal phase defect and infertility associated with marathon running. Lancet 1982; 2:269.

11. Prior JC: Luteal phase defects and anovulation: Adaptive alterations occurring with conditioning exercise. Semin Reprod Endocrinol 1985; 3:27.

12. Schweiger U, Laessle R, Schweiger M, et al: Caloric intake, stress, and menstrual function in athletes. Fertil Steril 1988; 49:447.

13. Ellison PT, Lager C: Moderate recreational running is associated with lowered salivary progesterone profiles in women. Am J Obstet Gynecol 1986; 154:1000.

14. Hoffman D, Villanueva A, Mezrow G, et al: Luteal phase abnormalities in elite eumenorrheic runners. Abstracts of the 35th Annual Meeting of the Society for Gynecologic Investigation. (Abstract #220). Baltimore, MD, March 17–20, 1988.

15. Beitins IZ, McArthur JW, Turnbull BA, et al: Exercise induces two types of luteal dysfunction: Confirmation by urinary free progesterone. J Clin Endocrinol Metab 1991; 72:1350.

16. Feicht CB, Johnson JS, Martin BJ, et al: Secondary amenorrhea in athletes. Lancet 1978; 2:1145.

17. Dale E, Gerlach DH, Whilhite AL: Menstrual dysfunction in distance runners. Obstet Gynecol 1979; 54:47.

18. Schwartz B, Cumming DC, Riordan E, et al: Exercise-associated amenorrhea: A distinct entity? Am J Obstet Gynecol 1981; 141:662.

19. Shangold MM, Levine HS: The effect of marathon training upon menstrual function. Am J Obstet Gynecol 1982; 143:862.

20. Feicht Sanborn C, Martin BJ, Wagner WW Jr: Is athletic amenorrhea specific to runners? Am J Obstet Gynecol 1982; 143:859.

21. Bullen BA, Skrinar GS, Beitins IZ, et al: Induction of menstrual disorders by strenuous exercise in untrained women. N Engl J Med 1985; 312:1349.

22. Bullen BA, Skrinar GS, Beitins IZ, et al: Induction of menstrual disorders by strenuous exercise in untrained women. N Engl J Med 1985; 312:1349.

23. Cumming DC, Vickovic MM, Wall SR, Fluker MR: Defects in pulsatile LH release in normally menstruating runners. J Clin Endocrinol Metab 1985; 60:810.

24. Cumming DC, Rebar RW: Hormonal changes with acute exercise and with training in women. Semin Reprod Endocrinol 1985; 3:55.

25. Pugliese MT, Lifshitz F, Grad G, et al: Fear of obesity: A cause of short stature and delayed puberty. N Engl J Med 1983; 309:513.

25a. Marcus R, Cann C, Madvig P, et al: Menstrual function and bone mass in elite women distance runners: Endocrine and metabolic features. Ann Intern Med 1985; 102:158.

26. Deuster PA, Kyle SB, Moser PB, et al: Nutritional intakes and status of highly trained amenorrheic and eumenorrheic women runners. Fertil Steril 1986; 45:636.

26a. Brooks-Gunn J, Warren MP, Hamilton LH: The relationship of eating disorders to amenorrhea in ballet dancers. Med Sci Sports Exerc 1987; 19:41.

26b. Burckes-Miller ME, Black DR: Male and female college athletes: Prevalence of anorexia nervosa and bulimia nervosa. Athletic Training 1988; 2:137.

26c. Rosen LW, Hough DO: Pathogenic weight-control behaviors of female college gymnasts. Physician Sports Med 1988; 16:141.

26d. Putukian M: The female athlete triad. Clin Sports Med 1998; 17:675.

27. Baker ER, Mathur RS, Kirk RF, Williamson HO: Female runners and secondary amenorrhea: Correlation with age, parity, mileage, and plasma hormonal and sex hormone–binding globulin concentrations. Fertil Steril 1981; 36:183.

28. Anderson JL: Women's sports and fitness programs at the US Military Academy. Physician Sports Med 1979; 7:72.

29. Rasmussen DD, Gambacciani M, Swartz W, et al: Pulsatile gonadotropin-releasing hormone release from the human mediobasal hypothalamus in vitro: Opiate receptor–mediated suppression. Neuroendocrinology 1989; 49:150.

30. Carr DB, Bullen BA, Skrinar GS, et al: Physical conditioning facilitates the exercise-induced secretion of beta-endorphin and beta-lipotropin in women. N Engl J Med 1981; 305:560.

31. McArthur JW, Bullen BA, Beitins IZ, et al: Hypothalamic amenorrhea in runners of normal body composition. Endocr Res Commun 1980; 7:13.

32. Dixon G, Eurman P, Stern B, et al: Hypothalamic function in amenorrheic runners. Fertil Steril 1984; 42:377.

33. Rogol AD, Veldhuis JD, Williams FT, Johnson ML: Pulsatile secretion of gonadotropins and prolactin in endurance-trained men: Relation to the endogenous opiate system. J Androl 1984; 5:21.

34. Villanueva AL, Schlosser C, Hopper B, et al: Increased cortisol production in women runners. J Clin Endocrinol Metab 1986; 63:126.

35. Ding J-H, Sheckter CB, Drinkwater BL, et al: High serum cortisol levels in exercise-associated amenorrhea. Ann Intern Med 1988; 108:530.

36. Baldwin DM, Sawyer CH: Effects of dexamethasone on LH release and ovulation in the cyclic rat. Endocrinology 1974; 94:1397.

37. Liptrap RM: Effect of corticotropin and corticosteroids on oestrus, ovulation and oestrogen excretion in the sow. J Endocrinol 1970; 47:197.

38. Stoebel DP, Moberg GP: Effect of ACTH and cortisol on estrous behavior and the luteinizing hormone surge in cows. Fed Proc 1979; 38:1254.

39. Matteri RL, Watson JG, Moberg GP: Stress and acute adrenocorticotropin treatment suppresses LHRH-induced LH release in the ram. J Reprod Fertil 1984; 72:385.

40. Cunningham GR, Goldzieher JW, de LaPena A, Oliver M: The mechanism of ovulation inhibition by triamcinolone acetonide. J Clin Endocrinol Metab 1978; 46:8.

41. Rivier C, Vale W: Influence of corticotropin-releasing factor on reproductive functions in the rat. Endocrinology 1984; 114:914.

42. Ono N, Lumpkin MD, Samson WK, et al: Intrahypothalamic action of corticotropin-releasing factor (CRF) to inhibit growth hormone and LH release in the rat. Life Sci 1984; 35:1117.

43. Olster DH, Ferin M: Corticotropin-releasing hormone inhibits gonadotropin secretion in the ovariectomized rhesus monkey. J Clin Endocrinol Metab 1987; 65:262.

44. Petraglia F, Sutton S, Vale W, Plotsky P: Corticotropin-releasing factor decreases plasma luteinizing hormone levels in female rats by inhibiting gonadotropin-releasing hormone release into hypophysial-portal circulation. Endocrinology 1987; 120:1083.

45. Gambacciani M, Yen SSC, Rasmussen DD: GnRH release from the mediobasal hypothalamus: *in vitro* inhibition by corticotropin-releasing factor. Neuroendocrinology 1986; 43:533.

46. Rivier C, Rivier J, Vale W: Stress-induced inhibition of reproductive functions: Role of endogenous corticotropin-releasing factor. Science 1986; 231:607.

47. Petraglia F, Vale W, Rivier C: Opioids act centrally to modulate stress-induced decrease in luteinizing hormone in the rat. Endocrinology 1986; 119:2445.

48. Almeida OFX, Nikolarakis KE, Herz A: Evidence for the involvement of endogenous opioids in the inhibition of luteinizing hormone by corticotropin-releasing factor. Endocrinology 1988; 122:1034.

49. Gindoff PR, Ferin M: Endogenous opioid peptides modulate the effect of corticotropin-releasing factor on gonadotropin release in the primate. Endocrinology 1987; 121:837.

50. Xiao E, Luckhaus J, Niemann W, Ferin M: Acute inhibition of gonadotropin secretion by corticotropin-releasing hormone in the primate: Are the adrenal glands involved? Endocrinology 1989; 124:1632.

51. Barbarino A, DeMarinis L, Folli G, et al: Corticotropin-releasing hormone inhibition of gonadotropin secretion during the menstrual cycle. Metabolism 1989; 38:504.

52. Barbarino A, De Marinis L, Tofani A, et al: Corticotropin-releasing hormone inhibition of gonadotropin release and the effect of opioid blockade. J Clin Endocrinol Metab 1989; 68:523.

53. Thomas MA, Rebar RW, LaBarbera AR, et al: Dose-response effects of exogenous pulsatile human corticotropin-releasing hormone on ACTH, cortisol and gonadotropin concentrations in agonadal women. J Clin Endocrinol Metab 1991; 72:1249.

54. Cumming DC, Rebar RW: Exercise and reproductive function in women: A review. Am J Ind Med 1983; 4:113.

55. Cumming DC, Brunsting LA III, Strich G, et al: Reproductive hormone increases in response to acute exercise in men. Med Sci Sports Exerc 1986; 18:369.

56. Rebar RW, Benson M, Stern B, et al: Hormonal responses to acute exercise in oophorectomized and normal menstruating women. Abstracts of the 67th Annual Meeting of The Endocrine Society. (Abstract #977). Baltimore, Md, 1985.

57. Baker ER: Menstrual dysfunction and hormonal status in athletic women: A review. Fertil Steril 1981; 36:691.

58. Bremer B, Cumming D, Stern B, et al: Hormonal responses to acute exercise in women with psychogenic hypothalamic amenorrhea (HA) and exercise-associated amenorrhea. Abstracts of the 31st Annual Meeting of the Society for Gynecologic Investigation. San Francisco, California, 1984: Abstract #281, p. 165.

59. Vigersky RA, Loriaux DL, Andersen AE, et al: Delayed pituitary hormone response to LRF and TRF in patients with anorexia nervosa and with secondary amenorrhea associated with simple weight loss. J Clin Endocrinol Metab 1976; 43:893.

60. Vigersky RA, Andersen AE, Thompson RH, Loriaux DL: Hypothalamic dysfunction in secondary amenorrhea associated with simple weight loss. N Engl J Med 1977; 297:1141.

61. Cann CE, Martin MC, Genant HK, Jaffe RB: Decreased spinal mineral content in amenorrheic women. JAMA 1984; 251:626.

62. Drinkwater BL, Nilson K, Chestnut CH III, et al: Bone mineral content of amenorrheic and eumenorrheic athletes. N Engl J Med 1984; 311:277.

63. Marcus R, Cann C, Madvig P, et al: Menstrual function and bone mass in elite women distance runners. Ann Intern Med 1985; 102:158.

64. Wolman RL: Bone mineral density levels in elite female athletes. Ann Rheum Dis 1990; 49:1013.

65. Drinkwater BL, Nilson K, Ott S, Chesnut CH III: Bone mineral density after resumption of menses in amenorrheic athletes. JAMA 1986; 256:380.

66. Warren MP, Brooks-Gunn J, Hamilton LH, et al: Scoliosis and fractures in young ballet dancers. Relation to delayed menarche and secondary amenorrhea. N Engl J Med 1986; 314:1348.

67. Wolman RL, Harries MG: Menstrual abnormalities in elite athletes. Clin Sports Med 1989; 1:95.

67a. Carroll MD, Abraham M, Dresser CM: Dietary Source Intake Data: United States 1976–1980. Hyattsville, Md: U.S. Department of Human Services Publication No. 83-168, 1983.

67b. Fagan KM: Pharmacologic management of athletic amenorrhea. Clin Sports Med 1998; 2:327.

68. Rebar RW: Effects of exercise on reproductive function in female. *In* Givens JR (ed): The Hypothalamus. Chicago: Year Book, 1984; pp 245–262.

69. Rebar RW: The reproductive age: Chronic anovulation. *In* Serra G (ed): Comprehensive Endocrinology. The Ovary. New York: Raven Press, 1983; pp 241–256.

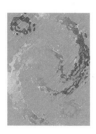

Chapter 30

Reproductive Health Care Needs of the Developmentally Disabled

David Muram and Thomas E. Elkins

The professional approach to caring for and supporting (in this case) females who live with developmental disabilities has witnessed significant changes since the 1970s. Patients who then were residents in hospitals and chronic care institutions are now integrated into the community (Tables 30–1, 30–2). The presence in communities of the former patients has necessitated a major reorganization of rehabilitation and training services. This rehabilitation effort has extended beyond vocational training, in an attempt to incorporate means of addressing these persons' social and emotional needs. Those who have moved into the community have realized a significant improvement in their quality of life. By acquiring new skills, disabled persons can take advantage of previously unavailable education and employment opportunities that enable them to lead as normal a life as possible. Studies have shown, however, that, for persons with disabilities, holding a job is often more difficult than getting one.[1]

The healthcare system must also adjust to these changes. The care provided in an institution may be very different from that provided in the community. Previously, preventive care, routine examinations, immunizations, and treatment of minor illnesses were provided by most institutions, and contracts with hospitals provided acute care for serious illness; minimal involvement on the part of patients or their families was needed to secure adequate health care. Today, as residents in the community, they must seek their own care, participate in the decision making, and be partially responsible for complying with prescribed treatment. Some communities may not be equipped to provide medical services that

are as accessible or as comprehensive as some residents need, especially those with complex conditions. A survey of community medical care for persons with mental retardation revealed that 89% of the study group had found a medical practitioner, and 90% were receiving adequate medical care.[2] Preventive gynecologic care was notably wanting: 60% of women had had no examination in the preceding 3 years.[3]

The healthcare needs of persons with developmental disabilities vary with the disability, so generalizations cannot be made (Table 30–3). Whereas some are only physically limited, others may be both physically and mentally disabled. Those with minor impairments have healthcare needs similar to those of the general population and thus do not require special consideration. Those at the other end of the spectrum require

Table 30–1. Prevalence of Disability According to Degree of Limitation for Adolescents 10 to 18 Years of Age, United States, 1984*

Degree of Limitation	% Distribution	Estimated Prevalence (thousands)
Unable to conduct major activity	0.5	165
Limited in kind or amount of major activity	3.7	1,185
Limited in other activities	2.0	629
Not limited	93.8	29,862

*Original tabulations from public use tapes, National Health Interview Survey.

From Newacheck PW: Adolescents with special health needs: Prevalence, severity and access to health services. Pediatrics 1989; 84:872–881.

Table 30–2. Prevalence of Mental Retardation in Urban and Rural Areas

Area	Age (yr)	Prevalence/1000 population		Comments
		Urban	*Rural*	
England and Wales	0–16	3.51	4.88	
	17–60+	3.20	5.61	
	Total°	6.71	10.49	
Onondaga County, NY	0–17	36.8	33.4	
New York State	5–15	2.9 (New York City)	2.3 (villages)	Includes only severe mental retardation.
		3.7 (other cities)	3.0 (rest of state)	
Wessex, England	15–19	3.54 (county boroughs)	3.84 (counties)	Includes only severe mental retardation.
Northeast Scotland	0–80+	3.63	3.02	For mild mental retardation.
		2.02	2.25	For severe mental retardation.
Netherlands	19	34.2	26.7	Schooling as the criterion for mild mental retardation.
		52.1	62.4	Raven matrices as the criterion for mild mental retardation.
		56.6	66.8	ICD† code as the criterion for mild mental retardation.
		0.63	0.63	Men with severe mental retardation with diagnosis of Down syndrome.
		3.13	3.34	All men with severe mental retardation except those with Down syndrome.

°Totals are not age-adjusted.
†ICD, *International Classification of Diseases* (1948).
From Kiely M: The prevalence of mental retardation. Epidemiol Rev 1987; 9:194–218.

very sophisticated and specialized care. The healthcare delivery system must be sensitive and responsive to these different needs to be able to provide not only basic care, but also the very special services required by those with severe disabilities.

Furthermore, the healthcare needs of persons with disabilities are constantly changing (Table 30–4). With improved medical technology and care, their life expectancy is greater today than ever before, as exemplified by a survey of persons with Down syndrome.[4] Many of them live a long life and, therefore, require different services and medical care. The older persons in this population who have multiple disabilities present an even greater challenge to the community service system.

ACCESS TO CARE

How healthcare is delivered is directly shaped by how it is financed. Many disabled persons rely on Medicaid to defray healthcare costs (Table 30–5). The disincentives to integrating these persons into the "mainstream" are compounded by inefficient payment mechanisms.[5] If the special

Table 30–3. Leading Causes of Disability Among Adolescents 10 to 18 Years of Age, United States, 1984*

Main Cause of Disability	Estimated Prevalence (thousands)
Mental disorders	634
Diseases of the respiratory system	406
Diseases of the musculoskeletal system and connective tissue	295
Diseases of nervous system	115
Diseases of the ear and mastoid process	80

*Original tabulations from public use tapes, National Health Interview Survey.
From Newacheck PW: Adolescents with special health needs: Prevalence, severity and access to health services. Pediatrics 1989; 84:872–881.

Table 30–4. Reproductive Health Care Needs of the Developmentally Disabled

Accessibility to care
Care providers' ability to listen to family members
Coordination of professional services
Specific medical problems that interfere with the gynecologic examination
Communication with the patient
Obtaining an adequate cervical smear for cytologic examination
Menarche and subsequent menstrual hygiene

Table 30–5. Health Care Coverage Characteristics According to Disability Status for Adolescents 10 to 18 Years of Age, United States, 1984*

Coverage Status of Adolescents With Known Coverage Status†	Distribution (%)		
	All Adolescents	*Adolescents With Disabilities*	*Adolescents Without Disabilities*
	100.0	100.0	100.0
Private only	74.0	64.6	74.7
Public only	10.0	18.6	9.4
Both private and public	1.9	3.0	1.8
None reported	14.1	13.8	14.1

*Original tabulations from public use tapes, National Health Interview Survey.
†Persons with unknown health care coverage status excluded.
From Newacheck PW: Adolescents with special health needs: Prevalence, severity and access to health services. Pediatrics 1989; 84:872–881.

requirements of persons with disabilities are not taken into account, certain problems can be expected:

- Attempts to provide periodic examinations for prevention, screening, and health maintenance programs will be curtailed.
- Choices among providers will be restricted.
- The quality of healthcare services will be inferior to the modal quality of services in the community.
- Healthcare will become increasingly crisis oriented.

Even so, persons with disabilities are more likely to require hospitalization, and their total hospital charges are almost twice the rate for the general population.[6]

Availability of medical and mental health services is essential to ensure delivery of appropriate care. Healthcare professionals are expected to be not only competent but also understanding, sensitive, and empathetic. They should be skilled in listening to family members and care providers and willing to include them in the decision-making process. Above all, professional services delivered by various specialists and agencies must be well-coordinated.[7]

Like the general population, persons with disabilities require the services of an identified primary healthcare provider who assumes longitudinal responsibility for their overall well-being, furnishes general medical and preventive care, and makes referrals to specialty care when appropriate. In such a setting, the person's health status is well-known, an up-to-date and comprehensive medical record exists, and a long-term relationship can be developed with the patient and the family. Compliance with appointments and therapy is better when patients are in an appropriate setting.[8–10]

REPRODUCTIVE HEALTH CARE NEEDS

The reproductive healthcare needs of a disabled child or adolescent are no different from those of the general population. The disability, however, may create difficulties for healthcare providers. Even young girls with disabilities may suffer from multiple health problems requiring consultation with specialists and continuous medical attention. In one study, investigators found associated medical conditions in 80% of children with mental retardation.[11] Children with lower intelligence quotients had more complicated medical problems, that resulted in more significant disability.

From a medical perspective, persons with severe physical disabilities also have specific concerns that require constant monitoring and, frequently, intervention:

1. Seizure disorders are common and may be complex. Multidrug anticonvulsant therapy may be required for optimal management and may cause medication interactions, interfere with the menstrual cycle, and even impair the child's ability to interact with others.
2. Multiple joint contractures, which often preclude ambulation, cause impaired sitting posture and render a conventional pelvic examination impossible.
3. Nutrition is often compromised by feeding difficulties. Gastroesophageal reflux with vomiting further aggravates the situation.

An additional complication is that many of these patients have only limited ability to communicate. An alteration in behavior may be the only sign of a physical ailment. Although many care providers are attuned to this fact, particularly those who have known the person for some-

Table 30–6. Ability to Perform Pelvic Examination in 150 Mentally Handicapped Females

Complete pelvic exam	26
Bimanual/cotton swab	91
Complete pelvic exam with sedation	
Chloral hydrate	0/8
Ketamine/Midazolam	21/25
Exam under general anesthesia	12

From Rosen DA, Rosen KR, Elkins TE, et al: Outpatient sedation: An essential addition to gynecologic care for persons with mental retardation. Am J Obstet Gynecol 1991; 164:825–828.

time, the severity of the problem may not be recognized and provision of the appropriate medical attention is sometimes delayed. This is a serious issue and should be addressed regularly in training and supervision.

THE GYNECOLOGIC EXAMINATION

The gynecologic examination can create significant anxiety for any adolescent girl. A girl with mental retardation may have only a limited understanding of the examination and its purpose and may refuse to be examined (Table 30–6). Obtaining a cervical smear for cytologic examination may be impossible. Nevertheless, these periodic examinations are required as part of the routine preventive care recommended for all patients (Table 30–7). The physician may wish to modify the method of collection, but a smear may identify patients with cytologic abnormalities.[12, 13]

Patients with disabilities are sensitive to healthcare professionals' attitude. They tend to withdraw if the caregiver is hurried, brusque, or indifferent, but they react positively to a clinician who is kind, warm, and patient. The presence of the mother or the care provider in the examina-

Table 30–7. The Gynecologic Examination

Physician should be sensitive, warm, and kind
Preexamination education
Use of lifelike dolls and a slide presentation
Encourage patient to help with the examination
Patient should have a sense of control over the examination process
Cytosmear with a cotton-tipped swab over a finger inserted into the vagina and directed toward the cervix
Bimanual (rectal) examination
Vaginoscopy when indicated
Periodic sonogram in lieu of pelvic examination
Sedation only when required

tion room often provides a sense of security. Preexamination education is key to a successful examination. Lifelike dolls and slide presentations that describe the examination process have been helpful when performing pelvic examinations in difficult-to-examine patients.[14, 15] The patient should be encouraged to help with the examination, to gain a sense of control and alleviate apprehension. Satisfactory palpation of the pelvic organs is usually accomplished by performing a rectal examination and should not cause pain. Samples for cytologic smears may be obtained by inserting a cotton-tipped swab over a finger into the vagina and directing it toward the cervix. When the vagina requires evaluation, special instruments (e.g., vaginoscope, Huffman-Graves virginal speculum.) may be required. As for any young patient, familiarizing her with the instrument before insertion usually reduces apprehension. Allowing her to touch the instrument is encouraged. She should notice that it feels slippery and cool. The instrument is then placed against the inner thigh, as the examiner reminds the patient that it feels cool, slippery, and unusual. Only then is the instrument passed through the hymenal orifice. Vaginoscopy should not be attempted without sedation or general anesthesia if the aperture is too small for an instrument to be passed without discomfort or if the patient is uncooperative. Periodic sonograms may be substituted for routine pelvic assessment for certain patients, especially when a Pap smear is not required. Oral ketamine and midazolam (used alone or together) have provided enough sedation to allow outpatient pelvic examinations in more than 80% of patients who otherwise would have required general anesthesia for routine care (see Table 31–6).[16] Occasionally, some patients do not tolerate a gynecologic examination. In one large series, the investigators reviewed 574 charts, for a total of 1235 pelvic examinations. Of these, 845 examinations were completed initially, 177 required sedation (14%), and 213 (17%) could not be completed.[13]

SEXUALITY

Although many physicians are familiar with the unusual medical requirements of the developmentally disabled, some are still uncomfortable dealing with issues of sexuality in this population. It is widely accepted that every human needs to develop his or her sexual feelings and be able to express these feelings freely. Because disabled persons today live in the community, their sexuality is no longer a hidden matter (Ta-

Table 30–8. Percentage of Mentally Retarded Individuals Who Had Experienced Various Sexual Activities More Than Two Times

Sexual Activity	% of Females	% of Males
Masturbation	30	60
Kissing a nonrelative of the opposite sex	60	70
Hugging and kissing for a long time	50	50
Going further than hugging and kissing	20	50

Modified from Ousley OY, Mesibov GB: Sexual attitudes and knowledge of high-functioning adolescents and adults with autism. J Autism Dev Disord 1991; 21:471–481.

ble 30–8; Figs. 30–1, 30–2). Although the accepted sociosexual model is to find a partner, marry, and have children, many perceive the expression or acting out of these desires by a disabled person as abnormal. Lack of proper education has caused even those people who approve of sexual expression to voice concerns that such sexual activity might increase the number of handicapped children.

When these patients were cared for in an institutional setting, physicians and other healthcare professionals were responsible for all their needs. A high standard of conduct was imposed on all patients, and any expression of sexuality was regarded as a potential public scandal that could damage the image of the institution. Sexual expression was regarded as a problem for which a solution must be found. The solution often was interdiction of the behavior and, thus, suppression of sexual expression, but this form of control cannot be exerted on patients who reside in the community. The fact that disabled people are sexual beings and have the right to express their feelings must be accepted. Instead of attempting to control their sexual behavior, professionals must help them to express it through accepted social channels.

Like other parents, many parents of disabled children are uncomfortable discussing sexuality. Although they would very much like their child to be "like everyone else," many do not wish that child to receive sex education. Some parents believe that ignorance makes children innocent and therefore less likely to have sexual experiences in the future. Many are convinced that the child has no interest in sexual expression and would have a sexual experience only because someone else would exploit their disability.

The concerns of parents vary as the child grows. Parents of a young girl with disabilities want to know how to prepare the girl for the physical changes of puberty. As the child matures, the major concepts are menstruation, personal hygiene, dating, possible sexual activity, avoidance of sexual abuse, and contraception. Parents of older patients are more concerned with the possibility of pregnancy, and many request that their daughters be surgically sterilized (Table 30–9).

A counseling program on sexuality should be offered to parents of children and adolescents with disabilities. Often, parents are alarmed when their child exhibits sexual behavior deemed inappropriate by them or other caregivers, such as teachers. Such counseling may also address other issues, such as sexual abuse, socialization education, and family stress.[16, 17] A man with mental disabilities may commit sex offenses against others.[18]

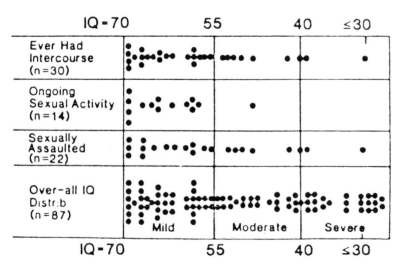

Figure 30–1. Sexual activity of mentally retarded subjects by intelligence level. (From Chamberlain A, Rauh J, Passer A, et al: Issues in fertility control for mentally retarded female adolescents: I. Sexual activity, sexual abuse, and contraception. Pediatrics 1984; 73:445–450.)

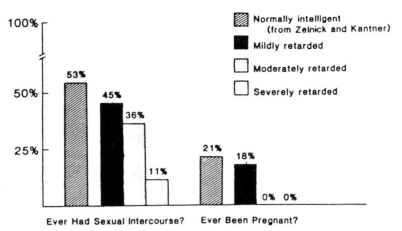

Figure 30–2. Sexual activity of mentally retarded subjects aged 15 to 19 years, and a sample of 15- to 19-year-old females of normal intelligence. (From Chamberlain A, Rauh J, Passer A, et al: Issues in fertility control for mentally retarded female adolescents: I. Sexual activity, sexual abuse, and contraception. Pediatrics 1984; 73:445–450.)

MENSTRUATION

For any girl, the first menstrual period can be a startling and frightening experience, and for a girl who is mentally disabled and inadequately prepared, it can be traumatic. Thus, many parents seek medical advice as pubertal changes become apparent. Almost all patients with developmental disabilities are evaluated either just before menarche or immediately after the first menstrual period. In some instances, menarche raises fears of initiation of sexual activity and, with it, the potential for unintended pregnancy. When parents feel that the child's supervision is insufficient (e.g., in school or a special program), they often request contraceptive advice. Like all school-aged children, those with developmental disabilities should be offered sex education appropriate for their level of understanding. Likewise, appropriate programs should be offered to the parents. Patients who are considered able to manage their own hygiene during menstruation should be provided with menstrual hygiene classes, and those who are sexually active should be given contraception.

Girls who are severely handicapped may not be able to provide proper perineal hygiene. For them, the menstrual blood sometimes causes significant problems, and they are often isolated from their normal environment during menstruation. Some who have had difficulty mastering toilet control may decompensate at this time. Others who are not toilet trained have an added problem to cope with. Many parents become frustrated and request that a hysterectomy be performed to abolish the menstrual cycle. In some clinics, poor menstrual hygiene is a leading indication for hysterectomy in girls with severe disabilities.

Anovulation and dysfunctional uterine bleeding are common in young adolescents after menarche, and adolescents with developmental disabilities are no exception. Many present with complaints of irregular and often heavy menstrual flow. Anovulatory cycles are common for the first year after menarche. Periods are often irregular, and the bleeding may be heavier than the flow in ovulatory cycles. Irregularity and heavy flow create additional difficulties for the patient and her family. The menstrual cycle may cause other problems as well. Some patients who suffer from epilepsy or emotional instability may notice a significant increase in the frequency of seizures or marked impairment of social behav-

Table 30–9. Parent Response to "Ever Thought of Sterilization?"

	No. of Parents Interviewed	Have you ever thought of sterilization for your daughter?			
		No	Yes, but decided against it	Yes, and still seeking	Yes, and obtained procedure
Mildly mentally retarded (MR)	33	24	3	6	0
Moderately MR	16	6	5	5	0
Severely MR	20	7	5	7	1
Total	69 (100%)	37 (54%)	13 (19%)	18 (26%)	1 (1%)

From Passer A, Rauh J, Chamberlain A, et al: Issues in fertility control for mentally retarded female adolescents: II. Parental attitudes toward sterilization. Pediatrics 1984; 73:451–454.

ior. Some are kept home from school during menstruation. This disruption in special educational efforts may increase isolation. To address this problem, a nursing staff or social worker is employed to conduct home training sessions for menstrual hygiene. This behavior modification program is often successful when the parents are supportive and the patient is toilet trained. When properly prepared, many parents are willing to let the menstrual cycle establish its own pattern.

Abolishing the menstrual cycle altogether, either medically or surgically, is another solution. Menstrual control can often be achieved using medroxyprogesterone acetate (DMPA). Adequate menstrual control is usually achieved and surgical intervention is seldom necessary. However, many centers perform endometrial ablation or hysterectomy as initial therapy to abolish the menstrual cycle in developmentally disabled patients.[19] Because the long-term risks and benefits of hysterectomy and those of DMPA have not been established, a specific treatment modality should be selected jointly by the individual physician and the patient's family.

CONTRACEPTION

Despite recent developments, options for contraception in this population continue to be quite limited. Barrier methods, which are highly effective when used properly by a well-motivated patient, may be suited for certain mentally disabled individuals. In addition, condoms protect against sexually transmitted diseases. These methods are particularly suitable for patients who infrequently have sexual exposure. Using a barrier method requires motivation and a supportive partner, and even normal healthy adolescents tend to use such methods haphazardly. The relationship is sometimes casual, and the long-term consequences are no deterrent to contraceptive failure.

Another option is an intrauterine contraceptive device (IUD). Once inserted, the IUD is quite effective, has a low failure rate, and requires no patient compliance. However, IUDs are in general not suitable for mentally disabled women, who may not recognize symptoms of the potential complications (e.g., pelvic inflammatory disease and ectopic pregnancy). Furthermore, the increased bleeding often associated with the IUD compounds hygiene problems.[20]

Oral contraceptives (OCs) are very effective, having a theoretical failure rate of less than 0.5%. The patient is required to take the medication daily, but in most instances the parents are supportive and can be trusted to ensure compliance.

OCs are obviously not suitable for women who cannot swallow pills or who live alone and may be noncompliant, or who experience severe side effects.

Long-term injectable contraceptives have been developed and are in use throughout the world. The agent most often used, DMPA, is a very effective method of contraception (failure rate 0.7 per 100 women-years for 12 months of use).[21] The medication has a low incidence of side effects, the most common complaint being breakthrough bleeding, which may, however, be quite disconcerting. Concerns have been raised that long-term use of DMPA may result in bone loss and thus predispose patients to osteoporosis.[22] Similarly, some physicians are concerned that DMPA, like other progestins, may cause weight gain and adversely affect blood lipids.[23] It is recommended that a baseline lipid profile be obtained so that patients at higher risk may be provided another contraceptive modality. Even so, long-term injectable contraceptives are widely used by persons with disabilities (Table 30–10).

Other injectable contraceptives include the levonorgestrel implants (Norplant). Although the implant is effective for 5 years, the high prevalence of breakthrough bleeding and the need for surgical insertion limit its usefulness in many patients with developmental disabilities. For some, however, Norplant can ensure long-term contraception with minimal reliance on patient compliance. (Contraception is discussed further in Chapter 19.)

STERILIZATION

Parents of adolescents or adults with mental retardation often consider sterilization of their offspring because of fear of sexual abuse, unwanted pregnancy, and failure of birth control methods.[24] Sterilization of mentally disabled persons must comply with the constraints designed to protect the patient. U.S. Public Health Service regulations that govern sterilization programs supported in part by federal funding agencies state that these programs shall not perform or arrange for the sterilization of any mentally incompetent or institutionalized person.[25] Although other authorities feel that sterilization of the mentally handicapped is a decision for the courts,[26] successful litigation by handicapped persons has called into question court ordered sterilization.[27–29] Such limitations may be frustrating to a physician who wishes to perform a hysterectomy or tubal sterilization when, for the patient

Table 30–10. The Use of Contraceptives by Individuals with Mental Retardation*

	Medroxyprogesterone Acetate (DMPA)	Oral Contraceptive Agents (OCA)	Intrauterine Device (IUD)	Total
Mildly mentally retarded (MR)	6	11	6	23
Moderately MR	9	3	1	13
Severely MR	13	5	0	18
Total	28	19	7	54

*Some subjects used more than one method.

From Chamberlain A, Rauh J, Passer A, et al: Issues in fertility control for mentally retarded female adolescents: I. Sexual activity, sexual abuse, and contraception. Pediatrics 1984; 73:445–450.

in question, such a procedure is reasonable or even essential.

Each facility that cares for mentally handicapped patients must establish its own protocol. It must allow for the delivery of appropriate care, and take into consideration legal precedents to ensure the rights of the disabled and "due process."[30] The physician must allow the parents to participate in decisions about the sterilization of their disabled child. These constraints do not apply to patients who are physically disabled but otherwise mentally competent, but similar guidelines for physically disabled persons are desirable.

SEXUAL ABUSE

Sexual exploitation is a major problem for mentally disabled persons and their families. Although the actual incidence of sexual abuse is not known, it appears that sexual abuse of children is widespread. The National Center on Child Abuse and Neglect estimates the number of child victims to be more than 200,000 per year.[31]

Children of all ages, from infancy to young adulthood, have been victims of sexual abuse. The average reported age at first incident ranges from 8 to 11 years.[32, 33] One report suggests that younger children (aged 4 to 9) may be at higher risk because of their naive and trusting attitude toward adults. They are easily misled about the meaning of various sexual activities.[34] Developmentally disabled persons are also at higher risk to be victims of sexual abuse. Many parents believe that a severely retarded girl is at the greatest risk and that the assailant is often a stranger or another retarded person; however, studies have shown that *mildly* retarded patients are at greatest risk and that assailants are more likely to be family members or persons well known to the victim.[35] Boys with mental disabilities appear to be at greater risk for physical and sexual abuse. In one study, boys represented a significantly larger proportion of physically abused, sexually

abused, and neglected children with disabilities than would be expected from the respective proportions of abused and neglected children without disabilities.[36] Unfortunately, even when physical findings of abuse are present, in some cases the perpetrators cannot be identified.[37] In that particular study, a child abuse medical team examined a group of 35 mentally retarded females from a residential treatment facility. Genital findings consistent with vaginal penetration were found in 13 (37%) patients, but, for lack of a credible history, in many of these cases the investigation did not proceed.

In another study, patients were able to provide information about the abuse. The study reviewed 461 cases of sexual abuse of adults with mental retardation. The investigators confirmed 37% of these cases. The victims, for the most part, had no problem communicating verbally. The majority of the perpetrators were men (88%) and included other adults with mental retardation, paid staff, family members, and others. Most sexual abuse occurred in the victim's residence, and in 92% of the cases the victim knew the abuser.[38]

Not only patients with mental disabilities are at risk. A recent study suggests that women with physical disabilities also are at risk for abuse by attendants or healthcare providers. In addition, the abuse is more likely to go on longer than for women without physical disabilities.[39]

Special effort is required to develop effective prevention programs in the community if sexual exploitation of the disabled is to be controlled. In addition, these educational programs should be specially designed for disabled persons of different mental capacities.

OTHER FAMILY MEMBERS

Although the crucial role of the family is beyond dispute, the needs of other family members are often forgotten. Most parents do well with their disabled children, but they require a variety of support mechanisms. They need training and advice on how to manage daily problems without creating a crisis atmosphere. Common examples of unnecessary confrontation are punishment or reprimand for masturbation or overprotection that leads to isolation, low self-esteem, and depression. It is important to help these families learn to foster their children's success and achieve gratification from them. Most important, the parents need to participate in the decision-making process, and, in fact, the family should make the final decision about medical care for a disabled person. The healthcare professional's role is often limited to providing detailed information about the various treatment options and helping the family to make the appropriate choice.

REFERENCES

1. Becker DR, Drake RE, Bond GR, et al: Job terminations among persons with severe mental illness participating in supported employment. Commun Mental Health J 1998; 34:71–82.
2. Minihan PM, Dean DH: Meeting the needs for health services of persons with mental retardation living in the community. Am J Public Health 1990; 80:1043–1048.
3. Crocker AC: Medical care in the community for adults with mental retardation (Editorial). Am J Public Health 1990; 89(9):1037–1038.
4. Thase ME: Longevity and mortality in Down's syndrome. J Mental Defic Res 1982; 26:177–179.
5. Master RJ: Medicaid after 20 years: Promise, problem, and potential. Mental Retard 1987; 25:211–214.
6. Walsh KK, Kastner T, Criscione T: Characteristics of hospitalizations for people with developmental disabilities: Utilization, costs, and impact of care coordination. Am J Mental Retard 1997; 101:505–520.
7. Ryan R, Neligh GL, Aderman S: A state-university collaboration to serve persons with developmental disabilities and mental health needs. Commun Mental Health J 1997; 33:445–454.
8. Muram D, Dorko B, Gold JJ, Golden J: Clinic coordinators for persons with developmental disabilities. Adolesc Pediatr Gynecol 1990; 3;47–48.
9. Brasic JR, Will MV, Ahn SC, et al: A review of the literature and a preliminary study of family compliance in a developmental disabilities clinic. Psychol Reports 1998, 82:275–286.
10. Shah R: Improving services to Asian families and children with disabilities. Child Care Health Development 1997; 23:41–46.
11. Smith DC, Decker HA, Herberg EN, Rupke LK: Medical needs of children in institutions for the mentally retarded. Am J Public Health 1969; 8:1376–1384.
12. Ware L, Muram D, Gale CL: Q-tip Pap smear: Should it be done routinely in patients who have developmental disabilities? Sexuality Disability 1992; 10:189–192.
13. Quint EH, Elkins TE: Cervical cytology in women with mental retardation. Obstet Gynecol. 1997; 89:123–126.
14. Elkins TE, McNeeley SG, Rosen D, et al: A clinical observation of a program to accomplish pelvic exams in difficult-to-manage patients with mental retardation. Adolesc Pediatr Gynecol 1988; 1:195–198.
15. Rosen DA, Rosen KR, Elkins TE, et al: Outpatient seda-

tion: An essential addition to gynecologic care for persons with mental retardation. Am J Obstet Gynecol 1991; 164:825–828.
16. Elkins TE, Kope S, Ghaziuddin M, et al: Integration of a sexuality counseling service into a reproductive health program for persons with mental retardation. J Pediatr Adolesc Gynecol 1997; 10:24–27.
17. Elkins TE, Gafford LS, Wilks CS, et al: A model clinic approach to the reproductive health concerns of the mentally handicapped. Obstet Gynecol 1986; 68:185–189.
18. Brown H, Stein J: Sexual abuse perpetrated by men with intellectual disabilities: A comparative study. J Intellect Disabil Res. 1997; 41:215–224.
19. Fraser IS, Holck S: Depo-medroxyprogesterone acetate. In Mishell DR Jr (ed): Long-Acting Steroid Contraception. New York: Raven Press, 1983.
20. American College of Obstetricians and Gynecologists: The Intrauterine Contraception Device. Washington, DC: ACOG Technical Bulletin no. 164, 1992.
21. Cundy T, Evans M, Roberts H, et al: Bone density in women receiving depo-medroxyprogesterone acetate for contraception. Br Med 1991; 303:13–16.
22. Sheth S, Malpani A: Vaginal hysterectomy for the management of menstruation in mentally retarded women. Int J Gynecol Obstet 1991; 35:319–321.
23. American College of Obstetricians and Gynecologists: Oral contraception. Washington, DC: ACOG Technical Bulletin no. 106, 1987.
24. Patterson-Keels L, Quint E, Brown D, et al: Family views on sterilization for their mentally retarded children. J Reprod Med. 1994; 39:701–706.
25. 42 OFR, [section]50.201–210, 1979
26. Annas GJ: Sterilization of the mentally retarded: Is a decision for the courts. Hastings Center Rep 1981; August: 18–19.
27. *Stump v Sparkman*, 435 US 349, 1978.
28. *Downs v Sawtelle*, 574 F2d l(Cal 1978).
29. In re: Gloria Sue Lambert 1976.
30. Elkins TE, Hoyle D, Darnton T, et al: The use of a societally-based ethics/advisory committee to aid in decisions to sterilize mentally handicapped patients. Adolesc Pediatr Gynecol 1988; 1:190–194.
31. National Center on Child Abuse and Neglect (NCCAN): Child Sexual Abuse: Incest, Assault and Eploitation. Special Report. Washington, DC: HEW, Children's Bureau, 1978.
32. Kemp CE: Sexual abuse, another hidden pediatric problem. Pediatrics 1978; 62:382–389.
33. Kemp CE: Incest and other forms of sexual abuse. In Kemp CE, Helfer RE (eds): The Battered Child. Chicago: University of Chicago Press, 1980.
34. Gelinas DJ: The persisting negative effects of incest. Psychiatry 1983; 46:312–332.
35. Chamberlain A, Rauh J, Passer A, et al: Issues in fertility control for mentally retarded female adolescents: I. Sexual activity, sexual abuse, and contraception. Pediatrics 1984; 73:445–450.
36. Sobsey D, Randall W, Parrila RK: Gender differences in abused children with and without disabilities. Child Abuse Neglect 1997; 21:707–720.
37. Elvik SL, Berkowitz CD, Nicholas E, Sexual abuse in the developmentally disabled: Dilemmas of diagnosis. Child Abuse Neglect 1990; 14(4):497–502.
38. Furey EM: Sexual abuse of adults with mental retardation: Who and where. Mental Retard 1994; 32(3):173–180.
39. Young ME, Nosek MA, Howland C, et al: Prevalence of abuse of women with physical disabilities. Arch Phys Med Rehabil 1997; 78:S34–S38.

Chapter 31

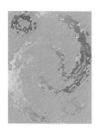

Legal Issues in Treating Minors

STEVEN R. SMITH

The practice of medicine is increasingly influenced by the law. Perhaps in no area of practice is this more apparent than in pediatric and adolescent gynecology. Legal issues arise from the formation of the physician-patient relationship and consent to treatment, the obligations of confidentiality, termination of treatment, and payment for services. The emotionally charged and politically difficult questions of adolescent abortion and contraception rights have created a complex set of regulations in most states.[1, 2] Very broad reporting laws (including sexual abuse–reporting statutes) have imposed additional obligations on physicians.

It is imperative that healthcare professionals who treat children and adolescents be well versed in the legal principles affecting their patients and their practice. In this chapter I introduce these basic principles, describe certain legal issues involving pediatric and adolescent patients, and present some statutes that illustrate a number of states' approaches to these issues. Space does not permit me to detail all of the many legal issues that involve obstetrics and gynecology, including professional liability, artificial insemination, in vitro fertilization, and genetic counseling; these are not unique to adolescents and are considered in texts on general obstetrics and gynecology.

In addition to understanding the general legal principles involved in adolescent obstetrics and gynecology, professionals should maintain a relationship with an organization or attorney who can keep them abreast of the laws that affect their treatment of patients. This is critical for three reasons. First, laws governing pediatric and adolescent gynecologic care are changing rapidly and can be expected to continue to do so. Second, legal principles vary somewhat from state to state, and no generalization can describe the law in all. Third, the law of reproductive issues is a particularly complex tangle of overlapping and inconsistent state and federal statutes and

constitutional provisions, federal and state court decisions, executive orders, and regulations.[3, 4]

UNDERLYING PRINCIPLES

Several basic common law and constitutional concepts serve as the basis for virtually all of the current legal issues and principles of reproductive health care for minors.[5, 6] Next, I will briefly consider several of them.

STATE AND FEDERAL LAW

Traditionally, state laws have regulated medical care, the definition of the legal rights of minors, and the relationships between parents and minors. (*Law*, in this sense, means not only statutes, but also constitutions, case law, and administrative regulations and directives.) Federal law has played an increasingly important role in these areas, however. Three factors have contributed to this: (1) The United States Supreme Court's interpretations of the provisions of the Constitution that limit state law (e.g., limit the ability of a state to prohibit abortions); (2) federal funds, which have become increasingly important in the delivery of health care services (e.g., Medicaid and federally funded family planning agencies); and (3) Congress's use of federal authority to control interstate commerce to regulate medical care (e.g., drugs and medical devices).[7] While this increasing federal role is important, state law still plays the dominant role in defining and regulating the provision of medical care to minors.

THE LAW ON PARENT-CHILD RELATIONSHIPS

Under traditional common law, children were virtually the property of their parents and thus

513

subject to parental decisions, direction, and discipline.[8] Throughout the 20th century, however, the concept of parental ownership and control of children increasingly has come under legal attack. Although parents still have wide latitude in raising their children, minors are currently recognized as separate legal entities who have their own rights and interests.[9] As a result of these changes, child abuse statutes limit the physical and mental abuse inflicted on children in the name of discipline, and mature minors, despite parental objection, may consent to medical procedures such as abortion.[10]

LEGAL RIGHTS OF MINORS

Children are protected from their own immature judgment by their limited ability both to enter into contracts (except for necessities) and to consent to medical care (except under very limited circumstances). The law generally considers minors to be incapable of making binding legal decisions until the age of majority. State law defines the age of majority, and most states use 18 years for general decision-making capacity.[11]

There have been some common exceptions to minors' being forbidden to make legally binding decisions. The most common is the *emancipated minors rule*. Emancipated minors may make legally binding decisions, because they are viewed as formally free of the control and responsibility of their parents, usually as a result of marriage, military service, or (in some states) economic independence coupled with parental approval.[12] Some states also have recognized that *mature minors* may make legally binding decisions. The concept of the mature minor is somewhat vague, but it generally refers to those who are able to understand and make complex decisions even though they have not yet reached the age of majority.[13]

The legal tendency during the 1970s and 1980s, consistent with studies of the decision-making ability of older minors,[14, 15] was to give minors the legal authority to make legally binding decisions at an earlier age.[16, 17] In areas such as abortion, for example, the Supreme Court indicated a fairly broad authority for mature minors to make their own decisions. More recently, however, the trend seems to have reversed and currently may be tending to expand parental control over fundamental decisions, at least for adolescents younger than 18.[18]

LEGAL PRINCIPLES OF CONSENT

Ordinarily, medical care may be provided only when the patient has given consent.[19] This is part of the general right of autonomy, the right of all adults to decide for themselves what will be done to their bodies.[20] When the treatment is important or invasive—surgery, for example—the patient must be informed of the risks and benefits and of alternative treatments and their consequences. That is, the patient must give *informed consent*.[21]

One exception is an emergency when no one is available to give consent. For example, when an adult is unconscious or when a minor has an emergency and there is no family available to give consent, treatment may be undertaken. Another exception to the requirement of informed consent is the so-called *therapeutic privilege*. When it is deemed that providing information would be quite harmful to the patient, that information may be withheld from the patient, although in many circumstances it should be revealed to others, for example the patient's family.[20] State statutes and court decisions have provided additional exceptions to the usual consent rules.[22]

PATIENT CONFIDENTIALITY

Physicians have an obligation to respect patient confidentiality. Failure to protect confidential information revealed during treatment may result in civil lawsuits based on negligence or invasion of privacy and may subject the physician to discipline by licensing agencies. There are, of course, exceptions to this requirement, as when the patient has waived the right to secrecy or when the law specifically permits or requires the physician to release information about the patient.* There are many reasons for breaching confidentiality, ranging from attempts to obtain insurance (or other third-party) payment for services to the requirement to report a communicable disease under state law.[23] Any breach of confidentiality should be carefully considered by the physician in light of the legal standards in the state where the patient is seen.

Under common law it was assumed that parents were entitled to any important information

---

*The obligation of maintaining confidentiality should not be confused with physician-patient privilege. The *privilege* permits physicians and patients to refuse to reveal, even to courts, the communications that occurred during treatment. *Confidentiality* is a broader obligation to maintain the secrets of the patient.

about their children, and this attitude probably colors current law. Because of individual state statutes and the constitutional privacy rights of minors, some exceptions may hold in the areas of psychiatric, obstetric, and gynecologic care. In many states, however, the right of minors and physicians to withhold general medical information from parents is not currently supported by state laws. The physician treating an adolescent patient should reach a clear understanding about confidentiality, including any communication with the patient's parents, *before treatment begins*.[23] When the treatment would raise issues of sexuality or substance abuse, such an understanding is especially important.[24]

CONSTITUTIONAL PRIVACY RIGHTS AND MINORS

RIGHTS TO MAKE CHILD-BEARING DECISIONS

In 1965, the Supreme Court, in *Griswold v. Connecticut*, first recognized a specific constitutional right of privacy.[25] In *Griswold* the Court struck down a Connecticut statute prohibiting married couples from using contraceptives. The Court noted the private nature of the relationship between the couple and their physician as well as the intimate relationship between husband and wife. The Court indicated that the constitutional right of privacy protects the right of the individual to make fundamentally important personal decisions without substantial government interference. Among the areas that the Court has identified as fundamentally important, and thus protected under the Constitution, are procreation decisions, marriage, child rearing, and family life.

Much of the constitutional privacy doctrine affects obstetric and gynecologic care, because procreation and child rearing decisions are involved. After *Griswold*, the Court recognized the constitutional right of unmarried persons to obtain contraceptives without governmental interference.[26] The Court stated "[if] the right of privacy means anything, it is the right of the *individual*, married or single, to be free from unwarranted governmental intrusion into matters so fundamentally affecting a person as the decision whether to bear or beget a child."[17]

In *Roe v. Wade*, the Supreme Court struck down criminal abortion laws that prohibit abortion except to save the mother's life.[2] The Court noted that such laws interfere with a woman's right to privacy. It also held, however, that the

right of privacy is not absolute and may be limited if there is a compelling state interest. The Supreme Court subsequently held that the right to have an abortion extends to minors,[12] that a minor cannot absolutely be required to have parental permission before undergoing an abortion,[27] that states may require parental notification before a minor receives an abortion,[28, 29] and that a minor has the right to at least some types of contraception without parental consent.[30] These decisions are obviously of direct concern to those who provide reproductive health services to adolescents, and they are discussed in detail later in this chapter.

PERSONAL INFORMATION

In addition to autonomy privacy, the right of privacy may include the right to withhold from others certain kinds of private information.[31, 32] The extent of this type of privacy is very ill-defined.[33] Thus far, the Supreme Court has permitted states to collect very personal information, such as the names of women who have abortions, as long as it ensures the confidentiality of such information.[18] In the future, the right to information privacy may be a determinant of when a state may require the release of private information about abortions, contraception, or other personal matters.[34] The Court has permitted states to pass laws that require that parents be notified that their minor child seeks to have an abortion.[28, 29] (This parental notification issue is considered in more detail later in this chapter.)

LIMITATIONS ON THE RIGHT OF PRIVACY

The nature and extent of the right of privacy are not fully defined, but it is clear that privacy rights are not absolute. The state may interfere with the right of privacy in a number of ways, as I describe in this section.

Compelling State Interests

The right of privacy may be limited to protect a compelling state interest. For example, in *Roe v. Wade*, the Supreme Court indicated that, after the first trimester, the state may regulate abortions for the protection of the mother's health. After a fetus is *viable* (i.e., able to live outside the mother's body with or without artificial assistance), the state may regulate abortion, because at that time it has a compelling interest in the life of that fetus.[2] Relatively few legitimate compelling state interests can be identified. The protection of human life, preventing violent overthrow of the government, and preserving democracy are some of them.[24] The Court will permit a state to regulate abortion more broadly under a claim that the regulation does not unduly burden the right to choose an abortion. Thus, the Court has upheld 24-hour waiting periods for abortions but has struck down *husband's consent* laws.[1]

Conflicting Rights

Another potential limitation on a minor's rights comes from the conflict between the minor's right to privacy to make procreation and child-bearing decisions and the parents' child-rearing privacy rights. Although the Supreme Court initially tended to favor the procreation decisions of the "mature minor" over the parents' child-rearing rights,[27,35] more recently it has seemed to place a higher constitutional value on parents' child-rearing rights than on minors' child-bearing rights.[28] Thus, a state cannot provide blanket authority for a parent to veto an adolescent's decision to have an abortion or to use contraceptives.[17] Nevertheless, the state has some latitude in limiting a minor's obstetric and reproductive health care. Some states, for example, may require that parents be informed of the decision of a minor child to have an abortion.[28, 36, 37]

Promotion of Privacy Rights

Federal and state governments are not required to promote or encourage the exercise of privacy rights. For example, the federal government may refuse to fund abortions for women through the Medicaid system, even though it pays for other forms of obstetric care.[38] Furthermore, the Court has upheld federal regulations that prevent family planning centers from discussing the possibility of an abortion, even when that part of the counseling center's activities is not paid for by federal funds.[39] The Court has only *permitted* such restrictions; neither the states nor the federal government is *required* to limit abortions or contraception. Because of the political nature of such regulation of abortion, it seems destined to change in the next decades, as the political winds do.

State Action and Private Institutions

Private institutions have much greater latitude than public facilities to prohibit procedures such as abortions and sterilizations. This is because the constitutional right of privacy essentially applies to governmental action. Thus, private hospitals may be able to prohibit abortions or sterilizations if they so choose. The receipt of federal or state funds may, however, be the basis for some regulation, even of "private" hospitals.

Nonsubstantial Burdens on Privacy

To violate constitutional privacy, the government must significantly interfere with the ability of the individual to exercise privacy interests. An incidental or minor impediment is not considered an unconstitutional invasion, even though some particularly sensitive people might object to it. State record keeping of abortion information, for example, does not unconstitutionally burden the abortion decision.[27] On the other hand, a state law permitting only pharmacists to sell contraceptives does unconstitutionally burden the individual's right to make fundamental decisions concerning child bearing, because it unnecessarily reduces access.[29] The U.S. Supreme Court has shown willingness to accept limitations on abortion that are not an "undue" interference with abortion.[1]

The Court has upheld a state requirement that second-trimester abortions be performed in licensed facilities (including outpatient hospitals),[40] but it has said that state statutes requiring all second-trimester abortions to be performed in general hospitals are unconstitutional.[35, 41] It has upheld 1- and 2-day waiting periods for abortions, very strong ("shock") abortion informed consent presentations, and laws requiring that physicians report to the state the names of patients on whom they have performed an abortion.[1] The Court has also permitted states to require parental notifications or consent for abortion (with a judicial bypass, discussed subsequently), but it has struck down a state law requiring spousal (husband's) consent to abortion, because that was deemed "undue interference" with a woman's abortion decision.[1] No clear line separates the insignificant from the impermissible burden, but the mere fact that a state regulation has some impact on obstetric or gynecologic care does not automatically invalidate it.

INFORMED CONSENT TO OBSTETRIC AND GYNECOLOGIC CARE

Consider Joan N., a 15-year-old living with her mother, who is not particularly supportive of Joan. Joan's father is seldom home but has been abusive to Joan and her mother from time to time. Joan is pregnant, and, at the prodding of a friend, she goes to see Dr. Snyder. She wants to have an abortion and to be given contraceptives to prevent future pregnancies. It also appears that she may have a sexually transmitted disease (STD). In this section we consider the following questions: May Dr. Snyder perform the abortion? Must Dr. Snyder inform Joan's parents of the abortion? Must Joan's parents consent to it? May he provide advice on contraception or prescribe a contraceptive? May he provide treatment for the STD? Should Dr. Snyder report the possible abuse by Joan's father? To begin to answer these questions, we must look at the "minor consent" statutes, and then consider some constitutional questions.

Except in emergencies, consent must be given before medical treatment is rendered. Unless the risks are minimal, some form of informed consent is necessary. Physicians who provide medical care to minors without parental consent could be held liable in tort (negligence or battery) and run the risk of not being paid for their services.[12] Generally, parents must consent to treatment for their unemancipated children. Some modifications of these general rules have been provided, however, for adolescent obstetric and gynecologic care,[42] by statute in some states and by federal court decisions.[43] In addition to the care discussed in this section, emergency care generally can be provided to minors without parental consent, and life-saving care may be undertaken on the intervention of state social service agencies or courts.[9, 44, 45]

SPECIAL STATE STATUTES GOVERNING CONSENT

Virtually all states allow adolescents to consent to some obstetric and gynecologic care, most often for treatment of STDs, pregnancy, and contraception. Several states, as part of the increased concern over child abuse, expressly allow the victims of abuse to consent to treatment for the abuse. Other changes have permitted adolescents to seek treatment without parental consent for drug or alcohol dependence. In most states, an effort has been made to limit the scope of these minor consent laws so that they do not apply to abortion.

These statutes often came about as a result of recognition, during the 1970s and 1980s, of the increased sexual activity and maturity of adolescents. The movement toward such statutes abated and reversed in the 1990s, and some states are considering modification or repeal. This phenomenon may reflect both a change in public attitude and the fact that the courts have implemented some of the policies that the statutes promoted.

The following excerpts from a few statutes illustrate the approaches of several states.

California

6920–6929 (portions): Subject to the limitations provided in this chapter, notwithstanding any other provision of law, a minor may consent to the matters provided in this chapter, and the consent of the minor's parent or guardian is not necessary. A consent given by a minor under this chapter is not subject to disaffirmance because of minority.

A minor may consent to the minor's medical care or dental care if [he or she is 15, living apart from parents and managing his own financial affairs]. The parents or guardian are not liable for medical care or dental care provided pursuant to this section. A physician may, with or without the consent of the minor patient, advise the minor's parent or guardian of the treatment given. . . .

A minor may consent to medical care related to the prevention or treatment of pregnancy. This section does not authorize a minor: To be sterilized without the consent of the minor's parent or guardian, [or] to receive an abortion without the consent of a parent or guardian. . . .

A minor who is 12 years of age or older and who may have come into contact with an infectious, contagious, or communicable disease may consent to medical care related to the diagnosis or treatment of the disease, if the disease or condition is one that is required by law or regulation adopted pursuant to law to be reported to the local health officer, or is a related sexually transmitted disease, as may be determined by the State Director of Health Services. The minor's parents or guardian are not liable for payment for medical care provided pursuant to this section.

A minor who is 12 years of age or older and who is alleged to have been raped may consent to medical care related to the diagnosis or treatment of the condition and the collection of medical evidence with regard to the alleged rape.

A minor who is 12 years of age or older may consent to medical care and counseling relating to the diagnosis and treatment of a drug- or alcohol-related problem.

The minor's parents or guardian are not liable for payment for any care provided to a minor pursuant to this section, except that if the minor's parent or guardian participates in a counseling program pursuant to this section, the parent or guardian is liable for the cost of the services provided to the minor and the parent or guardian. . . .

Notwithstanding any other provision of law, in cases where a parent or legal guardian has sought the medical care and counseling for a drug- or alcohol-related problem of a minor child, the physician shall disclose medical information concerning such care to the minor's parents or legal guardian upon their request, even if the minor child does not consent to disclosure, without liability for such disclosure.

Colorado

13-22-105 Except as otherwise provided . . . birth control procedures, supplies, and information may be furnished by physicians . . . to any minor who is pregnant, or a parent, or married, or who has the consent of his parent or legal guardian, or who has been referred for such services by another physician, a clergyman, a family planning clinic, a school or institution of higher education, or any agency or instrumentality of this state or any subdivision thereof, or who requests and is in need of birth control procedures, supplies, or information.

13-22-106 (1) Any physician licensed to practice in this state, upon consultation by a minor as a patient who indicates that he or she was the victim of a sexual assault, with the consent of such minor patient, may perform customary and necessary examinations to obtain evidence of the sexual assault and may prescribe for and treat the patient for any immediate condition caused by the sexual assault.

(2) (a) Prior to examining or treating a minor pursuant to subsection (1) of this section, a physician shall make a reasonable effort to notify the parent, parents, legal guardian, or any other person having custody of such minor of the sexual assault.[47]

Florida

381.0051 Maternal health and contraceptive information and services of a non-surgical nature may be rendered to any minor by persons licensed to practice medicine . . . as well as by the Department of Health and Rehabilitative Services through its family planning program, provided the minor:

1. Is married;
2. Is a parent;
3. Is pregnant;

4. Has the consent of a parent or legal guardian; or
5. May, in the opinion of the physician, suffer probable health hazards if such services are not provided.

Application of nonpermanent internal contraceptive devices shall not be deemed a surgical procedure.

[Permits physicians to refuse to furnish contraceptives or services for "medical or religious reasons."][48]

Kentucky

214.185 (1) Any physician, upon consultation by a minor as a patient, with the consent of such minor may make a diagnostic examination for venereal disease, pregnancy [or alcohol or drug abuse], and may advise, prescribe for, and treat such minor regarding [these conditions], all without the consent of or notification to the parent, parents, or guardian of such minor patient, or to any person having custody of such minor patient. Treatment under this section does not include inducing of an abortion or performance of a sterilization operation.

[(2) permits those 16 and older to consent to mental health counseling.

(3) permits emancipated minors to consent to treatment.]

(6) The professional may inform the parent or legal guardian of the minor patient of any treatment given or needed where, in the judgment of the professional, informing the parent or guardian would benefit the health of the minor patient.

[(7) exempts parents from paying for most services for which they have not given consent.][49]

Dr. Snyder's treatment of Joan N., the case described at the beginning of this section, would be influenced directly by the minor consent statute in the state where treatment was provided. Most state statutes would permit Dr. Snyder to provide treatment for the STD and to give advice on contraceptives and would not require that he notify Joan's parents of these actions, assuming, of course, that the contraception is not permanent sterilization.[50] These statutes would not, however, specifically permit a minor like Joan to consent to abortion. We will consider the issue of abortion in a subsequent section. First, however, we consider the question of Dr. Snyder's treatment of Joan when there is no statute that permits such treatment without parental consent.

THE CONSTITUTION AND CONTRACEPTION

In *Carey v. Population Services*,[30] the Supreme Court held that the right of privacy includes the right of minors to have access to some contraceptives. It struck down a New York statute that limited access by minors younger than 16 years. A state may not, therefore, completely prohibit the use or availability of nonprescription contraceptives to minors.[51] This is an exception to the general requirement of parental consent. The issue of whether a state may require that parents be informed of their child's use of contraceptives is another matter and is discussed later.

Informed consent for the use of intrauterine contraceptive devices (IUDs) and other prescription drugs and U.S. Food and Drug Administration (FDA)–controlled devices should be obtained from the adolescent and, when state law requires, from the parents. The constitutional right of a mature minor to prescription contraceptives without parental consent is not completely clear. It is likely, therefore, that minors who can demonstrate "maturity" (competence) would not be required to have their parents' permission to use contraceptives. As always, practitioners must provide to the patient reasonable information about the benefits and risks of the proposed treatment and about contraceptive alternatives.[52]

THE CONSTITUTION AND ABORTIONS

Since the *Roe v. Wade* decision, many states have tried to limit abortions by imposing a variety of fairly restrictive consent and other requirements. The federal courts have ruled many of these to be unconstitutional.[53] The states have then tried other approaches, the result being something of a cat-and-mouse game.[54]

In *Planned Parenthood v. Danforth*,[28] the Court held that the right of privacy to decide to have an abortion extends to minors and the state does not have the constitutional authority to delegate to a third party the decision of a "competent and mature minor" to have an abortion. In *Bellotti v. Baird*,[17] the Court held that a state statute permitting a judicial veto of a mature minor's decision to have an abortion was unconstitutional. The statute allowed the state courts considerable latitude in deciding whether to consent to the abortion.[55] The Court held unconstitutional an ordinance that provided that all minors younger than 15 were too immature to make abortion decisions,[35] but in *Planned Parenthood Association of Kansas City v. Ashcroft*,[41] the Court upheld a state statute requiring all minors to obtain either parental or judicial consent for

an abortion. This statute was constitutional because the state courts were *required* to give consent to the abortion if the minor was mature enough to make the decision or if the abortion was in her best interest. This is known as a *judicial bypass*, because it authorizes courts to bypass the usual family participation requirements. The Court believes that such provisions do not impose an undue burden on any right of a minor who wants or needs an abortion.[1]

The Supreme Court has upheld state laws that require graphic informed consent, including information about the fetus.[1] Such laws, the Court held, do not unduly burden the abortion decision. An increasing number of states have adopted such laws.[56] They probably will—and generally are intended to—reduce and restrict the availability of abortions to adolescents and the practice of obstetricians and gynecologists.[57] Professionals treating pregnant minors in states where parental or judicial consent is required may find it necessary to establish some way to assist them in obtaining judicial consent to abortion, a daunting task for a minor to undertake alone. When the bypass was used, courts overwhelmingly have approved abortions.

The fact that a state is constitutionally *permitted* to require judicial or parental consent does not, of course, mean that it is *required* to pass such a law. Many states have moved in this direction. As a consequence, most states require parental consent or a court order determining either (1) that the minor is sufficiently mature to make the decision or (2) that the abortion is in the best interest of the minor. States will also probably require "shock" informed consent and impose waiting periods between the time of consent and the abortion.

Apart from special abortion informed consent statutes, the physician should remember that abortion is a significant medical procedure and that informed consent of the minor is essential. Except in the most extraordinary circumstances, an abortion should not be done when the minor objects, and then should be done only with court approval.

Although the *Roe v. Wade* decision and subsequent cases have provided considerable protection for the right of adolescents to have an abortion, that right has been reduced considerably for minors. In 1992, the Supreme Court reaffirmed *Roe* but permitted considerable state regulation of abortion. Efforts in Congress to provide a national statutory abortion right have so far failed, and states have considerable latitude in formulating the abortion laws. As a result, inconsistent and shifting limits on abortion can be expected to occur.[58, 59]

CONSENT TO OTHER MEDICAL PROCEDURES

There are a limited number of cases that address minor consent to other obstetric and gynecologic treatments. As noted earlier, many states have adopted statutes that permit treatment of a minor without parental consent in a number of circumstances. Furthermore, it is likely a court would order consent, even over parental objection, to treatment for contagious conditions such as STD or an exceptionally harmful or life-threatening condition.[9, 60] Thus, Dr. Snyder would probably be safe in treating Joan N.'s STD.

CONFIDENTIALITY OF MINOR PATIENTS

The law may prohibit the release of certain information, require its release, or leave the release to the physician's discretion.[61] The usual obligation of a physician to maintain patient confidentiality is modified with a minor so that parents have access to the information.[62] This is not an absolute parental right, and there are a number of instances in which the parents do not have a right to medical information about a child. In this section I address the release of information to parents.

SPECIAL RULES REGARDING ABORTION

Some states have defined by statute physicians' obligations regarding the release of obstetric and gynecologic information.[63, 64] These statutes vary considerably. Compare, for example, the Colorado[48] statute with sections of the Kentucky[49] statute, excerpted earlier. Physicians are required to notify parents only in those states with a specific statute that mandates such disclosure.[65, 66] Most states with specific statutory provisions on the release of abortion information either permit or require release of the information to parents.[5] The trend appears to be to require its release, and even to require the physician to notify parents when a child requests an abortion or contraceptives.[6, 67] In *Ohio v. Center for Reproductive Health* and *Hodgson v. Minnesota*,[29] the Court held that a state may constitu-

tionally require the notification of one or even both parents when a minor seeks an abortion as long as the state also provides for a "judicial bypass." A bypass permits the minor to apply to a court to proceed with the abortion without parental notification if she is sufficiently mature to make the decision on her own or has been subjected to abuse by her parents, or if it is in her best interest not to inform the parents.[29]

The judicial bypass exception is so complicated that it is unlikely that most minors would be able to negotiate it by themselves.[68, 69] In some areas of the country, there are organizations that assist adolescents with the bypass procedures, and patients may know of these from their friends. Physicians who treat minors who may need or want to have an abortion, however, should determine whether a parental consent or notification statute exists[70] and whether they are permitted to help the minor to complete the bypass. Several studies suggest that courts overwhelmingly approve abortions when application is made through the bypass process, but the adolescent patient is likely to need assistance in going through the court process.[71–73]

Returning to our hypothetical Dr. Snyder, it is apparent that he will have a difficult time providing abortion services to Joan N. As we have seen, Dr. Snyder's obligations will depend on the state where he practices. In most states, he will be required to notify or obtain the consent of at least one parent. If there are good reasons not to have parental notification or consent, before proceeding, Dr. Snyder will need a court determination that Joan is sufficiently mature to make the abortion decision herself or that it is in her best interest. The vast majority of such judicial bypass efforts are granted by courts, but Joan (and perhaps Dr. Snyder) will probably have to appear before a judge to receive judicial consent. The state may also require "shock" informed consent and a 1- or 2-day waiting period between the consent and the abortion. Finally, in some states Dr. Snyder may be required to report to the state information about the abortion and about Joan N. It should also be noted that, if Dr. Snyder is employed in some state or federally funded institutions, he may not be permitted to participate in the abortion or to directly refer Joan for an abortion.

INFORMING ADOLESCENTS OF THE LIMITS OF CONFIDENTIALITY

The stated purpose of parental notification rules is to encourage parents to counsel their pregnant or sexually active children and help them through a difficult time. In fact, notifying the parents only increases some families' problems. A few clinics have, therefore, refused to inform parents of their children's treatment. It remains doubtful that such a position can be maintained in the face of specific state or federal laws requiring notification.[74]

The difficulty presented is illustrated by the Joan N. case described earlier. If Dr. Snyder tells Joan's parents about her desire to have an abortion or receive contraception, it is unlikely that Joan will receive parental counseling. Indeed, it is possible that such information will set off an abusive response by Joan's father. *Requiring* parental consent would be even more problematic. At the same time, seeking a judicial bypass would be extremely burdensome to Joan and to Dr. Snyder.

In jurisdictions where parental notification is required for certain types of obstetric and gynecologic care, the practitioner should inform minors of this reporting obligation at the beginning of treatment. This is another area where significant changes may be expected in the future, so particularly careful monitoring of changes in federal, state, and local law is important.[75]

As a general matter, even in states where parents have a right to their child's medical records, practitioners need not seek out parents to inform them of the therapy. That is not an option, of course, where the law specifies, as an increasing number of state abortion laws do, that parents must be notified before treatment is undertaken.[28] Often, parents do not know that their child is being treated. When the right of parents to information on the treatment of their child is in question, practitioners may choose to refuse to release the information unless the parents obtain a court order or other judicial determination that the information must be released.

If the release of information to parents is optional, physicians usually should release confidential information about treatment only when the patient has consented to the release or when such release is clearly in the best interest of the minor. Ordinarily, the minor should be told that the information is being released. Practitioners also may be asked to release information to an insurance company or another third party for payment of services. In such instances, that information should be released only with the consent of the patient or of a minor patient's parents.

In our hypothetical Joan N. case, it is very unlikely that Dr. Snyder will be able to avoid providing Joan N.'s parents with some very private information, if he agrees to treat her. That is, unless Joan and Dr. Snyder are willing to go to court to receive judicial consent via judicial bypass, Joan's parents will probably be informed of the abortion.

REPORTING ABUSE AND DISEASE

In a number of circumstances, practitioners are required by law to report certain diagnoses or findings to state authorities.[76] Reporting statutes vary from state to state, but obligations to report child abuse, neglect or sexual exploitation, and STDs are common. Some states require that records be kept or that reports be made to state authorities concerning abortions, certain prescription drugs, miscarriages, and infant deaths.

ABUSE AND NEGLECT

All states require that child abuse be reported, although statutes vary from state to state. The Colorado statute, excerpts of which are reprinted below, is a fair representation of the scope of many state statutes.[77]

Colorado

19-1-103 As used [here], unless the context otherwise requires: (1) (a) "Abuse" or "child abuse or neglect" means an act or omission in one of the following categories which threatens the health or welfare of a child:

(I) Any case in which a child exhibits evidence of skin bruising, bleeding, malnutrition, failure to thrive, burns, fracture of any bone, subdural hematoma, soft tissue swelling, or death, and either such condition or death is not justifiably explained; the history given concerning such condition is at variance with the degree or type of such condition or death; or the circumstances indicate that such condition may not be the product of an accidental occurrence;

(II) Any case in which a child is subjected to sexual assault or molestation, sexual exploitation, or prostitution;

(III) Any case in which a child is a child in need of services because the child's parents, legal guardian, or custodian fails to take the same actions to provide adequate food, clothing, shelter, medical care, or supervision that a prudent parent would take. . . .

(b) In all cases, those investigating reports of child abuse shall take into account accepted child-rearing practices of the culture in which the child participates. Nothing in this subsection (1) shall refer to acts which could be construed to be a reasonable exercise of parental discipline. . . .

19-3-304 (1) Any person specified in subsection (2) of this section who has reasonable cause to know or suspect that a child has been subjected to abuse or neglect or who has observed the child being subjected to circumstances or conditions which would reasonably result in abuse or neglect shall immediately report or cause a report to be made of such fact to the county department or local law enforcement agency.

(2) Persons required to report such abuse or neglect or circumstances or conditions shall include any [medical or mental health professional, school official, peace officer or film processor].

(3) In addition to those persons specifically required by this section to report known or suspected child abuse or neglect and circumstances or conditions which might reasonably result in child abuse or neglect, any other person may report known or suspected child abuse or neglect . . . to the local law enforcement agency or the county department.

(4) Any person who willfully violates the provisions of subsection (I) of this section:

(a) Commits a class 3 misdemeanor . . .

(b) Shall be liable for damages proximately caused thereby.

Note the broad definitions of *abuse* and *neglect* in the Colorado statute. This is a common definition, and many states currently require that emotional or mental abuse also be reported[75, 78]; sexual assault or molestation is specifically included. In addition, abuse must be reported, whether it is known or only suspected, and in cases where conditions would reasonably be expected to result in abuse or neglect.[79]

Most states provide immunity against liability for those who report suspected child abuse.[80, 81] Failure to report known or suspected abuse, neglect, or sexual exploitation is a criminal offense in most states and may also give rise to civil liability.[76, 82]

Claims of child abuse have been made against women who abuse a "child" (fetus) during pregnancy.[83] For example, women who continue to ingest illegal drugs during pregnancy, knowing that such conduct is seriously harmful to the fetus, may be seen as child abusers.[84, 85] Critics of this approach suggest that such prosecutions interfere with women's ability to control their own bodies.[86] It is not clear what direction the law will take, but some states are likely to consider the harmful use of illegal drugs (e.g., cocaine) by pregnant women to be child abuse.[85, 86] Those treating pregnant adolescents should be aware of legal developments in this area, as they

may become responsible for reporting pregnant patients who are abusing their unborn children.

SEXUALLY TRANSMITTED DISEASES

States commonly require that professionals report cases of STDs to a state or local board of health. The following portion of the Iowa statute is typical:

Iowa

140.4 Immediately after the first examination or treatment of any person infected with any venereal disease, the physician performing the same shall transmit to the Iowa department of health a report stating the name, age, sex, marital status, occupation of patient, name of the disease, probable source of infection, and duration of the disease; except, when a case occurs within the jurisdiction of a local health department, such a report shall be made directly to the local health department which shall immediately forward the same information to the Iowa Department of Health. Such reports shall be made in accordance with rules adopted by the State Department of Health. Such reports shall be confidential. Any person in good faith making a report of a venereal disease shall have immunity from any liability, civil or criminal, which might otherwise be incurred or imposed as a result of such report.[87]

As with child abuse reporting statutes, failure to report cases may subject the professional to criminal prosecution. A report made in good faith is immune from liability.[75]

Dr. Snyder, in the case of Joan N., would almost surely be required by the laws of his state to make two kinds of reports to state agencies. First, if Joan N. told him of physical or sexual abuse by her father, Dr. Snyder would be required to report this to a child protective services agency. Failure to do so is a criminal offense in most states. Second, Dr. Snyder would probably be required to report the STD to a health department.

OTHER LEGAL ISSUES

PAYMENT FOR SERVICES

Under common law, a minor cannot be held to contracts except for necessities, and a parent is obligated to provide the fundamentals of life. Thus, in most cases, a parent is required to pay for the minor's medical services, although when a minor legally contracts for necessary medical services, the minor can be held to that contract. It is not uncommon for states that permit minors to obtain medical treatment without parental consent to also release parents from financial responsibility for treatment to which they did not consent (e.g., see the Colorado and Kentucky consent statutes reprinted earlier). Ordinarily, the minor would be responsible for paying for such services.[60] Successfully securing payment, of course, may be difficult, even when it is legally due.

INVOLUNTARY STERILIZATION

Permanent sterilization of competent minors generally should not be undertaken unless it is necessary to save a life or is incidental to other essential treatment.[88] Some states by statute specifically do not allow minors to consent to sterilization. A troublesome question has been whether it is appropriate for minors to be sterilized when parents or guardians consent. Sterilization is usually sought because profoundly incompetent female minors are unable to understand their own sexuality and the consequences of sexual contacts and would be unable to care for any children they might bear.[89] On the other hand, courts are reluctant to remove the fundamental right to procreation and are concerned about the potential for abuse.[90]

Courts currently permit sterilization of profoundly incompetent minors in limited cases after a process to determine that such a step is justified. This usually follows a formal hearing during which a guardian *ad litem* (for this legal process) is appointed for the minor. If she is judged to be permanently incompetent because of profound mental deficiency and it is determined that sterilization is in her best interest, the court may approve the procedure. Even in the absence of express statutory authority, some courts have utilized their "inherent" judicial authority to order sterilization.[91] These court-ordered sterilizations are, appropriately, limited to a narrow group of severely mentally retarded minors.[92] A physician performing a sterilization pursuant to a court order ordinarily may do so without incurring civil liability. When the court issuing the order does not have authority to do so, it is possible that the physician will be liable. This has led one expert to suggest some caution in implementing these orders.[60]

HIV/AIDS

HIV and AIDS present the practitioner with legal and medical challenges.[93] This is another area where laws vary considerably from state to state and are likely to change periodically. The prudent practitioner will, therefore, establish mechanisms to stay abreast of new legal developments.

In most states, testing for HIV cannot be undertaken without consent. This sets HIV testing apart from minimally invasive, run-of-the-mill medical testing. In some areas, HIV testing of a minor may be undertaken without parental consent.

The level of confidentiality of test results also depends on the locale. Depending on the jurisdiction, physicians may be prohibited from disclosing HIV status without the patient's consent or be required to report it to health authorities. The extent to which physicians may or must inform parents of minor patients' HIV status also varies, and in some states so far remains undetermined.

Treatment may in a few instances pose thorny legal problems. For example, the question of whether parents need to consent to medication may arise. Because these medications carry more than a small risk and are quite costly, physicians may well feel the need to consult with parents about treatment.

Additional problems arise when treatment is refused either by the minor patient or her parents. On the one hand, refusal of treatment does not pose an immediate life-threatening situation. On the other hand, in the longer run, refusal of the medication represents a significant health risk. The degree to which HIV treatment for a minor may be given over the objection of a parent has not yet been established.

Recent studies suggesting that treatment for HIV during pregnancy may reduce substantially the risk of infection to the fetus will inevitably raise questions about involuntary medication of HIV-infected, pregnant women, a question analogous to the involuntary caesarean section. To date, courts and legislatures have not resolved the issue of whether it is appropriate to require a woman to undertake HIV treatment during pregnancy to reduce the risk of fetal infection.

As the treatment and prevention of HIV change, the legal issues facing practitioners who treat minor patients will change as well. In the long run, the law will probably move toward encouraging prevention and early treatment. In the short run, public policy is likely to be less certain, and that will create difficulties for physicians.

DISCUSSION

Current lawmakers should be more realistic about the ability of older minors to consent to treatment. Adolescents 14 years of age and older—except those who are not mentally competent—should be permitted to consent to most forms of medical treatment. Even without a general minor consent law, all states should adopt laws permitting minors to consent to treatment for pregnancy, contraception, abortion, and STDs. The Supreme Court's decisions, which apparently permit states to require that minors seeking abortions be judicially determined competent, are both unrealistic and likely to be a real burden to many minors.[29, 41] States should avoid adopting statutes that mandate such determinations.[94]

The confidentiality of the adolescent-physician relationship should be more clearly defined. Minors seeking contraceptive advice, treatment for STDs, or abortions should be urged to confide in their families, and the majority do.[95] Ordinarily, the decision of whether or not to involve parents should be left to the adolescent. Parental notification statutes are often based on idealized notions of what families are like.

Required parental consent or notification exacts a significant price. One study estimated that parental notice requirements might result in approximately 125,000 minors who use family planning agencies to stop using effective methods of contraception. This would result in 33,000 additional pregnancies, leading to 14,000 abortions, 9000 out-of-wedlock births, 6000 forced marriages, and 4000 miscarriages. A parental notice requirement for abortions would mean that 42,000 minors would not have had legal abortions, the result of which would have been 19,000 illegal abortions, 18,000 unwanted births, and 5000 runaways. These figures are speculative, but they do indicate the magnitude of the problem presented by parental notification laws. Restricting the rights to abortion and contraception may injure the weakest members of society.[96, 97]

State reporting statutes can serve an important social function by eliminating and preventing disease and injury. It is essential, however, that the confidentiality of these reports be maintained. It is equally essential that the statutes be reasonably narrow and clear; some child abuse statutes are broad to the point of being vague, and such breadth may defeat the purpose

of the statute. The law should recognize the ability of most "mature minors" to make treatment decisions and realistically face the fact that the failure of some parents and their teenagers to communicate makes it difficult or impossible for these issues to be discussed openly.

It is important that practitioners who treat pediatric and adolescent patients participate in the legal system to promote rational rules for the obstetric and gynecologic care of these patients. Sensible reform in the areas of minors' consent, parental notice of obstetric care, confidentiality of treatment, and involuntary sterilization depends on the participation of physicians who understand the medical issues and are willing to share their expertise with lawmakers.

REFERENCES

1. Planned Parenthood of Southeastern Pennsylvania v Casey, 505 US 833 (1992).
2. Roe v Wade, 410 US 113 (1973).
3. Cohn SD: The evolving law of adolescent health care. NAACOGs Clin Issues Perinatal Womens Health Nurs 1991; 2:201–208.
4. Silber TJ: Ethical and legal issues in adolescent pregnancy. Clin Perinatol 1987; 14:265–270.
5. Greydanus DE, Patel DR: Consent and confidentiality in adolescent health care. Pediatr Ann 1991; 20:80–84.
6. Rosenthal SL, Cohen SS, Burklow KA, Hillard PA: Family involvement in the gynecologic care of adolescents. J Pediatr Adolesc Gynecol 1996; 9:59–65.
7. Maher L: Government funding in Title X projects: Circumscribing the constitutional rights of the indigent: Rust v. Sullivan. Calif Western Law Rev 1992; 29:143–182.
8. Ewald LS: Medical decision making for children: An analysis of competing interests. St Louis Univ Law J 1982; 25:689–733.
9. Rosato JL: The ultimate test of autonomy: Should minors have a right to make decisions regarding life-sustaining treatment? Rutgers Law Rev 1996; 49:1–102.
10. Smith SR: Disabled newborns and the federal child abuse amendments: Tenuous protection. Hastings Law J 1986; 37:765–825.
11. Holder AR: Legal Issues in Pediatrics and Adolescent Medicine. New Haven, CT: Yale University Press, 1985.
12. Haynes B: The 'mature minor' doctrine: Medical-legal aspects of treating mature minors. Med Trial Technique Q 1995; 42:107–135.
13. Sigman GS, O'Connor L: Exploration for physicians of the mature minor role. J Pediatr 1991; 119:520–525.
14. Melton G: Children's participation in treatment planning: Psychological and legal issues. Prof Psychol 1981; 12:246–252.
15. Ambuel B, Rappaport J: Development trends in adolescents' psychological and legal competencies to consent to abortion. Law Human Behav 1992; 16:129–154.
16. American Academy of Pediatrics: A model act providing for consent of minors to health services. Pediatrics 1973; 51:293–299.
17. Bellotti v Baird (Bellotti II), 443 US 622 (1979).
18. Melton GB: Judicial notice of "facts" about child development. In Melton GB (ed): Reforming the Law: Impact

of Child Development Research. New York: Guilford Press, 1987.

19. Schloendorff v Society of New York Hospital, 211 NY 125 (1914).

20. Canterbury v Spence, 464 F2d 772 (DC Cir 1972).

21. Rozovsky FA: Consent to Treatment: A Practical Guide, 2nd ed. Boston: Little, Brown, 1990.

22. Costello J: Making kids take their medicine: The privacy and due process rights of de facto competent minors. Loyola of Los Angeles Law Rev 1998; 31:907–927.

23. Smith SR: Medical and psychotherapy privileges and confidentiality: On giving with one hand and removing with the other. Ky Law J 1986; 75:473–557.

24. Kelly KP: Abandoning the compelling interest test in free exercise cases. Catholic Univ Law Rev 1991; 40:929–965.

25. Griswold v Connecticut, 381 US 479 (1965).

26. Eisenstadt v Baird, 405 US 438 (1972).

27. Planned Parenthood of Missouri v Danforth, 428 US 52 (1976).

28. Ohio v Akron Center for Reproductive Health, 497 US 502 (1990).

29. Hodgson v Minnesota, 497 US 417 (1990).

30. Carey v Population Services, 431 US 678 (1977).

31. Nixon v Administrator of General Services, 433 US 425 (1977).

32. Whalen v Roe, 429 US 589 (1977).

33. Leigh LJ: Informational privacy: Constitutional challenges to the collection and dissemination of personal information by government agencies. Hastings Constitutional Law Q 1976; 3:229–259.

34. Smith SR: Constitutional privacy in psychotherapy. George Washington Law Rev 1980; 49:1–60.

35. Akron v Akron Center for Reproductive Health, 462 US 416 (1983).

36. H. L. v Matheson, 450 US 398 (1981).

37. Moore SA: Constitutional law: Right of privacy. *H. L. v Matheson.* Cincinnati Law Rev 1981; 50:867–881.

38. Harris v McRae, 448 US 297 (1980).

39. Rust v Sullivan, 500 US 173 (1991).

40. Simopoulos v Virginia, 462 US 506 (1983).

41. Planned Parenthood of Kansas City v Ashcroft, 462 US 476 (1983).

42. Holder AR; Disclosure and consent problems in pediatrics. Law Med Health Care 1988; 16:219–228.

43. Traugott I, Alpers A: In their own hands: Adolescents' refusals of medical treatment. Arch Pediatr Adolesc Med 1997; 151: 922–927.

44. Rice MM: Medicolegal issues in pediatric and adolescent emergencies. Emerg Med Clin North Am 1991; 9:677–695.

45. Pieranunzi VR, Freitas LG: Informed consent with children and adolescents. Child Adolesc Psychiatr Mental Health Nurs 1992; 5:21–27.

46. California Family Code (sections 6920–6929) (Deering 1998).

47. Colorado Revised Statutes (sections as cited in text) (1999).

48. Florida Statutes (sections as cited in text) (1999).

49. Kentucky Revised Statutes (sections as cited in text) (Baldwin 1998).

50. English A, Simmons PS: Legal issues in reproductive health care for adolescents. Adolesc Med 1999; 10:181–194.

51. Brown RT, Cromer BA, Fischer R: Adolescent sexuality and issues in contraception. Obstet Gynecol Clin North Am 1992; 19:177–191.

52. Schuster MA, Bell RM, Petersen, LP, Kanouse DE: Communication between adolescents and physicians about sexual behaviors and risk prevention. Arch Pediatr Adolesc Med 1996; 150:906–913.

53. Wildey LS: Legal issues in the management of the pregnant adolescent. Pediatr Health Care 1992; 6:93–111.

54. Melton GB: Legal regulation of adolescent abortion. Am Psychologist 1987;42:79–83.

55. Stuhlbarg SF: When is a pregnant minor mature? When is an abortion in her best interest? Univ Cincinnati Law Rev 1992; 60:907–961.

56. O'Shaughnessy M: The worst of both worlds? Parental involvement requirements and the privacy rights of mature minors. Ohio State Law J 1996; 57:1731–1765.

57. Benshoof J: The chastity act: Government manipulation of abortion information and the First Amendment. Harvard Law Rev 1988; 101:1916–1937.

58. Interdivisional Committee on Adolescent Abortion: Adolescent abortion. Am Psychologist 1987; 42:73–76.

59. Acquavella AP, Braverman P: Adolescent gynecology in the office setting. Pediatr Clin North Am 1999; 46:489–503.

60. Clark HH Jr: Children and the Constitution. Univ Illinois Law Rev 1992; 1–40.

61. Ford CA, Millstein SG: Delivery of confidentiality assurances to adolescents by primary care physicians. Arch Pediatr Adolesc Med 1997; 151:505–509.

62. Smith SR, Meyer RG: Law, Behavior, and Mental Health: Policy and Practice. New York: New York University Press, 1987.

63. Embree MG, Dobson TA: Parental involvement in adolescent abortion decisions: A legal and psychological critique. Law Inequality 1991; 10:53–79.

64. American Academy of Pediatrics Committee on Adolescence: Contraception and adolescents. Pediatrics 1990; 86:134–138.

65. May JW: Legal issues in pediatric gynecology. Clin Obstet Gynecol 1997; 40:241–253.

66. Thompson HA: Consent requirements for treatment of minors. Tex Med 1989; 85:56–59.

67. Marcaravage LT: Limiting minors' abortion rights. Ohio Nor Univ Law Rev 1991; 18:169–178.

68. Crosby ML, English A: Mandatory parental involvement/judicial bypass laws: Do they promote adolescents' health? J Adolesc Health 1991; 12:143–147.

69. Worthington EL Jr, Larson DB, Lyons JS, et al: Mandatory parental involvement prior to adolescent abortion. J Adolesc Health 1991; 12:138–142.

70. American Academic of Pediatrics: The adolescent's right to confidential care when considering abortion. Pediatrics 1996; 97:746–751.

71. Rogers JL, Boruch RF, Stoms GB, DeMoya D: Impact of the Minnesota parental notification law on abortion and birth. Am J Public Health 1991; 81:294–298.

72. Ehrlich JS, Sabino JA: A minor's right to abortion—the unconstitutionality of parental participation in bypass hearings. N Engl Law Rev 1991; 25:1185–1209.

73. Council on Ethical and Judicial Affairs, American Medical Association: Mandatory parents' consent to abortion. JAMA 1993; 269:82–86.

74. Bridge B: Parent versus child: *H. L. v Matheson* and the new abortion litigation. Wisc Law Rev 1982; 1982:75–116.

75. Simons PS: Legal issues in reproductive health care for adolescents. Adolesc Med 1999; 10:181–194.

76. Smith SR, Meyer RG: Child abuse reporting laws and psychotherapy: A time for reconsideration. Int J Law Psychiatry 1984; 7:351–366.

77. Marrus E: Please keep my secret: Child abuse reporting statutes, confidentiality, and juvenile delinquency. Georgetown J Legal Ethics, 1998; 11:509–546.

78. Appelbaum PS: Child abuse reporting laws: Time for reform? Psychiatr Serv 1999; 50:27–29.

79. Jones JTR: Kentucky tort liability for failure to report family violence. North Kentucky Law Rev 1999; 26:43–65.

80. Fraser BG: A glance at the past, a gaze at the present, a glimpse at the future: A critical analysis of the development of child abuse reporting statutes. Chicago-Kent Law Rev 1978; 54:641–686.

81. Steinberg KL, Levine M, Doueck HJ: Effects of legally mandated child-abuse reports on the therapeutic relationship: A survey of psychotherapists. Am J Orthopsychiatry 1997; 67:112–122.

82. Smith SR: Mental health malpractice in the 1990s. Houston Law Rev 1991; 28:209–283.

83. Leonard AM: Fetal personhood, legal substance abuse, and maternal prosecutions: Child protection or "gestational Gestapo"? N Engl Law Rev 1998; 32:615–660.

84. Parks KT: Protecting the fetus: The criminalization of prenatal drug use. William & Mary J Women & the Law 1998; 5:245–271.

85. Roberts DE: Punishing drug addicts who have babies: Women of color, equality, and the right of privacy. Harvard Law Rev 1991; 104:1419–1482.

86. Glink SB: Note: The prosecution of maternal fetal abuse: Is this the answer? Univ Ill Law Rev 1991; 1991:533–580.

87. Iowa Code Annotated (sections as cited in text) (1998).

88. Marcus J: Sterilization and competency. Denver Univ Law Rev 1991; 68:106–118.

89. Bambrick M, Roberts GE: The sterilization of people with mental handicaps: The view of parents. J Ment Res 1991; 35:353–363.

90. Small MA: Involuntary sterilization of mentally retarded minors in Nebraska. Nebraska Law Rev 1989; 68:410–429.

91. Lachance D: In re *Grady*: The mentally retarded individual's right to choose sterilization. Am J Law Med 1981; 6:559–590.

92. American Academic of Pediatrics, Committee on Bioethics: Sterilization of minors with developmental disabilities. Pediatrics 1999; 104:337–340.

93. Felsman JP: Eliminating parental consent and notification for adolescent HIV testing: A legitimate statutory response to the AIDS epidemic. J Law & Policy 1996; 5:339–383.

94. Lundberg S, Plotnick RD: Effects of state welfare, abortion and family planning policies on premarital childbearing among white adolescents. Fam Plann Perspect 1990; 22:246–291.

95. Ellertson C: Mandatory parental involvement in minors' abortions: Effects of the laws in Minnesota, Missouri, and Indiana. Am J Public Health 1997; 87:1367–1374.

96. Berger LR: Abortions in America: The effects of restrictive funding. N Engl J Med 1978; 298:1474–1477.

97. Harrison LK, Naylor KL: The laws that affect abortion in the United States and their impact on women's health. Nurse Pract 1991; 16:53–59.

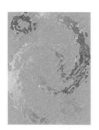

Chapter 32
Pubertal Aberrancy in the Third World

Geeta N. Pandya

A plethora of female adolescent problems have been manifested in recent years in the Third World. This is due largely to the fact that age-old inhibitions against seeking medical care for young girls are rapidly disappearing. In the past, such problems as abnormal genitalia and menstrual irregularities were kept hidden by family members because of a rigid pattern of arranged marriages in which the family's primary concern remained the possibility of not finding a mate for the girl in question. Only if all family members were in agreement would they venture a consultation with the family physician; this, of course, was done under oath of complete secrecy. That was usually as far as the family was willing to go; however, the suffering patient would continue to be denied the services of a trained specialist. Consequently, specialists in large communities currently are having to deal with the aftereffects of long-time pubertal neglect. When going through the history of many postadolescent cases, the origin of the problem can often be pinpointed to a period in the patient's pubertal or prepubertal age. Since the 1970s, the enhanced awareness of availability of specialized centers in large cities has reduced the neglect and mismanagement of pediatric and adolescent problems. This in turn has led to a reduction in iatrogenic female reproductive abnormalities.

Tuberculosis (TB) is responsible for a large percentage of chronic diseases in India. Apart from TB, other conditions seen with increasing incidence include malnutrition associated with chronic gastrointestinal conditions caused by amebiasis and resultant anemia, chronic renal disease, cardiac problems from childhood rheumatic fever, and congenital abnormalities.

Menstrual disturbances occur because of hematopoietic conditions such as thalassemia and purpura. These chronic conditions affect young girls before the prepubertal phase and become even more evident at puberty. They can produce a variety of menstrual irregularities, such as primary amenorrhea resulting from delayed puberty, polymenorrhea, menorrhagia, and secondary amenorrhea. Because the basic problem in thalassemia and purpura is anemia resulting from hemoglobinopathy, it becomes especially difficult to manage polymenorrhea and menorrhagia in this patient population.

CASE STUDY: ANEMIA ASSOCIATED WITH HELMINTHS. A 17-year-old female from Adhikari, India, presented as a very thin, weak, short adolescent with no secondary sex characteristics, primary amenorrhea, and the body habitus of a child of 10. On general examination, the girl had characteristic findings associated with anemia. She was found to be infested with worms and had a hemoglobin level of 6 gm/dl. After being treated for helminths and anemia, her growth and general condition improved, with resulting menarche and cyclic menses, confirming that the patient's delayed puberty was caused by anemia and malnutrition (Fig. 32–1).

CASE REPORTS. *Chronic Renal Disease.* A girl of 3 years started to develop pubic hair and slight enlargement of the clitoris, a few months after beginning steroid therapy for chronic renal failure. Her parents were reassured, and the nephrologist advised stopping steroids as soon as possible. Later on she underwent a kidney transplant (Fig. 32–2). Dialysis-dependent adolescent girls frequently have heavy menstrual periods with resultant anemia.

Metabolic Disorder. An adolescent girl, age 15 years, had primary amenorrhea and absent secondary sexual development. Her bone age was much lower than her chronologic age. FSH and total estrogen levels were very low, thus confirming delayed puberty. She also had hepatosplenomegaly with early cirrhosis due to her underlying metabolic disorder, for which she is followed by her pediatrician. Except for reassurance and multivitamins, no hormonal treatment was given. After one year she has had slight breast develop-

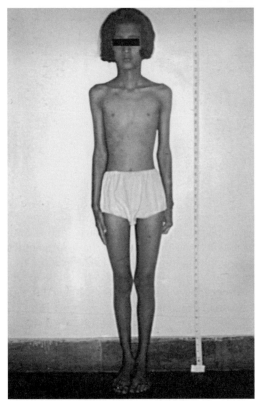

Figure 32–1. Adolescent with delayed puberty caused by anemia and malnutrition.

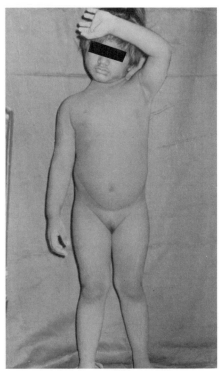

Figure 32–2. A 3-year-old girl a few months after being put on steroids for chronic renal failure.

ment but no menarche as yet. She is being followed at 3-month intervals.

Obesity. A young adolescent girl, 15 years of age and weighing 246 lb, presented with the chief complaint of sudden weight gain after she attained menarche at age 12 years. She has had regular menstrual cycles. Hormonal evaluation showed no abnormality. Her weight gain started following a change in environment. She was advised diet control and exercise (Fig. 32–3).

GENITAL TUBERCULOSIS

Information on the extent and magnitude of TB in Third World countries is difficult to gauge, but it is known to be a significant factor contributing to gynecologic problems. Statistics on incidence, morbidity, and mortality rates are available only from government or municipal hospitals or at institutes where TB is treated. Since the 1940s, the incidence of TB has been described by many authors and it varies with the particular case load and the type of institution and location (urban or rural) where the data were collected.[1]

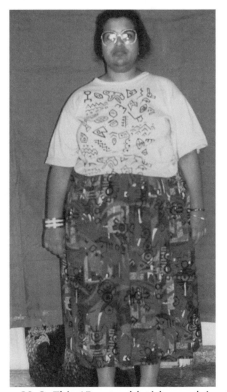

Figure 32–3. This 15-year-old girl complained of sudden weight gain after menarche.

In 1990 it was estimated that 1.7 billion people, or one third of the world population, have been infected with the tubercle bacillus.[1] However, such infection is responsible for 0.76%[2] to 9.8%[3] of all gynecologic admissions among infertile women. A patient with TB may be seen by a pediatrician or, in the case of an adult, by a chest physician or general or orthopedic surgeon, gynecologist, neurologist, or nephrologist. Thus, practitioners in associated disciplines may be able to document the incidence and type of TB.[1]

The incidence of TB among adolescents is extremely difficult to determine, because young girls at puberty are usually seen by general practitioners or gynecologists with inadequate statistical reporting techniques. Most of the time, parents do not like to acknowledge any history, and repeated interrogation may be necessary to find out whether the girl ever suffered from TB. Invariably, the physician must determine indirectly whether the girl has had episodes of repeated fever, cough, and coldlike symptoms or was ever prescribed 3 to 6 months of continuous medication. The prevalence of infection with pulmonary TB increases with age, from 2.1% to 16.5% in the pediatric age group to about 50% in those older than age 15.[4] The incidence of genital TB in children is fairly high (Table 32–1). When pulmonary TB is treated, it remains in a dormant state, often until puberty, when the primary infection of the lung or intestines, which has been silent for a long time, tends to flare up and manifest as a genital infection. It also can present as a new infection spread via the bloodstream from a different primary source. The result is genital TB occurring as a secondary infection with the primary focus lying elsewhere and the infection spreading in the early stages of the disease (frequently in adolescence or early maturity). Thus, in most cases, the primary infection not only has healed but also is "inconspicuous." Even so, genital TB can be associated with impaired fertility (Table 32–2).[4]

The pathophysiology of the disease must be understood. Bacteriologically, in approximately 95% of all cases, genital TB is caused by a human bacillus (*Mycobacterium tuberculosis*) rather than a bovine type.

Table 32–1. Types of Genital Tuberculosis

1. *Primary.* Very rarely, genital tuberculosis is of primary origin.
2. *Secondary.* Genital tuberculosis is nearly always secondary to pulmonary or lesions in extrapulmonary sites, such as lymph nodes, intestines, urinary tract, gonads, and joints.

Table 32–2. Routes of Infection of Genital Tuberculosis

1. *Bloodstream*—the most common mode (although the primary extragenital focus is somewhere else, usually the lungs).
2. *Lymphatic spread*—possible from tuberculosis involving the mesenteric lymph nodes and/or peritoneum.
3. *Direct spread*—possible through peritonitis, although direct adhesion of a tuberculous lesion with the genital tract is an important means of direct spread.

PRIMARY AMENORRHEA

CASE REPORTS. *Patient M.P.* presented at 16 years of age. The patient's mother was particularly worried about her primary amenorrhea, because she herself had experienced menarche at age 13. Physical findings included a tall, thin, cachectic adolescent with Tanner stage IV breasts (Fig. 32–4A). She had long, thin fingers with clubbing of the nails (Fig. 32–4B). A lower gastrointestinal series revealed typical findings of tuberculosis of the cecum (Fig. 32–4C). The patient was given antituberculosis therapy; during the third month of treatment menarche occurred.

Patient K., age 17, was an obese young woman who had developed tuberculous meningitis at age 15. She then developed secondary hypopituitarism and was placed on thyroid and corticosteroid replacement. On psychiatric evaluation, the patient's intelligence quotient (IQ) was found to be low, and her parents were not eager for her to continue sex steroid replacement, allowing her to menstruate cyclically.

Although a debated topic, many scientists are of the opinion that primary infection of the reproductive organs does not occur. Tuberculosis of the vulva or the vagina without any infection in the upper genital tract has been reported,[5] but such lesions appear to occur in association with a primary infection elsewhere in the body. Coitus is the most common method of transmission of primary infection.[5]

Tuberculous Meningitis. Patient A. A girl aged 5½ years had started thelarche and menarche while she was hospitalized for the diagnosis and treatment of tuberculous meningitis. Hormonal evaluation showed increased total serum estrogen and serum prolactin levels and pelvic ultrasound revealed a uterus of adult size. The patient was treated with bromocriptine daily, and depomedroxy/progesterone acetate every 3 weeks to suppress ovarian function and menstruation. She is now 8 years of age and growth appears normal.

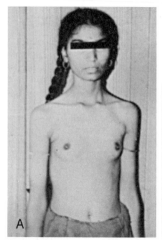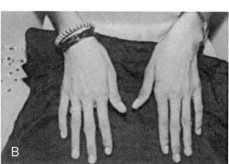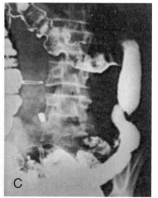

Figure 32–4. *A,* Adolescent with genital tuberculosis with primary amenorrhea. *B,* Long, thin fingers with clubbing. *C,* Barium enema shows changes in cecal area secondary to tuberculosis.

Treatment will continue until she is 9 years of age.

SITES OF TUBERCULOSIS LESIONS

Fallopian tubes. M. tuberculosis has high affinity for the fallopian tubes.[6] In 90% of cases of tubercular salpingitis, both tubes are affected.[6] From the fallopian tubes, the infection spreads to other pelvic organs.

Corpus uteri. In 50% of these cases, TB manifests itself as tubercular endometritis.[7] Contiguous spread occurs from the affected tubes. Only in very rare cases is the uterus involved without significant infection in the tubes.[7]

Cervix. The infection coming down from the fallopian tubes to the uterus affects the cervix in about 5% of cases.[8]

Vagina and vulva. Infection of the vagina or vulva sometimes can be traced to tubercular cervicitis.

Ovaries. In about 20% of patients, the ovaries are affected secondary to infection involving the fallopian tubes.[9]

Unusual presentations. Some patients with TB present with infertility, nonspecific menstrual disturbances, pain, or abdominal distention.[10] The infection appears to occur via hematogenous spread from a distant focus, the fallopian tubes being involved most often.[10] Another complication associated with TB was an abdominal pregnancy 10 years after treatment for pelvic TB.[11] Characteristic endoscopic findings have been identified.[12]

DIAGNOSIS OF TUBERCULOSIS IN ADOLESCENTS

In adolescent girls, diagnosis of TB is not a simple matter, as certain investigative procedures (e.g., vaginal examination with a speculum or sampling of the endometrium for confirmation) often are not possible. Therefore, whenever a young woman presents with menstrual irregularities, a detailed history of past illnesses, as well as a family history—especially when looking for a history of TB, treated or untreated—becomes essential. This must be followed by a general investigation to rule out other chronic illnesses. Genital TB is suspected when menstrual irregularities are associated with one or more of the following symptoms: weakness, general malaise, evening increase in temperature, repeated history of cough, repeated urinary tract infections, persistent high sedimentation rate, or leukopenia. In 69% of cases, a history of extragenital TB is documented;[13] 20% have a family history of TB.[14]

Generally, the investigations for confirmation of genital TB consist of histopathologic and bacteriologic examinations of endometrial scrapings or menstrual blood. A hysterosalpingogram identifying a typical tuberculous pattern and sometimes sonographic evidence of a tuboovarian mass provide confirmation of genital TB. Diagnostic tests are somewhat problematic in adolescent girls, except for ultrasonography because, according to cultural norms, virginity must be preserved unless a dire condition prevails (e.g., therapeutic curettage may be necessary for treatment of severe menorrhagia).

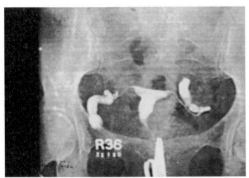

Figure 32–5. *A,* Hysterosalpingogram showing hydrosalpinx with tuberculous involvement.

Pediatric TB, when suspected, is easily diagnosed and cured. Adolescent girls at puberty (when various hormonal changes occur) are at higher risk in countries where TB is widely prevalent.

Pathology of Tuberculous Tubes

The classic gross description of tubes involved by TB is that of a long, thin, beaded, obstructed tube or a short, thick, pocketed one with associated hydrosalpinx (Fig. 32–5). Many times, the condition goes undiagnosed at puberty. As time goes by, they mature and marry; the damage done at the time of pubertal infection may then present as infertility.

TUBERCULAR SALPINGITIS. In a few cases, the mucosa of the tubes is first affected (endosalpingitis) and the infection then spreads to the remainder of the tube.

ADHESION FORMATION. The tubes thicken and dense "plastic" adhesions form around them. The distal ostia may be adherent or open, and fimbria may be destroyed. Tubercles may be visible on the surface.

TUBERCULOUS PYOSALPINX. Fallopian tubes are enlarged as a result of accumulation of caseous material that causes distention. The walls become thick and hard, surrounding adhesions are dense, and the distal ostium is occluded. Tubercles are seen on the surface of the pyosalpinx.

MILIARY FORM. The surfaces of the tubes are covered with tubercles. Microscopically, the endosalpinx and the subserous segments have tubercles with giant cells, a characteristic of tuberculosis. In advanced cases, caseation may occur, a condition that can result in a tuboovarian mass or ovarian abscess.

Menstrual Aberrations Secondary to Tuberculosis

Frequently, a young girl with TB begins menarche spontaneously and subsequently develops secondary amenorrhea. In other cases, menarche is delayed.

Primary amenorrhea is usually diagnosed relatively early, when the patient is taken to a physician because she has not started menstruating. Primary amenorrhea stemming from generalized or chronic disease is not unknown; it is quite common for menstruation to begin after 2 or 3 months of antituberculosis treatment.

In cases of secondary amenorrhea, the patient may cease menstruating after a few periods. This may be succeeded by menorrhagia, often with a flow so heavy that curettage becomes necessary to stop the abnormal bleeding. If intense curettage is not performed and the tissue is not sent for histopathologic examination, there is a chance that the correct diagnosis will not be made and the patient will not receive appropriate treatment. Indeed, this may lead to uterine synechiae resulting in secondary amenorrhea (Fig. 32–6). It appears that when a patient marries early, curettage is more readily performed for menorrhagia or oligomenorrhea as a result of TB infection. This is done to "rule out suspected pregnancy." Before the availability of laparoscopy, the diagnosis of endometrial TB was established by histopathologic investigation of the endometrium. With diagnostic laparoscopy the clinician is able to identify the fine tubercles on the tubes and to note any characteristics of the tubes that are typical of TB. Many times, in patients with secondary amenorrhea or oligomenorrhea associated with infertility, hysterosalpingography will identify the typical picture of TB. TB affecting the meninges (TB meningitis) may lead to disturbance of the hypothalamic-pituitary axis, some-

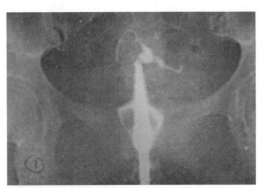

Figure 32–6. Hysterosalpingogram showing uterine synechiae.

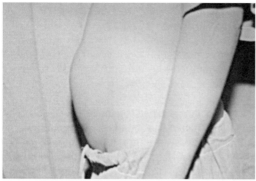

Figure 32–7. Abdominal distention associated with secondary amenorrhea in a patient with a large, caseating, tuboovarian abscess.

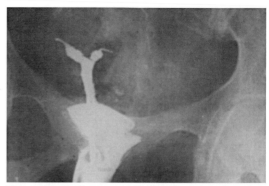

Figure 32–9. Hysterosalpingogram showing double uterus with occluded fallopian tubes.

times resulting in hypopituitarism. Genital TB per se leading to menorrhagia, oligomenorrhea, or secondary amenorrhea is associated with tuberculous salpingo-oophoritis or tuberculous endometritis, as well as a caseating tuboovarian mass.

In the Third World it is very common for patients to go unevaluated for long periods of time owing to lack of adequate medical facilities. Examples of such cases are described here.

CASE STUDIES: SECONDARY AMENORRHEA. *Patient D.*, aged 15, presented with abdominal distention and secondary amenorrhea (Fig. 32–7). Menarche occurred at 12½ years. Her menses were initially regular, but at age 14, one episode of very heavy menses occurred. Gradually her cycles became oligomenorrheic, and ultimately, secondary amenorrhea of 6 months' duration developed. At laparotomy, a large caseating tuboovarian mass was noted (Fig. 32–8).

Patient P., aged 19, had been married for 2 years and presented with a chief complaint of primary infertility and oligomenorrhea. Since 4 to 5 years of age, a cyclic scanty flow for 1 to 1½ days had been the pattern. Menarche occurred at age 12, with initially regular cycles that gradually became "scanty." Hysterosalpingography showed a septate uterus with occluded fallopian tubes (Fig. 32–9). A diagnosis of Asherman syndrome

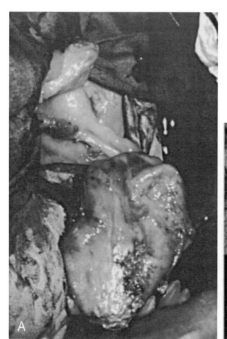

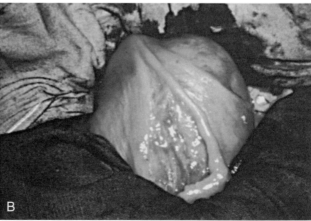

Figure 32–8. *A, B,* Tuboovarian mass with caseation.

secondary to tuberculous endometritis was established. (The condition had probably developed several years earlier.) On inquiry, the patient reported a history of intermittent fever between ages 13 and 15, a condition that was neither evaluated nor treated.

Patient S. was a 19-year-old who became amenorrheic and hirsute over an 11-month period. She presented with hirsutism of rapid onset and clinical evidence of an androgen-producing tumor. Sertoli-Leydig cell tumor (arrhenoblastoma) was detected (Fig. 32–10).

Hematologic disorders can result in pubertal delay. A 16-year-old girl with transfusion-dependent thalassemia had not attained menarche. Serum follicle-stimulating hormone, luteinizing hormone, and prolactin were normal. She was reassured and observed closely. After a year she started menstruating. After the onset of menses dysfunctional uterine bleeding developed that further worsened her anemia. Her condition has been controlled with oral progesterone to counterbalance the unopposed estrogen.

Similar problems have also been noted in patients with idiopathic thrombocytopenic purpura. Both the above-mentioned hematologic problems are common in the Third World.

FEMALE CIRCUMCISION

Female circumcision is a ritual peculiar to certain cults in India and Nigeria (Fig. 32–11). In Nigeria, the Edo tribe has been known to have the highest proportion of circumcised females (76.7%), followed by the Ibos (61%).[15] Circumcision is usually performed during infancy; only 5.9% are circumcised as adults.[15] Statistics on morbidity and mortality from this procedure are difficult to compile.

Two types of circumcision are performed. Shaving of the clitoris, practiced by certain sects of Muslims in India, is done when a girl is 8 years of age. In complete excision of the clitoris, the sutured skin covers the urethra and upper part of the introitus, which is narrowed.

Obstetric sequelae of female circumcision have been reported, the most apparent problems being increased maternal morbidity and fetal loss. No apparent long-term complications were noted in the series reported by DeSilva.[16]

Two types of complications, immediate and delayed, were noted by El-Dareer.[17] Immediate complications (noted in 25% of patients) included difficulty with urination, wound infection, and bleeding. Delayed complications included urinary tract infection, chronic pelvic infection, and "tight circumcision."

FEMALE GENITAL MUTILATION

Female genital mutilation presents a significant hazard to a woman's emotional and psychological health.[18] Female circumcision is included in the concern over genital mutilation. More than 25% of women subjected to severe forms of circumcision such as "pharonic rituals" suffer serious physical complications (Fig. 32–12).[18]

Figure 32–13A shows a 15-year-old girl who was attacked by a water buffalo and suffered a complete perineal and a partial vaginal tear. Plastic surgery restored normal genital function (Fig. 32–13B). Five months later, she married and after 1 year delivered a child by cesarean section.

MALE CASTRATION

Indian culture is permeated with many religious cults. Among these are a group of eunuchs known as *Hijras*, who used to serve as harem guards in the Indian Royal Palaces.[19] They are feminized in outward appearance by the use of female attire, makeup, jewelry, and the swinging gait of a dancing girl. The individuals who join this cult are usually born with ambiguous genitalia or are normal adult men who have chosen castration, often because of homosexual tendencies. Figures 32–14 to 32–16 are representative of these castrated males who behave as females.

CASE STUDIES: PUBERTAL ABERRATION. *Two sisters, aged 18 and 19,* complained of hirsutism and acne along with primary amenorrhea. Figure 32–17 shows the outward appearance of their genitalia. They were found to have male external genitalia; both had testicles, and one had an undescended testicle and perineal hypospadias. They had one older sister and six brothers. At birth, both patients had had undescended testicles and a slightly enlarged, clitoral-type penis, and thus they were reared as girls. Their hirsutism was diagnosed as normal male hair growth along with pubertal acne. They underwent plastic surgery for hypospadias and were reidentified as boys.

A 19-year-old recently married woman presented with ambiguous genitalia (Fig. 32–18). She had Tanner stage I breast development and had recently undergone surgery for removal of bilateral undescended testicles from the lower inguinal region. She had perineal hypospadias and was unaware of being a male. She was the

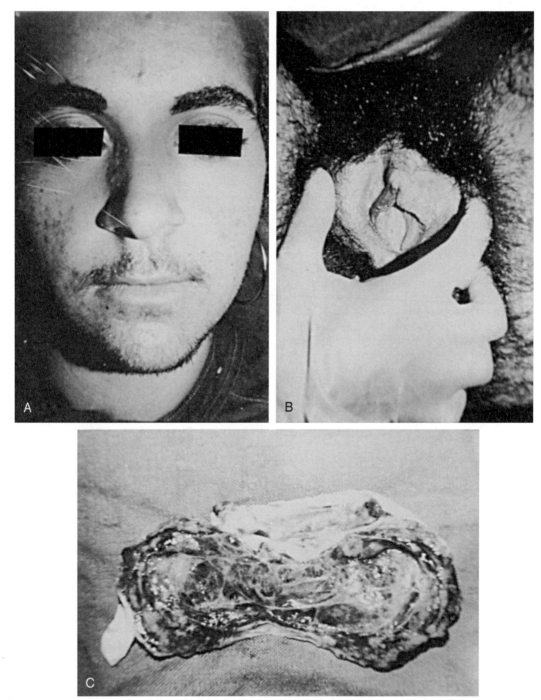

Figure 32–10. *A*, Face of 19-year-old female showing acne and hirsutism. *B*, Vulva of the same patient showing excessive hair and an enlarged clitoris (changes that developed over 11 months). *C*, Gross appearance of Sertoli-Leydig cell tumor from the same patient.

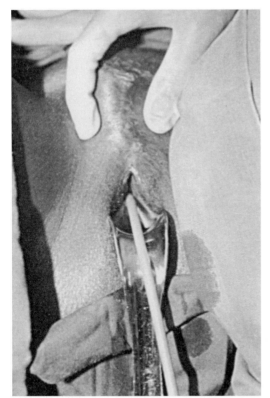

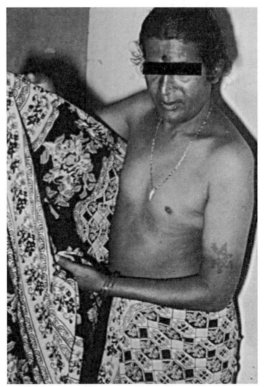

Figure 32–11. Typical appearance of a circumcised female.

Figure 32–14. A castrated Indian male, known as a *Hijras*.

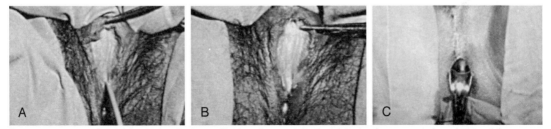

Figure 32–12. *A* through *C*, Genital mutilation in a patient subjected to extensive circumcision.

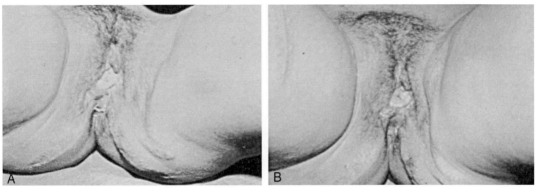

Figure 32–13. *A*, A 15-year-old female sustained a complete perineal and partial vaginal tear from the horn of a water buffalo. *B*, The perineal area of that patient after surgical reconstruction.

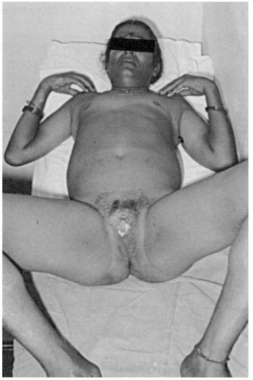

Figure 32–15. Eunuch showing no breasts or genitalia.

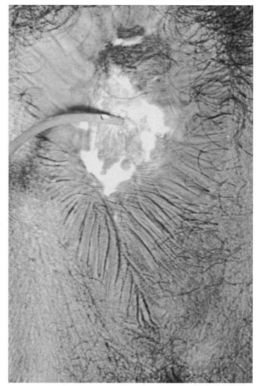

Figure 32–16. Scar tissue with a small opening for a catheter, for passage of urine, in a castrated male.

third wife of an Arab man and claimed to be having anal coitus.

Recently, a fair number of East Indian families have migrated to the Persian Gulf countries, for economic betterment. Many pubertal girls in these families suddenly start gaining weight because of changes in lifestyle—shorter school hours, afternoon naps, lack of exercise, little outdoor life. Also, higher economic status is associated with overeating rich, fatty foods and abnormal dietary habits (e.g., snacking between meals, especially during long hours spent in front of the television). All these factors contribute to rapid

weight gain, and a significant number of girls develop oligomenorrhea.

In contrast, young female students from well-to-do Indian families living in dormitories cannot avail themselves of the luxuries they had at home. As a result, they initially lose weight rapidly and develop menstrual abnormalities, mainly secondary amenorrhea.

47,XXY/46,XY MOSAIC WITH OVOTESTES. An 18-year-old girl with well-developed breasts, primary amenorrhea, a vaginal dimple, and a tall, thin habitus was diagnosed upon laparoscopy to

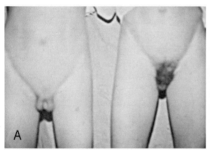
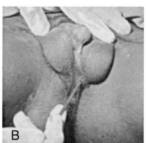
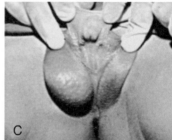

Figure 32–17. *A,* Siblings reared as females show male external genitalia. *B, C,* Their genitals appear similar.

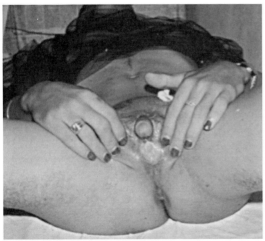

Figure 32–18. A 19-year-old married woman shows ambiguous genitalia. She had Tanner stage I breast development and undescended testes.

have ovotestes. Diagnostic laparoscopy confirmed gonads and no uterus. The fimbria of the fallopian tubes showed an abnormality, and the patient's genotype was 46 XX,XY. When removed, the gonads showed tissue of 40% testicular origin and 60% ovarian origin (Pandya G. Unpublished data; Fig. 32–19).

IATROGENIC TRAUMA TO THE PENIS. A young monk, during his training period, performed the ritual of rolling his penis on a stick (Fig. 32–20).

This is done in an effort to stretch and destroy nerve endings and elastic tissue, preventing an erection and eliminating sexual desire.

PERSPECTIVES, PAST AND FUTURE

As age-old inhibitions against seeking medical care for young girls break down, many unique problems relating to abnormal genitalia and menstrual irregularities that previously remained hidden are being identified at regional medical centers throughout India and other underdeveloped countries. The reluctance of parents to seek medical care in the past was largely due to their fears of being unable to effect the customary "arranged marriage" for their daughter.

TB continues to be responsible for a significant degree of chronic disease in India. It can manifest as exclusively genital TB with associated pubertal aberration and sometimes impaired fertility. Many unique problems have been presented.

The rituals associated with female circumcision in India and Africa remain a challenge for pediatric/adolescent gynecologists caring for such patients. Genital mutilation, with its associated emotional and psychological sequelae, is currently being identified more often as these patients are evaluated. Appropriate means of evaluation and treatment, including the psychosocial

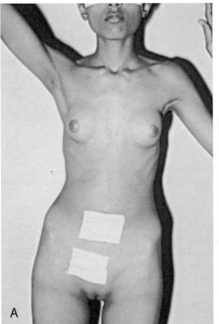

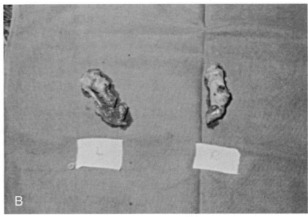

Figure 32–19. *A*, An 18-year-old female, tall and with well-developed breasts. *B*, Gross appearance of the gonads: 40% testicular and 60% ovarian.

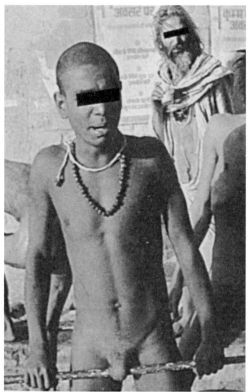

Figure 32–20. A young monk whose penis shows trauma from ritualistic rolling of his penis onto a stick.

aspects of these disease processes, are paramount in the management of this patient population.

In both the United States and Canada, it is predicted that clinicians will be seeing patients who have undergone female circumcision or female genital mutilation with increasing frequency. This reflects an increasing migration of such patients to North America as racial and ethnic demographics change. Canada and the United States have introduced legislation prohibiting the practice of female circumcision as well as genital mutilation. Specifically, in 1997 it became a federal crime to perform medically unnecessary surgery on the genitalia of a female less than 18 years of age. Punishment can include imprisonment for up to five years. Clinicians should be apprised that the United States Immigration and Naturalization Service provides information to all immigrants issued visas to the United States on the adverse health consequences associated with female circumcision and female genital mutilation, including the legal consequence of performing such surgery in the United States.

The American College of Obstetricians and Gynecologists has identified the need to inform clinicians of these practices and provide education in management. A slide series has been compiled entitled "Female Circumcision/Female Genital Mutilation: Clinical Management of Circumcised Women."[20] This series communicates diagnosis and management aspects of the problem and is extremely useful when dealing with this challenging clinical problem.

REFERENCES

1. Kochi A: Government intervention programs in HIV tuberculosis infection. Outline of guidelines for national tuberculosis control programs in view of the HIV epidemic. Bull Int Union Tuberc Lung Dis 1991; 66(1):33–36.
2. Bhaskara Rao KJ: Clinical aspect of genital tuberculosis in the female. J Obstet Gynaecol India 1959; 10:26–31.
3. Malkani P, Banerji A: The role of tuberculosis in pathogenesis of sub-acute and chronic adnexitis. J Obstet Gynaecol India 1959; 10:32–42.
4. Oosthuizen A, Wessels P, Herfer J: Tuberculosis of the female genital tract in patients attending an infertility clinic. South Afr Med J 1990; 77(11):562–564.
5. Naik R, Srinivas C, Balachandran C, et al: Esthiomene resulting from cutaneous tuberculosis of external genitalia. Genitourin Med 1987; 63(2):133–136.
6. Tang L, Cho H, Wong T: Atypical presentation of female genital tract tuberculosis. Eur J Obstet Gynaecol Reprod Biol 1984; 17(4):355–363.
7. Tripathy S, Tripathy S: Endometrial tuberculosis. J Indian Med Assoc 1987; 85(5):136–140.
8. Kumar N, Kapila K, Verma K: Cervical tuberculosis—case report. Aust NZ J Obstet Gynaecol 1989; 29(3pt 1):270–272.
9. Kalogirou D, Mantzavinos T, Zourlas P, Deligiorgi E: Primary adenocarcinoma of the fallopian tube with tuberculosis. Short communication. Eur J Gynaecol Oncol 1989; 10(5):307–309.
10. Carter J: Unusual presentations of genital tract tuberculosis. Int J Gynaecol Obstet 1990; 33(2):171–176.
11. Durukan T, Urman B, Yarali H, et al: An abdominal pregnancy ten years after treatment for pelvic tuberculosis. Am J Obstet Gynaecol 1990; 163(2):594–595.
12. Merchant R: Endoscopy in the diagnosis of genital tuberculosis. J Reprod Med 1989; 34(7):468–470.
13. Shah Hansa M: Genital tuberculosis—a study of 30 cases. J Obstet Gynaecol Naecol India 1963; 13:374–381.
14. Stalworthy J: Genital tuberculosis in females. J Obstet Gynaecol Br Emp 1952; 59:729–749.
15. Odujinrin O, Akitoye C, Oyediran A. A study of female circumcision in Nigeria. West Afr J Med 1989; 8(3):183–192.
16. DeSilva S: Obstetrical sequelae of female circumcision. Eur J Obstet Gynaecol Naecol Reprod Biol 1989; 32(3):233–240.
17. El-Dareer A: Complications of female circumcision in the Sudan. Trop Doct 1983; 13(3):131–133.
18. Cutner LP: Female genital mutilation. Obstet Gynaecol Surv 1985; 40(7):437–443.
19. Mukherjee J: Castration—a means of induction into the Hijras group of the eunuch community in India. A critical study of 20 cases. Am J Forens Med Pathol 1980; 1(1):61–65.
20. American College of Obstetricians and Gynecologists: Female Circumcision/Female Genital Mutilation: Clinical Management of Circumcised Women. Slide lecture kit. Washington, DC, ACOG, 1999.

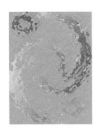

Chapter 33

Genital Injuries in Pediatric and Adolescent Girls

DIANE F. MERRITT, MARY E. RIMSZA, AND DAVID MURAM

Ideally, every obstetrician-gynecologist in general practice should have the ability to evaluate and manage genital injuries. The most likely cause of such injury in postpubertal women is childbirth trauma. In children and adolescents, accidental genital injuries (not iatrogenic) may be associated with falls, straddle injuries, chemical or thermal burns, pelvic fractures, high-pressure liquid injection, or penetrating injuries of a sexual or nonsexual nature.[1] Many injuries are minor and do not require hospitalization; however, serious coitus-related and accidental injuries do occur.

Because the external genitalia have a rich blood supply, relatively minor injuries can bleed profusely, particularly when lacerations involve the tissues of the vagina, the hymen, and adjacent structures. While there is a need for prompt recognition, diagnosis, and definitive repair of genital injuries, it is important to seek concomitant injuries and to stabilize the patient. To be able to recognize injuries and posttraumatic changes, the clinician must be cognizant of normal prepubertal genital anatomy and congenital variants.[2, 3] As always, a detailed history should be obtained, to determine how the trauma occurred (Table 33–1). If the child is preverbal or unable to speak for herself, a responsible caregiver or eyewitness should be able to provide the necessary information. Inconsistencies in the history may alert the physician and increase suspicion of physical or sexual assault.

INCIDENCE

The incidence of genital trauma in children and adolescents is difficult to assess. Much of the

literature on genital trauma consists of anecdotal case reports[4–8] or has been drawn from biased population samples, such as children who were evaluated for suspected sexual abuse.[9–14] A more accurate estimate of the true incidence of genital trauma would require study of an unbiased population group, for instance, all children and adolescents who present to an emergency department or to a pediatrics clinic.

VULVAR INJURIES

Vulvar injuries are deceleration injuries, commonly the result of straddle injuries sustained in a fall upon the crossbars of a bicycle (Fig. 33–1), as when climbing a fence or on playground equipment or entering or exiting a bathtub or swimming pool (especially above-ground pools).

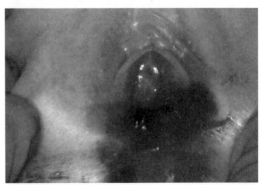

Figure 33–1. Straddle injury. Ecchymoses and abrasions were sustained in a fall onto a bicycle crossbar. Note, injury does not involve hymen. (See Color Fig. 33–1.)

Figures 33–1, 33–4 to 33–6, 33–8, 33–9, 33–11, and 33–12 are courtesy of Dr. Diane Merritt; all other illustrations in this chapter are courtesy of Dr. David Muram.

Table 33–1. Questions to Ask the Trauma Victim

What happened?
Where and how did the trauma occur?
Were there any witnesses?
Are there any other injuries?
How much bleeding has occurred?
Is the lesion stable, increasing, or decreasing?
Has the child been able to urinate since the traumatic incident?

In such accidents, the vagina, urethra, and hymenal areas are usually spared, because of the protection provided by the overlying labia. Nevertheless, the external genitalia of a child are less protected against injury than those of an adult. With most blunt injuries caused by a fall, the most prominent bruising is on the surface that bore most of the impact (i.e., the labia majora, mons pubis, and buttocks).[15] Bruising, abrasions, and hematomas are the most common injuries; lacerations are unusual unless the child falls on a sharp object. Usually, less superficial areas, including the urethra, the hymenal area, and the vagina, are not injured as severely by blunt trauma; however, a child who accidentally falls on a pointed object sometimes sustains a penetrating injury of the fourchette, hymen, and vagina or the rectum in addition to lacerations.

Figure 33–2 shows the kind of straddle injury that can result from blunt trauma. In that case, an 8-year-old girl was brought to the pediatrics clinic for evaluation after falling on the edge of the bathtub as she was attempting to get out of the tub. She sustained a straddle-type injury with prominent bruising on the buttocks. Figure 33–2 demonstrates extensive bruising on the external aspect of the labia majora that extends onto the buttocks. A small, clinically insignificant tear of the posterior fourchette was also observed, but no vaginal or hymenal injuries. For this child, these traumatic lesions are consistent with the history provided.

West and colleagues reported on a series of 13 children who had sustained accidental vulvar injuries.[16] Eight of them had a straddle injury; three, a penetrating injury; and one, a stretch injury. The children with straddle injuries often had linear bruising like that shown in Figure 33–2, usually over the anterior aspect of the labia. Straddle injuries are crush injuries of soft tissue overlying bone or tendon and are more likely to be anterior, perhaps because children are more likely to fall forward and because they have less superficial fat over the mons pubis than over the buttocks.

VULVAR HEMATOMAS

Vulvar hematomas can be so painful as to prevent a child or adolescent from urinating, as a result of pain and swelling. When the hematoma is not very large and the perineal anatomy is not distorted, the lesion can be managed with immediate application of ice packs to reduce local swelling (Fig. 33–3). Dysuria and local swelling may lead to urinary retention, and in some cases it may be necessary to place a urethral or suprapubic catheter. Bladder drainage should be continued until the swelling resolves. Very large vulvar hematomas sometimes dissect into the loose areolar tissue along the vaginal wall and along the fascial planes overlying the symphysis pubis and lower abdominal wall (Fig.

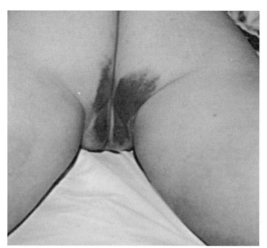

Figure 33–2. Labial bruising extending onto the buttocks secondary to a straddle injury.

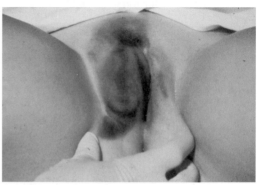

Figure 33–3. This vulvar hematoma does not distort the perineal anatomy. If the patient can void spontaneously, she can be managed conservatively with ice packs and bed rest. (See Color Fig. 33–3.)

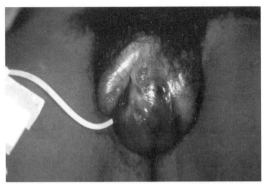

Figure 33–4. A large expanding vulvar hematoma distorts the anatomy and should be drained. (See Color Fig. 33–4.)

33–4). Pressure from the expanding hematoma can cause necrosis of the skin overlying the hematoma (Fig. 33–5). Evacuating the hematoma eases the pain, hastens recovery, and prevents necrosis, tissue loss, and secondary infection. Large vulvar hematomas should be incised at the medial mucosal surface, near the vaginal orifice. The wound should be cleaned of all devitalized tissue and irrigated. Ligation of bleeding vessels and placement of absorbable mattress sutures to control bleeding may hasten the patient's convalescence. Placement of a Jackson Pratt or Blake

(closed-system) drain to remove transudates, exudates, and blood (and, thereby, relieve local pressure) reduces pain and removes media for potential bacterial growth (Fig. 33–6).

Usually, vulvar lacerations do not bleed profusely, but it should be remembered that even minor periurethral injuries can cause urethral spasm that could lead to urinary retention. Therefore, before any child with vulvar injuries is discharged home, the physician should confirm that the child is able to void. Because injuries can extend into the urethra and bladder, examination of the urine for blood is also necessary. Perineal abrasions and tears can cause dysuria, even in patients with no direct injury to the urethra. In these cases, an analgesic agent such as phenazopyridine (Pyridium) given for 2 to 3 days until the superficial abrasions have healed, may be beneficial. Sitz baths may help to relieve local pain, and increasing fluid intake may also be useful. When pain is persistent or severe, the possibility of a pelvic fracture should be considered.

PERINEAL INJURIES

Perineal injuries sometimes extend to the anus and rectum. Black and colleagues[7] reviewed 16 cases of anorectal trauma in children seen in an emergency department. Most of the injuries were due to sexual abuse, but one child who fell astraddle a baton sustained a rectovaginal tear that extended through the anal sphincter and distal rectal mucosa and across the perineum into the distal posterior vagina.[7] Similar injuries can

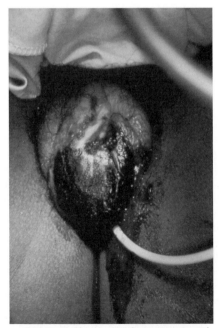

Figure 33–5. Failure to decompress the expanding hematoma can lead to tissue necrosis and eschar formation. This can be avoided by surgical drainage. (See Color Fig. 33–5.)

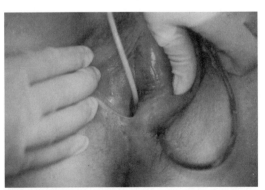

Figure 33–6. Vulvar hematoma that has been incised and drained. Note incision on medial aspect of left labium, which has been closed with absorbable sutures. A urethral catheter is in place for bladder decompression and a closed suction drain exits the most dependent aspect of vulva. (See Color Fig. 33–6.)

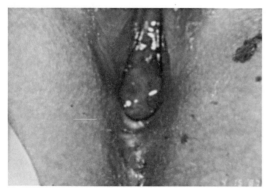

Figure 33–7. Scarring of the posterior fourchette secondary to accidental trauma.

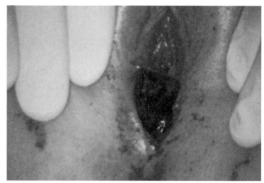

Figure 33–9. Impalement injury. This young girl leapt into a swimming pool and impaled herself on a broom handle. The entry wound is seen here, just beneath the introitus; the exit wound was in the rectum. (See Color Fig. 33–9.)

also result from severe motor vehicle trauma. A 3-year-old girl suffered scarring of the posterior fourchette after a complete tear that extended from the introitus through the rectal mucosa. She had fallen under a moving car, and tire marks were visible on her abdomen at the time of the initial examination. The photograph in Figure 33–7 was taken 1 year after the injuries had been repaired. Other reported anorectal injuries have resulted from impalement on vacuum cleaner handles or fence posts.[17]

VAGINAL INJURIES

Accidental vaginal injuries are usually penetrating injuries. They can be due to falls, especially falls on a pointed or sharp object such as a fence post. (Fig. 33–8). Crush injuries from motor vehicle accidents and falls are sometimes associated with pelvic fractures. Sharp bony spicules may penetrate the vagina and lower urinary tract. Hymenal injuries are uncommon but can

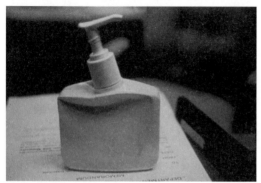

Figure 33–8. This soap dispenser was on the floor of the shower when a young girl fell onto the dispenser and impaled herself and sustained injuries to the hymen and vagina.

occur.[18] The hymenal ring may be torn by penetrating injuries, but the bleeding that follows such hymenal injuries is usually minimal and requires no treatment. When, however, the history or external genital examination findings suggest a penetrating injury, the possibility of other serious injuries to the upper vagina and pelvic viscera must be investigated. This requires examination under anesthesia and appropriate repair.

Case Report: A 9-year-old leapt from the side of a swimming pool just as her sister was retrieving a submerged pool broom. The child landed with such force that she impaled herself on the broom handle, sustaining lacerations of her hymen, vagina, and rectum (Fig. 33–9).

Most vaginal injuries are the result of an object's penetrating the vagina through the hymenal opening and producing a laceration or a tear of the hymenal ring. In general, in a very young girl, penetration is associated with a significant vaginal injury. The thin vaginal mucosa, because of its limited distensibility, is often lacerated along with the hymen. Penile pressure on the introitus is directed toward the posterior vaginal wall, and the hymen often tears between 4 and 8 o'clock. Secondarily, the laceration enlarges to involve the posterior vaginal wall and the perineum. The pattern of injury most often seen in these victims is a linear laceration of the hymen, usually in the posterior aspect. With deeper penetration, the rectovaginal septum is torn and the tear extends into the rectum.[19]

In rare instances, a large retroperitoneal hematoma develops when a penetrating vaginal injury tears a major vessel above the pelvic floor. Such tears can lead to massive hemorrhage into the retroperitoneal space. The injured child may present in shock because of the blood loss. These patients require close observation and fluid replacement. Large hematomas sometimes compress the ureters, leading to urinary retention. As pressure increases, large retroperitoneal hematomas usually stop bleeding spontaneously. Exploratory laparotomy is rarely necessary to identify and control bleeding.[20]

Consensual intercourse or sexual assault should be considered when an adolescent presents with vaginal trauma. Predisposing factors for intercoital injury include first experience of coitus, first coitus after long abstinence, congenital anomalies of the vagina, coital positions that permit deep penetration, and inebriation or drug use (on the part of either partner), brutality, violence, and insertion of foreign objects. The patient may have been threatened or feel awkward or self-conscious explaining her injuries. Initially, a spurious clinical history may be offered. Failure to perform a proper pelvic examination to evaluate vaginal bleeding compounds the error and leads to delay in diagnosis and treatment. Patients who sustain vaginal lacerations after coitus may give a history of sharp vaginal pain, profuse or prolonged vaginal bleeding or hypovolemic shock. Digital vaginal examination is inadequate to assess injuries; a proper speculum-guided inspection of the vagina is in order and must be performed. With initial coitus, minor lacerations of the introitus and lower vagina may occur. The most frequent type, and site, of injury in adolescent and adult victims of confirmed rape include tears and abrasions of the posterior fourchette, tears and abrasions of the labia minora, tears of the fossa navicularis, and lacerations and ecchymosis of the hymen.[21] Superficial lacerations without active bleeding may be managed with vaginal packing. Minor lacerations can be repaired under local anesthesia.

Adolescents subjected to blunt, forceful, penetrating, vaginal trauma usually sustain lacerations of the posterior portion of the hymen, between the 3:00 and 9:00 o'clock positions (Fig. 33–10). As compared with adults who have been sexually assaulted, adolescents are 4.5 times more likely to sustain hymenal lacerations.[21] Deep lacerations must be evaluated and treated with the patient under general anesthesia.

High-pressure insufflation injuries have been described that resulted from falling off Jet-Skiis or water skiis, sliding down waterchutes, and direct contact with pool or spa jets.[22–24] As water enters the vagina under pressure, the vagina may overdistend, and perhaps sustain lacerations that can extend into the vaginal fornices. Such injuries produce vaginal bleeding but may show no sign

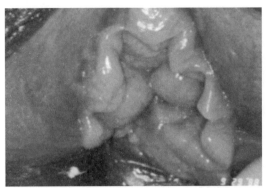

Figure 33–10. Vaginal-hymenal tear secondary to sexual abuse. Note the disruption of the hymen at the lower margin of the photograph.

of external trauma. Only by careful vaginal examination (often under anesthesia) can the true extent of injury and cause of bleeding be determined. Young children and women who participate in these water sports should be counseled about safeguards such as protective clothing for water-or Jet-skiing (wetsuits or cut-off jeans) and keeping the feet together when entering the water via a water slide.

Quite rarely, tampon insertion, especially with a plastic applicator produces vaginal lacerations that require repair.[25] Insertion of foreign objects, whether by the girl or someone else, can produce injuries, during placement or removal.[26]

EVISCERATION INJURIES

If the penetration is brutally forceful or if the penetrating object is larger in diameter or longer in length than the vagina, lateral vaginal wall and fornix lacerations may occur. In serious cases, the cervix may be avulsed from its attachment to the vagina, and the peritoneal cavity may be entered. The bowel, omentum, or fallopian tubes may protrude through the laceration. These patients all present with vaginal bleeding and may be at risk of morbidity or death from peritonitis or exsanguination.

Once it has been determined that an injury extends above the hymen in a child, or into the peritoneal cavity in any patient, a full examination under general anesthesia must be conducted. Details of such assessment and the repair of vaginal injuries are discussed elsewhere in this chapter.

Case Report: A 12-year-old seventh grader, who had menarche at age 11, was walking home from the neighborhood store in the early evening when she was seized by an assailant, taken into a

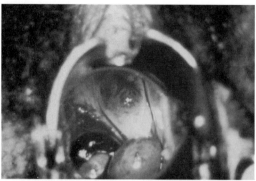

Figure 33–11. Evisceration injury. Lacerations of the posterior fornix may extend into the peritoneal cavity. In this young patient, loops of small bowel are seen in the vagina. (See Color Fig. 33–11.)

vacant house, and forced to withstand vaginal penetration. She then was released, and she staggered home. Her mother noted vaginal bleeding and took her to the emergency department of the local hospital. The patient denied any previous sexual encounters. According to the emergency physician, the patient was bleeding briskly and was unable to tolerate a vaginal examination. She was taken to the operating room and, by examination under general anesthesia, was found to have a laceration of the posterior fornix from the 5:00 o'clock to the 8:00 o'clock position and evisceration of small bowel into the vagina (Fig. 33–11). The patient then underwent a transabdominal exploratory laparotomy and transabdominal and transvaginal repair of her injuries. She was discharged on the second postoperative day and healed well.

Adequate assessment and repair of extensive vaginal injuries frequently is not possible in the emergency department. The necessity for prompt triage and comprehensive assessment of the vaginal injuries under general anesthesia is critical to the care of such patients.

SEXUAL ABUSE

Accidental hymenal and vaginal injuries are rare, and, although they can occur, injuries to the vagina of a child should always be suspected to be the result of abuse.[27] Prepubertal children subjected to blunt, forceful, penetrating vaginal trauma usually sustain lacerations of the posterior portion of the hymen, which can extend into the vagina and rectum. The unestrogenized tissues of the introitus, hymen, and vagina tend to tear on forceful penetration. With the onset of puberty, the effect of estrogen upon these tissues is to render them more pliable and elastic.

The medical evaluation of suspected child sexual abuse is described in Chapter 24 and has been extensively discussed in the pediatric literature.[28–31] Children who may have been sexually abused should not be further traumatized with a painful physical examination. The genital examination should take place in the context of a thorough pediatric examination, including assessments of developmental, behavioral, and emotional status. All children who have been molested or assaulted deserve a careful examination and referral for further care. For questionable cases, consultation can be sought with physicians expert in sexual abuse evaluation. Most states mandate reporting of any suspected sexual assault of a minor.

SPORTS INJURIES

Although a traditional argument against women's participation in sports has been concern for injuries of the genitalia and reproductive organs, such injuries are rare. Statistically, the genital area sustains the fewest injuries in women athletes,[32] and women's reproductive organs are obviously much better protected from injury than those of males who participate in sports. Garrick and Requa prospectively studied sports injuries in adolescent girls who participated in high school athletics over a 2-year period. Among 870 participant-seasons in nine girls' sports, 192 injuries were reported, none that involved the breasts or genitalia. Gymnastics and softball had the highest injury rates.[33] Although vulvar hematomas and straddle injuries sometimes occur in noncontact sports such as gymnastics, they are not common. Caine and associates conducted a prospective study of 50 highly competitive female gymnasts over a period of 1 year. During this period, the 50 gymnasts amassed more than 40,000 hours of training and sustained 147 injuries, but no genital or groin injuries.[34]

Bicycle-related genital injuries are also uncommon. In a retrospective study of 520 children between ages 1 and 18 years who presented to an emergency department because of bicycle-related injuries, Selbst and colleagues[35] noted that only 4% sustained primary injuries to the genital area.

URETHRAL INJURIES

In contrast to the male urethra, the female urethra is short and not rigidly fixed on the pelvic floor and is usually protected from injury. High-speed motor vehicle accidents are the most common cause of pelvic fractures and deceleration injuries that lead to bladder and urethral injuries in children and adolescents. Indicators of urethral disruption are blood at the introitus or urethral meatus, inability of a conscious patient to void, or gross hematuria. Every female patient with a pelvic fracture should have a careful vaginal examination during the initial resuscitation, in an effort to detect vaginal and or urethral injury as soon as possible. Digital palpation of the vagina is not adequate. A speculum examination, or vaginoscopy, using saline irrigation and a cystoscope in young patients reveals any lacerations in the anterior vaginal wall that might be associated with urethral injuries. In women, urethrography is a waste of valuable time and is not a useful diagnostic tool, even though it is an important diagnostic study in male patients suspected to have a urethral disruption. Urethroscopy should be used to investigate suspected disruption of the urethra based on physical examination. When the urethra is intact, a Foley catheter should be placed. When it is disrupted, primary repair of the injury by an experienced urogynecologist or pediatric urologist is preferred to delayed repair. Failure of prompt diagnosis may delay repair of a urethral injury and result in urinary incontinence, urethral stricture, or vesicovaginal or urethrovaginal fistula. Female patients who experience difficulty voiding or who develop vulvar edema (secondary to extravasation of urine) after removal of a urinary drainage catheter placed for pelvic fracture should be promptly examined by cystoscopy for partial urethral injury.[36]

BLADDER INJURIES

The child's bladder is predominately an intra-abdominal organ. When it is full, it is more vulnerable to blunt abdominal trauma. Injuries to the lower urinary tract may not be detected immediately. A patient with a bladder injury may have the classic complaints of suprapubic or pelvic pain, dysuria, inability to void, hematuria, or shock. Anyone who presents with severe abdominal trauma and hematuria should be assessed with retrograde cystography (after it is first determined that the urethra is intact). Contrast material should be instilled into the bladder through an indwelling catheter. Unless the bladder is distended to capacity, a small perforation could be missed. Anteroposterior and lateral views are taken, and a postevacuation film, which can demonstrate small extravasations that had been

masked by the bladder shadow. If the bladder can be adequately distended, computed tomography may be used to demonstrate bladder rupture and pelvic fractures.

Microscopic or gross hematuria occurs in up to 60% of patients with pelvic fractures.[36a] Injuries to the bladder or urethra are less common. A contused bladder can bleed profusely without being ruptured. The passage of clear urine, on the other hand, does not rule out a ruptured bladder. Extraperitoneal bladder rupture is most common. Uncomplicated tears may be managed by bladder drainage, but suprapubic exploration may be advisable in some cases. Intraperitoneal rupture at the dome of the full bladder follows lower abdominal impact from blunt force or a lap restraint during motor vehicle accidents. Bone spicules, knives, and bullets have all been reported to cause penetrating injuries. Intraperitoneal rupture requires surgical exploration, débridement, closure in multiple layers, and bladder decompression. Drains should be left in the space of Retzius and in the lateral recesses of the pelvis.

EVALUATION OF GENITAL INJURIES

Before performing a genital examination, the clinician should take a thorough history (see Table 33–1). The genital examination should be performed in the context of a complete physical examination. It should be preceded by a careful explanation of the purpose of the examination, what the patient may experience, and assurances to the patient and her parents that she is in control of what takes place during the examination. Genital injuries are likely to create tremendous anxiety for a child or adolescent and her parents, because concerns are raised about future reproductive capability. Parental education, consent, and supportive involvement are crucial to optimizing the success of examination of a young girl. The option of examination under sedation or general anesthesia should also be offered when appropriate.

A meticulous physical examination must be conducted under the proper conditions. There is a tendency, among clinicians, to underestimate the extent and severity of genital injuries, especially in a young, frightened or uncooperative patient. A cursory examination without benefit of sedation, proper positioning of the patient, and proper lighting, may miss the diagnosis and lead to improper treatment.[37, 38] Absolute indications for an examination requiring general anesthesia include extension of the injury through or above the hymen in a prepubertal child, vaginal lacerations that extend into the rectum or peritoneal cavity, unexplained vaginal bleeding, other injuries that require surgical management, or any obstacle to determining the full extent of the injury.

Once it has been determined that an injury extends above the hymen in a prepubertal child, or into the peritoneal cavity, or if the true extent of the injury cannot be assessed or repaired, a comprehensive pelvic examination must be conducted under general anesthesia. Each hospital should have a formal protocol for documentation and collection of forensic evidence. A detailed description of the extent of the injuries is important. Videocystoscopy and saline irrigation may be used to visualize a child's vagina to determine the extent of vaginal injuries. The labia may be held together gently to allow distention of the vagina with saline and careful inspection. This technique distends the walls of the vagina, rinses away blood, and is invaluable for affording optimal visualization of a young child's vagina. All specimens for vaginal cultures should be collected before saline irrigation. For adolescents, a vaginal speculum of appropriate size may be used.

REPAIR OF VAGINAL INJURIES

The importance of proper patient positioning, a suitable light source, and complete cooperation of the patient (which may require sedation or general anesthesia) cannot be overstated. Extension of lacerations into the peritoneal cavity mandates exploratory laparotomy or laparoscopy especially if the penetrating object was sharp or if the object causing the injury is known, to determine whether other structures (bowel, blood vessels) have been injured. If the caliber of the vagina of a young patient is small, the deepest (i.e., most distal from the introitus) vaginal lacerations should be repaired first and the introital lacerations last, to allow maximum working space and better visualization. The anal sphincter should be identified, and repaired if injured. Some lacerations extend into the rectum and must be closed in layers. Vaginal injuries that are not bleeding may be packed with moistened sterile gauze in lieu of suturing. The clinician must keep in mind that removal of the packing may be very painful to a conscious patient. Postoperative application of topical estrogen cream to injuries of the mucosal surfaces of the vagina and introitus may limit formation of granulation tissue and promote healing without stricture. In-

troital application of estrogen cream should suffice for most prepubertal children. No attempt should be made to utilize vaginal applicators designed for adults to place intravaginal medication in a prepubertal child.

Primary repair of injuries of the vagina that extend into the anal mucosa and sphincter are preferred when, on palpation and proctoanoscopy, the rectum seems intact. Such injuries can result from accidental impalement, coital trauma, or penetration by a bullet or knife.[39] A diverting colostomy may be necessary when the injury is high.[40] Pediatric and general surgeons usually recommend a diverting colostomy when the bowel of a patient with a penetrating injury to the rectum has not been prepared for surgery. This approach is controversial. Obstetricians and gynecologists who have experience in the repair of fourth-degree episiotomies in parturients whose bowel is not "prepped" would argue that primary repair of low anogenital injuries carries only a small risk of break-down and fistula formation. In all likelihood, the patient might be spared a colostomy. If a postoperative rectovaginal fistula were to develop, a diverting colostomy could be electively undertaken for repair.

GENITAL BURNS

Because the perineum is hidden between the thighs, it is generally protected from burns. Burns of the female genitalia and perineum are most often associated with extensive burns involving a third to half of the total body surface, injury that carries a 30% to 70% risk of death. Adults are most often burned by flames; children are generally scalded by spilled fluid or by immersion. Chemical burns of the vagina from carbolic acid, formaldehyde, sulfuric acid, iodine, and ammonia have been associated with illegal abortion, attempted contraception, and self-medication for a sexually transmitted disease or vaginal infection. Patients have been described who attempted suicide by inserting explosives, mercuric chloride, or drain cleaner into the vagina. Radiation, podophyllin, trichloracetic acid, and laser therapy have produced iatrogenic burns, as has the (now obsolete) high-pressure steam treatment for menorrhagia.[41] ThermaChoice is an intrauterine balloon device used to treat menorrhagia in adults with circulating saline at 87°C (187°F) and balloon pressure of 160 to 180 mm Hg, and to date has not been associated with injuries like those from high-pressure steam.

Case Report: An 11-year-old girl was brought to the emergency department of a community hospital by her mother, who became concerned

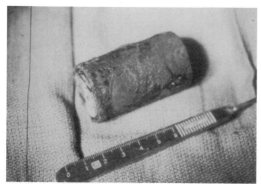

Figure 33–12. This D-cell battery was removed from the vagina of an 11-year-old, having been in place for 9 days. The corrosive chemicals produced full-thickness burns in the vagina.

upon seeing a black, foamy substance in the toilet after assisting her daughter in the bathroom. In the previous week, the child had developed lower abdominal pain and a low-grade fever. Her last menstrual period had also occurred in the previous week. Menarche occurred at age 10. The examining physician detected a foreign object in the vagina. A 1.5-volt battery (D cell) was extracted, and on examination the vagina was grossly abnormal. It was only then that the child revealed that she had placed the battery into her vagina "to see what would happen," and, when she couldn't remove it, was too afraid to tell anyone. It was estimated that the battery had been in place for at least 9 days. The battery casing was buckled and it appeared to be leaking (Fig. 33–12). Examination under anesthesia included colposcopy, cystoscopy, vaginoscopy, proctoscopy, and laparoscopy. Burns were noted at the introitus and involving the vaginal walls. The vaginal mucosa was stained black, and patches of full-thickness tissue loss were observed. Vaginal cultures grew *Escherichia coli*, *Klebsiella* sp., *Enterococcus* organisms, and *Bacteroides fragilis*. The posterior walls of the bladder trigone appeared inflamed at cystoscopy. Findings of proctoscopy to 20 cm were negative. At laparoscopy, the cul de sac was involved by an acute inflammatory process. Purulent yellow fluid was aspirated for culture, and the pelvis was copiously irrigated. There was no evidence of peritoneal-vaginal, rectovaginal, or vesicovaginal fistula. The burn was managed with intravaginal sulfadiazine and estrogen cream, débridement, and antibiotics. The veracity of the girl's story was supported by consultations with social services and psychology professionals. Over the course of 3 weeks, the vagina epithelialized, but a stricture developed in the lower vagina. Initially, dilators were utilized to the stenosis, but later a reconstructive operation was necessary to resect the stenotic portion of the vagina (in the same way one would a transverse septum).

The management of genital and perineal burns includes short-term urinary diversion for comfort and hygiene, and a topical antimicrobial (silver sulfadiazine). Skin grafting is utilized only for full-thickness loss, and, typically, when it comes to grafting, the genitalia take low priority as compared with the face, hands, and trunk. Long-term consequences of internal genital burns can include fistula formation, stenosis, agglutination, and scarring of the vagina. In girls who have external perineal burns, contractures may be prevented by thigh abduction, hip exercises, early ambulation, and pressure garments. Scarring as a result of perineal burns affects skin texture, pigmentation, and pliability. The burn victim's ability to clean the area after micturition and defecation may be compromised, a complication that can have a devastating effect on sexuality and body image.

PSYCHOLOGICAL FACTORS

The ability in the future to bear children and to have sexual relations should be addressed with young victims of genital injuries and their families. When appropriate, reassurance of reproductive capacity should be provided by the clinician, because patients and parents do not always verbalize their concerns. Victims of sexual assault may suffer sleep disturbances, nightmares, flashbacks, anxiety, and anger. Depression, common in these victims, is compounded by feelings of guilt and shame. Specific referrals for professional counseling should be offered to all victims of sexual assault.[42]

GENITAL DISORDERS THAT MAY BE CONFUSED WITH TRAUMA

A number of genital conditions can be mistaken for trauma, among them, dermatologic conditions, congenital anomalies, infections, and normal variations in the genitals (Table 33–2).[5, 43–47] The skin condition most often confused with genital trauma is lichen sclerosus. It most often

Table 33–2. Genital Lesions Confused with Trauma

Lichen sclerosus
Chronic dermatitis
Urethral prolapse
Urethral caruncles
Other bullous and ulcerative lesions

involves the vulvar and perianal areas of prepubertal children and postmenopausal women. The cause is unknown, although some researchers think it may be an autoimmune disease.[44, 47] The initial lesions consist of ivory-colored macules that coalesce to form homogeneous, white, atrophic plaques. The affected skin is sharply demarcated from the surrounding normal skin. Because this atrophic skin is fragile and easily traumatized, petechiae, bruises, and hemorrhage are noted after minimal pressure.[47] Affected girls may present for evaluation of possible sexual abuse because of vulvar bleeding or the unusual appearance of the vulvar skin.

Chronic dermatitis involving the vulvar area can also be mistaken for trauma. If the skin is pruritic, self-induced excoriations may be mistaken for trauma, and in some cases the chronic changes associated with eczema, seborrhea, or psoriasis may be mistaken for scarring. Vulvar hemangiomas (Fig. 33–13) have also been confused with traumatic lesions of the external genitalia.[5]

Since the advent of hymenal colposcopy, many genital lesions that previously went unrecognized have been reported. Because these lesions were first noted in a group of children who were examined for suspected sexual abuse, there was a tendency to attribute the findings to trauma. Fortunately, new studies have determined the incidence of a number of these findings in a normal population of girls who were carefully selected for "nonabuse".[43] Periurethral bands are one common normal variant that can be confused with trauma. These bands extend from the urethral meatus, creating a false pocket on either side of the urethra (Fig. 33–14). The periurethral pits created by these bands can be distinguished from traumatic penetrating wounds by their location adjacent to the urethra, their symmetry, and the absence of bruising and bleeding. McCann

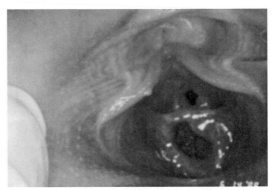

Figure 33–14. Periurethral bands.

noted that these periurethral bands can be found in 50% of nonabused children with the aid of colposcopy.[43] Other anatomic variations that can be confused with trauma include congenital pits of the perineal body,[5] epispadias,[6] and perineal grooves.[48]

Urethral abnormalities may also be confused with genital trauma. Urethral prolapse and periurethral caruncles have been misdiagnosed as genital trauma.[5] Both of these conditions sometimes first present as vaginal bleeding, which can add to the diagnostic confusion.[46, 49]

CONCLUSION

The spectrum of genital injuries is broad and identifying them correctly requires a detailed history and physical examination. The pelvic examination of a child or adolescent should be conducted in a sensitive manner that does not traumatize the young patient. Parental consent and supportive involvement are important components of this evaluation. Frequently, the correct diagnosis can be achieved only with a more comprehensive examination under anesthesia conducted by a suitably qualified physician.

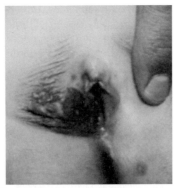

Figure 33–13. Vulvar hemangioma.

REFERENCES

1. Nsau A, Dhar KK, Dhall GI: Nonobstetric lower genital tract trauma. Aust NZ J Obstet Gynaecol 1993; 33(4):433–435.
2. Berenson AB: The prepubertal genital examination: What is normal and abnormal. Curr Opin Obstet Gynecol 1994; 6:526–530.
3. Berenson AB, Heger AH, Hayes JM, et al: Appearance of the hymen in prepubertal girls. Pediatrics 1992; 89:387–394.
4. Baker RB: Seat belt injury masquerading as sexual abuse. Pediatrics 1986; 77:436.
5. Bays J, Jenny C: Genital and anal conditions confused

with child sexual abuse trauma. Am J Dis Child 1990; 144:1319.

6. Reinhart MA: Sexual abuse of battered young children. Pediatr Emerg Care 1987; 3:36.
7. Black CT, Pokorny WJ, McGill CW, Harberg FJ: Anorectal trauma in children. J Pediatr Surg 1982; 17:501.
8. Finkel MA: Anogenital trauma in sexually abused children. Pediatrics 1989; 84:317.
9. Rimsza ME, Niggemann EH: Medical evaluation of sexually abused children: A review of 311 cases. Pediatrics 1982; 69:8.
10. Muram D: Child sexual abuse: Relationship between sexual acts and genital findings. Child Abuse Neglect 1989; 13:211.
11. Paul DM: The medical examination in sexual offenses against children. Med Sci Law 1977; 17:251.
12. Teixeira WRG: Hymenal colposcopic examination in sexual offenses. Am J Forensic Med Pathol 1981; 2:209.
13. Lindblad F, Ormstad K, Elinder G: Child sexual abuse: Physical examination. Acta Paediatr Scand 1989; 78:935.
14. Cartwright PS: The Sexual Assault Study Group: Factors that correlate with injury sustained by survivors of sexual assault. Obstet Gynecol 1987; 70:44.
15. Bond GR, Dowd MD, Landsman I, Rimsza M: Unintentional perineal injury in prepubescent girls: A multicenter, prospective report of 56 girls. Pediatrics. 1995; 95(5):628–631.
16. West R, Davies A, Fenton T: Accidental vulval injuries in childhood. Br Med J 1989; 298:1002.
17. Fox PF: Impalement injuries of the perineum. Am J Surg 1951; 82:511.
18. Hostetler BR, Jones CE, Muram D: Sharp penetrating injuries of the hymen. Adolesc Pediatr Gynecol 1994; 7:94–96.
19. Muram D: Child sexual abuse—genital findings in perpubertal girls. I. The unaided medical examination. Am J Obstet Gynecol 1989; 160:328–333.
20. Muram D: Genital tract injuries in the prepubertal child. Pediatr Ann 1986; 15:616.
21. Slaughter L, Brown CRV, Crowley S, et al: Patterns of genital injury in female sexual assault victims. Am J Obstet Gynecol 1997; 176:609–616.
22. Niv J, Lessing JB, Hartuv J, et al: Vaginal injury resulting from sliding down a water chute. Am J Obstet Gynecol 1992; 166(3):930–931.
23. Perlman SE, Hertweck SP, Wolfe WM: Water-ski douche injury in a premenarcheal female. Pediatrics 1995; 96:782–783.
24. Haefner HK, Anderson F, Johnson MP: Vaginal laceration following a Jet-Ski accident. Obstet Gynecol 1991; 78:986–988.
25. Gray MJ, Norton P, Treadwell K: Tampon-induced injuries. Obstet Gynecol 1981; 58:667–668.
26. Elam AL, Ray VG: Sexually related trauma: A review. Ann Emerg Med 1986; 15:576–584.
27. Heger A, Emans SJ: Evaluation of the Sexually Abused Child. A Medical Textbook and Photographic Atlas. New York: Oxford University Press, 1992.
28. Adams JA: Medical evaluation of suspected child sexual abuse. In Pokorny SF (ed): Pediatric and Adolescent

Gynecology. New York: Chapman and Hall, 1996, pp 1–14.
29. Paradise JE: The medical evaluation of the sexually abused child. Pediatr Clin North Am 1990; 37:830–862.
30. Muram D: Child sexual abuse. In Stenchever M, Goldfarb AF (eds): Atlas of Clinical Gynecology, Vol I. Pediatric and Adolescent Gynecology. Philadelphia: Appleton and Lange, 1998, pp 11.1–11.14.
31. AAP Guidelines for the Evaluation of Sexual Abuse of Children. Pediatrics 1991; 87:254–260.
32. Roy S, Irvin R: Sports Medicine. Englewood Cliffs, NJ: Prentice-Hall, 1983.
33. Garrick JG, Requa RK: Girls sports injuries in high school athletics. JAMA 1978; 239:2245.
34. Caine D, Cochrane B, Caine C, Zemper E: An epidemiologic investigation of injuries affecting young competitive female gymnasts. Am Sports Med 1989; 17:811.
35. Selbst SM, Alexander D, Ruddy R: Bicycle-related injuries. Am J Dis Child 1987; 141:140.
36. Perry MO, Husmann DA: Urethral injuries in female subjects following pelvic fractures. J Urol 1992; 147:139–143.
36a. Morgan DE, Nallamala LK, Kenney PJ, et al: CT cystography: Radiographic and clinical predictors of bladder rupture. AJR 174:89–95, 2000.
37. Lynch JM, Gardner MJ, Albanese CT: Blunt urogenital trauma in prepubescent female patients: More than meets the eye! Pediatr Emerg Care 1995; 11:372–375.
38. Pokorny SF, Pokorny WJ, Kramer W: Acute genital injury in the prepubertal child. Am J Obstet Gynecol 1992; 166:1461–1466.
39. Orr CJ, Clark MA, Hawley DA, et al: Fatal anorectal injuries: A series of four cases. J Forensic Sci 1995; 40:219–221.
40. Elkins TE, Arrowsmith S: Repair of urogenital and rectovaginal fistulas. Vol 1, part 75. In Sciarra JJ (ed): Gynecology and Obstetrics (CD-ROM). Philadelphia: Harper & Row, 1998.
41. Weiler-Mithoff EM, Hassal ME, Burd DA: Burns of the female genitalia and perineum. Burns 1996; 22(5):390–395.
42. Hampton H: Care of the woman who has been raped. N Engl J Med 1995; 332:234–237.
43. McCann J, Wells R, Simon MD, Voris J: Genital findings in prepubertal girls selected for nonabuse: A descriptive study. Pediatrics 1990; 86:428.
44. Handfield-Jones SE, Hinde FRJ, Kennedy CTC: Lichen sclerosus et atrophicus in children misdiagnosed as sexual abuse. Br Med J 1987; 294:1404.
45. McCann J, Voris J, Simon M, Wells R: Perianal findings in prepubertal children selected for nonabuse: A descriptive study. Child Abuse Neglect 1989; 13:179.
46. Esposito JM: Circular prolapse of the urethra in children: A cause of vaginal bleeding. Obstet Gynecol 1968; 31:363.
47. Jenny C, Kirby P, Fuquay D: Genital lichen sclerosus mistaken for child sexual abuse. Pediatrics 1981; 83:597.
48. Shaw A, DeWitt GW: Picture of the month: Perineal groove. Am J Dis Child 1977; 131:921.
49. Merritt PF: Evaluation of vaginal bleeding in the preadolescent child. Semin Pediatr Surg 1998; 7:35–42.

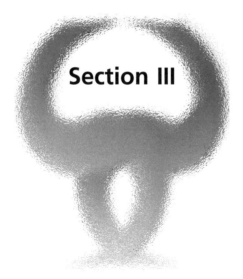

Section III

Surgical Problems

EDITOR: JOSEPH S. SANFILIPPO

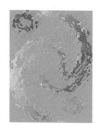

Chapter 34

Sexual Developmental Anomalies and Their Reconstruction: Upper and Lower Tracts

D. KEITH EDMONDS AND DAVID MURAM

The development of the genital tract is a complex process that involves (1) tissue differentiation into various structures—fallopian tubes, uterus, cervix, and vagina—all of which develop from the wolffian, or paramesonephric, ducts, and subsequently, (2) union of this embryonic process with the vulva, which develops from the cloaca. Congenital anomalies of this system are more common than most clinicians realize, and detailed knowledge of the embryology of this process is paramount to reaching an accurate anatomic diagnosis and, subsequently, managing the disorder. Before considering the management outlined in this chapter, readers should refer to Chapters 1 and 2. Only by understanding the anatomic malformations and their psychological and sexual implications can the physician expect to achieve a successful outcome. Surgery alone is inadequate for treating these patients. A team of professionals trained in psychosexual counseling and psychological and social support is necessary to achieve a successful long-term outcome.

EMBRYOLOGY

In the presence of the testicular determining factor (TDF), the undifferentiated gonadal tissue develops into a testis. In the absence of a TDF, the indifferent gonad develops into an ovary. Once gonadal development is established, genital and ductal differentiation proceeds predictably. In the presence of a testis, the ducts and external genitalia develop along male lines, and in the absence of a testis, the development proceeds

Figures 34–2 to 34–7, 34–9 to 34–17, 34–19, and 34–21 to 34–27 are Courtesy of Dr. David Muram

along female lines. The testicular stroma contains two discrete cell lines, Sertoli and Leydig cells. Both Leydig cells and Sertoli cells function in dissociation from testicular morphogenesis.[1, 2] They secrete hormones that direct subsequent genital differentiation along male lines. Fetal Leydig cells produce an androgen, probably testosterone, that stabilizes wolffian ducts and permits differentiation of the vas deferens, epididymis, and seminal vesicles. Testosterone is converted by 5α-reductase to dihydrotestosterone, which virilizes the external genitalia. These actions were first demonstrated in rabbits.[3] Fetal Sertoli cells produce a different hormone, a glycoprotein that diffuses locally to cause regression of the müllerian duct. The gene that controls anti-müllerian hormone (AMH) production has been isolated and localized to chromosome 19.[5] In the absence of AMH, the internal genitalia develop along female lines, the müllerian ducts develop into uterus and fallopian tubes, and wolffian ducts regress. In the absence of testosterone and dihydrotestosterone, the external genitalia develop along female lines.

From the müllerian ducts develop most of the structures of the female genital tract. On each side, the cranial-longitudinal segment forms the fallopian tube and its coelomic opening develops into fimbriae. The caudal longitudinal parts fuse and form the uterus and cervix. Fusion and incorporation may be incomplete, in which case vaginal and uterine malformations result. Subsequent development of the vagina is considered in detail in Chapter 1, but extension of the vaginal plate toward the normally developing female vulva eventually leads to canalization that creates the vagina.

UPPER TRACT ANOMALIES

UTERUS

Classification

Many classification systems have been devised for uterine abnormalities.[6-8] All of these classifications are descriptive, and their necessity becomes apparent when comparing the management of different anomalies. The classification system of Buttram and Gibbons[9] appears to be the most enduring (Fig. 34–1). It describes six classes of müllerian anomalies but fails to take into account communicating uteri. A new classification for this type of uterus (Fig. 34–2) is a subclass of Buttram and Gibbons' classes III and IV.[10, 11] Thus, the classification scheme is complex, but using the two systems in combination affords a somewhat standardized nomenclature for uterine anomalies.

The American Society for Reproductive Medicine (formerly the American Fertility Society) in 1988 developed a classification system organized according to the principal anatomic types of uterus (see Fig. 34–1). It was developed to facilitate collection of data on the prevalence of different anomalies and takes into account the degree of failure of development of the müllerian structures. An additional class contains anomalies related to exposure to diethylstilbestrol (DES) in utero.

Incidence

The true incidence of müllerian duct anomalies is not known. Many estimates have been published, but how many uterine abnormalities are reported depends on the diligence of the investigator and the techniques used in the study population. In obstetric patients, the incidence of abnormalities ranges from 1 in 7 to 1 in 625, but, in an infertile population, the incidence is 1 in 100 and 1 in 20.[8, 13–15] In patients who have recurrent abortions, the incidence of uterine abnormalities is approximately 12%.[16, 17] Almost certainly, the incidence of uterine malformations is grossly underestimated, as the majority of patients are asymptomatic and fertility potential is not affected.

GENETICS

Most forms of isolated müllerian duct and urogenital sinus abnormalities are inherited in a polygenic or multifactorial fashion, some by mendelian inheritance. Such abnormalities are sometimes a component of a mendelian multiple-malformation syndrome.[18] The recurrent risk for disorders acquired by polygenic multifactorial inheritance is between 1% and 5%.[19]

Associated Abnormalities

The association between müllerian abnormalities and defects of other organ systems is well-known, but, often, in the literature reference to this association is omitted. Renal abnormalities occur in patients with a didelphic uterus in about 9% to 12.5% of cases,[20, 21] but multiple-malformation syndromes are also associated with incomplete müllerian fusion. Hand-foot dysplasia,[22] Meckle syndrome,[23] and Rudiger syndrome,[24] are sometimes associated; therefore extragenital malformations must alert the physician to the possibility of uterine abnormalities.

Presentation

Uterine anomalies are usually asymptomatic, but, often, they are discovered in the course of disorders such as recurrent abortions, primary infertility, menstrual disorders, and in utero exposure to DES. Recurrent pregnancy wastage and primary infertility are not considered here, as clinicians with an interest in pediatric and adolescent gynecology rarely see them.

Menstrual disorders may well present in patients with uterine anomalies. Oligomenorrhea was reported by 56% of patients with mild uterine abnormalities,[25] and some have suggested that it may be the result of an abnormality of steroid receptor development in the malformed uterus. Dysmenorrhea can also present as a uterine abnormality in patients who have the obstructive anomaly rudimentary horn.

A wide variety of anomalies have been described in girls who were exposed in utero to DES.[26] The drug was frequently prescribed to pregnant women until the early 1970s with the intention of preventing miscarriages and other pregnancy complications. Many daughters born to women who took DES have demonstrable structural changes in the genital tract that are attributable to DES. Most of these changes are benign and have no clinical significance. In some "DES daughters," the vagina and cervix exhibit structural changes such as cervical "collar" or "hood" or "cockscomb." This hood, an extra ridge of cervical tissue that many DES daughters have,

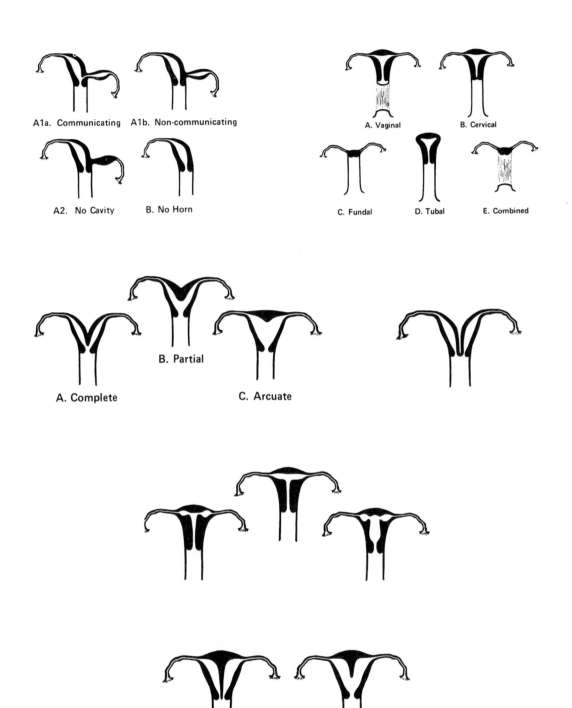

Figure 34–1. Classification of uterine abnormalities. (From Buttram VC Jr, Gibbons WE: Müllerian anomalies: A proposed classification [an analysis of 144 cases]. Fertil Steril 1979; 32:40–6. Reproduced with permission of the publisher, The American Society for Reproductive Medicine.)

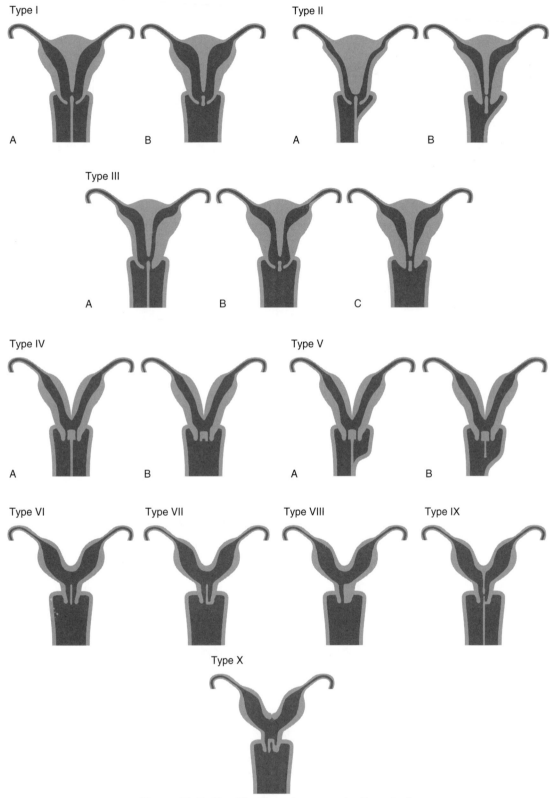

Figure 34–2. Classification of communicating uteri.

is benign and may eventually disappear. Sometimes a woman with a cervical hood finds it difficult to use a diaphragm, but, since DES was discontinued in the 1970s, it is no longer a problem in today's adolescents.

Fertility and pregnancy outcomes are sometimes adversely affected by uterine structural abnormalities. Fertility rates are lower among those who have structural abnormalities as compared with DES-exposed women whose hysterosalpingographic findings are normal (4% and 44%, respectively).[27] In vitro fertilization data indicate that implantation rates are lower for women who have structural abnormalities.[28] DES-exposed women may also be at increased risk for ectopic pregnancy.[29] In addition, the overall risk of preterm delivery is two to three times greater for DES-exposed women with structural uterine abnormalities.[30]

Diagnosis

An accurate diagnosis is essential to determine whether surgical intervention is necessary and to appropriately counsel the patient on the long-term outcome. Several radiographic techniques have been useful for detecting müllerian anomalies.

Pelvic sonography is a convenient, noninvasive first modality to consider. The sonogram may show a large, blood-filled vagina (hematocolpos), uterus (hematometra), or fallopian tube (hematosalpinx). A fluid collection, representing a hydrometrocolpos or hydrocolpos, is sometimes visualized in a fetus with an obstructive anomaly.[31]

Hysterosalpingography (HSG) can be helpful in identifying patency—and, possibly, complex communications—in cases of genital tract anomalies, but, because the external uterine contour is not demonstrated, it cannot be relied on to distinguish a septate uterus from a bicornuate one. Obstructed, atretic, or noncommunicating segments may also be missed by HSG, and laparoscopy may be necessary if making that distinction is very important. The role of laparoscopy remains unclear, because the necessary information can be obtained radiographically.

Diagnosis of uterine anomalies by ultrasonography has been described in detail. In a study comparing real-time ultrasound with HSG to surgery for identifying uterine abnormalities,[32] ultrasonography was as accurate as HSG and provided a more complete assessment of the uterine cavity. Findings were enhanced by hydrosonography, sonography with saline infused into the uterine cavity.

HYSTEROSCOPY

The use of hysteroscopy in the diagnosis of uterine abnormalities has become more popular. It provides an excellent view of the internal anatomy of the uterus, and, thus, allows direct assessment of any septum that may exist.

MAGNETIC RESONANCE IMAGING

Magnetic resonance imaging (MRI) is becoming increasingly popular because it is noninvasive and provides excellent anatomic information.[33]

Surgical Management

Surgical management of uterine anomalies is rarely necessary during adolescence, because the clinical manifestations are usually related to reproductive capability. The only reason for treatment of uterine abnormalities in this age group is dysmenorrhea.[34]

RUDIMENTARY UTERINE HORN

Failure of fusion of the müllerian ducts sometimes results in two separate uterine bodies. Maldevelopment of one creates a small rudimentary uterine horn. Sometimes, this rudimentary horn does not communicate with the other uterine cavity or the vagina. Menstrual blood trapped in the rudimentary cavity causes severe dysmenorrhea, hematometra, or pyometra (Fig. 34–3). When a zygote implants in a rudimentary horn, the horn sometimes ruptures; that is a potentially fatal complication, for both mother and fetus.

A rudimentary horn should be resected. The tube on the affected side should be removed, but the ovary can be preserved, provided its blood supply is not compromised. Should the endometrial cavity of the remaining horn be entered during the operation, in subsequent pregnancies, cesarean section is a reasonable option.

METROPLASTY

Three basic procedures have been described for treatment of the bicornuate or the septate uterus. The Strassman procedure uses a transverse incision on the superior aspect of the fundus that is extended inferiorly until the inner surface of both uterine horns is exposed. The

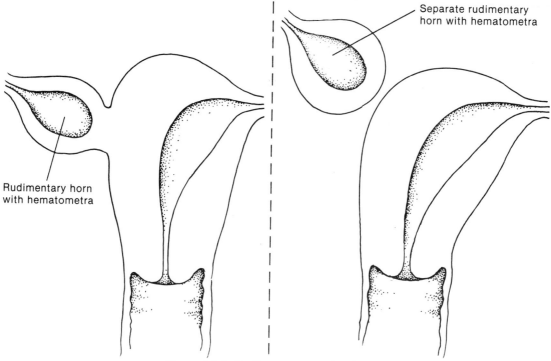

Figure 34–3. Rudimentary uterine horns.

septum is then excised and the uterine horns reunited (Fig. 34–4).

In the Jones metroplasty, a wedge-shaped incision is made; the uterine septum is removed with the remaining edges of the uterus reunited (Fig. 34–5). This operation has not become popular, however, because identifying the correct line of incision is difficult. Often, the result is a considerable reduction in the size of the intrauterine cavity.

The third procedure, described by Tompkins (Fig. 34–6), uses a vertical incision in the fundus of the uterus extending down the center of the septum to the cavity. This incision is relatively bloodless, and the cavities can then be exposed through lateral incisions and the uterus reunited.

The Strassman procedure is the most feasible operation for bicornuate uterus. If the decision is for a laparotomy to correct the septate uterus, the Tompkins procedure is often used.

HYSTEROSCOPIC METROPLASTY

The capability of the hysteroscope to visualize the uterine cavity allows it to be used as an operating instrument to incise the uterine septum. This is best done with either an operating resectoscope[35] or a laser.[36] The septum is incised from below, and, as it is removed, it retracts, leaving the cavity united. Resectoscopic scissors[36] have also been used to divide the septum in the

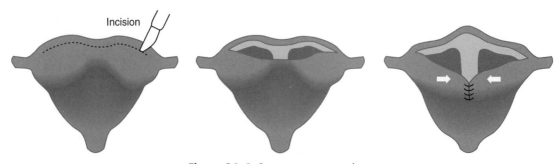

Figure 34–4. Strassman operation.

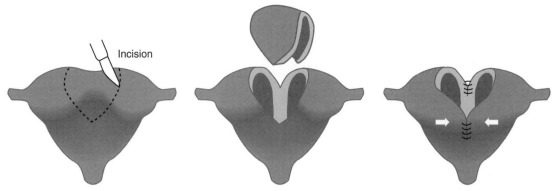

Figure 34–5. Jones metroplasty.

midline to allow it to retract. The hysteroscopic approach to metroplasty is useful when the septum is no more than 1 cm thick.

CERVIX

Congenital absence of the cervix, an extremely rare condition, consists of a functional uterus whose cervix has failed to develop. In true cervical atresia, no vagina forms, as, embryonically, the upper part of the vagina cannot develop unless the cervix also develops. In the literature are many reports of an absence of the cervix in a girl with a vagina. In one series, a normal vagina was present in 75% of cases.[37] It would seem, therefore, that there is some debate about whether the term *absent cervix* should be used to describe aplasia or agenesis of the cervix. Complete absence would seem to indicate a hypoplastic or rudimentary cervix, whereas the term *cervical atresia* should be used to describe *total absence* of the cervix.

The incidence of cervical atresia is not known; only 58 cases have been described.[37, 38] Because, traditionally, the treatment has been hysterectomy, it may well be underreported. Affected patients primarily present with cyclic abdominal pain in the absence of menstruation, usually between age 13 and 17 years (although one patient was reported to have presented at age 31).[37, 38]

A number of other malformations have been described in association with cervical atresia. The extragenital anomalies are similar to those associated with Rokitansky syndrome and affect primarily the renal system (e.g., renal agenesis, hypoplasia, and duplication of the collecting system).[39]

The diagnosis is often difficult to establish. In most cases, diagnosis is made at laparotomy on discovery of hematometra in a person with no definitive cervix and complete absence of the vagina and transverse vaginal septum. Currently, preoperative ultrasonography can determine the absence or presence of a cervix and can easily demonstrate the upper transverse vaginal septum and the open cervix. Absence of the cervix produces an image of an echogenic uterus but no cervix or vagina. One report[40] describes the use of MRI in the diagnosis of cervical atresia concomitant with vaginal agenesis. Again, both ultrasonography and MRI can be used to assess the anomaly before a surgical procedure is performed.

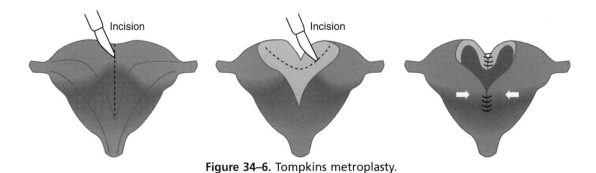

Figure 34–6. Tompkins metroplasty.

Management

When cervical atresia is present in conjunction with a functioning endometrium, surgical treatment is paramount: the hematometra must be drained and the development of pelvic endometriosis avoided. A number of authors have advocated hysterectomy, conserving the ovaries, as the primary procedure.[38, 41] For women so affected, the possibility of pregnancy is remote, and successful outcomes from procedures to preserve the uterus have been negligible. Rock and colleagues[41] cite hysterectomy as the absolute treatment of choice. This stance has been disputed by a number of authors, however,[39, 42] and adaptation of techniques that preserve a functional uterus and create a persistent fistula from the endometrial cavity into the neovagina has been described. The procedure uses a combined abdominal and vaginal approach, and the neovagina may be created in a number of ways.

An abdominal Pfannenstiel incision is made to expose the hematometra and the (absent) cervix. When the cervix is absent, the two uterine arteries lie essentially in apposition; thus, great care must be taken to identify them before the fistula is created. The bladder is reflected inferiorly and the upper part of the vagina exposed from above. The vaginal wall is then incised to create a vaginal orifice. The uterus is incised longitudinally on its anterior surface, and the incision extended between the uterine arteries to create the fistula space. A stent is placed from the fundus of the uterus, through the fistulous aperture, into the vagina. A number of different stents have been used; a No. 14 Foley catheter is ideal. The stent is sutured in place with a slow-dissolving suture material, and the uterus is reconstructed over the stent. The paracervical fascia is brought forward so that the fistulous space is covered. Trauma to the bladder base is prevented with this technique. The suturing of the upper part of the vagina to the lower part of the uterus demands great care, to avoid the major vessels. The abdomen is then closed in the traditional manner. The catheter is left in place for 6 to 8 weeks and, usually, is expelled spontaneously as the suture dissolves. Menstruation may occur through the fistulous space before the catheter is removed. This operation has been performed in 11 patients with congenital absence of the cervix, and regular menstruation was achieved in nine.[43] The other two patients subsequently required hysterectomy.

Outcome

For any woman, conservation of the uterus provides a major psychological boost, and reports of pregnancies in women treated with this procedure justify attempts at preservation. The first two cases of pregnancy[44, 45] were reported some time ago, but, in 1990, a third case was reported of spontaneous pregnancy and delivery by cesarean section.[46] Another report[47] describes successful use of zygote intrafallopian tube transfer (ZIFT) in a patient with congenital cervical atresia after a fistula-drainage procedure. Thus, the newer assisted reproduction techniques may further enhance the ability of these women to conceive, as their ovaries are totally normal.

LOWER TRACT ANOMALIES

VAGINA

Most developmental abnormalities of the vagina can be classified in one of three groups: (1) disorders marked by congenital absence of the vagina, with or without a functional uterus; (2) disorders caused by failure of vertical fusion; and (3) anomalies caused by failure of lateral fusion. (Some rare, complex anomalies may not fit into any of these groups.)

Congenital Absence of the Vagina

INCIDENCE

The incidence of vaginal malformation has been variously estimated between 1 in 4000 and 1 in 20,000 female births.[48, 49] It is second only to gonadal dysgenesis as a cause of primary amenorrhea.[50]

ETIOLOGY

The exact etiology of congenital absence of the vagina remains a matter of speculation. In its most common presentation (i.e., remnants of the müllerian duct and no vagina), it is known as the *Mayer-Rokitansky-Küster-Hauser syndrome*. Affected girls have no vagina, have (1) no uterus at all, (2) an extremely rudimentary organ, or (3) rudimentary uterine horns on the lateral pelvic side walls. The ovaries and distal fallopian tubes arise from a different embryonic tissue and are normal and functional. Ovarian steroid production and puberty progress normally, with the exception of amenorrhea. Two aspects of etiology deserve comment.

1. Whether any familial trait is involved in the mechanism of vaginal atresia remains to be

determined, but congenital absence has been described in 46XX siblings[51] and in one set of monozygotic twins.[52]

2. It is more likely that the mechanism of inheritance of this disorder is polygenic and multifactorial.

The suggestion that congenital absence of the vagina is an autosomal-dominant trait limited to females[53] was the impetus for studies to determine whether probands would, in fact, manifest the same abnormalities. The study[54] failed to report on affected relatives and, so, disproved the previous theory. The polygenic multifactorial inheritance theory is much more likely to hold, as the reported recurrence risk in first-degree relatives with these abnormalities is 1% to 5%. The additive effects of several genes' interacting with genetic and environmental factors (and, therefore, leading to this mode of inheritance) is most likely the cause.

ASSOCIATED ANOMALIES

As many as 40% of cases of vaginal atresia are associated with urinary tract defects. Some 15% of patients with the Mayer-Rokitansky-Küster-Hauser syndrome have major defects of the urinary tract, including renal agenesis, or a pelvic kidney. In view of the high incidence of urinary tract abnormalities, all patients found to have no vagina should be investigated by abdominal ultrasound to determine whether two kidneys are present. Intravenous pyelography (IVP) identifies abnormalities of the collecting system as well.

Skeletal abnormalities are common in patients with Mayer-Rokitansky-Küster-Hauser syndrome (some 12% of cases).[55] Two thirds of such abnormalities involve the spine, and limb and rib abnormalities account for the majority of the remainder. The vertebral abnormalities include wedge vertebrae, rudimentary vertebral bodies, and supernumerary or asymmetric vertebrae. There is an association with Klippel-Feil syndrome (i.e., congenital fusion of the cervical spine, short neck, low nuchal hairline, and painless limitation of cervical motion), although the incidence is low.[56] Among the other abnormalities that have been described in association with vaginal atresia are conduction deafness and other mesodermal defects. Their low incidences suggest, however, that they are incidental, rather than associated.

OVARIAN FUNCTION

Studies of patients with congenital absence of the cervix have failed to demonstrate any endocrine dysfunction. Endocrinologically, the menstrual cycle is of normal length, and hypothalamic control of gonadotropin release is also normal.[57] One report describes successful stimulation and retrieval of oocytes from a patient with the Mayer-Rokitansky-Küster-Hauser syndrome with transfer of fertilized oocytes into a surrogate uterus.[58]

DIAGNOSIS

Congenital absence of the vagina is not usually suspected until puberty, when primary amenorrhea occurs. Secondary sexual characteristics develop normally and at the appropriate time, because ovarian function is normal; as a result, detection of the absence of a vagina may be delayed, because clinicians would not suspect vaginal absence in an adolescent who exhibits normal secondary sexual characteristics. The diagnosis is confirmed by clinical examination, which reveals a vaginal dimple in an otherwise normal vulva. Diagnostic imaging can identify a rudimentary uterus, absence of a uterus, or small, nonfunctional uterine horns on the lateral pelvic wall. A case of functional anlage has been described in which the two hemiuteri lay on the lateral pelvic sidewalls but a normal appearing uterus was absent.[59] Fibroids have been described in a rudimentary uterus[60]; should they enlarge, excision might be necessary. Operative procedures such as examination under anesthesia and diagnostic laparoscopy are not necessary to establish the diagnosis.

MANAGEMENT

The goal of treatment is to create a vagina adequate to allow sexual activity. Both surgical and nonsurgical approaches have been utilized. The timing of the intervention is generally elective, but immediate intervention may be necessary if the patient is in pain. The first description of a simple nonsurgical technique was published by Frank,[61] who used glass dilators to create a vagina large enough for coitus. Currently, new grafting techniques,[62] tissue expanders,[63] and endoscopic procedures are being used for this purpose.

Frank Procedure

The technique of choice in all cases of congenital absence of the vagina in a girl who does not have a functional uterus is the Frank procedure. Ingram modified it to facilitate the process by using a bicycle seat mounted on a stool. These nonsurgical techniques involve insertion of incrementally larger vaginal dilators over a period of 6 to 12 weeks (Fig. 34–7). It is important for the patient to be familiar with her own anatomy. Most affected girls have never explored their anatomy because they have never menstruated and, therefore, it has never been necessary. They are completely unfamiliar with the position of the vagina in relation to the vulva and need to be taught digital exploration before a dilator is used. Once they are familiar with this, the tip of the smallest dilator is placed in the appropriate position on the dimple of the vagina as the patient presses it steadily in the direction of the normal vagina (i.e., 30 degrees posteriorly). This is done for 20 minutes, three times a day, with pressure that should not cause any pain. Occasionally, a lubricant may be used to facilitate insertion of the vaginal dilator and make it more comfortable. It is extremely important that instruction be given by persons who are totally familiar with the technique and in an atmosphere of empathy and commitment.

Close supervision is necessary for the first 3 or 4 days, and, with such guidance, patients are able to progress through dilators of the first three sizes within 4 to 5 days of commencement. A modified bicycle seat has been recommended to facilitate the procedure (Fig. 34–8).[64a] The patient should then be seen regularly, at least every 2 weeks, to ensure that she is continuing to use the dilators. Sexual intercourse may be attempted at any stage during therapy, and patients are encouraged to involve themselves, with their partners, in sexual discovery. The results are usually very gratifying; over 6 to 8 weeks girls progress to a No. 5 dilator, which creates a neovagina adequate for most sexual practices. Rare cases of prolapse of the neovagina after the Frank procedure have been described.[64] This may be managed by sacrocolpopexy in the manner used for recurrent enterocele, since the "prolapse" is actually an enterocele.

In the largest series reported so far,[65] 78 patients used this dilator regimen, and 80% were sexually functional within 3 months of commencing therapy. With provision of good psychological management and encouragement in the use of dilators, this can be a highly successful (and perhaps the most appropriate) form of therapy for patients with the Mayer-Rokitansky-Küster-Hauser syndrome.

Girls who fail to achieve a functional vagina with this technique require surgery. The most common type of vulvovaginoplasty is the McIndoe split-thickness skin graft technique.

McIndoe Vaginoplasty

This technique was first described in 1938 by McIndoe and Banister,[66] although split-thickness skin grafts had been used earlier by Abbe.[67] In the first part of the procedure the patient is placed in the lithotomy position and a transverse incision is made in the middle of the vaginal dimple. A neovaginal space is created digitally in the connective tissue lying between the bladder and the rectum (Fig. 34–9). It is imperative that digital exploration be performed with the fingers moving in a lateral and posterior direction, *not* in the direction of the bladder or the rectum, since damaging these structures is extremely easy. As the peritoneum of the pouch of Douglas is approached, a median raphe is encountered; it

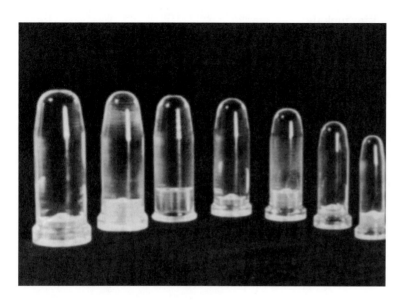

Figure 34–7. Frank dilators.

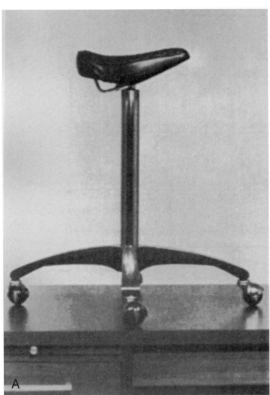
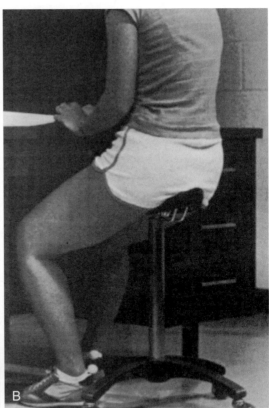

Figure 34–8. *A,* A bicycle seat stool. *B,* For at least 2 hours each day, the patient sits on the stool, learning forward slightly with the dilator held in place by a light girdle. (From Ingram JM: The bicycle seat stool in the treatment of vaginal agenesis and stenosis: A preliminary report. Am J Obstet Gynecol 1981; 140:867–871.)

is imperative that this structure be divided, so that subsequent retraction of the vagina does not occur in the midline. When the neovaginal space is deep enough, hemostasis must be achieved. A soft vaginal mold (stent) of foam rubber is then made (each custom-tailored). This use of a soft mold, rather than a solid mold, is known as the *Counsellor and Flor modification* of the McIndoe technique.[68] A split-thickness skin graft is obtained from a donor site using an electroderma-tome (Fig. 34–10). The vaginal mold is covered with a condom, and the skin graft is placed, skin side down, over the mold and sutured to fit (Fig. 34–11). The mold is then inserted in the neovagina (Fig. 34–12), and interrupted silk sutures are placed between the labia to hold the mold in place (Fig. 34–13). An indwelling catheter is placed in the urethra to prevent pressure build-up and allow free urine drainage. The mold is removed 7 days later with the patient under general anesthesia, and the vaginal cavity is irrigated. A second soft rubber mold is then put in place, and the patient is taught to remove the mold to douche and then to replace it daily for

6 weeks (Fig. 34–14). Now, she is taught to use vaginal dilators until the healing is complete, usually for 3 months.

While the use of a amnion to line the neovagina may prevent pain and scarring at a skin graft donor site, recently, the prevalence of HIV has rendered this method unsafe. To overcome this problem, some surgeons are experimenting with artificial membranes to line the newly created cavity. Oxidized regenerated cellulose, for example, was shown to be effective in achieving complete and quick epithelialization of the cavity.[69]

The results of the McIndoe vaginoplasty seem very satisfactory. About 85% to 95% of all procedures result in a sexually functional vagina.[70–72] Before the introduction of the self-mold technique, some serious complications resulted from the pressure produced by the solid mold and associated necrosis. With the introduction of the soft mold, these complications were eliminated, and, today, 75% of patients can expect a 100% graft take. To avoid infection, antibiotics are routinely used during the operation and in the postoperative period.

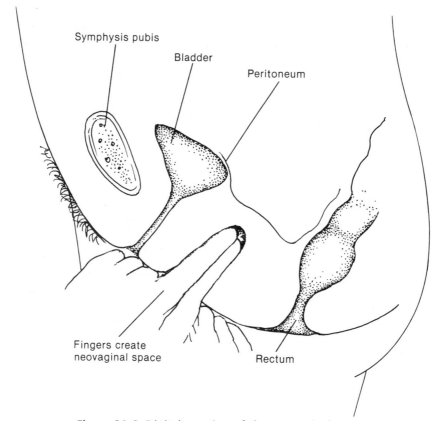

Figure 34–9. Digital creation of the neovaginal space.

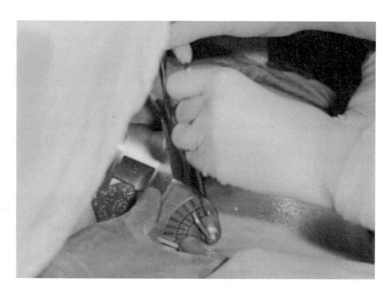

Figure 34–10. Split-thickness skin graft.

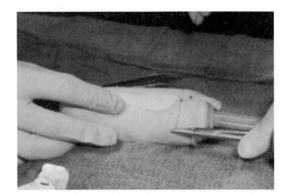

Figure 34–11. Vaginal mold.

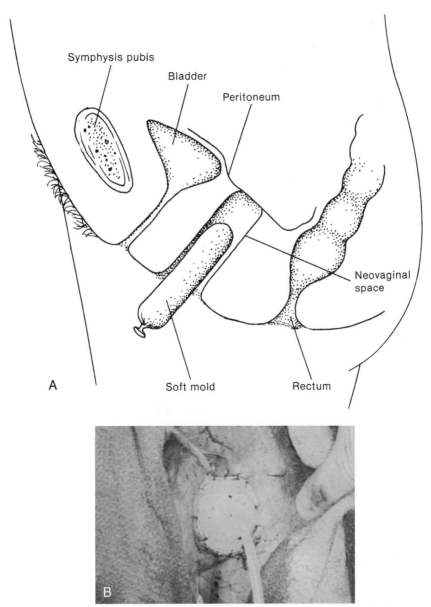

Symphysis pubis

Bladder

Peritoneum

Neovaginal space

Soft mold

Rectum

A

B

Figure 34–12. *A*, Schematic view of a soft mold inserted into the neovaginal space. *B*, At the completion of the procedure, the mold is shown within the neovagina.

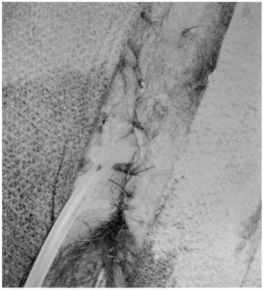

Figure 34–13. Neovagina showing interrupted silk sutures placed between the labia to hold the mold in place.

An international collaborative study that evaluated patients with congenital absence of the vagina found that the overall success rate for primary surgical procedures was 68.2%[73]; however, 25% of patients reported dyspareunia secondary to scarring of the upper margin of the vagina. Similar instances of dyspareunia have been reported in nearly all series of vaginoplasties, and that seems to occur regardless of what technique is used. The artificial vagina created in this way takes on the characteristics of normal vaginal epithelium, although the number of es-

trogen receptors at the new site does not increase.[74]

The artificial vagina is susceptible to malignant change: intraepithelial neoplasia[75] and squamous cell carcinoma[76, 77] have been described. Girls who are sexually active after vaginoplasty have a risk of malignant change equal to that of those with a functional cervix. It is, therefore, recommended that a vault smear, similar to a Pap smear, be obtained regularly, every 3 years. Condylomata acuminata have also been described in the neovagina.[78]

OTHER OPERATIVE PROCEDURES

Use of Bowel

Using bowel to construct a vagina has been extremely popular since the early 1900s. New skin-grafting techniques have replaced this procedure to some extent, but it is still the procedure of choice when the space between the rectum and the urethra is too small to create an adequate neovagina using traditional techniques. Various parts of the ileum and colon have been used, but cecum or sigmoid colon is used most often. The segment of bowel to be used is dissected free with its vascular pedicle and, after the neovaginal space is created, is transected and swung on its pedicle to lie in apposition to the vulva at one end. It is then sutured in place, along with the upper cut edge. Reanastomosis of the remaining bowel concludes the procedure. A number of authors have reported success,[79] but all accept the complication of excessive mucus discharge in a considerable proportion of pa-

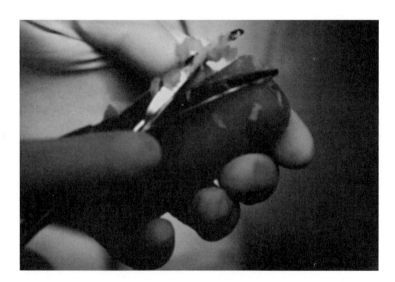

Figure 34–14. Soft rubber mold in situ.

tients. Functionally, however, it is an extremely useful technique in a number of circumstances.

Davydov Operation

The procedure described by Davydov and Zhvitiashvili[80] uses pelvic peritoneum to line the neovaginal space (Fig. 34–15). The neovaginal space is created in the traditional way (see Fig. 34–9), and the peritoneum is identified. Then, an abdominal incision is made, the peritoneum is dissected from its interstitial pelvic tissue and pulled down through the neovagina (Fig. 34–16), and sutured to the introitus. The upper portion is then closed, creating a peritoneal lining to the neovagina (Fig. 34–17). Subsequently, dilators must be used to avoid constriction.

Williams Vulvovaginoplasty

This procedure, first described in 1964[81] is still useful when dissection of a neovagina is impossible.[82] The technique involves the creation of a vulvar pouch from the labia majora (Fig. 34–18) that makes possible coitus and orgasm. It also disrupts a previously normal vulva, however, and, consequently, has psychological drawbacks. The operation has been reported to be very successful.[82]

Flap Vaginoplasty

Flap vaginoplasty has two techniques. The first is a simple flap technique,[83] (Fig. 34–19) in which two flaps of skin are mobilized from the labia through incisions and swung on their bases into the neovaginal space, a tubular structure having previously been created by the union of the anterior and posterior surfaces of the flaps.

The second technique involves the use of a donor site in the scapular region and mobilization of this skin flap and its vascular supply. It is then formed into a skin-lined tube and transferred to the neovagina, the vascular supply being anasto-

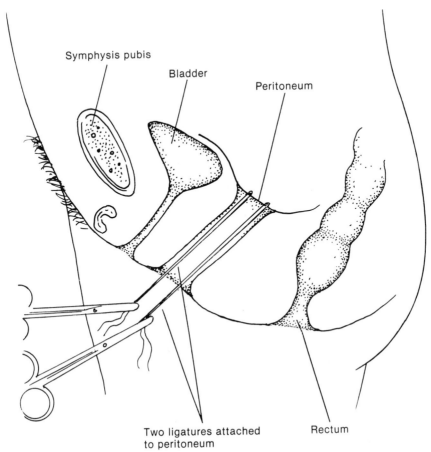

Symphysis pubis

Bladder

Peritoneum

Two ligatures attached to peritoneum

Rectum

Figure 34–15. The use of peritoneum in the Davydov operation.

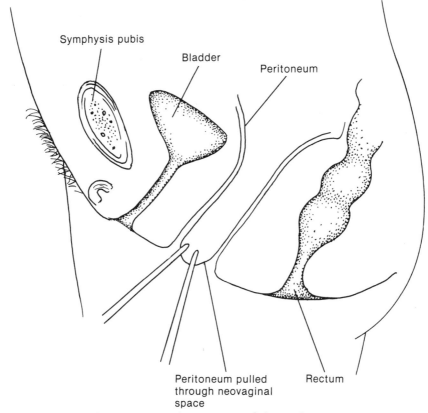

Symphysis pubis

Bladder

Peritoneum

Peritoneum pulled
through neovaginal
space

Rectum

Figure 34–16. Advancement of the peritoneum.

mosed to the major vessels in the inguinal region.[84]

Tissue Expansion Techniques

Use of subcutaneous balloons to increase and stretch the surface of the skin in the vulvar region has resulted in a modified flap vaginoplasty.[63, 85] This procedure requires placement of subcutaneous balloons in the region of the vulva whose size is gradually increased by introducing more and more fluid over a 3-month period. The result is a large area of skin to be used as a flap to create a vagina, as described in the flap vaginoplasty. This procedure, although it creates a larger amount of skin, causes considerable discomfort to patients during the tissue expansion.

The Vecchetti Technique

A modification of the Frank procedure, the Vecchetti technique uses a sphere placed in the blind vagina. Two wires attached to it are guided through the potential neovaginal space to exit on the anterior vaginal wall. An apparatus is then strapped to the anterior vaginal wall, to which the wires are attached, and pressure on the ball is increased daily, to continuously stretch the blind vaginal pouch. After 2 to 3 months, the skin is stretched sufficiently and the apparatus and ball are removed, leaving behind a functional vagina. This elaborate technique has become popular in Europe.

Perineal Reconstruction

Nikolaev and others presented a surgical approach for hematocolpos in adolescent girls with high vaginal atresia.[86] The procedure was described for five girls aged 12 to 14 years. The distance from the perineal skin to the hematocolpos ranged from 4 to 7 cm. The introitus was no longer than 2 cm. A perineal approach included surgery of the distal portion of the vagina using a U-shaped mucous-submucous vaginal flap and introital and labial flaps. Dilators and estrogen cream were used postoperatively. A limited number of patients enjoyed excellent results,

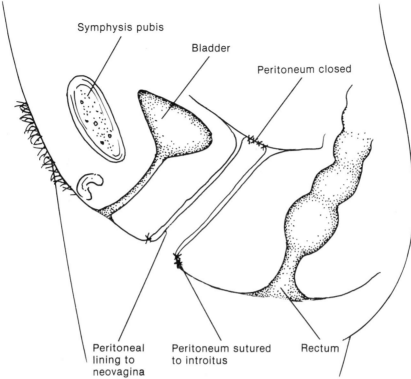

Figure 34–17. Completion of the Davydov operation.

without stenosis for as long as 6 months. Long-term success has not been reported.

PSYCHOLOGICAL ASPECTS

The psychological impact of absence of the vagina is immense, for both the patient and her parents. The initial period of shock is followed by a prolonged period of depression, when many patients question their femininity. They have serious doubts about their ability to maintain a heterosexual relationship, even though they have been told that sexual intercourse will almost certainly be possible. The most difficult challenge they have to cope with is their sterility. Often, they never come to terms with it entirely. They resent the fact that they are unable even to try to conceive. Thus, their situation is completely different from that of infertile couples who fail in their attempts to conceive, despite their best efforts.

The parents feel guilty, and responsible for their daughter's anomaly. They often consider whether difficulties during the pregnancy might have caused the problem. They should be assured that there is no evidence for this. They also need to be reassured of their daughter's ability to have a normal sex life.

Cultural problems may arise that make management difficult. For some ethnic groups, the ability to procreate is fundamental to marriage and social acceptance, and the absence of a vagina and its associated sterility can mean total isolation for the girl. These patients and their parents can be almost impossible to console; they sometimes refuse to accept the situation—and in some cases contemplate suicide.

It is not surprising that patients and their parents often request immediate surgery to return the girl to "normal." That is a major mistake as adequate psychological and physical preparation cannot yet have been provided. The minimum recommended preparation time before any attempt at vaginal surgery is 6 months. Ideally, the patient should establish a heterosexual relationship. It is extremely important that these patients, and their parents, have adequate psychological support before they embark on any therapy.

During the period of adjustment, counseling can be extremely difficult. Patients may be normally reactionary adolescents, and the impact of this major congenital abnormality on their sexuality can be immense. Managing their loss of self-

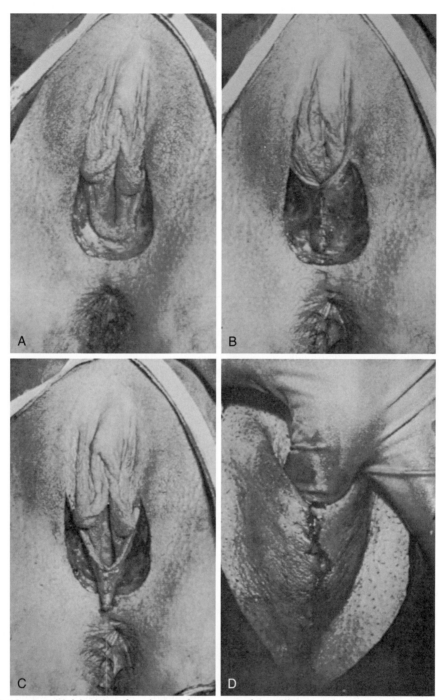

Figure 34–18. *A*, Initial incision for the performance of a Williams vulvovaginoplasty. (The anterior limbs of this incision are more medial than is desirable.) *B*, After freeing and undercutting the deeper tissues, the inner skin layer is being brought together to form a tube that will be the new vagina. *C*, Suturing the inner skin layer has almost been completed. *D*, The outer skin layer has been brought together over the inner, and two fingers are inserted into the introitus of the new vagina. A satisfactory functional result occurred in this case. (From Edmonds DK. Dewhurst's Practical Paediatric and Adolescent Gynaecology. 2nd ed. London: Butterworth & Co [Publishers] Ltd, 1989, p 42.)

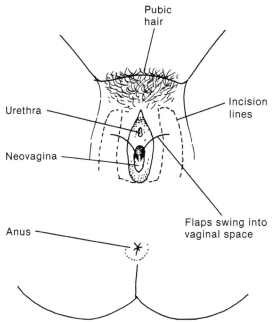

Pubic hair

Urethra

Neovagina

Anus

Incision lines

Flaps swing into vaginal space

Figure 34–19. Incisions for creation of the flap vaginoplasty.

esteem and inevitable depression requires counseling from properly trained professionals who are familiar with the problems of patients who lack a vagina. Unfortunately, because few psychologists have the necessary experience and expertise, the counseling girls receive is sometimes inadequate or inappropriate. It is important that gynecologists who care for these patients have meaningful discussions with the counselors to make them fully conversant with the situation and to enable them to manage the patients appropriately.

A second problem is psychosexual counseling and dealing with the difficulties associated with sexual activity in the absence of a vagina. Counseling these girls involves reestablishing the belief that a sex life will be possible, and they must be advised and reassured that they have a normally functioning clitoris and, so, are quite capable of orgasm. Words must be chosen very carefully, however, and the word *artificial* must be avoided in referring to the vagina. It is important that these girls understand the normality of their created vagina and the fact that they will experience the same feelings that females with a normally formed vagina do. Equally difficult to inculcate is the understanding that their vagina will feel normal to their partner. Therefore, counseling should involve the sexual partner, so that he also understands the difficulties associated with a neovagina.

The fear of failure, both sexual and reproductive, may take years, or even a lifetime, to overcome. Thus, psychological counseling must begin before any attempt is made to form a vagina, and the best results accrue from therapy that occurs during a stable relationship. Girls who are counseled and managed appropriately can have a completely normal sex life, one comparable to that of any woman in the "normal" population.[65]

Disorders of Longitudinal Fusion

As the two müllerian ducts fuse, a single vagina usually develops, but when fusion is incomplete, a duplex system is sometimes created. Duplication of the vagina, an extremely rare condition, is often associated with duplication of the vulva, bladder, and uterus. Each part of the vagina is encircled with a separate muscle layer.

LONGITUDINAL VAGINAL SEPTUM

Longitudinal septa develop when the distal ends of the müllerian ducts fail to fuse properly. The result is a vagina divided by a longitudinal septum, both parts being encircled by the same muscle layer. Failure to fuse may be limited to the vagina, or may affect the uterus as well, forming a bicornuate, septate, or didelphic uterus. Patients may be asymptomatic, in which case no therapy is required. Indications for division of the septum are dyspareunia, obstruction of drainage from one half of the vagina, and suspicion that a septum might interfere with vaginal delivery. The surgeon should inspect the entire length of the vagina on both sides of the septum to determine whether the patient has one cervix or two (i.e., one on each side of the septum). Next, the surgeon places the septum on tension by pushing the posterior vaginal wall downward. With scissors the septum is cut in the middle, at a point of equal distance from the anterior and the posterior vaginal walls. Because the septum represents the line of fusion of two tubular structures, it is thinnest, and least vascular, at its midpoint. In addition, the incised edges tend to retract, and, should the septum be divided too close to the vaginal mucosa, a defect of the vaginal mucosa will result. Hemostasis is secured by placing a continuous locking suture, absorbable (00) on each edge of the divided septum.

IMPERFORATE UNILATERAL VAGINA

Outflow obstruction of menstrual flow may result if blood collects in the blind vagina. It can cause severe dysmenorrhea and the development of a cystic swelling that bulges into the side of the vagina and that may be large enough to be palpable abdominally. This imperforate unilateral vagina is treated by excising the septum between the two vaginas, allowing one to drain into the other. The incision should be large enough to create a large opening. Failure to create an adequate ostium will result in contraction and sealing of the sinus and, subsequently, retention of menstrual fluid, which may become infected.

Disorders of Vertical Fusion

Transverse vaginal septa are the result of faulty canalization of the embyonic vagina. These septa may have no opening (a *complete septum*) or a small central aperture *(incomplete septum)*. Usually, they are found in the mid-vagina, but they can be found at any level. When the septum is located in the upper vagina, it is more likely to be patent (incomplete), whereas those located in the lower part of the vagina are often complete.

An incomplete septum is usually asymptomatic and, therefore, does not have to be corrected during childhood or early adolescence. The central aperture allows egress from the vagina of vaginal secretions and menstrual flow. A complete septum or an imperforate hymen gives rise to a hematocolpos. Patients present with amenorrhea and abdominal pain. The hematocolpos may be so large that it is palpable abdominally.

IMPERFORATE HYMEN

Typically, imperforate hymen is seen in 14- to 16-year-old girls with normal secondary sexual development who have not menstruated. The intermittent lower abdominal pain is due to accumulation of blood in the vagina. If the hematocolpos grows large enough it exerts pressure on the urinary tract that leads to urine retention. Vulvar examination reveals a tense, bulging, bluish membrane at the introitus. The blue color is attributable to retained menstrual fluid. On rectal examination, the distended vagina is palpable as a large cystic mass. The diagnosis is straightforward, and treatment involves a stellate incision of the membrane and removal of any redundant segments. No additional surgery may be required, and any impulse to swab or irrigate the vagina should be resisted. Alternatively, the surgeon may grasp the central portion of the hymen

with forceps, and, using scissors, remove the central portion. Bleeding is minimal and no sutures are required. Further inspection of the vagina should be delayed 4 to 6 weeks to reduce the risk of introducing infection. In addition, the significant distention of the uterus limits the examiner's ability to evaluate the pelvic organs properly. Endometriosis and vaginal adenosis are known, but not inevitable, complications in such patients.

TRANSVERSE VAGINAL SEPTUM

A transverse septum is most often found at the junction of the middle and the upper third of the vagina (Fig. 34–20).[87] Before any attempt at surgical treatment, the amount of vagina must be determined, either clinically or with the aid of ultrasonography or magnetic resonance imaging (MRI). It is extremely important to perform intravenous pyelography to exclude renal abnormalities, especially a pelvic kidney, and the status of the urinary tract must be clearly defined before any surgical procedure is performed. In general, the less residual vagina that is present, the more difficult the surgery becomes, and success may be hampered by the presence of endometriosis[88] and concurrent hematosalpinges.

When the transverse vaginal septum is in the lower two thirds of the vagina, dissection may be performed from below. The surgeon incises through the septum. After the initial incision, dissection should be performed along the track of the absent vagina into the hematocolpos above. This is probably best accomplished by blunt dissection until the hematocolpos is reached, at which point it is incised and the retained menstrual blood released. The vaginal septum is then excised with scissors, and the upper and lower parts of the vagina are reanastomosed (Fig. 34–21). The importance of complete excision of the septum cannot be overstated, as failure to do so will leave a stenotic vaginal ring, owing to the creation of a fibrous band. This complication makes subsequent sexual function difficult and painful.

When the transverse septum is high and it is difficult to confirm the presence of an hematocolpos, an approach from both the vagina and the abdomen may be required. The abdomen is opened and the hematometra or hematocolpos identified. The hematocolpos is then incised and the menstrual blood aspirated. While another surgeon operates through the vagina, a probe can then be passed from above to permit identification of the upper vagina from below. The septum

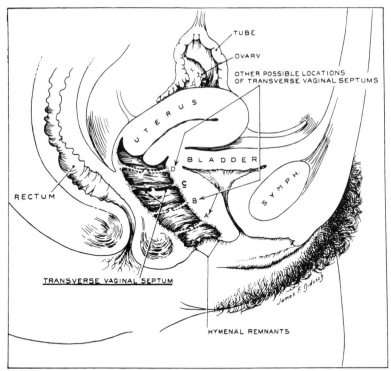

Figure 34–20. Sketch of a congenital transverse vaginal septum showing the possible locations of the vagina. (From Bowman JA, Scott RB. Transverse vaginal septum. Report of four cases. Obstet Gynecol 1954; 3:444. Reprinted with permission from The American College of Obstetricians and Gynecologists.)

may then be incised and removed, from either above or below, but anastomosis of the upper vagina to the lower is usually best performed from above. Closing the drainage incision in the vagina completes the operation. A mold is usually left in place and removed 1 week later.

When a large portion of vagina is absent, drainage of the hematocolpos may be necessary after removal of the septum and anastomosis or, alternatively, the creation of a neovagina may be delayed by 1 week, to reduce the risk of infection. A mold is usually left in situ for 3 to 4 months, to ensure that the upper vagina does not contract and that there is a drainage channel through the middle to allow passage of menstrual blood. The prospects for fertility after these procedures are difficult to predict.

For patients with an imperforate hymen, the fertility potential is probably normal, but those with a transverse vaginal septum may be less fortunate, as they present later and their rates of endometriosis and adhesions are much greater, so fertility is adversely affected. An overall pregnancy rate of 47% is reported.[87] All patients with lower-third obstruction conceived; of those with middle-third obstruction, 43%, but only 25% of those with high obstruction did. Thus, prompt diagnosis and treatment are necessary to preserve these patients' reproductive capacity.

Vulva

Problems that arise in the vulva in pediatric and adolescent patients are those associated with intersex and the androgenization of the female vulva during development. In this section female intersex induced by congenital adrenal hyperplasia, endogenous and exogenous androgen production, incomplete androgen insensitivity, and 5α-reductase deficiency are discussed.

CONGENITAL ADRENAL HYPERPLASIA

The endocrine problems produced by congenital adrenal hyperplasia are discussed in Chapter 7. The end result of this disorder is overproduction of androgen, which is converted peripherally to dihydrotestosterone, resulting in cloacal virilization. The degree of virilization depends on the amount of androgen; thus, the range of physical changes is wide as is the degree of masculinization.

Two aspects of the cloaca deserve attention: those related to the vulva per se and those related to clitoral or phallic growth. In normal development, the urogenital sinus allows the urethra to exit in the midvulvar position, between the clitoris and the vaginal opening. As masculinization increases, the urethra is more likely to be

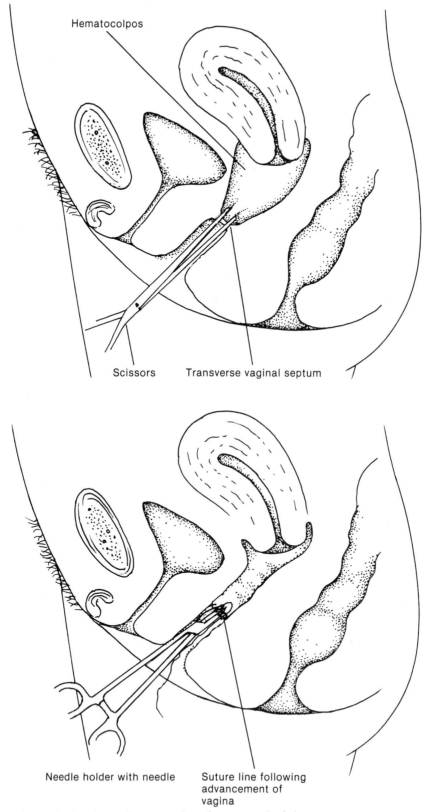

Figure 34–21. Operative procedure for removal of the transverse septum.

enclosed and to open at the base of the phallus (a gross appearance almost like hypospadias; Fig. 34–22). More often, as the vulva becomes occluded by labial fusion, the urethra opens high on the anterior vaginal wall (Fig. 34–23). The increasing degree of androgenization is associated with increasing thickening of the lower vagina, which in severe cases opens into the urethra, forming a urogenital sinus. A vagina is always present in congenital adrenal hyperplasia, and drainage of menses through the sinus is always possible. The genetic aspects of the various types of congenital adrenal hyperplasia are considered in Chapter 7.

PRENATAL DIAGNOSIS. Prenatal diagnosis of congenital adrenal hyperplasia is possible, and for women who are known to be at risk, either chorionic villus sampling (CVS) or amniocentesis can identify the condition. CVS is preferred, as the direct DNA probe for congenital adrenal hyperplasia can be used and intrauterine treatment of the fetus commenced. Treatment is steroids (dexamethasone) administered to the mother, which are then transferred across the placenta to suppress adrenocorticotropin (ACTH) release, preventing excessive androgen production in utero.

DIAGNOSIS. When a child is born with an intersex problem, it is extremely important to establish the diagnosis as quickly as possible. The most important and appropriate endocrinologic assessment techniques are discussed in Chapter 6. Pelvic ultrasonography is recommended to determine the presence of a normal uterus and vagina, which makes the diagnosis of congenital adrenal hyperplasia most likely. Chromosome studies can be obtained very quickly on blood, and a sample should be drawn for the measurement of serum 17-hydroxyprogesterone. These two serum tests should be performed simultaneously. Thus, in the first 2 or 3 days of life both gender and sex of rearing can be established. The most common abnormality is 21-hydroxylase deficiency. If it is the salt-wasting type, management of water and sodium intake must be considered. There are two forms of congenital adrenal hyperplasia: the salt-wasting and the non–salt-wasting classic forms. The former causes the most severe virilization problems, which, of themselves, lead to long-term difficulties of management in the adolescent years.

SURGICAL MANAGEMENT. Once the diagnosis of congenital adrenal hyperplasia has been confirmed, the child should be reared as a female,

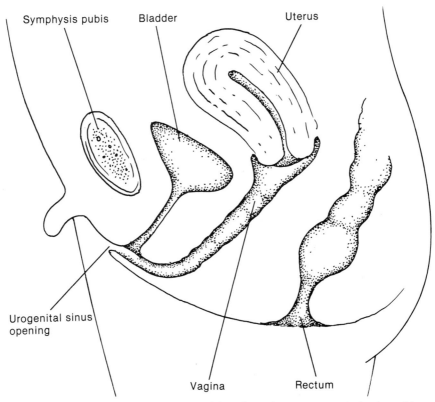

Figure 34–22. Urogenital sinus opening in mild and moderate congenital adrenal hyperplasia.

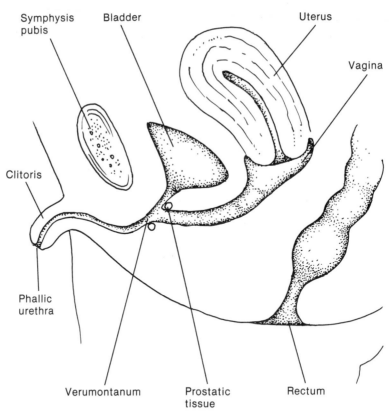

Figure 34–23. Severe congenital adrenal hyperplasia with clitoral hypertrophy and the vagina entering into the urethra.

regardless of the degree of masculinization of the external genitalia, which can always be corrected surgically. The ovaries are normal and function at puberty for the initiation of normal female puberty and subsequent fertility. Having been established that the child is female, any enlargement of the clitoris and excessive fusion of the labial folds must be addressed. If the degree of clitoral enlargement is sufficient to cause parental distress, reduction clitoroplasty should be undertaken and the labial folds divided at the same time to expose the vaginal opening, giving the vulva a more normal female appearance. Reduction clitoroplasty is best performed during the neonatal period, as the parents are eager to take a child home with no visible evidence of masculinity, to avoid mental anguish. The procedure is shown in Figure 34–24.

A V-shaped incision is made, and the skin over the anterior wall is reflected downward and excised to reveal the body of the phallus. The principle behind the reduction clitoroplasty is to maintain the neurovascular bundle supplying the glans of the clitoris with its sensory and vascular supply, to preserve its function. Two lateral inci-

sions must be made along the corpora to allow dissection of the connective tissue on the lateral walls. Dissection is then carried dorsally, identifying the vascular bundle lying on the dorsal surface of the phallus and separating the body of the phallus from the vascular bundle. When this has been achieved, the corpora is transected at its base and just below the level of the glans. Two major arteries are always present at its base, and these must be suitably ligated. Hemostasis is extremely important; once it has been achieved, the glans of the phallus is then sutured with interrupted absorbable sutures to its base and the skin closed over the new clitoris. Bruising is reasonably common after this procedure, but the anatomic outcome is excellent. It is difficult to ascertain whether this procedure has resulted in improved sexual function as compared with total clitoridectomy; studies have not yet been published. A vulvoplasty, if performed at the same time, is done in the manner shown in Figure 34–25. It is imperative that the urethra be identified and catheterized before any procedure is performed, as it can easily be damaged. After the patient is catheterized, an instrument is placed

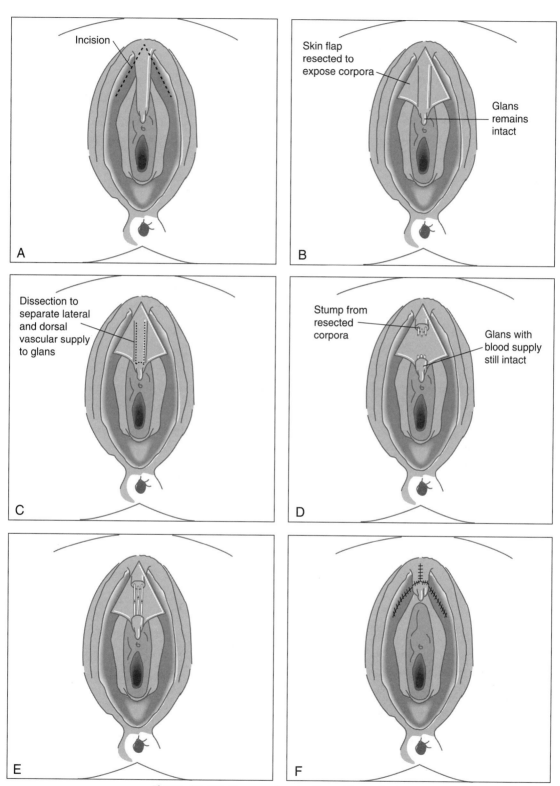

Figure 34–24. Stages of reduction clitoroplasty.

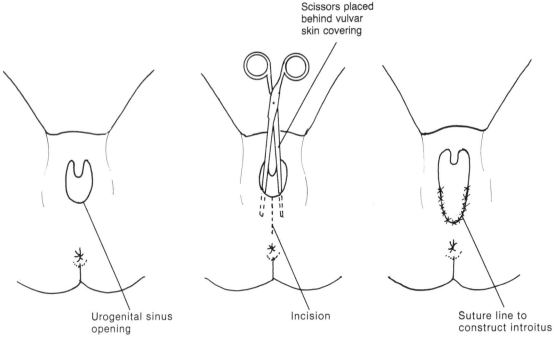

Scissors placed
behind vulvar
skin covering

Urogenital sinus
opening

Incision

Suture line to
construct introitus

Figure 34–25. The cutback vulvoplasty for congenital adrenal hyperplasia.

behind the vulvar skin and opened to stretch the fused labia and, so, to identify the line of fusion. An incision is then made in the midline and the cut edges of the labia are sutured, as illustrated. The vagina is always visible behind this, but the necessity for further introital surgery should be decided when puberty has passed and adult maturation has been achieved.

When the patient presents in adolescence and the vulva must be reconstructed, the procedure may be approached in a slightly different way if the degree of masculinization is much greater. In this case a flap vaginoplasty is required, which may be carried out in one of two ways: as described in Figure 34–25 or, if the degree of masculinization is greater, as described in Figure 34–26. In the latter procedure, a perineal flap is created by incisions, as shown in the diagram, and the skin is reflected posteriorly, revealing the posterior vaginal wall. As can be seen, before any incisions are made the urethra must be catheterized. The posterior vaginal wall must be dissected away from the interstitial tissue, and an instrument is often required to identify the vaginal orifice. That orifice having been identified, the vagina is then incised longitudinally, and the lateral walls are sutured. The defect in the posterior wall is repaired by inserting the flap of vulvar skin. This procedure allows opening of the introi-

tus with minimal subsequent scarring and contraction (Fig. 34–27).

The outcome of these surgical procedures is generally very good, although successful sexual function is more likely in the non–salt-wasting form. Menstruation generally is delayed slightly beyond the norm.[89] Fertility rates in patients with congenital adrenal hyperplasia are also related to (1) compliance with therapy, which influences the onset of menstruation and subsequent normal hypothalamic-pituitary-ovarian function, and (2) the degree of androgenization. In the largest review reported thus far,[90] 80 women were assessed with respect to fertility. In those with simple virilization, satisfactory surgical correction was achieved in 73%, but 56% of those in the salt-losing group had an inadequate introitus. Among 15 of 25 patients with the simple virilizing form, 25 pregnancies resulted in 20 normal children; only 1 of 15 women with the salt-wasting form became pregnant. Thus, achieving adequate medical control and using good surgical technique to ensure normal sexual function are imperative.

ENDOGENOUS ANDROGEN PRODUCTION

Androgenization of the vulva has been described in various circumstances. The most com-

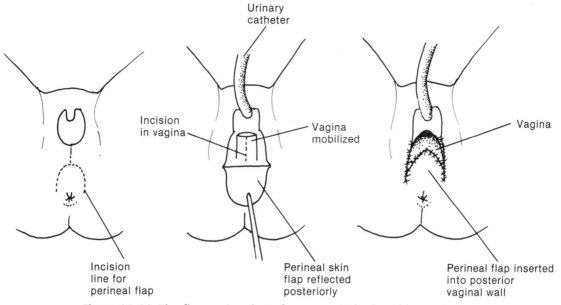

Figure 34–26. The flap vaginoplasty for congenital adrenal hyperplasia.

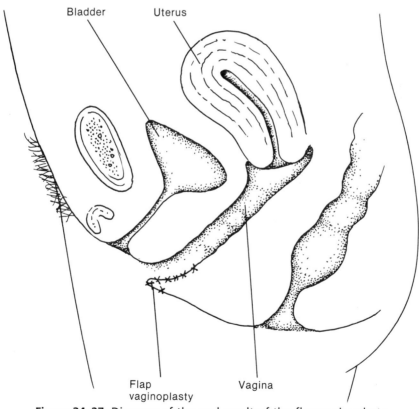

Figure 34–27. Diagram of the end result of the flap vaginoplasty.

Table 34–1. Clinical Features of Androgen Resistance Syndromes

Feature	5α-Reductase Deficiency	Androgen Receptor Disorder				
		Complete Testicular Feminization	Incomplete Testicular Feminization	Reifenstein Syndrome	Infertile Male Syndrome	Undervirilized Male Syndrome
Inheritance	Autosomal-recessive	X-linked recessive	X-linked recessive	X-linked recessive	X-linked recessive	X-linked recessive
Hormone profile	Normal male androgen and estrogen production	Increased androgen and estrogen (usually)	Increased androgen and estrogen (usually)	Increased androgen and estrogen (usually)	Increased androgen and estrogen (usually)	Increased androgen and estrogen (usually)
Phenotypic features						
Spermatogenesis	Decreased	Absent	Absent	Absent	Absent or decreased	Normal or decreased
Müllerian derivatives	Absent	Absent	Absent	Absent	Absent	Absent
Wolffian derivatives (epididymis, vas deferens, seminal vesicle)	Male	Absent	Male	Male	Male	Male
Urogenital sinus derivatives (prostate and urethra)	Female	Female	Female	Underdeveloped male	Male	Male
External genitalia (penis and scrotum)	Female (may virilize at puberty)	Female	Posterior fusion and clitoromegaly	Perineoscrotal hypospadias	Male	Male
Breasts	Male	Female	Female	Gynecomastia	Gynecomastia in some	Gynecomastia

Modified from Griffin JE: Androgen resistance—the clinical and molecular spectrum. N Engl J Med 1992; 326(9):611–618. Reprinted, by permission of The New England Journal of Medicine.

mon conditions are adrenal adenomas, luteomas, and virilization in pregnancy associated with polycystic ovarian disease. These are extremely rare phenomena, and the degree of virilization depends on the amounts of androgen. Surgical management is similar to that described for congenital adrenal hyperplasia.

EXOGENOUS ANDROGEN PRODUCTION

Exogenous androgen production is also rare, and there seems to be no reason for it to occur. One case of a female infant with virilization following administration of danazol to the mother has been described.[91] Again, surgical management is that described for congenital adrenal hyperplasia.

INCOMPLETE ANDROGEN INSENSITIVITY

Incomplete androgen insensitivity, though extremely rare, covers a wide spectrum of disorders, ranging from gynecomastia with azoospermia to a pseudovagina (Table 34–1). The most common presentation is perineoscrotal hypospadias and associated cryptorchidism in a male neonate. The testes are small but contain normal Leydig cells. Endocrinologically, these persons exhibit normal postpubertal development, have levels of testosterone in the normal male range, and are similar to 46,XY females. Psychosexually, most subjects' behavior is "masculine." This is almost certainly because they have a quantitative defect in androgen receptors, and the incomplete androgen insensitivity leads to varying degrees of masculinization. It can also be difficult to determine the gender role, because the patients are psychosexually male and androgen receptors exist in the brain to influence psychological sex. The options are (1) a male role and a microphallus that may not be reconstructible or (2) a female role and removal of the gonads and subsequent perineal reduction. The latter is most often chosen, because creation of a vagina is almost always feasible, whereas construction of a penis is extremely difficult. Vaginoplasty may be performed in a manner similar to that described for the absent vagina, although creation of labial folds is very difficult, since the perineum in these patients is generally flat.[92]

5α-Reductase Deficiency. Children with this rare condition are born with a markedly bifid scrotum that appears similar to labia, but the phallus is enlarged, and there is a urogenital sinus with a blind vaginal pouch. The testes are usually found in the abdomen but may be located in the inguinal canal or in the scrotum. No müllerian structures are present, and the wolffian ducts are normally developed. It is important to establish this diagnosis soon after birth, because, at puberty, rising levels of testosterone will cause rapid virilization and deepening of the voice and phallus growth. Failure to remove the gonads before puberty will result in testicular descent and even ejaculation from the urethral orifice. This is a familial condition and is almost certainly an autosomal-recessive disorder found only in males. Surgical management may involve reduction clitoroplasty and subsequent development of a vagina, as described earlier for vaginoplasty.

CONCLUSION

Successful management of congenital anomalies of the genital tract demands both intensive psychological support and great surgical skill. All patients should be referred to specialized centers where such expertise is available. Otherwise, results may be less than optimal—and traumatic for the patient.

REFERENCES

1. Patsavoudi E, Magre S, Castinior M, et al: Dissociation between testicular morphogenesis and functional differentiation of Leydig cells. J Endocrinol 1985; 105:235–238.
2. Magre S, Jost A: Dissociation between testicular morphogenesis and endocrine differentiation of Sertoli cells. Proc Natl Acad Sci USA 1984; 81:7831.
3. Jost A: Recherches sur la differenciation sexuelle de l'embryon de lapin. II. Action des androgenes de synthese sur l'histogenese genitale. Arch Anat Microscop Morphol Exp 1947; 36:242–270.
4. Cates RL, Mattaliano RJ, Hession C, et al: Isolation of the bovine and human genes for müllerian inhibiting substance and expression of the human gene in animal cells. Cell 1986; 45:685–698.
5. Cohen-Haguenauer O, Picard JY, Mattei MG, et al: Mapping of the gene for anti-müllerian hormone to the short arm of human chromosome 19. Cytogenet Cell Genet 1987; 44:2–6.
6. Jarcho J: Malformations of the uterus. Am J Surg 1946; 71:106.
7. Jones WS: Obstetric significance of female genital anomalies. Obstet Gynecol 1957; 10:113.
8. Semmens JP: Congenital anomalies of female genital tract. Obstet Gynecol 1962; 19:328.
9. Buttram VC, Gibbons WE: Müllerian anomalies: A proposed classification. Fertil Steril 1979; 32:90.
10. Toaff ME, Lev-Toaff AS, Toaff R: Communicating uteri: Review and classification with introduction of two previously unreported types. Fertil Steril 1984; 41:661.

11. Fedele L, Vercellini P, Marchini M, et al: Communicating uteri: Description and classification of a new type. Int J Fertil 1988; 33:168.

12. The American Fertility Society Classifications of Adnexal Adhesions, Distal Tubal Occlusion, Tubal Occlusion Secondary to Tubal Ligations, Tubal Pregnancies, Mullerian Anomalies, and Intrauterine Adhesions. Fertil Steril 1988; 49:944–955.

13. Bennett MJ, Berry JVJ: Preterm labor and congenital malformations of the uterus. Ultrasound Med Biol 1979; 5:83.

14. Strassman EO: Fertility and unification of double uterus. Fertil Steril 1966; 17:165.

15. Sanfilippo JS, Yussman MA, Smith O: HSG in the evaluation of infertility. A six year review. Fertil Steril 1978; 30:636.

16. Sandler SW: Spontaneous abortion in perspective. S Afr Med J 1977; 52:1115.

17. Stray-Petersen B, Stray-Petersen S: Etiologic factors and subsequent reproductive performance in 195 couples with a prior history of habitual abortion. Am J Obstet Gynecol 1984; 148:140.

18. Shulman LP, Elias S: Developmental abnormalities of the female reproductive tract: Pathogenesis and nosology. Adolesc Pediatr Gynecol 1988; 1:230–238.

19. Elias S, Simpson JL, Carson SA, et al: Genetic studies in incomplete müllerian fusion. Obstet Gynecol 1984; 63:276.

20. Gurin J, Lester E: Associated anomalies of müllerian and wolffian duct structures. South Med J 1981; 74:805.

21. Rock JA, Zacur HA: The clinical management of repeated early pregnancy wastage. Fertil Steril 1983; 39:123.

22. Stem AM, Gall JC, Perry BL, et al: The hand-foot-uterus syndrome. J Pediatr 1970; 77:109.

23. Winter JSD, Kohn G, Mellman WJ, Wagner S: A familial syndrome of renal, genital and middle ear anomalies. J Pediatr 1968; 71:88.

24. Rudiger RA, Schmidt W, Loose DA, Passarge E: Severe developmental failure with coarse facial features, distal limb hypoplasia, thickened palmar creases, bifid vulva and ureteral stenosis. J Pediatr 1971; 79:977.

25. Sorenson SS: Minor müllerian anomalies and oligomenorrhoea in infertile women. Am J Obstet Gynecol 1981; 140:636.

26. Kaufman RH, Binder GL, Gray PM, Adam E: Upper genital tract changes associated with exposure in utero to diethylstilbestrol. Am J Obstet Gynecol 1977; 128:51.

27. Berger M, Alper M: Intractable primary infertility in women exposed to diethylstilbestrol in utero. J Reprod Med 1986; 31:231–235.

28. Karande VC, Lester RG, Masher SJ, et al: Are implantation and pregnancy outcome impaired in diethylstilbestrol exposed women after in vitro fertilization and embryo transfer? Fertil Steril 1990; 54:287–291.

29. Barnes AB, Colton T, Gundersen J, et al: Fertility and outcome of pregnancy in women exposed in utero to diethylstilbestrol. N Engl J Med. 1980; 302:609–613.

30. Kaufman RH, Irwin JF: DES exposure and reproductive performance. In Bennett MJ, Edmonds DK (eds): Spontaneous and Recurrent Abortion. Chicago, Blackwell Scientific Publications, 1987.

31. Manzella A, Borba P: Hydrocolpos, uterus didelphys and septate vagina in association with ascites: Antenatal sonographic detection. J Ultrasound Med 1998; 17(7):465–468.

32. Malini S, Valdes C, Malinaki LR: Sonographic diagnosis and classification of anomalies of the genital tract. J Ultrasound Med 1984; 3:397.

33. Pellerito J, McCarthy S, Doyle M, et al: Diagnosis of uterine anomalies: Relative accuracy of MR imaging, endovaginal sonography, and hysterosalpingography. Radiology 1992; 103:795–800.

34. Sanfilippo JS: Strassman operation for the correction of a class II anomaly in an adolescent. J Adolesc Health 1991; 12:63.

35. Daly DC, Maier D, Soto-Albors C: Hysteroscopic metroplasty: Six years experience. Obstet Gynecol 1989; 73:201.

36. Candiani GB, Vercellini P, Fedele L, et al: Argon laser versus microscissors for hysteroscopic incision of uterine septa. Am J Obstet Gynecol 1991; 164:87.

37. Jacob JH, Griffin WT: Surgical reconstruction of the congenitally atretic cervix: Two cases. Obstet Gynecol Surv 1989; 44:556.

38. Regan L, Dewhurst J: Atresia of the cervix. Pediatr Adolesc Gynecol 1985; 3:83.

39. Farber M: Congenital atresia of the uterine cervix. Semin Reprod Endocrinol 1986; 4:33.

40. Markham SM, Parmley TH, Murphy AA, et al: Cervical agenesis combined with vaginal agenesis diagnosed by MRI. Fertil Steril 1987; 48:143.

41. Rock JA, Schlaff WD, Zacur HA, Jones HW: The clinical management of congenital absence of the uterine cervix. Int J Gynaecol Obstet 1984; 22:231.

42. Edmonds DK: Congenital malformations of the vagina and their management. Semin Reprod Endocrinol 1988; 6:91.

43. Edmonds DK (ed): Practical Paediatric and Adolescent Gynaecology. London: Butterworths, 1988, p 37.

44. Zarou GS, Espesito JM, Zarou DM: Pregnancy following surgical correction of congenital atresia of the cervix. Int J Obstet Gynecol 1973; 11:143.

45. Singh J, Devi YL: Pregnancy following surgical correction of nonfused müllerian bulbs and absent vagina. Obstet Gynecol 1983; 61:267.

46. Hampton HL, Meeks GR, Bates W, Wiser WL: Pregnancy after successful vaginoplasty and cervical stenting for partial atresia of the cervix. Obstet Gynecol 1990; 76:900.

47. Thijssen RFA, Hollanders JMG, Willemsen P, et al: Successful pregnancy after ZIFT in a patient with congenital cervical atresia. Obstet Gynecol 1990; 76:902.

48. Bryan AL, Nigro JA, Counsellor VS: One hundred cases of congenital absence of the vagina. Surg Gynecol Obstet 1949; 88:79.

49. Evans TN, Poland ML, Boving RL: Vaginal malformations. Am J Obstet Gynecol 1981; 141:910.

50. Reindollar RH, Byrd JR, McDonough PG: Delayed sexual development: A study of 252 patients. Am J Obstet Gynecol 1981; 140:371.

51. Jones HW, Mermut S: Familial occurrence of congenital absence of the vagina. Obstet Gynecol 1974; 42:38.

52. Lischke JH, Curtis CH, Lamb EJ: Discordance of vaginal agenesis in monozygotic twins. Obstet Gynecol 1973; 41:920.

53. Shokeir MHK: Aplasia of the müllerian system: Evidence of possible sex limited autosomal dominant inheritance. Birth Defects 1978; 14:147.

54. Carson SA, Simpson JL, Malinak LR, et al: Heritable aspects of uterine anomalies II: Genetic analysis of müllerian aplasia. Fertil Steril 1983; 40:86.

55. Griffin JE, Edwards C, Madden JD: Congenital absence of vagina. Ann Intern Med 1976; 85:224.

56. Willemson WNP: Combination of Mayer-Rokitansky-Kuster and Klippel-Feil syndromes. A case report and review of literature. Eur J Obstet Gynecol Reprod Biol 1982; 13:229.

57. Shane JM, Wilson EA, Schiff L, Naftolin F: A preliminary report on gonadotrophin release in the Rokitansky syndrome. Am J Obstet Gynecol 1977; 127:326.

58. Egarter CH, Huber J: Successful stimulation and retrieval of oocytes in a patient with Mayer-Rokitansky-Kuster syndrome. Lancet 1988; i:1283.

59. Rock JA, Baramki TA, Parmley TH, Jones HW: A functioning unilateral uterine anlage with müllerian duct agenesis. Int J Gynaecol Obstet 1980; 18:99.

60. Farber M, Stein A, Adashi E: Rokitansky-Kuster-Hauser syndrome and leiomyoma uteri. Obstet Gynecol 1978; 51:70S.

61. Frank RT: The formation of an artificial vagina without operation. Am J Obstet Gynecol 1938; 35:1053.

62. Lilford RJ, Johnson N, Batchelor A: A new operation for vaginal agenesis: Construction of a neovagina from a rectus abdominus musculocutaneous flap. Br J Obstet Gynaecol 1989; 96:1089.

63. Lilford RJ, Sharpe DT, Thomas DFM: Use of tissue expansion techniques to create skin flaps for vaginoplasty. Br J Obstet Gynaecol 1988; 95:402.

64. Peters WA, Uhlir JK: Prolapse of the neovagina created by self-dilatation. Obstet Gynecol 1990; 76:904.

64a. Ingram J: The bicycle seat stool in the treatment of vaginal agenesis and stenosis: A preliminary report. Am J Obstet Gynecol 1981; 140:867–873.

65. Edmonds DK, Rose GL: Non-surgical technique to create a neovagina in the Rokitansky syndrome. In press.

66. McIndoe AH, Banister JB: An operation for the cure of congenital absence of the vagina. J Obstet Gynaecol Br Commonw 1938; 45:490.

67. Abbe R: New method of creating a vagina in a case of congenital absence. Med Record 1898; 54:836.

68. Counsellor VS, Flor FS: Congenital absence of the vagina. Surg Clin North Am 1957; 37:1107.

69. Sauer-Ramirez R, Carranza-Lira S, Romo-Aguirre C, et al: Modification of the Abbe-Wharton-McIndoe technique using regenerated oxidized cellulose instead of a skin graft. Ginecol Obstet Mex 1995; 63:112–114.

70. McIndoe AH: Discussion on treatment of congenital absence of the vagina with emphasis on long term results. Proc R Soc Med 1959; 52:952.

71. Cali RH, Pratt JH: Congenital absence of the vagina. Am J Obstet Gynecol 1968; 100:752.

72. Rock JA, Reeves LA, Retto H, et al: Success following vaginal creation for müllerian agenesis. Fertil Steril 1983; 39:809.

73. Goerzen J, Gidwani G, Bailez M, et al: Outcome of surgical reconstructive procedures for the treatment of vaginal anomalies. Adolesc Pediatr Gynecol 1994; 7:76.

74. Smith MR: Vaginal aplasia: Therapeutic options. Am J Obstet Gynecol 1983; 146:488.

75. Lathrop JC, Ree HJ, McDuff HC: Intraepithelial neoplasia of the neovagina. Obstet Gynecol 1985; 65:91S.

76. Hopkins MP, Morley GW: Squamous cell carcinoma of the neovagina. Obstet Gynecol 1987; 69:525.

77. Baltzer J, Zander J: Primary squamous cell carcinoma of the neovagina. Gynecol Oncol 1989; 35:99.

78. Buscema J, Rosensheim NB, Shah K: Condylomata acuminata arising in a neovagina. Obstet Gynecol 1987; 69:528.

79. Burger RA, Riedmiller H, Knapstein PG, et al: Ileocecal vaginal construction. Am J Obstet Gynecol 1989; 161:162.

80. Davydov SN, Zhvitiashvili OD: Formation of vagina from peritoneum of Douglas pouch. Acta Chir Plast 1974; 16:35.

81. Williams EA: Congenital absence of the vagina: A simple operation for its relief. J Obstet Gynaecol Br Commonw 1964; 71:511.

82. Williams EA: Uterovaginal agenesis. Ann R Coll Surg Engl 1976; 58:266.

83. Morton KE, Davies D, Dewhurst CJ: The use of the fasciocutaneous flap in vaginal reconstruction. Br J Obstet Gynaecol 1986; 93:970.

84. Johnson N, Lilford RJ, Batchelor A: The free flap vaginoplasty; a new surgical procedure for the treatment of vaginal agenesis. Br J Obstet Gynaecol 1991; 98:184.

85. Muram D, Rau FJ, Shell DH III: Modified Williams' vulvovaginoplasty: The role of tissue expanders. Adolesc Pediatr Gynecol 1992; 5:81–83.

86. Nikolaev V, Bizhanova D: Perineal reconstruction in girls with high vaginal atresia. J Urol 1998; 159(6):2140–2142.

87. Rock JA, Zacur HA, Dlugi AM: Pregnancy success following surgical correction of imperforate hymen and complete transverse vaginal septum. Gynecology 1982; 59:448.

88. Sanfilippo JS, Wakim NG, Schikler KN, Yussman MA: Endometriosis in association with uterine abnormalities. Am J Obstet Gynecol 1986; 154:39.

89. Grant D, Muram D, Dewhurst CJ: Menstrual and fertility patterns in patients with congenital adrenal hyperplasia. Pediatr Adolesc Gynecol 1983; 1:97.

90. Mulkaikal RM, Migeon CJ, Rock JA: Fertility rates in female patients with congenital adrenal hyperplasia due to 21-hydroxylase deficiency. N Engl J Med 1987; 316:178.

91. Duck SC, Katayama KP: Danazol may cause female pseudohermaphroditism. Fertil Steril 1981; 35:230.

92. Rock JA, Jones HW: Construction of a neovagina for patients with a flat perineum. Am J Obstet Gynecol 1989; 160:845.

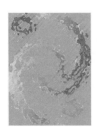

Chapter 35

Urologic Problems

ANTHONY J. CASALE AND PAUL F. AUSTIN

Many common pediatric urinary tract problems seem at first to be due to gynecologic problems. This is due to the proximity of the urinary and genital tracts and their interrelationship during embryonic development. The clinician must be aware of this association, and in this chapter we review the most common urologic abnormalities encountered in this age group and how they relate to gynecologic problems.

Children with urologic problems may present with a variety of complaints, and they often seem to have little relationship to the urinary tract. The problems may be anatomic, developmental, or functional. Not only is it important to define the anatomy of the urinary tract; behavior must also be observed. Children often cannot adequately identify or communicate the nature of their problem. The parents must recount the history of voiding patterns, frequency and urgency, quality of stream, day and night wetting, and urinary tract infection (UTI). The physical examination should include assessment of the abdomen and external genitalia; a brief neurologic examination that includes assessment of reflexes, perineal sensation, and sphincter tone; and inspection of the lower back for evidence of sacral dimpling or cutaneous anomalies suggestive of spinal abnormality.

Adolescents present with their own unique urinary tract problems, essentially of two broad categories: childhood abnormalities that have failed to resolve and abnormalities related to the initiation of sexual activity. When sexual activity is initiated, an increase in the incidence of urinary tract infections is common.

Many congenital genitourinary anomalies are first detected in adolescence primarily because of their association with menstrual abnormalities that are manifested with menarche. Overall, the structure and function of the adolescent urinary tract do not differ significantly from the adult's.

It is important for any physician who cares for children and adolescents to understand UTIs, voiding dysfunction, enuresis, incontinence, vesicoureteral reflux (VUR), hematuria, and other conditions such as pelvic pain, sexual abuse, and sexually transmitted diseases (STDs).

URINARY TRACT INFECTION

HOST RISK FACTORS

Perineal colonization by intestinal flora is the source of most primary and recurrent UTIs. Colonization of the introitus occurs by epithelial attachment of bacteria, and the relatively short female urethra provides relatively easy access to the urinary tract. Resident bacterial strains in the fecal flora of girls with UTIs are more likely pathogenic. These bacteria from the intestinal flora more commonly express P-fimbriae, cause mannose-resistant hemagglutination, and are one of the uropathogenic serotypes, as compared to *Escherichia coli* isolated from unaffected girls.[1] Most UTIs are ascending infections from these colonized bacteria at the perineum and introitus, and hematogenous seeding of the urinary tract is an uncommon source.

ASYMPTOMATIC BACTERIURIA

The prevalence of asymptomatic bacteriuria in childhood is influenced by age, sex, and the method of diagnosis. In a 3-year prospective study conducted in Sweden of infants younger than 1 year, 0.9% of girls were found to have asymptomatic bacteriuria.[2] In school screening studies, the prevalence of bacteriuria has ranged from 0.7% to 1.7% in girls.[3-6] In this age group, the risk of developing acute upper UTI with untreated bacteriuria is low.[2, 7-9] Asymptomatic bacteriuria is usually associated with low-virulence bacterial strains that lack the ability to adhere to the uroepithelium and thus are less pathogenic.[10, 11] In addition, it has been suggested that colonization by a low-virulence bacterial strain is prophylactic and prevents invasion from more virulent organisms.[12, 13] In a follow-up of 252 schoolgirls with asymptomatic bacteriuria for

5 years, the Newcastle Covert Bacteria Research group reported that 40% of the girls randomly allocated to no treatment demonstrated spontaneous resolution of their bacteriuria.[14] Furthermore, the incidence of symptomatic UTIs and renal growth were no different between the girls randomized to antibiotic prophylaxis and untreated controls. Ironically, patients with asymptomatic UTIs often report lower urinary tract symptoms when carefully questioned. Symptoms of urgency, frequency, squatting, and enuresis are often present—and a history of a UTI in 20%.[15, 16] Because asymptomatic bacteriuria in children may be a marker for underlying renal abnormality, it is recommended that young children with asymptomatic bacteriuria be investigated and appropriately managed.

CLINICAL PRESENTATION

UTIs are commonly divided into lower tract (cystitis) and upper tract (pyelonephritis) infections. There is some overlap in the clinical presentations, but proper identification is necessary to ensure proper treatment (Table 35–1).

Cystitis

In very young patients, the classic signs and symptoms of cystitis are often absent, and such infants may present with irritability, poor feeding, failure to grow, vomiting, or abdominal distention. Fever may be absent in neonates but is usually present in older infants and children. Unsuccessful toilet training, at an age when the child should be toilet trained, primary or secondary enuresis, incontinence, urgency, frequency, and dysuria are the more common symptoms of UTI. Recurrent UTIs are common, and Winberg showed that the risk of developing a UTI within a year is proportional to the number of earlier infections: the risk for a second UTI is 25%, for

a third 50%, and over 75% for those who have had three UTIs.[17]

Adolescents with cystitis present with the same symptoms as adults; however, clinical presentation may be more severe, and hemorrhagic cystitis is more common. Most girls complain of low back pain that does not lateralize and may be associated with irritable bladder symptoms. Within 24 hours, the infection causes severe dysuria and is often accompanied by nausea and low-grade fever. The variability in the severity of symptoms is striking, ranging from mild discomfort to a severe illness.

Bacterial vaginitis and contact vaginitis are part of the differential diagnosis in children thought to have a lower UTI. A common misconception is that bubble baths and soaps predispose a child to a UTI, but the dysuria actually stems from the local meatal or vaginal irritation. Vaginal discharge can lead to contamination of voided urine specimens with white blood cells, and in children the symptoms of vaginitis may be identical to those of UTI.

Pyelonephritis

Patients with pyelonephritis usually are quite ill, with a high, spiking fever, flank pain, nausea, chills, vomiting, and myalgia. They often require hospitalization. Lower tract symptoms often precede upper tract symptoms by hours or days; however, the symptoms are not always obvious in young infants, who usually present with nonspecific findings. Unlike patients with cystitis, patients with pyelonephritis demonstrate leukocytosis on blood counts with a marked leftward shift.

VUR is the single most common risk factor for pyelonephritis, as it affords infecting organisms access to the renal parenchyma. In fact, Rushton and Majd reported that, when VUR is present, approximately 80% to 85% of children with febrile UTIs have acute abnormalities on DMSA renal scans.[18] An important point, however, is

Table 35–1. Symptoms of Urinary Tract Infection

	Cystitis	Pyelonephritis
Very young children	Irritability, poor feeding, failure to grow, vomiting or distended abdomen.	Nonspecific findings associated with high fever.
Young children	Failure to be toilet-trained, enuresis, incontinence, urgency, frequency, dysuria.	High fever, abdominal or flank pain, nausea, vomiting; symptoms of cystitis may or may not be present.
Older children	Urinary frequency, dysuria, enuresis, low back pain, low-grade fever.	

that they also demonstrated that, despite the importance of VUR, the majority of cases of acute pyelonephritis in children documented by DMSA scan are not associated with VUR.

In a prospective study, Rushton and coworkers followed 33 children with acute pyelonephritis documented by DMSA renal scan at infection.[19] At a mean follow-up of nearly a year, renal scarring occurred in approximately 40% of patients with VUR and 40% of those without VUR. Interestingly, new renal scarring developed in approximately 85% of children with neuropathic bladder or obstruction. When neuropathic bladders and obstructed patients were excluded, only 30% of kidneys demonstrated new scarring. Obstruction and severe malformation of the urinary tract are also significant predisposing factors for pyelonephritis. Inefficient emptying of urine compromises the renal defenses and allows bacteria to multiply and initiate infection.

The acute inflammatory response is the most important step in the subsequent development of renal scarring. When the bacteria are phagocytosed, they simultaneously release enzymes, superoxide, and oxygen free radicals that directly affect the renal tubular epithelium and result in permanent renal scarring.[20] Renal scarring also tends to occur at the renal poles, owing to abnormal flattened renal papillae which allow reflux of urine into the parenchyma (intrarenal reflux).[21, 22]

A clear association between the number of episodes of pyelonephritis and the incidence of renal scarring has been reported by Jodal.[23] Children with renal scarring have approximately a 10% incidence of subsequent hypertension, and there is also the risk of progressive deterioration of renal function.[24, 25] Because scarring is worse when treatment is delayed, early intervention is very important.[26] Finally, studies have demonstrated that aggressive early antibiotic treatment may prevent or diminish renal scarring.[27, 28]

DIAGNOSIS

The only reliable method of diagnosing UTI is by urine culture. Although urinalysis may provide guidance for initiating treatment, the association of inflammatory cells in urine is not completely reliable. Because it takes 24 hours or more for the urine culture results to come back, however, urinalysis findings can certainly direct the diagnosis along with the medical history. Aspects of the urinalysis that are important include the presence of white blood cells (pyuria), bacteria, urinary leukocyte esterase, and urinary nitrite.

The method of collection varies with the age of the child. When a child is still in diapers, a collecting bag is frequently applied to obtain the urine specimen. The perineum and surrounding skin is associated with a high level of contamination, and this method of urine collection is only reliable when the culture is negative. The most reliable urine specimen for culture is obtained either by suprapubic bladder aspiration or by urethral catheterization. The significant level of bacterial growth was established in 1956 by Kass and Finland, who demonstrated that more than 95% of cultures growing in children with UTI grew 10^5 colonies per milliliter.[29] Others have shown that clinically significant infections may occur with lower colony counts on culture, but these findings are related to the child's hydration status and pattern of voiding, and the bacterial growth characteristics.[30]

Bacteriology

The majority of UTIs are caused by Enterobacteriaceae species. These gram-negative organisms are most often represented by *E. coli*, which is present in 60% to 80% of cases. The most common gram-positive organisms identified are *Staphylococcus* and *Enterococcus*. The majority of uncomplicated UTIs are caused by a single pathogen. Lactobacilli, corynebacteria, and streptococci rarely cause UTI and should be considered contaminants unless the specimen was obtained by suprapubic aspiration or catheterization.

Stamey has demonstrated that the majority of UTI pathogens originate in the gut, are present in the flora of the vaginal vestibule, and surround the urethral meatus.[31] They gain access to the bladder by ascending the relatively short female urethra. In adolescents, bacteria may access the urethra through minor trauma at the onset of sexual activity. As the female urogenital tract becomes more accustomed to sexual activity, the frequency of infection decreases.

EVALUATION OF THE CHILD WITH URINARY TRACT INFECTION

Current standards of care dictate evaluation of the child after the first documented UTI. Epidemiologic studies have revealed that infection recurs within 18 months in as many as 40% to 60% of all children.[4] All patients with evidence of upper UTI should have a complete radiographic evaluation, including an upper and lower urinary tract examination, after the initial infection.

Radiologic Evaluation

Imaging can be helpful in determining the site of infection and is necessary to define the anatomy of the urinary tract. The upper and lower urinary tract should be evaluated in children with documented febrile UTI. Renal ultrasonography (US) is the most common study of the upper urinary tract. Renal US is an ideal method of initially inspecting the kidneys because it is painless and noninvasive and visualizes the renal parenchyma and collecting system effectively. In children, US has been found to be as sensitive as intravenous pyelography (IVP) for the detection of significant renal abnormalities, except for uncomplicated duplication anomalies and focal scarring.[32]

Since the early 1980s there has been a drastic reduction in the use of IVP. The iodinated contrast agents used in IVP concentrate poorly in infant kidneys and often produce a washed-out image hidden by a sea of intestinal gas. On the other hand, adolescents with recurrent UTIs are better evaluated by IVP than by US because of the better imaging of the collecting system and ureters with IVP and problems in visualizing kidneys in some large patients with US. Cystoscopy often replaces or augments voiding cystourethrography (VCUG) and is more sensitive for finding bladder stones and the rare neoplasm.[33]

Although US is helpful in evaluating the kidneys, it does not reliably identify lower urinary tract conditions and cannot effectively rule out reflux. VCUG is necessary to evaluate children with UTI when reflux is suspected.[34] In fact, VCUG is the most important single imaging study in the evaluation of children with a febrile UTI. VCUG is also useful in determining the size, shape, and function of the bladder. Because it requires the insertion of a urethral catheter, it should not be performed when the child is infected because of the risk of introducing bacteria into the kidneys under pressure should reflux be present.

A number of centers utilize nuclear cystography to test for reflux. Radionuclide cystography has the advantage over VCUG in that it exposes the child to less radiation but it cannot adequately grade the degree of VUR nor does it provide adequate imaging of the bladder anatomy. Newer techniques and equipment have significantly decreased the radiation dose of the radiographic VCUG, and it remains the mainstay for the evaluation of bladder in children.

Once diagnosed by US, IVP, or any other modality, hydronephrosis is best evaluated by diuretic renography to assess both renal function and drainage of the upper tracts. The two most common nucleotides used to assess renal drainage are technetium-99m-mercaptoacetyltriglycine (MAG III) and technetium-99m-diethylenetriamine pentaacetic acid (DTPA). DTPA is freely filtered and MAG III is both filtered and secreted by the tubules. Each provides quantitative assessment of both renal function and drainage of the dilated collecting system. Dimercaptosuccinic acid (DMSA) is a radionucleotide that is fixed in the renal tubules with only minimal excretion and provides optimal visualization of the renal parenchyma. DMSA is useful for demonstrating renal scarring and has become the gold standard for imaging renal cortical defects resulting from pyelonephritis.[35]

TREATMENT

Treatment of pediatric UTIs is dependent on the child's age, the severity of the illness, and the susceptibility of the organism. Initial treatment should be a broad-spectrum antibiotic until the urine culture and sensitivity results are received and then adjusted accordingly.

Cystitis

Agents that are successful in the treatment of acute, uncomplicated, lower UTI are sulfonamide, trimethoprim, nitrofurantoin, and cephalosporins. Trimethoprim has the added benefit of diffusing into the vaginal fluid and subsequently decreasing bacterial colonization.[36] The combination of trimethoprim-sulfamethoxazole (TMP-SMX) is synergistic and probably is the most common antibiotic prescribed for UTI. TMP-SMX (Bactrim or Septra) should not be used in the first 3 months of life because the sulfonamide competes for bilirubin binding and may cause neonatal bilirubinemia and kernicterus.

Ampicillin and amoxicillin are often administered but are not the best choice, as high intestinal levels of these medications result in development of resistant bacteria in the gastrointestinal tract, which then become sources of reinfection.[37] This problem can be corrected with the combination of amoxicillin and clavulanate potassium (Augmentin), which inhibits the β-lactamase–resistant enzymes but is more expensive and more often causes gastrointestinal side effects. Because of their safety, ampicillin and amoxicillin are the antibiotics of choice for neonates and young infants.

The fluoroquinolones have a wide spectrum of activity against most gram-positive and gram-negative organisms, including *Pseudomonas* and *Proteus* species. They are widely used in adult women and may be used in older adolescents. Fluoroquinolone studies in animals, however, have demonstrated toxicity to developing cartilage, so they are best avoided in children and growing adolescents.[38]

There is controversy about the ideal duration of treatment. Several randomized controlled studies have compared the efficacy of single-dose and short-course (3 to 5 days) antibiotic treatment in children.[39, 40] The advantages with the former are obvious: lower cost, better compliance, and fewer side effects. Because it is not always easy to distinguish lower UTI from pyelonephritis, most pediatric urologists still recommend treatment for 7 to 10 days because of the higher risk of anatomic anomalies. After the first UTI, the child should continue taking prophylactic antibiotics until the radiographic evaluation, usually within 2 to 3 weeks. Short-term treatment has also been associated with increased recurrence of UTIs, even though the first treatment was initially effective, in 93.5% of patients.[39]

Pyelonephritis

Treatment must be instituted as soon as the diagnosis is suspected, since the extent of renal damage is related to how quickly effective therapy is provided.[26] Oral medications can be given to older children who are not toxic, provided there is close follow-up and compliance with medication is expected. TMP-SMX or cephalosporins are effective in these cases.

For a younger or very sick child, immediate parenteral therapy should be initiated. After appropriate culture specimens are obtained, combination therapy that includes broad-spectrum antibiotics such as aminoglycosides or cephalosporins should be prescribed until the sensitivity is known. Parenteral treatment should be continued until the child has been afebrile for at least 48 hours and full-dose oral therapy has been administered for 10 to 14 days. Material for control cultures should be obtained, and the child should be maintained on low-dose prophylaxis until radiologic evaluation is completed.

PROPHYLAXIS

Long-term antibiotic prophylaxis is recommended for children with reflux, recurrent UTI, or voiding dysfunction. Antimicrobials of choice are nitrofurantoin or TMP-SMX and are taken at half to a quarter of the daily dose.[30, 41] Nitrofurantoin is a good choice for prophylaxis because it achieves high urinary levels and low serum levels with subsequent minimal effect on the gut flora.[42] Nitrofurantoin, however, should not be given to children with glucose-6-phosphate dehydrogenase deficiency because it can cause hemolysis.[30] Urine culture should be repeated to assess the effectiveness of therapy.

Sexually active adolescents with postcoital cystitis are a special category of patients. Culture material should be obtained, and the patients should be treated as adult women and kept on either low-dose prophylaxis or postcoital antibiotics for several months. Immediate postcoital voiding may also reduce recurrent infections.

Urethral manipulation in young girls is rarely, if ever, necessary. In the absence of significant abnormalities that require further diagnostic evaluation, there is no routine role for cystoscopy, dilatation, or urethrotomy.

VESICOURETERAL REFLUX

INCIDENCE

VUR is retrograde flow of urine from the bladder into the ureters and kidneys. Its prevalence in healthy children is estimated at 1%. The incidence increases in persons with UTI and can be 70% in those younger than 1 year, 25% at 4 years, 15% at 12 years, and 5.2% for adults. VUR is also less common in black children.[43]

DIAGNOSIS

Because of prenatal US, urinary tract anomalies are being diagnosed much earlier in life. Gunn and coworkers reported that prenatal US after 28 weeks' gestation identified significant renal tract abnormalities with a frequency of 14.3 per 1000 births. After obstruction, VUR was the next most common cause at 3.6 per 1000 births.[44] Zerin and colleagues reported that VUR was the most common urinary tract diagnosis (37%) found on postnatal examination of 130 neonates with abnormal prenatal US findings. Most of these cases of reflux were transient and insignificant.[45] Despite the increased diagnosis of VUR by prenatal US, the majority of children still present with UTI, and many have signs of cystitis or pyelonephritis. Reflux affects 90% of children with UTIs whose fever exceeds 38.5° C.[46]

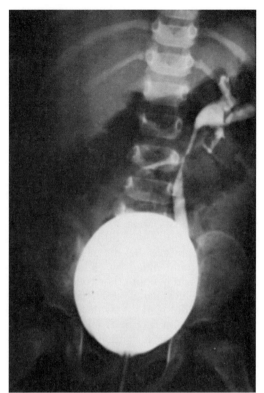

Figure 35–1. A voiding cystouretogram reveals grade III vesicoureteral reflux.

EVALUATION

The diagnosis of reflux is established with a VCUG or nuclear cystography (Fig. 35–1). Reflux may occur either during bladder filling or voiding and images should be obtained throughout the study. The dynamic VCUG is preferred when the child is awake, as this allows an approximation of bladder capacity and bladder dynamics.

Ultrasound should be used to evaluate the kidneys and a renal scan may be helpful to evalu-

ate renal scarring and function. Other anomalies and conditions associated with VUR can be identified, such as ureteropelvic junction obstruction, ureteral duplication, and bladder diverticula.

CLASSIFICATION

The grading system used by the International Reflux Study Group offers a standard classification that allows more accurate comparison of treatment modalities. Reflux is graded from I though V according to severity and is based on the appearance of contrast in the ureter and upper collecting system during VCUG (Fig. 35–2).

CAUSES

Reflux occurs because of an abnormality of the ureterovesical junction (UVJ). In a normal UVJ the ureter enters the bladder at an oblique angle. A section of the ureter typically lies within a tunnel between the mucosa and the detrusor muscle of the bladder. Good detrusor muscle backing is essential because, with bladder filling, the ureteral lumen is flattened between the bladder mucosa and the detrusor, creating a flap valve effect that prevents reflux. Classically, a 5:1 ratio of tunnel length to ureteral diameter is considered necessary to prevent VUR.

In the vast majority of children with reflux, the cause is a congenital maldevelopment of the UVJ. In children with severe bladder dysfunction, a normal valve mechanism may be overwhelmed by high pressure and lead to reflux. Acute cystitis may produce transient reflux on the VCUG secondary to irritative bladder contractions leading to high bladder pressures. VUR in the setting of a normal bladder and without

Figure 35–2. International scale for grading vesicoureteral reflux.

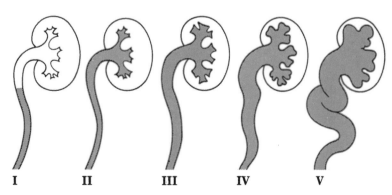

I   II   III   IV   V

infection is a benign condition. Reflux and infection, however, can lead to renal scarring.[41, 47]

CLINICAL FEATURES

Renal scars caused by reflux and infection more often develop during the first 5 years of life. Reflux may affect renal growth, and its effect is directly proportional to the presence of an abnormal kidney on the contralateral side, recurrent UTI, and the grade of reflux.[48] Scarring at the renal poles in patients with VUR is associated with hypertrophy of the remaining normal parenchyma and of the contralateral kidney.

Reflux occurs in conjunction with a neuropathic bladder in 15% to 60% of patients.[49] VUR may also occur in neurologically intact children with uninhibited bladder contractions due to a UTI.[50] Taylor demonstrated that as many as 75% of girls with reflux had evidence of voiding dysfunction with uninhibited bladder contractions.[51] Most low-grade reflux in these patients resolves spontaneously with improved bladder dynamics and treatment of infection. Anticholinergic therapy, however, is often necessary to treat the bladder dysfunction and has demonstrated dramatic resolution in VUR.[52, 53]

TREATMENT

Medical Management

The main goal in management of reflux is to prevent ascending infection and renal scarring. Low-grade reflux has a tendency to resolve spontaneously over time. In a large prospective study of low-grade and moderate reflux (grades I to III) followed medically, Arant reported reflux resolution in 82% of grade I and 80% of grade II by 5 years.[54] The International Reflux Study in Children prospectively randomized children with high-grade reflux (grades III to IV) to surgery or medical management. Cessation of VUR with medical management was significantly more common in unilateral reflux, and approximately 40% of grades III and IV unilateral VUR resolved at 5 years, as compared with only 10% of bilateral VUR with similar grades. Overall, surgery was significantly more effective than medical therapy in preventing pyelonephritis, although the incidences of UTI, renal scarring, and renal growth were the same in both groups.[55, 56]

To establish treatment guidelines in the United States, the Pediatric Vesicoureteral Re-

Table 35–2. Chance of Reflux Persistence for 5 Years After Presentation

Reflux Grade	Chance of Reflux Persistence > 5 Years %
I	10
II	20
IV—Unilateral	40
IV—Bilateral	90

Based on American Urological Association Pediatric Vesicoureteral Reflux Guidelines Panel Summary Report. J Urol 1997; 157:1846.

flux Guidelines Panel was created by the American Urological Association. The panel has recommended that, for most children, continuous antibiotic prophylaxis be the initial treatment. Surgery is recommended for children with persistent reflux and certain other conditions.[57] The Reflux Guidelines Panel also compiled results from these studies and others on the chances of reflux persisting for 5 years (Table 35–2).

Most spontaneous resolutions occur within the first few years after diagnosis, and the rate of reflux resolution remains constant, during and after childhood, at approximately 10% to 15% per year.[58] Puberty is associated with neither an increase nor a decrease in resolution rates. The absence of renal scarring is beneficial for medical management because it is associated with the ability to concentrate and maintain sterile urine with prophylactic antibiotics.[59]

Reflux nephropathy is the most common disorder that predisposes children to renal hypertension and is related to the degree of parenchymal damage that resulted in renal insufficiency. It may develop in as many as 10% to 20% of children with reflux and renal scarring.[58] Reflux is observed in 30% to 40% of children who experience renal failure before 16 years of age.

Medical management must emphasize prevention of UTI with daily antibiotic prophylaxis, frequent voiding, and forestalling constipation. Antibiotic prophylaxis should be taken at bedtime, because the child goes longest without voiding overnight and infection is most likely to develop. The best choices of antibiotics for prophylaxis are TMP-SMX and nitrofurantoin. Routine urine culture should be performed every 3 to 4 months for the first year and annual radiographic evaluation of the upper and lower urinary tracts until the reflux disappears.

Surgical Management

Ureteral reimplantation is highly successful in more than 95% of children. Various techniques have been described, but the goal of the procedure remains the construction of a one-way flap valve mechanism at the UVJ by creating an adequate submucossal tunnel for the reimplanted segment of ureter.

Indications for surgery are (1) persistent or recurrent infection despite antibiotic prophylaxis, (2) noncompliance with medical treatment, (3) development of new scarring or failure of renal growth, or (4) persistent and significant reflux in adolescent girls. Surgery in older adolescents is technically more difficult and has higher morbidity (pain) when compared with younger children.

VOIDING DYSFUNCTION AND DAYTIME INCONTINENCE

Most children with minor voiding disturbances do not have underlying malformations and, therefore, usually do not need invasive urologic investigation. Although wetting problems are "benign," the resulting social stigma, humiliation, and low self-esteem cause real suffering for some children and families. Most of these functional problems are attributable to either a delay in maturation or learned abnormal toilet habits.

EVOLUTION OF NORMAL URINARY CONTROL

In infants a simple reflex governs bladder emptying. When enough urine collects in the bladder, it stimulates a reflex moderated by the spinal cord, and bladder contraction occurs. Simultaneously, reflex relaxation of the external sphincter allows the bladder to empty. During gradual bladder filling, the sphincter tightens to maintain continence. In infancy, there is no conscious or voluntary mediation of this voiding reflex.

Development of an adult pattern of voiding or urinary control depends on three separate events. First, the capacity of the bladder must increase if it is to act as a reservoir. Second, voluntary control over the external sphincter must be gained to allow initiation and termination of micturition. This step is usually mastered by age 3 years and first operates during daytime. Third, direct voluntary control over the voiding reflex must develop to initiate or inhibit bladder contraction. By about age 4 years, the adult pattern—no involuntary or uninhibited bladder contractions during bladder filling—is usually acquired.

NONNEUROPATHIC VOIDING DYSFUNCTION IN CHILDREN

In the majority of children with voiding dysfunction the underlying problem is an unstable bladder whose detrusor contractions occur before children have learned to voluntarily inhibit them.[60] This is not a pathologic or neurologic disorder; rather it is due to a delay in central nervous system maturation. Because these contractions are involuntary and not suppressible, a child attempting to maintain continence must constrict the sphincter to stay dry. This results in dyssynergia, or a lack of coordination, between the bladder and the sphincter, leading to high bladder pressures. In fact, the sphincter acts as an outflow obstruction, and the high intravesical pressures may damage the entire urinary tract, leading to thickening, trabeculation, and diverticula of the bladder, as well as reflux and upper urinary tract damage.

Children with uninhibited bladder contractions and a weak sphincter experience urgency, frequency, and urge incontinence. Those with contractions and a strong sphincter maintain continence despite urgency and frequency. Reflux occurs in as many as 50% of this patient population. UTIs are also common, especially when residual urine volume is large. In such children, the most important diagnostic aid is the description of the voiding pattern on clinical history.

Little girls often describe "tricks" that they use to stay dry (Fig. 35–3). Vincent's curtsey is a sign of voiding dysfunction: the child squats with her heel pressed against the perineum; this position helps to obstruct the urethra and prevent leakage. Other girls cross their legs, shuffle, or dance around. Children trying to hold their urine when they have strong bladder contractions often complain of abdominal or suprapubic pain, which is related to the bladder pressure generated against an obstructed outlet.

Sexual abuse can have significant effects on the voiding pattern.[61] Little girls who have been abused can regress to an immature pattern of voiding (either enuresis or daytime wetting). They can also develop voiding dysfunction when they hold urine, either to avoid going to the bathroom (and having to undress) or to try to regain some control over their body, which the abuser has usurped.

At the most severe end of the voiding dysfunction spectrum are children with day and night wetting, recurrent UTIs, constipation, and encopresis. These rare patients often have abnormal findings on imaging evaluation, such as trabeculated bladder, residual urine, VUR, hydronephrosis, and renal scarring. Their bladders closely

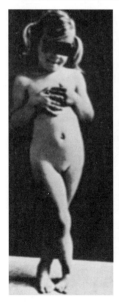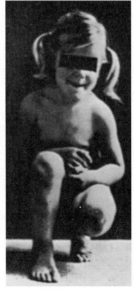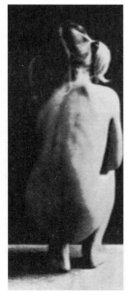

Figure 35–3. Examples of postures assumed by children trying to avoid urination. The two photographs on the right show Vincent's curtsey. Note the heel placed to compress the perineum.

resemble true neurogenic bladders, and the condition has been termed *nonneurogenic neurogenic bladder*, or Hinman syndrome.[62]

CONSTIPATION

A frequent problem that has not been given adequate consideration in the past is the role of constipation in bladder instability. O'Regan and associates have shown evidence of stabilization of bladder dysfunction after aggressive management of constipation with enemas.[63] Koff and colleagues recently coined the term *dysfunctional elimination syndrome* to describe functional bowel and bladder disturbances, including bladder instability, infrequent voiding, and constipation.[64] Among 143 children with primary VUR, Koff reported that 66 (46%) had dysfunctional elimination syndrome. Of these 66 children, 50% had constipation. Seventy children had breakthrough infections, and dysfunctional elimination syndromes were present in 54 patients (77%). Finally, dysfunctional elimination syndrome prolonged the average interval until reflux was "outgrown" by 1.6 years.

DAYTIME WETTING

Daytime wetting, or diurnal enuresis, that persists into childhood is never normal and suggests an organic or neurologic cause. Daytime wetting may be episodic and associated only with recurrent UTIs. In adolescent girls with borderline

continence from underlying neurologic disorders, intermittent continence may be related to periurethral changes related to the menstrual cycle. This problem is not common, however, and warrants thorough evaluation.[65]

For complicated cases of diurnal enuresis, a complete urologic evaluation should be performed, including cystography and, in some adolescents, cystoscopy to examine the anatomy of the lower urinary tract. The upper urinary tract should be imaged with intravenous pyelography (IVP) or US. Finally, a complete urodynamic evaluation, including cystometrography with electromyography, may be necessary.

Neurogenic dysfunction of the bladder is often due to some form of spinal dysraphism. The more overt types of spinal abnormalities, including myelomeningocele and sacral agenesis, are usually discovered early in childhood. Occult types of spinal dysraphism, such as lipoma of the cord, tethered cord, neurenteric cyst, diastematomyelia, and dermal sinus tract, may present in adolescence.[66] These lesions alter the sacral nerve roots, and the first sign of the neurologic condition is often bladder dysfunction. Patients may also complain of weakness, pain, and numbness of the lower extremities. Physical examination reveals that as many as 90% of patients with significant lower spinal anomalies have a skin lesion (e.g., discoloration, a hairy patch, a small fat pad, or sinus tract) over the base of the spine, just above the lateral cleft.[66] Spinal radiography, computed tomography (CT), or magnetic resonance imaging (MRI), and, occasionally, myelography are necessary to conclusively document lower spinal cord lesions.

TREATMENT

The primary goal is resolution of the incontinence, which is usually achieved by eliminating uninhibited bladder contractions. The basics of treatment are combined therapy with anticholinergic medication, reduction of fluid intake, and control of voiding and constipation.

Anticholinergic medications are used to reduce the intensity of bladder contractions or eliminate them and to increase functional bladder capacity. The most commonly used medication is oxybutynin chloride (Ditropan), a moderately potent anticholinergic with strong smooth-muscle antispasmodic activity. Oxybutynin is also known to have analgesic properties, which may reduce bladder sensation and, therefore, urgency. Children treated with anticholinergics can exhibit increased bladder capacity and decreased frequency and intensity of uninhibited bladder contractions. The usual dosage for children is 0.2 mg/kg/24 hours in two or three divided doses. Common side effects are dry mouth and flushing, and the dosage may need to be adjusted accordingly. Because of the anticholinergic effects, intestinal motility is slowed, which can exacerbate constipation.

Constipation has a profound effect on bladder function in children and needs full evaluation and treatment concurrent with any bladder treatment. Some patients' severe constipation and wetting can be cured by successful treatment of the constipation alone. To eliminate possible compression of the bladder by a large fecal mass it may be necessary to increase the daily dietary fiber intake (e.g., fiber grams/day = age (years) + 2) or provide therapy with laxatives and stool softeners. In fact, control of the child's constipation and voiding frequency are perhaps the most important measures in improving bladder and bowel function.

Frequent and complete bladder emptying is critical to the elimination of bacteria. We begin by having the parents keep a voiding and stooling diary for the child for at least two 24-hour periods. In these elimination diaries, they record the volume voided, the time of voiding, and whether the child was wet or dry. We also have the parents observe and record the child's bowel movements and watch for encopresis. The parents also record "holding behavior" intended to prevent voiding, such as squatting and dancing.

Once the child's toilet habits have been determined and described to all parties, we begin a timed voiding and stooling schedule and provide "goals" for amounts voided. Establishing a voiding schedule in a young child may be difficult and sometimes provokes conflicts between parent and child. Nevertheless, children should be expected to adhere to the schedule, even though they may not feel the urge to void. Results of this approach are generally good when combined with anticholinergics and bowel programs, as needed.

Acute urinary retention in adolescents is unusual. Urinary retention may be caused by urethritis, vaginitis, trauma, or genital herpes. Also, it is often psychogenic.[66] Hysteria of this type can be the result of family, school, or social problems, in which case the patient should undergo psychological evaluation and treatment. The urinary tract is best managed with either intermittent or short-term catheterization, which is basically a temporizing measure until the underlying psychological cause of the disorder is resolved.[66]

Some adolescents have deep-seated psychic fears of either "the bathroom" or of the act of voiding or defecating. Such children may have been severely punished by their parents for either wetting or fecal soiling and usually have other manifestations of psychological disturbances. The family situation usually is problematic, and social counseling is most important.[67]

NOCTURNAL ENURESIS

Enuresis is defined as involuntary voiding of urine beyond the anticipated age of control. The diagnosis of *primary enuresis* is reserved for children who have never been dry for extended periods; *secondary enuresis* applies to those who were dry for at least 6 months before enuresis developed. Nocturnal enuresis involves only nighttime wetting; daytime continence and voiding are normal.

Nocturnal enuresis occurs in approximately 15% of 5-year-olds (Table 35–3).[67] Of these, 15% more achieve nocturnal continence each year and, by age 15, only 1% to 2% remain enuretic. *Secondary enuresis* accounts for approximately 25% of all enuresis and occurs more frequently in people of lower socioeconomic means, in larger families, and in children from discordant families.[68]

Enuresis causes enormous stress and anxiety for the adolescent patient. It is an embarrassing

Table 35–3. Facts About Enuresis

Prevalence at 5 years of age: 15%–20%
Patients achieving control each year: 15%–20%
Patients with associated diurnal enuresis: 15%–20%
Patients with secondary enuresis: 20%–25%

problem that inhibits the development of confidence and a positive self-image. Adolescents may secretly believe that there is a relationship between the bladder and sexual function, which can alter future fertility. Furthermore, they may be too embarrassed to seek medical attention.

CAUSES

Many causes have been proposed for enuresis. The theory of delayed functional maturation remains the most popular. Genetic or hereditary factors also play a role and are supported by the high incidence of a family history of enuresis in affected children. When both parents have a history of nocturnal enuresis, 77% of their children are likely to be enuretic. When only one parent was enuretic, 44% of their children have enuresis, and when neither parent was enuretic, nocturnal enuresis occurs in only 15% of children.[69] Genetic studies have corroborated these findings by localizing familial primary nocturnal enuresis to chromosome 13q.[70] Development of functional micturition depends on attaining adequate bladder capacity, voluntary control of the urethral sphincter, and direct volitional control over the spinal micturition reflex.

Enuretic children have been noted to have significantly lower peaks of serum antidiuretic hormone (ADH) levels as compared with controls.[71] Higher mean nocturnal urine production has also been observed in children with enuresis. Total diurnal urinary volume, osmolality, or water reabsorption are the same in enuretic and normal children.

Why these children do not wake up to empty the bladder is not known. Enuretics have been labeled "deep sleepers," but sleep studies show that enuresis is independent of sleep stage.[72] Despite these findings, parents consistently observe that children who wet the bed sleep more soundly and are unusually difficult to awaken.

Although a higher proportion of enuretic children are maladjusted and exhibit behavioral symptoms as compared with nonenuretic children, only a few have any underlying psychiatric problem. Some studies have demonstrated that enuretic children tend to be more immature and less secure and to have less ambition. Children who seek help for enuresis are under more stress and have more behavioral symptoms than those who do not.[73]

An uncommon, but important, cause of secondary enuresis is UTI. Frequently an otherwise dry child begins to wet the bed when a UTI develops and regains continence, once the infection is treated. The increased incidence of bacteriuria in the enuretic population may be related to unstable bladder and associated with a voiding disorder.

EVALUATION

After a careful history that focuses on the parents' and child's motivations has been collected, enuresis can be categorized as complicated or uncomplicated. The vast majority of children with only nighttime wetting, normal physical examination findings, and normal urine cultures have uncomplicated enuresis. The incidence of associated urinary tract anomalies is so low that it does not justify further investigation unless the child is older than 15 years. When underlying disease is suspected, enuretic children should be studied with VCUG, ultrasound, and spinal radiographs as basic investigations.

TREATMENT

Therapy must be individualized to the child and parents and is largely determined by their interest in treatment and motivation to comply. Therapy is rarely necessary before age 5 or 6 years. Often, the physician does well to leave the choice to treat or not to treat enuresis to the patient and parents.

Behavioral Modification

The behavioral modification approach requires greater commitment and involvement of the parents, the child, and the physician. Conditioning therapy relies on a signal alarm device that is triggered when the child begins to void. Use of this treatment is limited by the difficulty of awakening the child and the parent or caregiver. *The cure rate is superior to that of drug therapy in controlled studies and averages 60 to 80%.*[68] Success depends on a cooperative and motivated child, and, therefore, treatment is inappropriate before age 7 to 8 years. Results are not as good when there are associated behavioral (psychological) disturbances. Some children fail to awake to the alarm, whereas others are frightened and stressed by it. Adjunctive measures include rewarding after a predetermined number of dry nights. The child is also encouraged to keep a record of progress by placing stickers on a calendar for every dry night. Relapse occurs in 20% to 30% of the children, but this can also be expected with treatment.[68] Transistorized alarm modifications are popular and utilize a small sensor that is attached to the child's underwear with an alarm attached to the wrist or pajama.

Pharmacologic Therapy

No benefit has been demonstrated from sedatives, stimulants, or sympathomimetic agents. Imipramine (Tofranil) is a widely used tricyclic antidepressant. It exerts multiple effects, including an antidepressant effect, alterations in arousal and sleep mechanisms, and anticholinergic effects. It is not usually used before adolescence, and success rates approach 50%.[68] The recommended dose is 0.9 to 1.5 mg/kg per day, or 25 mg for children 5 to 8 years old and 50 mg/day for older children. Imipramine is given 1 to 2 hours before bedtime for 3 to 6 months, at which point in time, the child should be weaned by reducing the dose, and then the frequency (every 2 to 3 nights over 3 to 4 weeks). Side effects that often limit its use include daytime sedation, anxiety, insomnia, dry mouth, nausea, and adverse personality changes. Overdose can induce fatal cardiac arrhythmias, hypotension, respiratory distress, or convulsions. The use of this drug has decreased dramatically because of its side effects and dangers. It should be used only after careful consideration and in certain circumstances, with proper warnings and precautions.

An analogue of arginine vasopressin (AVP), 1-deamino-[8-D-arginine]-vasopressin (DDAVP), is a common medication used to treat nocturnal enuresis and produces a marked increase in antidiuretic activity similar to AVP. DDAVP has a longer duration of action and is readily absorbed through the nasal mucosa. DDAVP also does not affect endogenous secretion of AVP. Although DDAVP is considerably more expensive than imipramine, its effects are usually immediate and it can be used as needed for sleepovers and summer camps. The proposed mechanism of action is a reduction in nocturnal urine output.[71] DDAVP is particularly effective in a subgroup of enuretic patients who do not exhibit the normal circadian rhythm of vasopressive excretion. Response varies from an 80% reduction in wetting to a 50% cure rate.[68] Eller and coworkers investigated the predictive value of bladder capacity, age, and urine osmolality to DDAVP response and found that only functional bladder capacity was a significant predictor.[74] Hogg and Husman also reported a high rate of success (91%) when DDAVP was used in patients with a family history of enuresis.[75] The commercially available spray delivers a dose of 10 μg of DDAVP per spray, and the initial recommended dose is 20 μg (one spray in each nostril) at bedtime. In nonresponders and partial responders, the dosage can be increased to 40 μg per day. The relapse rate after discontinuation of medication is high. The optimal duration is not known, but it is rare for treatment to extend beyond 6 months, and it is preferable to taper the dose when discontinuation is planned. Side effects, which are rare and appear to be dose related, include transient headache, nausea, and mild abdominal cramps.

Dose delivery of DDAVP with the nasal spray will be variable, depending on the child's coordination. DDAVP has recently been developed as an oral form to optimize and provide consistent delivery. Initially a 0,2 mg tablet is started nightly and may be titrated up to 0.6 mg nightly to achieve the desired response.

Other Treatment

Anticholinergics such as oxybutynin reduce or abolish uninhibited bladder contractions and may be particularly beneficial for patients who have daytime frequency or diurnal enuresis associated with an unstable bladder. Prophylactic antibiotics may be added to this regimen for girls with recurrent UTI[68] until they have better control of the bladder.[69]

OTHER "SUSPECTED" VOIDING DYSFUNCTIONS

True stress incontinence is rare in neurologically normal children, and urodynamic study findings are generally normal. Bladder emptying before exertion may be helpful in children with mild symptoms of stress incontinence. The daytime urinary frequency syndrome is characterized by daytime-only urgency and frequency in a previously toilet-trained child.[76] Bladder emptying may occur as often as every 20 minutes without any infection or anomaly. Affected children are usually young, and as many as 40% have a history of enuresis. The cause is unknown, but stressful situations are usually noticed. Left untreated, symptoms usually disappear after 2 days to 16 months; the recurrence rate is approximately 3%.

The "lazy bladder" syndrome applies to "busy" girls who hold their urine as long as they can, for as long as 8 to 12 hours or longer. The bladder enlarges, and the emptying capacity is often insufficient, leaving a fair amount of residual urine. Urinary retention develops, reflecting bladder decompensation without obstruction. Investigation is mandatory to rule out an underlying neurologic condition, but results are usually normal. Treatment consists of patient education, voiding on schedule, double or triple voiding (repeat voiding a few minutes after initial void), and catheterization for large postvoid residuals.[77]

When urinary incontinence is reported as dribbling just after voiding when the child stands up, pooling of urine into the vagina should be suspected. Unless labial adhesions are present, the problem can be solved by having the child void while sitting with her knees far apart over the commode. On the other hand, continuous dribbling should raise the suspicion of a more complicated problem, such as an ectopic ureter, and demands further investigation.

HEMATURIA

Gross hematuria is rare in neonates and children. The implications of gross hematuria in children are very different from those in adults, as neoplasia is rarely the cause in children (Table 35–4). In adolescents, stress hematuria is occasionally encountered in association with sports. Gross hematuria in children must be evaluated seriously and thoroughly.

In children presenting to the emergency department with gross hematuria, Ingelfinger and coworkers found that 49% had an associated UTI.[78] Urine cultures may be negative in children with gross hematuria and signs of cystitis. In such cases, a viral infection may be the cause, and, when it is, adenovirus is the most common cause of acute hemorrhagic cystitis in children.[79]

Microscopic hematuria is even more common

Table 35–4. Causes of Gross Hematuria in 150 Children

	Number (%)
Readily Apparent Causes	
Documented urinary tract infection	39 (26)
Perineal irritation	16 (11)
Meatal stenosis with ulcer	11 (7)
Trauma	10 (7)
Coagulopathy	5 (3)
Stones	3 (2)
Other Causes	
Suspected urinary tract infection	35 (23)
Unknown	13 (9)
Recurrent gross hematuria	7 (5)
Acute nephritis	6 (4)
Ureteropelvic junction obstruction	2 (1)
Cystitis cystica	1 (<1)
Epididymitis	1 (<1)
Tumor	1 (<1)

and has been reported in 5% of asymptomatic school-aged children on screening urinalysis.[80] This figure was further reduced to 0.5% to 1% after repeat screening over 6 to 12 months. Hypercalciuria is the most frequent cause of isolated hematuria in healthy white children and is reported to occur in 5% of this population.[81]

The initial evaluation of hematuria in children should include a urine culture and studies to localize the bleeding if the culture result is negative. Urinalysis of a freshly voided specimen that demonstrates proteinuria, oval fat bodies, dysmorphic red cells, or RBC casts is strongly suggestive of renal parenchymal disease, and a nephrologic workup should be initiated. When gross hematuria is present in the absence of UTI or renal parenchymal damage, however, a complete urologic evaluation is necessary to rule out neoplasms, urolithiasis, a foreign body, or other anatomic causes of hematuria. In every unexplained case of hematuria, the possibility of sexual abuse must also be ruled out.

URINARY CALCULI

Urinary stones or calculi are quite rare in adolescents and children. The vast majority of stones in the pediatric population are either struvite or calcium oxalate.[82] UTI, immobilization, and associated inborn errors of metabolism are important causes to consider. Calculi are sometimes associated with congenital obstructive abnormalities of the urinary tract, which need surgical correction. If urinary calculi are identified, these should be eliminated and any underlying metabolic condition treated medically to prevent further stone formation.

URINARY TRACT MALIGNANCIES

Urinary tract malignancies are quite rare in children and adolescents. In children, Wilms tumor is the most common malignant neoplasm of the genitourinary system. Renal cell carcinoma is the most frequent malignant tumor in adolescents and adults. Transitional cell carcinoma has been reported in the bladder of children, but rhabdomyosarcoma is the most common pelvic tumor of childhood. The presentation of these tumors is variable and depends on the location and size of the tumor.[83] Pelvic rhabdomyosarcoma may present as recurrent painless hematuria, stranguria, abdominal pain, recurrent UTI, or as an abdominal mass.

TRAUMA

Trauma is the leading cause of death in children.[84] Renal trauma is classified as blunt or penetrating. Blunt trauma is more common in children and is usually associated with other significant injuries. Preexisting renal abnormalities such as hydronephrosis or abnormal position increase the potential for renal damage. Physical findings such as abdominal tenderness, flank mass, ecchymosis or hematoma over the flank, or fractured ribs can be important markers for possible renal injury. Hematuria is usually the first and the most reliable indicator of injury. Blood at the urethral meatus suggests severe urethral injury.

There is controversy with respect to the amount of hematuria considered indicative of severe renal injury. Stalker and coworkers reported that more than 50 red blood cells per high-power field (RBC/hpf) is significant, whereas Lieu and coworkers agreed that 20 RBC/hpf is significant.[85, 86] Recently Morey and colleagues reported that significant renal injury is unlikely in pediatric patients who exhibit no gross or substantial microscopic hematuria.[87] In contrast, Abou-Jaoude and associates demonstrated that a cutoff point greater than 20 RBC/hpf would have missed 28% of 100 patients with genitourinary trauma.[88] The need for urinary tract evaluation in pediatric trauma patients should be based as much on clinical judgment as on the presence of hematuria.

Complications of renal trauma can be early—delayed bleeding, infection, abscess, sepsis, urinary fistulae, extravasation or urinoma—or late—strictures, hydronephrosis, hypertension.

In infants and young children, the full bladder sits farther cephalad and is primarily an abdominal organ not protected by the bony pelvis. Blunt lower abdominal trauma, with or without pelvic fracture, may cause bladder rupture. When rupture occurs, urine seeps into either the peritoneal or the extraperitoneal space. Treatment depends on the location of the bladder rupture, and the diagnosis is established with cystography. Extraperitoneal bladder ruptures are managed with Foley catheter drainage, whereas intraperitoneal ruptures are managed surgically.

Straddle-type injuries, not uncommon in the pediatric population, usually affect the anterior urethra as it is compressed against the ischial ramus. When injury is significant, the patient may present with blood at the meatus or difficulty voiding with suprapubic bladder distention.

ANOMALIES OF THE URINARY TRACT

Anomalies of the urogenital tract are among the most common malformations of any organ system. A thorough understanding of the embryonic development of the urinary tract is a prerequisite for the evaluation and management of a child with a congenital defect.

RENAL AGENESIS

Renal agenesis results from failure of induction of the metanephric blastema by the ureteral bud. The clinical incidence (found in school children by sonographic screening) was 1 in 1200.[89] There is a slight male predominance, and the condition more often occurs on the left side.

In most cases, renal agenesis is associated with other anomalies (e.g., absence of the ipsilateral ureter), including anomalies of the contralateral kidney such as malrotation and ectopia. The genital tract is by far the most common system involved in associated anomalies.[90] Such anomalies usually involve the uterus and vagina and are represented by either a unicornuate or a bicornuate uterus with a rudimentary ipsilateral fallopian tube, or none. Complete duplication of the vagina, cervix, and uterus with imperforate hemivagina are rare conditions caused by müllerian and mesonephric duct abnormalities. *Mayer-Rokitansky-Küster-Hauser syndrome* describes a group of associated findings that includes unilateral renal agenesis or renal ectopia, ipsilateral müllerian defects, and vaginal agenesis.[91]

Renal agenesis is frequently found incidentally on US, excretory urography, or CT. In the absence of a kidney compensatory contralateral renal hypertrophy frequently occurs. US may be helpful for screening parents or siblings. Bilateral agenesis or Potter syndrome is a rare condition and incompatible with life. Many of these infants are stillborn, and the remainder succumb to pulmonary hypoplasia.

ASSOCIATED ANOMALIES

Malrotation or abnormal rotation is associated with ectopic or fused kidney. The condition is usually an incidental finding and can be unilateral or bilateral. Most patients are asymptomatic unless urinary drainage is obstructed by an anomalous accessory vessel.

Failure of the kidney to complete its ascent (i.e., renal ectopia) can be secondary to a number of factors, including an abnormality of the ureteral bud, a teratogen, or a vascular anomaly. The incidence of renal ectopy is higher at autopsy (1 in 500 to 1 in 1200) than in clinical studies, a finding that suggests that many cases go unrecognized.[92] The most common position is at the sacrum, immediately below the aortic bifurcation.

Most ectopic kidneys are asymptomatic but pain is still the most common symptom. Pelvic kidneys may be difficult to visualize, but excretory urography and US confirm the location of the anomaly. Hydronephrosis, present in approximately 50% of ectopic kidneys, is due to ureteropelvic junction (UPJ) obstruction, ureterovesical obstruction, VUR, or to malrotation alone. Besides agenesis, the contralateral kidney may also be hydronephrotic (25%) owing to obstruction or reflux.[93] Other anomalies associated with renal ectopia affect the genitalia, cardiovascular system, and skeleton.

Horseshoe kidney is the most common type of renal fusion defect (incidence 1 in 400).[92] The isthmus joining the kidneys may consist of either renal parenchyma or fibrous tissue, and the blood supply of horseshoe kidneys is quite variable. Other conditions, such as UTI and urinary calculi, often lead to the diagnosis. UPJ obstruction with hydronephrosis is present in as many as a third of these patients. Finally, the incidence of renal tumors is higher than normal in these patients, particularly Wilms tumor.

URETHRAL PROLAPSE

Urethral prolapse most often affects African-American girls younger than 10 years (Fig. 35–4). Affected patients usually present with dysuria and bloody spotting. Frank hematuria and urinary retention may also occur. On physical examination, a rather typical-looking, everted, hemor-

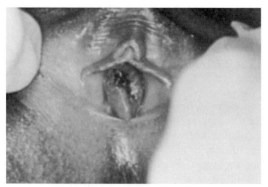

Figure 35–4. Urethral prolapse.

rhagic, doughnut-shaped mass is seen superior to, but often obscuring, the hymenal ring.

Nonsurgical approaches (e.g., application of an antimicrobial ointment and a conjugated estrogen cream in association with sitz baths) are effective and should be tried first. Excision of the prolapsed epithelium and securing the edge with a suture is reserved for persistent or recurrent cases.

OTHER ABNORMALITIES RELATED TO THE URINARY TRACT

SEXUALLY TRANSMITTED DISEASES

Urethritis, or inflammation of the urethra, is manifested as urethral discharge, burning, or pain on initiation of urination. The symptoms of urethritis are similar in adolescents and in adults. In children, additional symptoms include urethral discharge, meatal inflammation (e.g., erythema, edema), pyuria, and urethral tenderness. The most common cause of urethritis is infection with *Chlamydia trachomatis*, but *Neisseria gonorrhoeae*, *Mycoplasma* species, *Trichomonas vaginalis*, herpes simplex virus, or coliform bacteria are sometimes implicated.

Dysuria affects 20% of women with chlamydial or gonococcal infection, but this symptom often prompts diagnosis of UTI. Urinalysis often shows pyuria with a nonsignificant growth on culture.[4] Pyuria (10 white blood cells per high power field) in the absence of significant bacteria is the hallmark of underlying urethritis. Treatment, of course, is based on the particular pathogen.

ABNORMALITIES IN ADOLESCENTS WITH SPECIAL NEEDS

Upper and lower urogenital tract dysfunction often afflicts children and adolescents with neurologic handicaps. Patients with special needs include those with central nervous system lesions (e.g., cerebral palsy, mental retardation) or spinal cord lesions from either congenital anomalies (spina bifida, myelomeningocele, or sacral agenesis) or acquired lesions (trauma, neoplasms).

In a child or adolescent with such abnormalities the principal concerns are management of bladder and bowel control and of sexual functioning. A program of urologic surveillance (radiographic and urodynamic) should therefore be instituted early in newborns with spinal disorders and should continue throughout childhood and adolescence. Patients who exhibit high intravesical pressures secondary to neurogenic bladder should be identified and treated as soon as possible, to prevent irreversible lower and upper urinary tract damage. A program of intermittent catheterization, along with anticholinergic medications, may be needed to reduce persistently elevated intravesical pressure. This resolves upper urinary tract changes such as reflux and hydronephrosis in the majority of cases. Clean intermittent catheterization can be accomplished in newborns and can be mastered by some 6-year-olds when they are taught by a supportive multidisciplinary team. This approach has virtually revolutionized the care of these patients.

SUMMARY

Physicians who treat children and who have an interest in the gynecologic problems of children and adolescents should be familiar with the urologic conditions common in these age groups. Because of a child's limited ability to identify the source of symptoms and to express her problems to caregivers, the physician should search for urologic lesions that are seemingly manifested as gynecologic complaints and conversely. The close physical association and common embryonic origin of the urinary and reproductive tracts make it mandatory to have a working knowledge of both if the physician is to provide the best care for children.

REFERENCES

1. Wold AE, Caugant DA, Lidin-Janson G, et al: Resident *E. coli* strains frequently display uropathogenic characteristics. J Infect Dis 1992; 165:46.
2. Wettergren B, Jodal U, Jonasson G: Epidemiology of bacteriuria during the first year of life. Acta Paediatr Scand 1985; 74:925–933.
3. Lindberg U, Claésson I, Hanson LÅ, Jodal U: Asymptomatic bacteriuria in schoolgirls. I. Clinical and laboratory findings. Acta Paediatr Scand 1975; 64:425–431.
4. Kunin CM, Deutscher R, Paquin A Jr: Urinary tract infection in school children: An epidemiologic, clinical and laboratory study. Medicine 1964; 4:91.
5. Savage DC, Wilson MI, McHardy M, et al: Covert bacteriuria of childhood. Arch Dis Child 1973; 48(1):8–20.
6. McLachlan MSF, Meller ST, Verrier-Jones ER, et al: Urinary tract infection in children. Br Med J 1984; 289:299–303.
7. Savage DCL: Natural history of covert bacteriuria in schoolgirls. Kidney Int 1975; 8:S90–95.
8. Lindbergh U, Claesson I, Hanson LÅ, Jodal U: Asymp-

tomatic bacteriuria in schoolgirls. VIII. Clinical course during a 3-year follow-up. J Pediatr 1978; 92:194–199.
9. Verrier-Jones ER, Meller ST, McLachlan MSF, et al: Treatment of bacteriuria in schoolgirls. Kidney Int 1975; S4:93–103.
10. Lindbergh U, Hanson LÅ, Jodal U, et al: Asymptomatic bacteriuria in school-girls. II. Differences in *E. coli* causing asymptomatic and symptomatic bacteriuria. Acta Paediatr Scand 1975; 64:432–436.
11. Hansson S, Caugant D, Jodal U, Svanborg-Edén C: Untreated asymptomatic bacteriuria in girls: I—stability of urinary isolates. Br Med J 1989; 298:853–855.
12. Kemper KJ, Avner ED: The case against screening urinalyses for asymptomatic bacteriuria in children. Am J Dis Child 1992; 146:343–346.
13. Linshaw M: Nephrology forum: Asymptomatic bacteriuria and vesicoureteric reflux in children. Kidney Int 1996; 50:312–329.
14. Newcastle Asymptomatic Bacteriuria Research Group: Covert bacteriuria in schoolgirls in Newcastle-upon-Tyne. A 5-year follow-up. Arch Dis Child 1981; 56:585.
15. Kunin CM, Zacha E, Paquin A: Urinary-tract infections in schoolchildren: I. Prevalence of bacteriuria and associated urologic findings. N Engl J Med 1962; 266: 1287–1296.
16. Savage DCL, Howie G, Adler K, Wilson MI: Controlled trial of therapy in covert bacteriuria of childhood. Lancet 1975; 1:358–361.
17. Winberg J, Anderson HJ, Bergström T, et al: Epidemiology of symptomatic urinary tract infection in childhood. Acta Paediatr Scand 1974; S252:1–20.
18. Rushton HG, Majd M: Dimercaptosuccinic acid renal scintigraphy for the evaluation of pyelonephritis and scarring: A review of experimental and clinical studies. J Urol 1992; 148 (5 Pt 2):1726–1732.
19. Rushton HG, Majd M, Jantausch B, et al: Renal scarring following reflux and nonreflux pyelonephritis in children: Evaluation with ^{99m}Technetium–dimercaptosuccinic acid scintigraphy. J Urol 1992; 147:1327–1332.
20. Roberts JA, Roth JK, Dominue GJ: Immunology of pyelonephritis. J Urol 1982; 129:193–196.
21. Ransley PG, Risdon RA: Renal papillae and intrarenal reflux in the pig. Lancet 1974; ii:1114.
22. Hannerz L, Kikstad I, Johansson L, et al: Distribution of renal scars and intrarenal reflux in children with a past history of urinary tract infection. Acta Radiol 1987; 28:443–446.
23. Jodal U: The natural history of bacteriuria in childhood. Infect Dis Clin North Am 1987; 1:713–729.
24. Wallace DMA, Rothwell DL, Williams DI, et al: The long-term follow-up of surgically treated vesicoureteric reflux. Br J Urol 1978; 50:479.
25. Goonasekera CD, Shah V, Wade AM, et al: 15-Year follow-up of renin and blood pressure in reflux nephropathy. Lancet 1996; 347(9002):640–643.
26. Jakobsson B, Nolstedt L, Svensson L, et al: ^{99m}Technetium–dimercaptosuccinic acid scan in the diagnosis of acute pyelonephritis in children: Relation to clinical and radiological findings. Pediatr Nephrol 1992; 6:328–334.
27. Miller T, Phillips S: Pyelonephritis: The relationship between infection, renal scarring, and antimicrobial therapy. Kidney Int 1981; 19:654–662.
28. Slotki IN, Asscher AW: Prevention of scarring in experimental pyelonephritis in the rat by early antibiotic therapy. Nephron 1982; 30:262.
29. Kass EH, Finland M: Asymptomatic infections of the urinary tract. Trans Assoc Am Physicians 1956; 69:56–64.
30. Shortliffe LM: Urinary tract infections in infants and children. *In* Walsh PC, Retik AB, Vaughan ED, Wein

AJ (eds): Campbell's Urology, 7th ed. Philadelphia: WB Saunders, 1998, pp 1681–1707.

31. Stamey TA, Sexton CC: The role of vaginal colonization with Enterobacteriaceae in recurrent urinary infections. J Urol 1975; 113:214–217.

32. Johnson CE, DeBaz EP, Shurin PA, et al: Renal ultrasound evaluation of urinary tract infections in children. Pediatrics 1986; 78:871–878.

33. Berdon WE: Contemporary imaging approach to pediatric urology problems. Radiol Clin North Am 1991; 29(3):605–618.

34. Blane CE, DiPietro MA, Zerin JM, et al: Renal sonography is not a reliable screening examination for vesicoureteral reflux. J Urol 1993; 150 (Pt 2):752–755.

35. Pohl HG, Rushton HG: The diagnosis and management of urinary tract infection in children. AUA Update Series 1998; Vol. XVII, lesson 31.

36. Stamey TA, Condy M: The diffusion and concentration of trimethoprim in human vaginal fluid. J Infect Dis 1975; 131:261.

37. Roberto U, d'Eufenua P, Martino F, et al: Amoxicillin and clavulanic acid in the treatment of urinary tract infection in children. J Int Med Res 1989; 17:168.

38. Ball P: Ciprofloxacin: An overview of adverse experiences. J Anti Chemother 1986; 18(Suppl D):187.

39. Madrigal G, Ohio CM, Mohs E, et al: Single-dose antibiotic therapy is not as effective as conventional regimens for management of acute urinary tract infections in children. Pediatr Infect Dis J 1988; 7:316.

40. Bailey R: Review of published studies on single dose therapy of urinary tract infections. Infection 1990; 18(Suppl 2):53.

41. Smellie JM, Normand ICS, Kaz G: Children with urinary infection: A comparison of those with and those without vesicoureteric reflux. Kidney Int 1981; 20:717.

42. Winberg J, Bergström T, Lidin-Janson G, Lincoln K: Treatment trials in urinary tract infection (UTI) with special reference to the effect of antimicrobials on the fecal and periurethral flora. Clin Nephrol 1973; 1:142.

43. Baker R, Moxted W, Majlath J, et al: Relation of age, sex and infection to reflux and data indicating high spontaneous cure rate in pediatric patients. J Urol 1966; 95:27.

44. Gunn TR, Mora JD, Pease P: Antenatal diagnosis of urinary tract abnormalities by ultrasonography after 28 weeks' gestation: Incidence and outcome. Am J Obstet Gynecol 1995; 172:479–486.

45. Zerin JM, Ritchey ML, Chang AC: Incidental vesicoureteral reflux in neonates with antenatally detected hydronephrosis and other renal abnormalities. Radiology 1993; 187:157.

46. Woodard JR, Holden S: The prognostic significance of fever in childhood urinary infections: Observations in 350 consecutive patients. Clin Pediatrics 1976; 15:1051.

47. Ransley PG, Risdon RA: Reflux and renal scarring. Br J Radiol 1978; 14(Suppl):1.

48. Hannerz K, Wikstad I, Celsi G, et al: Influence of vesicoureteral reflux and urinary tract infection and renal growth in children with upper urinary tract duplication. Acta Radiol 1989; 30:391.

49. Sidi AA, Perry W, Gonzalez R: Vesicoureteral reflux in children with myelodysplasia: Natural history and results of treatment. J Urol 1986; 136:239.

50. Koff SA, Lapides J, Piazza DH: Association of urinary tract infection and reflux with uninhibited bladder contractions and voluntary sphincteric obstruction. J Urol 1979; 122:373.

51. Taylor CM: Unstable bladder activity and the rate of resolution of vesicoureteric reflux. Contrib Nephrol 1984; 39:238.

52. Koff SA, Murtagh DS: The uninhibited bladder in children: Effect of treatment on recurrence of urinary infection and on vesicoureteral reflux resolution. J Urol 1983; 130:1138–1141.

53. Homsy YL, Nsouli N, Hamburger B, et al: Effects of oxybutynin on vesicoureteral reflux in children. J Urol 1985; 134:1168–1171.

54. Arant BS Jr: Medical management of mild and moderate vesicoureteral reflux: Follow-up studies of infants and young children. A preliminary report of the Southwest Pediatric Nephrology Group. J Urol 1992; 148:1683.

55. Tamminen-Mobius T, Brunier E, Ebel KD, et al: Cessation of vesicoureteral reflux for 5 years in infants and children allocated to medical treatment. The International Reflux Study in Children. J Urol 1992; 148:1662.

56. Weiss R, Duckett J, Spitzer A, et al: Results of a randomized clinical trial of medical vs. surgical management of infants and children with grades III and IV primary vesicoureteral reflux (United States). J Urol 1992; 148:1667.

57. Elder JS, Peters CA, Arant BS, et al: Pediatric Vesicoureteral Reflux Guidelines Panel summary report on the management of primary vesicoureteral reflux in children. J Urol 1997; 157:1846–1851.

58. Smellie JM, Edwards D, Normond IC, et al: Effect of vesicoureteral reflux on renal growth in children with urinary tract infection. Arch Dis Child 1981; 56:593–600.

59. Olbing H, Claesson I, Ebel KD, et al: Renal scars and parenchymal thinning in children with vesicoureteral reflux: A 5-year report of the international reflux study in children. J Urol 1992; 148:1653.

60. Koff SA: Relationship between dysfunctional voiding and reflux. J Urol 1992; 148:1703.

61. Klevan JL, De Jong AR: Urinary tract symptoms and urinary tract infection following sexual abuse. Am J Dis Child 1990; 144: 242–244.

62. Hinman F: Non-neurogenic neurogenic bladder (the Hinman syndrome)—15 years later. J Urol 1986; 136:769.

63. O'Regan S, Yazbeck S, Schick E: Constipation, bladder instability, urinary tract syndrome. Clin Nephrol 1985; 23:152.

64. Koff SA, Wagner TT, Jayanthi VR: The relationship among dysfunctional elimination syndromes, primary vesicoureteral reflux and urinary tract infections in children. J Urol 1998; 160:1019–1022.

65. Koff SA: Evaluation and management of voiding disorders in children. Urol Clin North Am 1988; 15(4):769.

66. Reshef E, Casale AJ, Sanfilippo JS: Age specific urinary tract problems: Young adult female. In Buchsbaum HJ, Schmidt JD (eds): Gynecologic and Obstetric Urology, 3rd ed. Philadelphia: WB Saunders, 1993.

67. Forsythe WI, Redmond A: Enuresis and spontaneous cure rate: Study of 1129 enuretics. Arch Dis Child 1974; 49:259.

68. Koff SA: Enuresis. In Walsh PC, Retik AB, Vaughan ED, Wein AJ (eds): Campbell's Urology, 7th ed, Vol 2. Philadelphia: WB Saunders, 1998, pp 2055–2068.

69. Bakwin H: The genetics of enuresis. In Kolvin I, MacKeith RC, Meadow SR (eds): Bladder Control and Enuresis. London: W Heinemann, 1973, pp 73–77.

70. Eiberg H: Assignment of dominant inherited nocturnal enuresis (ENUR1) to chromosome 13q. Nature Genet 1995; 10:354–356.

71. Norgaard JP, Rittig S: Recent studies of the pathophysiology of nocturnal enuresis. In Meadow SR (ed): Desmopressin in Nocturnal Enuresis. Proceedings of an International Symposium. Conwell, Sutton, Coldfield, England: Horus Medical, 1989.

72. Norgaard JP, Hansen JH, Nielsen JB, et al: Simultaneous

registration of sleep stages and bladder activity in enuresis. Urology 1985; 26:316–319.

73. Moffatt MEK: Nocturnal enuresis: Psychologic implications of treatment and nontreatment. J Pediatrics 1989; 114(Suppl):697.

74. Eller DA, Austin PF, Tanguay S, et al: Daytime functional bladder capacity as a predictor of response to desmopressin in monosymptomatic nocturnal enuresis. Eur Urol 1998; 33 (Suppl 3):25–29.

75. Hogg RJ, Husmann D: The role of family history in predicting response to desmopressin in nocturnal enuresis. J Urol 1993; 150:444–445.

76. Koff SA, Byard MA: The daytime urinary frequency syndrome of childhood. J Urol 1988; 140:1280–1282.

77. Homsy YL: Dysfunctional voiding syndromes and vesicoureteral reflux. Pediatr Nephrol 1994; 8:116–121.

78. Ingelfinger JR, Davis AE, Grupe WE: Frequency and etiology of gross hematuria in a general pediatric setting. Pediatrics 1977; 59:557.

79. Mufson MA, Belshe RB, Horrigan TJ, Zollar LM: Cause of acute hemorrhagic cystitis in children. Am J Dis Child 1973; 26:605–608.

80. Vehaskari VM, Rapola J, Koskimies O, et al: Microscopic hematuria in school children: Epidemiology and clinicopathologic evaluation. J Pediatr 1979; 95:676–684.

81. Stapleton FB, Roy S III, Noe HN, Jerkins GR: Hypercalciuria in children with hematuria. N Engl J Med 1984; 310:1345–1348.

82. Gearhart JP, Herzberg GZ, Jeffs RD: Childhood urolithiasis: Experiences and advances. Pediatrics 1991; 87:445–450.

83. Hays DM: Pelvic rhabdomyosarcoma in childhood: Diagnosis and concepts of management reviewed. Cancer 1980; 45:1811.

84. Fingerhut LA, Annest JL, Baker SP, et al: Injury mortality among children and teenagers in the United States, 1993. Inj Prev 1996; 2:93–94.

85. Stalker HP, Kaufman RA, Stedje K: The significance of hematuria in children after blunt abdominal trauma. AJR 1990; 154:569.

86. Lieu TA, Fleischer GR, Mahboubi S, Schwatz JS: Hematuria and clinical findings as indications for intravenous pyelography in pediatric blunt renal trauma. Pediatrics 1988; 82:216.

87. Morey AF, Bruce JE, McAninch JW: Efficacy of radiographic imaging in pediatric blunt renal trauma. J Urol 1996; 156:2014–2018.

88. Abou-Jaoude WA, Sugarman JM, Fallat ME, Casale AJ: Indicators of genitourinary tract injury or anomaly in cases of pediatric blunt trauma. J Pediatr Surg 1996; 31:86–89.

89. Shieh CP, Hung CS, Wei CF, Lin CY: Cystic dilatations within the pelvis in patients with ipsilateral renal agenesis or dysplasia. J Urol 1990; 144:324.

90. Anderson KA, McAninch JW: Uterus didelphia with left hematocolpos and ipsilateral renal agenesis. J Urol 1982; 127:550–553.

91. Glassberg KI: Renal dysplasia and cystic disease of the kidney. In Walsh PC, Retik AB, Vaughan ED, Wein AJ (eds): Campbell's Urology, 7th ed, Vol 2. Philadelphia: WB Saunders, 1998, pp 1757–1813.

92. Bauer SB: Anomalies of the kidney and ureteropelvic junction. In Walsh PC, Retik AB, Vaughan ED, Wein AJ (eds): Campbell's Urology, 7th ed, Vol 2. Philadelphia: WB Saunders, 1998, pp 1708–1755.

93. Gleason PE, Kelalis PP, Husmann DA, Kramer SA: Hydronephrosis in renal ectopia: Incidence, etiology, and significance. J Urol 1994; 151:1660.

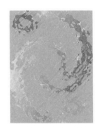

Chapter 36
Breast Disorders

Patricia S. Simmons

It is common in medical practice to apply principles to the care of children and adolescents that have been derived from experience with adult patients. This is not surprising, as many diseases are more common in adults and many of the studies in the medical literature have been derived from adult populations, for humanitarian and practical reasons. The ethics and the technical aspects of research in minors are necessarily complex and limit data generation. However, caution is in order when applying principles and lessons derived from adult medicine to young persons. Nowhere is this more true than in physiologic and pathologic conditions of the female breast. This chapter on the breast of female children and adolescents represents a synthesis of the relevant pediatric and adolescent medical literature and the impressions of physicians who frequently deal with these issues. Specific topics include congenital anomalies of the breast, normal and abnormal development, and breast masses in children and adolescents.

In addition, the issue of adolescent breast self-examination will be explored, with discussions of the value and potential hazards of this health maintenance practice. One of the most important developments in breast disease has been imaging techniques for the pediatric and adolescent population. While mammograms are the mainstay of evaluation of the adult female breast, they are less useful in young girls. The role of other forms of breast imaging, as well as mammography, in pediatric and adolescent patients is explored.

EXAMINATION OF THE BREAST IN THE CHILD AND ADOLESCENT

INFANTS AND YOUNG CHILDREN

The breasts should first be examined in the neonatal period for the presence of normal breast buds and to rule out a congenital anomaly.

The Mayo Foundation retains copyright for all figures in this chapter.

Examination of the breast is part of the gestational age assessment, as the amount of tissue varies with maturation. Polymastia may be detectable in a newborn but may not be recognized until the child is older. Examining the infant with the parent present provides an opportunity to educate the family about normal breast appearance and related concerns. Well-child examinations and general medical evaluations through childhood provide the physician with an opportunity to monitor the normal stages of breast development and to detect any developmental or structural abnormality. Simple inspection and palpation of the juvenile breast should not be emotionally traumatic, as it can be readily accomplished during anterior chest inspection and auscultation. Just as in adults, it is imperative to respect the child's or the adolescent's modesty.

PUBERTAL GIRLS

Examination of the pubertal girl should include Tanner staging of the breast and the pubic hair.[1] Reassuring the patient that she is developing normally and some discussion of what that means are appropriate and encouraged. Many young girls question their own normalcy, including their degree or lack of breast development. Breasts should be checked for asymmetry and for masses, congenital anomalies, developmental abnormalities, and nipple discharge.

ADOLESCENTS

Breast examination should be performed as part of routine health care for and general examination of the adolescent female. Tanner staging should be accomplished along with visual inspection and palpation of the breasts to exclude abnormality. The technique for examination of the adolescent breast is not dissimilar to that for adults. In this chapter the subject of adolescent breast self-examination is addressed. If self-examination is to be taught, this point in the patient's visit is an appropriate time to do so. If the breast self-examination is not to be taught, the rationale for deferring it could be addressed instead. Most adolescents prefer to have their breasts examined with parents out of the room and should be given that option. This provides an opportunity to explain normal development, address any abnormalities, and review any concerns the patient has. With the adolescent, the physician must determine who should be present during the breast examination—the parent, another trusted person, and/or a chaperone.

INFANCY AND EARLY CHILDHOOD

The presence of palpable, and often visible, breast tissue in a term newborn infant is normal and expected. Premature infants are less likely to have neonatal breast buds, a fact that has been incorporated into the assessment of gestational age system defined by Dubowitz and Dubowitz.[2] The amount of breast tissue in normal newborns varies and may be associated with milk production ("witch's milk"). The presence of breast tissue in the newborn has been attributed to maternal hormone stimulation, but there is reason to believe that another mechanism may be involved, as breast buds may persist for months, long after the direct effect of maternal hormones should be gone.[3] In fact, the natural history of neonatal breast development is incompletely understood. Persistence of neonatal breast buds through age 10 months has been documented in normal infants by McKiernan and Hull[4]; however, persistence of breast tissue in normal female children through the first 2 years of life has been observed. This observation is complicated by the fact that in this age group breasts could signal an abnormal condition, precocious puberty. Defining the normal amount of breast tissue present through early life is important, as it may help to understand when it is appropriate to be concerned about the presence of breast tissue in young children and embark on an evaluation to rule out true, incomplete, or pseudoprecocious puberty. A study currently in progress is looking at normal degrees of breast tissue during the first 2 years of life and possible modifying factors. For the present, in an individual patient, it can be useful to document breast tissue on well-child evaluations, as new appearance versus persistence may distinguish an abnormality from normal development.

CONGENITAL ANOMALIES OF THE BREAST

The most common congenial anomaly of the breast is polythelia (Fig. 36–1). In this condition,

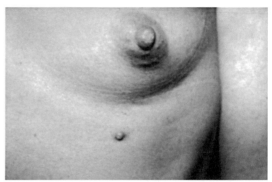

Figure 36–1. Polythelia.

accessory nipples and areolae appear somewhere along the milk ridge from the axillae to the groins. Most often, an incomplete nipple/areola appears within a few centimeters inferior to the breast on one or both sides. Polymastia (i.e., accessory breast tissue) is less common and may become a significant problem at puberty or during pregnancy and lactation. Sometimes surgical excision of the extra mammary tissue is indicated.

Congenital amastia is extremely rare (Fig. 36–2). Occasionally concern arises over what appears to be poor nipple/areolar development in a child with hypopigmentation; however, at puberty development of the breasts can be expected.

MASTITIS

Mastitis in the newborn presents as erythema, tenderness, and sometimes swelling of the affected breast; it is usually unilateral but may be bilateral. The underlying mechanism may involve obstruction of a mammary duct. Treatment with warm compresses is generally effective, but if there is engorgement in the newborn's breast,

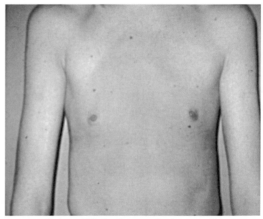

Figure 36–2. Congenital amastia.

the physician may express some milk to relieve pressure, increase comfort, and hasten resolution. Antibiotics are not usually necessary, but these infants must be watched carefully for signs of infection in the breast. If infection is suspected, antibiotic therapy, as well as close observation and local care, may be indicated. Mastitis, although uncommon, also occurs in older infants and children. Management includes warm compresses to the affected breast, antibiotics, and monitoring for signs of systemic infection.

BREAST ENLARGEMENT AND MASSES IN THE PREPUBERTAL CHILD

UNILATERAL BREAST MASSES

The presence of a breast mass in a young child provokes anxiety in parents—and often in physicians (Fig. 36–3). Fortunately, breast malignancy is extremely rare in this age group, and most of these masses are benign. A variety of types of masses have been identified in children's breasts, including hemangioma, lipoma, papilloma, lymphangioma, benign cyst, fibrosis, localized mastitis, hematoma, fat necrosis, and other benign tumors (Table 36–1). Of these, breast hemangioma is probably the most common, and the diagnosis is usually obvious on inspection. A breast hemangioma is most often found superior and lateral to the areola and is soft, freely movable, nontender, and the consistency of hemangiomas that occur elsewhere in humans. A superficial vascular pattern on the breast may be apparent, which is actually a hemangioma of the connective tissue superficial to the breast paren-

Table 36–1. Differential Diagnosis of Breast Enlargement in Prepubertal Girls

Unilateral
  Hemangioma
  Lipoma
  Papilloma
  Lymphangioma
  Cyst
  Fibrosis
  Mastitis
  Hematoma
  Fat necrosis
  Tumors of adjacent structures
  Thelarche
  Breast cancer (extremely rare)
Bilateral
  Premature thelarche
  Precocious puberty
    True precocious puberty
    Exogenous estrogen exposure
    Endogenous estrogen hyperproduction
      (usually an ovarian source)
    Hypothyroidism ("overlap syndrome")

chyma. Breast hemangiomas in children are best left alone and observed only. Surgical excision is not necessary and in fact can destroy the underlying breast bud and lead to iatrogenic unilateral amastia. The hemangioma may persist for years and becomes less apparent with pubertal breast development.

Cysts are rare in this age group, being more likely to occur in pubertal or adult females. Transillumination, ultrasonography, and transdermal aspiration may be useful in the diagnosis, just as in older patients, but, again, care should be taken to avoid trauma, and follow-up is very important.

A mass lesion underlying the area of the breast but not truly in the breast may also mimic

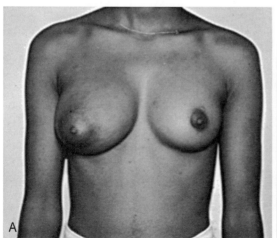
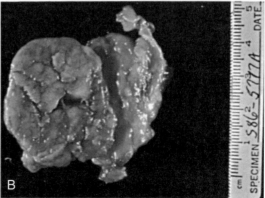

Figure 36–3. *A,* Unilateral fibroadenoma. *B,* Surgical specimen of a fibroadenoma.

a breast mass. This differentiation tends to be more difficult in pubertal girls or adolescents with more breast tissue; however, specific imaging techniques may help to localize a mass and suggest its cause.

When breast development is asynchronous at thelarche, the first breast bud may be mistaken for a neoplasm. With either precocious or normal puberty a unilateral breast bud can be the first sign. Development of the second breast or other secondary sex characteristics may not be apparent for as long as 6 months. Again, biopsy should be avoided.

Malignancy of the breast is extremely rare in children, and although case reports exist, it is difficult to determine its incidence or prevalence. Only 17 cases of primary carcinoma of the breast have been reported in children 15 years old or younger.[5]

When the clinical assessment suggests a benign process leading to development of a mass in the breast, observation is preferred over surgical excision or biopsy for most children. When a malignancy or infection refractory to medical management alone is suspected, surgery must be undertaken and extreme care exercised to protect the breast bud.

EARLY BREAST DEVELOPMENT

The normal breast buds present in newborn infants of both sexes resolve over the early weeks and months of life. Breast development before age 8 years in girls is considered abnormal. Bilateral breast enlargement may result from premature thelarche or precocious puberty. Differentiation of these two conditions is important, as the former is a self-limited process without significant underlying disease or sequelae and the latter a progressive process that may have a serious underlying cause and adverse sequelae.

PREMATURE THELARCHE AND PRECOCIOUS PUBERTY

By definition, premature thelarche is isolated breast development in girls before age 8. It was first described in 1946 and named in 1965.[6] Its prevalence is calculated to be 2%.[7] This common cause of breast development in young girls represents an incomplete, transient, and benign form of precocious puberty. The most common age for presentation is 15 months, and most girls are younger than 2 years. There is another peak of incidence between 6 and 8 years, but this is less common. Premature thelarche is characterized

by isolated bilateral breast development. Otherwise, the girls' growth is normal and no other clinical signs of estrogen or androgen effect are apparent (i.e., no sex hair, axillary sweat, acne, virilization, gross vaginal mucosa estrogenization, or menses). This is not a familial condition, and it is not associated with central nervous system gross pathology or other symptoms or findings. The medical history is usually unremarkable, although some data suggest that premature infants may be at risk for premature thelarche.[8] Others have failed to show this association.[9] It is important to obtain a thorough history to rule out exogenous estrogen exposure. Presently, the most common form of exogenous estrogen may be the oral contraceptive. Estrogen creams and other preparations may also result in breast development and other hormonal effects. Some "health foods" or "alternative medicines" may also contain estrogens. Pseudoprecocious puberty has been linked to meat treated or contaminated with sex steroids.[10]

If the patient meets the clinical criteria for premature thelarche, certain studies are recommended to exclude precocious puberty, as breast development may be its first sign. Radiographic imaging to determine bone age is recommended. With premature thelarche, the bone age should be within two standard deviations of the chronologic age. Bone age may be greater than normal in precocious puberty, and less than expected bone age may result from hypothyroidism. An assessment of estrogen is also recommended. This can be obtained either through venous sampling for estradiol levels or with a vaginal maturation index. This index is determined from samples collected atraumatically by swabbing the vaginal wall with a saline-moistened urethral swab, taking care to avoid touching the hymen.[11] Contact with the hymen can cause pain and can falsely elevate the percentage of superficial cells, leading to overestimation of estrogen effect. Often, serial serum estradiol levels are necessary to detect or rule out hyperestrogenemia. Mild elevations of estradiol have been described in premature thelarche[12, 13]; higher elevations suggest another diagnosis. Table 36–2 shows the results of vaginal maturation index and serum estradiol for normal girls and for those with premature thelarche and precocious puberty. Assessment of thyroid function is also appropriate. Serum total thyroxine and thyroid-stimulating hormone (TSH) levels should be normal and are assessed to exclude the "overlap syndrome." Sexual precocity can occur with severe hypothyroidism, although this is rare. Patients with hypothyroidism associated with breast development should have low serum thyroxine levels, elevated

Table 36–2. Hormonal Activity in Normal Prepubertal Girls Compared with That in Girls with Premature Thelarche and Precocious Puberty

	Normal	Premature Thelarche	Precocious Puberty
Serum estradiol[12] (pg/ml)	4 ± 0.6	5.5 ± 0.32	38 ± 9
VMI[12]	60–90/10–20/0–3	60/30/5–10	20/50/30
Bone age	Normal	Normal	Usually advanced
Serum prolactin	Normal	Normal	Normal
Stimulated prolactin	Normal	Normal	Elevated°
Serum LH	Normal	Normal	Normal or elevated
Stimulated LH	Normal	Normal	Elevated
Serum FSH	Normal	Normal or elevated	Normal or elevated
Stimulated FSH	Normal	Elevated	Elevated

°Greater than 2 S.D. above the mean.

FSH, Follicle-stimulating hormone; LH, Luteinizing hormone; VMI, Vaginal maturation index, expressed as a percentage of basal/intermediate/superficial cells.

thyroid-stimulating hormone levels, short stature and/or decreased growth rate, and delayed bone age.

Random or basal levels of luteinizing hormone (LH) and follicle-stimulating hormone (FSH) generally are not useful in diagnosing premature thelarche. Levels of these hormones should be in the prepubertal normal range, but similar levels may also be seen in precocious puberty and thus do not rule out the latter possibility. Provocative testing with gonadotropin-releasing hormone is used to document LH and FSH elevations of precocious puberty. Assessment of serum prolactin also contributes nothing to the diagnosis. Basal levels of both prolactin and thyrotropin-releasing hormone–stimulated prolactin are normal in premature thelarche and precocious puberty.

In general, except to determine bone age, imaging studies are not necessary to make the diagnosis of premature thelarche. Brain imaging using computerized tomography or magnetic resonance imaging is indicated in patients with suspected precocious puberty or central nervous system abnormality. Pelvic ultrasound may also be useful if the diagnosis of premature thelarche is questionable. The sonogram should show a normal prepubertal uterus as compared with the estrogen-stimulated uterus of larger size and different proportions expected in either normal or precocious pubertal females. Pelvic ultrasound is useful if an ovarian lesion is suspected (i.e., hormonally active ovarian cyst or tumor leading to pseudoprecocious puberty). One author reported that ovarian cysts in girls with premature thelarche look different from those of girls with precocious puberty. In premature thelarche, cysts are isolated or nonexistent, whereas in precocious or normal puberty, cysts are multiple.[14]

This observation has not been applied to a large number of patients, and its clinical utility has not been established.

The prognosis for patients with premature thelarche is excellent. If the child is younger than 2 years, the breast tissue regresses. In an older child, breast development may regress or persist.[15] In either case, normal puberty occurs at the appropriate age.

The mechanism of premature thelarche is intriguing. A number of theories have been put forward, including increased breast sensitivity to estrogen, transient estrogen-secreting follicular cysts of the ovaries, increased estrogen from adrenal precursors, increased dietary estrogen, and transient partial activation of the hypothalamic-pituitary-ovarian axis with excessive FSH secretion. This last theory appears most likely and is supported by a number of studies.[13, 14, 16–18]

It is important to differentiate premature thelarche from precocious puberty in girls who present with early breast development. Premature thelarche is a transient and benign condition that is diagnosed by exclusion. Precocious puberty is progressive and may have a serious underlying origin and sequelae. Clinically, these conditions may be distinguished by examining growth, bone age, vaginal maturation index and/or serum estradiol levels, course, presence of other hormonal effects, and clinical or laboratory exclusion of primary hypothyroidism. The laboratory findings in normal young girls are compared with those in girls with premature thelarche and precocious puberty in Table 36–2. When precocious puberty is suspected from clinical and/or laboratory findings, further evaluation is indicated to look for an underlying cause. Which studies are indicated depends on the results of the initial clinical assessment. In isosexual precocity, brain imaging using computerized tomography (coronal views) or magnetic resonance should be performed to rule out a central nervous system mass lesion. Signs of virilization mandate evaluation for excessive androgen production, which is nearly always of adrenal or ovarian origin. Patients suspected of having precocious puberty should be appropriately evaluated and followed closely (see Chapter 6). Although most cases of isosexual precocious puberty in girls are idiopathic, the psychological manifestations of early pubertal development, as well as the potential for short stature from prematurely fused epiphyses, demand careful follow-up by a physician familiar with this condition. In addition, malignant or benign tumors (more often of the ovary than of the adrenal) may present as precocious puberty and require surgical intervention for diagnosis and therapy.

THE BREAST AT PUBERTY

Thelarche is defined as the onset of breast development in females. The normal age range for thelarche is 8 to 14 years, with a mean age of 11 years. Thelarche is usually the first sign of puberty and is followed within 6 months by pubarche and within 2 to 4 years by menarche. It is not uncommon for asynchronous breast development to occur, in which case the second breast may not begin to develop until as long as 6 months after the first. Appearance of sex hair before thelarche is also normal and not uncommon. The stages of breast development have been described by Marshall and Tanner, who provide an excellent classification system for evaluating pubertal progress.[1] The Tanner staging criteria are presented in Appendix B. Absence of breast development at age 13 years is of concern and at 14 years is abnormal and should be evaluated. Family history is pertinent to predicting the age of thelarche in girls.

When delayed thelarche is diagnosed, the initial evaluation should be directed toward determining whether this is an isolated abnormality or is associated with other delays and abnormalities in puberty. Specifically, height, growth velocity, presence of sex hair, body habitus, and virilization should be assessed. In addition, associated congenital anomalies, particularly those of the cardiovascular and genitourinary systems, should be sought. Stigmata of syndromes, particularly Turner's syndrome or other forms of gonadal dysgenesis and karyotypic abnormalities, must be sought. This initial evaluation should lead to a more extensive and directed evaluation for disorders of puberty. Referral to a pediatric endocri-

nologist is recommended. For a more extensive discussion of delayed puberty, the reader is referred to Chapter 6.

ABNORMALITIES OF THE ADOLESCENT FEMALE BREAST

Congenital anomalies of the breast, as described in the section on infancy and childhood, may first be recognized in an adolescent. This is a time when the patient is usually quite aware of her anatomy, particularly secondary sex characteristics. It is important to address the psychological and the physical aspects of developmental or congenital abnormalities of the breast.

ANATOMIC ABNORMALITIES

Asymmetry of the breast is common and may be clinically detectable in most patients (Fig. 36–4). Most often the larger breast is ipsilateral with the patient's dominant hand. After examination to exclude any pathologic explanation for the asymmetry (e.g., a breast mass or unilateral hypoplasia), most adolescents simply need reassurance if the asymmetry is apparent to them. Improvement may occur with maturation. When the degree of asymmetry and the patient's body image are of great concern, instruction to improve cosmetic appearance is appropriate. For many, a padded bra and a swim suit with a padded bra often are adequate to achieve the desired result. Others may require a breast prosthesis in the form of a foam insert. Patients with significant asymmetry should be followed through puberty, and, once breast development is complete (Tanner stage 5), surgery may be a consideration. Either unilateral reductive mammoplasty or augmentative mammoplasty may be

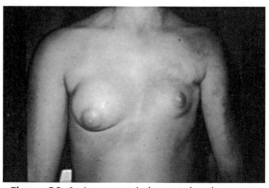

Figure 36–4. Asymmetric breast development.

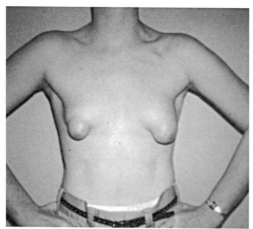

Figure 36–5. Tuberous breasts.

preferred. Some of the prostheses used in augmentation mammoplasty can be inserted relatively early and, using a valve device, enlarged to correspond to the growth of the nonoperative breast. This is particularly useful in managing patients with unilateral breast hypoplasia or aplasia. Bilateral breast hypoplasia, with normal maturation but insufficient final breast volume, may also be amenable to bilateral augmentative mammoplasty. These patients should be allowed to achieve adequate maturation before surgery is undertaken so that natural growth can be optimized.

Another developmental abnormality is tuberous breast deformity (Fig. 36–5). These patients have a small breast volume and appear to have a protuberant and overdeveloped areola. Depending on the severity of the deformity and the patient's perception, plastic surgery may be indicated. These patients are not readily staged using the Tanner system, so other criteria may be applied to determine the optimal time for surgery (i.e., course, pubertal staging, menarche, growth, bone age).

Inverted nipples can occur, and diagnosis can be made once the breasts are Tanner stage 5. Although this can be a cosmetic problem, surgical correction may prevent the ability to breast feed. The decision for surgically addressing a breast anomaly must carefully take into account not only the risks and cost of surgery and anesthesia but the realistic limitations of the result and the potential psychological advantages of improved appearance.

BREAST ATROPHY

Breast size and shape are controlled by a number of variables, including genetic factors.

Because breasts are composed largely of fatty tissue, there is an association between breast size and weight. Significant weight loss may result in decreased breast volume. Breast atrophy can also result from other causes, including hypoestrogenism and virilization syndromes. When systemic disease results in breast atrophy, it is because of associated weight loss, catabolic state, or hypoestrogenism. Scleroderma may produce localized changes leading to atrophy of the breast.

JUVENILE OR VIRGINAL HYPERTROPHY

The terms *virginal hypertrophy* and *juvenile hypertrophy* are used interchangeably and refer to pathologic overgrowth of the breast (Fig. 36–6). This condition may involve one or both breasts and may be familial. Deciding when breasts are too large is subjective, but some patients with juvenile or virginal hypertrophy develop enlargement so extreme that they suffer physical as well as psychological consequences. Massive and rapid enlargement of the breasts may result in pain, hypovascularization, tissue necrosis, and even rupture of the skin. Even without these serious physical consequences, the psychosocial aspects of massive breast enlargement can be significant, and these patients often require sympathetic and expert psychological intervention. Of 24 patients with juvenile hypertrophy who underwent reductive mammoplasty in one published series, 10 had more than 500 gm of breast tissue excised.[19]

Clinically, virginal or juvenile hypertrophy is a subjective diagnosis, but there are distinctive histologic changes in the breasts of these pa-

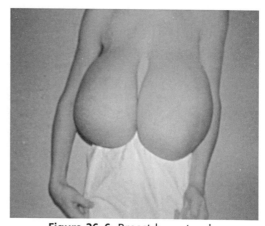

Figure 36–6. Breast hypertrophy.

tients. Interestingly, the histopathologic findings are similar to those of gynecomastia in males. Some patients have benefited from medical treatment with danazol,[20] but experience is limited. Reductive mammoplasty can be an important therapeutic modality for these patients to prevent or treat the physical or psychological consequences of massive breast enlargement.

BREAST PAIN

Breast pain (mastalgia or mastodynia) may occur in adolescents. Causes include puberty, estrogen therapy, trauma, hypertrophy, infection, and mammary dysplasia. Sometimes, breast pain is the result of physical activity, particularly running, which produces discomfort from friction and jarring. Pain, injuries, and other problems of the breast are particularly common in adolescent athletes and are reviewed in *Adolescent Medicine*.[21] Oral contraceptives, especially higher-dose preparations, have stimulated breast growth and caused pain. Sometimes it is necessary to discontinue or decrease the dose of estrogen. Symptomatic relief of breast pain may be provided with analgesics, nonsteroidal antiinflammatory medications, and supportive measures. A properly fitted bra that provide good support can be useful. Nonspecific breast pain has been treated with oral vitamin E preparations, but there are few data to demonstrate the efficacy of this therapy. Some have even noted improvement in mastalgia when vitamin E was discontinued. Danazol and avoiding caffeine and dairy products have had some success in reducing the pain associated with mammary dysplasia.

MASTITIS AND BREAST ABSCESS

Although mastitis is most common in lactating women, this bacterial infection can also occur in nonlactating individuals, including adolescents. Breast trauma can result in infection. Plucking of areolar hair or sexual activity involving the breasts may lead to infection. Infection presents as erythematous, tender, warm induration of the breast. Fluctuance or failure of mastitis to resolve on medical management suggests an associated abscess. Systemic signs of infection may indicate the need for study, including blood cultures. The patient should be tested for pregnancy. When an abscess is suspected, breast ultrasound may be useful for diagnosis and has been used to guide therapeutic needle aspiration. Treatment of mastitis consists of warm compresses, supportive measures, and antibiotics. When outpatient antibiotic therapy is indicated, amoxicillin–clavulanate potassium (Augmentin), 500 mg orally tid for 10 days, provides good coverage of the most likely bacterial pathogens. Surgical drainage may be necessary when an abscess is present.

GALACTORRHEA AND NIPPLE DISCHARGE

When a patient presents with a breast discharge, galactorrhea (production of breast milk) may be confirmed with a Sudan stain of the discharge for fat. The differential diagnosis of milk production includes pregnancy, lactation, hyperprolactinemia, hypothyroidism, and benign galactorrhea. Patients with hyperprolactinemia should have a magnetic resonance head study with pituitary views to look for pituitary adenoma. Other causes of idiopathic nipple discharge include pus-producing infection; intraductal papillomatosis, which usually produces a bloody serous fluid; breast cyst; and secretions from areolar glands. When a breast discharge in a nonlactating female presents with concerning features (e.g., blood, underlying mass, skin changes, or history of neoplasia or chest radiation), further evaluation is indicated. The color of the breast discharge is not a good predictor of histologic findings.[22] A nonbloody discharge without an underlying mass and no apparent endocrine-related cause may eventually resolve spontaneously.

BREAST MASSES IN ADOLESCENTS

The detection of a breast mass by an adolescent or her physician provokes significant anxiety. Single or multiple fibroadenomas are the most common mass lesions of the breast. Fibrocystic disease is the second most common one—cysts, sclerosing adenosis, parenchymal fibrosis, and duct ectasia. Proliferative breast disease may also present as one or more masses and includes the diagnoses of papillomatosis and intraductal papillomas. Other causes of breast masses include hemangioma, intramammary lymph node, fat necrosis, abscess, localized mastitis, hematoma, and malignant neoplasm. Relative frequencies of breast disease treated surgically are listed in Table 36–3.

A variety of benign tumors can involve the breasts of adolescent females. Neoplasms and

Table 36–3. Incidence of Breast Disease of Various Causes Based on Surgical Diagnoses

	No.	Age (yr)	Fibroadenoma (%)	Fibrocystic or Proliferative Disease (%)	Infection (%)	Malignancy (%)
Goldstein and Miller[23]	51	8–20	81	12	1	0
Ligon et al.[24]	249	11–30	67	15		2
Bower et al.[25]	134	0–16	76	3	7	1
Stone et al.[26]	143	11–20	72	6	3	1
Gogas et al.[27]	63	10–20	67	14	8	5
Daniel and Mathews[28]	95	12–21	94	2	2	0
Turbey et al.[29]	42	12–18	71		19	0
Simmons and Wold[19]	185	11–17	54	24	1	2

Totals do not equal 100%, because not all diagnoses are reported here.

cysts may originate from the breast tissue itself or from anatomically related tissues such as lymph nodes.

FIBROADENOMA

Fibroadenomas account for more than half of breast masses in adolescent females. In surgical series, as many as 95% of breast masses have been fibroadenomas. Clinically, this benign neoplasm is well-defined, nontender, mobile, and most often found in the upper outer quadrants of the breasts. Although most often solitary, 10% to 15% are multiple. When followed through one or more menstrual cycles, they may remain constant in size or increase slightly to moderately. Occasionally these tumors will grow extremely large (>500 gm) and are then called *giant fibroadenomas*, which can result in changes of the overlying skin, including a prominent venous pattern, pressure necrosis, and even ulceration. When the mass is large or growing, surgical excision is recommended to rule out a malignancy and to prevent significant cosmetic consequences of the fibroadenoma's replacing and compressing breast tissue. Adolescents with a fibroadenoma tend to have very good recovery of breast size and shape after surgery, as the previously compressed breast tissue tends to fill in the defect with time. For that reason, breast prostheses are not generally recommended after excision of a fibroadenoma.

History of fibroadenoma in adults has been shown to increase later risk for breast cancer, but only for patients with complex fibroadenoma (adjacent benign proliferative disease, cysts, sclerosing adenosis, epithelial calcifications, or papillary apocrine changes), where the risk was about three-fold greater. No increased risk for breast cancer was found in two thirds of the patients, those with simple fibroadenoma.[30] It is not known whether a fibroadenoma in adolescence confers increased risk of breast carcinoma later in life, nor whether excision of the fibroadenoma affects that risk. At present, there are no data to support excision of a fibroadenoma from an adolescent's breast to lower later risk of breast cancer.

CYSTOSARCOMA PHYLLOIDES

A less common condition that is sometimes clinically confused with fibroadenoma is cystosarcoma phylloides. Like fibroadenoma, this tumor tends to be firm, nontender, and well-defined; it is usually slow-growing. Imaging may not distinguish cystosarcoma phylloides.[31] When it is suspected or cannot be differentiated from a fibroadenoma, excision is indicated. Although most such lesions are benign, some are malignant and some metastasize. Malignant phylloides tumors vary in their biologic behavior, and this behavior cannot be entirely predicted by histologic finding. Infiltrative tumor borders and positive surgical margins have been shown to be the best histologic predictors of local recurrence, and mitotic activity the most important predictor of metastatic potential.[32]

FIBROCYSTIC AND PROLIFERATIVE DISEASE

Fibrocystic and proliferative disease may also be manifested as a breast mass in adolescents. After fibroadenoma, these are the most common surgical diagnoses in adolescent breast disease (Fig. 36–7). Clinically, these patients sometimes present with an otherwise asymptomatic breast mass, but they often complain of pain or tenderness of the breast, particularly premenstrually. Disease may be focal or diffuse and bilateral.

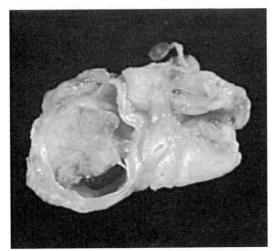

Figure 36–7. Biopsy of a fibrocystic lesion.

Following these patients through one or two menstrual cycles often demonstrates resolution of the mass. Papillomatosis may present as a large mass that is clinically indistinguishable from cystosarcoma phylloides or fibroadenoma.[33] If a cystic mass is suspected and persists, fine-needle aspiration (FNA) is useful. Aspiration is discussed further in the section on evaluation of breast masses in adolescents. The proliferative disease of intraductal papilloma or papillomatosis may be associated with a bloody discharge from the nipple. Although usually benign, these proliferative diseases can be premalignant.

BREAST MALIGNANCY IN ADOLESCENT FEMALES

Most clinical experience with breast neoplasms is with adult women who have breast carcinoma. Only 0.2% of patients with carcinoma of the breast are younger than 25 years.[28, 34] The incidence of breast cancer in females younger than 20 years is 0/1,000,000 per year.[35] Medical knowledge of primary carcinomas of the breast of adolescents consists of only a few case reports. Therefore, when considering an adolescent with a breast mass, it is important to keep in mind the very low incidence of breast cancer in this population and not to translate experience from adult women directly to younger females.

Risk factors for breast carcinoma (based predominantly on studies of adults) include chest radiation[36] and chronic anovulation.[37] The issue of whether unopposed estrogen therapy may increase the risk of breast cancer is the subject of a number of studies and remains unresolved.[38–41]

Breast cancer has been reported in two women in their twenties who had received chest radiation as children.[36] Even if the risk is increased with unopposed estrogen, the latency period for breast cancer after unopposed estrogen is 15 to 20 years, so presentation during adolescence is not likely. However, controversial data from postmenopausal women on the protective effect of progestin added to estrogen therapy[42] may be applicable to young patients requiring estrogen therapy to reduce the risk of endometrial or breast carcinoma later in life.

In the rare child or adolescent with breast carcinoma, the lesion tends to present as an asymptomatic nodule adjacent to, but discrete from, the nipple (Fig. 36–8).[43] Only 17 cases of breast carcinoma have been reported in patients 15 years old or younger.[5] The natural history of these tumors is not well-defined because of their rarity. Both disseminating carcinoma and carcinomas in young patients that seemed less aggressive than expected have been reported.[44]

Malignant phylloides tumors have been reported in adolescents. Although these neoplasms are usually benign, they can be malignant and can disseminate via hematogenous spread, most often to the lungs. Because this neoplasm is rare in young persons, little is known about its natural history. Its biologic behavior cannot reliably be predicted from its histologic appearance. Malignant cystosarcoma phylloides tumors are treated aggressively with surgery, radiation, chemotherapy, and sometimes hormonal manipulation.

Malignancies of the breast in adolescents are more likely to be something other than carcinoma. Rhabdomyosarcoma, lymphoma, neuroblastoma, acute leukemia, and other primary ma-

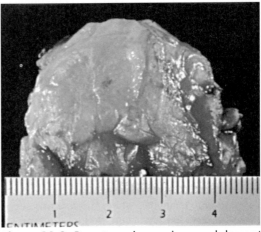

Figure 36–8. Breast carcinoma in an adolescent female.

lignant neoplasms have been reported. Alveolar rhabdomyosarcoma may pose a particular risk for metastasis to the breast.[45, 46] In the Mayo Clinic experience of four adolescents with malignancies of the breast, none were primary carcinoma. The breast mass was the presenting complaint and the source of tissue diagnosis in three of the four. In the fourth patient, the breast mass appeared 3 years after metastatic rhabdomyosarcoma had been diagnosed.[19]

The presentation of malignancies other than carcinoma in the breast of the adolescent can be dramatic. The mass is usually nontender, fixed, and associated with overlying skin changes, including prominent vascularity, dimpling, or ulceration. In addition, there may be other clinical features suggestive of malignancy, including constitutional symptoms (i.e., fever, weight loss, malaise), lymphadenopathy, hepatosplenomegaly, or masses elsewhere. However, these associated findings and mass characteristics are not universally present in breast cancer; so, an enlarging mass should arouse concern and consideration for biopsy.

Intraductal papilloma or papillomatosis of the breast is rare in young persons. A benign condition, it can be premalignant. The variant of juvenile papillomatosis has been reported to be linked with a high risk of breast carcinoma in the patient's family.[47] These masses may be associated with a bloody discharge from the nipple, which is often the presenting complaint. Patients with papilloma or papillomatosis should be followed carefully for malignant transformation.

Most breast disease in adolescence does not require surgery, as it is benign and self-limited; however, in cases of abscess, hypertrophy, or mass resulting in destruction of breast architecture, or suspected malignancy, surgery is indicated.

Although breast cancer is rare in adolescents and is less likely to be carcinoma than another malignant neoplasm, it does occur and should influence the evaluation and management of breast masses and the health maintenance practices and education for this population.

EVALUATION OF BREAST MASSES IN ADOLESCENT FEMALES

Careful history taking and physical examination by an experienced clinician generally lead to the correct diagnosis of a breast mass in an adolescent female. When the diagnosis is questionable or the extent of the disease requires

better definition, imaging techniques can be extremely useful, and when these findings are coupled with the clinical examination, nearly all patients can be diagnosed without—or before—operative intervention. Key features of the clinical evaluation are listed in Table 36–4.

HISTORY

The history for an adolescent female with a breast mass should include questions about previous or intercurrent malignancy, as malignant breast disease may be metastatic or a second primary lesion. Other risk factors for breast cancer include chest radiation, and, in adults at least, chronic anovulation. The association between unopposed estrogen therapy and breast cancer in adults is not entirely resolved. A history of constitutional symptoms—weight loss, fever, sweats, pain elsewhere, malaise, nausea, anorexia—suggests malignancy or infection. The menstrual history should be obtained and the possibility of pregnancy investigated. Any history of trauma should be elicited, as trauma may lead to mastitis, breast abscess, hematoma, or fat necrosis. Occasionally, the history of trauma is a "red her-

Table 36–4. Clinical Evaluation of Breast Masses in Adolescent Females

History
  Previous breast disease
    Previous or intercurrent malignancy
    Chest radiation
    Unopposed estrogen
    Chronic anovulation
    Constitutional symptoms
  Menstrual history
  Pregnancy
  Trauma
  Mass history
    Duration
    Size change
    Precipitating factors
  Nipple discharge
  Family history
Physical examination
  Complete, general
  Visual breast inspection
  Expressible nipple discharge
  Mass characteristics
    Location
    Consistency
    Mobility
    Cystic/fluctuance
    Tenderness
    Warmth
  Lymph nodes
  Hepatosplenomegaly
  Signs of malignancy

ring" and has just called attention to a preexisting mass. Areolar hair follicle disruption may lead to mastitis or abscess formation. A history of hair plucking, sexual activity involving the areola, or other areolar trauma should be obtained. With respect to the mass itself, it is important to ask about duration, size change, and any precipitating factors. A history of nipple discharge raises the possibility of galactorrhea, lactation, malignancy, papillomatosis, or infection. Family history is important in that patients with close relatives, especially the mother or sister, with breast carcinoma are at greater risk and may develop the disease earlier in life than the relative did.[48]

PHYSICAL EXAMINATION

The physical examination should be a complete, general evaluation. The breasts should be inspected visually for asymmetry, mass effect, and overlying skin changes. Dimpling of the skin, a prominent venous pattern, and ulceration are worrisome and raise the likelihood of malignancy. Pressure should be applied to the breast to express nipple discharge. A clear or mucoid discharge from the nipple can be studied with a Sudan stain for fat to identify milk. The presence of breast milk (galactorrhea) may suggest pregnancy, lactation, hypothyroidism, hyperprolactinemia, or benign galactorrhea. Although, with the exception of mastitis in a lactating female, conditions resulting in galactorrhea would not be expected to result in a breast mass, it is important to rule out an intercurrent condition when galactorrhea is present. A serosanguineous nipple discharge may be associated with breast infection, inflammation, papillomatosis, or malignancy. Examination of the mass itself provides much useful information about its cause. Palpation to distinguish a cystic lesion from a solid one may be augmented by transillumination of the mass. The location of the mass in the breast may also give a clue to its cause. The most common breast mass, fibroadenoma, is usually located in the upper outer breast quadrant. Most breast abscesses appear under or extend from the area under the areola. It can be difficult to localize precisely a mass palpated during breast examination. For instance, a mass lesion of an underlying rib or the anterior chest wall may appear to be a breast mass.

Imaging techniques and palpation both may be necessary to define the structure of origin of a breast mass. Most benign breast masses are well defined, discrete, and mobile. Fibroadeno-

mas, in particular, may seem encapsulated. Tenderness of the mass should also be assessed by history and physical examination. Most fibroadenomas are nontender, as are most malignant lesions. Tissue involved with mastitis, with or without abscess formation, is likely to be tender, as are areas that were recently traumatized. Warmth and erythema also suggest mastitis. Fluctuance on palpation suggests abscess or cyst.

Examination of the lymph nodes is very important and should not be limited to the axillas, as malignancies of the breast may be associated with lymphatic spread elsewhere, including to the supraclavicular area. The abdomen should be palpated for hepatosplenomegaly, and the patient should be examined for any signs of malignancy elsewhere, including mass lesions.

When a cystic lesion of the breast is suspected, consideration should be given to diagnostic aspiration. This can usually be accomplished atraumatically in the office setting. A simple cyst, most likely associated with fibrocystic disease, should diminish with aspiration. When aspiration does not result in disappearance of the cyst or when other findings suggest malignancy, the aspirated breast fluid should be sent for cytologic analysis. Sometimes, these cysts are complex or multiple, and simple aspiration does not result in complete resolution. Persistence or recurrence of a mass after aspiration or obtaining fluid that is bloody or cytologically abnormal mandates excisional biopsy because of the risk of cancer.

Fine-needle aspiration (FNA) of breast masses in adolescents was recently studied and appears to offer some value in reducing the need for open surgery.[49] Particularly in patients with large, persistent, or growing masses, FNA and ultrasound may be useful in establishing the diagnosis. The physician should consider, though, whether the results of the FNA would not obviate surgical excision or determine therapy. In a patient with known malignancy who develops a breast mass, FNA may be useful for establishing the nature of the mass if surgery is not indicated or possible. However, in this situation a negative biopsy result may not be considered definitive.

Further study, particularly long-term studies, are needed to establish specific recommendations about the indications, sensitivity, and specificity of FNA in the evaluation of adolescents' breast masses. Growing experience with imaging techniques in young patients is encouraging.

Other diagnostic studies may be indicated if malignancy is suspected; these should be tailored to the individual patient.

IMAGING IN THE ADOLESCENT WITH A BREAST MASS

Imaging of the adolescent with a breast mass varies from that of the mature woman because of the extremely uncommon occurrence of breast malignancy in this younger population.[50] The need to diagnose or exclude malignancy is not as compelling as in older women. If a breast mass appears clinically benign by examination and history, the clinician may elect to follow the patient closely but conservatively without imaging studies. Imaging studies are indicated in the diagnostic workup of a breast mass that is persistent, growing, painful, fixed, hard, associated with overlying skin changes, or otherwise clinically worrisome. Even in an adolescent with a breast mass and a positive family history of breast cancer, imaging should be based on the clinical examination because of the rare occurrence of breast carcinoma in this age group.

Various imaging modalities may be helpful in the diagnostic evaluation of breast masses. These include mammography, ultrasonography, plain radiography, and computed tomography.

MAMMOGRAPHY

The type and sequence of imaging studies depend on the clinical presentation. Mammography is usually the initial imaging choice in most adult women. It has proven very useful in the detection of clinically occult lesions and has helped to characterize palpable masses. Because breast malignancies are rare in adolescents, there is no reason to perform breast screening in this age group. Mammography is also of limited value in adolescents with a breast mass. The developing breast is usually dense on mammograms,[51] and a discrete mass in an adolescent may be obscured on mammography by this surrounding dense, normal tissue. Breast tissue in developing adolescents is composed primarily of dense fibroglandular tissue with a minimal component of fatty tissue (Fig. 36–9). Fatty tissue supplies low-

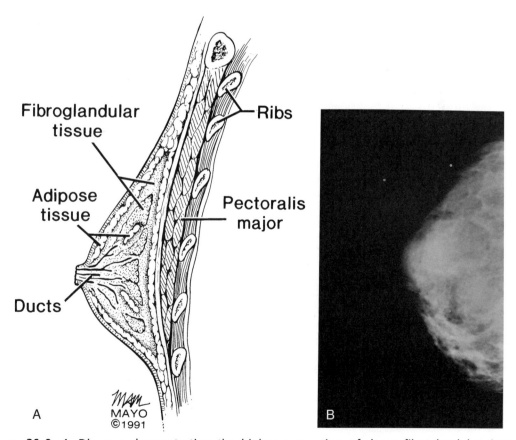

Figure 36–9. *A,* Diagram demonstrating the higher proportion of dense fibroglandular tissue in relation to the scant adipose tissue in the adolescent breast. *B,* Mammogram demonstrating the diffusely dense breast of the adolescent.

density contrast to the denser fibroglandular tissue. During a woman's lifetime, the proportion of adipose tissue increases, making mammography useful for mature women.

Adolescents with breast masses in whom mammography may be helpful include those with large breasts that are difficult to examine and image using other modalities, patients with diffuse breast disease, and patients at high risk for developing breast cancer or breast metastasis. This last group includes patients who have undergone high-dose chest irradiation for previous malignancy and those with a known or history of malignancy.[19]

If a mass can be visualized mammographically, it is evaluated by the same criteria used for adults. Signs of a benign lesion include a well-defined border, round or oval shape, and uniform density. Signs suggesting malignancy include an irregular, poorly defined border that fades into the surrounding normal breast tissue, a stellate or spiculated shape, and clusters of punctate, irregular calcifications. Secondary signs of malignancy include skin thickening and retraction, architectural distortion of the parenchyma, and enlarged regional lymph nodes.

State-of-the-art mammography using high-resolution film/screen combination delivers a mean glandular dose of 200 mrad to each breast for a two-view study. This is a low level of exposure, equivalent to the amount of background radiation to the breast received by women living in the upper elevations of Colorado for a year.

For asymptomatic adolescent girls, mammography is not an appropriate screening tool. There may be a few patients for whom mammography might contribute to the diagnosis, those with a high risk of breast cancer (including metastasis to the breast) whose breast size and maturity are amenable to mammographic examination.

ULTRASONOGRAPHY

Breast sonography is valuable for determining the cystic or solid nature of a palpable mass. The density of the developing breast does not affect the sensitivity of ultrasound in identifying masses. The sonographic characteristics of a simple cystic mass are smooth, sharp margins; absence of internal echoes; and posterior acoustic enhancement (i.e., increased echoes beneath the mass; Fig. 36–10).[52] Cysts may be multiple in number, round or lobular, or contain internal septations. Complex cystic masses meet some but not all of the criteria for simple cysts. They may be partly solid and partly cystic or contain inter-

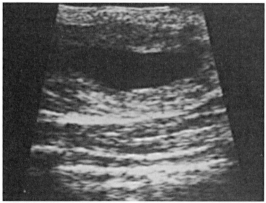

Figure 36–10. Ultrasonogram of a simple cyst. The wall is smooth, with no internal echoes and enhancement of the posterior echoes.

nal echoes (Fig. 36–11). The differential diagnosis of complex cystic masses includes cysts with internal debris, pus, or blood; intracystic papilloma; hematoma; and abscess.

If the mass meets the criteria for a cyst, whether simple or complex, aspiration may be helpful. Percutaneous aspiration can be performed under ultrasound guidance. The needle can be visualized and guided accurately into the cyst, and the cyst can be imaged as it is evacuated.[52] Ultrasound is also helpful in defining the extent of breast abscess.

Fibroadenomas, the most common breast mass in adolescents, often have a typical sonographic appearance. They tend to be hypoechoic and homogeneous, with smooth margins (Fig. 36–12).[53] They are usually 2 to 3 cm in size and are multiple in 10% to 15% of patients (Fig. 36–13). Some fibroadenomas seen on ultrasound may not be detected on mammograms because of the normally increased density of the adolescent's breast. The diagnosis of fibroadenoma can be suggested, but not confirmed, by the sonographic appearance. There is significant overlap

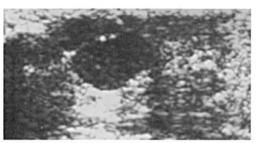

Figure 36–11. Ultrasonogram of a complex cyst. There are multiple internal echoes, thought to represent a focal area of fat necrosis.

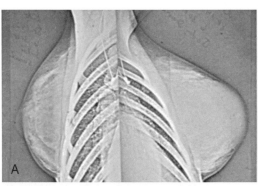
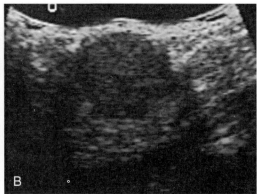

Figure 36–12. *A,* Fibroadenoma. *B,* Ultrasonogram of a partially defined, homogeneous, hypoechoic mass in the subareolar region. At surgery this was found to be a fibroadenoma.

between the sonographic appearances of benign and malignant solid masses.

Assessment of breast masses in patients known to have cancer is another potential use of ultrasound. The sonographic characteristics of lesions metastic to the breast may differentiate them from benign breast lesions. Ultrasound appears to be more helpful than mammography in patients with known malignancy when metastasis to the breast is suspected.[54]

Sonography may help to predict whether the mass will resolve spontaneously or persist. In one small series, teens found to have a solid breast mass on ultrasound did not experience resolution on follow-up examination at mean 7 months; whereas half of those with a normal ultrasound or fibrocystic changes had resolution of the mass on follow-up.[55]

Ongoing developments in ultrasonographic technology may add to the value of this modality for the evaluation of breast masses in adolescents. Particular forms of ultrasound may prove

to be more accurate than others for establishing the type of mass.[56]

PLAIN RADIOGRAPHY AND COMPUTED TOMOGRAPHY

Breast masses may, in fact, be chest wall lesions, particularly in thin adolescents. When the mass is found to be fixed to the chest wall on clinical examination, chest radiographs or high-resolution rib films may help to identify rib lesions. These lesions may be benign (e.g., an enchondroma or healing rib fracture), infectious (e.g., osteomyelitis), or malignant. Thin-section, high-resolution computed tomography (CT) is helpful in evaluating bony rib lesions and the overlying soft tissue (Fig. 36–14). Calcifications within the soft tissue may represent myositis ossificans from previous trauma. Extension of the CT through the chest and abdomen may reveal the full extent of an inflammatory or other lesion in a patient with a malignant-looking process. Biopsy can also be attempted under CT or fluoroscopic guidance.

COMPARISON OF BREAST IMAGING TECHNIQUES AND THEIR CLINICAL APPLICATION

Management of breast masses in adolescents is conservative and is based on clinical diagnosis and careful follow-up.[50, 57] Imaging studies are not routinely indicated but may be of use in diagnosis and management. Mammography is less useful than in adult women because of the nature of the dense fibroglandular tissue in adolescents and the low risk of breast cancer. Mam-

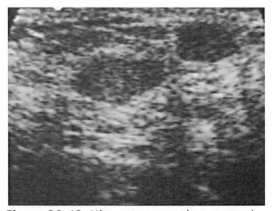

Figure 36–13. Ultrasonogram demonstrating multiple fibroadenomas.

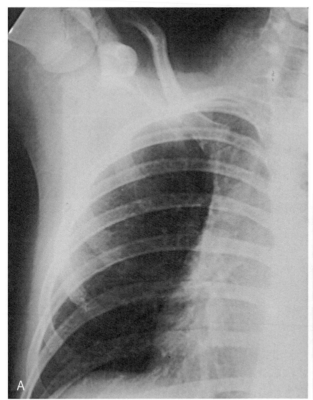
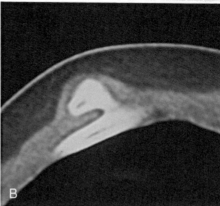

Figure 36–14. *A,* Radiograph demonstrating a subtle irregularity and increased density in the anterior fourth rib. *B,* Thin-section computed tomographic scan through the fourth rib demonstrates a small bony protuberance of the anterior rib. This is an enchondroma, a benign bone lesion.

mography plays a role in patients who have a mass and are at high risk for primary malignancy or metastasis. Ultrasonography is perhaps the most useful imaging modality for adolescent breast disease. It is easy to perform, is sensitive, and avoids radiation exposure. It is used most to confirm the cystic or solid nature of a mass. A chest wall mass is better evaluated with plain films, CT, or magnetic resonance imaging.

TEACHING THE ADOLESCENT BREAST SELF-EXAMINATION

The advent of routine breast self-examination has been important to the health of adult women. In well-intentioned efforts to improve the health of adolescents, many clinicians have advocated and practiced teaching the breast self-examination to their adolescent female patients. There are many reasons, in addition to detecting breast cancer, for promoting this practice. Proponents cite teaching the adolescent this technique as an opportunity to teach her about her own body, increase her level of comfort with her body, en-

hance her perception of the examiner as contributing to her health care, and provide a basis for discussion of a number of puberty- and sexuality-related issues. Although efforts to improve adolescent self-knowledge and health maintenance are admirable, data do not currently exist to support the utility of the breast self-examination in this population. There are no data to show that adolescents who have been taught or who practice breast self-examination detect breast tumors, including malignancy, more frequently or earlier. In a review of the reports on malignant tumors of the adolescent breast, there is no information to show that these tumors were detected by patients practicing breast self-examination. Breast self-examination in adults is designed primarily to detect breast carcinoma, and the incidence of carcinoma under age 20 is zero in 1,000,000.[35] Physicians must also consider any potential negative outcome of the breast self-examination in adolescents. Goldbloom has warned of the potential for increased anxiety, unnecessary physician visits, and more unnecessary surgery if breast self-examination is taught to a population of such low risk.[58] Because there are no long-term studies, the compliance during the higher-risk adult years in women who were taught breast self-examination during adolescence cannot reliably be predicted. Certainly, patients seen during adolescence may not receive ongoing care and may not have another opportunity to learn the technique and benefits of breast self-examination in her higher-risk, later years. It is also not known whether patients taught the breast self-examination during adolescence will maintain compliance or, after 20 years of detecting no disease, will discontinue the practice before they enter their higher-risk years.

At present, there are no data sufficient to establish the validity of teaching breast self-examination to the general population of adolescent females. While there is no established position or standard of care for breast self-examination for adolescents in the United States, both the World Health Organization[59] and the Canadian Task Force[60] do not recommend teaching women younger than 20 years to do breast self-exams.

There are certain high-risk patients who should be taught breast self-examination. Patients with a strong family history of breast carcinoma should be taught the breast self-examination in their late adolescent years, as they have a risk of developing carcinoma earlier in life than their affected relative did.[48] However, even in the presence of familial risk, onset of breast cancer is not expected in the teen years. Patients with a history of breast malignancy or a cancer that may metastasize to the breast should also be taught self-examination. Other high-risk patients include those with a history of radiation to the chest, breast papillomatosis, or breast cystosarcoma phylloides.

Given that many adolescents already have or will hear about self-examination of the breast, and in fact be counseled to practice it, when it is not to be taught or encouraged to the adolescent patient, an explanation for delaying the recommendation may well be warranted. Girls who have been taught the self-examination are unlikely to comply during adolescence.[61, 62] Supplying our patients with information on the rationale for and recommended time to institute the self-examination along with data about their risk of breast cancer may help them not only to anticipate their future health care needs but allay unnecessary anxiety. Women aged 18 years and older at least, overestimate their risk of breast cancer.[63] Encouraging ongoing primary or preventive health care may serve them better than premature instruction in self-examination, since having a source of routine medical care does correlate with breast cancer screening in adult life.[64]

REFERENCES

1. Marshall WA, Tanner JM: Variations in pattern of pubertal changes in girls. Arch Dis Child 1969; 44:291.
2. Dubowitz L, Dubowitz V: Gestational age of the newborn. Reading, Mass: Addison-Wesley, 1977.
3. McKiernan JF, Hull D: Prolactin, maternal estrogens, and breast development in the newborn. Arch Dis Child 1981; 56:770.
4. McKiernan JF, Hull D: Breast development in the newborn. Arch Dis Child 1981; 56:525–529.
5. Sutow WW, Fernbach DJ, Vietti TJ: Clinical Pediatric Oncology, 3rd ed. St. Louis: CV Mosby, 1984.
6. Speroff L, Glass RH, Kase NG: Clinical Gynecologic Endocrinology and Infertility, 4th ed. Baltimore: Williams & Wilkins, 1988.
7. VanWinter JT, Noller KL, Zimmerman D, Melton LJ III: Natural history of premature thelarche in Olmsted County, Minnesota, 1940–1984. J Pediatr 1990; 116(2):278–280.
8. Nelson KG: Premature thelarche in children born prematurely. J Pediatr 1983: 103(5):756.
9. D'Ambrosio F, Angiolillo M, Flauto U, et al: La mortalita pernatale e neonatale in Lombardia. Notizie Sanita 1981; 32:7.
10. Sa'enz de Rodriguez CA, Bongiovanni AM, Conde de Borrego L: An epidemic of precocious development in Puerto Rican children. J Pediatr 1985; 107(3):393–396.
11. Emans Herriott SJ, Goldstein DP: Pediatric and Adolescent Gynecology, 3rd ed. Boston: Little, Brown, 1990.
12. Radfar N, Ansusingha K, Kenny FM: Circulating bound and free estradiol and estrone during normal growth and development and in premature thelarche and isosexual precocity. J Pediatr 1976; 89(5):719.
13. Ilicki A, Prager Lewin R, Kauli R, et al: Premature thelarche—natural history and sex hormone secretion in 68 girls. Acta Paediatr Scand 1984, 73:756.
14. Stanhope R, Abdulwahid NA, Adams J, Brook CGD: Studies of gonadotrophin pulsatility and pelvic ultrasound examinations distinguish between isolated premature thelarche and central precocious puberty. Eur J Pediatr 1986; 145:190.
15. Pasquina AM, Tebaldi L, Cioschi L, et al: Premature thelarche: A follow-up study of 40 girls. Arch Dis Child 1985; 60:1180.
16. Beck W, Stubbe P: Pulsatile secretion of luteinizing hormone and sleep-related gonadotropin rhythms in girls with premature thelarche. Eur J Pediatr 1984; 141:168.
17. Pescovitz OH, Hench KD, Barnes KM, et al: Premature thelarche and central precocious puberty: The relationship between clinical presentation and the gonadotropin response to luteinizing hormone-releasing hormone. J Clin Endocrinol Metab 1988, 67(1):474.
18. Forest MG: Sexual maturation of the hypothalamus: Pathophysiological aspects and clinical implications. Acta Neurochir 1985; 75(104):23–42.
19. Simmons PS, Wold LE: Surgically treated breast disease in adolescent females: A retrospective review of 185 cases. Adolesc Pediatr Gynecol 1989; 2:95.
20. Taylor PJ, Cumming DC, Corenbluem B: Successful treatment of D-penicillamine–induced breast gigantism with danazol. Br Med J 1981; 282:362.
21. Greydanu DE, Patel DR, Baxter TL: The breast and

sports: Issues for the clinic. Adolesc Med 1998; 9(3):533–550.

22. Hou MF, Huang CJ, Huang YS, et al: Evaluation of galactography for nipple discharge. Clin Imaging 1998; 22(2):89–94.

23. Goldstein D, Miller V: Breast masses in adolescent females. Clin Pediatr 1982; 21:17.

24. Ligon R, Stevenson D, Diner W, et al: Breast masses in young women. Am J Surg 1980; 140:770.

25. Bower R, Bell M, Ternberg J: Management of breast lesions in children and adolescents. J Pediatr Surg 1976; 11:337.

26. Stone A, Shenker J, McCarthy K: Adolescent breast masses. Am J Surg 1977; 134:275.

27. Gogas J, Sechas M, Skalkeas G: Surgical management of diseases of the adolescent female breast. Am J Surg 1979; 137:634.

28. Daniel WA, Mathews MD: Tumors of the breast in adolescent females. Pediatrics 1968; 41(4):743.

29. Turbey W, Buntain W, Dudgeon D: The surgical management of pediatric breast masses. Pediatrics 1975; 56:736.

30. DuPont WD, Page DL, Fritz FP, et al: Long-term risk of breast cancer in women with fibroadenoma. N Engl J Med 1994; 331(1):10–15.

31. Iau PT, Lim TC, Png DJ, Tan WT: Phylloides tumour: An update of 40 cases. Ann Acad Medi Singapore 1998; 27(2):200–203.

32. Rajan PB, Cranor ML, Rosen PP: Cystosarcoma phylloides in adolescent girls and young women: A study of 45 patients. Am J Surg Pathol 1998; 22(1):64–69.

33. Farid MK, Sarma HN, Ramesh K, et al: Giant juvenile papillomatosis of the breast: Report of two cases. East Afri Med J 1997; 74(2):116–167.

34. Haagensen CD: Diseases of the Breast, 2nd ed. Philadelphia: WB Saunders, 1971.

35. Simmons PS, Melton JL: Presented at World Congress of Pediatric and Adolescent Gynecology, Helsinki, Finland, June 2–3, 1998. Incidence of breast cancer in female children and adolescents.

36. Ivins JC, Taylor WF, Wold LE: Elective whole-lung irradiation in osteosarcoma treatment: Appearance of bilateral breast cancer in two long-term survivors. Skeletal Radiol 1987; 16:133.

37. Coulam C, Annegers J, Kranz J: Chronic anovulation syndrome and associated neoplasia. Obstet Gynecol 1983; 61:403–407.

38. Korenman SG: The endocrinology of breast cancer. Cancer 1980; 46:876–878.

39. Hulka BS: Hormone-replacement and the risk of breast cancer. CA 1990; 40(5):289–296.

40. Dupont WD, Page DL: Menopausal estrogen replacement therapy and breast cancer. JAMA 1991; 265(15):1985–1990.

41. Steinberg KK, Thacker SB, Smith SJ, et al: A meta-analysis of the effect of estrogen replacement therapy on the risk of breast cancer. JAMA 1991; 265(15):1985–1990.

42. Gambrell RD, Maier R, Sanders B: Decreased incidence of breast cancer in postmenopausal estrogen-progestogen users. Obstet Gynecol 1983; 62:534–443.

43. Capraro VJ, Gallego MB: Breast disorders. Pediatr Ann 1975; 47:82.

44. McDevitt RW, Stewart FW: Breast carcinoma in children. JAMA 1966; 195:144.

45. Hays DM, Donaldson SS, Shimada H, et al: Primary and metastatic rhabdomyosarcoma in the breast: Neoplasms of adolescent females, a report from the Intergroup Rhabdomyosarcoma Study. Med Pediatr Oncol 1997; 29(3):181–189.

46. Kwan WH, Choi PH, Li CK, et al: Breast metastasis in adolescents with alveolar rhabdomyosarcoma of the extremities: Report of two cases. Pediatr Hematol Oncol 1996; 13(3):277–285.

47. Rosen PP, Kimmel M: Juvenile papillomatosis of the breast: A follow-up study of 41 patients having biopsies before 1979. Am J Clin Pathol 1990; 93:599–603.

48. Lynch HT, Guirgis H, Brodkey F, et al: Early age of onset in familial breast cancer. Arch Surg 1976; 111:126.

49. Pacinda SJ, Ramzy I: Fine-needle aspiration of breast masses. A review of its role in diagnosis and management in adolescent patients. J Adolesc Health 1998; 23(1):3–6.

50. Ferguson CM, Powell RW: Breast masses in young women. Arch Surg 1989; 124:1338–1341.

51. Hart BL, Steinbock RT, Mettler FA, et al: Age and race related changes in mammographic parenchymal patterns. Cancer 1989; 63:2537–2539.

52. Hackelor BJ, Dudo V, Lanth G: Ultrasound Mammography. New York: Springer-Verlag, 1989.

53. Fornage BD, Lorigan JG, Andry E: Fibroadenoma of the breast: Sonographic appearance. Radiology 1989; 172:671–675.

54. Chateil JF, Arboucalot F, Perel Y, et al: Breast metastases in adolescent girls: US findings. Pediatr Radiol 1998; 28(11):832–835.

55. Neinstein LS, Atkinson J, Diament M: Prevalence and longitudinal study of breast masses in adolescents. J Adolesc Health 1993; 13:277–281.

56. Wilkens TH, Burke BJ, Cancelada DA, Jatoi I: Evaluation of palpable breast masses with color Doppler sonography and gray scale imaging. J Ultrasound Med 1998; 17(2):109–115.

57. Diehl T, Kaplan DW: Breast masses in adolescent females. J Adolesc Health Care 1985; 6:353–357.

58. Goldbloom R: Self-examination by adolescents. Pediatrics 1985; 76(1);126.

59. World Health Organization: Self-examination in the Early Detection of Breast Cancer: A Report on a Consultation on Self-examination in Breast Cancer Early Detection Programmes. Geneva: World Health Organization, 1983.

60. Canadian Task Force on Periodic Health Examination: The periodic health examination: 2, 1998 update. Can Med Assoc J 1988; 138:617–626.

61. Cromer BA, Frankel ME, Hayes J, Brown RT: Compliance with breast self-examination instruction in high school students. Clin Pediatrics 1992; 31(4):215–220.

62. Cromer BA, Frankel ME, Keder LM: Compliance with breast self-examination instruction in healthy adolescents. J Adolesc Health Care 1989; 10(2):105–109.

63. McCaul KS, O'Donnell SM: Naïve beliefs about breast cancer risk. Womens Health 1998; 4(1):93–101.

64. Ettner SL: The timing of preventive services for women and children: The effect of having a usual source of care. Am J Public Health 1996; 86(12):1748–54.

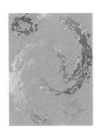

Chapter 37
Oncologic Problems

MICHAEL L. HICKS AND M. STEVEN PIVER

Advances in the management of childhood gynecologic malignancies have improved survival and have made possible less radical surgery and, in some instances, better preservation of fertility as compared with the 1970s. Malignancies, specific to pediatic and adolescent patients include pelvic rhabdomyosarcoma (RMS), diethylstilbestrol (DES)-related adenocarcinoma of the vagina and cervix, and germ cell and juvenile granulosa cell tumors of the ovary.

RHABDOMYOSARCOMAS

Sarcomas of gynecologic origin in the pediatric population are primarily RMS. These tumors, the most common soft tissue neoplasms of children, account for 4% to 8% of all malignant disease in children under 15, and they are the seventh leading cause of death among children.[1, 2] Genital and urinary tract RMS accounts for 20% of the cases in children and is the most common malignancy of the lower genital tract in young girls.[3, 4]

RMS originates from primitive or incompletely differentiated mesenchyme of the urogenital ridge.[5] There are five types: pleomorphic, embryonal, botryoid, alveolar, and undifferentiated. The embryonal variant botryoid sarcoma is the most common subtype of RMS presenting as a genital lesion.

Primary lesions of RMS can originate from the vagina, cervix, vulva, perineum, or uterus. All of the various sites of origin have different peaks of incidence during childhood; the lower genital lesions of the perineum, vulva, and vagina occur early in childhood, usually before age 2 years, and cervical or uterine lesions occur more frequently in the adolescent age group.

The clinical presentation in a pediatric or adolescent patient with RMS can be an enlarging vulvar, perineal, or vaginal lesion or a large polypoid mass protruding from the introitus of the vagina and resembling a bunch of grapes (Fig. 37–1). These lesions are usually clinically visible, but occasionally the only symptom the patient may present with is unexplained vaginal bleeding or, on examination, an abdominopelvic mass.

Before the 1970s, prognosis for those with this rare malignancy was extremely dismal. Initial approaches were individualized, but it was not until 1950 that Shackman reported the first successful use of total pelvic exenteration in a patient with RMS, followed by 2.5-year disease-free interval.[6] This report marked the beginning of the use of radical pelvic surgery for the treatment of RMS. However, even with ultraradical surgery, the survival rate before 1970 rarely exceeded 20%.[7] Attempts were made to improve survival using radiation, alone or in combination with radical pelvic surgery, but this was success-

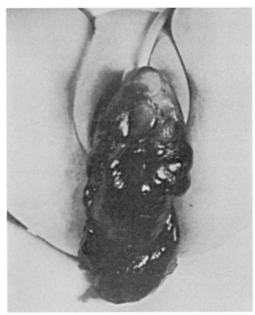

Figure 37–1. Response of vaginal botryoid sarcoma to preoperative combination therapy. This is a large hemorrhagic mass staged as nonresectable vaginal tumor (stage IIB). (From Kumar APM, Wrenn EL, Fleming ID, et al: Combined therapy to prevent complete pelvic exenteration for rhabdomyosarcoma of the vagina or uterus. Cancer 1976; 37:120.)

Table 37–1. Survival Rates Utilizing Multimodality Therapy for Rhabdomyosarcoma

Authors	No. of Patients	Treatment Regimen	Survival Rate	
Grosfeld et al.[13]	5	Surgery, RT, VAC	5/5	(100%)
Pratt et al.[17]	20	Surgery, RT, VAC	9/20	(45%)
Kilman et al.[15]	31	Surgery, RT, VA	28/31	(90%)
Piver et al.[16]	3	Surgery, RT, VA, VC	3/3	(100%)
Rivard et al.[18]	9	Surgery, RT, VAC	5/9	(56%)
Donaldson et al.[12]	19	Surgery, RT, VAC	14/19	(74%)
Heyn et al.[14]	28	Surgery, RT, VA	24/28	(86%)

RT, Radiation therapy; VA, vincristine, actinomycin D; VAC, vincristine, actinomycin D, cyclophosphamide.
From Hicks ML, Piver MS: Conservative surgery plus adjuvant therapy for vulvovaginal rhabdomyosarcoma, DES/clear cell adenocarcinoma of the vagina and unilateral germ cell tumors of the ovary. Obstet Gynecol Clin North Am 1992; 19(1):219.

ful only for microscopic disease limited to the margins of the resected lesion.[7–11]

Multimodality therapy began in the mid 1970s; this combined radical surgery, radiotherapy, and adjuvant chemotherapy and was noted to improve survival significantly (Table 37–1).[12–18] Later, the Intergroup Rhabdomyosarcoma Study Group evaluated the response to chemotherapy and radiotherapy in early stages of RMS (stages I and II) and the response to chemotherapy alone in advanced stages of RMS (stages III and IV) (Table 37–2). The authors concluded the following:

1. Combined vincristine, actinomycin D, and cyclophosphamide (VAC) therapy was an effective adjuvant for stage I disease with or without radiotherapy, resulting in 92% survival with no evidence of disease at 2 years in both groups.
2. VAC given over 2 years or vincristine and actinomycin D (VA) therapy given over 1 year, both with localized radiotherapy, were equally effective in patients with stage II disease (microscopic residual disease after surgery), with 85% of patients having no evidence of disease at 2 years.
3. Of patients with gross residual disease after surgery (stage III) or metastatic disease at the time of diagnosis (stage IV), 81% to 82% responded favorably to chemotherapy.[19]

Table 37–2. Staging Classification System for Rhabdomyosarcoma After Surgery for Primary Lesion

Stage I	Local disease only
Stage II	Microscopic residual disease in regional lymphatic or positive margins after surgery
Stage III	Gross residual disease after surgery
Stage IV	Distant metastasis

Although survival improved with multimodality therapy, young patients with RMS still underwent radical surgery requiring the removal of the uterus, fallopian tubes, ovaries, vagina, and rectum and occasionally a portion of the vulva (Figs. 37–2, 37–3). With the development of successful multimodality therapy and improvement in the survival rate, new approaches were explored in an attempt to avoid radical pelvic surgery and thus preserve the bladder, rectum, and reproductive organs of these young children.

The introduction of preoperative chemotherapy with VAC was initially reported by Kumar and associates, who were able to obtain complete regression of tumor when preoperative chemotherapy with VAC was followed by localized resection of vaginal RMS, with preservation of the bladder and rectum.[20] Later, Voute and associates reported their experience with 24 patients; 7 patients (29%) experienced complete remission after chemotherapy alone, requiring no surgical intervention, and 10 patients (42%) had no evidence of disease after preoperative chemotherapy and limited pelvic surgery, again showing the chemosensitivity of these tumors.[21] Other studies have shown the value of preoperative chemotherapy with the objectives of less radical surgery and organ preservation.[22, 23]

If complete regression of tumor is not obtained after VAC chemotherapy, with or without limited resection of the genital lesion, radical pelvic surgery may still be avoided. Flamant and colleagues reported that 15 of 17 young girls were cured of RMS of the vagina and vulva after treatment with incomplete excision followed by localized brachytherapy (intracavitary application or interstitial) and 18 months of alternating VAC and vincristine and adriamycin therapy. Twelve of the pubescent or postpubescent girls were followed for long-term sequelae; 11 had normal puberty, 11 had normal menses, and two eventu-

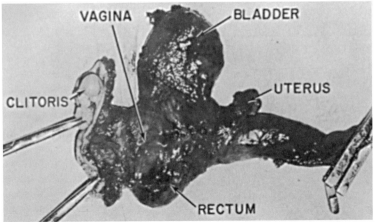

Figure 37–2. Specimen from a total pelvic exenteration in a 10-month-old patient with rhabdomyosarcoma of the vagina. A tumor involving the clitoris can be seen. (From Piver MS, Barlow JJ, Wang JJ, Shah NK: Combined radical surgery, radiation therapy and chemotherapy in infants with vulvovaginal embryonal rhabdomyosarcoma. Obstet Gynecol 1973; 42(4):524. Reprinted with permission from the American College of Obstetricians and Gynecologists.)

ally had a total of three healthy children.[24] Metastatic disease from rhabdomyosarcoma in a gynecologic presentation is rare; however, for more advanced stages of rhabdomyosarcomas, multiple agent chemotherapy with the incorporation of ifosfamide and etoposide are being utilized with some success.[25]

Currently, treatment for RMS should begin with tissue confirmation and staging to rule out systemic disease; this should include a chest ra-diograph and bone marrow aspiration. Primary therapy should consist initially of combination chemotherapy with VAC, and the response to chemotherapy should be monitored closely (Table 37–3). After rapid tumor regression with chemotherapy, conservative surgery can be attempted without compromising survival. In this way, most young children with the diagnosis of RMS will be able to experience preservation of the function of the rectum, bladder, vagina, and

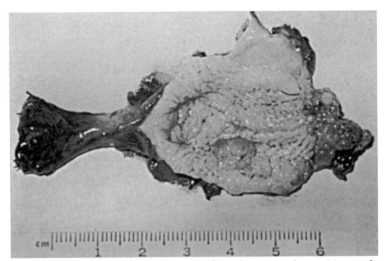

Figure 37–3. Specimen from a hysterectomy and total vaginectomy in an 11-month-old patient with rhabdomyosarcoma of the vagina and cervix. The entire vagina was involved with grapelike lesions of rhabdomyosarcoma. (From Piver MS, Barlow JJ, Wang JJ, Shah NK: Combined radical surgery, radiation therapy and chemotherapy in infants with vulvovaginal embryonal rhabdomyosarcoma. Obstet Gynecol 1973; 42(4):525. Reprinted with permission from the American College of Obstetricians and Gynecologists.)

Table 37–3. VAC Chemotherapy Regimen for Vulvovaginal Rhabdomyosarcoma

Drug	Dosage
Vincristine	2 mg/m² IV weekly × 12 courses
Actinomycin D	0.015 mg/kg/day IV × 5 courses at 12-week intervals
Cyclophosphamide	2.5 mg/kg/day PO daily × 90 weeks, beginning on the 7th week

From Hicks ML, Piver MS: Conservative surgery plus adjuvant therapy for vulvovaginal rhabdomyosarcoma, DES/clear cell adenocarcinoma of the vagina and unilateral germ cell tumors of the ovary. Obstet Gynecol Clin North Am 1992; 19(1):219.

ovaries, thereby allowing conservation of reproductive function.

CLEAR-CELL ADENOCARCINOMA OF THE VAGINA/CERVIX

Primary adenocarcinoma of the vagina or cervix has been reported infrequently in the pediatric age group.[26–29] In 1971, Herbst and associates reported eight cases of adenocarcinoma of the vagina, six in adolescents (ages 9 to 15).[30] This single report of vaginal adenocarcinoma exceeded the total of all documented cases in the world literature before 1945. More significantly, this report was the first to show the association of vaginal clear cell adenocarcinoma with intrauterine exposure to DES, which became commercially available in 1938 and was used principally in pregnant patients at high at risk for spontaneous abortion. Four months after the original report by Herbst, Roswell Park Cancer Institute reported five additional cases of adenocarcinoma of the vagina in daughters exposed to DES or other synthetic estrogens in utero.[31] After these two reports linking DES exposure to clear-cell adenocarcinoma of the vagina, the use of DES was banned by the U.S. Food and Drug Administration in 1971, and a registry was established to centralize and study epidemiologic, clinical, and pathologic findings of patients who develop adenocarcinoma of the vagina or cervix.

Herbst and Anderson have summarized their most recent findings from the Registry for Research on Hormonal Transplacental Carcinogenesis, which are as follows:[32]

1. Currently there are 594 reported cases of clear-cell adenocarcinoma of the vagina and cervix.
2. Of these patients, 80% were exposed to DES or similar synthetic estrogens in utero.
3. Patient age ranges from 7 to 34, with a median age of 20.
4. Seventy-five percent of the primary lesions are vaginal, and 25% are cervical.
5. Cervical lesions are located primarily on the exocervix, and vaginal lesions are mainly located on the upper third of the anterior vaginal wall.
6. Ninety percent were in early stages (stage I and stage II) at the time of diagnosis.
7. The risk of developing adenocarcinoma of the cervix or vagina in an exposed female from birth to 34 years of age is approximately 0.1% (or one case per 1000 women exposed), implying that these tumors are extremely rare among DES-exposed females and that DES is not a complete carcinogen.[32]

Treatment for early-stage clear-cell adenocarcinoma of the vagina and cervix has traditionally been with radical pelvic surgery (radical hysterectomy, pelvic lymphadenectomy, partial or total vaginectomy, and replacement of the vagina with a split-thickness skin graft). Radiation therapy (whole-pelvis radiotherapy and vaginal brachytherapy) has been used for more advanced stages, large bulky lesions, and in cases with extension to the lymphatic systems.[33–35]

The majority of cases (90% or more) of clear-cell adenocarcinoma of the vagina and cervix present as stage I or stage II disease, and the survival rate usually exceeds 90% (Fig. 37–4). To date, treatment has become more conservative. Wharton and colleagues reported on five patients with stage I or II clear-cell adenocarcinoma of the vagina or cervix who were treated entirely with transvaginal cone or interstitial irradiation. Four of the five were reported to be living without any evidence of disease 2 to 8 years after completion of therapy. The one nonsurvivor's death was related to pulmonary embolism, not to progression of disease.[36] Senekjian and associates reported on 219 cases of stage I vaginal clear-cell adenocarcinoma; 176 had radical therapy, and 43 had only localized therapy (wide local excision and/or local irradiation). The 5- and 10-year survival rates were equivalent in the two groups. In addition, a subgroup of patients receiving localized irradiation had a recurrence experience equal to that of the conventional therapy group (radical therapy), which was more favorable than that of patients undergoing local excision alone.[37] The authors concluded that to preserve reproductive function in young patients, the combination of wide local excision with retroperitoneal pelvic lymphadenectomy to rule out lymph node metastasis, followed by local radia-

Figure 37–4. Survival for each International Federation of Gynecology and Obstetrics stage for vaginal and cervical clear-cell adenocarcinoma over a span of 10 years. Stage I, n = 323; stage II, n = 79; stage IIA, n = 70; stage IIB, n = 26; stage III, n = 34; stage IV, n = 9. (From Herbst AL, Anderson D: Clear cell adenocarcinoma of the vagina and cervix secondary to intrauterine exposure to diethylstilbestrol. Semin Surg Oncol 1990; 6:345. Copyright © 1990. Reprinted by permission of Wiley-Liss, a division of John Wiley and Sons, Inc.)

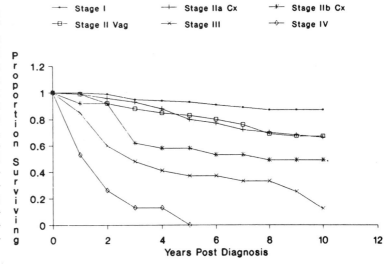

tion, is effective treatment for small (<2 cm) vaginal clear-cell adenocarcinomas.

OVARIAN GERM CELL TUMORS

Malignant germ cell tumors are a segment of human solid tumors in which there has been a significant improvement in survival with the introduction of combination chemotherapy. Although these tumors are rare, 60% to 70% of childhood gynecologic malignancies originate in the ovaries.

For purposes of therapy, these tumors can be divided into two classifications: pure dysgerminomas and nondysgerminomas (Table 37–4).

DYSGERMINOMAS

Of all the germ cell tumors of the ovaries, dysgerminomas are the most common. Dysgerminomas are the female homologue of seminomas of the testes. Microscopically, these tumors show sheets of polygonal cells with clear cytoplasm in a fibrous stroma infiltrated with lymphocytes (Fig. 37–5). They represent approximately 3% to 5% of all ovarian malignancies and occur primarily before age 30 (median age at occurrence, 17) years.

Dysgerminomas are usually unilateral but bilateral in approximately 15% of cases, in contrast to all other germ cell tumors of the ovaries, which are bilateral in only 1% of patients.[38–41] Although almost all patients with dysgerminomas have normal sexual development, in rare instances dysgerminomas have been associated with phenotypic females with dysgenetic gonads in such disorders as pure gonadal dysgenesis, testicular feminization, Turner's syndrome, and hermaphroditism.[42–46]

Tumor markers for dysgerminomas are usually absent. However, levels of human chorionic gonadotropin (hCG) have been noted to be elevated in isolated cases, in which they may contain syncytial giant cells that produce histochemically detectable amounts of hCG. Rarely, hCG production results in precocious puberty, and virilization may also occur, although infrequently, when dysgerminomas are admixed with gonadoblastomas owing to hormonal stimulation by the surrounding stroma. Lactic dehydrogenase (LDH) levels, especially fractions of LDH 1, 2, and 3, have been noted to be elevated in many cases of dysgerminoma.[42, 47–50]

Treatment of suspected dysgerminomas begins with complete exploration of the abdomen and pelvis followed by unilateral salpingo-oophorectomy. A frozen section sample should be obtained at the time of laparotomy to confirm the

Table 37–4. Germ Cell Tumors of the Ovary

Dysgerminoma
Nondysgerminoma tumors
  Endodermal sinus tumors
  Embryonal carcinoma
  Immature teratoma
  Choriocarcinoma
  Mixed germ cell tumors (any combination of
    dysgerminoma and nondysgerminoma)

From Hicks ML, Piver MS: Conservative surgery plus adjuvant therapy for vulvovaginal rhabdomyosarcoma, DES/clear cell adenocarcinoma of the vagina and unilateral germ cell tumors of the ovary. Obstet Gynecol Clin North Am 1992; 19(1):219.

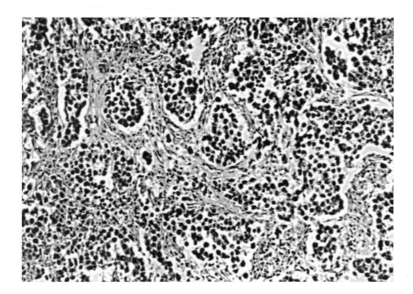

Figure 37–5. Dysgerminoma composed of islands of tumor cells surrounded by connective tissue stroma containing lymphocytes. (From Talerman A. Germ cell tumors of the ovary. *In* Kurman RJ [ed]: Blaustein's Pathology of the Female Genital Tract, 3rd ed. New York: Springer-Verlag, 1987, p. 663.)

diagnosis. Dysgerminomas have a greater propensity than other ovarian malignancies to spread to the retroperitoneal regional lymph nodes.[38, 39, 51–62] Therefore, appropriate surgical staging should be done using paraaortic and ipsilateral pelvic lymphadenectomy, pelvic and paracolic washings, diaphragmatic sampling, and omentectomy to determine the extent of disease. At the time of laparotomy, the surgeon must keep in mind the possibility of contralateral ovarian involvement. If the contralateral ovary is grossly negative, a biopsy can be performed to rule out occult microscopic involvement; if the result is negative, the ovary should be left in situ.[58] If there is bilateral ovarian involvement (gross and microscopic), after bilateral salpingo-oophorectomy, the uterus can be preserved for future child bearing via assisted reproductive technologies. For more advanced-stage disease (stages II through IV), cytoreduction should be performed. This has been shown to improve the response to adjuvant chemotherapy; if the remaining ovary is not involved, the contralateral ovary and uterus should be preserved.

Adjuvant therapy after conservative surgery with unilateral salpingo-oophorectomy has been a controversial issue with regard to preservation of fertility in these young patients. It has been shown that nearly 100% cure can be achieved with postoperative radiation to the pelvis and abdomen, but this leads to loss of fertility.[39, 54, 57, 59] Gordon and coworkers reported a 92% 10-year actual survival rate for patients who underwent conservative surgery with unilateral salpingo-oophorectomy without adjuvant postoperative radiotherapy.[56] With this conservative treatment, there was a 17% recurrence rate and

a 6% mortality rate in these young children, which calls into question its validity. The high recurrence rates can be partially explained by inadequate surgical staging.

Adjuvant ipsilateral hemipelvic and paraaortic lymph node radiation, with shielding of the contralateral ovary and uterus, after conservative surgery with unilateral salpingo-oophorectomy has been reported by DePalo and associates. In this series of 13 patients with stage I dysgerminoma, there have been no reported relapses, with a median follow-up of 77 months.[63] Although, historically, postoperative, radiation has been associated with excellent outcomes, as indicated above, it is associated with infertility. Currently, chemotherapy is the main modality of therapy for dysgerminomas.

To this date we do not have any long-term observational trials to determine the survival outcome of patients properly staged with stage I-A dysgerminomas. In a report by Gershenson and colleagues, five patients with dysgerminomas underwent conservative surgery (unilateral salpingo-oophorectomy), followed by adjuvant chemotherapy with bleomycin, etoposide, and cisplatinum (BEP) (Table 37–5). At median follow-up of 22.4 months, there were no recurrences, indicating that adjuvant chemotherapy

Table 37–5. BEP Combination Chemotherapy Regimen

Drug	Dosage
Cisplatin	20 mg/m², days 1–5
Etoposide	100 mg/m², days 1–5
Bleomycin	30 U/m²/wk

may be just as effective as adjuvant radiotherapy.[64] It is still very controversial whether to institute chemotherapy or to observe the patient with stage I-A dysgerminoma. Dark and associates reported in a surveillance study for stage I ovarian germ cell tumors that three of nine patients with stage I-A dysgerminoma recurred at 9, 11 and 16 months after diagnosis. However, all three of these patients were salvaged with chemotherapy.[65]

Because of the infrequency of this disease, we have no long-term observational data on stage I-A dysgerminomas. With a 30% recurrence rate and no long-term studies comparing observation and treatment, perhaps a more conservative approach with treatment with BEP would be appropriate.

Combination chemotherapy has also been shown to be effective in the treatment of the more advanced stages (II through IV) of dysgerminoma. Gershenson and colleagues reported seven cases of advanced stages of dysgerminoma and two cases of recurrent dysgerminoma treated with BEP, resulting in complete remission of disease in all instances with a median follow-up time of 22.4 months.[64] Williams and coworkers, reporting for the Gynecologic Oncology Group, used two consecutive protocols cisplatinum, vinblastine, bleomycin (PVB) and BEP, to treat metastatic dysgerminomas. Of 20 evaluable patients with stage III or IV disease (most with large residual disease), 19 were disease-free at a median follow-up of 26 months.[66]

The management of dysgerminomas has completely evolved. Chemotherapy has currently replaced radiation therapy as the primary treatment modality for dysgerminomas. BEP has resulted in excellent survival rates, but more importantly, preservation of fertility.

ENDODERMAL SINUS TUMOR

Endodermal sinus tumors of the ovary account for approximately 5% of all malignant ovarian tumors and are the second most common germ cell tumor. They are usually unilateral.

These tumors were originally thought to be of mesonephric origin but later were found to originate from extraembryonic germ cells.[67–69] The median age at presentation is 19 years.[70, 71] Histologically, endodermal sinus tumors are noted to have papillary projections with a peripheral lining of neoplastic cells associated with blood vessels (Schiller-Duval bodies; Fig. 37–6).

Endodermal sinus tumors produce a very specific tumor marker, α-fetoprotein (α-FP), which

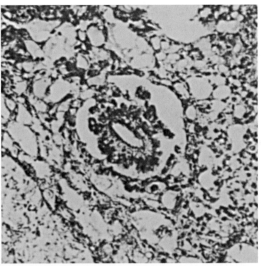

Figure 37–6. Endodermal sinus tumor showing a typical perivascular formation (Schiller-Duval body). (From Talerman A: Germ cell tumors of the ovary. *In* Kurman RJ [ed]: Blaustein's Pathology of the Female Genital Tract, 3rd ed. New York: Springer-Verlag, 1987, p. 673.)

is present in virtually 100% of all cases of endodermal sinus tumors.[71] This tumor marker gives the clinician a parameter to follow during the course of therapy.

Endodermal sinus tumors usually present with abdominal pain, fever, vaginal bleeding, or an abdominal pelvic mass. Treatment should begin with surgical exploration, unilateral salpingo-oophorectomy, and frozen section for tissue confirmation, followed by appropriate staging, as discussed earlier. Cytoreductive surgery should be performed for disease of more advanced stages. The most frequent stage at the time of laparotomy is stage I.[70, 71] Several researchers analyzing the management of endodermal sinus tumors reported 2-year survival rates of 25%, 18%, and 9% with the use of conservative surgery (unilateral salpingo-oophorectomy) alone for stage I patients and a 100% mortality rate with adjuvant radiotherapy, indicating (unlike dysgerminomas) the radioresistance of endodermal sinus tumors.[70–72]

Survival rates for endodermal sinus tumors did not improve until the institution of VAC combination chemotherapy. Kurman and Norris and Gershenson and associates, respectively, reported 75% and 92% 2-year survival rates for stage I endodermal sinus tumor after postoperative administration of VAC.[70, 71] In a follow-up study, Gershenson and colleagues reported a 94% sustained remission rate in stage I endodermal sinus tumor patients with a median follow-up of 100 months[73]; however, that same year, the Gynecologic Oncology Group reported only 50% sustained remission for such patients.[74]

Subsequent to the development of VAC chemotherapy, the cisplatin-based PVB regimen has been shown to achieve a 74% complete remission rate in nonseminomatous testicular carcinomas.[75] In an effort to improve remission rates in ovarian germ cell tumors, investigators began to evaluate the effectiveness of PVB. For stage I endodermal sinus tumors treated with PVB, the sustained remission rate was 100% in the 11 reported series,[76–86] as compared with 72% complete remission in the collective series reporting the use of VAC.

With more advanced-stage endodermal sinus tumors (II through IV), remission rates were even more dismal. Gershenson and colleagues reported a 30% complete remission rate with VAC chemotherapy, with the Gynecologic Oncology Group reporting a 56% sustained remission rate. In an attempt to improve remission rates in the advanced-stage group, PVB was evaluated, with a collective series noting a remission rate of 68%. However, although PVB seemed to be slightly more efficacious for endodermal sinus tumor of advanced stages, it was also clearly more toxic than VAC chemotherapy. Myelosuppression, nephrotoxicity, neurotoxicity, and pulmonary fibrosis have been reported, and deaths have been attributed to PVB therapy.

In an attempt to achieve a more active and less toxic combination of chemotherapy, Williams and associates compared PVB and BEP in the treatment of disseminated germ cell tumors.[87] The authors concluded that BEP was superior in inducing remission: 83% of patients were reported disease free after BEP therapy, as compared with 74% after therapy with PVB. Also, the BEP group had significantly less toxicity. Gershenson and colleagues in 1990 reported 100% sustained remission when BEP was used as primary therapy for endodermal sinus tumor in all stages with minimal toxicity.[64] In 1990, Hicks and coworkers reported dose intensification with BEP induction followed by VAC maintenance chemotherapy in stage III endodermal sinus tumor patients, resulting in complete resolution of disease, as documented by second-look laparotomy, and minimal toxicity.[88] The Gynecologic Oncology Group reported on their experience with BEP in stage I, II and III disease; 89 of 93 patients (96%) were disease-free as confirmed by second-look laparotomy for a duration of follow-up of 4 to 90 months.[89]

Adjuvant chemotherapy is absolutely neces-

sary in the treatment of all stages of endodermal sinus tumor. Therapy using BEP for endodermal sinus tumors has shown excellent progression-free survival rates as compared with all other regimens of chemotherapy (VAC or PVB). Therefore, to achieve complete remission and preserve fertility in young girls with the diagnosis of endodermal sinus tumor, conservative surgery in early stages of the disease or conservative surgery and cytoreductive surgery in more advanced stages of disease should be followed by BEP chemotherapy.

EMBRYONAL CARCINOMA

Embryonal carcinoma of the ovary is analogous to embryonal carcinoma of the testis (Fig. 37–7). This is a very rare tumor, and until the report by Kurman and Norris[90] classifying these tumors as a separate entity, they were routinely confused with choriocarcinoma and endodermal sinus tumors of the ovary. Embryonal carcinoma of the ovaries is rarely found in a pure form but is usually is part of a mixed germ cell tumor. The median age at presentation is 13, and the tumor primarily presents as a stage I lesion and is usually exclusively unilateral. Embryonal carcinomas have totipotential cells capable of extraembryonic or embryonic differentiation. Sixty percent of embryonal carcinomas produce hormonal manifestations consistent with precocious puberty in premenarchal girls, abnormal vaginal bleeding in postmenarchal women, and a positive pregnancy test.[90] All pure embryonal carcinomas produce hCG, and occasionally α-FP levels are elevated.

Treatment for suspected embryonal carci-

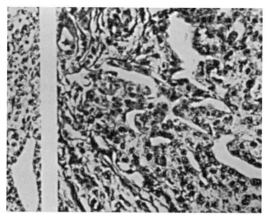

Figure 37–7. Embryonal carcinoma forming clefts and spaces. (From Talerman A: Gonadoblastoma associated with embryonal carcinoma. Obstet Gynecol 1974; 43:138.)

noma of the ovary should begin with exploration of the abdomen, appropriate staging, unilateral salpingo-oophorectomy, and, for advanced disease, cytoreduction as described for other germ cell tumors.

Reports evaluating the efficacy of adjuvant chemotherapy for embryonal carcinomas are limited because of the rarity of the tumor. Williams and associates have reported sustained remissions after therapy with etoposide and cisplatin with or without bleomycin for advanced stages of testicular embryonal carcinomas.[87, 91]

Currently, embryonal carcinomas of the ovary should be treated essentially the same as endodermal sinus tumors of the ovary (i.e., with BEP combination chemotherapy).

IMMATURE TERATOMAS

Immature teratomas represent the third most common germ cell tumor of the ovary, accounting for approximately 15% of all germ cell tumors and 1% of all teratomas. These tumors are composed of elements from all three germ cell layers (ectoderm, mesoderm, and endoderm; Fig. 37–8). Immature teratomas are usually exclusively unilateral, and the median age at presentation is 19 years.[92, 94] This neoplasm is usually without evidence of tumor marker production, although Gershenson's group reported elevated levels of α-FP in 5 of 16 (31%) immature teratoma cases.[93] These tumors usually present primarily as stage I lesions.[93, 95]

Treatment of suspected immature teratomas also begins with surgical exploration, unilateral salpingo-oophorectomy, appropriate staging, and,

Table 37–6. Survival Rates for Stage I Immature Teratoma According to Grade

Grade	No. of Patients	No. Survived
I	14	13 (93%)
II	30	11 (55%)
III	6	2 (33%)

From Hicks ML, Piver MS: Conservative surgery plus adjuvant therapy for vulvovaginal rhabdomyosarcoma, DES/clear cell adenocarcinoma of the vagina and unilateral germ cell tumors of the ovary. Obstet Gynecol Clin North Am 1992; 19(1):219.

in advanced stages of disease, cytoreduction. Norris and associates noted a clear relationship between the grade of immature teratomas and ultimate survival. The authors noted that, in patients treated with conservative surgery (i.e., unilateral salpingo-oophorectomy only), those with a grade I lesion had a 93% survival rate, as compared with 33% survival for those with grade III lesions (Table 37–6). For all stage I disease, reported survival was 76%, as compared with 38% for advanced stage disease (stages II and III).[94] Gallion and colleagues noted an 83% 2-year disease-free survival rate in patients with grade I immature teratoma lesions, as compared with a 33% rate in patients with grade III lesions; the 2-year disease-free survival rate was 63% for stage I disease, but 30% for stage III lesions.[92] Both of these studies indicate the importance of adequate exploration and sampling of all lesions in the abdomen and pelvis, as prognosis is related to the grade of the most advanced lesion in the abdominal cavity.

Adjuvant chemotherapy is necessary to ensure complete remission and improve survival. In

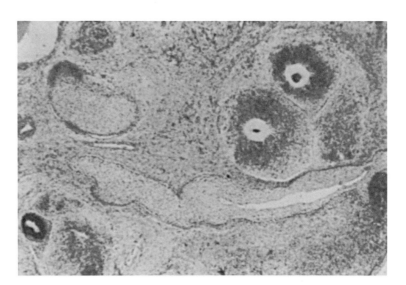

Figure 37–8. Immature neural elements evident along with squamous epithelium and cartilage. (From DiSaia PJ, Creasman WT: Germ cell, stromal and other ovarian tumors. *In* Clinical Gynecologic Oncology, 3rd ed. St. Louis: CV Mosby, 1989, p 433.)

1986, Gershenson and associates treated 21 patients with VAC; 18 of 21 (85%) (all stages) had sustained remission. Of stage I patients, 91% treated with VAC had sustained remission, versus 9% treated with surgery alone; for advanced stages, an 80% remission rate was noted in the chemotherapy-treated group versus 0% in those treated otherwise.[93] Slayton and colleagues reported a 100% sustained remission rate in stage I immature teratomas treated with VAC and a 58% sustained remission rate for advanced stage disease so treated.[74]

Until recently, VAC chemotherapy was thought to be the best adjuvant therapy, especially in stage I disease; however, the Gynecologic Oncology Group showed that 89 of 93 patients who had a tumor other than dysgerminoma were alive without disease (96%). This report encompassed all stages, stage I-III, and there were 42 immature teratomas. Of the 4 patients who did not survive, two had immature teratomas. Thus, the disease-free survival rate for patients with immature teratomas was 95%.[89] Additionally, Gershenson reported complete remission with BEP chemotherapy and two cases of stage I and one case of recurrent immature teratoma with 22.4-month median follow-up. Again, the BEP regimen was superior.[64] There are no large reports on the management of stage I-A, grade I, pure immature teratomas. For this group of patients the reported survival rate is 93% with observation alone.

Because of the infrequency of the disease and no long-term observational trials, the management of stage I-A, grade I, immature teratoma is controversial; however, it appears that the recurrence rate is exceptionally low and observation alone may be an option. Patients with stage I, grade II and III and more advanced-stage immature teratomas should be treated with BEP chemotherapy.

MIXED GERM CELL TUMORS

Mixed germ cell tumors have more than one malignant germ cell component. These tumors present primarily as stage I lesions, and the mean age at presentation is 16 years.[96, 97] These tumors are usually unilateral and often produce hCG and α-FP and occasionally LDH. Most often, mixed germ cell tumors are composed of dysgerminomas and endodermal sinus tumors, but any combination of germ cell tumors may be present. Treatment of mixed germ cell tumors begins with exploration of the abdomen, unilateral salpingo-oophorectomy (with contralateral ovarian biopsy in the presence of dysgerminoma), appropriate staging, and cytoreduction in advanced stages of disease. Survival after surgery alone has been poor; adjuvant chemotherapy is needed.[72, 96, 97] Gershenson and associates and Slayton and colleagues reported 75% and 83% remission rates, respectively, with VAC chemotherapy in stage I disease, but for advanced-stage disease, the remission rates were 33% and 22%, respectively.[73, 74] PVB has not been used frequently in the treatment of mixed germ cell tumors but has shown some activity in early and advanced-stage tumors.[76, 78, 82, 84, 85]

The Gynecologic Oncology Group represents the largest series of patients treated for mixed germ cell tumors. After three cycles of BEP chemotherapy, 89 of 93 patients (96%) were noted disease-free. BEP appears to be the most effective regimen for this subcategory of germ cell tumors.[89]

NONGESTATIONAL OVARIAN CHORIOCARCINOMA

Pure ovarian choriocarcinomas are extremely rare tumors (Fig. 37–9). These neoplasms are usually a component of mixed germ cell tumors. They are primarily unilateral and are associated with elevated hCG levels.

Treatment, as for all germ cell tumors, begins with surgical exploration and appropriate staging, followed by unilateral salpingo-oophorectomy. Experience with adjuvant chemotherapy has been limited because of the rarity of this tumor. Methotrexate, actinomycin D, and chlorambucil have been successful in achieving long-term remission.[98] PVB has also been shown to have some activity in the treatment of ovarian choriocarcinoma. The Gynecologic Oncology Group also noted that BEP is an effective adjuvant for nongestational ovarian choriocarcinoma.[89]

JUVENILE GRANULOSA CELL TUMORS

Juvenile granulosa cell tumors (JGCTs) account for approximately 5% of all ovarian tumors in children (Fig. 37–10). More than 80% occur in the first two decades of life; 5% are diagnosed in the prepubertal period. Eighty percent of patients with JGCT present with isosexual precocity, but in the postpubertal period, menstrual irregularities (i.e., dysfunctional uterine bleeding) may be the only presenting sign.[99–105] In addition to hormonal abnormalities, the patient

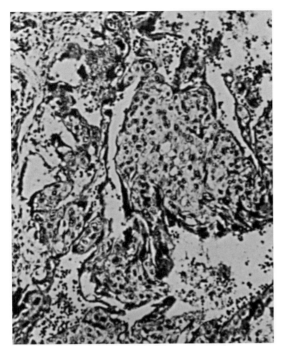

Figure 37–9. Choriocarcinoma showing a cytotrophoblast composed of medium-sized cells situated centrally and a syncytiotrophoblast composed of very large multi-nucleate cells situated peripherally. (From Talerman A: Germ cell tumors of the ovary. *In* Kurman RJ [ed]: Blaustein's Pathology of the Female Genital Tract, 3rd ed. New York: Springer-Verlag, 1987, p 685.)

with JGCT may present with signs of peritonitis, ascites, or an abdominopelvic mass.

JGCT differs from adult granulosa cell tumor in its recurrence pattern, age of onset, and histologic characteristics (Table 37–7).[99] These tumors occur bilaterally only very infrequently, and in most cases the tumor is confined to the ovary at the time of laparotomy (stage IA).

Table 37–7. Differences Between Adult and Juvenile Granulosa Cell Tumors

	Adult	Juvenile
Age	Infrequently prepubertal	Primarily prepubertal
	Presents at >30 years of age	Presents at <30 years of age
Microscopic findings	Call-Exner bodies common	No Call-Exner bodies
	No mucin	Irregular follicles
	Pale nuclei and grooved	Dark nuclei and nongrooved
	No luteinization	Luteinization present
Recurrence	Late	Early

Treatment of JGCT begins with exploration of the abdomen and appropriate staging (pelvic and right and left paracolic washings; diaphragmatic sampling; omentectomy; and pelvic and paraaortic lymph node sampling). Because the majority of these lesions are unilateral, conservative surgery (unilateral salpingo-oophorectomy only) is usually all that is necessary, but, in the presence of advanced disease, cytoreductive surgery should be performed.

After limited surgery (unilateral salpingo-oophorectomy only), disease confined entirely to the ovary (stage IA) requires no further therapy, and survival rates range from 80% to 100% (Table 37–8). Less than 100% survival can be explained by the fact that patients were sometimes improperly staged, and some cases represent more advanced stages of disease.

For more advanced stages of JGCT, no effective modality of therapy has been determined. Radiotherapy and various combinations of chemotherapy have yielded poor results in terms of sustained clinical remissions.[99, 106–108] For advanced and recurrent adult granulosa cell tumors, the PVB regimen has been shown to be of

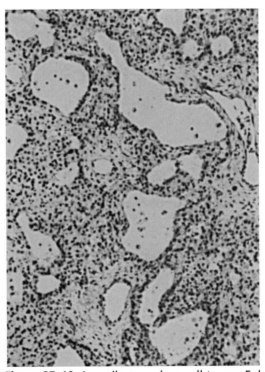

Figure 37–10. Juvenile granulosa cell tumor. Follicles of varying sizes and shapes are separated by cellular areas. (From Young RH, Dickersin GR, Scully RE: Juvenile granulosa cell tumor of the ovary. A clinicopathological analysis of 125 cases. Am J Surg Pathol 1984; 8:575–596.)

Table 37–8. Survival Rates for Stage I Juvenile Granulosa Cell Tumors of the Ovary Treated with Surgery Alone

	Number	%	Median Follow-up
Zaloudek and Norris[106]	24/26	92	19 yr
Lack et al.[107]	10/10	100	21 yr
Young et al.[99]	87/95	92	5 yr
Vassal et al.[108]	4/5	80	6 yr
Total	125/136	92	

some therapeutic efficacy in improving survival.[109] However, PVB is also associated with severe hematologic and neurologic toxicity, and treatment-related deaths have been reported. Reports have shown some benefits with methotrexate, actinomycin-D, and chlorambucil (MAC), and another report has shown success with carboplatinum and etoposide.[110,111] Because JGCT is a rare tumor, the small numbers of advanced JGCT cases do not permit adequate evaluation of chemotherapeutic agents in the treatment of this disease.

REFERENCES

1. Bartholomew TH, Gonzales ET, Starling KA, et al: Changing concepts in management of pelvic rhabdomyosarcoma in children. Urology 1979; 13:613.
2. Sutow WW, Sullivan MP, Ried HL, et al: Prognosis in childhood rhabdomyosarcoma. Cancer 1970; 25:1384–1390.
3. Maurer HM: The Intergroup Rhabdomyosarcoma Study: Update, November 1978. Natl Cancer Inst Monogr 1981; 56:61–68.
4. Maurer HM: The Intergroup Rhabdomyosarcoma Study (NIH): Objectives and clinical staging classification. J Pediatr Surg 1975; 10:977–978.
5. Dehner LP: Soft tissue sarcomas of childhood: The differential diagnostic dilemma of the small blue cell. Natl Cancer Inst Monogr 1981; 56:43.
6. Shackman R: Sarcoma botryoids of the genital tract in female children. Br J Surg 1950; 38:26–30.
7. Hilgers RD, Malkasian GD, Soule EH: Embryonal rhabdomyosarcoma (botryoid type) of the vagina. A clinicopathologic review. Am J Obstet Gynecol 1970; 107:484–501.
8. Hilgers RD: Pelvic exenteration for vaginal embryonal rhabdomyosarcoma. A review. Obstet Gynecol 1975; 45:175–180.
9. Cassady JR, Sagerman RH, Tretter P, et al: Radiation therapy for rhabdomyosarcoma. Radiology 1968; 91:116–120.
10. Edland RW: Embryonal rhabdomyosarcoma. Am J Roentgenol Rad Ther Nucl Med 1965; 93:671–685.
11. McNeer GP, Cantin J, Chu F, et al: Effectiveness of radiation therapy in the management of sarcomas of the soft somatic tissues. Cancer 1968; 22:391–397.
12. Donaldson SS, Castro JR, Wilbur JR, et al: Rhabdomyosarcoma of head and neck in children. Combination treatment by surgery, irradiation, and chemotherapy. Cancer 1973; 31:26–35.
13. Grosfeld JL, Smith JP, Chatworthy HW: Pelvic rhabdomyosarcoma in infants and children. J Urol 1972; 107:673–675.
14. Heyn RM, Holland R, Newton WA, et al: The role of combined chemotherapy in the treatment of rhabdomyosarcoma in children. Cancer 1974; 34:2128–2142.
15. Kilman JW, Clatworthy HW, Newton WA, et al: Reasonable surgery for rhabdomyosarcoma. A study of 67 cases. Ann Surg 1973; 178:346–351.
16. Piver MS, Barlow JJ, Wang JJ, et al: Combined radical surgery, radiation therapy and chemotherapy in infants with vulvovaginal embryonal rhabdomyosarcoma. Obstet Gynecol 1973; 42:522–526.
17. Pratt CB, Hustu HO, Fleming ID, et al: Coordinated treatment of childhood rhabdomyosarcoma with surgery, radiotherapy and combination chemotherapy. Cancer Res 1972; 32:606–610.
18. Rivard G, Ortega J, Hittle R, et al: Intensive chemotherapy as primary treatment for rhabdomyosarcoma of the pelvis. Cancer 1975; 36:1593–1597.
19. Maurer HM, Moon T, Donaldson M, et al: The Intergroup Rhabdomyosarcoma Study. A preliminary report. Cancer 1977; 40:2015–2026.
20. Kumar APM, Wrenn EL, Fleming ID, et al: Combined therapy to prevent complete pelvic exenteration for rhabdomyosarcoma of the vagina or uterus. Cancer 1976; 37:118–122.
21. Voute PA, Vos A, deKraker J, Behrendt H: Rhabdomyosarcomas: Chemotherapy and limited supplementary treatment program to avoid mutilation. Natl Cancer Inst Monogr 1981; 56:121–125.
22. Andrassy RJ, Hays DM, Raney B, et al: Conservative surgical management of vaginal and vulvar pediatric rhabdomyosarcoma: A report from the intergroup rhabdomyosarcoma study III. J Pediatr Surg 1995; 30:1034–1037.
23. Raney RB, Gehan EA, Hays DM, et al: Primary chemotherapy with or without radiation therapy and/or surgery for children with localized sarcoma of the bladder, prostate, vagina, uterus and cervix. Cancer 1990; 66:2072–2081.
24. Flamant F, Gerbaulet A, Nihoul-Fekete C, et al: Long term sequelae of conservative treatment by surgery, brachytherapy, and chemotherapy for vulvar and vaginal rhabdomyosarcoma in children. J Clin Oncol 1990; 8:1847–1853.
25. Ruymann F, Crist W, Wiener E, et al: Comparison of two doublet chemotherapy regimens and conventional radiotherapy in metastatic rhabdomyosarcoma: Improved overall survival using ifosfamide/etoposide compared to vincristine/melphalan in IRSG-IV. Proc Am Soc Clin Oncol 1997; 16:521a.
26. Nix HG, Wright HL: Mesonephric adenocarcinoma of the vagina. Am J Obstet Gynecol 1967; 99:893–899.
27. Novak E, Woodruff JD, Novak ER: Probable mesonephric origin of certain female genital tumors. Am J Obstet Gynecol 1952; 68:1222–1242.
28. Scannel RC: Primary adenocarcinoma of the vagina. Am J Obstet Gynecol 1939; 38:331–333.
29. Studdiford WE: Vaginal lesions of adenomatous origin. Am J Obstet Gynecol 1957; 73:641–656.
30. Herbst AL, Ulefelder H, Poskanzer DC: Adenocarcinoma of the vagina. Association of maternal stilbestrol therapy with tumor appearance in young women. N Engl J Med 1971; 284:878–881.
31. Greenwald P, Barlow JJ, Nasca PC, et al: Vaginal cancer after maternal treatment with synthetic estrogens. N Engl J Med 1971; 285:390–392.

32. Waggoner SE, Mittendorf R, Biney N, et al: Influence of in Utero Diethylstilbestrol Exposure on the Prognosis and biologic behavior of vaginal clear-cell adenocarcinoma. Gynecol Oncol 1994; 55:238–244.

33. Herbst AL, Kurman RJ, Scully RE, et al: Clear cell adenocarcinoma of the genital tract in young females. Registry report. N Engl J Med 1972; 287:1259–1264.

34. Herbst AL, Norusis MJ, Rosenow PJ, et al: An analysis of 346 cases of clear cell adenocarcinoma of the vagina and cervix with emphasis on recurrence and survival. Gynecol Oncol 1979; 7:111–122.

35. Robboy SJ, Herbst AL, Scully RE: Clear cell adenocarcinoma of the vagina and cervix in young females. Analysis of 37 tumors that persisted or recurred after primary therapy. Cancer 1974; 34:606–614.

36. Wharton JT, Rutledge FN, Gallagher HS, Fletcher G: Treatment of clear cell adenocarcinoma in young females. Obstet Gynecol 1975; 45:365–368.

37. Senekjian EK, Frey AW, Anderson D, et al: Local therapy in stage I clear cell adenocarcinoma of the vagina. Cancer 1987; 60:1319–1324.

38. Asadourian LA, Taylor HB: Dysgerminoma. An analysis of 105 cases. Obstet Gynecol 1969; 33:370–379.

39. DePalo G, Pilotti S, Kenda R, et al: Natural history of dysgerminoma. Am J Obstet Gynecol 1982; 143:799–807.

40. Gershenson DM, Wharton JT: Malignant germ cell tumors of the ovary. In Alberts D, Surwit E (eds): Ovarian Cancer. Norwell, Mass: Kluwer Publishing, 1985, pp 227–269.

41. Santesson L: Clinical and pathological survey of ovarian tumors treated at the Radium-Hemmet. 1. Dysgerminoma. Acta Radiol (Stockholm) 1947; 28:643–668.

42. Hart WR, Burkons DM: Germ cell neoplasms arising in gonadoblastomas. Cancer 1979; 43:669–678.

43. Schellhas HH, Trujillo JM, Rutledge FN: Germ cell tumors associated with XY gonadal dysgenesis. Am J Obstet Gynecol 1971; 109:1197–1204.

44. Schwartz IS, Cohen CJ, Deligdisch L: Dysgerminoma of the ovary associated with true hermaphroditism. Obstet Gynecol 1980; 56:102–106.

45. Talerman A, Jarabak J, Amarose AP: Gonadoblastoma and dysgerminoma in a true hermaphrodite with a 46, XX karyotype. Am J Obstet Gynecol 1981; 140:475–477.

46. Teter J, Bozkowski K: Occurrence of tumors in dysgenetic gonads. Cancer 1967; 20:1301–1310.

47. Friedman M, White RG, Nissenbaum MM, et al: Serum lactic dehydrogenase—a possible tumor marker for an ovarian dysgerminoma: A literature review and report of a case. Obstet Gynecol Surv 1984; 39:247–265.

48. Lippert MC, Javadpour N: Lactic dehydrogenase in the monitoring and prognosis of testicular cancer. Cancer 1981; 48:2274–2278.

49. Sheiko MC, Hart WR: Ovarian germinoma (dysgerminoma) with elevated serum lactic dehydrogenase: Case report and review of literature. Cancer 1982; 49:994–998.

50. Zondag HA: Enzyme activity in dysgerminoma and seminomas. A study of lactic dehydrogenase isoenzymes in malignant diseases. The 1963 Fiske essay. RI Med J 1964; 47:273–281.

51. Afridi MA, Vongtama V, Tsukada Y, et al: Dysgerminoma of the ovary. Radiation therapy for recurrence and metastases. Am J Obstet Gynecol 1976; 126:180–194.

52. Boyes DA, Pankratz E, Galliford BW, et al: Experience with dysgerminomas at the Cancer Control Agency of British Columbia. Gynecol Oncol 1978; 6:123–129.

53. Burkons DM, Hart WR: Ovarian germinomas (dysgerminomas). Obstet Gynecol 1978; 51:221–224.

54. Buskirk SJ, Schray MF, Podratz KC, et al: Ovarian dysgerminoma: A retrospective analysis of results of treatment, sites of treatment failure and radiosensitivity. Mayo Clin Proc 1987; 62:1149–1157.

55. Freel JH, Cassir JF, Pierce VK, et al: Dysgerminoma of the ovary. Cancer 1979; 43:798–805.

56. Gordon A, Lipton D, Woodruff D: Dysgerminoma: A review of 158 cases from the Emil Novak Ovarian Tumor Registry. Obstet Gynecol 1981; 58:497–504.

57. Krepart G, Smith JP, Rutledge F, et al: The treatment for dysgerminoma of the ovary. Cancer 1978; 41:986–990.

58. Kurman RJ, Norris HJ: Malignant germ cell tumors of the ovary. Hum Pathol 1977; 8:551–564.

59. Lucraft HH: A review of thirty-three cases of ovarian dysgerminoma emphasizing the role of radiotherapy. Clin Radiol 1979; 30:585–589.

60. Muller CW, Topkins P, Lapp WA: Dysgerminoma of the ovary. An analysis of 427 cases. Am J Obstet Gynecol 1950; 60:153–159.

61. Pedowit P, Felmus LB, Grayzel DM: Dysgerminoma of the ovary. Prognosis and treatment. Am J Obstet Gynecol 1955; 70:1284–1297.

62. Talerman A, Huyzinga WT, Kuipers T: Dysgerminoma clinicopathologic study of 22 cases. Obstet Gynecol 1973; 41:137–147.

63. DePalo G, Lattuada A, Kenda R, et al: Germ cell tumors of the ovary: The experience of the National Cancer Institute of Milan. I. Dysgerminoma. Int J Radiat Oncol Biol Phys 1987; 13:853–860.

64. Gershenson DM, Morris M, Cangir A, et al: Treatment of malignant germ cell tumors of the ovary with bleomycin, etoposide, and cisplatin. J Clin Oncol 1990; 8:715–720.

65. Dark GG, Bower M, Newlands ES, et al: Surveillance policy for stage I ovarian germ cell tumors. J Clin Oncol 1997; 15:620–624.

66. Williams SD, Blessing JA, Hatch KD, Homesley HD: Chemotherapy of advanced dysgerminoma: Trials of the Gynecologic Oncology Group. J Clin Oncol 1991; 9:1950–1955.

67. Schiller W: Mesonephroma ovarii. Am J Cancer 1939; 35:1–21.

68. Teilum G: Gonocytoma: Homologous ovarian and testicular tumors, with discussion of "Mesonephroma Ovarii" (Schiller W: Am J Cancer 1939). Acta Pathol Microbiol Scand 1946; 23:242.

69. Teilum G: Endodermal sinus tumors of the ovary and testes, comparative morphogenesis of the socalled mesonephroma ovarii (Schiller) and extra embryonic (yolk-sac allantoic) structure of the rat's placenta. Cancer 1959; 12:1092–1105.

70. Gershenson DM, DelJunco G, Herson J, et al: Endodermal sinus tumor of the ovary. The M.D. Anderson experience. Obstet Gynecol 1983; 61:194–202.

71. Kurman RJ, Norris HJ: Endodermal sinus tumor of the ovary. A clinical and pathologic analysis of 71 cases. Cancer 1976; 38:2404–2419.

72. Jimerson GK, Woodruff JD: Ovarian extraembryonal teratoma II. Endodermal sinus tumor mixed with other germ cell tumors. Am J Obstet Gynecol 1977; 127:302–304.

73. Gershenson DM, Copeland LJ, Kavanagh JJ, et al: Treatment of malignant nondysgerminomatous germ cell tumors of the ovary with vincristine, dactinomycin and cyclophosphamide. Cancer 1985; 56:2756–2761.

74. Slayton RE, Park RC, Silverberg SG, et al: Vincristine, dactinomycin and cyclophosphamide in the treatment of malignant germ cell tumors of the ovary. A Gynecologic

Oncology Group Study (a final report). Cancer 1985; 56:243–248.

75. Einhorn LH, Donohue J: Cis-diaminedichloroplatinum, vinblastine, and bleomycin combination chemotherapy in disseminated testicular cancer. Ann Intern Med 1977; 87:293–298.

76. Carlson RW, Sikic BI, Turbow MM, et al: Cisplatin, vinblastine and bleomycin (PVB) therapy for ovarian germ cell tumors. J Clin Oncol 1987; 1:645–651.

77. Davis TE, Loprinzi CL, Buchler DA: Combination chemotherapy with cisplatin, vinblastine, and bleomycin for endodermal sinus tumor of the ovary. Gynecol Oncol 1984; 19:46–52.

78. Gershenson DM, Kavanagh JJ, Copeland LJ, et al: Treatment of malignant nondysgerminomatous germ cell tumors of the ovary with vinblastine, bleomycin and cisplatin. Cancer 1986; 57:1731–1737.

79. Julian CG, Barrett JM, Richardson RL, et al: Bleomycin, vinblastine and cisplatin in the treatment of advanced endodermal sinus tumor. Obstet Gynecol 1979; 56:396–401.

80. Lockey JL, Baker JJ, Prince NA, et al: Cisplatin, vinblastine and bleomycin for endodermal sinus tumor of the ovary. Ann Intern Med 1981; 94:56–57.

81. Sawada M, Okudaira Y, Matsui Y, et al: Cisplatin, vinblastine and bleomycin therapy of yolk sac (endodermal sinus) tumor of the ovary. Gynecol Oncol 1985; 20:162–169.

82. Schwartz PE: Combination chemotherapy in the management of ovarian germ cell malignancies. Obstet Gynecol 1984; 64:564–572.

83. Sessa C, Bonazzi C, Landoni F, et al: Cisplatin, vinblastine and bleomycin combination chemotherapy in endodermal sinus tumor of the ovary. Obstet Gynecol 1987; 70:220–224.

84. Taylor MH, DePetrillo AD, Turner AR: Vinblastine, bleomycin and cisplatin in malignant germ cell tumors of the ovary. Cancer 1984; 56:1341–1349.

85. Vriesendorp R, Aalders JG, Sleijfer DT, et al: Treatment of malignant germ cell tumors of the ovary with cisplatin, vinblastine, and bleomycin (PVB). Cancer Treat Rep 1984; 68:779–781.

86. Wiltshaw E, Stuart-Harris R, Barker GH, et al: Chemotherapy of endodermal sinus tumor (yolk-sac tumor) of the ovary. Preliminary communication. J R Soc Med 1982; 75:888–892.

87. Williams SD, Birch R, Einhorn EH, et al: Treatment of disseminated germ-cell tumors with cisplatin, bleomycin, and either vinblastine or etoposide. N Engl J Med 1987; 316:1435–1440.

88. Hicks ML, Maxwell SL, Kim W: Management of advanced endodermal sinus tumor of the ovary with preservation of reproductive function. Henry Ford Hosp Med J 1990; 38:76–78.

89. Williams S, Blessing JA, Liao SY, et al: Adjuvant therapy of ovarian germ cell tumors with cisplatin, etoposide and bleomycin: A trial of the Gynecologic Oncology Group. J Clin Oncol 1994; 12:701–706.

90. Kurman RJ, Norris HJ: Embryonal carcinoma of the ovary. A clinicopathologic entity distinct from endodermal sinus tumor resembling embryonal carcinoma of the adult testis. Cancer 1976; 38:2420–2433.

91. Williams SD, Einhorn LH, Greco A, et al: VP-16–213

salvage therapy for refractory germinal neoplasms. Cancer 1980; 46:2154–2158.

92. Gallion H, VanNagell JR, Donaldson ES, et al: Immature teratoma of the ovary. Am J Obstet Gynecol 1983; 146:361.

93. Gershenson DM, DelJunco G, Silva EG, et al: Immature teratoma of the ovary. Obstet Gynecol 1986; 68:624.

94. Norris HJ, Zerkin HJ, Benson WL: Immature (malignant) teratoma of the ovary. Cancer 1976; 37:2359.

95. Perrone T, Steeper TA, Dehner LP: Alpha-fetoprotein localization in pure ovarian teratoma. An immunohistochemical study of 12 cases. Am J Clin Pathol 1987; 88:713.

96. Gershenson DM, DelJunco G, Copeland LJ, et al: Mixed germ cell tumors of the ovary. Obstet Gynecol 1984; 64:200–206.

97. Kurman RJ, Norris HJ: Malignant mixed germ cell tumors of the ovary. Obstet Gynecol 1976; 48:459–589.

98. Wider JA, Marshall JR, Bardin CW, et al: Sustained remissions after chemotherapy for a primary ovarian cancer containing choriocarcinoma. N Engl J Med 1969; 280:1439.

99. Young RH, Dickersin GR, Scully RE: Juvenile granulosa cell tumor of the ovary. A clinicopathological analysis of 125 cases. Am J Surg Pathol 1984; 8:575–596.

100. Morris JM, Scully RE: Endocrine Pathology of the Ovary. St. Louis: CV Mosby, 1958.

101. Scully RE: Ovarian tumors with endocrine manifestations. In DeGroot LJ (ed): Endocrinology. Vol 3. New York: Grune & Stratton, 1979.

102. Scully RE: Ovarian tumors. A review. Am J Pathol 1977; 87:686–720.

103. Scully RE: Sex cord stromal, lipid cell and germ cell tumors. In Sciarra JJ (ed): Gynecology and Obstetrics. Vol 4: Gynecologic Oncology. Hagerstown, MD: Harper & Row, 1980.

104. Scully RE: The ovary. In Wolfe HJ (ed): Endocrine Pathology. New York: Springer-Verlag, 1986.

105. Scully RE: Tumors of the ovary and maldeveloped gonads. In Atlas of Tumor Pathology, 2nd ser. Fasc. 16. Washington, DC: Armed Forces Institute of Pathology, 1979.

106. Zaloudek C, Norris HJ: Granulosa tumors of the ovary in children. A clinical and pathologic study of 32 cases. Am J Surg Pathol 1982; 6:513–522.

107. Lack EE, Perez-Atayde AR, Murthy ASK, et al: Granulosa theca cell tumors in premenarchal girls: A clinical and pathologic study of ten cases. Cancer 1981; 48:1846–1854.

108. Vassal G, Flamant F, Caillaud JM, et al: Juvenile granulosa cell tumor of the ovary in children: A clinical study of 15 cases. J Clin Oncol 1988; 6:990–995.

109. Colombo N, Sessa C, Landoni F, et al: Cisplatin, vinblastine and bleomycin combination chemotherapy in metastatic granulosa cell tumor of the ovary. Obstet Gynecol 1986; 67:265–268.

110. Powell JL, Johnson NA, Bailey CL, et al: Case report: management of advanced juvenile granulosa cell tumor of the ovary. Gynecol Oncol 1993; 48:119–123.

111. Powell JL, Otis NO: Case report: management of advanced juvenile granulosa cell tumor of the ovary. Gynecol Oncol 1997; 64:282–284.

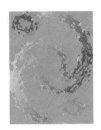

Chapter 38
Rectovaginal Fistulas and Associated Anomalies

John Dewhurst

On rare occasions the gynecologist may be consulted about an anomaly that affects both the lower bowel and the genital tract. A number of these defects can be treated simply, whereas others require one or more major surgical procedures and the cooperation of a surgical team with expertise in pediatric patients, complemented by considerable ingenuity. Guidelines for the gynecologist unexpectedly confronted with one of these abnormalities are of utmost importance. Outcomes of reconstructive surgery have been reported elsewhere.[1-7] An International Classification was proposed by Stephens and Smith[7] and modified in 1985.[8]

It is not always possible to determine how such defects arise, since all malformations are, by definition, "abnormal," but, in general terms, they derive from errors in division of the primitive cloaca, exteriorization of the vagina onto the vestibule, and posterior migration of the anal opening.

EMBRYOLOGY

In the very early embryo (4 weeks; 4 mm in size) the allantois and primitive gut come together to form a common cavity, the cloaca, which at this point has no external opening. By 6 weeks (16 mm), this cavity has been divided by the urorectal septum; shortly after, the cloacal membrane breaks down. As development proceeds, the anus moves backward with the formation of the perineum, while the phallic and pelvic portions of the urogenital sinus flatten out to bring the vaginal introitus to the vestibule. Development may be arrested at any stage. If this happens early, the infant will be left with a primitive cloaca into which the bladder, genital tract, and bowel open. Arrest soon after this stage (i.e., after formation of the urorectal septum) may leave the bowel opening into the upper vagina as a high rectovaginal fistula; whereas subsequent arrest may result in a fistula entering low into the vagina or vestibule or to a more normally formed anal opening situated in front of the usual site, sometimes immediately alongside the vagina. This is a very simplistic explanation of these anomalies; other abnormalities, far more bizarre (e.g., when an accessory phallic urethra is found in association with a cloaca), defy explanation.

THE LOW RECTOVAGINAL FISTULA AND PERINEAL ANUS

The simplest of the anogenital anomalies are a low rectovaginal fistula and a perineal anus. The bowel may open at some point on the perineum in front of its usual situation, at the fourchette, or into the lowest part of the vagina. The important point to understand about all these abnormalities is that the bowel passes through the levator sling, whose contraction can produce an effective sphincteric action and close the opening (Fig. 38-1). Despite this, the normal process of defecation may be disrupted by the size of the external opening, which is frequently contracted (Fig. 38-2). This leads to a condition that was referred to many years ago as the *syndrome of rectal inertia*. Because of the greater resistance to defecation, the rectum becomes filled with more and more impacted fecal matter, and soon the rectal reflex is lost. This impaction may extend into the descending or even the transverse colon. There is much straining at stool, but despite this the child still soils her clothes, as fluid fecal matter from a high level flows past the solid rectal masses.

In most instances, an abnormality is evident at birth. Sometimes absence of the anal opening is noticed, and the labia have to be parted to allow the fistula to be identified with a probe (Fig. 38-3). If the child is older and no treatment has been given, it may be possible to palpate the feces-filled colon on abdominal examination. A

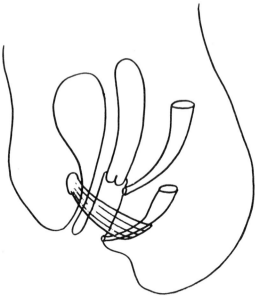

Figure 38–1. Diagram illustrating the position of low and high rectovaginal fistulae relative to the levator sling. Contraction of the sling can control egress of fecal matter from a low fistula, but not from a high one.

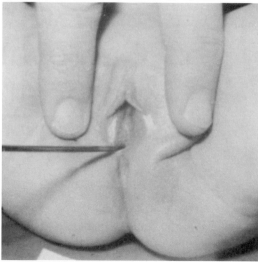

Figure 38–3. A low rectovaginal fistula in a newborn. The anus is absent from its normal site, but the abnormal opening can be identified by a probe. (From Dewhurst J: Surgery to repair disorders of development. In Nichols D [ed]: Gynecologic Obstetric Surgery. St. Louis, Mosby–Year Book, 1993.)

suggested approach to such a problem encountered in a newborn is set out in Table 38–1.

TREATMENT

In most cases, treatment should be instituted early to avoid the rectal inertia syndrome. Management can be approached in two ways:

1. The anal opening may be left where it lies, close to the vagina, but the contracted opening enlarged by a "cutback" or by anal dilatation (Fig. 38–4).[9]
2. Some form of pull-through procedure may be carried out, an option currently preferred by many pediatric surgeons for all but the most superficial abnormalities. The fistulous opening is dissected off the vagina and the bowel pulled through to the normal position, taking infinite care not to damage sphincteric action in the process. This is a difficult and delicate maneuver.

The gynecologist is not, as a rule, involved in early management but may be consulted later, especially if a cutback or dilatation has been performed. In most cases of an anteriorly placed anus, good bowel control can be expected from

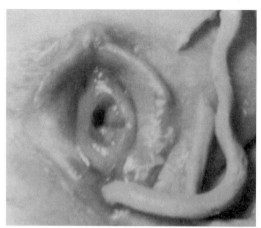

Figure 38–2. A rectovestibular fistula in a newborn. Note the contraction of the abnormal opening.

Table 38–1. Anus Absent or Anteriorly Displaced at Birth

Is an external anal opening visible?
Is this opening constricted and to what degree?
If not visible, is meconium issuing from the vagina?
Does inspection of the lower vagina reveal a fistulous opening?
Are other genital anomalies present? Double vagina? Hydrocolpos? Bladder or urethral anomalies?
Are more general anomalies evident? Cardiac? Respiratory? Sacral? Other?
Consult with a pediatrician and pediatric surgeon at the earliest opportunity.

When a pull-through procedure has been carried out, the process of dissecting the bowel off the vagina and closing the ostium may lead to vaginal contraction at that point. This is a more likely problem with the high rectovaginal fistula (discussed later).

The most formidable gynecologic problem associated with a rectovestibular fistula or perineal anus is congenital absence of the vagina. The customary procedure for dealing with vaginal absence, which involves the use of a mold after a space has been dissected between bladder and bowel (McIndoe procedure), is not appropriate in this situation, as the use of a mold would almost certainly lead to pressure necrosis of the immediately adjacent rectum and anus and development of another fistula. A successful alternative is to mobilize an isolated loop of cecum between the bowel and the bladder, which requires no molds.[10] However, this operation is a surgical *tour de force* and should be attempted only by the most experienced surgeons.

HIGH RECTOVAGINAL FISTULA

When the abnormal rectal opening is situated in the upper or middle vagina, it lies above the levator sling, so that contraction of the levator cannot prevent the flow of fecal matter into the vagina (see Fig. 38–1). These are much more serious anomalies and inevitably require major surgery. In most instances a preliminary colostomy is necessary initially, with a pull-through procedure a short time later, when the child is well enough. Freeman and Bulut[11] performed immediate sigmoid loop colostomy in 18 patients with high fistulas; this was followed with a sacroperineal or abdominosacroperineal pull-through operation at the age of 1 to 14 days in seven patients, at 15 to 40 days in another seven, and not until 60 to 120 days in the remainder. Longer delays may be necessary.

Cases managed in this fashion are unlikely to involve the gynecologist at first but may subsequently. Many patients with a congenital rectovaginal defect, whether major or minor, have associated genital tract anomalies that may also require subsequent intervention. Fleming and colleagues[12] identified uterine anomalies in 18 of 51 female adolescents whose upper genital tract had been examined. In eight of these, the uterus was bicornuate; eight others, had a didelphic uterus; and two, a hypoplastic uterus. Vaginal anomalies, in addition to the fistula, were present in 22 of 71 girls; in 13 there was a septate vagina; in five the vagina was absent; and distal

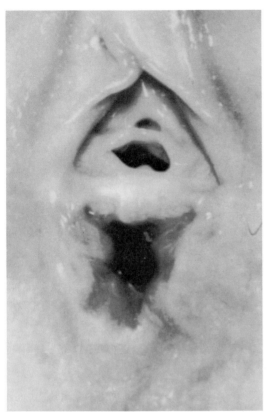

Figure 38–4. Appearance of the vulva in a child treated by a "cutback." The anus, although immediately adjacent to the vagina, functioned well, and vaginal soiling did not occur. (From Dewhurst J: Surgery to repair disorders of development. In Nichols D [ed]: Gynecologic and Obstetric Surgery. St. Louis, Mosby–Year Book, 1993.)

a cutback procedure carried out early in life. A surgeon asked to see a pediatric patient whose anal opening lies close to the vaginal introitus or even just within it may fear the risk of genital tract infection as a result of vaginal soiling with fecal matter or of dyspareunia later in life. Perineorrhaphy may be contemplated to build up a thicker septum between the two openings; however, this procedure is neither necessary nor advisable, since neither vaginal soiling nor dyspareunia is likely to occur. Moreover, the surgical procedure might compromise rectal continence, which must be avoided at all costs. This need for preservation of sphincter control makes cesarean section desirable when the patient gives birth.

These recommendations should be discussed with the parents when they are counseled about their daughter's future. They must understand that sexual function and fertility are unlikely to be affected.

vaginal stenosis, absence of the lower one third of the vagina, an imperforate hymen, and a bifid hymen each occurred once. Abnormalities of the urinary tract were also frequent and included bladder exstrophy, unilateral renal agenesis, hydronephrosis, and ectopic and malformed kidneys. A number of these associated genital tract developmental abnormalities (e.g., bicornuate uterus or didelphic uterus) require no treatment, and others (e.g., hymenal abnormalities or a septate vagina) can be treated without difficulty. However, congenital absence of the vagina along with a vestibular fistula or perineal anus is a formidable problem, as discussed earlier.[13–18]

An acquired defect that may result from dissection of the fistula from the vagina and closure of the opening is vaginal narrowing at the surgical site. Constriction of this type may lead to dyspareunia later in life, but no attempt should be made to correct this surgically during childhood or adolescence. Division of the constricting fibrous tissue may need to be carried out widely to restore normal vaginal capacity; in a child this is exceedingly difficult. More important, a vaginal mold must be worn until epithelialization is complete, and then must be inserted and removed from the vagina several times each day lest the vagina contract. A younger, less mature patient may not be able to cooperate with this regimen,

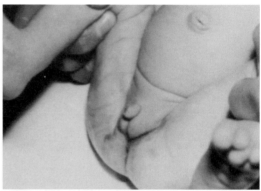

Figure 38–6. A complex case in which a newborn female with a cloaca had, in addition, a second filiform urethra that extended to the tip of an enlarged phallus.

and thus intervention must be postponed until she reaches emotional maturity.

CLOACAL AND OTHER GROSS ABNORMALITIES

The high rectovaginal fistula usually occurs when development in this area is abnormal. In its earliest expression, the child may be born with a cloaca, a single opening into which bladder, genital tract, and bowel all open (Fig. 38–5). As in high fistula cases, an immediate colostomy is generally required, after which an attempt may be made to determine the best way to manage the genitourinary aspects of the case. Again, other malformations affecting the uterus and upper renal tracts may coexist. One of the most serious, which may defeat all attempts to establish urinary control, is sacral agenesis, a rare accompaniment. Affected patients may have difficulty establishing urinary control. Despite the dismal prognosis for many of them, some degree of success is often achieved by the pediatric surgeon, and a gynecologist may be consulted later, when the patient reaches adolescence or adulthood. The variations are so considerable that management is beyond the scope of this discussion. Pregnancy has occasionally been achieved.[19]

A most curious form of anomaly rarely described in the literature is a cloaca or urogenital sinus defect associated with an enlarged phallus with a second filiform urethra running down from the tip.[20–23] No convincing explanation for this enlargement of the phallus has been advanced, and it does not seem to be related to the more common forms of phallic enlargement, such as congenital adrenal hyperplasia, androgen

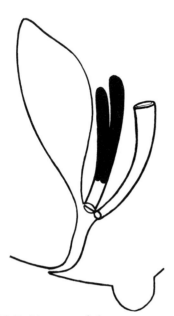

Figure 38–5. Diagram of the appearances found in a newborn girl with a cloaca. Note that the bladder, genital tract, and bowel share a single opening; note also the double uterus and bifid short vagina.

stimulation in utero, or true hermaphroditism. Several cases have been reported in the literature, although even among these, variation is great (Fig. 38–6).

REFERENCES

1. Stephens FD: Congenital Malformation of the Rectum, Anus, and Genitourinary Tracts. London: Churchill Livingstone, 1963.
2. Stephens FD, Smith ED: Anorectal Malformations in Children. Chicago: Year Book, 1971.
3. Nixon HH, Puri P: The results of treatment of anorectal anomalies. J Pediatr Surg 1977; 12:27–37.
4. Smith EI, Tunel WP, Williams GR: Clinical evaluation of the surgical treatment of anorectal malformation. Ann Surg 1978; 187: 583–592.
5. de Vries PA: The surgery of anorectal anomalies. Curr Probl Surg 1984; 21(5):1–75.
6. Iwai N, Yanagihara J, Tokiwa K, et al: Results of surgical correction of anorectal malformation. Ann Surg 1984; 207:219–222.
7. Stephens FD, Smith ED: Anorectal Anomalies (Proposed International Classification). Chicago: Year Book, 1971.
8. Stephens FD, Smith ED: Classification identification and assessment of surgical treatment of anorectal anomalies. Report of a workshop meeting, Racine, WI, March 1984. Cited in de Vries PA, Cox KL: Surgery of anorectal anomalies. Surg Clin North Am 1985; 65(5):1139–1169.
9. Dewhurst CJ: Gynaecological Disorders of Infants and Children. London: Cassell, 1963.
10. Morton K, Dewhurst J: The use of bowel to create a vagina. Pediatr Adolesc Gynecol 1984; 2:51–61.
11. Freeman NV, Bulut M: High anorectal anomalies treated by early (neonatal) operation. J Pediatr Surg 1986; 21:218–220.
12. Fleming SE, Hall R, Gysler M, McLorie GA: Imperforate anus in females: Frequency of genital tract involvement, incidence of anomalies and functional outcome. J Pediatr Surg 1986; 21:146–150.
13. Escobar LF: Urorectal septum malformation sequence. Am J Dis Child 1987; 141:1021–1031.
14. Hendren WH: Urogenital sinus and anorectal malformation: Experience of 22 cases. J Pediatr Surg 1980; 15:628–634.
15. Nakayama DK, Snyder HW, Schnaufer L, et al: Posterior sagittal exposure for reconstructive surgery for cloacal anomalies. J Pediatr Surg 1987; 22:588–592.
16. Pena A: Anorectal malformations. Semin Pediatr Surg 1995; 4:35–47.
17. Hendren WH: Urogenital sinus and cloacal malformations. Semin Pediatr Surg 1996; 5:72–79.
18. Smith EA, Woodard JR, Broecker R, et al: Current urological management of cloacal exstrophy: Experience of 11 patients. J Pediatr Surg 1997; 32:263–267.
19. Water EG: Cloacal dysgenesis: Related anomalies and pregnancies. Obstet Gynecol 1982; 59:398–402.
20. Belis JA, Hrabovsky EE: Idiopathic female intersex with clitoromegaly and urethral duplication. J Urol 1979; 122:805–809.
21. Belinger MF, Duckett JW: Accessory phallic urethra in the female patient. J Urol 1982; 127:1159–1163.
22. Hurwitz RS, Fitzpatrick TJ: Vaginal urethra, clitoral hypertrophy and accessory phallic urethra. J Urol 1982; 127:1165–1170.
23. Gale DH, Stocker JT: Cloacal dysgenesis with urethral vaginal outlet and anal agenesis and functioning internal genitourinary excretion. Pediatr Pathol 1987; 7:475–466.

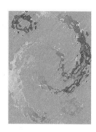

Chapter 39

Chronic Pelvic Pain—Medical and Surgical Approaches

Betsy Schroeder and Joseph S. Sanfilippo

Chronic pelvic pain in an adolescent girl continues to challenge clinicians. By definition, chronic pelvic pain is persistent lower abdominal pain of at least 6 months' duration.[1] The typical scenario involves distraught parents making multiple visits to a clinic or physician's office with their child in frantic efforts to identify the underlying cause of the pain. At the same time, the girl may use chronic pelvic pain as a means of attracting attention, which makes it imperative that the physician observe interactions between the patient and her family and consider whether a psychological component might be contributing to the pelvic pain.

Initial evaluation requires a thorough history and physical examination. The history should gather specific information on multiple organ systems (Table 39–1), including any gastrointestinal problems such as spastic colon or regional enteritis. The clinician evaluating the genitourinary system should look for evidence of recurring cystitis or a gynecologic disorder (e.g., persistent vaginal discharge) that might lead to upper or lower reproductive tract infections. The patient should be questioned about dysmenorrhea. Abnormal uterine bleeding is important in the overall assessment of pelvic pain, because the discomfort can be secondary to a menstrual aberration, often including passage of clots. In addition, endomyometritis can be associated with pelvic pain and abnormal uterine bleeding. This infectious-inflammatory problem is associated principally with pregnancy. The pattern of pubertal development and any problems associated with obstruction to the outflow tract that could cause pelvic pain, must also be documented. Although childhood diseases rarely cause pelvic pain, infections such as mumps oophoritis must be ruled out during history taking.[2]

A general physical examination must be performed as well as a pelvic examination to determine whether the pelvic area is tender or harbors a mass. If endometriosis is suspected, a rectovaginal examination also is useful because nodular areas along the uterosacral ligaments and cul de sac regions or cul de sac masses, although rare in adolescents, may be discovered. Thus, the essential components of pelvic pain assessment are (1) ruling out significant pelvic abnormality, (2) thorough history taking, and (3) a detailed pelvic examination, including rectovaginal assessment.

What are the appropriate laboratory tests is determined by the symptoms and pelvic findings. It may be necessary to assess the gastrointestinal (GI) tract radiologically (upper GI studies, small bowel follow-through) and to perform barium enema and gallbladder studies if the pelvic pain is associated with specific GI symptoms. Sigmoidoscopy may be indicated when there is evidence of lower GI tract symptoms such as hematochezia.

In this age group, diagnostic laparoscopy is an integral study in the assessment of pelvic pain. Goldstein and coworkers[3] used laparoscopy to examine 109 adolescent girls between the ages of 10½ and 19 years who had unexplained chronic pelvic pain. Of interest is the finding that the youngest documented patient to have endometriosis was 10.8 years old and had reached menarche 5 months earlier.[3]

PSYCHOLOGICAL ASPECTS

The psychological aspects of chronic pelvic pain have been evaluated by Gross and coworkers[4] in a multidisciplinary study of 25 "gynecology patients." Although each patient's pelvic examination findings were normal, psychiatric assess-

Table 39–1. Causes of Chronic Pelvic Pain

Reproductive System
   Noncyclic
      Adhesions
      Endometriosis
      Salpingo-oophoritis
      Ovarian remnant syndrome
      Pelvic congestion syndrome (varicosities)
      Ovarian neoplasms
      Pelvic relaxation
   Cyclic
      Primary dysmenorrhea
      Secondary dysmenorrhea
         Imperforate hymen
         Transverse vaginal septum
         Cervical stenosis
         Uterine anomalies (congenital
           malformation—bicornuate uterus, blind uterine
           horn)
         Intrauterine synechiae (Asherman syndrome)
         Endometrial polyps
         Uterine leiomyoma
         Adenomyosis
Gastrointestinal Tract
   Irritable bowel syndrome
   Ulcerative colitis
   Granulomatous colitis (Crohn disease)
   Carcinoma
   Infectious diarrhea
   Recurrent partial small bowel obstruction
   Diverticulitis
   Hernia
   Abdominal angina
   Recurrent appendiceal colic
Genitourinary System
   Recurrent or relapsing cystourethritis
   Urethritis
   Interstitial cystitis
   Ureteral diverticuli or polyps
   Carcinoma of the bladder
   Ureteral obstruction
   Pelvic kidney
Nervous System
   Nerve entrapment syndrome
   Neuroma
Musculoskeletal System
   Low back pain syndrome
   Congenital anomaly
   Scoliosis and kyphosis
   Spondylosis
   Spondylolisthesis
   Spine injuries
   Inflammation
   Tumors
   Osteoporosis
   Degenerative changes
   Coccydynia
   Myofascial syndrome
Systemic Disease
   Acute intermittent porphyria
   Abdominal migraine
   Systemic lupus erythematosus
   Lymphoma
Neurofibromatosis

Adapted from Rapkin AJ, Reading AE: Chronic pelvic pain. Curr Probl Obstet Gynecol Fertil 1991; XIV:110.

ment determined that the most frequent diagnosis was "significant pathology with borderline syndrome, and hysterical character disorder." A significant incidence of early childhood family dysfunction and incest also was noted. Psychological testing corroborated the high incidence of psychopathology.

Differences between organic and psychogenic functional pelvic pain have been identified.[1] Organic pain is frequently sharp and "crampy," and awakens the patient at night with intermittent radiation of the pain, whereas psychogenic pain usually is absent during sleep. Some authors suggest that women with chronic pelvic pain are mentally or emotionally disturbed. Often, the onset of pelvic pain can be linked to a stressful event or life crisis.[1]

Treatment of chronic pelvic pain often involves reassuring the patient that she has no organic pelvic abnormality. She must be apprised of the contribution of stress to her pain, and she must be afforded a safe forum where she can express anger or frustration.

PELVIC PAIN OF MUSCULOSKELETAL CAUSES

Causes of pelvic pain that originate in the musculoskeletal system or abdominal wall have received little attention in the gynecologic literature, but often musculoskeletal dysfunction is the primary factor or a contributing condition. Aftimos[5] describes two girls, aged 11 and 13, whose musculoskeletal pelvic and abdominal pain was misdiagnosed as conversion disorder and constipation, respectively. Peters and co-workers[6] evaluated 106 women with chronic pelvic pain and found trigger points in 26 (24%). Among 177 patients referred to a pelvic pain clinic, Slocumb[7] identified trigger points in 74%. Clearly, this diagnosis should be considered when girls complain of pelvic pain.

Trigger points are areas of hyperirritability that are locally tender on compression and cause referred pain and tenderness; the myofascial pain syndrome occurs within taut bands of skeletal muscle that cause the pain.[8] Most of the theories about the development of trigger points implicate noxious stimuli to the affected fascia and muscles. Sustained muscle contraction, like that caused by poor posture or in response to an injury, may be a trigger. Cold or damp weather (especially after a viral illness), or a new physical activity in an unconditioned person can also be causal factors.[5]

Both acute and chronic pelvic pain can be associated with trigger points in the abdominal wall, the vagina, or the sacrum. The referred pain is often visceral, resembling dysmenorrhea, or, alternatively, presents as dyspareunia or with urinary tract or gastrointestinal symptoms. While the trigger points are quite distinctive areas on physical examination, the referred pain is often poorly localized and may not follow dermatome patterns.

It is very difficult to distinguish musculoskeletal pain from visceral pain by history. In each case, the pain may be sharp and stabbing or achy and dull. The pain may improve with nonsteroidal antiinflammatory drugs (NSAIDs) or application of heat. It may worsen with activity and subside with rest, and, in each case, changing position may "change" the discomfort. The patient may be awakened from sleep by visceral pain, but likely not by musculoskeletal pain, though paresthesias and muscle weakness are more common with musculoskeletal dysfunction. Although it might be expected that changes in the quality or severity of the pain associated with menstruation would not occur in musculoskeletal pain, it may be due to increased relaxin production in the luteal phase.[9]

A thorough physical examination is paramount in identifying trigger points, as they are easy to miss. Techniques for diagnosis have been described by Slocumb.[7] First, the abdominal skin should be gently pinched in each dermatomal region from T10 to L1, and it should be compared to that in the contralateral region, looking for a sharper sensation in one or more areas to identify regions of hypersensitivity. Next, to look for trigger points, single-finger pressure is applied over the abdominal wall, beginning in the dermatome closest to the area of pain and systematically exploring all dermatomes in the abdomen. When the patient's pain is reproduced, the examiner asks her to contract the rectus muscles by elevating her legs off the table and then applies pressure at the same point. With this maneuver, visceral pathology is rarely reproduced by abdominal wall palpation, and pain from single-finger pressure is the most valuable tool for identifying abdominal wall trigger points.[10, 11] Finally, trigger points may also be detected on examination of the vaginal wall. Trigger points can be detected by applying gentle pressure with a cotton-tipped applicator or a single finger lateral to the cervix at the 3:00 to 4:00 o'clock position and at 8:00 to 9:00 o'clock, as well as along the lateral wall at the mid-vagina.

Treatment involves injecting 0.25% bupivacaine or 1% procaine into the trigger points. Relief may last weeks to months, though, initially, the injection may reproduce the pain, which may be extreme for a few moments. Eighty-nine percent of 122 patients who received trigger point injections with 3 to 5 ml of 0.25% bupivacaine had positive responses—relief or improvement

in the pain such that no further treatment was required.[7] Gallegos[12] reported similar results: improvement in 80% of 20 patients. Another study documented significant improvement with chiropractic flexion-distraction in combination with trigger point injections.[13] Other investigators have suggested that injection of saline[14, 15] or dry needling alone[16] results in improvement; however, only local anesthetic injections provide relief consistently, for months to years.

The use of vasocoolants and stretching has been advocated by some physicians, particularly for children who fear needles. The affected area is first sprayed with a local anesthetic; then fluoromethane or ethyl chloride is applied via a nozzle that produces a "jet stream." It is applied from a distance of approximately 50 cm and at a tangent to the skin. A unidirectional sweep parallel to the muscle fibers, beginning proximal to the trigger point, ending distal to it, and encompassing the entire pain zone is the preferred technique. The muscle is massaged and passively stretched, but not to the point that it is painful.[17] This technique provided complete relief within 1 to 3 days for three of five children who had trigger points. The other two responded within 6 weeks when transcutaneous electrical nerve stimulation was used as an adjunct.[5]

For patients with pelvic pain of musculoskeletal causes, physical therapy may also be beneficial, but it is important that the physical therapist be familiar with pelvic pain. Of 150 patients seen in a chronic pelvic pain clinic, 132 had twice weekly physical therapy for 2 to 3 months. Complete relief of symptoms was reported by 19.6%, significant improvement by 50%, and no change by 10.6%. The rest were lost to follow-up. No one's symptoms worsened. Half of the patients had undergone gynecologic and psychological treatment (without improvement in their pain) before initiation of physical therapy; the other half underwent gynecologic, psychological, and physical therapy evaluations simultaneously. Seventy-five percent of these patients had a common faulty posture pattern, which investigators called *typical pelvic pain posture*.[18] Another study comparing multidisciplinary treatment to standard treatment for chronic pelvic pain found that physical therapy was appropriate for 49% of the patients in the multidisciplinary group, an approach that also included psychosocial intervention, dietary and nutritional management, and medical and surgical gynecologic treatment, as indicated.[6]

Although literature is scant, musculoskeletal causes of both acute and chronic pelvic pain should be considered in the adolescent population. Because of differences in activities, teens may in fact be more likely than adults to benefit from investigation, and diagnosis is straightforward and noninvasive.

ENDOMETRIOSIS

In the past, endometriosis, (endometrial glands and stroma outside the normal intrauterine endometrial cavity) was not considered a common disorder in teenagers. Its true incidence in adolescents is difficult to discern because surgical exploration is required and physicians have been hesitant to operate on this age group. With the availability of laparoscopy and the growing awareness of the possibility of endometriosis in this population, more accurate assessments are becoming available. Still, asymptomatic cases go undiagnosed. Among teens with chronic pelvic pain, reported rates have ranged from 19% to 65%.[19–24] More recent studies have addressed the incidence of endometriosis in adolescents with chronic pelvic pain that was unresponsive to oral contraceptive pills (OCPs) or nonsteroidal antiinflammatory drugs, (NSAIDs), and findings range from 69.6% to 73%.[25, 26]

DEVELOPMENT

In 1946, Fallon[27] suggested that the development of endometriosis requires at least 5 years of menstrual cycles with ovulation; however, there are reports of endometriosis occurring within 5 years of menarche, such as the 10.8-year-old girl diagnosed only 5 months after menarche.[3] Yamamoto and coworkers[28] reported a case of endometriosis within 1 month after menarche. It is not even clear that menarche is required for endometriosis to develop. Whitehouse[29] reported endometriosis in a 22-year-old with primary amenorrhea, and Seitz[30] reported endometriomas in a 21-year-old with primary amenorrhea. Reese and colleagues[26] more recently reported on two premenarcheal girls, aged 12 and 13, with endometriosis. Although older teens are more likely to seek gynecologic care than younger adolescents, clinicians must also realize that the disease can and does exist in the preteens and younger adolescents.

The exact mechanism of development of endometriosis continues to challenge our understanding. The current theories apply to both adults and adolescents and include coelomic metaplasia (Myer's theory),[31] endometrial tissue transplanted via hematogenous and lymphatic spread,[32] and retrograde menstruation (theory of Sampson).[33] Although no single theory provides an adequate explanation, epidemiologic evidence supports retrograde menstruation, as patients with endometriosis have shorter cycle lengths, longer duration of flow, and heavier flow than controls,[34] and many adolescents with obstructive müllerian anomalies have endometriosis. This does not explain premenarcheal patients with endometriosis[26] or endometriosis at sites remote from the pelvis such as the lung, however. Immune system susceptibility may be involved, and there is strong evidence of a genetic influence. Simpson and associates[35] reported that 6.9% of women who have a close relative with endometriosis have endometriosis themselves, as compared with only 1.0% of those with no family history.

A major distinction between adolescents and adults in the development of endometriosis is its association with anomalies of the reproductive system. Several müllerian anomalies, particularly those with obstruction of the outflow tract, have been associated with endometriosis. In a series reported by Schifrin and coworkers,[36] six of 15 patients (40%) younger than 20 with endometriosis had a genital tract anomaly. Goldstein's group[3] found congenital anomalies of the reproductive tract in 11% of 74 teenagers with endometriosis, and Reese and coworkers[26] reported obstructive anomalies in four of 49 teens with endometriosis.

The clinical course of endometriosis associated with reproductive tract anomalies appears to be different from that of other cases. Sanfilippo and colleagues[37] described a 12-year-old patient with outflow tract obstruction who had endometriosis. Once the obstruction was surgically corrected, the endometriosis also resolved.

Others have found no association between endometriosis and reproductive tract anomalies in teenagers. Laufer and associates[25] found müllerian anomalies in 6.5% of teens with pelvic pain that did not respond to conventional therapy for dysmenorrhea, and only one of those had associated endometriosis; thus, only one of 31 patients in this group with endometriosis had a müllerian anomaly. Davis and coworkers,[38] Vercellini and colleagues,[21] and Emmert[39] found no anomalies among 36, 18, and 37 adolescents, respectively, with endometriosis. Furthermore, a study of infertile women by Fedele's group[40] found no difference in the frequency of endometriosis in those with nonobstructive müllerian anomalies, as compared with those without, suggesting that the pathogenic factor of müllerian anomalies and endometriosis is different in the two conditions.

CLINICAL PRESENTATION

Adolescents' symptoms often differ from adults'. Characteristic symptoms in adults include dysmenorrhea, pelvic pain, infertility, or adnexal masses from endometriomas. Infertility is rarely an issue in teens, and endometriomas are infrequent. One study, though, describes endometriomas in 13 of 16 adolescents with endometriosis who underwent laparotomy.[41] Pelvic pain, with or without dysmenorrhea, is the most common presentation of endometriosis. Symptoms are typically worse around the time of menses and, in contrast to primary dysmenorrhea, appear to be refractory to NSAIDs and OCPs. Other common symptoms include dyspareunia (29%), menstrual irregularity (25%), and abdominal pain or nausea (43%).[26] Forty-six patients younger than 22 years who for more than 3 months had chronic pelvic pain that did not respond to OCPs or NSAIDs and who underwent laparoscopy were reviewed by Laufer's group.[25] Thirty-two (69.6%) had endometriosis. Presenting symptoms are listed in Table 39–2.

Physical examination findings are also different from those of adults. Due to adhesions, the uterus may be fixed and retroflexed in adults, and ovaries are often tender and enlarged by endometriomas. Nodularity of the cul de sac and uterosacral ligaments are other classic findings. In contrast, they are uncommon in adolescents, whose pelvic examination findings are often normal, with only mild to moderate tenderness. The adnexa are usually without masses.

It is important to look for anomalies of the hymen, vagina, and cervix during the pelvic examination. This may be difficult, as in adolescents, these examinations are often challenging. A rectal exam may provide valuable information, such as cul de sac nodularity or adnexal masses that could otherwise be missed. Analgesia, or even anesthesia, may be required for adequate examination. Ultrasonography can be helpful in looking for endometriomas or reproductive tract anomalies.

DIAGNOSIS

It is important that diagnosis not be delayed, not only for symptomatic relief but also to preserve fertility and arrest progression of the disease. Symptomatic patients should be evaluated laparoscopically when the condition is refractory to standard treatment for primary dysmenorrhea. In a prospective study, Stovall and coworkers[42] found worse pain at follow-up in those whose disease was more advanced at the time of diagnosis (mean interval from initial treatment to follow-up was 15.7 years). Unfortunately, in teenagers laparoscopy is often deferred for several years after the onset of symptoms.[26, 38]

Adolescents are more likely to have early or atypical lesions than the classic blue-black, powder-burn lesions seen frequently in adult women. Red lesions appear to be the most common in this age group (prevalence 82% to 86%[26, 38]), but white and clear, vesicular lesions are also common, as are peritoneal pockets. These findings are supported by Redwine,[43] who found that patients with atypical endometriosis lesions are, on average, 10 years younger than those who have black lesions, and by Martin and coworkers,[44] who reported evolution from subtle lesions in adolescence to classic lesions 10 years later.

Owing to the subtle presentation of vesicular lesions, they may be difficult to identify laparoscopically, in part because of light reflected from the endoscope. Laufer[45] described a technique that assists in the identification of this form of the disease. Filling the pelvis with irrigation fluid and submerging the laparoscope into the fluid-filled pelvis eliminates light reflection, and the clear vesicles can be appreciated in three dimensions.

When there is evidence of endometriosis at laparoscopy, biopsy specimens should be collected to provide histologic confirmation of the disease. If the pelvis is normal in appearance, random peritoneal biopsy specimens may still reveal the disease. Among infertile women without visible pelvic lesions, Nisolle and colleagues[46] found microscopic endometriosis in 6%, whereas among teens with chronic pelvic pain that did not respond to conventional therapy, Laufer's group[25] found biopsy-proven endometriosis in one of five who had a grossly normal pelvis.

Staging of endometriosis should follow the

Table 39–2. Prevalence of Symptoms of Endometriosis

Symptoms	Prevalence (%)
Cyclic and noncyclic pain	62.5
Noncyclic pain	28.1
Cyclic pain	9.4
Gastrointestinal tract pain	34.3
Urinary tract symptoms	12.5
Irregular menses	9.4

Adapted from Laufer MR, Goitein L, Bush M, et al: Prevalence of endometriosis in adolescent girls with chronic pelvic pain not responding to conventional therapy. J Pediatr Adolesc Gynecol 1997; 10:199.

Table 39–3. Sites of Endometriosis Lesions in Adolescent Girls

Sites	Prevalence (%)
Pouch of Douglas	64.8
Uterosacral ligaments	37.8
Ovarian fossa	24.3
Parametrium	8.1
Appendix area	2.7
Cardinal ligaments	2.7
Bladder	2.7

Emmert C, Romann D, Riedel HH: Endometriosis diagnosed by laparoscopy in adolescent girls. Arch Gynecol Obstet 1998; 261:89–93.

American Fertility Society (now American Society for Reproductive Medicine) classification.[47] Most adolescents have stage I (77% to 92%) or stage II (8% to 22.6%) disease.[25, 26, 39] Emmert and coworkers[39] described types and locations of endometriotic implants in 37 adolescents who had endometriosis diagnosed laparoscopically. All had stage I or II disease, 67% of lesions being pinhead sized, 27% rice sized, and 2.7% pea sized. The sites of the lesions are described in Table 39–3.

TREATMENT

It is important to note that there are no published studies of treatment modalities in adolescents. Consequently, adolescents are treated in the same manner as adults, although it is possible that outcomes may be different in teenage patients. Treatment may be medical, surgical, or a combination of the two. In teenagers, surgical treatment is usually conservative, consisting of laparoscopic ablation of endometrial implants with laser or cautery. This is generally followed with medical management.

Studies comparing medical therapy after laparoscopic ablation of endometriosis with placebos after surgery have found that recurrence of symptoms is delayed in those who receive hormonal therapy. Hornstein and colleagues,[48] in a randomized, prospective, placebo-controlled, multicenter clinical trial, administered nafarelin or placebo for 6 months to 105 patients after laparoscopic diagnosis of endometriosis. The group treated with the gonadotropin-releasing hormone (GnRH) agonist did not seek alternative treatment (repeat medical or surgical treatment) for a median interval of more than 24 months after surgery, whereas, for the placebo group, the median was 11.7 months. Similarly, Telima and colleagues[49] demonstrated fewer clinical symptoms and smaller implants at second-look laparoscopy in patients who were treated medically after laparoscopy, as compared with those treated with a placebo. Clearly, medical therapy after laparoscopy for endometriosis is warranted.

Medical treatment consists of hormone suppression. A number of regimens are available, including OCPs, danazol, depomedroxyprogesterone acetate (DMPA), and GnRH agonists.

Adolescents tolerate OCPs well. They may be administered in a cycle of 21 days of hormonally active pills followed by 7 days of placebo pills, which will allow a withdrawal bleed, or continuously, without the placebo pills, to create a "pseudopregnancy." Breakthrough bleeding is a frequent side effect when active pills are taken continuously. Because estrogen stimulates endometrial implants and androgens result in atrophy, progestin-dominant pills should be used. In spite of clinical improvement, there is no evidence for regression of endometrial implants with use of OCPs.[50]

Danazol treats endometriosis by creating a low-estrogen, high-androgen environment. Although it is very efficacious, it is rarely used in adolescents because of its side effects, which include both androgenic and hypoestrogenic side effects, such as acne, irregular menses, weight gain, decreased breast size, fluid retention, hot flushes, atrophic vaginitis, hirsutism, and deepening of the voice. Some of the masculinizing side effects may not be reversed on discontinuation of the medication.

Intramuscular DMPA, administered in a dose of 150 mg every 4 to 12 weeks, is an effective alternative. Vercellini and coworkers[51] showed that progestins are as effective as danazol or GnRH agonists for pelvic pain in patients with endometriosis. Pelvic pain at the end of follow-up (mean 6 months) was 50%, and the odds ratio for nonresponders in the progestin group (as compared with the danazol or GnRH agonist group) was 1.1 (CI 0.4 to 3.1). In a prospective study, the same group[52] demonstrated that DMPA was as effective as birth control pills in combination with low-dose danazol. At the end of 1 year of treatment, 29 of 40 (72.5%) of those who received DMPA, 150 mg IM every 3 months, were satisfied, as compared with only 23 of 40 (57.5%) of those who received ethinyl estradiol, 0.02 mg, desogestrel 0.15 mg, and danazol, 50 mg, 21 of 28 days per month. Relief of dysmenorrhea was significantly greater among the DMPA group.

Potential side effects of DMPA must be discussed with patients before therapy is instituted.

Breakthrough bleeding is common at the beginning of treatment; however, once endometrial atrophy has been achieved, bleeding is unusual. By the end of 1 year of use, 57% have amenorrhea, and by 2 years, 68%.[53] Other common side effects include weight gain, hair loss, and headaches. Another concern is the fact that bone mineral density (BMD) had been reported to be lower among women using DMPA,[54] and this finding has also been observed in adolescents.[55, 56] In a study by Cromer and colleagues,[56] dual photon absorptiometry (DEXA) was performed on controls (not using hormonal contraception) and on patients using DMPA, Norplant, or OCPs, at baseline and after 1 and 2 years of therapy. Among those using DMPA, after 1 year BMD had decreased by 1.5% and after 2 years by 3.1%. In controls, BMD had increased by 2.9% at 1 year and 9.5% at 2 years. BMD increased among the users of Norplant and OCPs as well, but to a lesser extent. It is not known whether this bone loss will be recovered after the medication is discontinued.

GnRH agonists are considered the treatment of choice for endometriosis. Traditionally, they have been administered as an intramuscular injection in doses of 3.75 mg every 4 weeks for 6 months, but recent literature[57] suggests that 11.25 mg every 12 weeks for a total of 6 months is equally efficacious. These agents have been shown to be as effective as danazol[58, 59] but have much more tolerable side effects. The hypoestrogenic environment created by the agonist creates pseudomenopause, with the typical side effects, such as hot flushes and vaginal dryness. GnRH agonists, like DMPA, carry the risk of trabecular bone loss;[60, 61] thus, traditionally they have been used no more than 6 months. The evidence about recovery of bone loss after discontinuation of therapy is equivocal.[62–66] To minimize bone loss and other hypoestrogenic side effects, "addback" therapy has been advocated.[67, 68] Hornstein and associates[67] found that depoleuprolide acetate, 3.75 mg IM every 4 weeks, supplemented with norethindrone acetate, 5 mg, with or without conjugated equine estrogen, 0.625 mg daily, provided effective suppression of pelvic pain and protected adult women from bone loss.

LAPAROSCOPY IN PEDIATRIC AND ADOLESCENT PATIENTS

Both pediatric and adolescent patients represent the "neophyte" of technological advances. Now that operative laparoscopy has been performed in preterm infants, neonates, and young children, the surgical horizon appears to be one continuum of exploration that begins soon after birth.

Improvements in instrumentation have afforded children endoscopic surgical intervention. Gans and Berci are given the primary credit for convincing pediatric surgeons and gynecologists who deal in this subspecialized area that laparoscopy has a major role in the management of surgical abnormalities in children.[69]

The questions remain, which procedures can be performed endoscopically, and how. Laparoscopy is possible in both infants and children because of technologic advances, such as the Hopkins rod lens telescopes, which have revolutionized pediatric laparoscopic procedures. These instruments range from smaller than 2 to 10 mm in diameter and are used most often in 0-degree or 30-degree lens configurations. Most surgeons who treat pediatric and adolescent patients prefer to use 0-degree endoscopes because they are less disorienting for the operating surgeon. The 30-degree lenses are useful for certain applications, such as endoscopic suturing or when a structure must be assessed at an angle and placing a second port is not desired. The right-angle or operating laparoscope is of little use for most of the endoscopic procedures in this age group, and if a new system is to be purchased, it is probably not worth the additional expense. Lightweight video camera systems have also facilitated surgical procedures in young patients. Three-chip cameras and systems with the chip on the end of the scope further expedite laparoscopic procedures in this age group. Ideally, a camera system with controls on the camera head makes it possible to obtain still photographs and allows the operating surgeon to control the video printer and recorder.

Laparoscopic equipment for infants and children must have smaller port sets and more delicate instrumentation. The ideal trocar for an infant or small child is one that is about 2.5 cm long and remains fixed in the peritoneal cavity until it is no longer needed. Several disposable devices approach this configuration, being shorter than most adult cannulas and having an expandable flange that keeps them from slipping out of the abdomen after insertion. The standard screw-type fixation device tends to tear a child's skin and often slips out easily because the child's abdominal wall is thin. Adhesive rings show promise for holding cannulas in place.

There has been a logarithmic expansion in the development of instrumentation for endoscopic surgery. Many of the disposable devices are still too crude to be used in small children. Reusable instruments enable delicate dissection; 3- or 5-mm instruments appear to be most appropriate.

Most laparoscopy of infants and children is performed under general anesthesia with endotracheal intubation. Prophylactic antibiotics are administered preoperatively. All infants and children should have their stomach and bladder emptied before beginning the procedure. The stomach can be emptied with a suction catheter, and in most instances the bladder by the Credé method.

The abdominal wall of a child is thin and elastic. It is easy to mistake the subcutaneous space for the peritoneal cavity and to introduce a Veress needle or port into this layer. It is also easy to injure abdominal viscera with secondary port entrance.

A Veress needle can be used to establish a pneumoperitoneum in even the smallest infant. First, in the skin of the inferior rim of the umbilicus, a stab wound is made whose length equals the diameter of the trocar to be introduced. The abdominal wall is then elevated by grasping it on either side of the umbilicus as the Veress needle is introduced. The needle is introduced at an angle perpendicular to the long axis of the patient to avoid inserting it into the loose areolar subcutaneous tissue. The needle is best held by its shaft, and the maneuver is a quick shallow thrust into the peritoneal cavity until the retractable blunt end of the needle is felt to pop free into the abdomen. When the insufflation tubing is connected, the flow rate of gas should be at least 0.5 L per minute. A slower rate of flow suggests that the needle is not in the proper location. In adolescents, the technique is similar. For any patient it is strongly recommended that aspiration of the needle occur with use of irrigation solution to ensure appropriate placement of the Veress needle.

The total volume of gas introduced into the abdomen varies with the patient's size, so it is difficult to establish specific rules. It is preferable to set the pressure limits on pressure-regulated automatic insufflators: for infants, the pressure is 6 to 8 mm Hg; for children, most procedures can be accomplished using pressures of 8 to 10 mm Hg, and for adolescents 10 to 12 mm Hg is recommended.

After the abdomen is insufflated, the umbilical trocar is introduced. Ideally, a trocar and laparoscope no larger than 5 mm are used. Caution should be exercised while introducing the trocar. The path of entry should be monitored, and the operative note should document the information accordingly. Twisting the trocar while introducing

it permits better control and tends to reduce the probability of injuring the viscera.

In children, the port sites are sutured postoperatively. Because of the thinness of the abdominal wall, a hernia could develop in a port site. Therefore, closure of the fascia in a separate layer and then the skin with interrupted absorbable sutures is recommended. Steri-Strips or a transparent occlusive dressing at each port site is recommended. Patients are given postoperative medication to prevent nausea. In general, children complain of postoperative shoulder pain less often than do adults. Postoperative analgesic requirements vary.

CONCLUSIONS

Dysmenorrhea and pelvic pain are common complaints in adolescent girls. Although most cases are primary dysmenorrhea, which is usually easily treated with NSAIDs or OCPs, other diseases should be considered, especially when standard medical management does not produce the desired results. Endometriosis is the most common finding in teenagers who do not respond to this regimen, but müllerian anomalies and musculoskeletal lesions must also be considered.

REFERENCES

1. Glinter K: Chronic pelvic pain. J Am Osteopath Assoc 1974; 74:335–341.
2. Cramer D, Welch W, Cassell S, et al: Mumps, menarche, menopause and ovarian cancer. Am J Obstet Gynecol 1983; 147:1–6.
3. Goldstein D, DeCholnoky C, Leventhal J, et al: New insights into the old problem of chronic pelvic pain. J Pediatr Surg 1979; 14:675–680.
4. Gross R, Doerr H, Caldirola D, et al: Borderline symptom and incest in chronic pelvic pain patients. Int J Psychiatr Med 1980; 10:79–96.
5. Aftimos S: Myofascial pain in children. N Z Med J 1989; 102:440.
6. Peters AAW, van Dorst E, Jellis B, et al: A randomized clinical trial to compare two different approaches to women with chronic pelvic pain. Obstet Gynecol 1991; 77(5):740.
7. Slocumb JC: Neurological factors in chronic pelvic pain: Trigger points and the abdominal pelvic pain syndrome. Am J Obstet Gynecol 1984; 149(5):536.
8. Ling FW, Slocumb JC: Use of trigger point injections in chronic pelvic pain. Obstet Gynecol Clin North Am 1993; 20(4):809.
9. Myers CA, Baker PK, Ling F: Musculoskeletal screening in the pelvic pain patient. *In* Sanfilippo JS, Smith RP (eds): Primary Care in Obstetrics and Gynecology: A Handbook for Clinicians. New York: Springer-Verlag, 1998, pp 339–352.
10. Carnett JB: Intercostal neuralgia as a cause of abdominal pain and tenderness. Surg Gynecol Obstet 1926; 42:625.

11. Thomson H, Francis DMA: Abdominal wall tenderness: A useful sign in the acute abdomen. Lancet 1977; 1:1053.

12. Gallegos NC, Hobsley M: Recognition and treatment of abdominal wall pain. J R Soc Med 1989; 82:343.

13. Hawk C, Long C, Azad A: Chiropractic care for women with chronic pelvic pain: A prospective single-group intervention study. J Manipulative Physiol Ther 1997; 20(2):73.

14. Frost FA, Jesson B, Siggard-Anderson J: A controlled double blind comparison of mepivacaine injection versus saline injection for myofascial pain. Lancet 1980; 1:499.

15. Theobald GW: The relief and prevention of referred pain. J Obstet Gynecol Br Eur 1949; 56:447.

16. Gunn CC: Dry needling of muscle motor points for chronic low back pain. Spine 1980; 5:279.

17. Bates T, Grunwaldt E: Myofascial pain in childhood. J Pediatr 1958; 53:198.

18. King PM, Myers CA, Ling FW, et al: Musculoskeletal factors in chronic pelvic pain. J Psychosom Obstet Gynecol 1991; 12:87.

19. Bandera CA, Brown LR, Laufer MR: Adolescents and endometriosis. Clin Consult Obstet Gynecol 1995; 7:200.

20. Chatman D, Ward A: Endometriosis in adolescents. J Reprod Med 1982; 27:156.

21. Vercellini P, Fedele L, Arcaini L, et al: Laparoscopy in the diagnosis of pelvic pain in adolescent women. J Reprod Med 1989; 34(10):827.

22. Wolfman W, Kreutner K: Laparoscopy in children and adolescents. J Adolesc Health Care 1984; 5:261.

23. Goldstein DP, de Cholnoky C, Emans SJ: Adolescent endometriosis. J Adolesc Health Care 1980; 1:37.

24. Goldstein DP, de Choloky C, Emans SJ, et al: Laparoscopy in the diagnosis and management of pelvic pain in adolescents. J Reprod Med 1980; 24:251.

25. Laufer MR, Goitein L, Bush M, et al: Prevalence of endometriosis in adolescent girls with chronic pelvic pain not responding to conventional therapy. J Pediatr Adolesc Gynecol 1997; 10:199.

26. Reese KA, Reddy S, Rock JA: Endometriosis in an adolescent population: The Emory experience. J Pediatr Adolesc Gynecol 1996; 9(3):125.

27. Fallon J: Endometriosis in youth. JAMA 1946; 131:1405.

28. Yamamoto K, Mitsuhashi Y, Takaike T, et al: Tubal endometriosis diagnosed within one month after menarche: A case report. Tohoko J Exp Med 1997; 181:385–387.

29. Whitehouse H: Endometriosis invading the bladder removed from a patient who had never menstruated. Proc R Soc Med 1925–1926; 19:15.

30. Seitz L: Uber Genese, Klinik und Therapie der Endometriosis. (Heterotopein der Uterus-Schleimhaut). Arch Gynaekol 1932; 149:529.

31. Myer R: Ueber Endometrium in der Tube sowie uber die hieraus entstehenden wirkichen un vermeintlichen Folgen. Zentralbl Gynaekol 1927; 51:1482–1491.

32. Haney A: Endometriosis: Pathogenesis and pathophysiology. In Wilson E (ed): Endometriosis. New York: Alan R. Liss, 1987.

33. Sampson J: The development of the implantation theory for the origin of peritoneal endometriosis. Am J Obstet Gynecol 1940; 141:49.

34. Vercellini P, De Georgi O, Aimi G, et al: Menstrual characteristics in women with and without endometriosis. Obstet Gynecol 1997; 90(2):264.

35. Simpson JL, Elias J, Malinak LR, et al: Heritable aspects of endometriosis. Am J Obstet Gynecol 1980; 137:327.

36. Schifrin B, Erez S, Moore J: Teenage endometriosis. Am J Obstet Gynecol 1973; 116:973.

37. Sanfilippo JS, Wakim NG, Shickler K, et al: Endometriosis in association with uterine anomaly. Am J Obstet Gynecol 1986; 154(1):39–43.

38. Davis DD, Thillet E, Lindemann J: Clinical characteristics of adolescent endometriosis. J Adolesc Health 1993; 14:362.

39. Emmert C, Romann D, Riedel HH: Endometriosis diagnosed by laparoscopy in adolescent girls. Arch Gynecol Obstet 1998; 261:89–93.

40. Fedele L, Bianchi S, Di Nola G, et al: Endometriosis and nonobstructive müllerian anomalies. Obstet Gynecol 1992; 79(4):515–517.

41. Liang CC, Soong YK, Ho YS: Endometriosis in adolescent women. Chang Gung Med J 1995; 18(4):315.

42. Stovall DW, Bowser LM, Archer DF, et al: Endometriosis-associated pelvic pain: Evidence for an association between the stage of disease and a history of chronic pelvic pain. Fertil Steril 1997; 68:13.

43. Redwine DB: Age-related evolution in color appearance of endometriosis. Fertil Steril 1987; 48:1062.

44. Martin DC, Hubert GD, Vander Zwagg R, et al: Laparoscopic appearances of peritoneal endometriosis. Fertil Steril 1989; 51:63.

45. Laufer MR: Identification of clear vesicular lesions of atypical endometriosis: A new technique. Fertil Steril 1997; 68:739–740.

46. Nisolle M, Berliere M, Paindaveine B, et al: Histologic study of peritoneal endometriosis in infertile women. Fertil Steril 1990; 53:984.

47. American Society for Reproductive Medicine: Revised American Society for Reproductive Medicine classification of endometriosis: 1996. Fertil Steril 1997; 67:817–821.

48. Hornstein MD, Hemmings R, Yuzpe AA, et al: Use of naferelin versus placebo after reductive laparoscopic surgery for endometriosis. Fertil Steril 1997; 68:860–864.

49. Telima S, Ronnberg L, Kauppila A: Placebo-controlled comparison of danazol and high dose medroxyprogesterone acetate in the treatment of endometriosis after conservative surgery. Gynecol Endocrinol 1987; 1:363–371.

50. Lu P, Ory SJ: Endometriosis: Current management. Mayo Clin Proc 1995; 70:453–463.

51. Vercellini P, Cortesi I, Crosignani PG: Progestins for symptomatic endometriosis: A critical analysis of the evidence. Fertil Steril 1997; 68(3):393.

52. Vercellini P, De Georgi O, Oldani S, et al: Depomedroxyprogesterone acetate versus an oral contraceptive combined with very–low-dose danazol for long-term treatment of pelvic pain associated with endometriosis. Am J Obstet Gynecol 1996; 175(2):396.

53. Emans SJ: Contraception. In Emans SJ, Laufer MR, Goldstein DP (eds): Pediatric and Adolescent Gynecology, 4th ed. Philadelphia: Lippincott-Raven, 1998, p 646.

54. Cundy T, Evans M, Roberts H, et al: Bone mineral density in women receiving depomedroxyprogesterone acetate for contraception. Br Med J 1991; 303:13.

55. Edwards CP, Hertweck SP, Perlman SE, et al: A prospective study evaluating the effects of Depo-Provera on bone mineral density in adolescent females: A preliminary report. J Pediatr Adolesc Gynecol 1998; 11(4):201.

56. Cromer BA, Blair JM, Mahan JD, et al: A prospective comparison of bone density in adolescent girls receiving Depo-medroxyprogesterone acetate (Depo-Provera), levonorgestrel (Norplant), or oral contraceptives. J Pediatr 1996; 129:671.

57. Crosignani PG, De Cecco L, Gastaldi A, et al: Leuprolide in a 3-monthly versus a monthly depot formulation for the treatment of symptomatic endometriosis: A pilot study. Hum Reproduction 1996; 11(12):2732–2735.

58. Shaw RW: An open randomized comparative study of the effect of goserelin depot and danazol in the treatment of endometriosis. Fertil Steril 1992; 58:265.

59. Wright S, Valdes CT, Dunn RC, et al: Short-term Lupron or danazol therapy for pelvic endometriosis. Fertil Steril 1995; 63:504.
60. Dawood MY: Hormonal therapies for endometriosis: Implications for bone metabolism. Acta Obstet Gynecol Scand 1994; 159(Suppl):22.
61. Nencioni T, Penotti M, Barbieri-Carones M, et al: Gonadotropin-releasing hormone agonist therapy and its effect on bone mass. Gynecol Endocrinol 1991; 5:49.
62. Paoletti AM, Serra GG, Cagnacci A, et al: Spontaneous reversibility of bone loss induced by gonadotropin-releasing hormone analogue treatment. Fertil Steril 1996; 65:707.
63. Whitehouse RH, Adams JE, Baucroft K, et al: The effects of nafarelin and danazol on vertebral trabecular bone mass in patients with endometriosis. Clin Endocrinol 1990; 33:365.
64. Taga M, Mineguchi H: Reduction of bone mineral density by gonadotropin-releasing hormone agonist, nafarelin, is not completely reversible at 6 months after the cessation of administration. Acta Obstet Gynecol Scand 1996; 75:162.
65. Revilla R, Revilla M, Hernandez ER, et al: Evidence that the loss of bone mass induced by GnRH agonists is not totally recovered. Maturitas 1995; 22:145.
66. Matta WH, Shaw RW, Hesp R, et al: Reversible trabecular bone density loss following induced hypoestrogenism with the GnRH analogue buserelin in premenopausal women. Clin Endocrinol 1988; 29:45.
67. Hornstein MD, Surrey EC, Weisberg GW, et al: Leuprolide acetate depot and hormonal add-back in endometriosis: A 12-month study. Obstet Gynecol 1998; 91:16.
68. Lubianca JN, Gordon CM, Laufer MR: "Add-back" therapy for endometriosis in adolescents. J Reprod Med 1998; 43:164.
69. Gans SL, Berci G: Advances in endoscopy of infants and children. J Pediatr Surg 1971; 6:19.

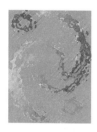

Chapter 40

Future Perspectives

Leo Plouffe, Jr., and Keith Hansen

It has been more than 5 years since our last attempt at predicting the future, in a chapter by the same title from the previous edition of this text book.[1] It may be interesting to look back at our predictions to see how well we fared. While it may be of interest, it would also provide the reader with a solid justification to skip this chapter altogether, in view of our skills at clairvoyance (or lack thereof). A thorough statistical analysis of the accuracy of our previous predictions places us in the same accuracy range as your least favorite investment advisor or the Sunday professional football oddsmaker. For these reasons, the main focus in this chapter will be newly evolving diagnostic and treatment techniques and their applications in pediatric and adolescent gynecology.

MOLECULAR MEDICINE LEADING THE WAY

THE HUMAN GENOME PROJECT

The completion of the Human Genome Project will constitute an unparallalled milestone in modern scientific and medical achievement.[2] The project is expected to be completed ahead of schedule, i.e., in 2001. In addition, a number of private interests are competing with the primarily government-sponsored multinational project and may further speed the completion of the project.[3, 4]

While much data will be acquired through the Human Genome Project, one must understand that, in some ways, the output will be akin to a random collection of all the words contained in a book (such as the Bible) with a few hints as to the order of the words, sentences, paragraphs, and chapters.[5] The formidable challenge of transforming this wealth of nucleotide sequences into clinically applicable information will no doubt be met but is likely to take a decade or more. A number of techniques to accomplish these tasks are already under exploration.[6, 7] Ultimately, all of the current data consecrate the mapping of the human genome as a revolutionary step in the

history of medicine, with direct applications for all fields of medicine, including pediatric and adolescent gynecology.[8]

SPECIFIC GENETIC DISORDERS

In parallel to the efforts of the Human Genome Project, ongoing investigations will provide further insights into specific disorders. This includes a broadening of the knowledge around the mechanisms of sexual differentiation and related problems.[9] Comparable advances are expected for a broad range of conditions, such as müllerian development and disorders of gonadotropin regulation.[10–13]

The recent explosion of knowledge around receptor systems, including the estrogen and androgen receptors,[14–16] should provide new insights into disorders linked to dysfunctions of these specific receptors. Furthermore, a number of new therapeutic opportunities should evolve from the newly acquired knowledge.

Last, but not least, research techniques are constantly evolving. For example, the ultraviolet laser microbeam is allowing investigators literally to perform "microsurgery" on genetic material.[17] Another technique that has just recently come of age and is opening new frontiers is the so-called DNA chip technology or, more accurately, gene expression microarrays.[18, 19] The technique allows for extremely rapid and efficient screening, at one time, of several thousand genetic polymorphisms, events linked to gene regulation, and may ultimately lead to new therapeutic opportunities.[20] A description of the technique is beyond the scope of the current chapter, but recent references are provided for the interested reader.[21–23]

THE ROLE OF MOLECULAR BIOLOGY IN CLINICAL DIAGNOSIS

There is little doubt that molecular techniques offer great promise for reaching a clinical diagnosis in a large number of cases, for common disorders and rare ones. For years, many opinion leaders have predicted that the current standard biochemical techniques will soon be replaced by molecular biology techniques.[24] While this is already a reality for the diagnosis of a number of common conditions, certain inherited disorders and infectious diseases, the real question is how soon this shift from traditional biochemical or immunochemical assays to molecular techniques will occur and how widespread it will be.[25, 26] A large number of developments will be required before molecular techniques supplant our current diagnostic tools, including the resolution of serious legal and ethical issues.[27, 28]

Techniques are rapidly evolving that will expedite and facilitate molecular diagnosis. A recent report suggests that DNA diagnostic material could be retrieved from a standard urine specimen, even after a prolonged period of storage at room temperature or freezing.[29] Such advances could greatly facilitate the steps patients have to go through to achieve a diagnosis. Other technical breakthroughs in the area of molecular diagnosis include single nucleotide polymorphisms (SNP), which may have wide applications for individual diagnosis and for population-based studies.[30]

In summary, there is little doubt that molecular diagnostic techniques will eventually become the standard approach to the diagnosis of most disorders. This evolution has lagged severely behind the predictions of many. It continues to be unclear when the much anticipated conversion will actually take place. The authors cannot help but think of the analogy to the conversion from older units to the *Système International*; all agree it will occur at some point but all predictions are off. It may be that, ultimately, a main driver to switch to molecular techniques will be the greater ease to learn about a new test than convert to the SI unit system.

NONINVASIVE DIAGNOSTIC TECHNIQUES

Development of minimally invasive diagnostic techniques has continued principally in radiology. The two areas that we feel hold the greatest promise are three-dimensional ultrasonography and fast magnetic resonance imaging (MRI). Both of these techniques should assist clinicians in reaching a correct diagnosis while avoiding the need for a diagnostic surgical procedure. These techniques may also allow for the development of guided surgeries.

A role for three-dimensional ultrasound imaging has already been suggested in the study of müllerian anomalies.[31] While successful, these early attempts relied upon rather primitive technology. New advances have greatly improved the resolution and accuracy of three-dimensional ultrasound imaging and expanded its role to a number of areas, including studies of the central nervous system and urogenital tract.[32, 33] The technique appears to be well-suited as well for the study of the fetus or newborn.[34]

The new MRI techniques permit the assessing of rapidly moving organs, including the heart, and require only a few minutes to be completed.[35, 36] The techniques also allow the monitoring of dynamic physiologic changes in a number of target areas, such as the brain.[37, 38] Such techniques could provide new insights into conditions involving the central nervous system, such as hypothalamic amenorrhea, anorexia nervosa, bulimia, or even the polycystic ovary syndrome.

MEDICAL THERAPEUTICS

Of all areas, the most challenging to predict is the therapeutic venue. While there is much promise on the horizon, the eventual development of therapeutic approaches must rely not only on technological advances but also on the conduct of appropriate double-blind randomized clinical trials. The latter has proven to be rather challenging, especially given the current environment of litigation and the increasing scrutiny around clinical research involving minors.

We have selected three areas of therapeutics that hold the greatest promise: gene therapy, pharmacogenetics, and new drug delivery systems.

GENE THERAPY

Gene therapy has evolved from dream to reality during the 1990s. Current gene therapy targets focus on a small number of inherited genetic conditions, such as hemophilia and immune deficiency syndromes, and several malignancies.[39–41] Gene therapy is expanding in scope to include prenatal therapeutics.[42] The indications for gene therapy are expected to broaden considerably during the next decade.[43–45]

The techniques available for gene therapy are expanding rapidly. A number of controlled delivery systems are being explored, including implantable polymer matrices and injectable microspheres.[46] New host-vector delivery systems are also being developed, which should make gene therapy safer and more practical.[47]

Despite the great scientific interest in gene therapy, relatively few conditions in the field of pediatric and adolescent gynecology may lend themselves to such an approach. One can predict a few target disorders. The adrenal hyperplasias, with their known enzymatic defects, lend themselves to such an approach. One could conceive of gene therapy for gonadal dysgenesis, where full ovarian function and other developmental functions might be preserved or restored. Developmental disorders affecting secretion of the gonadotropins would be another target. While all of these are potential areas of investigation, the relatively non–life-threatening nature of these conditions and the ability to manage them currently with medical therapy makes it seem unlikely that they will lead the charge in the field of gene therapy.

PHARMACOGENETICS

Pharmacogenetics may produce major advances in pediatric and adolescent gynecology. Pharmacogenetics is the rapidly expanding science of studying genetic polymorphisms relative to the treatment response to a specific drug.[48–51] Differences in individual, racial, or ethnic response to medications can be elucidated through pharmacogenetics.[52–54]

Pharmacogenetics may hold the key to predicting how well or poorly a given patient will respond to a specific treatment.[55] This would be of great assistance, for example, in predicting whether the response pattern of an adolescent to contraceptive steroids would include such side effects as acne, weight gain, or irregular bleeding. It will have major implications in the quality of care, the risk-benefit ratio, and cost-effectiveness of treatment.[56, 57]

NEW DRUG DELIVERY SYSTEMS

Few areas are likely to evolve quicker than novel therapeutic techniques—currently used medications, newer therapeutics, and molecular biology–based therapies. Some improvements will be refinements of currently used techniques, such as transdermal delivery systems.[58] More significant progress is expected through a variety of new techniques and greatly enhanced insights into drug absorption and metabolism.

A number of novel systems are being developed for delivery of medications across the skin, most of them still in the early stages of development.[59] Most of these systems involve some mechanical action on the epidermis and dermis with concurrent transfer of medication in the tissues, which act as a reservoir.[59, 60, 61] In parallel, investigations are under way for new delivery systems, such as ceramic-based implants.[61] Work is also continuing on other modes of delivery, such as transbuccal (across the oral mucosa) or pulmonary (delivery of medication to the alveoli[62] and subsequent systemic absorption).[63] Last but not least, a fascinating new area of investigation is using autologous tissues as drug delivery systems. Recent reports have demonstrated that erythrocytes loaded with a therapeutic agent allow highly efficient systemic delivery.[63, 64] All of these systems would improve delivery of steroid preparations (estrogens, progestins, corticosteroids) and proteins (growth hormone, GnRH, insulin).

Selective delivery of therapeutic agents to the primary target tissue(s) is a major area of current research. For now, the focus is on cancer therapy but the findings are likely to be expanded to include pediatric and adolescent gynecology. Excipients (e.g. lactose, wax) in most oral preparations (pills or tablets) have until now been largely used to help stabilize the active ingredient, but recent discoveries have shown that their role can be greatly enchanced. For example, B_{12} conjugates may allow many protein drugs (such as GnRH) to be given by the oral route.[65] The use of folic acid as an excipient may also help to target activity in certain highly metabolically active tissues.[66] Many other inert compounds or food-based products are being studied for their ability to selectively deliver medication.[67–69] Developments in this arena would provide novel therapies for conditions which target specific organs, such as McCune-Albright syndrome, with its ovarian, skeletal, and dermal targets.

In summary, the spectrum of available drug delivery techniques will be greatly expanded in the coming years. This will, hopefully, result in better patient compliance and minimize the negative impact of therapeutic intervention on the quality of life of our patients. More important, many of these novel delivery modalities may enhance our ability to treat a wide range of conditions. Ultimately, a combination of improved delivery systems and targeted delivery may open wide the frontier of fetal therapeutics and allow effective therapies for a number of genetic conditions, such as gonadal dysgenesis.

SURGICAL THERAPEUTICS

The amazing evolution of surgical techniques in the past decade makes it very difficult to predict the future. On the one hand, the evolution may continue at an exponential rate and bring about surgical approaches nearly impossible to imagine today. On the other hand, we may see a leveling off of progress and a focus on refinement of current techniques. We favor the latter at present, mostly because of our intellectual limitations in conceiving of more futuristic approaches.

IMPROVING THE PRESENT

Intraoperative ultrasound has been of limited use up to now.[70] We foresee that it will gain in popularity and become nearly routine in the operative management of müllerian anomalies. Another technical advance that is likely to gain in popularity is three-dimensional laparoscopy.[71] Current investigations are also under way into concurrent use of MRI and endoscopic surgery (Rodolphe Maheux, personal communication, 1996). In parallel, we would expect continued improvement in telemedicine techniques that should afford more patients access to highly specialized centers.[72]

DREAMING OF THE FUTURE (PAST TENSE)

The movie *Fantastic Voyage* was a favorite with the authors. While we are not proposing that surgeons be miniaturized (some believe that managed care organizations have already done this), there are foreseeable technical options for "intracorporeal satellite surgery." Microprobes could be injected into the vascular tree or into body cavities. They could be directed to a specific operative site, either by blood flow–mediated navigation or through external magnetic field focusing. At that point, they could provide a therapeutic intervention by delivering a drug or producing a mechanical disruptive effect (microexplosion). This may be the future of truly minimally invasive surgery.

YOUR OWN PREDICTIONS

Any reader could easily have written this chapter. We therefore invite you to note here your own predictions for the next 10 years. You may enjoy looking back at this page once this book has reached the historical register status, and compare your score to ours.

1. _____
2. _____
3. _____
4. _____
5. _____

CONCLUSION

The corresponding chapter in the previous edition of this textbook highlighted the fact that, despite all of our technologic advances, a key element in achieving true medical progress was to increase access to medical care.[1] While this is a reality in a number of countries, it is still a distant goal in many areas of the world, including the United States. Paradoxically, in many countries where there is ready access to medical care, the latest technologic and therapeutic breakthroughs are not available, whereas only a small percentage of pediatric and adolescent patients can access the state-of-the-art care available in countries such as the United States.

We have primarily focused on exciting technical developments likely to occur in the near future, yet, we truly hope that our readers will remember the critical importance of securing health care access for all newborns, infants, children, and adolescents. The challenge is immense, but the goal is fully within our reach.

REFERENCES

1. Plouffe L Jr, McDonough PG: Future perspectives. *In* Sanfilippo JS, et al (eds): Pediatric and Adolescent Gynecology. Philadelphia: WB Saunders 1994, pp 654–664.
2. Collins FS: Shattuck lecture—medical and societal consequences of the Human Genome Project. N Engl J Med 1999; 341(1):28–37.
3. Putman L: US firm claims it can "sequence human genome in 3 years." Lancet 1998; 23; 351:1566.
4. Pennisi E: Academic sequencers challenge Celera in a sprint to the finish. Science 1999; 19; 283:1822–1823.
5. Collins FS: The human genome project and the future of medicine. Ann NY Acad Sci 1999; 882:42–55.
6. Clark MS: Comparative genomics: The key to understanding the Human Genome Project. Bioessays 1999; 21(2):121–130.
7. van Ommen GJ, et al: The human genome project and the future of diagnostics, treatment, and prevention. Lancet 1999; 354(Suppl 1):SI5–10.
8. McCabe ER: The new biology enters the generalist pediatrician's office: Lessons from the human genome project. Pediatr Rev 1999; 20(9):314–319.
9. Parker KL, Schimmer BP, Schedl A: Genes essential for early events in gonadal development. Cell Molec Life Sci 1999; 55:831–838.
10. Jacob M, Konrad K, Jacob HJ: Early development of the müllerian duct in avian embryos with reference to the human. An ultrastructural and immunohistochemical study. Cells Tissues Organs 1999; 164(2):63–81.

11. Roberts LM, Hirokawa Y, Nachtigal MW, Ingraham HA: Paracrine-mediated apoptosis in reproductive tract development. Develop Biol 1999; 208:110–122.

12. Parr BA, McMahon AP: Sexually dimorphic development of the mammalian reproductive tract requires Wnt-7a. Nature 1998; 395(6703):707–710.

13. Layman LC, Cohen DP, Jin M, et al: Mutations in gonadotropin-releasing hormone receptor gene cause hypogonadotropic hypogonadism. Nat Genet 1998; 18:14–15.

14. Reynolds T: New estrogen receptor adds complexity, recasts drug strategies. J Natl Cancer Inst 1999; 91:1445–1447.

15. Ikeuchi T, Todo T, Kobayashi T, Nagahama Y: cDNA Cloning of a novel androgen receptor subtype. J Biol Chem 1999; 274:25205–25209.

16. Couse JF, Korach KS: Reproductive phenotypes in the estrogen receptor–alpha–knockout mouse. Ann Endocrinol (Paris) 1999; 60:143–148.

17. Schutze K, Posl H, Lahr G: Laser micromanipulation systems as universal tools in cellular and molecular biology and in medicine. Cell Mol Biol 1998; 44:735–746.

18. Kurian KM, Watson CJ, Wyllie AH: DNA chip technology. J Pathol 1999; 187:267–271.

19. Case-Green SC, Mir KU, Pritchard CE, Southern EM: Analyzing genetic information with DNA arrays. Curr Opin Chem Biol 1998; 2:404–410.

20. Gerhold D, Rushmore T, Caskey CT: DNA chips: Promising toys have become powerful tools. Trends Biochem Sci 1999; 24:168–173.

21. Schena M: Genome analysis with gene expression microarrays. Bioessays 1996; 18:427–431.

22. Duggan DJ, Bittner M, Chen Y, et al: Expression profiling using cDNA microarrays. Nat Genet 1999; 21(1 Suppl):10–14.

23. Johnston M: Gene chips: Array of hope for understanding gene regulation. Curr Biol 1998; 8:R171–174.

24. Bertholf RL: The expanding role of molecular biology in clinical chemistry. Cell Vision 1998; 5:67–69.

25. Vnencak-Jones CL: Molecular testing for inherited diseases. Am J Clin Pathol 1999; 112(1 Suppl 1):S19–32.

26. Lairmore TC, Norton JA: Advances in molecular genetics. Am J Surg 1997; 173:37–41.

27. Leonard DG: The future of molecular genetic testing. Clin Chem 1999; 45:726–731.

28. Plomin R, Rutter M: Child development, molecular genetics, and what to do with genes once they are found. Child Dev 1998; 69:1223–1242.

29. Vu NT, Chaturvedi AK, Canfield DV: Genotyping for DQA1 and PM loci in urine using PCR-based amplification: Effects of sample volume, storage temperature, preservatives, and aging on DNA extraction and typing. Forensic Sci Internat 1999; 102:23–34.

30. Brookes AJ: The essence of SNPs. Gene 1999; 234:177–186.

31. Raga F, Bonilla-Musoles F, Blanes J, Osborne NG: Congenital müllerian anomalies: Diagnostic accuracy of three-dimensional ultrasound. Fertil Steril 1996; 65:523–528.

32. Nelson TR, Pretorius DH: Three-dimensional ultrasound imaging. Ultrasound Med Biol 1998; 24:1243–1270.

33. Liu JB, Goldberg BB: 2-D and 3-D endoluminal ultrasound: Vascular and nonvascular applications. Ultrasound Med Biol 1999; 25:159–173.

34. Ebel KD: Uroradiology in the fetus and newborn: Diagnosis and follow-up of congenital obstruction of the urinary tract. Pediatr Radiol 1998; 28:630–635.

35. Keller PJ: Fast(er) MR imaging. Neuroimag Clin North Am 1999; 9:243–252.

36. Jakob PM, Griswold MA, Edelman RR, Sodickson DK: AUTO-SMASH: A self-calibrating technique for SMASH imaging. SiMultaneous Acquisition of Spatial Harmonics. MAGMA 1998; 7:42–54.

37. Werring DJ, Clark CA, Parker GJ, et al: A direct demonstration of both structure and function in the visual system: Combining diffusion tensor imaging with functional magnetic resonance imaging. Neuroimage. 1999; 9:352–361.

38. Crelier GR, Hoge RD, Munger P, Pike GB: Perfusion-based functional magnetic resonance imaging with single-shot RARE and GRASE acquisitions. Magn Reson Med 1999; 41:132–136.

39. Kay MA, et al: Gene therapy for the hemophilias. Proc Natl Acad Sci USA. 1999; 31:9973–9975.

40. Romano G et al: Gene transfer technology in therapy: Current applications and future goals. Stem Cells 1999; 17(4):191–202.

41. Smith AE: Gene therapy—where are we? Lancet 1999; 354(Suppl 1):SI1–4.

42. Walsh CE: Fetal gene therapy. Gene Ther 1999; 6:1200–1201.

43. Rodriguez R, et al: Urologic applications of gene therapy. Urology 1999; 54:401–406.

44. Lernoine N, et al: Gene therapy for the millennium: In with the new. Gene Ther 1999; 6:1199.

45. Russell CS, et al: Recombinant proteins for genetic disease. Clin Genet 1999; 55:389–394.

46. Luo D, Woodrow-Mumford K, Belcheva N, Saltzman WM: Controlled DNA delivery systems. Pharm Res 1999; 16:1300–1308.

47. Soubrier F, Cameron B, Manse B, et al: pCOR: A new design of plasmid vectors for nonviral gene therapy. Gene Ther 1999; 6:1482–1488.

48. Kalow W: Pharmacogenetics in biological perspective. Pharmacol Rev 1997; 49:369–379.

49. Krynetski EY, Evans WE: Pharmacogenetics as a molecular basis for individualized drug therapy: The thiopurine S-methyltransferase paradigm. Pharmaceut Res 1999; 16:342–349.

50. Nebert DW, Ingelman-Sundberg M, Daly AK: Genetic epidemiology of environmental toxicity and cancer susceptibility: Human allelic polymorphisms in drug-metabolizing enzyme genes, their functional importance, and nomenclature issues. Drug Metab Rev 1999; 31:467–487.

51. Bailey DS, Bondar A, Furness LM: Pharmacogenomics—it's not just pharmacogenetics. Curr Opin Biotechnol 1998; 9:595–601.

52. Bell J: Medical implications of understanding complex disease traits. Curr Opin Biotechnol 1998; 9:573–577.

53. Wood AJ: Ethnic differences in drug disposition and response. Ther Drug Monit 1998; 20:525–526.

54. Caraco Y: Genetic determinants of drug responsiveness and drug interactions. Therap Drug Monit 1998; 20:517–524.

55. Erickson RP: From "magic bullet" to "specially engineered shotgun loads": The new genetics and the need for individualized pharmacotherapy. Bioessays 1998; 20:683–685.

56. Lichter JB, Kurth JH: The impact of pharmacogenetics on the future of healthcare. Curr Opin Biotechnol 1997; 8:692–695.

57. Leeder JS, Kearns GL: Pharmacogenetics in pediatrics. Implications for practice. Pediatr Clin North Am 1997; 44:55–77.

58. Good WR, John VA, Ramirez M, Higgins JE: Double-masked, multicenter study of an estradiol matrix transdermal delivery system (Alora) versus placebo in postmenopausal women experiencing menopausal symptoms. Clin Ther 1996; 18:1093–1105.

59. Bareille P, MacSwiney M, Albanese A, et al: Growth hormone treatment without a needle using the Preci-Jet 50 transjector. Arch Dis Child 1997; 76:65–67.

60. Svedman P, Lundin S, Hoglund P, et al: Passive drug diffusion via standardized skin mini-erosion; Methodological aspects and clinical findings with new device. Pharmaceut Res 1996; 13:1354–1359.

61. Lasserre A, Bajpai PK: Ceramic drug-delivery devices. Crit Rev Ther Drug Carrier Sys 1998; 15:1–56.

62. Chetty DJ, Chien YW: Novel methods of insulin delivery: An update. Crit Rev Ther Drug Carrier Sys 1998; 15:629–670.

63. Magnani M, Rossi L, d'Ascenzo M, et al: Erythrocyte engineering for drug delivery and targeting. Biotechnol Appl Biochem 1998; 28:1–6.

64. Fraternale A, Rossi L, Magnani M: Encapsulation, metabolism and release of 2-fluoro-ara-AMP from human erythrocytes. Biochimi Biophys Acta 1996; 1291:149–154.

65. Russell-Jones GJ: Use of vitamin B_{12} conjugates to deliver protein drugs by the oral route. Crit Rev Therapeutic Drug Carrier Syst 1998; 15:557–586.

66. Reddy JA, Low PS: Folate-mediated targeting of therapeutic and imaging agents to cancers. Crit Rev Therapeutic Drug Carrier Syst 1998; 15:587–627.

67. Wirth M, Hamilton G, Gabor F: Lectin-mediated drug targeting: Quantification of binding and internalization of wheat germ agglutinin and *Solanum tuberosum* lectin using Caco-2 and HT-29 cells. J Drug Targeting 1998; 6:95–104.

68. Tsuji A: [Strategies for drug delivery to the brain across the blood-brain barrier]. Nippon Rinsho – Japanese J Clin Med 1998; 56:613–618.

69. Hope MJ, Mui B, Ansell S, Ahkong QF: Cationic lipids, phosphatidylethanolamine and the intracellular delivery of polymeric, nucleic acid–based drugs. Molec Membrane Biol 1998;15:1–14.

70. Makuuchi M, Torzilli G, Machi J: History of intraoperative ultrasound. Ultrasound Med Biol 1998; 24:1229–1242.

71. Herron DM, Lantis JC 2nd, Maykel J, et al: The 3-D monitor and head-mounted display. A quantitative evaluation of advanced laparoscopic viewing technologies. Surg Endos 1999; 13:751–755.

72. Takeda H, Matsumura Y, Okada T, et al: Functional evaluation of telemedicine with super–high-definition images and B-ISDN. Medinfo 1998; 9:311–314.

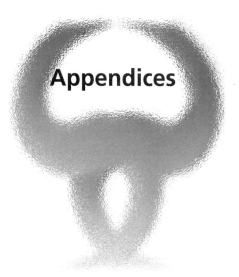

Appendices

Appendix A BARBARA R. HOSTETLER
Growth Charts

BOYS: BIRTH TO 36 MONTHS
PHYSICAL GROWTH
NCHS PERCENTILES*

NAME_____ RECORD #_____

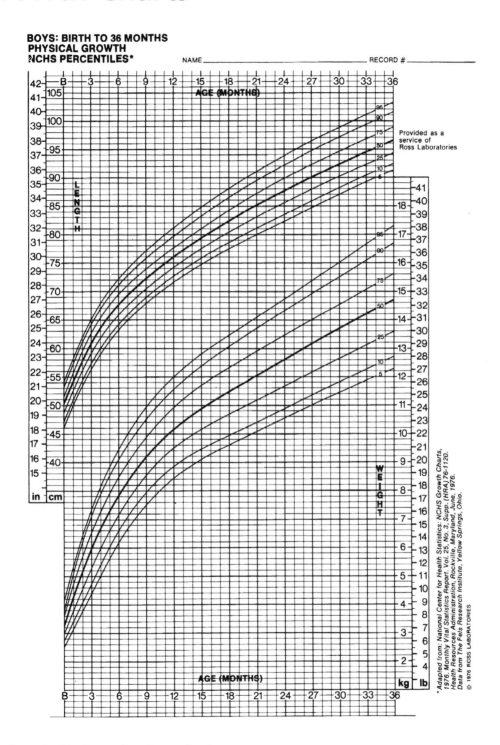

From Summitt RL. Comprehensive Pediatrics. St. Louis: C.V. Mosby, 1990, pp. 14–22. Modified from National Center for Health Statistics: NCHS growth charts, 1976; Monthly vital statistics report, vol 25, no 3, suppl (HRA) 76-1120, Health Resources Administration, Rockville, MD, June 1976; Data from The Fels Research Institute, Yellow Springs, OH. Published by Ross Laboratories, Columbus, OH, 1976.

GIRLS: BIRTH TO 36 MONTHS
PHYSICAL GROWTH
NCHS PERCENTILES*

NAME_____   RECORD #_____

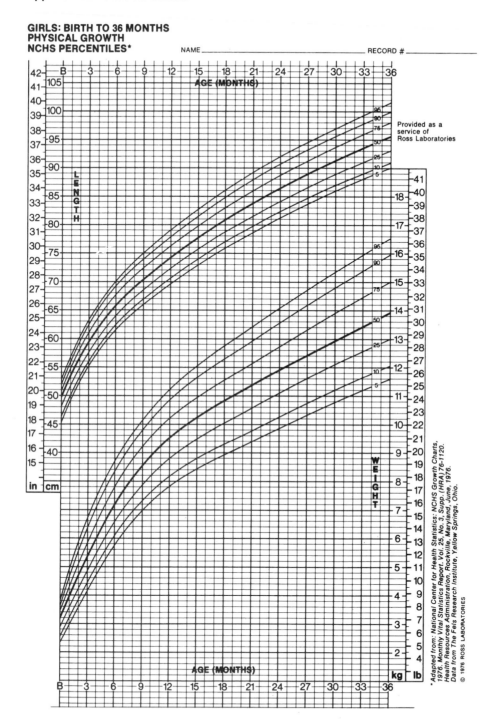

Provided as a
service of
Ross Laboratories

* Adapted from: National Center for Health Statistics: NCHS Growth Charts, 1976. Monthly Vital Statistics Report. Vol. 25, No. 3, Supp. (HRA) 76-1120. Health Resources Administration, Rockville, Maryland, June, 1976. Data from The Fels Research Institute, Yellow Springs, Ohio.

© 1976 ROSS LABORATORIES

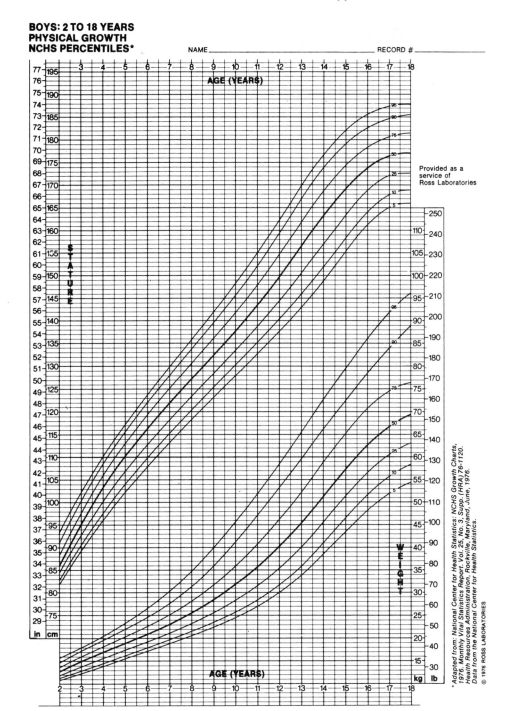

**GIRLS: 2 TO 18 YEARS
PHYSICAL GROWTH
NCHS PERCENTILES***

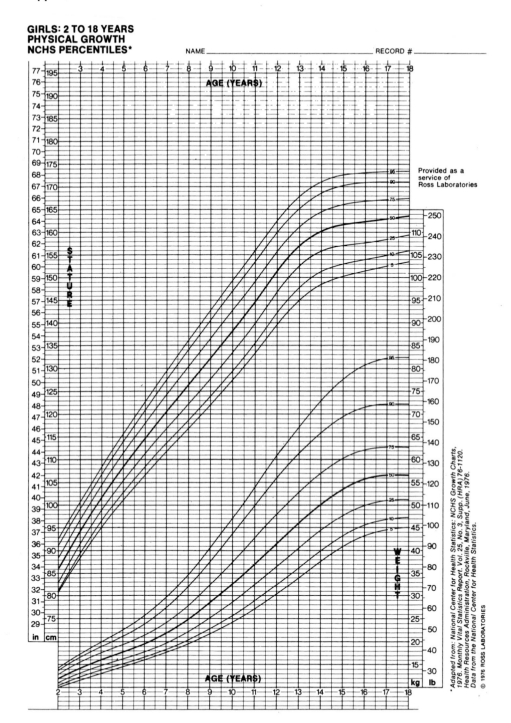

NAME _____   RECORD # _____

Provided as a
service of
Ross Laboratories

*Adapted from: National Center for Health Statistics: NCHS Growth Charts,
1976. Monthly Vital Statistics Report. Vol. 25, No. 3, Supp. (HRA) 76-1120.
Health Resources Administration, Rockville, Maryland, June, 1976.
Data from the National Center for Health Statistics.

© 1976 ROSS LABORATORIES

Name... Date of Birth............................. Reg. No. ....

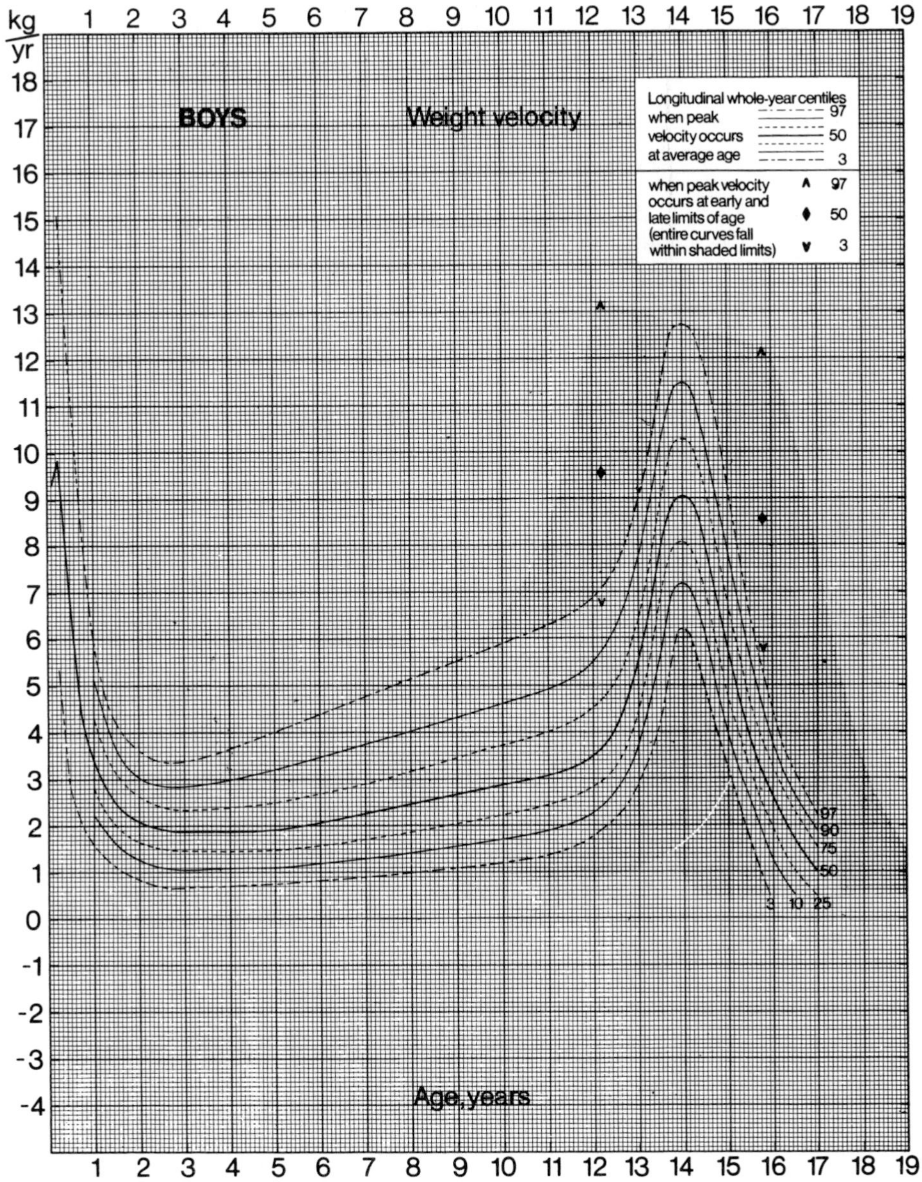

BOYS   Weight velocity

Longitudinal whole-year centiles
when peak 97
velocity occurs 50
at average age 3

when peak velocity ^ 97
occurs at early and ♦ 50
late limits of age
(entire curves fall v 3
within shaded limits)

Age, years

Name.. Date of Birth............................. Reg. No. ....

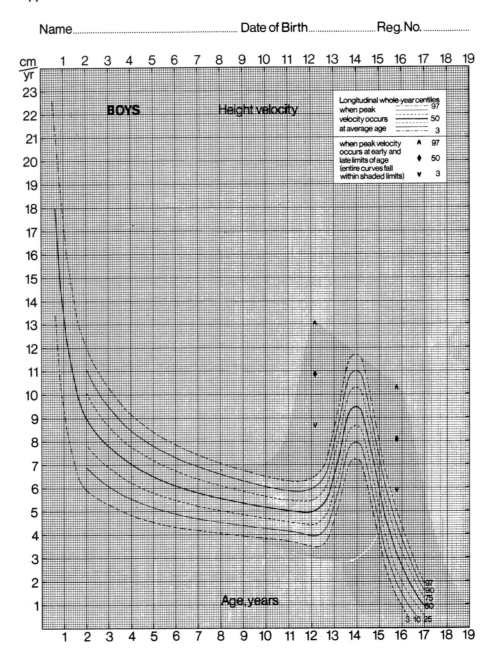

Name... Date of Birth............................ Reg. No. ....

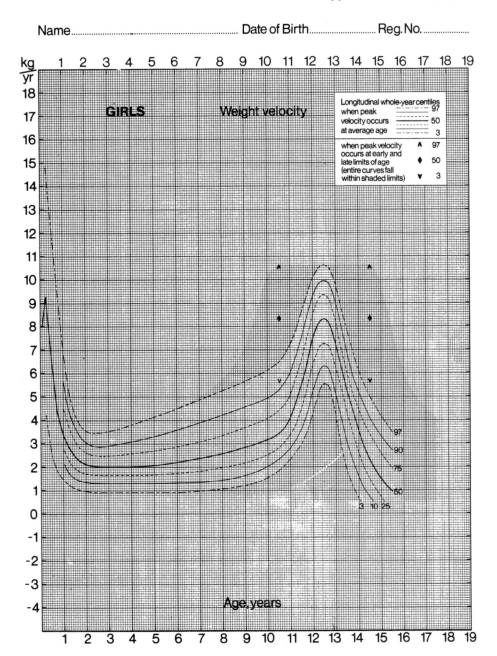

Name... Date of Birth............................ Reg.No.......................

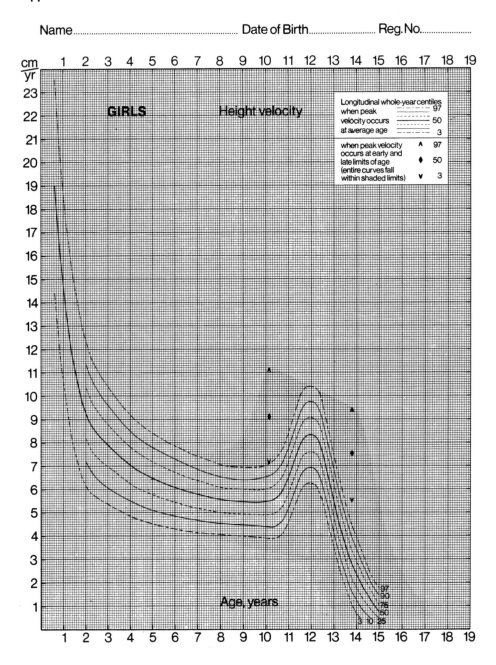

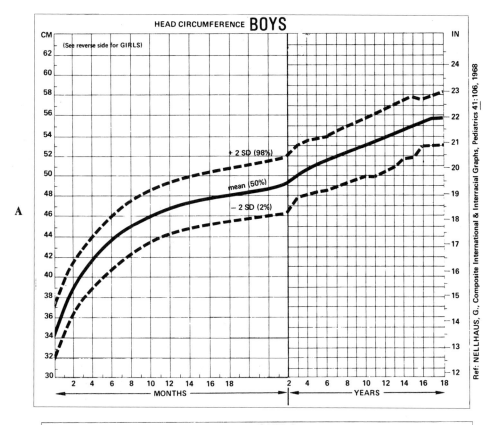

A

HEAD CIRCUMFERENCE **BOYS**

(See reverse side for GIRLS)

+ 2 SD (98%)

mean (50%)

− 2 SD (2%)

MONTHS — YEARS

Ref: NELLHAUS, G., Composite International & Interracial Graphs, Pediatrics 41:106, 1968

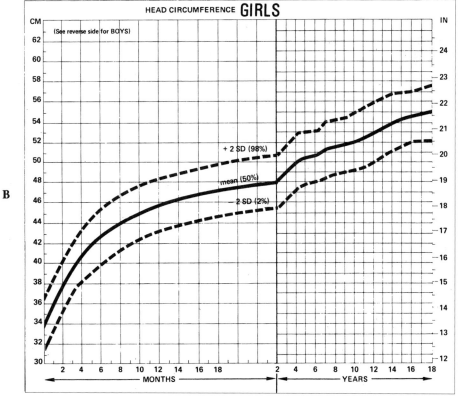

B

HEAD CIRCUMFERENCE **GIRLS**

(See reverse side for BOYS)

+ 2 SD (98%)

mean (50%)

2 SD (2%)

MONTHS — YEARS

Appendix B   BARBARA R. HOSTETLER
Tanner Staging

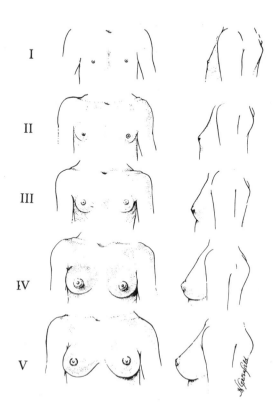

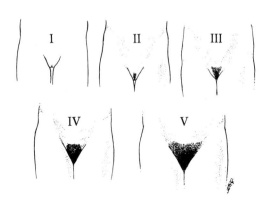

Both Sexes: Pubic Hair

Stage I   Preadolescent. The vellus over the pubes is not further developed than that over the abdominal wall; that is, no pubic hair.

Stage II   Sparse growth of long, slightly pigmented downy hair, straight or curled, chiefly at the base of the penis or along the labia.

Stage III   Considerably darker, coarser, and more curled. The hair spreads sparsely over the junction of the pubes.

Stage IV   Hair now adult in type, but area covered is still considerably smaller than in the adult. No spread to the medial surface of the thighs.

Stage V   Adult in quantity and type with distribution of the horizontal (or classically "feminine") pattern. Spread to medial surface of thighs but not up linea alba or elsewhere above the base of the inverse triangle (spread up linea alba occurs late and is Stage VI).

Girls: Breast Development

Stage I   Preadolescent. Elevation of papilla only.

Stage II   Breast bud stage. Elevation of breast and papilla as small mound. Enlargement of areolar diameter.

Stage III   Further enlargement and elevation of breast and areola with no separation of their contours.

Stage IV   Projection of areola and papilla to form a secondary mound above the level of the breast.

Stage V   Mature stage. Projection of papilla only caused by recession of the areola to the general contour of the breast.

Figures adapted from Marshall WA, Tanner JM. Variations in patterns of pubertal changes in girls. Arch Dis Child 1969; 44:291. Reprinted from Ross GT, Vande Wiele RL, Frantz AG. The normal ovary. In: Williams RH (ed). Textbook of Endocrinology. 6th ed. Philadelphia: W.B. Saunders, 1981, p 362.

Appendix C   *Barbara R. Hostetler*

Normal Laboratory Values

Test	Specimen	Reference Range		Factor	Reference Range International
Androstenedione	Serum		*ng/dl*	× 0.0349	*nmol/L*
		Child:	8–50		3–18
		Adult, M:	75–205		26–72
		Adult, F:	85–275		30–96
Creatinine clearance	Serum or plasma and urine	Newborn: 40–65 ml/min/1.73 m² <40 yr., M: 97–137 F: 88–128 Decreases 6.5 ml/min/decade			
Dehydroepiandrosterone (DHEA)	Serum		*ng/ml*	× 3.467	*nmol/L*
		Cord:	5.6–20.0		19.4–69.3
		Child:	1.0–3.0		3.5–10.4
		Adult, M:	1.7–4.2		5.9–14.6
		Adult, F:	2.0–5.2		6.9–18.0
		Pregnancy:	0.5–12.5		1.7–43.3
	Urine, 24-hr		*mg/ml*	× 3.467	*µmol/dL*
		Child, 0–1 yr:	<0.1		<0.35
		10–15 yr:	<0.4		<1.4
		Adult, M:	0–2.3		0–8.0
		Adult, F:	0–1.2		0–4.2
Dehydroepiandrosterone sulfate (DHEAS)	Serum or plasma (heparin or EDTA)		*µg/ml*	× 2.608	*µmol/L*
		Newborn,	<300		<780
		1–4 d:	<20		<52
		Child:	0.60–2.54		1.6–6.6
		Adult, M:	1.99–3.34		5.2–8.7
		Adult, F:			
		Premenopausal:	0.82–3.38		2.1–8.8
		Pregnancy, term:	0.23–1.17		0.6–3.0

Test	Specimen	Reference Range				Factor	Reference Range International	
Dihydrotestosterone (DHT)	Serum		*ng/dl*			× 0.03443	*nmol/L*	
		Prepubertal:	<3.5				<0.12	
		Pubertal:	M	F			M	F
		stage I:	<10	<10			<0.34	<0.34
		II:	<20	<15			<0.7	<0.5
		III:	<35	<25			<1.2	<0.86
		IV–V:	<75	<25			<2.6	<0.86
		Adult:	<30–85	4–22			1.03–2.92	0.14–0.76
Estradiol	Serum or plasma (heparin or EDTA)		*pg/ml*			× 3.671	*pmol/L*	
		M. pubertal:						
		stage I:	2–8				7–29	
		II:	11				40	
		III:	>20				>73	
		Adult, M:	8–36				29–132	
		F, pubertal:						
		stage I:	0–23				0–84	
		II:	0–66				0–242	
		III:	0–105				0–385	
		IV:	20–300				73–1101	
		Follicular:	10–90				37–330	
		Midcycle:	100–500				367–1835	
		Luteal:	50–240				184–881	
	Urine, 24-hr		*µg/d*			× 3.671	*nmol/d*	
		Adult, M:	0–6				0–22	
		Adult, F:						
		Follicular:	0–3				0–11	
		Ovulatory peak:	4–14				15–51	
		Luteal:	4–10				15–37	

Modified from Behrman RE, Vaughan VC. Nelson Textbook of Pediatrics. 13th ed. Philadelphia: W.B. Saunders, 1987, pp 1537–1558.

Test	Specimen	Reference Range		Factor	Reference Range International
Estrogens, total	Serum		*pg/ml*	× 1	*ng/L*
		Child:	<30		<30
		M:	40–115		40–115
		F, cycle days			
		1–10 d:	61–394		61–394
		11–20 d:	122–437		122–437
		21–30 d:	156–350		156–350
		Prepubertal:	≤40		≤40
	Urine, 24-hr		*μg/d*	× 1	*μg/d*
		Child:	<10		<10
		Adult, M:	5–25		5–25
		Adult, F:			
		Preovulation:	5–25		5–25
		Ovulation:	28–100		28–100
		Luteal peak:	22–80		22–80
		Pregnancy:	<45,000		<45,000
		Postmenopausal:	<10		<10
Follicle-stimulating hormone (FSH)	Serum or plasma (heparin)		*mU/ml* (IRP-2-hMG)	× 1	*IU/L*
		Birth–1 yr, M:	<1–12		<1–12
		F:	<1–20		<1–20
		1–8 yr, M:	<1–6		<1–6
		F:	<1–4		<1–4
		9–10 yr, M:	<1–10		<1–10
		F:	2–8		2–8
		11–12 yr, M:	2–12		2–12
		F:	3–11		3–11
		13–14 yr, M:	3–15		3–15
		F:	3–15		3–15
		Adult, M:	4–25		4–25
		Adult, F:			
		Premenopausal:	4–30		4–30
		Midcycle peak:	10–90		10–90
		Pregnancy:	Low to undetectable		Low to undetectable
Growth hormone (hGH, somatotropin)	Serum of plasma (EDTA, heparin) Fasting, at rest	Cord:	*ng/ml* 10–50	× 1	*μg/L* 10–50
		Newborn:	10–40		10–40
		Child:	<5		<5
		Adult, M:	<5		<5
		Adult, F:	<8		<8
Hematocrit (HCT, Hct) Calculated from MCV and RBC (electronic displacement or laser)	Whole blood (EDTA)	% of packed red cells (V red cells/V whole blood × 100)		Volume (V) fraction (V red cells/V whole blood × 0.01)	
		1 d (cap):	48–69		0.48–0.69
		2 d:	48–75		0.48–0.75
		3 d:	44–72		0.44–0.72
		2 mo:	28–42		0.28–0.42
		6–12 yr:	35–45		0.35–0.45
		12–18 yr, M:	37–49		0.37–0.49
		F:	36–46		0.36–0.46
		18–49 yr, M:	41–53		0.41–0.53
		F:	36–46		0.36–0.46
17-Hydroxyprogesterone (17-OHP)	Serum		*ng/ml*	× 3.026	*nmol/L*
		M,			
		Pubertal stage I:	0.1–0.3		0.3–0.9
		Adult:	0.2–1.8		0.6–5.4
		F,			
		Pubertal stage I:	0.2–0.5		0.6–1.5
		Follicular:	0.2–0.8		0.6–2.4
		Luteal:	0.8–3.0		2.4–9.0
		Postmenopausal:	0.04–0.5		0.12–1.5

Test	Specimen	Reference Range		Factor	Reference Range International
Luteinizing hormone (LH)	Serum or plasma (heparin)		*mU/ml*	× 1	*IU/L*
		Child:	1–6		1–6
		M, 10–13 yr:	4–12		4–12
		12–14 yr:	6–12		6–12
		12–17 yr:	6–16		6–16
		15–18 yr:	7–19		7–19
		F, 8–12 yr:	2–12		2–12
		9–14 yr:	2–14		2–14
		12–18 yr:	3–29		3–29
		Adult, M:	6–23		6–23
		Adult, F,			
		Follicular phase:	5–30		5–30
		Midcycle:	75–150		75–150
		Luteal:	3–40		3–40
		Postmenopausal:	30–200		30–200
Progesterone	Serum		*ng/ml*	× 3.18	*nmol/L*
		M,			
		Pubertal stage I:	0.11–0.26		0.35–0.83
		Adult:	0.12–0.3		0.38–1
		F,			
		Pubertal stage I:	0–0.3		0–1
		II:	0–0.46		0–1.5
		III:	0–0.6		0–2
		IV:	0.05–13.0		0.16–41
		Follicular:	0.02–0.9		0.06–2.9
		Luteal:	6.0–30.0		19–95
Prolactin (PRL)	Serum		*ng/ml*	× 1	*µg/ml*
		Adult, M:	<20		<20
		Adult, F,			
		Follicular phase:	<23		<23
		Luteal phase:	5–40		5–40
		Pregnancy,			
		1st trimester:	<80		<80
		2nd trimester:	<160		<160
		3rd trimester:	<400		<400
		Newborn: >10-fold adult levels			>10-fold adult levels

Appendix D   *Barbara R. Hostetler*

Temperature Conversion

C	F	C	F	C	F	C	F
0	32.0	37.2	99	39.2	102.6	41.2	106.2
20	68.0	37.4	99.3	39.4	102.9	41.4	106.5
30	86.0	37.6	99.7	39.6	103.3	41.6	106.9
31	87.8	37.8	100.1	39.8	103.7	41.8	107.2
32	89.6	38.0	100.4	40.0	104	42	107.6
33	91.4	38.2	100.8	40.2	104.4	43	109.4
34	93.2	38.4	101.2	40.4	104.7	44	111.2
35	95.0	38.6	101.5	40.6	105.1	100	212
36	96.8	38.8	101.8	40.8	105.4		
37	98.6	39.0	102.2	41.0	105.8		

*To convert Celsius (centigrade) readings to Fahrenheit, multiply by 1.8 and add 32. To convert Fahrenheit readings to Celsius, subtract 32 and divide by 1.8.

From Behrman RE, Vaughan VC. Nelson Textbook of Pediatrics. 13th ed. Philadelphia: W.B. Saunders, 1987, p 1560.

Appendix E *Barbara R. Hostetler and S. Beth Edwards*

Commonly Used Medications

Drug	How Supplied	Dose and Route	Remarks
Acetaminophen (Panadol, Tempra, Tylenol, and others)	Tabs: 325, 500 mg Chewable Tabs: 80 mg Caplets: 160 mg Drops: 80 mg/0.8 ml Elixir: 160 mg/5 ml Syrup: 160 mg/5 ml	*Usual Dose:* 10–15 mg/kg/dose Q4h (**Max. dose:** 5 doses/d) *Alternative:* 0–3 mo: 40 mg/dose 4–11 mo: 80 mg/dose 12–24 mo: 120 mg/dose 4–5 yr: 240 mg/dose 6–8 yr: 320 mg/dose 9–10 yr: 400 mg/dose 11–12 yr: 480 mg/dose Adult: 325–650 mg Q4h (**Max. dose:** 65 mg/kg/d)	T½: 1–3 h. **Contraindicated** in patients with G6PD deficiency. Overdose may cause hepatotoxicity, often delayed. Some preparations contain alcohol.
Acyclovir (Zovirax)	Capsules: 200 mg Inj: 500 mg/10 ml Ointment: 5% (15 g)	*Herpes Simplex Virus:* Newborns: 30 mg/kg/d admin. Q8h IV Children (<12 yr): 750 mg/M²/d admin. Q8h IV; give over 1 hour. *Genital HSV:* 200 mg PO Q4h × 5 doses/d. Treat 10 d for first genital HSV infection, 5 d for recurrences. Topical Use: Apply oint. 5–6 ×/d Suppression: 200 mg PO QID for **max. dose** 6 months *Varicella Zoster:* 1500 mg/M²/d admin. Q8h IV	Can cause renal impairment; adequate hydration essential to prevent renal tubular crystallization. Encephalopathic reactions have been reported. Dose alterations necessary in preterm infants and in patients with reduced creatinine clearance. May cause nausea, vomiting, diarrhea, headache, dizziness, arthralgia, fatigue, rash, insomnia, fever.
Amoxicillin (Amcill, Amoxil, Larotid, Trimox, Wymox, Utimox)	Drops: 50 mg/ml (15, 30 ml) Susp: 125, 250 mg/5 ml (80, 100, 150, 200 ml) Caps: 250, 500 mg Chewable Tabs: 125 mg	*Child:* 20–40 mg/kg/d admin. Q8h PO *Adult:* 250–500 mg/dose Q8h PO *Gonorrhea* (acute uncomplicated): ≤45 kg: 50 mg/kg/single PO dose with 25 mg/kg probenecid (**Max. dose:** 1 g probenecid) >45 kg: 3 g as single PO dose with 1 g probenecid	Renal elimination. Achieves serum levels about twice those achieved with equal dose of ampicillin. Fewer GI effects, but otherwise similar to ampicillin. Side effects: rash and diarrhea.
Amoxicillin-Clavulanic Acid (Augmentin)	Tabs: 125, 250 mg Chewable Tabs: 125, 250 mg Susp: 125, 250 mg/5 ml (31.25, 62.5 mg clavulanate) (75, 150 ml)	*Child:* 20–40 mg/kg/d as amoxicillin admin. Q8h PO *Adult:* 250–500 mg/dose Q8h PO (**Max. dose:** 1.5 g/d)	Beta lactamase inhibitor extends the activity of amoxicillin to include beta-lactamase–producing strains of *H. influenzae, B. catarrhalis,* some *S. aureus.* Causes diarrhea more than amoxicillin.
Ampicillin (Omnipen, Polycillin, Principen)	Drops: 100 mg/ml (20 ml) Susp: 125, 250 mg/5 ml (80, 100, 150, 200 ml) 500 mg/5 ml (100 ml) Caps: 250, 500 mg Inj: 125, 250, 500 mg; 1, 2 g	*Neonate:* <7 days: 50–150 mg/kg/d admin. Q8h–12h >7 days: 75–200 mg/kg/d admin. Q6–8h IM or IV *Child:* Mild-moderate infections: 50–100 mg/kg/d admin. Q4–6 h PO, IM or IV (**Max. dose:** 2–4 g/d) Severe infections: 200–400 mg/kg/d admin. Q4–6h IM or IV (**Max. dose:** 10–12 g/d)	Use higher doses to treat CNS disease. Same side effects as penicillin, with cross-reactivity. Rash commonly seen at 5–10 days. May cause interstitial nephritis.
Aspirin (ASA, various trade names)	Tabs: 65, 75, 200, 300, 325, 500, 600, 650 mg Chewable Tabs: 65, 81 mg Caps: 325 mg Susp: 60, 120, 130, 195, 300, 325, 650 mg; 1.2 g	*Antipyretic:* 10–15 mg/kg/dose Q4h up to total 60–80 mg/kg/d (**Max. dose:** 3.6 g/d) *Antirheumatic:* 60–100 mg/kg/d admin. Q4h *Kawasaki Disease:* 80–100 mg/kg/d PO admin. QID during febrile phase until defervesces × 36 h then decrease to 5–10 mg/kg/d PO Q AM	Use with caution in platelet and bleeding disorders. Follow serum levels used as antirheumatic or with Kawasaki disease. May cause GI upset, allergic reactions, and liver toxicity. **Therapeutic levels: 20–100 mg/L antipyretic/analgesic; 10–30 mg/dL antiinflammatory.**

Drug	How Supplied	Dose and Route	Remarks
Azithromycin (Zithromax)	Tabs: 250 mg, 600 mg Inj: 500 mg/10 ml Susp: 100 (15 ml), 200 mg/5 ml (15, 22.5, 30 ml)	*Child:* Acute otitis media/community acquired pneumonia: 10 mg/kg as single dose on the first day (not to exceed 500 mg/d) followed by 5 mg/kg on days 2 through 5 (not to exceed 250 mg/d) Chlamydial infections (*C. trachomatis*): (≥ 45 kg and < 8 years of age or ≥ 8 years of age) − 1 g PO in single dose Pharyngitis/tonsillitis: 12 mg/kg qd for 5 days (max dose: 500 mg/d) *Adult:* 500 mg as a single dose on the first day followed by 250 mg qd on days 2 through 5 *Genital ulcer disease (H. ducreyi):* single 1 g dose *Nongonococcal urethritis/cervicitis (C. trachomatis):* Single 1 g dose *Gonococcal urethritis/cervicitis (N. gonorrhoeae):* Single 2 g dose *Gonococcal pharyngitis:* Single 1 g dose (plus a single dose of 125 mg ceftriaxone, 500 mg ciprofloxacin, or 400 mg ofloxacin) *Uncomplicated gonococcal infections of the cervix, uretha, rectum (N. gonorrhoeae):* 1 g single dose (plus a single dose of 125 mg ceftriaxone, 500 mg ciprofloxacin, or 400 mg ofloxacin) *Chlamydial infections (C. trachomatis):* Single 1 g dose *Parenteral:* Community acquired pneumonia: 500 mg as a single daily dose IV for ≥ 2 days Pelvic inflammatory disease: 500 mg as a single daily dose IV for 1 or 2 days. Give 1 mg/ml over 3 hours or 2 mg/ml over 1 hour	Do not administer oral suspension with food. Administer at least 1 hour before or 2 hours after a meal. Caution patients not to take aluminum- and magnesium-containing antacids and azithromycin simultaneously. Do not use in patients with pneumonia who are judged to be inappropriate for oral therapy. Rare serious allergic reactions, including angioedema, anaphylaxis, and dermatologic reactions including Stevens-Johnson syndrome and toxic epidermal necrolysis have occurred. Because azithromycin is eliminated via the liver, exercise caution when administering to patients with impaired liver function. Dosage adjustment does not appear to be necessary for older patients with normal renal and hepatic function. Pregnancy Category B. Safety and efficacy of IV injection in children or adolescents < 16 years have not been established. Safety and efficacy in children < 6 months of age have not been established for acute otitis media or community-acquired pneumonia. Safety and efficacy in children < 2 years of age have not been established for pharyngitis/tonsillitis. Local IV site reactions have been reported; avoid concentrations higher than 2 mg/ml.
Cefaclor (Ceclor) (2nd generation)	Caps: 250, 500 mg Susp: 125, 250 mg/5 ml (75 ml, 150 ml)	*Infant and Child:* 40 mg/kg/d admin. Q8h PO (**Max. dose:** 2 g/d) *Adult:* 250–500 mg/dose Q8h PO (**Max. dose:** 4 g/d)	Not recommended for infants <1 month old. Use with **caution** in patients with penicillin allergy or renal impairment. May cause positive Coombs or false-positive test for urinary glucose.
Ciprofloxacin (Cipro)	Tabs: 250, 500, 750 mg	*Adults:* 250–750 mg/dose Q12h PO (**Max. dose:** 2 g/d)	Like other quinolones, ciprofloxacin causes cartilage arthropathy in experimental animals. **Its use in children <16–18 yr is *not* recommended.**
Clindamycin (Cleocin)	Caps: 75, 150, 300 mg Oral Liquid: 75 mg/5 ml (100 ml) Inj: 150 mg/ml	*Neonates:* Preterm: 15 mg/kg/d admin. Q8h IV/IM Term: 20 mg/kg/d admin. Q6h IV/IM *Children:* 10–25 mg/kg/d admin. Q6–8h PO; 15–40 mg/kg/d admin. Q6–8h IM or IV *Adults:* 150–450 mg Q6h PO; 600–2700 mg/d admin. Q6–12h IM or IV (**Max. dose:** 4 g/d IV; 2 g/d PO)	Not indicated in meningitis. Use with caution in hepatic or renal insufficiency. Pseudomembranous colitis may occur up to several weeks after cessation of therapy but generally is uncommon in pediatric patients. May cause diarrhea, rash, Stevens-Johnson syndrome, granulocytopenia, thrombocytopenia, or sterile abscess at injection site.
Clotrimazole (Lotrimin, Mycelex)	Cream: 1% (15, 30, 45, 90 g) Solution: 1% (10, 30 ml) Vaginal Tabs: 100, 500 mg Vaginal Cream: 1% (45, 90 g) Oral Troche: 10 mg	*Topical:* apply to skin BID *Vaginal Candidiasis:* 1 tab per vaginal daily × 7 d *Thrush:* Dissolve one troche in the mouth 5 times/d	May cause erythema, blistering, or urticaria where applied.
Codeine (Various brands)	Tabs: 15, 30, 60 mg Inj: 15, 30, 60 mg/ml Oral Sol'n: 15 mg/5 ml Combination product with acetaminophen: Elixir: Acet 120 mg and codeine 12 mg/5 ml Tabs: (all contain 300 mg acetaminophen per tab) Tylenol #1–7.5 mg Codeine Tylenol #2–15 mg Codeine Tylenol #3–30 mg Codeine Tylenol #4–60 mg Codeine	*Analgesic:* Children: 0.5–1.0 mg/kg/dose Q4–6h IM, SC, or PO Adults: 30–60 mg/dose Q4–6h IM, SC, or PO *Antitussive:* Children (2–6 yr): 1 mg/kg/d admin. QID; (**Max. dose:** 30 mg/d) Adults: 15–30 mg/dose Q4–6 (**Max. dose:** 120 mg/d)	Side effects include CNS and respiratory depression, constipation, cramping. May be habit forming. For analgesia, use with acetaminophen orally. **Do not use in children <2 yr. Do not administer by IV route.**

Drug	How Supplied	Dose and Route	Remarks
Co-trimoxazole (Trimethoprim-sulfamethoxazole) (Bactrim, Septra, TMP-SMX)	Tabs (reg. strength): 80 mg TMP/400 mg SMX Tabs (double strength): 160 mg TMP/800 mg SMX Susp: 40 mg TMP/200 mg SMX per 5 ml Inj: 16 mg TMP/ml and 80 mg SMX/ml	**Doses based on TMP component.** *Minor infections:* (PO or IV): Child: 8–10 mg/kg/d admin. Q12h Adult (>40 kg): 160 mg/dose Q12h *UTI prophylaxis:* 2 mg/kg/d QD *Severe infections and Pneumocystis carinii pneumonitis* (PO or IV): 20 mg/kg/d admin. Q6–8h *Pneumocystis prophylaxis:* 10 mg/kg/d Q12h	Do not use in infants <2 months old. Available as a fixed combination of 5 mg of sulfamethoxazole to each 1 mg of trimethoprim. May cause kernicterus in newborns, blood dyscrasias, crystalluria, glossitis, renal or hepatic injury, GI irritation, allergy, or hemolysis in G6PD. Reduce dose in renal impairment.
Doxycycline (Vibramycin and other brand names)	Caps: 50, 100 mg Tabs: 50, 100 mg Syrup: 50 mg/5 ml (30 ml) Susp: 25 mg/5 ml (60 ml) Inj: 100, 200 mg	*Initial:* ≤45 kg: 5 mg/kg/d admin. BID PO or IV × 1 d to max. of 200 mg/d >45 kg: 200 mg/d admin. BID PO or IV × 1 d *Maintenance:* <45 kg: 2.5–5 mg/kg/d admin. QD-BID PO or IV >45 kg: 100–200 mg/d admin. QD-BID PO or IV (**Max. adult dose:** 300 mg/d PID)	Use with **caution** in hepatic and renal disease. May cause increased intracranial pressure. **Do not use in children <8 yr;** may result in tooth enamel hypoplasia and discoloration. May cause GI symptoms, photosensitivity, hemolytic anemia, hypersensitivity reactions. Infuse over 1–4 h IV. Avoid direct sunlight. See Tetracycline. Avoid use in pregnancy.
Erythromycin Preparations (Erythrocin, E-Mycin, EryPed, Pediamycin, and others)	*Erythromycin:* Caps: 125, 250 mg Tabs: 250, 333, 500 mg Topical Sol'n: 1.5%, 2% (60 ml) Ophth. Oint.: 0.5% (3.75 g) *E. Ethyl Succinate (EES):* Susp: 200, 400 mg/5 ml (60, 100, 200 ml) Drops: 100 mg/2.5 ml (50 ml) Tabs: 200, 400 mg *Erythro, Lactobionate:* Inj: 500, 1000 mg *Erythromycin Gluceptate:* Inj: 250, 500, 1000 mg	*Oral:* Children: 30–50 mg/kg/d admin. Q6–8h (**Max. dose:** 2 g/d) Adults: 1–4 g/d admin. Q6h (**Max. dose:** 4 g/d) *Parenteral:* Children: 20–50 mg/kg/d admin. Q6h IV or as continuous infusion. Adults: 15–20 mg/kg/d admin. Q6 IV or as continuous infusion (**Max. dose:** 4 g/d) *Rheumatic Fever Prophylaxis:* 500 mg/d admin. Q12h PO *Endocarditis Prophylaxis:* 20 mg/kg (**Max. dose:** 1 g) PO 1h before **and** 10 mg/kg. (**Max. dose:** 4 g) PO 6h after procedure *Ophthalmic:* Apply 0.5 inch ribbon to affected eye BID–QID *Pertussis:* Use estolate salt 50 mg/kg/d PO admin. Q6h	Avoid IM route (pain, necrosis). GI side effects common (nauses, vomiting, abdominal cramps). Give doses after meals. Use with **caution** in liver disease. Estolate may cause cholestatic jaundice, although hepatotoxicity is uncommon (2% of reported cases). May produce elevated digoxin, theophylline, carbamazepine, cyclosporine, methylprednisolone levels. Oral therapy should replace IV as soon as possible. Because of different absorption characteristics, higher oral doses of EES are needed to achieve therapeutic effects. **Note:** formulations other than the estolate have a high incidence of relapse in the treatment of pertussis.
Erythromycin Ethylsuccinate and Sulfisox-azole Acetyl (Prediazole)	Susp: 200 mg erythro and 600 mg sulfa/5 ml (100, 150, 200 ml)	*Otitis Media:* 50 mg/kg/d (as erythro) and 150 mg/kg/d (as sulfa) admin. Q6h PO (**Max. dose:** 6 g sulfisoxazole/d)	See adverse effects of erythromycin and sulfisoxazole. **Not recommended in infants <2 months old.**
Fludrocortisone Acetate (Florinef, 9a-Flu-orohydro-cortisone)	Tabs: 0.1 mg	*Infants:* 0.1–0.2 mg/d QD PO *Children and Adults:* 0.05–0.1 mg/d QD PO Titrate dose to suppress plasma renin activity to normal levels	Preferably administered in conjunction with cortisone or hydrocortisone. Has primarily mineralocorticoid activity. If BP rises, decrease dose to 0.05 mg/24 h. 0.1 mg 9a-fluorocortisol = 1 mg DOCA.
Gentamicin (Garamycin and others)	Inj: 10, 40 mg/ml Ophth. Oint.: 0.3% (3.5 g) Drops: 0.3% (5 ml) Topical Ointment: 0.1% Intrathecal Inj: 2 mg/ml	*Parenteral* (IM or IV): Neonates <7 days: <28 wks: 2.5 mg/kg/dose Q18h Term: 2.5 mg/kg/dose Q12h >7 days: <28 wks: 2.5 mg/kg/dose Q18h 28–34 wks: 2.5 mg/kg/dose Q12h Term: 2.5 mg/kg/dose/Q8h Children: 6–7.5 mg/kg/d admin. Q8h Adults: 3–5 mg/kg/d admin. Q8h (**Max. dose:** 300 mg/d) *Intrathecal/Intraventricular:* >3 mo: 1–2 mg daily Adults: 4–8 mg daily *Ophth. Oint:* apply Q6–8h *Ophth. Drops:* 1–2 gtts Q4h	Monitor levels (peak and trough). Monitor renal status; may cause proximal tubule dysfunction. Watch for ototoxicity. Intrathecal or intraventricular administration is adjunctive to parenteral administration. Arachnoiditis and phlebitis are uncommon. **Therapeutic levels: 6–10 mg/L (peak); <2 mg/L (trough).** Eliminated more quickly in patients with cystic fibrosis, multiple sclerosis, or neutropenia. **Neonatal doses are the same for gentamicin and tobramycin. Amikacin dose is 3 times higher.**

Drug	How Supplied	Dose and Route	Remarks
Ibuprofen (Motrin, Medipren, Pediaprofen)	Susp: 100 mg/ 5 ml Tabs: 200, 300, 400, 600, 800 mg	*Children:* Antipyretic: 20 mg/kg/d admin. Q8h PO JRA: 30–70 mg/kg/d admin. 6h–8h PO *Adults:* 400 mg/dose Q4–6h PO (**Max. adult dose:** 2.4 g/d)	Side effects include GI distress (lessened with milk), rashes, ocular problems. Inhibits platelet aggregation. Use **caution** with aspirin hypersensitivity or hepatic or renal insufficiency.
Iron Preparations	*Ferrous Sulfate (20% Elemental Fe):* Drops (Fer-In-Sol): 75 mg (15 mg Fe)/0.6 ml (50 ml) Syrup (Fer-In-Sol): 90 mg (18 mg Fe) 5 ml Elixir (Feosol): 220 mg (44 mg Fe)/5 ml (355 ml) Caps and Tabs: 195 mg (39 mg Fe) 300 mg (60 mg Fe) 325 mg (65 mg Fe) *Ferrous Gluconate (12% Elemental Fe):* Elixir: 300 mg (35 mg Fe)/5 ml Tabs: 320 mg (37 mg Fe), 325 mg (38 mg Fe) Sustained-Release Caps: 435 mg (50 mg Fe) Caps: 325 mg (38 mg Fe)	*Iron Deficiency Anemia:* 3–6 mg elemental Fe/ kg/d admin. TID PO *Prophylaxis:* Children: PO/QD–TID Premature: 2 mg elemental Fe/kg/d Full-term: 1–2 mg elemental Fe/kg/d (**Max. dose:** 15 mg/d elemental Fe) Adults: 60–100 mg elemental Fe/d PO/ QD–BID	Iron preparations are variably absorbed. **Do not** use in hemolytic disorders. Less GI irritation when given with or after meals. Vitamin C 200 mg per 30 mg iron may enhance absorption. Liquid iron preparations may stain teeth. Administer with dropper or straw. May produce constipation, dark stools, nausea, and epigastric pain. Iron and tetracycline inhibit each other's absorption. Antacids may decrease iron absorption.
Lidocaine 2.5% and prilocaine 2.5% (EMLA)	Cream: 5 g tube with *Tega-derm* dressings and 30 g tube Anesthetic disc: 1 g	*Topical anesthetic for local analgesia:* *Pediatric patients:* (see table below) *Adult patients:* Minor dermal procedures: Apply 2.5 g of cream over 20 to 25 cm² of intact skin surface, or 1 anesthetic disc for at least 1 hour. Cover cream with an occlusive dressing Major dermal procedures: Apply 2 g of cream per 10 cm² of intact skin for at least 2 hours. Cover with an occlusive dressing Adult male genital skin: Apply a thick layer of cream (1 g/10 cm²) to intact skin surface for 15 minutes	Dermal analgesia can be expected to increase for up to 3 hours under occlusive dressing and persist for 1 to 2 hours after removal of the cream. Care must be taken in young children to prevent accidental ingestion of EMLA, occlusive dressing, or the anesthetic disc. EMLA should not be used in neonates with a gestational age less than 37 weeks nor in infants under the age of 12 months who are receiving treatment with methemoglobin-inducing agents. Pregnancy Category B. Use is not recommended on mucous membranes. EMLA should be used with caution in patients receiving Class I antiarrhythmic drugs since the toxic effects are additive and potentially synergistic.
Magnesium Citrate	Solution: (300 mg) 5 ml = 4–4.7 mEq/mg	*Children:* 4 ml/kg/dose PO repeat Q4–6h until liquid stool results (**Max. dose:** 200 ml) *Adults:* 240 ml OD PO PRN	Use with caution in renal insufficiency. May cause hypermagnesemia, hypotension, respiratory depression; up to about 20% of dose is absorbed.
Meperidine HCl (Demerol)	Tabs: 50, 100 mg Elixir: 50 mg/5 ml Inj: 25, 50, 75, 100 mg/ml	*PO, IM, IV and SC* Children: 1–1.5 mg/kg/dose Q3–4h PRN (**Max. dose:** 100 mg) Adults: 50–150 mg/dose Q3–4h PRN	**Contraindicated** in cardiac arrhythmias, asthma, increased intracranial pressure. Potentiated by MAO inhibitors, phenothiazines, other CNS-acting agents, and isoniazid. Lower dose if IV. May cause nausea, vomiting, respiratory depression, smooth muscle spasm, constipation, and lethargy. **Caution:** in renal failure; accumulated metabolite has CNS effects. **75 mg IV meperidine = 10 mg IV morphine.**

EMLA Pediatric patients table:

Age and body weight requirements	Max total dose of EMLA	Max application area	Max application time
0 up to 3 months or < 5 kg	1 g	10 cm²	1 hour
3 up to 12 months and > 5 kg	2 g	20 cm²	4 hours
1 to 6 years and > 10 kg	10 g	100 cm²	4 hours
7 to 12 years and > 20 kg	20 g	200 cm²	4 hours

Drug	How Supplied	Dose and Route	Remarks

Metronidazole (Flagyl)	Tabs: 250, 500 mg
	Susp°: 100 mg/5 ml, or 50 mg/ml
	Inj: 500 mg or 50 mg/ml ready to use
		Amebiasis:
		  Children: 35–50 mg/kg/d PO admin. TID × 10 days
		  Adults: 750 mg/dose PO TID × 5–10 days
		Anaerobic Infection:
		  Neonates:
		   Loading dose: 15 mg/kg IV
		   Maintenance:
		    Pre-term: 7.5 mg/kg/dose IV Q12h beginning 48 h after loading dose
		    Term: 7.5 mg/kg/dose IV Q12h beginning 24 h after initial dose
		  Infants, Children, and Adults:
		   Loading dose: 15 mg/kg IV
		   Maintenance: 7.5 mg/kg/dose Q6h IV or PO. (**Max. dose:** 4 g/d)
		Gardnerella vaginalis Vaginitis:
		  500 mg PO BID × 7 d
		Giardiasis:
		  Children: 15 mg/kg/d PO admin. TID × 10 d
		Pelvic Inflammatory Disease:
		  1 g BID PO or IV
		Trichomonas Vaginitis:
		  Children: 15 mg/kg/d PO admin. TID × 7 d
		  Adults: 250 mg/dose PO TID × 7 d or 2 g PO × 1
		Clostridium difficile: (Adult) 0.75–2 g/d PO admin. TID–QID × 7–14 d
			Side effects include nausea, diarrhea, urticaria, dry mouth, leukopenia, vertigo. Candidiasis may worsen. Patients should not ingest alcohol for 24 h after dose (disulfuram-type reaction). Potentiates anticoagulants. IV infusion must be given slowly over 1 h. Except for amebiasis, safe use of metronidazole in children <12 yr has not been established.

Morphine Sulfate	Oral Sol'n: 2, 4, 20 mg/ml (30, 120 ml)
	Tabs: 10, 15, 30 mg
	Sustained-Release Tabs: 30 mg
	Inj: 1, 2, 4, 5, 8, 10, 15 mg/ml
		Analgesia/Tetralogy (Cyanotic) Spells:
		Child: 0.1–0.2 mg/kg/dose SC, IV, or IM Q2–4h PRN (**Max. dose:** 15 mg/dose)
		Adults:
		  PO: 10–30 mg Q4h PRN
		  IV: 2–15 mg dose Q2–6h PRN
		Continuous IV: 0.025–2 mg/kg/h; begin with lower dose and titrate to effect
			Causes dependence. CNS and respiratory depression, nausea, vomiting, constipation, hypotension, bradycardia, increased intracranial pressure, biliary or urinary tract spasm, allergy may occur. IM/IV dose equal to 6 × PO dose. Naloxone may be used to reverse effects, especially respiratory depression.

Naloxone (Narcan)	Inj: 0.4, 1 mg/ml Neonatal Inj: 0.02 mg/ml	*Children:* 5–10 μg/kg/dose IM or IV Repeat as necessary Q3–5 min *Adults:* 0.4–2.0 mg/dose Q2–3 min × 1–3. May give 10-fold higher dose if needed for diagnosis or therapy *Continuous Infusion:* After titrating initial dose to effectiveness, add 75–100% of last effective dose to 1 h of maintenance IV fluid to run over 1 h. May wean in 50% increments over next 6–12 h. (May need to wean over as long as 48 h for methadone.) If symptoms recur, rebolus at 100% of dose **Max. dose:** 2 mg	Does not cause respiratory depression. Short duration of action may necessitate multiple doses. For very large ingestions, 100–200 mcg/kg have been necessary. Will produce narcotic withdrawal syndrome in patients with chronic dependence. Use with **caution** in patients with chronic cardiac disease.
Penicillin G Preparations			

Potassium and Sodium	Potassium
	  Tabs: 250,000, 400,000, 500,000, 800,000 Units
	  Solution: 200,000, 400,000 Units/5 ml (100, 200 ml)
	  Inj: 0.2, 0.5, 1, 5, 10, 20 million Units
	Sodium
	  Inj: 5 million U
		Newborn: (IV or IM)
		  ≤7 days:
		   <2 kg: 50,000–100,000 U/kg/d admin. Q12h
		   >2 kg: 50,000–150,000 U/kg/d admin. Q8h
		  >7 days:
		   <2 kg 75,000–150,000 U/kg/d admin. Q8h
		   >2 kg: 100,000–200,000 U/kg/d admin. Q6h
		Children:
		  IV or IM: 100,000–300,000 U/kg/d admin. Q4–6h
		  PO: 40,000–80,000 U/kg/d admin. Q6h
		Adults:
		  IV or IM: 100,000–250,000 U/kg/d admin. Q4–6h
		  PO: 300,000–1.2 mil U/d admin. Q6h
			1 mg = approx 1600 units. Contains 1.7 mEq of Na or K per 1 million units. Penicillin G must be taken 1–2 h before or 2 h after meals. Side effects: anaphylaxis, hemolytic anemia, interstitial nephritis. T½ = 30 min, may be prolonged by concurrent use of probenecid. For meningitis use at shorter dosing intervals.

Benzathine (Permapen, Bicillin L-A)	Inj: 300,000, 600,000 U/ml	*Newborns:* 50,000 U/kg × 1 IM *Infants/Children:* 50,000 U/kg × 1 IM. (**Max. dose:** 2.4 mil U) *Adults:* 1.2 mil U × 1 IM *Rheumatic Fever Prophylaxis:* 600,000 U Q2 wks or 1.2 million U Q month IM	Provides sustained levels for 2–4 wks. Do **not** administer IV.

Drug	How Supplied	Dose and Route	Remarks
Procaine (Duracillin, Wycillin)	Inj: 300,000, 500,000, 600,000 U/ml	*Infants and Children:* 25,000–50,000 U/kg/d admin. Q12–24h IM (**Max. dose:** 4.8 million U/d) *Adults:* 600,000–1 mil U/d admin. Q12–24h IM	Provides sustained levels for 2–4 days. May cause sterile abscess at injection site. Contains 120 mg procaine/300,000 Units—this may cause allergic reactions, CNS stimulation, seizures. Use with **caution** in neonates. Do **not** use IV.
Bicillin C-R	Tubex: 300,000 U Pen G Procaine + 300,000 U Pen G Benzathine/ml, or 150,000 U Pen G Procaine + 450,000 U Pen G Benzathine/ml	*Acute Streptococcal Infections* <14 kg: 600,000 U × 1 IM 14–27 kg: 900,000–1.2 mil U × 1 IM >27 kg: 2.4 million U × 1 IM	Provides early peak levels in addition to prolonged levels of penicillin in the blood.
Penicillin V Potassium (Pen-Vee K, V-Cillin-K)	Tabs: 125 mg (200,000 U) 250 mg (400,000 U) 500 mg (800,000 U) Oral Sol'n: 125, 250 mg/5 mg (100, 200 ml)	*Children:* 25–30 mg/kg/d admin. Q6h **Max. dose:** 3 g/d *Adults:* 250–500 mg/dose PO Q6h *Rheumatic Fever/ Pneumococcal Prophylaxis:* <5 yr: 125 mg PO BID >5 yr: 250 mg PO BID	GI absorption is better than penicillin G. **Note:** Must be taken 1 h before or 2 h after meals.
Podofilox (Condylox)	Topical gel: 0.5% podofilox (alcohol; in 3.5 ml aluminum tubes) Topical solution: 0.5% podofilox (alcohol; in 3.5 ml bottles)	*Gel (anogenital warts) and solution (external warts):* Apply every 12 hours to completely cover the lesions with a finger (gel only) or the cotton-tipped applicator supplied with the drug. Allow to dry. Dispose of applicator and wash hands before and after use. Apply for 3 consecutive days, then withhold use for 4 consecutive days. Cycle can be repeated up to 4 times.	Limit treatment to < 10 cm² of wart tissue and to ≤ 0.5 ml of solution or ≤ 0.5 g of gel per day. If incomplete response after 4 treatment weeks, consider alternate treatment. Safety and effectiveness of > 4 treatment weeks have not been established. Not indicated in the treatment of mucous membrane or perianal (solution only) warts. Intended for cutaneous use only. Avoid contact with eyes. Pregnancy Category C. Safety and efficacy in children have not been established. Most common adverse reactions noted: burning, pain, inflammation, erosion, itching.
Tetracycline HCl (Many brand names: Achromycin, Aureomycin, Panmycin, Sumycin, Terramycin)	Tabs: 250, 500 mg Caps: 100, 250, 500 mg Susp: 125 mg/5 ml (473 ml) Ophth. Oint: 0.5%, 1% (3.5 g) Ophth. Susp: 1% (4 ml) Cream: 1% Oint: 3% (15, 30 g) Inj: (IV) 250, 500 mg; (IM) 100, 250 mg with 40 mg procaine/vial	**Do not use in children <8 yrs.** *Older Children:* (**Max. dose:** 2 g/d) PO: 25–50 mg/kg/d admin. Q6h IM: 15–25 mg/kg/d admin. Q8–12h (**Max. dose:** 250 mg/d) IV: 20–30 mg/kg/d admin. Q8–12h *Adults:* (**Max. dose:** 2 g/d) PO: 1–2 g/d admin. Q6h IM: 250–300 mg/d admin. Q8–12h IV: 250–500 mg/dose Q6–12h *Chlamydia Genital Infections:* 500 mg Q6h PO *Ophth:* 2 drops into affected eye BID-QID	**Not** recommended in patients <8 yr due to tooth staining and decreasing bone growth. Also **not** recommended for use in pregnancy because these side effects may occur in the fetus. May cause nausea and GI upset, hepatotoxicity, stomatitis, rash, photosensitivity, fever. **Do not give** with dairy products or with any divalent cations (i.e., Fe⁺⁺, Ca⁺⁺, Mg⁺⁺). Give 1 h before or 2 h after meals.
Vancomycin (Vancocin)	Inj: 500, 1000 mg Caps: 125, 250 mg Solution: 1, 10 g (reconstitute to 500 mg/6 ml)	*Neonates:* <7 days: <1 kg: 10 mg/kg Q24h IV 1–2 kg: 10 mg/kg Q18h IV >2 kg: 10 mg/kg Q12h IV >7 days: <1 kg: 10 mg/kg Q18h IV 1–2 kg: 10 mg/kg Q12h IV >2 kg: 10 mg/kg Q8h IV Give 15 mg/kg/dose if CNS involved. *Infants and Children:* CNS: 15 mg/kg/dose Q8h IV Other: 10 mg/kg/dose Q8h IV *Adults:* 2 g/d admin. Q6–12h IV *Colitis:* *Children:* 40–50 mg/kg/d admin. Q6h PO (**Max. dose:** 2 g/d) *Adults:* 0.5–2 g/d admin. Q6h PO	Ototoxicity, nephrotoxicity, allergy may occur. "Red man syndrome" associated with rapid IV infusion. Infuse over 60 minutes. **Note:** diphenhydramine is used to treat "red man syndrome." Therapeutic Levels: Peak 25–40 μg/ml Trough <10 μg/ml

*Suspensions are not commercially available; must be extemporaneously compounded by a pharmacist.

Appendix F   *David Muram and S. Beth Edwards*

Commonly Used Oral Contraceptives

Product	Manufacturer	Type	Estrogen (μg)	Progestin (mg)
Necon 1/50	Watson Labs	Monophasic	50 mestranol	1 norethindrone
Nelova 1/50M	Warner Chilcott	Monophasic	50 mestranol	1 norethindrone
Norinyl 1 + 50	Watson Labs	Monophasic	50 mestranol	1 norethindrone
Ortho-Novum 1/50	Ortho-McNeil	Monophasic	50 mestranol	1 norethindrone
Ovcon-50	Bristol-Myers Squibb	Monophasic	50 ethinyl estradiol	1 norethindrone
Demulen 1/50	Searle	Monophasic	50 ethinyl estradiol	1 ethynodiol diacetate
Zovia 1/50E	Watson Labs	Monophasic	50 ethinyl estradiol	1 ethynodiol diacetate
Ovral	Wyeth-Ayerst	Monophasic	50 ethinyl estradiol	0.5 norgestrel
Necon 1/35	Watson Labs	Monophasic	35 ethinyl estradiol	1 norethindrone
Nelova 1/35E	Warner Chilcott	Monophasic	35 ethinyl estradiol	1 norethindrone
Norinyl 1 + 35	Watson Labs	Monophasic	35 ethinyl estradiol	1 norethindrone
Ortho-Novum 1/35	Ortho-McNeil	Monophasic	35 ethinyl estradiol	1 norethindrone
Brevicon	Watson Labs	Monophasic	35 ethinyl estradiol	0.5 norethindrone
Modicon	Ortho-McNeil	Monophasic	35 ethinyl estradiol	0.5 norethindrone
Necon 0.5/35	Watson Labs	Monophasic	35 ethinyl estradiol	0.5 norethindrone
Nelova 0.5/35E	Warner Chilcott	Monophasic	35 ethinyl estradiol	0.5 norethindrone
Ovcon-35	Bristol-Myers Squibb	Monophasic	35 ethinyl estradiol	0.4 norethindrone
Ortho-Cyclen	Ortho-McNeil	Monophasic	35 ethinyl estradiol	0.25 norgestimate
Demulen 1/35	Searle	Monophasic	35 ethinyl estradiol	1 ethynodiol diacetate
Zovia 1/35E	Watson Labs	Monophasic	35 ethinyl estradiol	1 ethynodiol diacetate
Loestrin 21 1.5/30	Parke-Davis	Monophasic	30 ethinyl estradiol	1.5 norethindrone acetate
Loestrin Fe 1.5/30	Parke-Davis	Monophasic	30 ethinyl estradiol	1.5 norethindrone acetate
Lo/Ovral	Wyeth-Ayerst	Monophasic	30 ethinyl estradiol	0.3 norgestrel
Desogen	Organon	Monophasic	30 ethinyl estradiol	0.15 desogestrel
Ortho-Cept	Ortho-McNeil	Monophasic	30 ethinyl estradiol	0.15 desogestrel
Levlen	Berlex Labs	Monophasic	30 ethinyl estradiol	0.15 levonorgestrel
Levora 0.15/30	Watson Labs	Monophasic	30 ethinyl estradiol	0.15 levonorgestrel
Nordette	Wyeth-Ayerst	Monophasic	30 ethinyl estradiol	0.15 levonorgestrel
Alesse	Wyeth-Ayerst	Monophasic	20 ethinyl estradiol	0.1 levonorgestrel
Levlite	Berlex Labs	Monophasic	20 ethinyl estradiol	0.1 levonorgestrel
Loestrin 21 1/20	Parke-Davis	Monophasic	20 ethinyl estradiol	1 norethindrone acetate
Loestrin Fe 1/20	Parke-Davis	Monophasic	20 ethinyl estradiol	1 norethindrone acetate
Jenest-28	Organon	Biphasic	35 ethinyl estradiol (all 21 days)	0.5 norethindrone (days 1–7), 1 norethindrone (days 8–21)
Necon 10/11	Watson Labs	Biphasic	35 ethinyl estradiol (all 21 days)	0.5 norethindrone (days 1–10), 1 norethindrone (days 11–21)
Nelova 10/11	Warner Chilcott	Biphasic	35 ethinyl estradiol (all 21 days)	0.5 norethindrone (days 1–10), 1 norethindrone (days 11–21)
Ortho-Novum 10/11	Ortho-McNeil	Biphasic	35 ethinyl estradiol (all 21 days)	0.5 norethindrone (days 1–10), 1 norethindrone (days 11–21)
Mircette	Organon	Biphasic	20 ethinyl estradiol (days 1–21), 0.01 ethinyl estradiol (days 22–26)	0.15 desogestrel (days 1–21)
Ortho-Novum 7/7/7	Ortho-McNeil	Triphasic	35 ethinyl estradiol (all 21 days)	0.5 norethindrone (days 1–7), 0.75 norethindrone (days 8–14), 1 norethindrone (days 15–21)
Tri-Levlen	Berlex Labs	Triphasic	30 ethinyl estradiol (days 1–6, 12–21), 40 ethinyl estradiol (days 7–11)	0.05 levonorgestrel (days 1–6), 0.075 levonorgestrel (days 7–11), 0.125 levonorgestrel (days 12–21)
Tri-Norinyl	Searle	Triphasic	35 ethinyl estradiol (all 21 days)	0.5 norethindrone (days 1–7, 17–21), 1 norethindrone (days 8–16)
Triphasil	Wyeth-Ayerst	Triphasic	30 ethinyl estradiol (days 1–6, 12–21), 40 ethinyl estradiol (days 7–11)	0.05 levonorgestrel (days 1–6), 0.075 levonorgestrel (days 7–11), 0.125 levonorgestrel (days 12–21)

Table continued on following page

679

Product	Manufacturer	Type	Estrogen (µg)	Progestin (mg)
Trivora-28	Watson Labs	Triphasic	30 ethinyl estradiol (days 1–6, 12–21), 40 ethinyl estradiol (days 7–11)	0.05 levonorgestrel (days 1–6), 0.075 levonorgestrel (days 7–11), 0.125 levonorgestrel (days 12–21)
Ortho Tri-Cyclen	Ortho-McNeil	Triphasic	35 ethinyl estradiol (all 21 days)	0.18 norgestimate (days 1–7), 0.215 norgestimate (days 8–14), 0.25 norgestimate (days 15–21)
Estrostep 21	Parke-Davis	Triphasic	20 ethinyl estradiol (days 1–5), 30 ethinyl estradiol (days 6–12), 35 ethinyl estradiol (days 13–21)	1 norethindrone acetate (all 21 days)
Estrostep Fe	Parke-Davis	Triphasic	20 ethinyl estradiol (days 1–5), 30 ethinyl estradiol (days 6–12), 35 ethinyl estradiol (days 13–21)	1 norethindrone acetate (all 21 days)
Micronor	Ortho-McNeil	Progestin-only		0.35 norethindrone
Nor-Q.D.	Watson Labs	Progestin-only		0.35 norethindrone
Ovrette	Wyeth-Ayerst	Progestin-only		0.075 norgestrel

Index

Note: Page numbers followed by the letter f refer to figures; those followed by the letter t refer to tables.

ISBN 0-7216-8346-0

90038